PROFESSIONAL PARAMEDIC

MEDICAL EMERGENCIES, MATERNAL HEALTH & PEDIATRICS

VOLUME II

PROFESSIONAL PARAMEDIC

MEDICAL EMERGENCIES, MATERNAL HEALTH & PEDIATRICS

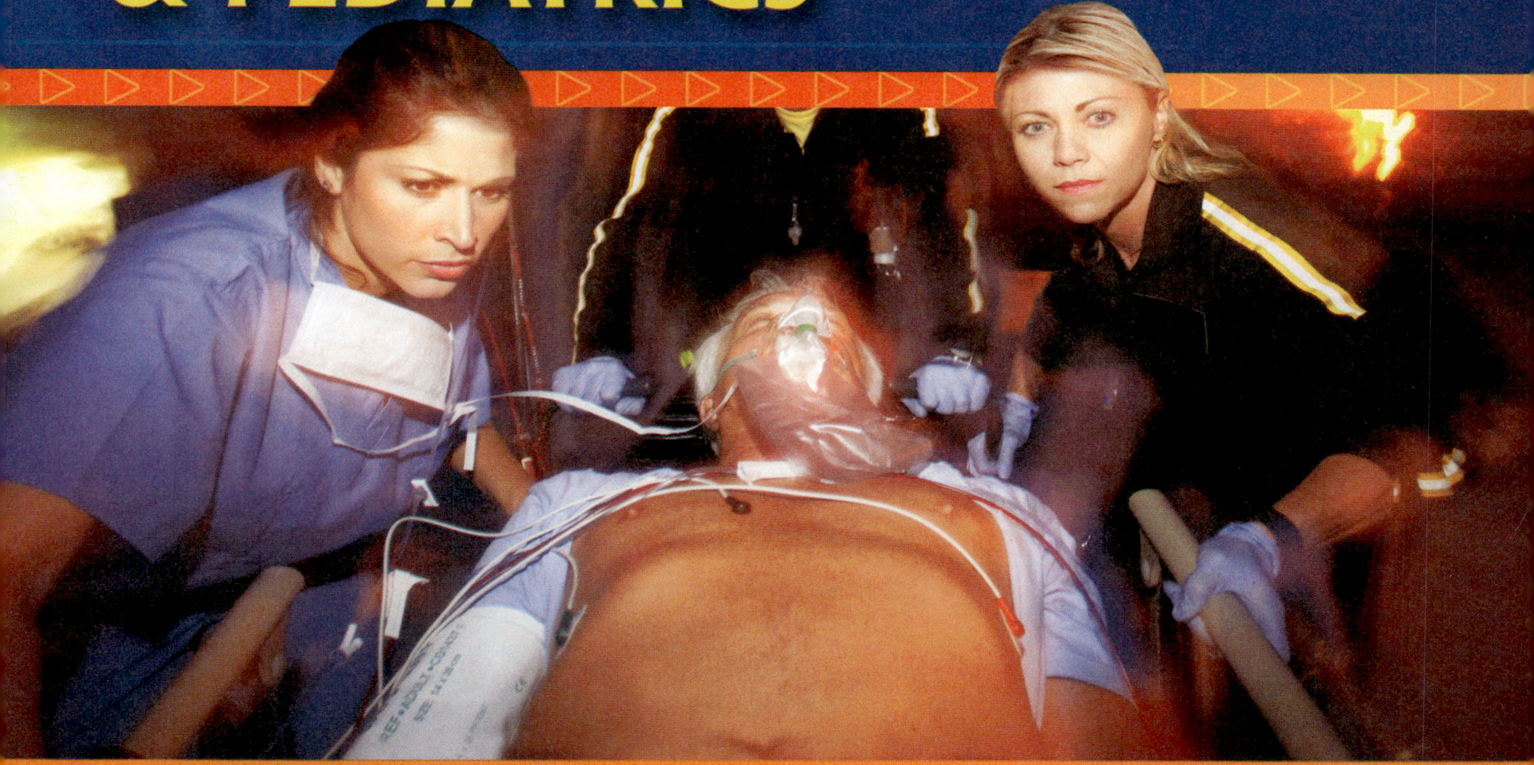

VOLUME II

RICHARD BEEBE | **JEFFREY MYERS, DO**

DELMAR
CENGAGE Learning

Australia • Brazil • Japan • Korea • Mexico • Singapore • Spain • United Kingdom • United States

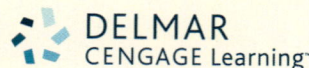

DELMAR
CENGAGE Learning™

Professional Paramedic: Medical Emergencies, Maternal Health, & Pediatrics
Richard Beebe and Jeffrey Myers, DO

Vice President, Career and Professional Editorial: Dave Garza

Director of Learning Solutions: Sandy Clark

Product Development Manager: Janet Maker

Managing Editor: Larry Main

Senior Product Manager: Jennifer A. Starr

Editorial Assistant: Amy Wetsel

Vice President, Career and Professional Marketing: Jennifer Baker

Executive Marketing Manager: Deborah S. Yarnell

Senior Marketing Manager: Erin Coffin

Marketing Coordinator: Shanna Gibbs

Production Director: Wendy Troeger

Production Manager: Mark Bernard

Senior Content Project Manager: Jennifer Hanley

Art Director: Benj Gleeksman

Technology Project Manager: Christopher Catalina

Library of Congress Control Number: 2009943113
ISBN-13: 978-1-4283-2351-3
ISBN-10: 1-4283-2351-1

Delmar
5 Maxwell Drive
Clifton Park, NY 12065-2919
USA

Cengage Learning is a leading provider of customized learning solutions with office locations around the globe, including Singapore, the United Kingdom, Australia, Mexico, Brazil and Japan. Locate your local office at: **international.cengage.com/region**

Cengage Learning products are represented in Canada by Nelson Education, Ltd.

To learn more about Delmar, visit **www.cengage.com/delmar**

Purchase any of our products at your local college store or at our preferred online store **www.cengagebrain.com**

NOTICE TO THE READER

Publisher does not warrant or guarantee any of the products described herein or perform any independent analysis in connection with any of the product information contained herein. Publisher does not assume, and expressly disclaims, any obligation to obtain and include information other than that provided to it by the manufacturer. The reader is expressly warned to consider and adopt all safety precautions that might be indicated by the activities described herein and to avoid all potential hazards. By following the instructions contained herein, the reader willingly assumes all risks in connection with such instructions. The publisher makes no representations or warranties of any kind, including but not limited to, the warranties of fitness for particular purpose or merchantability, nor are any such representations implied with respect to the material set forth herein, and the publisher takes no responsibility with respect to such material. The publisher shall not be liable for any special, consequential, or exemplary damages resulting, in whole or part, from the readers' use of, or reliance upon, this material.

Printed in the United States of America
1 2 3 4 5 6 7 14 13 12 11 10

DEDICATION

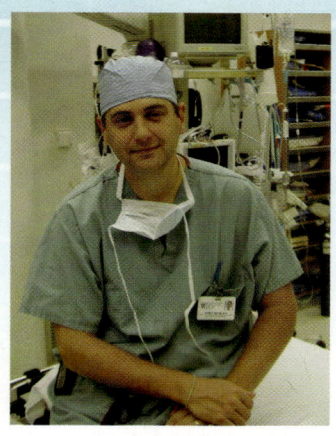

Dedicated to the memory of John Pryor: Paramedic, surgeon, father, husband, brother, and son.

On Christmas Day, 2008, while serving his country in Iraq, Dr. Pryor was tragically killed in the line of duty. Dr. Pryor felt compelled to join the U.S. Army Reserve after witnessing the effects of September 11, 2001, from the rubble pile at Ground Zero. As a member of the U.S. Forward Army Surgical Unit, Dr. Pryor volunteered for not one, but two tours of duty in Iraq, believing that he needed to be there to help others, especially his fellow soldiers. Dr. Pryor's history as a volunteer in medical service started at age 17 with the Clifton Park–Halfmoon Volunteer Ambulance Corp., where he became an Emergency Medical Technician and later a Paramedic. These early beginnings in EMS may have led Dr. Pryor to a career as a widely respected trauma surgeon in Philadelphia.

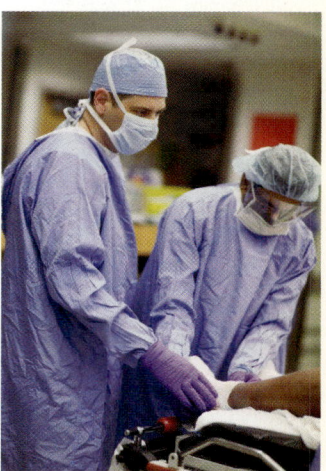

Dr. Pryor often wrote eloquently about his view of the human condition, whether he observed it in war-torn Iraq or the streets of Philadelphia. In one letter he wrote to the family of a mortally wounded Marine, he described his struggle to save the soldier. He expressed that he, his fellow physicians, and especially the Paramedics and EMTs who had the honor of serving with the dead Marine "more than anyone else, know he was a true American hero."

The life of service, love for others, and spirit of devotion of Dr. John Pryor is an example for us all. We, his fellow Paramedics, more than almost anyone else, know he was a true American hero.

TABLE OF CONTENTS

SECTION I: MEDICAL EMERGENCIES

1. DIAGNOSTIC ECG—THE 12-LEAD 2

2. ACUTE CORONARY SYNDROME 36

3. HEART FAILURE 64

8. DISORDERS OF OXYGENATION   212

9. DISORDERS OF VENTILATION   232

10. DISORDERS OF BRAIN FUNCTION   262

11. DISORDERS OF CEREBRAL CIRCULATION   282

17. PSYCHIATRIC DISORDERS   402

18. BEHAVIORAL DISORDERS   418

19. DISORDERS: ABDOMINAL HEMORRHAGE   432

20. DISORDER: ABDOMINAL PAIN   446

21. LOSS OF RENAL FUNCTION   462

SECTION II: MATERNAL HEALTH AND THE NEWLY BORN

SECTION IV: SPECIAL PATIENTS

FOREWORD

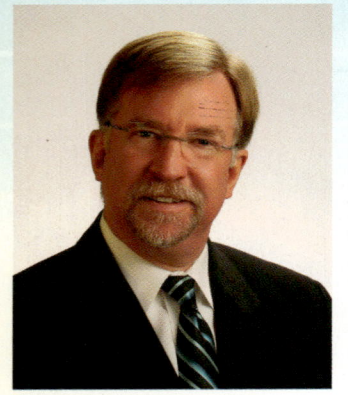

Edward M. Racht, MD

EMS is a practice of medicine. . . .

In medicine, there is an art and a science to everything. The science is *what* we need to do to improve our patient's condition. In its purest form, *what* we do is based on rigorous scientific scrutiny and all the available evidence applicable to the conditions we treat. The art of medicine is *how* we apply the science to our patients in a way that maximizes the potential for an improved outcome. Ironically, the science is often much easier to master than the art. This is perhaps no more pronounced than in the ever-changing, often unpredictable world of EMS.

One thing is very clear: A good practitioner must be accomplished at both the art and the science of medicine.

This is a fascinating time to work in emergency health care. EMS is undergoing tremendous evolution. Not only do we know more about the conditions we treat, but more and more of our clinical practices are now based on sound scientific evidence that applies specifically to our patient population. In the early days of EMS, we adapted evidence from inpatient studies or the laboratory environment and applied it to what we did in the field. While that was certainly appropriate for much of what we did, the challenges of the field and the unique environment of medical care outside the hospital created the need for very targeted research in out-of-hospital medicine. Fortunately, we have more academic initiatives focused on the field than ever before in our brief history. The more we study, the more we learn.

We also understand much more about the seemingly insignificant details that can have a dramatic impact on patient outcomes. Paying attention to those details and focusing on what's truly important in the field practice of medicine is another characteristic of the EMS evolution. For example, there are major changes in the way we attempt to resuscitate our patients. A very consistent, focused attention to perfusion is at the core of everything we do during resuscitation attempts. While many would say we've always believed that to be true, the fact is we didn't always focus on those details during patient care. During those critical moments of assessing and repairing altered physiology and broken anatomy, paying attention to details can often mean the difference between life and death.

As we learn more about the amazing science of the human body and how it behaves when it's "broken," we appreciate that the best approach to management of illness and injury requires more than just memorizing facts. It requires us to put together everything we know, use all our available resources, and develop a plan of action that incorporates clinical care, different modes of transport, and different receiving facilities that have different capabilities. EMS, as a unique practice of medicine, is charged with making complex decisions in short periods of time, often with only limited data. The educational toolbox you hold in your hand will follow you throughout your career and guide you in making the tough calls.

Our role in the Big Picture of Medicine is also evolving. The devastating and unfortunate events of September 11th and the emerging challenges of terrorism, intentional violence, and newer, unpredictable threats have forever focused the American public's attention on the importance of emergency medical care. EMS providers must have the knowledge and ability to deal with an entire spectrum of out-of-hospital problems, ranging from the simple to the unimaginable. Because of the potential for rapidly changing scenarios, we as Paramedics must now know where to go to get the right information and how to rapidly access data we need to make our decisions. Our ability to rapidly deploy our resources throughout a community has also highlighted the value of using EMS providers and systems to disseminate emergency medications and immunizations in the event of a need for rapid public health interventions.

As economic conditions change, our society is retooling healthcare delivery and our patients are using EMS in different ways than they have historically. While that creates some new stresses on EMS, it's a vitally important part of our EMS culture. We are the safety net for many communities suffering from inadequate healthcare resources. Regardless of the number of facilities, patients still get sick and hurt. We should be very proud of our collective ability to care for our fellow human beings regardless of their ability to afford it or our community's ability to provide it. It's who we are.

The newly promulgated Educational Standards are the result of thousands of hours of work from the most accomplished EMS educators, clinicians, and administrators in the profession. The standards provide us with a new approach to delivering the tools that perfect the out-of-hospital delivery of medical care. Rich Beebe, Jeff Myers, and their colleagues have done a spectacular job of presenting the latest evidence in a very comprehensible manner.

As you embark on your educational journey to master the art and science of field medicine, you will continuously discover the valuable educational approach of the *Professional Paramedic Series*. Volume I provides a solid foundation in the knowledge and clinical skills a Paramedic needs to expertly assess and treat patients. In Volumes II and III, the clinical material is presented in a unique way that facilitates the development of critical thinking skills (remember the art?). These volumes use an interrupted case format that narrows a patient's chief concern into a paramedical diagnosis. Volume III also discusses the wide range of operational issues faced by the Paramedic and presents students with the many niches within EMS. In addition, the accompanying student resources and instructor curriculum provide additional cases and avenues to test student knowledge, further refine critical thinking skills, and enhance the teaching and learning experience. Throughout the learning process, students will not only understand what's important, they will also learn how to think their way into the diagnosis and develop an approach that has the best opportunity to improve a patient's condition. *That* is critical thinking.

Enjoy. Enjoy this part of your journey. Enjoy taking care of people when they need you the most. Enjoy learning about the fascinating intricacies of the human body, and enjoy the impact you will have on people's lives every day.

Always remember how important your knowledge, skills, and compassion are for those at the other end of the 9-1-1 call.

Edward M. Racht, MD

PREFACE

THE INTENT OF THIS BOOK

Volume II: Medical Emergencies, Maternal Health, and Pediatrics, the next step in the *Professional Paramedic Series,* applies the knowledge and skills learned in Volume I to specific medical emergencies.

With a focus on both future Paramedics *and* the Paramedics of today, the *Professional Paramedic Series* was designed as a comprehensive resource for Paramedic students during their education and as a source for life-long learning. This series seeks to prepare aspiring Paramedic students in community colleges, universities, and other educational programs with not only the knowledge to become a Paramedic, but also the ability to think critically and decisively when seconds count. Beyond the basic foundation of paramedical knowledge and skills, this series helps the Paramedic student reach a higher level of understanding. For this reason, the series is also an essential resource for practicing Paramedics who are studying for recertification and continuing education.

In January 2009, the new National EMS Education Standards were released to the EMS community. This document serves to set an academic standard for all Paramedic education programs. The *Professional Paramedic Series* was specifically developed with the National EMS Education Standards in mind, yet can also be used in Paramedic programs that are not yet transitioned to the new standards. Each of the three volumes, as a series, meet *and exceed* these new education standards by not only teaching the essential knowledge and skills, but also by preparing each student to *think* like a Paramedic. As Paramedics who started in the streets and who continue to practice in the streets, we support the vision of the National EMS Education Standards, and have created this series, aptly named "Professional Paramedic."

WHY WE WROTE THIS SERIES

As educators, we *challenge* our learners—the students of this series—to be the best Paramedics possible. Although other Paramedic textbooks are available, we felt that the evolving nature of the Paramedic field demanded a fresh approach. We wanted our textbook to challenge Paramedic students to think about the application of medical knowledge to field practice. This approach changed the focus of a Paramedic textbook from being the center of a Paramedic's education to one in which it serves as an authoritative resource that implores the student to explore the current state of the science.

As part of our vision in writing this series, we wanted to recognize the practice of *paramedicine*. What is paramedicine? Paramedicine is a unique practice of emergency medicine that happens in the out-of-hospital setting. First described in the *EMS Agenda for the Future* in 1996, paramedicine is the result of the growth of EMS over almost one-half of a century. It encompasses the complete roles and responsibilities of the Paramedic within the domains of health care, public health, and public safety systems. We offer this series as a guide to prehospital emergency medical care and the practice of paramedicine, providing learners with a reference for the often complex, at times ambiguous, and always challenging field of emergency medicine.

We understand that often the best Paramedics are those who start with a natural curiosity about emergency medicine and inquisitiveness about how that medical knowledge could be practically applied in the streets. These students know it is important to be *street smart* as well as *book smart*. This book seeks to help answer their questions through a conversation with the student.

THE *PROFESSIONAL PARAMEDIC SERIES*

This series is designed to follow a logical progression of learning, in which knowledge and skills are presented first in Volume I, followed by the application of those skills in emergency situations in Volume II, and then trauma and special response considerations in Volume III. The framework of each book is practical in approach: introducing principles, skills, and terminology; presenting a typical case; walking through critical response steps; and again reviewing key concepts to ensure understanding for successful application on the job.

The series is inclusive of all of the content areas listed in the National EMS Education Standards and contains material on most of the critical and emergent disorders listed in the EMS core content, as well as many of the lower acuity conditions. This coverage helps ensure the student's preparation for the National Registry or state Paramedic certification examinations. More importantly, the series helps prepare the Paramedic student for professional Paramedic practice.

VOLUME I: FOUNDATIONS OF PARAMEDIC CARE

ISBN: 978-1-14283-2345-2

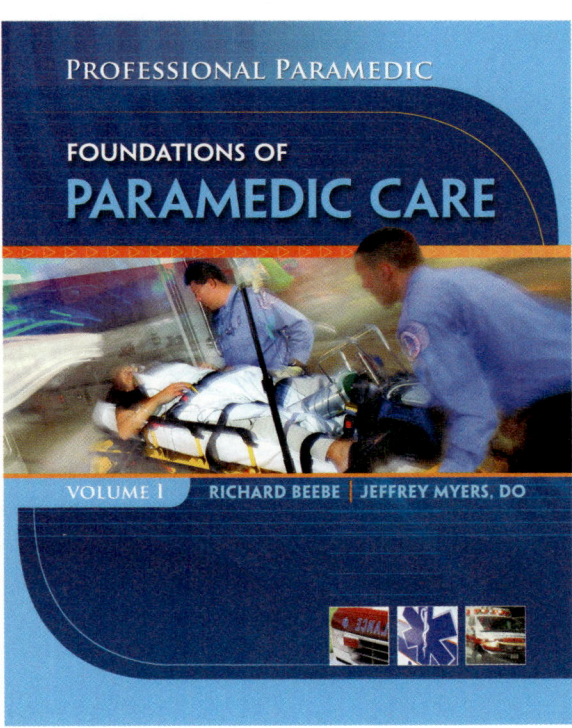

To be able to make a diagnosis, the Paramedic must be well grounded in the basics of medicine including anatomy and physiology as well as pathophysiology. *Volume I: Foundations of Paramedic Care* begins with the basics. This first volume in the series initiated this learning by introducing the fundamental knowledge and skills for success, as well as the necessary tools

to begin developing a professional approach to emergency medicine and Paramedic care.

Volume I is divided into six sections:

- **Section I:** Framework for Paramedic Practice
- **Section II:** Ethics and Law in EMS
- **Section III:** EMS and Public Health
- **Section IV:** Scientific Principles
- **Section V:** Principles of Clinical Practice
- **Section VI:** Clinical Essentials

VOLUME II: MEDICAL EMERGENCIES, MATERNAL HEALTH & PEDIATRICS

ISBN: 978-1-4283-2351-3

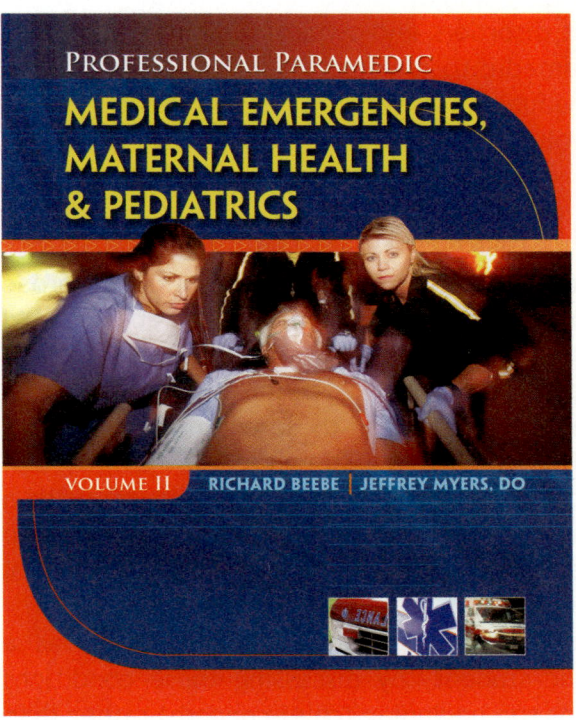

Volume II of the series introduces an *interrupted case* approach to discuss medical, maternal, and pediatric emergencies, as well as emergencies in special patient populations. This book walks the reader through a wide range of emergency response situations: from cardiac emergencies to various diseases and disorders; from gynecological concerns to neonatal resuscitation; from the chronically ill to the victims of domestic violence and sexual assault. Utilizing a typical emergency that a Paramedic might encounter in the field, each chapter includes a Case Study that relates to the subject of the chapter and presents critical information, leading the reader to develop a Paramedic's diagnosis from the information provided.

It should be understood that the case represented in each Volume II chapter is only one potential patient presentation for that chief concern. To that end, we have included additional cases in the accompanying *Study Guide*. It is the responsibility of both the student and the instructor to explore these other cases, as well as other real world examples, to fully appreciate other potential patient presentations. Even so, this cannot possibly cover the entire universe of potential patient presentations; this is the essence of what makes paramedicine exciting, challenging, and refreshing. The intention of these cases is to reinforce the commonalities of presentation for the different disorders and syndromes that will permit the Paramedic to make a diagnosis, regardless of the individual patient-specific conditions.

This volume is divided into four sections.

SECTION I: MEDICAL EMERGENCIES

The medical emergencies section covers the broad range of medical conditions the Paramedic will encounter in the field. This section is organized by the chief concern that is commonly elicited from a patient who has one of these conditions. Patients don't often provide a Paramedic with a final diagnosis, but they will provide the Paramedic with a chief concern and a set of symptoms that will help the Paramedic arrive at a paramedical differential diagnosis.

In this way, the organization helps you, as a Paramedic student, by discussing these conditions starting at the beginning (chief concern) rather than at the end (the diagnosis). Although the presentation in the chapter may be the same way a patient will present, the Professional Paramedic understands that many of these conditions may present with different chief concerns. For example, a patient who has an acute coronary syndrome may present with a chief concern of chest pain (common) or may present with a chief concern of syncope (not as common).

Chapters are cross-referenced with each other to help the Paramedic student build this framework as the course progresses. Each chapter is also based around a case, leading the student through the process of arriving at a paramedical diagnosis for the patient. The case-based approach found in this

volume is augmented by cases in the *Study Guide* and the instructor materials.

SECTION II: MATERNAL HEALTH AND THE NEWLY BORN

In the section on maternal health and the newly born, the discussion focuses on women's health issues that the Paramedic will encounter. This section covers conditions that can occur in the non-pregnant female as well as the pregnant female. The Paramedic is guided through the normal delivery process and walked through complicated childbirth. Finally, the section concludes with a review of newborn resuscitation.

SECTION III: PEDIATRICS

Children are neither just small adults nor patients that the Paramedic should be frightened of! In this section, the assessment, physiology, and pathophysiology of children is presented to allow the Paramedic student to become more confident in assessing and treating pediatric patients.

SECTION IV: SPECIAL PATIENTS

In the final section of this volume, the unique needs of several different types of patients are covered. These special patient populations include geriatric patients who have special considerations due to changes in physiology that come with aging as well as other potential impairments. Patients who are technology dependent, chronically ill, or have different cultural backgrounds from our own are all patient populations that may have special needs. Finally, the subject of domestic violence and sexual assault is covered, providing the Paramedic with the tools to sensitively handle these situations.

VOLUME III: TRAUMA CARE AND EMS OPERATIONS

ISBN: 978-1-4283-2348-3

Volume III highlights the care of patients with traumatic and environmental emergencies. Additionally, special response considerations and a broad range of operational medical topics are presented to prepare readers with the complete spectrum of knowledge required to succeed as a Paramedic. These aspects of Paramedic practice help to make paramedicine a unique profession with its own unique body of knowledge.

Topics in this volume include trauma care, environmental medicine, EMS operations, emergency incident management, and other topics in operational medicine.

Volume III is divided into four sections:

- **Section I:** Trauma Care
- **Section II:** Environmental Medicine
- **Section III:** EMS Operations
- **Section IV:** Emergency Incident Management

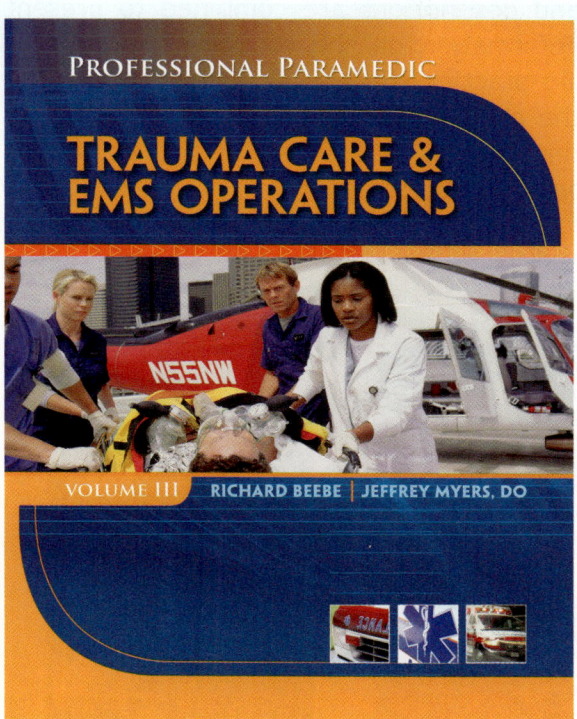

FEATURES

Along with an appealing design, the series has many features intended to motivate the student to read and learn the knowledge and skills presented in each volume.

COMPREHENSIVE COVERAGE

The complex depth and comprehensive breadth of information required for a working knowledge of Paramedic practice, for Paramedic certification, and ultimately for success on the job are all provided in an engaging and reader-friendly manner. Students will be properly prepared for these challenges with evidence-based information presented within the content that meets and *exceeds* National EMS Education Standards.

KEY CONCEPTS

Presented in the beginning of each chapter, the Key Concepts set learning goals for students and preview both the didactic and psychomotor skills presented in the chapter that they are expected to learn.

ANATOMY CONCEPTS

Following the Key Concepts at the beginning of the chapter, Anatomy Concepts outline the anatomy and physiology topics that students should be familiar with in order to gain a complete understanding of the subject matter discussed in the chapter.

INTERRUPTED CASE STUDIES

The interrupted case studies included in each chapter facilitate the *conversation*, both the internal dialogue within the student and the dialogue between the student and instructor within the classroom. The Case Study presented in each chapter relates to the chapter content and is carried through the entire chapter, with each new section providing further details on the emergency in order to encourage students to develop critical response skills. By portraying realistic emergency situations that a Paramedic is likely to encounter, the book introduces the student to the material in a meaningful manner. This presentation also encourages the decision-making process involved in making a field diagnosis, and outlines a plan of treatment that meets the standard of care within the scope of practice for the patient—for prehospital care and transport to the hospital.

Each case is designed to encourage a Paramedic's thought process and includes Critical Thinking Questions immediately following the sections where the case is discussed in the chapter.

CASE STUDY (CONTINUED)

During the course of the patient history, the patient's assistant relates that the professor had the flu, and suggests that maybe these symptoms are related to the virus she had. The Paramedic reassures her that, while that was a possibility, it would be more prudent to transport the professor to the emergency department for a medical evaluation.

CRITICAL THINKING QUESTIONS

1. What other conditions can mimic a stroke?
2. Why did the Paramedic suggest that the patient be transported?

CHEATED METHOD

This method follows the standard medical intelligence of a Paramedic (sometimes called "medic think") and encourages students to engage in the critical thinking process needed for a proper field diagnosis and treatment—Chief concern, History, Examination, Assessment, Treatment, Evaluation, and Disposition. Each is discussed, as applicable, in the chapters and follow the presentation of each case so that learners can think logically about these critical response steps.

PROFESSIONAL PARAMEDIC

Integrated throughout the book, this advice highlights the professional attitudes that signify the difference between a competent Paramedic and a proficient Paramedic—one fellow Paramedics respect and look to as a leader.

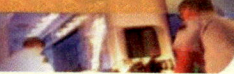

PROFESSIONAL PARAMEDIC

Most 12-lead monitors offer a printed computer interpretation. While this printout is accurate, the Paramedic must be capable of assessing, interpreting, and planning care based on the ECG.

STREET SMART

Consisting of lessons learned by the authors while in practice in the field, Street Smart tips focus on practical information that can help new Paramedic students perform in less-than-ideal or unusual situations.

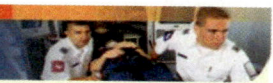

STREET SMART

Although the terms "convulsion" and "seizure" are commonly used interchangeably by the public, seizure connotes an epileptic seizure whereas convulsion would be any new and unexplained event. Although the public often uses the term "seizure" to describe any episode of unconsciousness, spasms, and even strokes, the Paramedic should not take that to mean that the patient has the diagnosis of epilepsy.

CULTURAL/REGIONAL DIFFERENCES

Important considerations are pointed out for responding to patients of different cultural backgrounds. This prepares students for the diverse patient population that the Paramedic will encounter in emergency situations. Understanding these cultural/regional differences will increase the Paramedic's effectiveness in the field.

CULTURAL/REGIONAL DIFFERENCES

Some cultures have specific death rituals. Providing that these rituals do not violate local regulation, the Paramedic should facilitate the performance of these rituals by the family.

STEP-BY-STEP SKILLS

Photos and descriptions are combined to present critical information on the fundamental skills of Paramedic practice. Each Skill is included at the end of the chapter to avoid interrupting the flow of learning, and is referenced in the applicable discussion within the chapter.

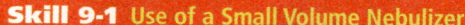

Skill 9-1 Use of a Small Volume Nebulizer

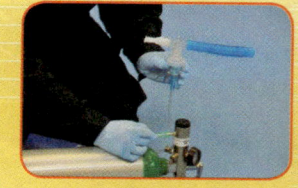

1 Assemble the nebulizer components and attach them to an oxygen source.

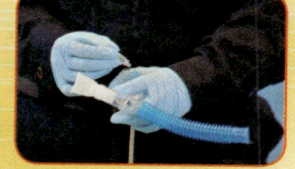

2 Instill the appropriate medication into the chamber.

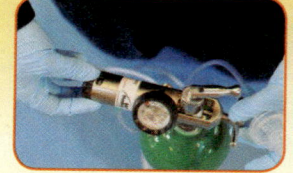

3 Set the oxygen flow rate to 8 liters per minute.

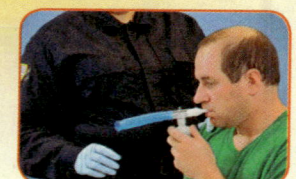

4 Instruct the patient to place the mouthpiece in the mouth with a good seal.

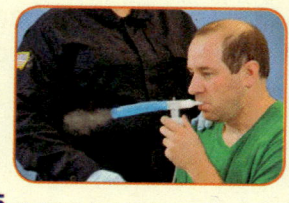

5 Instruct the patient to inhale as deeply as possible and fully exhale.

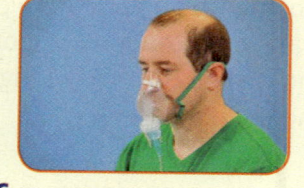

6 Some patients will perform better using a face mask rather than a mouthpiece for delivery of aerosolized medication, though its effectiveness is questionable.

CONCLUSION AND KEY POINTS

Critical points included in the chapter are covered and provide a basis of review for the student. Whereas the Conclusion provides an overall summary of the chapter's main theme, the Key Points provide a bulleted list of important information that is helpful for study or review.

REVIEW QUESTIONS

Questions at the end of each chapter are helpful for evaluating student knowledge of the concepts presented in the chapter.

CASE STUDY QUESTIONS

Following the Review Questions at the end of each chapter, the Case Study Questions focus on the Case Study that is presented throughout the chapter. Whereas the Critical Thinking Questions introduced in the Case Study sections focus on specific response steps, the Case Study Questions at the end of the chapter encourage learners to take a step back and review the entire case—from initial response to conclusion.

REFERENCES AND AN EVIDENCE-BASED APPROACH

Validation is essential to ensure the content discussed is substantiated by science and medicine. Each thoroughly researched chapter includes documentation of references that support the content presented in the chapter.

REFERENCES:

1. American Heart Association. Heart disease and stroke statistics: 2008 update at a glance. Available at: http://www.americanheart.org/downloadable/heart/1200082005246HS_Stats%202008.final.pdf. Accessed April 15, 2008.
2. White HD, Chew DP. Acute myocardial infarction. *Lancet.* 2008;372(9638):570–584.

THE *PROFESSIONAL PARAMEDIC SERIES* CURRICULUM PLAN

We are proud to present a robust curriculum plan for the Paramedic student and instructor. As part of this plan, we offer resources that work hand-in-hand with each volume in the series, serving to further enhance both the teaching and the learning experience. For the students, resources are available that will help them review important concepts through practical application, develop and practice critical thinking skills, and guide them toward further research and discovery. For the instructors, we offer tools that will help them efficiently prepare for classroom instruction, manage and track student progress of didactic and skill requirements, keep informed of new advances in the EMS field, and overall, engage students in learning both in and out of the classroom.

FOR THE STUDENT

STUDY GUIDES

Bridging the gap between knowledge and application, one *Study Guide* accompanies each volume to offer students additional case reviews for each chapter, along with multiple types of practice questions and activities required for comprehension of the material.

- Volume I Study Guide, ISBN: 978-1-4283-2346-9
- Volume II Study Guide, ISBN: 978-1-4283-2352-0
- Volume III Study Guide, ISBN: 978-1-4283-2349-0

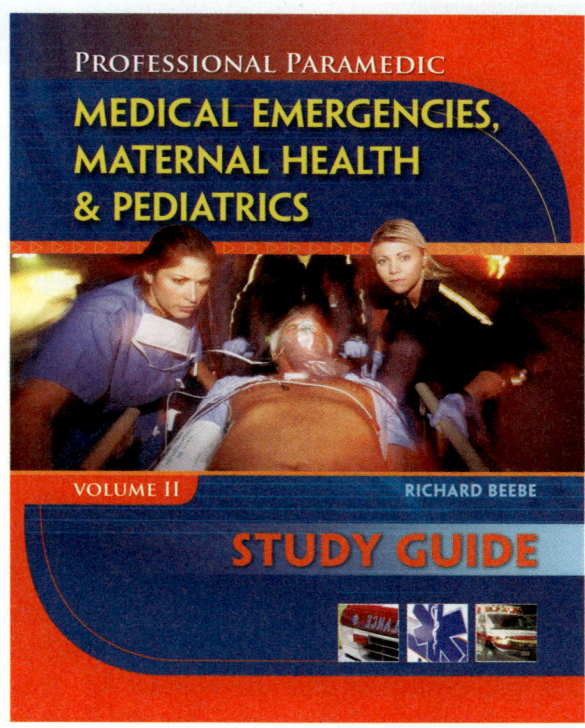

ONLINE COMPANIONS

Students are provided with FREE access to our website with an Online Companion to accompany each volume. This website invites students to further study and explore the concepts presented in each volume. The Online Companion includes articles and up-to-date information on the EMS field, related links to important industry organizations and resources, information related to national guidelines, illustrated glossaries, and bonus content. Each Online Companion is uniquely designed to the corresponding volume in the series, and contains information relevant to the topics covered within that volume.

Visit http://www.cengage.com/community/ems to access these Online Companions!

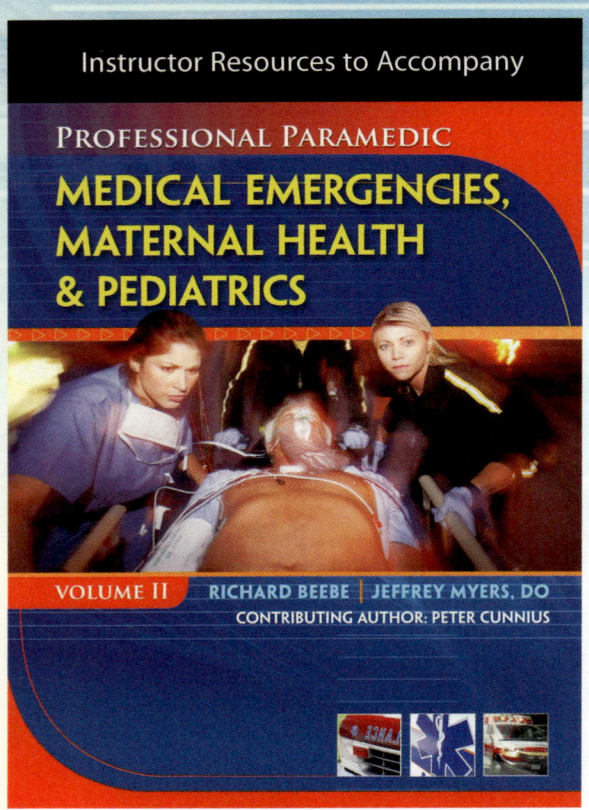

Instructor Resources to Accompany

PROFESSIONAL PARAMEDIC

MEDICAL EMERGENCIES, MATERNAL HEALTH & PEDIATRICS

VOLUME II   RICHARD BEEBE | JEFFREY MYERS, DO
CONTRIBUTING AUTHOR: PETER CUNNIUS

FOR THE INSTRUCTOR

INSTRUCTOR RESOURCES (CD-ROM)

Our instructor resources for each volume are designed to help you effectively prepare students to become well-rounded, street-smart Paramedics within the guidelines of the new National EMS Educational Standards. The Instructor Resources on CD-ROM includes tools that help instructors and administrators prepare their Paramedic program in a timely and efficient manner. Each CD-ROM includes the following features:

■ **Administration:** This section includes information on setting up the program, as well as practical advice for transitioning your program to the new National EMS Educational Standards. In addition, it includes the following tools:

● **Equipment Checklist:** The Equipment Checklist provides a resource for instructors to ensure that they have the necessary tools for classroom instruction and for setting up and running skill sequences.

● **Concept Maps:** Highlighting the decision-making process, these Concept Maps offer a way for instructors to help students conceptualize ideas in the classroom and help them develop the critical thinking skills necessary for determining a field diagnosis. Each Concept Map, utilizing a typical emergency scenario, walks students through the critical thinking steps used during a EMS response.

● **Correlation to National EMS Education Standards and D.O.T. Paramedic Curriculum:** These guides map out Paramedic content and indicate the volume, chapter, and pages where this content is covered in the *Professional Paramedic Series*.

■ **Lesson Plans:** Including an outline of each chapter with correlations to the accompanying PowerPoint® presentations, skill sheets, and helpful teaching tips, these Lesson Plans provide a helpful guide for classroom instruction. These plans are provided in Word format so that instructors may revise them according to local practice variations and regional/state medical protocols.

■ **PowerPoint® Presentations:** Correlated to the accompanying Lesson Plans, these presentations combine key points with photos, graphics, and video to serve as a basis for either interactive classroom instruction or as augmentation of an asynchronous distance learning program.

■ **Computerized Test Banks:** Containing over 1,000 questions and covering the content in each chapter, these Test Banks in ExamView format allow instructors to manage test administration in the classroom. Instructors may create or edit tests based on existing questions, edit questions, and add or delete questions to fit local practice variations and regional/state medical protocols—all in this user-friendly program.

■ **Teaching Sheets:** Highlighting the Paramedic skills necessary for Paramedic practice, these Teaching Sheets provide a baseline for skills learning. Each Teaching Sheet provides a breakdown of the critical principles for the skill, and is included in Word format to allow instructors to add specifics based on their local requirements and/or regional/state protocols and procedures.

■ **Clinical Logs:** Based on the Teaching Sheets, these Clinical Logs provide forms for tracking student accomplishment of prehospital (field) and in-hospital (clinical) skills. These forms, complete with a signature page, are provided in Word format to allow instructors to edit them in order to meet local requirements.

- ■ **Research and Discovery—Instructor Reference Guide:** Paramedicine, like medicine, has an ever-changing body of knowledge. To remain current, the Paramedic must be a life-long learner. In addition to the listing of references that appear at the end of chapters in each volume in the series, this Instructor Reference Guide provides additional resources—including articles, websites, organizations, and other reference materials—to find information on specific topics. This ensures that instructors remain informed of current practices in the EMS field.

ONLINE COMPANIONS

Linked to the student Online Companions, these resources provide instructors FREE access to bonus content, including podcasts, articles on new information and technology, links to EMS community websites, information related to national guidelines, and additional classroom materials. Each Online Companion is uniquely designed to the corresponding volume in the series, and contains information relevant to the topics covered within that volume.

WEB TUTOR ON WEBCT AND BLACKBOARD

Providing a content-rich, Web-based teaching and learning aid, this tool helps to emphasize and clarify complex concepts, provides a forum for discussion, and offers a venue for tracking course syllabus and other program-related activities.

WebTutor on Blackboard Course allows instructors to quickly and easily jump-start their on-line course development. Whether you want to Web-enable your class or put an entire course on-line, WebTutor delivers!

ABOUT THE AUTHORS

RICHARD BEEBE, MSED, BSN, RN, NREMT-P

Richard Beebe started his EMS career as an Explorer Scout with the Moyers Corners Volunteer Fire Department in upstate New York in 1974. Since obtaining his Emergency Medical Technician

certification in 1975, Mr. Beebe has continuously maintained his certification and his practice. During his career, Mr. Beebe has served in fire/EMS, commercial EMS, volunteer EMS, and as a municipal Paramedic. During that time, he has served as a volunteer crew chief, a squad captain, and a Paramedic supervisor. Mr. Beebe currently serves as a civilian Paramedic for the Guilderland Police Department, outside of Albany, New York.

Mr. Beebe has also been a critical care nurse since 1985, having practiced for 10 years in both the Emergency Department and the Intensive Care Unit. During these years, Mr. Beebe developed his knowledge of medicine and—perhaps, more importantly—an appreciation of the potential impact that prehospital advanced life support could have on patient morbidity and mortality.

Consistent with that belief, Mr. Beebe became a Paramedic in 1988 and, in hopes of advancing the practice of his fellow Paramedics, started his career as a Paramedic Educator.

During his tenure as a Paramedic Educator, Mr. Beebe has served in the capacity as lecturer, instructor-coordinator, and Paramedic program director. He continues to speak at local, regional, state, and national conferences on topics of importance to both the EMT and the Paramedic.

Mr. Beebe was a clinical assistant professor at the State University of New York at Cobleskill and Paramedic program director for Bassett Healthcare's Center for Rural Emergency Medical Services Education for over a decade.

Mr. Beebe has been published in several journals, including the *Journal of Emergency Medical Services and Fire-Engineering,* as well as being a co-author for Delmar/Cengage Learning's *Fundamentals of Basic Emergency Care,* now in its third edition.

Mr. Beebe has contributed to the previous editions of the National Standard Curriculum for Paramedic, Intermediate, and Basic; to the national EMS Education Agenda for the Future; to the National EMS Scope of Practice; and served as content leader for the National EMS Education Standards. Mr. Beebe is also a charter member of the National Association of EMS Educators.

JEFF MYERS, DO, EDM, NREMT-P, FAAEM

Dr. Myers has been involved in EMS for over 20 years, including 12 years in the prehospital environment and 18 years as an EMS educator. Dr. Myers began his EMS journey in 1988 in upstate New York by volunteering for his college ambulance (RPI Ambulance) and a local community ambulance (North Greenbush Ambulance Association). He began teaching in 1990 for the Rensselaer County Ambulance and Rescue Association, eventually becoming a state Certified Instructor Coordinator. Dr. Myers ran the EMT-Basic original course in Rensselaer County for three years before leaving to attend medical school. During the early 1990s, he also served as a Rensselaer County Deputy County EMS Coordinator for four years, responding to multi-ambulance and multi-agency incidents. His field experience includes volunteer, commercial, and combination paid-volunteer agencies as a Paramedic in upstate New York and in southern Maine.

Dr. Myers attended medical school at the University of New England College of Osteopathic Medicine in Biddeford, Maine. While in medical school, he continued to teach ACLS and BCLS classes through the local hospital.

Dr. Myers then moved to Buffalo, New York, completing his residency in Emergency Medicine at the State University of New York, University at Buffalo in 2004. In his final year of residency, he served as Chief Resident. He stayed in Buffalo for a two-year EMS Fellowship through the Erie County Medical Center and completed a Masters in Education at the University at Buffalo. He is board certified in Emergency Medicine and a Fellow of the American Academy of Emergency Medicine.

He is currently on faculty at the State University of New York, University at Buffalo as a clinical assistant professor and serves as the associate system EMS medical director and EMS fellowship director at the Erie County Medical Center. Dr. Myers is an active member of the Specialized Medical Assistance Response Team, western New York's physician response team, which is called upon to augment local EMS in MCIs, assist in special situations, and provide tactical medical support. He is also the Director of the Behling Simulation Center at the University at Buffalo Academic Health Sciences Center, New York. Dr. Myers has several publications in peer-reviewed journals and is an author for Delmar/Cengage Learning, writing *Automated Defibrillation for Professional and Lay Rescuers* and *Principles of Pathophysiology and Emergency Care*. He also produced and directed the *Techniques in Airway Management* DVD series. Dr. Myers has spoken at several regional and national conferences on a variety of topics.

For more information on topics or to provide feedback on the textbook, please check out Dr. Myers' website at http://ems-ed.photoemsdoc.com.

ACKNOWLEDGMENTS

As with all of our projects, the *Professional Paramedic Series* would not have been possible without the support, guidance, and participation of the contributors, reviewers, and advisory board members. We owe these individuals our sincere thanks.

CONTRIBUTORS

During the development of *Volume II: Medical Emergencies, Maternal Health & Pediatrics*, we were honored to have the following contributors participate in researching, writing, editing, and reviewing materials to ensure a comprehensive and accurate Paramedic guide.

Kyle David Bates, MS, NREMT-P, CCEMT-P, FP-C, Paramedic, Town of Tonawanda Police Emergency Medical Unit, Tonawanda, NY; Education Program Coordinator, Lake Plains Community Care Network, Batavia, NY

Karen M. Beckman, RN, MSN/Ed, SANE-A, Clinical Nurse Specialist of Emergency Services, Erie County Medical Center, Buffalo, NY

Sharon Chiumento, BSN, RN, EMT-P, EMS Quality Improvement Coordinator & Paramedic Educator, University of Rochester Medical Center, Rochester, NY

Heidi Cordi, MD, MS, MPH, EMT-P, Associate Medical Director, Emergency Medical Services, New York Presbyterian Hospital, New York, NY; Medical Director, Cordi Consultants, Inc.

William E. Gandy, JD, NREMT-P, Principle Paramedic Instructor, Cochise College, Sierra Vista, AZ; EMS Education and Consultation, Tuscon, AZ

Deborah Kufs, MS, RN, EMT-P, Director, Paramedic Program, Hudson Valley Community College (HVCC)

Gerald Maloney, DO, FACOEP, Associate Director, Northern Ohio Poison Control Center, Assistant Professor of Emergency Medicine and Environmental Health Sciences, Case Western Reserve University, Cleveland, OH

Jennifer Miller, RN, Albany Medical Center, Neonatal Intensive Care Unit (NICU), Albany, NY

Laura O'Shea, RD, CNM, MSN, Director of Nurse-Midwifery Services, Bassett Healthcare, Cooperstown, NY

Alexandre R. Picard, MD, NREMT-P, Pediatric Emergency Medicine Fellow, Clinical Instructor Emergency Medicine, State University of New York at Buffalo

Jeffrey Thompson, MD, Attending Physician, Professional Emergency Services, Clinical Instructor of Emergency Medicine, State University of New York at Buffalo

Robert Waddell, II, BS, BA, EMT-P (ret), Vice President, Think Sharp, Inc., Cheyenne, WY

Brett Williams, MD, Florida Emergency Physicians, Orlando, FL

For the development of the art program in this volume—the countless hours spent in preparation, set up, and shooting of the photography appearing in this book, as well as the extensive research, persistence, and acquisition of those "hard to find" photos and graphics—we express our gratitude to the following individuals:

Jon Behrens, AAS, EMT-P, Paramedic Instructor, State University of New York at Cobleskill

Liana Dypka, Art Manuscript Development

Mike Gallitelli, Photographer, Metroland Photo, Inc.

Abigail Reip, Photo Acquisition and Permission Coordinator

REVIEWERS

To the reviewers, who provided an honest evaluation of the content in the book and continual guidance throughout development of this volume, we express our appreciation:

Mike McLaughlin, Director of Health Occupations, Kirkwood Community College, IA

Barry Nicoson, Program Chair, Paramedic Science, Ivy Tech Community College, IN

M. Jane Pollock, Extension Education Training Specialist, Emergency Medicine, East Carolina University, NC

Don Royder, Emergency Medical Services Program Coordinator, Texas Engineering Extension Service, Emergency Services Training Institute, TX

Jason Segner, Program Director, EMS Education, Blinn College, TX

Shari Turner, EMS Program Director, Palm Beach Community College, FL

EMS ADVISORY BOARD

We offer special thanks to our Advisory Board Members, who take time out of their schedules to advise us on our training materials, the status of the EMS field, and to work with us as partners in striving to meet the needs of the students and instructors of today—and those of the future.

Scott Bourn, National Director of Clinical Programs, National Resource Center, American Medical Response, CO

Deb Cason, Associate Professor, University of Texas Southwestern Medical Center, TX

Don Collins, Captain, Massport Fire-Rescue, Logan International Airport, Boston, MA

Stephen Dean, Director, Corporate Training, Paramedic Plus, OK

Joe Grafft, President, Customized Safety Training

Art Hsieh, Chief Executive Officer and Director of Education, San Francisco Paramedic Association, CA

Mike Kennamer, Director of Workforce Development, Northeast Alabama Community College, AL

Guy Piefer, Paramedic Program Coordinator, Borough of Manhattan Community College, City of Yonkers Fire Department, NY

Ed Racht, Vice President of Medical Affairs and Chief Medical Officer, Piedmont Newnan Hospital, GA

Karla Rickards, EMS Training Coordinator, Unified Fire Authority, Salt Lake County

John Rinard, Training Coordinator, TEEX, Texas A&M University

John Sinclair, Fire Chief, Kittitas Valley Fire Rescue; Emergency Manager, City of Ellensburg, WA; Immediate Past Chair and International Director, International Association of Fire Chiefs, Emergency Medical Services Section

Mike Ward, Director of Emergency Health Services, George Washington Medical Center, Washington DC

FROM THE AUTHORS

BEEBE

First, I would like to acknowledge my friends and family, and particularly my wife Laura, whose support has sustained me over the 10 years that it took to write this book. Thank you for your love.

I would also like to thank the professionals at Delmar/Cengage Learning who have helped support this idea from its onset and continue to encourage me to greater accomplishments. I would like to thank Sandy, Benj, Erin, and particularly Jennifer, the backbone of this excellent team.

Finally, I would like to thank my students who, each and every year, challenge me to be the best Paramedic and educator that I can be and who, even to this day, continue to inspire me. In the 30-plus years I have been involved in EMS and EMS education, I have truly seen EMS in general—and Paramedics in particular—evolve into a caring profession that we all can be proud of.

MYERS

Thanks and love to my family. This textbook (and all my life's projects) would not be possible without their support.

DELMAR/CENGAGE LEARNING TEAM

For the team that always finds a way, every day, to turn an idea into a reality, we thank these extraordinary people for their hard work, dedication, support, and creativity:

Janet Maker, Product Development Manager

Jennifer Starr, Senior Product Manager

Amy Wetsel, Editorial Assistant

Jennifer Hanley, Senior Content Project Manager

Erin Coffin, Senior Marketing Manager

Shanna Gibbs, Marketing Coordinator

CLOSING THOUGHTS

In a time when the importance of quality improvement is understood and appreciated, we encourage students and instructors alike to communicate with us. Via these conversations, all parties can improve their understandings. We are all enriched through this communication.

Richard W. O. Beebe
MedicThink@gmail.com

Jeffrey W. Myers
http://ems-ed
.photoemsdoc.com

SECTION I

MEDICAL EMERGENCIES

This section covers the broad range of medical conditions the Paramedic will encounter in the field. The chapters within this section are organized by the various chief concerns commonly elicited from patients. Although patients don't often provide a Paramedic with a final diagnosis, they will provide the Paramedic with a chief concern and a set of symptoms that will help the Paramedic arrive at a paramedical differential diagnosis.

CHAPTER 1

DIAGNOSTIC ECG—THE 12-LEAD

KEY CONCEPTS:

Upon completion of this chapter, it is expected that the reader will understand these following concepts:

- Use of 12-lead ECG as the first step in a critical care pathway for patients with acute coronary syndrome
- The critical need for accurate acquisition of the 12-lead ECG
- How analysis of the 12-lead ECG permits the Paramedic to assess the patient and make a prognosis

ANATOMY CONCEPTS:

Prior to reading this chapter the Paramedic student should be familiar with the following anatomy and physiology concepts:

- Anatomical walls of the left ventricle
- Coronary arteries in relation to walls of the left ventricle
  - Right coronary artery
  - Left coronary artery
  - Left anterior descending coronary artery
  - Circumflex
  - Septal perforators
- Layers of the myocardium

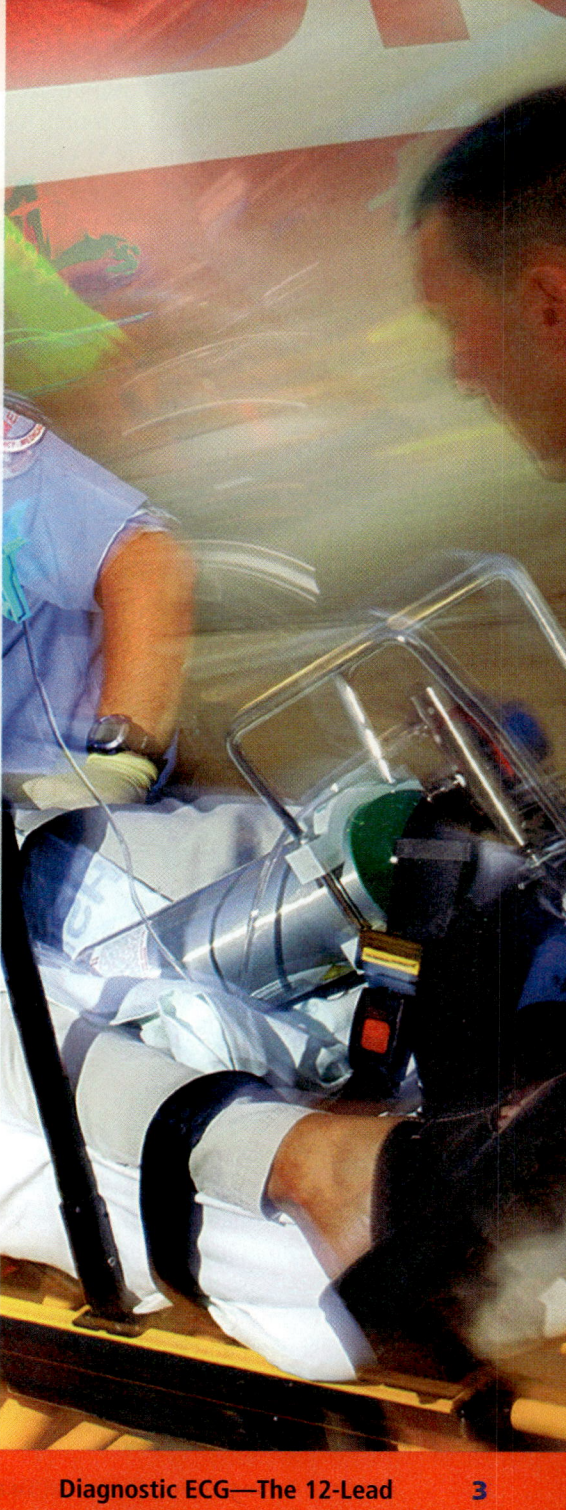

CASE STUDY:

The Paramedics were called to the home of Jennie Swinter. Mrs. Swinter is an 82-year-old widow, living alone on a small farm on which she still raises vegetables. She called EMS because she became exhausted and out of breath after walking to the bathroom. The inexperienced Paramedic commented that, at her age, Mrs. Swinter should be tired and out of breath. The more experienced Paramedic suggested that many acute processes could account for Mrs. Swinter's complaints.

As the ambulance arrived, the two Paramedics noted a large field of vegetables and flowers. The door was opened and the home was spotless. Mrs. Swinter was slouched in a chair in the living room.

CRITICAL THINKING QUESTIONS

1. Could Mrs. Swinter's shortness of breath and fatigue be cardiac related?
2. Why would Mrs. Swinter not have chest pain?
3. What diagnostic information might a 12-lead ECG yield in Mrs. Swinter's case?

OVERVIEW

Death from acute myocardial infarction remains a leading reason for mortality in the United States despite advances in medicine. If untreated, acute coronary syndrome can lead to fatal heart attacks. Nonetheless, it is estimated that only 50% of patients with acute coronary syndrome are transported by EMS and the majority of cardiac arrests occur in the prehospital setting. It is therefore important that Paramedics be able to identify and aggressively treat these patients.

Chief Concern

There are numerous causes of chest pain, which are discussed in detail in Chapter 2 on acute coronary syndrome. Of particular concern for the Paramedic is chest pain of a cardiac etiology. Patients with cardiac-related chest pain are at high risk for **acute myocardial infarction (AMI)** and sudden cardiac death.

The identification of the patient with potential for acute myocardial infarction is predicated on a clinical history which is suggestive of acute coronary syndrome and certain specific electrocardiographic findings on a 12-lead ECG. It has been estimated that upwards of 50% of patients who will develop an acute myocardial infarction had no confirmatory electrocardiographic (ECG) findings upon the initial ECG.[1–3]

The maxim "treat the patient, not the monitor" holds true for these patients. Treatment for suspected acute myocardial infarction—specifically morphine, oxygen, nitrates, and aspirin—should not be withheld because of a lack of electrocardiographic findings.

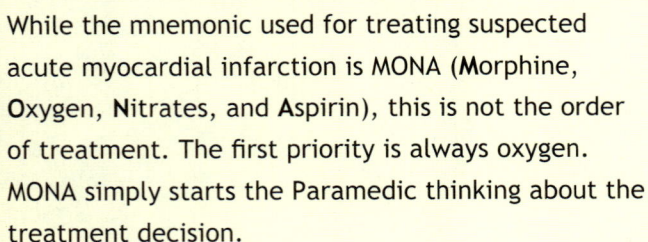

PROFESSIONAL PARAMEDIC

While the mnemonic used for treating suspected acute myocardial infarction is MONA (**M**orphine, **O**xygen, **N**itrates, and **A**spirin), this is not the order of treatment. The first priority is always oxygen. MONA simply starts the Paramedic thinking about the treatment decision.

However, that is not to dismiss the importance of obtaining a 12-lead ECG as soon as possible on a patient with suspected acute coronary syndrome. A 12-lead ECG can also help the Paramedic estimate the location of the coronary occlusion and ascertain the ventricular wall involved. Not only is this information valuable downstream, to the emergency physicians and cardiologists who will eventually treat the patient, but it is important for the Paramedic. By being able to estimate the location and extent of injury, the

Paramedic can predict, with relative confidence, the clinical course that the patient will take. This prognostic ability permits the Paramedic to prepare for predictable complications related to the acute coronary event.

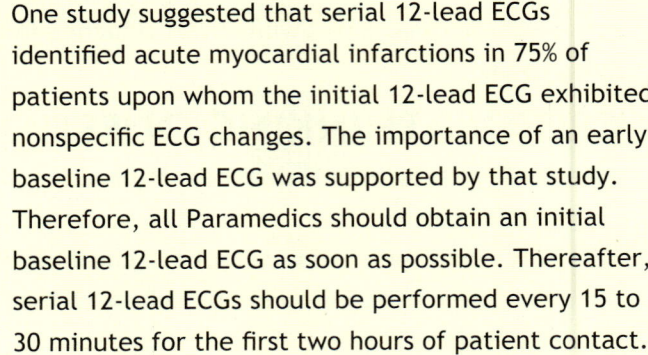

STREET SMART

One study suggested that serial 12-lead ECGs identified acute myocardial infarctions in 75% of patients upon whom the initial 12-lead ECG exhibited nonspecific ECG changes. The importance of an early baseline 12-lead ECG was supported by that study. Therefore, all Paramedics should obtain an initial baseline 12-lead ECG as soon as possible. Thereafter, serial 12-lead ECGs should be performed every 15 to 30 minutes for the first two hours of patient contact.

Atypical Presentations of Acute Coronary Syndrome

While it is obvious that patients with substernal chest pain (SSCP) should have a 12-lead ECG, other occasions when a 12-lead ECG may be necessary are sometimes less obvious. For example, perimenopausal females often do not present with chest pain. These patients tend to present with atypical presentations for acute coronary syndrome.[4,5]

These atypical presentations can include shortness of breath, unexplained weakness, and sudden diaphoresis. Unfortunately, some of these symptoms can be mistaken for menopausal signs, leading to delayed treatment. Compounding that mistake is the misconception that a patient with an acute coronary event must have concomitant substernal chest pain.

Another group of patients who can present with an atypical presentation is the elderly. This group of patients tends to have a higher frequency of acute myocardial infarction, even when identified early in the evolution, and complications such as heart and renal failure.

For these reasons, and others explained later, the Paramedic should have a low threshold of sensitivity for 12-lead ECG acquisition. The best support for this argument is found in the frequency that 12-lead ECG is obtained in the emergency department.

Rhythm Strip

The primary mission of all Paramedics has always been to prevent sudden cardiac death from dysrhythmia. This has been the essence of Paramedic care since the advent of Dr. Pantridge's "mobile coronary care units" in Belfast, Ireland, over half a century ago.[6] However, with the advent of fibrinolytics and invasive cardiology, the original mission has been expanded to include rapid acquisition and interpretation of 12-lead ECGs.

The 12-lead ECG stands at the center of the decision pathway in the management of patients with ischemic chest pain. Delays in obtaining the 12-lead ECG must be eliminated whenever possible in the field. The most effective means of obtaining a 12-lead ECG at the earliest point in time is to have a Paramedic obtain one.

The importance of obtaining a rapid and accurate 12-lead ECG is underscored by the American Heart Association's (AHA) statements. The AHA states that upon recognition of acute coronary syndrome and a suspected acute coronary event, a 12-lead ECG should be obtained as soon as possible but no later than ten (10) minutes upon arrival at the hospital.[7,8]

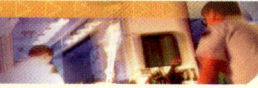

PROFESSIONAL PARAMEDIC

The importance of an early 12-lead ECG is underscored by the fact that in some states an EMT or advanced EMT may obtain and transmit a 12-lead ECG in the field. Multitasking on scene improves operational efficiency as well as patient care.

This rapid 12-lead ECG acquisition and interpretation will facilitate the patient's transfer to cardiac centers for interventional cardiology. This time frame has been demonstrated to decrease both morbidity and mortality.

The efficiency of this process can be substantially improved with 12-lead ECGs being obtained by Paramedics and the diversion of ambulances to cardiac centers. The American College of Emergency Physicians (ACEP) supports this process in their position paper entitled "Out-of-Hospital 12-Lead ECG."

While ACEP acknowledges that 12-lead ECG acquisitions will prolong scene times, many Paramedics have become very adept at obtaining 12-lead ECGs in minimal time. Studies have shown that Paramedics can obtain 12-lead ECGs at the point of care in the field in approximately five minutes.

The advent of Paramedic 12-lead ECGs has greatly affected physicians' opinions of Paramedics. Paramedics are now viewed as a part of the continuum of care that starts in the field and ends in the interventional cardiologist suite. It is recognized that aggressive Paramedic care can substantially impact cardiac patient morbidity and mortality.

Origins of the Electrokardiogram

The "electrokardiogram" has a long history that may have started with Italian physicist Carlo Matteucci. Matteucci, interested in the works of the noted physicist Luigi Galvani, continued Galvani's work on bioelectricity and started to investigate the role of electricity in the human body. Matteucci observed that with every heartbeat there was a passage of electrical current in the body. What Matteucci did not realize when he made that observation was that he was actually witnessing the birth of electrocardiography.

Following Matteucci's early lead, noted British physiologist Augustus Waller, of St. Mary's Medical School in London, created the first tracing of the heart's electrical activity in 1887, using his lab assistant, Thomas Goswell, as a patient. Subsequently, British physiologists William Bayliss and Edward Starling from the University College of London, following Waller's direction, attached a terminal to the right hand of a patient and to the skin overlying the apex of the heart. They observed a triphasic pattern to the electricity's flow.

Continuing the work of Bayliss and Starling, Willem Einthoven, who had also witnessed Waller demonstrate an ECG in 1889, used a silver string galvanometer to reproduce the triphasic waves that Bayliss and Starling had observed. Willem Einthoven named the deflections of these waves P, Q, R, S, and T, a convention that lasts to this day.[9]

Continuing his work with the "electrokardiogram" (EKG) in 1905, Einthoven transmitted his first EKG over 1.5 kilometers to another lab using a telephone cable. This was the first experience with telemetry. Einthoven also went on to standardize the electrocardiogram by referencing the body and using the designators leads I, II, and III. These first leads formed an equilateral triangle which is now referred to as "Einthoven's triangle." From this platform, Einthoven was able to distinguish normal "EKG" from abnormal, noting premature ventricular contractions, heart blocks, atrial flutter, and other forms of dysrhythmia. For this and other work, Einthoven was awarded the Nobel Prize in medicine in 1924 for "inventing the electrocardiogram." He is commonly referred to as the "father of electrocardiology."

Standard Limb Leads

Einthoven's standard limb leads (Figure 1-1) used two electrodes—one negative and one positive—and measured the electrical potential between these electrodes as it flowed from negative to positive. Because the limb leads required two leads which measured the current difference between the leads' electrodes, they were—and still are—referred to

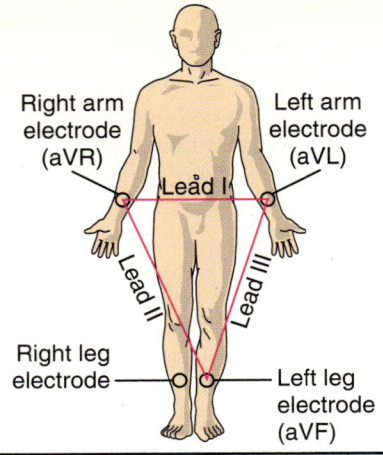

Lead	Right arm	Right leg	Left leg	Left arm
I	−			+
II	−		+	
III			+	−
aVR	+	−	−	−
aVL	−	−	−	+
aVF	−	−	+	−

Figure 1-1 The standard limb leads are used for tracing the body's electrical activity.

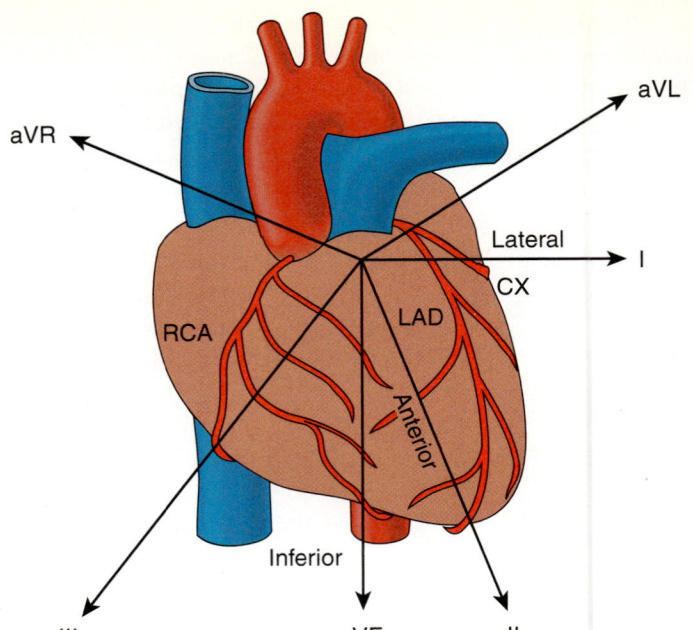

Figure 1-2 The frontal plane's relationship to the heart.

as **bipolar leads**. Einthoven's original bipolar limb leads provided electrical information relating to the heart's electrical activity along the body's frontal plane.

Perhaps the most useful of these bipolar leads was Lead II in that its orientation, from right shoulder to the left foot, was more or less in alignment with the heart's electrical conduction system. For this reason, Lead II provides the best view of the conduction system. It is often used to monitor patients for an irregular heart rhythm, a disturbance in conduction along the heart's electrical pathway, called a dysrhythmia.

Unfortunately, because of its orientation along the frontal plane, Lead II only permits a view of the inferior wall of the heart. However, the bulk of the ventricular mass is in the anterior wall.

Even with the use of three limb leads, the ECG was only able to view the frontal plane and the inferior and lateral wall of the heart. However, the majority of the ventricular mass lies along the transverse plane in the anterior wall. Thus, even with these additional leads, the electrical activity of the anterior wall was still not being captured by the ECG (Figure 1-2).

Precordial Leads

In an effort to obtain a more comprehensive view of the heart, researchers sought to create new leads. In 1931, researchers Wilson, MacLeod, and Barker devised a method for recording the heart's electrical activity along any of its surfaces. They continued to use the three limb leads but, through the use of

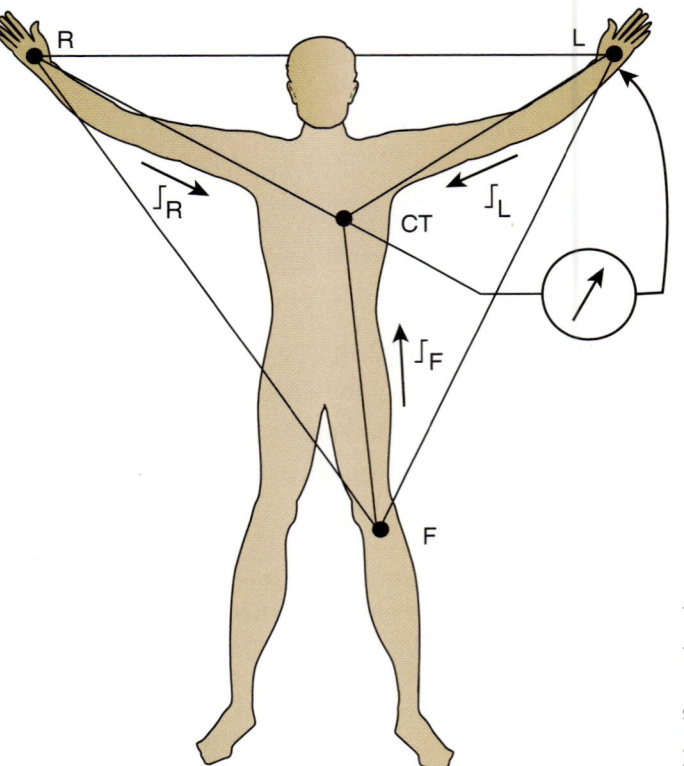

Figure 1-3 Wilson's central terminal (i.e., the virtual negative electrode) and the creation of the unipolar lead.

electrical resistors, were able to move the negative electrode to the center of the body, proximal to the right atria and the SA node, to form a central point called Wilson's central terminal (CT) (Figure 1-3).

Because the negative electrode is a "virtual" electrode, not an actual electrode, in the center of the body, the positive electrode is now available to become an "exploring" lead which can be placed anywhere on the thorax to view any angle of the heart. The use of a single positive electrode, using Wilson's central terminal, created the **unipolar lead**.

Using the central terminal concept, Wilson placed electrodes in a semicircle around the precordium, that portion of skin that overlies the heart. Wilson's unipolar precordial **chest leads** encircled the anterior ventricular wall from the septal wall on the right to the lateral wall on the left and permitted a complete view of the anterior myocardium.

These leads were originally called the V leads—V for voltage. In 1938 the American Heart Association standardized the precordial leads and called them V1, V2, V3, V4, V5, and V6. Adding these precordial (chest) leads to the standard limb leads gave nine views of the heart along both the frontal plane and the transverse plane.

Augmented Leads— A More Complete Picture

Although using six precordial chest leads gave physicians a better view of the anterior wall, the three bipolar limb leads did not give physicians the same view of the inferior wall. The origin of the standard limb leads, Einthoven's triangle, is an equilateral triangle and has, by definition, angles of 60 degrees. Use of these angles left wide gaps with the potential for much of the heart's electrical activity to be unrecorded by these standard limb leads.

Using Wilson's central terminal theory, Goldberger recorded the activity between each of the limb leads' positive electrodes and the central terminal, and added three additional limb leads. Unfortunately, when the signals were recorded, they were too small to be properly examined and required a boosting of the signal in order to identify any characteristics. In 1942 Goldberger devised a method to boost, or augment, the signal, hence the title **augmented leads**.

Combining the lead type and the positive electrode location gave rise to the names of Goldberger's augmented leads (i.e., augmented voltage right or aVR, then augmented voltage left or aVL and augmented voltage foot, now called aVF). The placement of the augmented leads, as well as their relationship to the standard limb leads, is crucial for the Paramedic to know (Figure 1-4).

Acquisition of the 12-Lead Electrocardiogram

The importance of the acquisition of a high-quality 12-lead ECG, as explained earlier, cannot be overstated. Clinical decisions regarding treatment and transportation of the patient are based, in part, on the 12-lead ECG. Therefore, it is imperative that the Paramedic know how to obtain a clear and concise 12-lead ECG.[10–13]

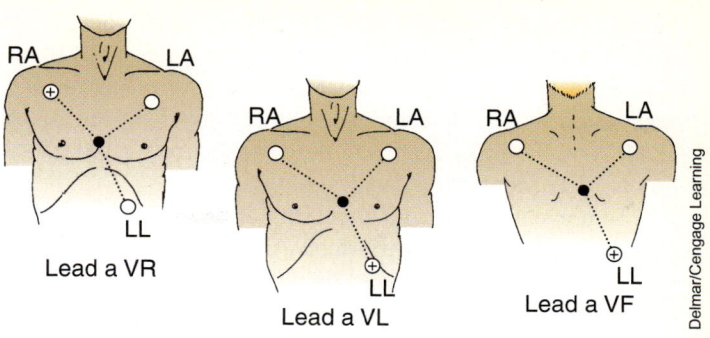

Figure 1-4 Augmented lead placement and the relationship of augmented limb leads to the standard limb leads.

Diagnostic 12-Lead Electrocardiogram versus Rhythm Monitoring

These early ECG machines were intended to monitor the rhythm only. Thus, tracings of early ECGs were often plagued with artifact and distortions that made reading the ECG difficult. To solve these problems, electrical engineers resorted to adjusting the frequency range, that area of the electric signal that is being recorded. They also used electronic filters such as common mode rejection.

In order to capture subtle changes in amplitude and duration which are necessary for the interpretation of a diagnostic 12-lead, the 12-lead ECG monitors require a wider frequency range than simple three lead ECG rhythm monitors. In the simple ECG rhythm monitor, a narrower frequency range between 0.5 Hz and 30 to 50 Hz removes distortions which interfere with correct analysis of the rhythm but does so at the cost of accuracy in the measurement of segments of the ECG complex. In the simple ECG rhythm monitor, an ST segment may appear far above (elevated) or below (depressed) the baseline, indicating potential ischemia or acute injury/infarct. Paramedics are generally directed to take patients with an ST segment above baseline to an interventional cardiology center as opposed to the local hospital. A false positive in this regard is not only an inconvenience to the patient and to the patient's family, but misuses critical cardiac services needed for more acutely ill patients.

To obtain a proper diagnostic 12-lead ECG that correctly shows all segments accurately, the American Heart Association recommends that a frequency range of 0.05 to 150 Hz be used. However, switching from monitoring mode to diagnostic mode raises the problems of artifact which were previously eradicated. Therefore, the Paramedic must take other measures to reduce artifact.

12-Lead Electrocardiogram Artifact

The common sources of ECG artifact can be broadly classified as physiologic and nonphysiologic. Physiologic artifact includes muscle artifact and skin artifact. The first, muscle artifact, is the result of muscle movement or muscle tension—muscle tension being the result of agonist and antagonist muscles competing to maintain a limb in one position. Any time a muscle contracts it produces an electrical current which will be detected as an **electromyographic signal (EMG)** by the ECG. An EMG is seen as narrow rapid spikes on the ECG monitor.

To prevent EMG from appearing on the ECG, the patient should be positioned comfortably, in an effortless position, with arms and legs supported by the stretcher. In some cases it may be more prudent for the Paramedic to perform the ECG in the patient's bed or couch rather than the stretcher because the patient's arms will hang off the stretcher. Folding of the arms across the chest only creates muscle tension and resultant EMG.

The other source of physiologic artifact is the result of skin movement. Whenever the skin is stretched under an electrode it will create an epidermal signal. For example, when a patient inhales and exhales the skin's movement will create baseline shifts (wandering baseline) as the electrodes move along with the chest wall. To prevent epidermal signal interference it is important for the Paramedic to properly place the electrodes on the patient's chest away from the thoracic cage.

An example of a nonphysiologic source of ECG artifact is **electromagnetic interference (EMI)**. Whenever alternating current (AC) electricity passes through a wire it produces an electromagnetic field; this is the premise for radio waves. Therefore, whenever a 12-lead ECG monitor is in the vicinity of a wire carrying AC electricity, the monitor will pick up the electromagnetic field as 60 cycle interference.[14–16] Examples of common sources of 60 cycle EMI are fluorescent lights, particularly those with a malfunctioning ballast, and poorly shielded ambulance convertors. Usually 60 cycle EMI will present on the 12-lead ECG as a fuzzy baseline.

Static electricity can also produce artifact on the ECG. The patient may build up an electrical charge (static electricity). When the patient, as the charged body, is in proximity of an uncharged body, such as the ECG monitor, then electricity will pass between the two and be recorded on the ECG. This occurs frequently in dry climates.

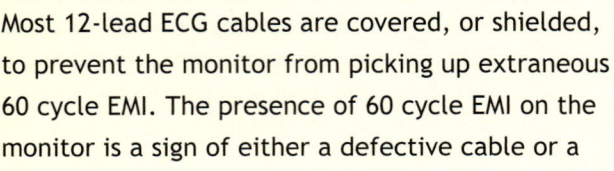

STREET SMART

Most 12-lead ECG cables are covered, or shielded, to prevent the monitor from picking up extraneous 60 cycle EMI. The presence of 60 cycle EMI on the monitor is a sign of either a defective cable or a broken lead.

One of the more common sources of artifact is electrode failure. Since the outer layer of skin is electrically "dead" an electrical signal cannot be transmitted across the skin without a conductive medium to act as a bridge between the inner body and the electrode. The typical ECG electrode uses silver chloride as the conductive medium. When a metal, such as silver chloride, is placed next to an electrolyte solution (i.e., the interstitial fluid), then an electromagnetic connection is created and an electromagnetic "signal" is sent to the ECG monitor.

If the skin is not prepared properly then the skin can create an impedance to this signal of approximately 100,000 to 200,000 ohms. Simple site preparation can reduce the skin's impedance to less than 10,000 ohms in 90% of patients and thereby markedly improve the quality of the ECG signal.

Patient Preparation

To prevent artifact, the Paramedic should first arrange the patient in a position of comfort. Preferably, the patient should be supine with arms at the sides and the entire body supported. If the patient is not relaxed, because of a painful condition such as arthritis, then the Paramedic might consider the use of analgesia or sedatives.

The Paramedic should then prepare the skin before the application of the electrodes. The Paramedic should remove any chest hair on the patient that might interfere with the close adherence of the electrode to the skin. Although it might be expeditious to use a straight razor to remove the hair, shaving the chest can create microlacerations that can bleed if the patient is given fibrinolytics later. Also, the hair follicles can become infected (folliculitis). Therefore, the patient's chest hair should be carefully trimmed using either a commercially available clipper or a pair of blunt-tipped bandage scissors.

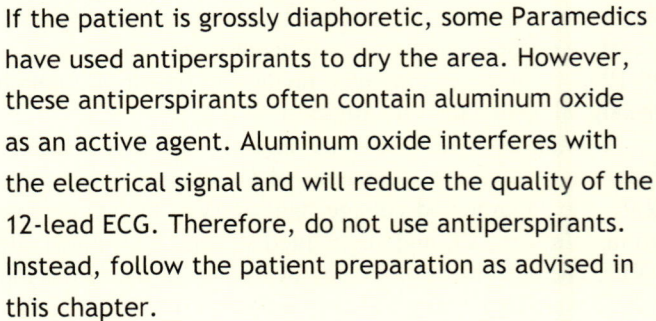

STREET SMART

If the patient is grossly diaphoretic, some Paramedics have used antiperspirants to dry the area. However, these antiperspirants often contain aluminum oxide as an active agent. Aluminum oxide interferes with the electrical signal and will reduce the quality of the 12-lead ECG. Therefore, do not use antiperspirants. Instead, follow the patient preparation as advised in this chapter.

Although wiping the contact surface with a gauze pad will reduce the pickup of 60 Hz EMI and motion artifact, it will only reduce the skin's resistance by 1,000 to 5,000 ohms. It is important to not only remove the dead cells of the stratum corneum but to also scratch the lower stratum granulosum of the epidermis.

Scratching the stratum granulosum improves the ECG signal by allowing the electrode gel to permeate the skin and contact the electrolyte solution (i.e., interstitial fluid).

Typically, either fine weight sandpaper (220 to 400 grit) or a commercially available gritty ECG preparation gel is used. Five to ten strokes of either a gel-soaked gauze pad or sandpaper is sufficient. The skin should be slightly reddened but not abraded.

The area immediately surrounding the electrode contact should be cleansed with an alcohol-soaked preparation pad. The alcohol helps to remove surface fats which can undermine the electrode's adhesive and prevent close skin contact with the electrode's gel.

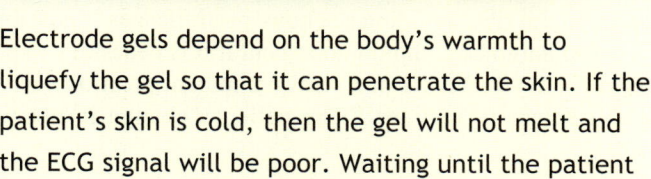
It is important that the gel on the electrode be moist. Most electrodes come prepackaged and have an expiration date. The Paramedic should first confirm that the electrodes are not expired before proceeding. Next, the Paramedic should remove the electrode from the package and remove the plastic protective cover over the gel. With one finger, the Paramedic should gently compress the gel. Moist electrode gel should have a little spring when gently compressed. In contrast, dried electrode gel will be stiff and unyielding. Dried electrodes should be discarded immediately as they are of no practical use.

After confirming that the gel on the electrode is still moist, the lead wire should be attached to the electrode. The gel under the electrode is formed into a pod so that the gel stays concentrated in an area when the electrode is placed on the skin. If the electrode is placed on the skin first and then the lead wire is attached, the pressure from attaching the lead wire can crush the pod, disperse the gel, and diminish the signal quality, as well as cause patient discomfort.

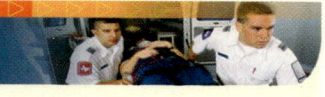
Electrode Placement

Accurate electrode placement is important. In some cases the prehospital 12-lead ECG may not display ischemic changes. However, when serial ECGs (obtained later) are compared against the initial 12-lead ECG, the differences become apparent.[17,18] These comparisons are only valid if the electrodes have been placed in the same position.

The American Heart Association emphasized proper lead placement in 1938 when it first standardized the placement of precordial leads. It continues to establish the standard for electrode placement in order to obtain a clinically relevant 12-lead ECG.

Standard Limb Leads

Traditionally limb leads are placed where Einthoven placed them, on the end of the extremities. One electrode should be placed on the ventral surface of the right and the left wrist and another placed on the ankle proximal to the medial malleolus. The electrode should be placed on the properly prepared skin overlying muscle, not bone. The resulting leads—Lead I, Lead II, and Lead III—are therefore a function of the polarity ascribed to them by the ECG monitor. Often these electrode wires are labeled for ease of application.

While technically correct, the placement of electrodes on the ankles and wrist of the patient is often mechanically inconvenient. Problems with resting tremors and clothing prevent the Paramedic from obtaining an accurate 12-lead ECG. This distortion can be minimized if the electrodes are moved more centrally. In 1966, Mason and Likar suggested moving the electrodes to the shoulders and the hip, known as the **Mason–Likar modification**. To properly place the limb electrodes in the Mason–Likar modification, the right arm electrode is moved to the right infraclavicular fossa, approximately 2 cm below the clavicle. The left arm electrode is similarly placed in the left infraclavicular fossa and the left leg electrode is moved next to the left iliac crest in the iliac fossa. This placement of the limb leads maintains the integrity of Einthoven's triangle without the inconvenience of distal limb lead electrodes.

Because the ECG machine electrically converts the bipolar limb leads into unipolar augmented leads using the same leads and electrodes, it is unnecessary to add additional electrodes for the augmented leads.

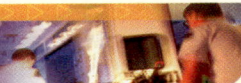
Precordial Leads

Wilson's precordial leads measure the ECG potentials across the anterior wall of the left ventricle. Precordial leads are to be placed according to specific landmarks. Variation in the placement of precordial electrodes can sometimes produce diagnostically significant changes in the 12-lead ECG.

The first electrodes, V1 and V2, are placed within the fourth intercostal space at the right and left sternal border, respectively. Mistakenly, Paramedics may palpate the space just below the clavicle, assume it is the first intercostal space, and start counting down three more spaces. This placement is incorrect and will cause V1 and V2 to be placed too high.

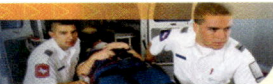
The Paramedic should first identify the suprasternal notch above the sternum and palpate inferiorly until a ridge is felt. The ridge on the bone is the connection of the manubrium to the body of the sternum (the angle of Louis). Moving laterally to the right, the Paramedic should palpate the second intercostal space along the sternal border and then palpate the spaces downward until the fourth intercostal space is palpated. The first precordial electrode, V1, is placed, and then V2 is placed immediately across from V1 on the left sternal border.

From the V2 position, the Paramedic should palpate the fifth intercostal space and move laterally to the midclavicular line to place the V4, the third electrode. The fourth electrode

placed, V3, is positioned midpoint along an imaginary line that runs between V2 and V4.

Continuing to palpate along the fifth intercostal space, the Paramedic should place V5 at the left anterior axillary line, in line with the iliac crest, and V6 at the fifth intercostal space along the left midaxillary line. These steps illustrate the proper placement of the precordial electrodes along the standard anatomical reference lines (Figure 1-5 and Table 1-1).

If the patient—male or female—has large breasts, place V4 under the breast and V3 over the breast. The V4 electrode should be placed flat against the chest and not partially on the breast and partially on the chest. This position would cause the electrode to fold over on itself and impair electrical reception. If the patient is small or thin, then place the electrodes between the ribs, avoiding the bony prominences if possible.

The Paramedic should document if it is necessary to perform the 12-lead ECG in a semi-recumbent position such as a wheelchair or recliner.[19] The patient's change in position

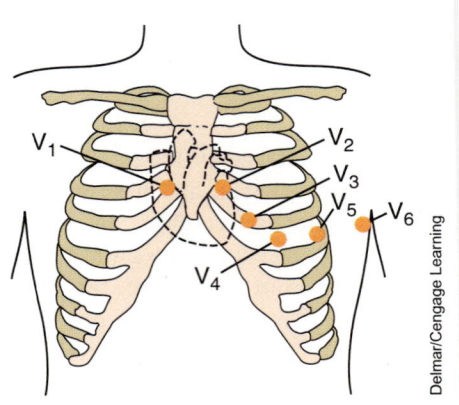

Figure 1-5 Precordial electrode placement.

Table 1-1 Lead Names with Correct Electrode Placement

LA		Left arm over muscle or flesh
RA		Right arm over muscle or flesh
LL		Left leg over muscle or flesh
RL		Right leg over muscle or flesh
V1	Fourth ICS RSB	Fourth right intercostal space at the sternal border
V2	Fourth ICS LSB	Fourth left intercostal space at the sternal border
V3		between V2 and V4
V4	Fifth ICS MCL	Fifth left intercostal space at the midclavicular line
V5	Fifth ICS LAAL	Fifth left intercostal space at the anterior axillary line
V6	Fifth ICS LMAL	Fifth left intercostal space at the midaxillary line

from Fowler's position, at a 45-degree angle, causes the heart to swing anterior and closer to the chest wall.

Dextrocardia

Some patients are born with their heart in the right side of their chest, a condition called **dextrocardia**. A small subset of these patients have **situs inversus**, a congenital condition in which the organs of the body are mirror opposite of normal. Situs inversus occurs in less than 1 in 10,000 patients but has been a documented medical phenomenon since 1643.

When the Paramedic initially places the patient on the monitor for a rhythm it will be noted that Lead I is inverted. An inversion in Lead I is suggestive of dextrocardia and a standard 12-lead ECG will support the diagnosis. The patient with dextrocardia will have a P wave axis greater than 90 degrees and a poor R wave progression, both discussed shortly.

If dextrocardia is suspected, or the patient confirms dextrocardia, then the Paramedic should proceed by placing the electrodes on the right side of the thorax. The Paramedic should make a note on the 12-lead ECG printout that dextrocardia is suspected and right-sided chest leads were placed.

12-Lead Electrocardiogram Tracing

Before reading a 12-lead ECG the Paramedic must understand the standard layout of the printout. Like a rhythm, a 12-lead ECG is never read off the monitor screen but instead is printed out for careful analysis.

A 12-lead ECG is printed in a standard four column format. The 12-lead ECG machine reads three leads simultaneously for 2.5 to 3 seconds until all 12-leads are obtained and then prints out the 12-lead ECG.

Beginning on the far left column, the printout contains the standard limb leads I, II, and III. The 12-lead ECG machine then uses the limb leads and, with the creation of Wilson's central terminal, creates the augmented leads: aVR, aVL, and aVF.

Moving from the limb leads to the precordial leads, the 12-lead ECG machine reads and records the precordial leads, starting within V1, V2, and V3, then reads and records V4, V5, and V6.

In some instances the 12-lead ECG machine will simultaneously record and print a single monitoring strip that may be found across the bottom of the 12-lead ECG. Although most machines will default to Lead II for the monitoring strip (Figure 1-6), the Paramedic may choose to record a different lead depending upon the patient's condition.

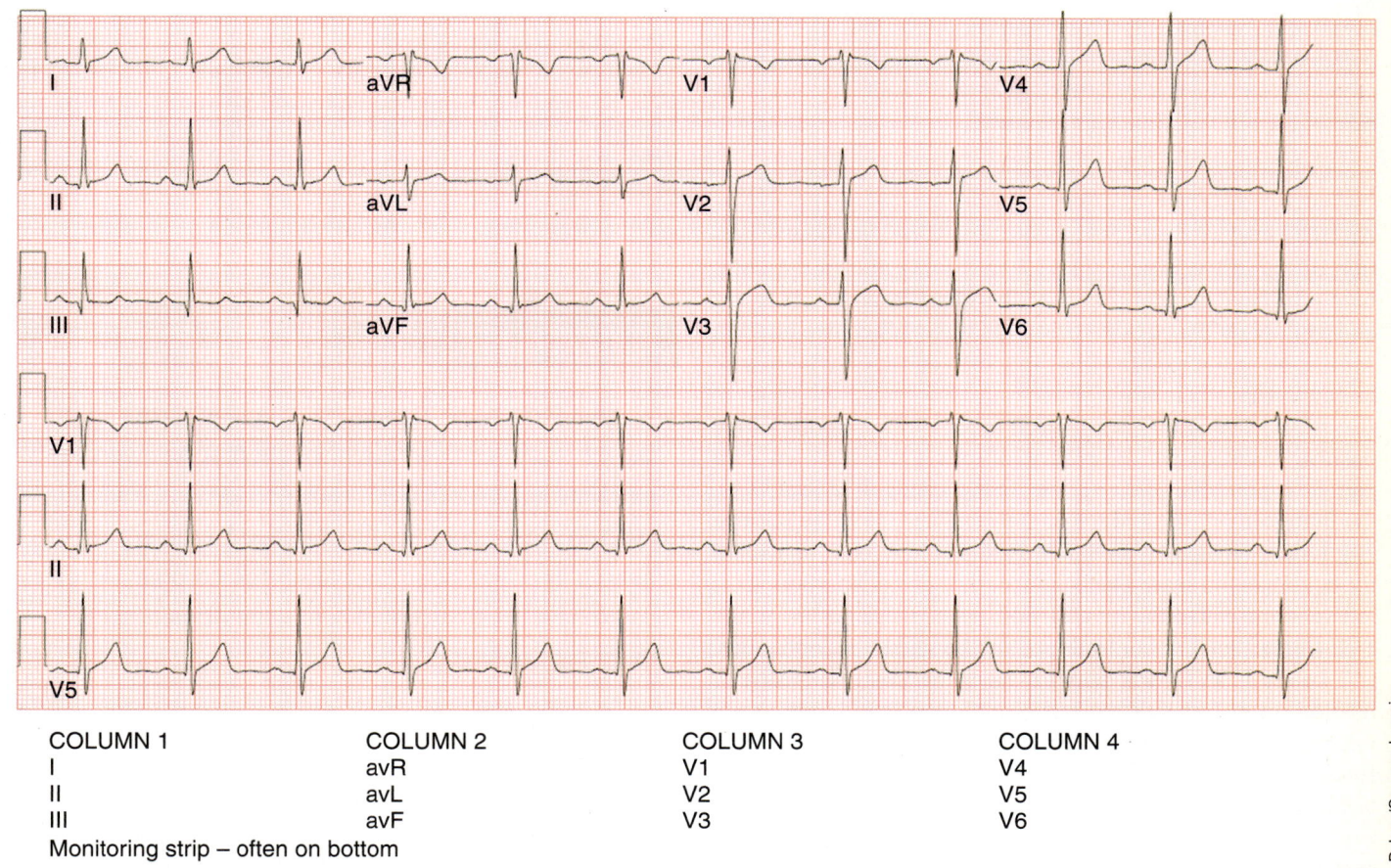

COLUMN 1	COLUMN 2	COLUMN 3	COLUMN 4
I	avR	V1	V4
II	avL	V2	V5
III	avF	V3	V6

Monitoring strip – often on bottom

Figure 1-6 The standard layout for a normal 12-lead ECG.

Electrocardiographic Assessment of Left Ventricular Function

The left ventricle is essential for cardiac output to the body, in general, and to the brain, in particular. All other portions of the heart—the atriums and the right ventricle—could be considered auxiliary to the left ventricle. In fact, loss of any one of these auxiliary portions of the heart is survivable, whereas loss of the left ventricle is usually fatal. For this reason the 12-lead ECG focuses on the left ventricle.

For ease of conceptualization, the left ventricle is said to have four walls—it is actually a cone-like shape with artificially contrived sides. The lower portion of the left ventricle, next to the epigastrium, is called the inferior wall. The portion of the left ventricle that is shared with the right ventricle, the septum, is called the septal wall. That foremost portion of the left ventricle, where the bulk of the myocardium exists, is called the anterior wall. The last wall, the lateral wall, is actually an extension of the left ventricle's anterior wall.

Contiguous Leads

An ECG lead gives the Paramedic a view of a particular portion of the left ventricle. The 12-lead ECG allows the Paramedic to have several views of the heart in an effort to try and capture evidence of myocardial injury. When two or more leads look at the same wall of the left ventricle they are said to be **contiguous leads**.

ECG leads are related to each other by the position of the positive electrode which, in turn, affords a specific view of a particular portion of the ventricle. In the standard 12-lead ECG, the limb leads II, III, and the augmented lead, aVF, the positive electrode is located on the lower extremity and looks up toward the bottom of the heart. The bottom of the heart is a portion of the left ventricle called the inferior wall. Thus, these leads—II and aVF—are called inferior leads and can be said to be contiguous.

Leads I, aVL, V5, and V6 have the positive electrode located on or beneath the left arm. These leads look at the lateral wall of the heart and are called lateral leads. Similarly, leads V1 through V4 have the positive electrode on the front of the chest. These leads look at the front portion or anterior wall of the left ventricle. The front of the chest is a large area and thus these leads are broken into subcategories. V1 and V2 have the positive electrode over the interventricular septum

Table 1-2 Contiguous Leads

• Pure changes		
II/III/aVF	=	Inferior
V1/V2	=	Septal
V3/V4/V5	=	Anterior
I/aVL/V5/V6	=	Lateral
• Mixed changes		
V1/V2/V3/V4	=	Anteroseptal
I/II/III/aVL/aVF/V5/V6	=	Inferolateral
I/aVL/V3/V4/V5/V6	=	Anterolateral
II/III/aVF/V1/V2	=	Inferoseptal
• Global changes		
V1/V2/V3/V4/V5/V6	=	Global anterior
I/II/III/aVL/aVF/aVR/V1–V6	=	Global

and are also referred to as septal leads. In contrast, V3 and V4 continue to be known as true anterior leads.

In some cases the evidence of myocardial damage spreads across two walls of the left ventricle. In those cases, both walls are used in the description. For example, injury to both the anterior wall and the septal wall, as evidenced by ECG changes in the contiguous leads V1, V2, V3, and V4, would be referred to as anteroseptal (Table 1-2). Similarly, myocardial damage to both the inferior and the lateral wall, as evidenced by ECG changes in the leads I, II, III, aVL, aVF, V5, and V6, would be called inferolateral. If there are changes suggestive of damage to the entire myocardium (i.e., ECG changes in all leads), then the term "global" is used. ECG changes in only two contiguous leads are necessary to make a presumption of myocardial injury.

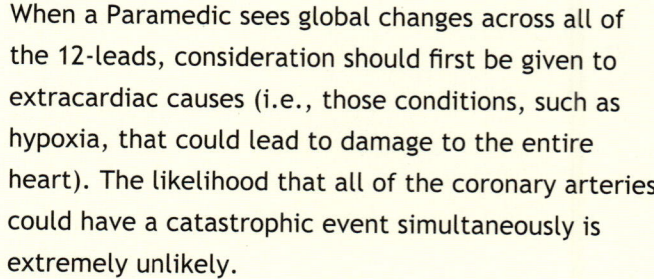
Relationship of Leads to the Coronary Arteries

The main coronary arteries perfuse specific areas of the heart and, in particular, the left ventricle. By evaluating the 12-lead ECG for evidence of myocardial injury in the contiguous leads, the Paramedic can infer that ECG changes in those contiguous leads raise a suspicion of involvement of specific coronary arteries.

The coronary arteries originate at the sinus of Valsalva and proximal to the aortic valve, with which they have a symbiotic relationship. There are two coronary arteries which are simply called the right coronary artery and the left coronary artery. The right coronary artery (RCA) runs the length of the heart and has a minor branch, called the marginal branch, toward its terminus. Conversely, the left coronary artery (LCA) divides almost immediately at its mainstem into the left anterior descending (LAD) coronary artery and the circumflex coronary artery (Cx).

The RCA provides blood to the inferior wall of the left ventricle and to the AV node in the majority of patients. Thus, ECG changes in the inferior leads of II, III, and/or aVF would suggest that the RCA may be involved.

The LCA serves the entire anterior wall including the septum. Occlusions of the left mainstem—referred to as "widow makers," thus emphasizing the importance of the LCA—can cause global anterior wall damage. ECG changes in the anterior leads of V1 to V4 and the lateral leads of I, aVL, V5, and V6, suggest that the LCA is affected.

The LCA almost immediately bifurcates, giving rise to the LAD coronary artery and the circumflex coronary artery. The LAD artery serves the central portion of the anterior wall of the left ventricle. Therefore, anterior wall ECG changes would be expected (V3 and V4).

Lesser branches off the LAD, called the septal perforators (SP), provide the septum with blood, including the bundle branches. Atherosclerotic involvement of the SP will injure the septum and may cause ECG changes in leads V1 and V2 and possible bundle branch blocks.

The LAD then continues to run along the anterior interventricular groove which separates the right and left ventricles toward the apex of the heart. Along its path another minor branch of the LAD, which cuts diagonally away from the anterior interventricular groove and toward the anterolateral wall and the apex of the heart, is the diagonal (Dx). Distal occlusions of the Dx can give rise to ECG changes in leads I, aVL, V5, and V6, or just as V4 and V5.

The circumflex coronary artery (Cx) was the second artery at the bifurcation of the left coronary artery. The Cx follows the atrioventricular groove to the lateral wall of the left ventricle. In approximately 85% of patients, the Cx stops at the left lateral wall. In the other 15% of patients, the Cx continues and provides perfusion to the AV node; normally blood for the AV node comes from the right coronary artery. In those cases, the patient is said to be "left dominant," indicating an alternative blood supply to the AV node as opposed to the normal blood supply. The difficulty for the patient who is left dominant arises when an occlusion of the left coronary artery occurs, hypoperfusing almost the total of the left ventricle's myocardium. A unique connection exists between the arteries in the coronary anatomy (Figure 1-7) and the relationship of those arteries to ECG leads (Table 1-3).

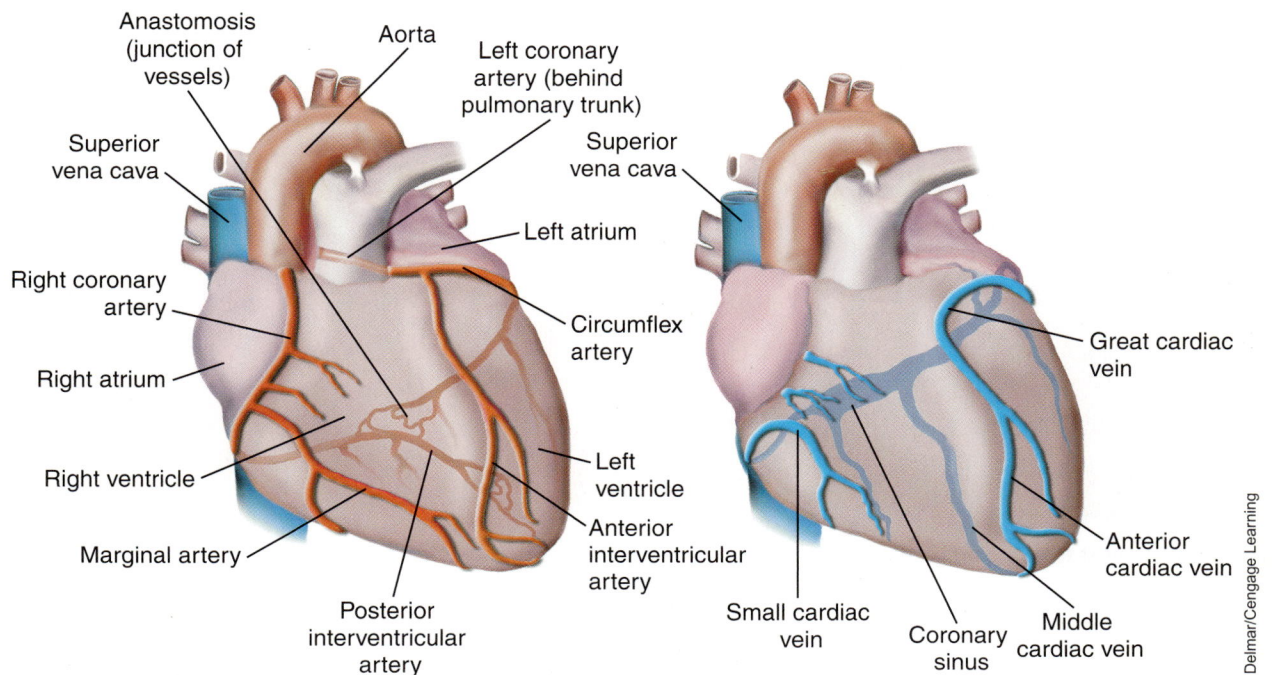

Figure 1-7 Coronary artery anatomy.

Table 1-3 Relationship of Leads to Walls of Coronary Arteries

II/III/aVF	=	Inferior	Right coronary artery (RCA)
V1/V2	=	Anteroseptal	Left anterior descending (LAD)/(SP)
V3/V4	=	Anterior	Left anterior descending (LAD)
V3/V4/V5/V6	=	Anterolateral	Diagonal (Dx)
I/aVL/V5/V6	=	Lateral	Circumflex (Cx)
V1–V6	=	Global anterior	Left mainstem (LCA)

Interpretation

The primary value of a Paramedic-obtained 12-lead ECG in the field is the identification of myocardial injury and the transportation of the patient to the definitive care center.[20–22] However, the value in a 12-lead ECG is not only in the identification of myocardial injury but also in the Paramedic's ability to make a prognosis based on that information. By having information about the location of the myocardial injury, the Paramedic can prepare for complications associated with that injury.

12-Lead Electrocardiogram Identification of Myocardial Injury

The era of the ECG identification of acute myocardial infarction may have started with Harold Pardee when he published the first ECG of an acute myocardial infarction, describing the T wave as "tall" and "starts from a point well up in the descent of the R wave." From that point physicians have had a keen interest in using the 12-lead ECG to identify the patient with acute coronary syndrome who is at risk for an acute myocardial infarction.

Normal Depolarization and Repolarization

Normal ventricular depolarization begins with the onset of the QRS complex. The first negative deflection, called a Q wave, represents the depolarization of the septum (Figure 1-8). A Q wave is not always visible in every patient, nor is it seen in every lead. The presence of a small Q wave, called a physiologic Q wave, is normal.

Following the depolarization of the septum, ventricular depolarization occurs (Figure 1-9). Normally, ventricular depolarization proceeds from the endocardium outward to the epicardium. The specific wave pattern (i.e., rS, Rs, etc.) is a function of the placement of the electrode. For example, since the energy is going away from V1, the QRS deflection should be negative. The energy is going toward V6 and the QRS deflection in V6 should be primarily positive.

Normally the segment between the QRS and the T wave, called the ST segment, is isoelectric as the Purkinje fibers start to repolarize (Figure 1-10).

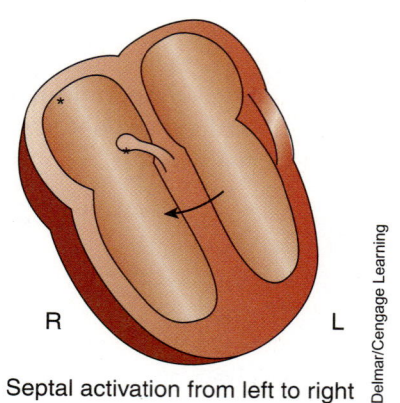

R   L

Septal activation from left to right

Delmar/Cengage Learning

Figure 1-8 Septal depolarization.

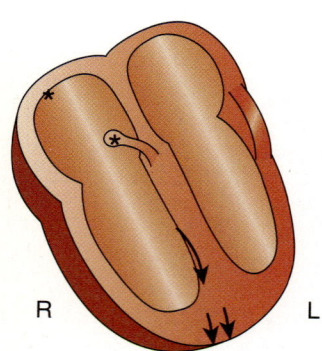

R   L

Activation of anteroseptal region of the ventricular myocardium

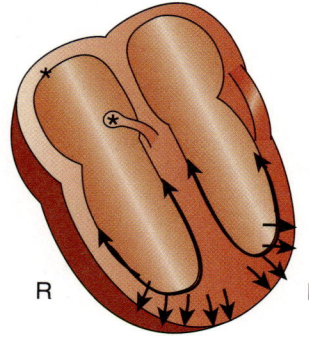

R   L

Activation of major portion of ventricular myocardium from endocardial to epicardial surfaces

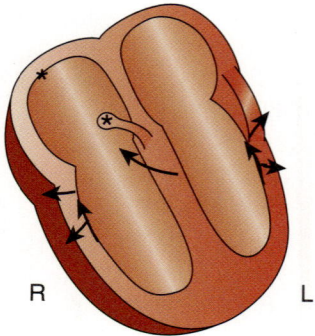

R   L

Late activation of posterobasal portion of the left ventricle, the pulmonary conus, and the uppermost portion of the interventricular septum

Delmar/Cengage Learning

Figure 1-9 Ventricular depolarization.

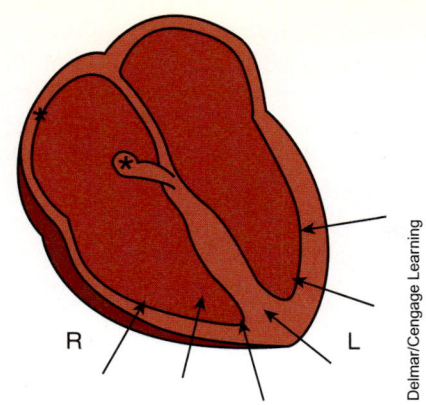

Figure 1-10 Ventricular repolarization.

R   L

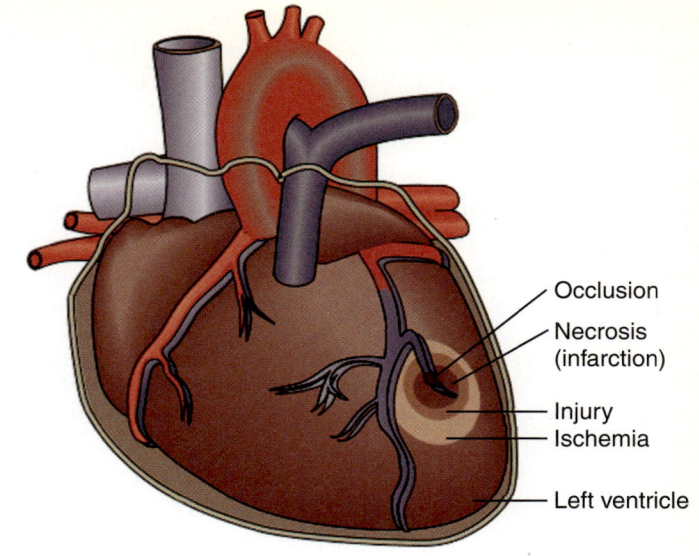

Occlusion
Necrosis
(infarction)
Injury
Ischemia
Left ventricle

Figure 1-11 Ischemic penumbra.

Ventricular repolarization is represented by the T wave. In a reverse process, normal repolarization begins at the epicardial surface and progresses through the ventricular walls to the endocardium. The process of repolarization is the resuming of a negatively charged interior of the cell compared to the outside. The combination of the interior of the cell becoming more negative while moving away from the positive electrode results in a positive deflection on the screen.[23] The T wave representing ventricular repolarization is positive or upright in all leads except aVR.

Ischemic Patterns

A healthy myocardial cell requires oxygen, glucose, and a balance of electrolytes in order to function; that is, to depolarize then repolarize. Abnormal depolarization/repolarization occurs whenever the myocardial cells lack these essential conditions. The most common cause of myocardial dysfunction is acute occlusion of the coronary arteries.

As a result of this occlusion, and subsequent hypoxia, the myocardial cells go through a predictable pathway to cell necrosis and myocardial infarction called **penumbra** (Figure 1-11). The cellular changes that occur during penumbra can be witnessed by the Paramedic as changes in the ECG called **ischemic patterns**. These ischemic patterns are the result of abnormal repolarization.

There are three successive stages that occur before myocardial cell death: ischemia, injury, and infarction. These stages are evolutionary and affect tissues incrementally, spreading out from a central point in a bull's eye fashion, and can be described as the three "I's" of acute coronary syndrome (ACS).

Ischemia

The first change is **myocardial ischemia**. During the ischemic phase myocardial cells are deprived of oxygen and hypoxia ensues. During this phase the myocardial cells convert to anaerobic metabolism to conserve energy. This decreased cellular activity slows myocardial repolarization. As coronary perfusion occurs from the surface, or epicardium, inwardly, the

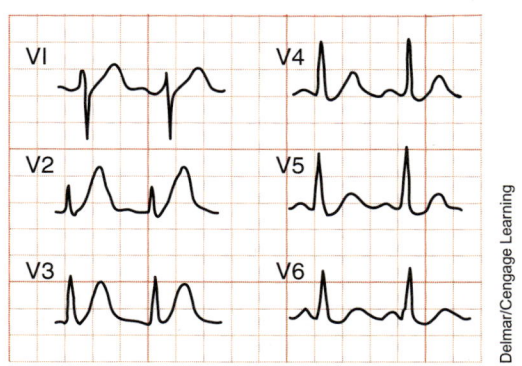

V1   V4
V2   V5
V3   V6

Figure 1-12 Hyperacute T waves in the anteroseptal leads.

deeper myocardial tissues become ischemic first. This limited ischemic involvement is called **subendocardial ischemia**.[24] This slowing of repolarization does not alter the direction of repolarization; therefore, the ECG will appear normal, but it does lengthen the time for repolarization. Accordingly, the first manifestation of myocardial ischemia can be a lengthening QT interval.

As the cell's sodium–potassium pump starts to falter, due to insufficient adenosine-5'-triphosphate (ATP), potassium leaks from the cell. The leaking potassium causes an increase in the amplitude of the T waves, called a **hyperacute T wave**, in the leads facing the damage (Figure 1-12).

Transmural ischemia occurs as the ischemia reaches a point in which it affects the entire thickness of the myocardium, from the endocardium to the epicardium. Then the deeper myocardial cells begin to malfunction.

Normally, when the repolarization occurs and the polarity changes as potassium is pumped back into the cell, thus reversing the current, the repolarization results in an upright T wave on the ECG. However, when the ischemic endocardial cells deeper in the myocardium fail to repolarize, the result is a loss of the change in direction of polarity which normally occurs during repolarization. This failure to change in direction causes a negative deflection in the T wave. Without repolarization and the subsequent negative polarity of the myocardium, the normally upright T waves become inverted in the ECG leads that overlay the ischemic area. In some cases, Paramedics will observe these **inverted T waves** as one of the first electrocardiographic changes.[25]

Injury

The unrelenting hypoxia causes the myocardial cells to change from ischemia to injury. The faltering sodium–potassium pump of the injured myocardial cells can no longer maintain polarization and the cell becomes electrically inert. At first the injured endocardial cells tend to draw the ST segment downward (**ST segment depression**). An ST segment, by definition, is a > 1 mm depression below the J point, from isoelectric baseline. To decide if the ST segment is depressed, the Paramedic must first ascertain the J point.

J Point

To decide if an ST segment is depressed or elevated, the Paramedic starts by identifying the J point. The **J point** is the start of the ST segment and is found at the juncture of the QRS and the ST segment, the point where the angle from the QRS changes. To find the J point, the Paramedic starts at the beginning of the P wave and draws a straight line across to where it crosses the T wave. If any portion of the ST segment is below that line, then there is an ST segment depression. If any portion of the ST segment is above this line, there is an ST segment elevation. If the Paramedic is unable to find the beginning of the P wave, then the line is drawn from the bottom of the calibration wave straight across.

ST Segment Elevation

As the injury continues and becomes full thickness (transmural), the ST segment starts to raise (**ST segment elevation**). Myocardial injury, as manifested by ST segment elevation in the ECG leads overlying the area, generally occurs after 20 to 40 minutes of ischemia.[26] ST segment elevation in the anterior leads may include some "tombstone" elevations in V2, V3, and V4 (Figure 1-13).

Patterns of Ischemia and Penumbra

At this point, the Paramedic may see a complex picture of T wave inversions, ST segment depressions, and ST elevations. These markings represent the process of ischemia and are manifestations of penumbra. The key is to focus on those

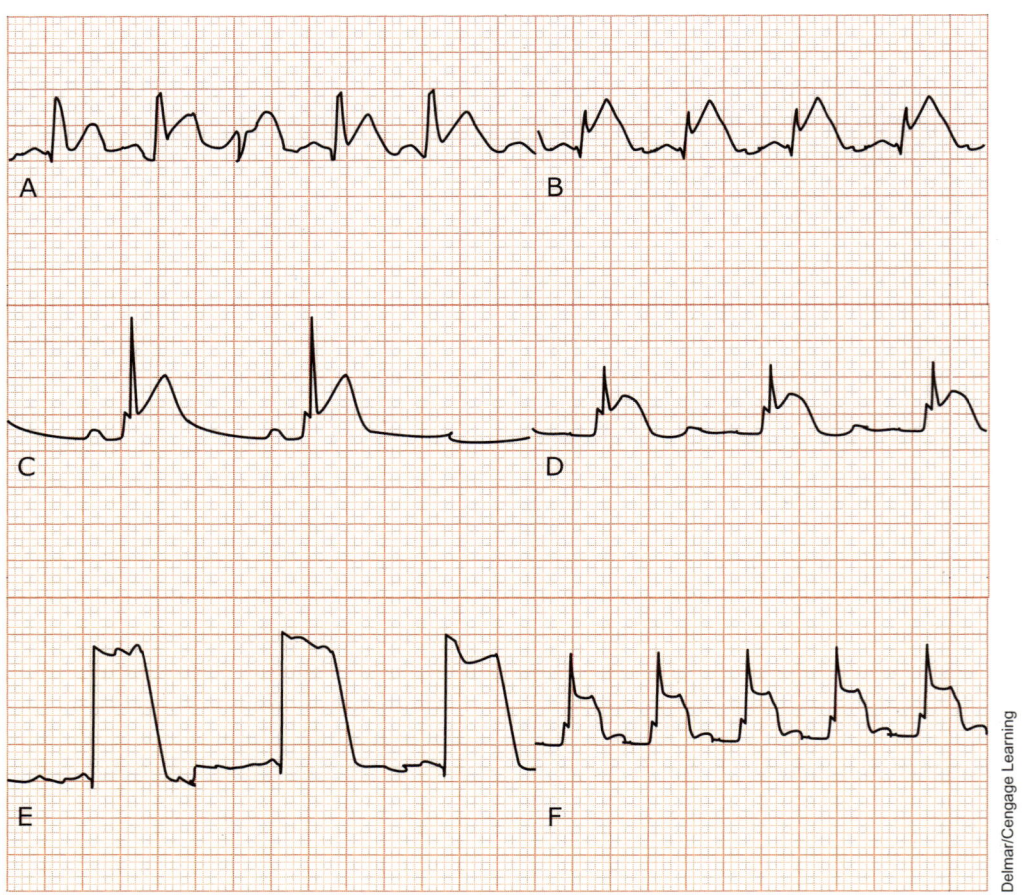

Delmar/Cengage Learning

Figure 1-13 ST segment elevation.

leads that indicate the greatest degree of damage. The other ECG changes should radiate away from the location of the primary event.

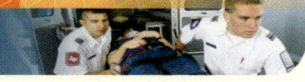

STREET SMART

In around 50% of initial ECGs, the Paramedic may not see ST segment elevations with the initial 12-lead ECG because the event has not evolved to that level. Nevertheless, it is important to obtain a baseline ECG for later analysis, particularly for QT intervals and T wave changes.

Infarction

Without oxygen the myocardial cells eventually die (myocardial infarction), and the area begins **necrosis**, a physiologic process where dead cells are replaced with new cells (i.e., scar tissue). The ECG hallmark of this change is the development of pathologic Q waves. Pathologic **Q waves** indicate electrical silence (i.e., no depolarization) in that portion of the ventricular wall. Because that portion of the ventricular wall is electrically silent, the depolarization in the opposite wall, going away from the electrodes in that lead, is the only signal present. It is recorded as a negative deflection on the ECG.

Q waves can also represent the depolarization of the intraventricular septum. As the septum depolarizes from left to right, any leads that are looking from the left (i.e., the lateral leads I, V5, and V6) will show a negative deflection. These physiologic or septal Q waves are normal.

While some Q waves are normal (physiologic), the Q waves associated with infarction (pathologic Q waves) are deep (greater than 25% of the R wave) and wide (typically 0.04 seconds). These characteristics, and the presence of Q waves in contiguous leads, suggest pathology and infarction.

The presence of a pathologic Q wave in a 12-lead ECG suggests that the patient has had a transmural myocardial infarction, also known as a Q wave infarction. This condition can remain for years, alerting the Paramedic to the presence of a previous acute myocardial infarction (AMI). In up to 30% of 12-lead ECGs with Q waves, the Q waves resolve, especially in the inferior wall, within one year (Figure 1-14).

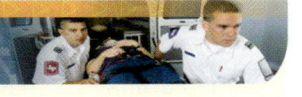

STREET SMART

An isolated pathologic Q wave in Lead III may be a normal finding and is not indicative of an inferior wall AMI unless it is accompanied by other ECG changes in the contiguous leads II and aVF.

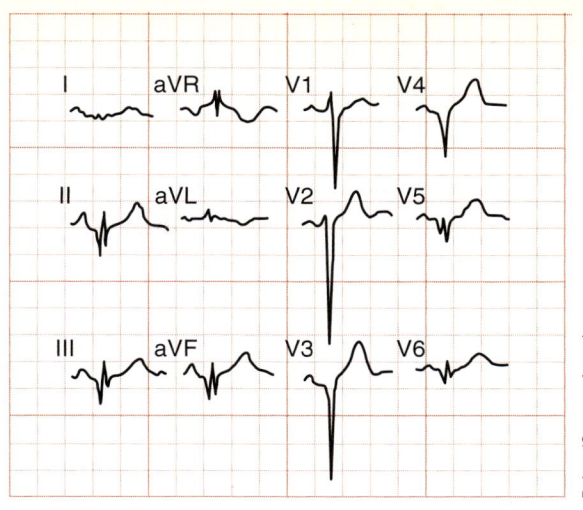

Figure 1-14 Q waves in both the anterior and inferior leads.

Electrocardiographic Diagnosis of Acute Myocardial Infarction

To make an electrocardiographic diagnosis of acute myocardial infarction, the Paramedic should look through all leads for hyperacute T waves, T wave inversions, ST segment depressions, and/or ST segment elevations as well as pathologic Q waves. When a pattern of ischemia is noted (ECG changes in contiguous leads), then the Paramedic may have a high index of suspicion that the artery which perfuses the corresponding wall is occluded.

The presence of Q waves in the face of concurrent ST elevation speaks to the evolution of the infarction and may indicate that this MI has been in progress for several hours (Figure 1-15). However, the presence of ST elevations indicates that there may be myocardium that can be salvaged with thrombolytic therapy or interventional cardiology.[27–30]

Reciprocal Changes

Supporting evidence of an acute myocardial infarction in progress is referred to as reciprocal changes. **Reciprocal changes** are concomitant ST segment depressions seen on the 12-lead ECG in leads that face the wall opposite of those with ST segment elevations. Reciprocal changes are more commonly seen in inferior wall MI (approximately 70%) versus anterior wall MI (about 30%). The presence of reciprocal changes is an excellent marker of acute myocardial infarction in progress and has a positive predictive value of 90%.[31]

These reciprocal ST segment depressions of reciprocal changes are thought to be due to "mirror reflections" of the electrical signal from the affected wall. The ST segment depression seen in a reciprocal change is more downsloping than those caused early in an AMI and is typically seen when the AMI is large.

**Myocardial wall
cross section**

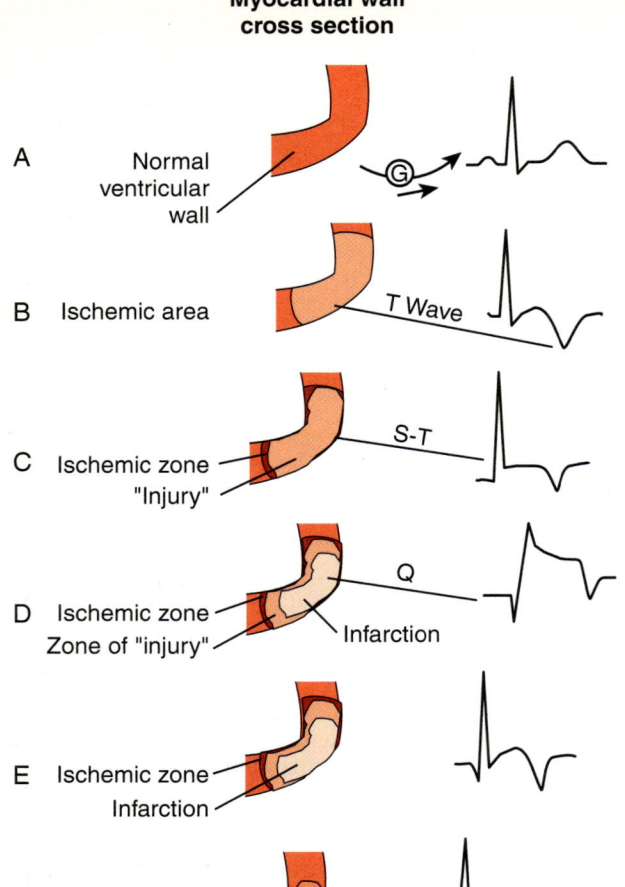

A Normal ventricular wall

B Ischemic area T Wave

C Ischemic zone "Injury" S-T

D Ischemic zone
Zone of "injury" Q
Infarction

E Ischemic zone
Infarction

F Infarct (healed) Scar

Figure 1-15 Wave changes during evolution of myocardial damage.

Delmar/Cengage Learning

As an example of the predictive value of reciprocal changes, ST depression in leads V1, V2, V3, and V4—all anterior leads—suggests an acute myocardial infarction in evolution in the posterior wall and an occlusion of the circumflex coronary artery (Cx) (Table 1-4).

Table 1-4 Reciprocal Changes between Leads, Walls, Coronary Arteries, and Reciprocal Leads

Wall	Artery	Lead	Reciprocal Wall	Reciprocal Leads
Inferior	RCA	II/III/aVF	Lateral	I/aVL
Anterior	LAD	V3/V4	Inferior	II/III/aVF
Lateral	Cx	I/aVL/V5/V6	Inferior	II/III/aVF

R Wave Progression

A normal 12-lead ECG contains a series of changes in the primary deflection of the QRS from negative in V1 to positive in V6, called an **R wave progression** in the precordial leads. Starting with the deep S wave in V1, the deflection in the precordial leads gradually changes direction, with a transition at approximately V3 or V4, until V6, where there is a tall R wave.

Whenever there is an electrical disturbance in the anterior wall, secondary to ischemia, then the R wave progression is disturbed. Specifically, this occurs when there is a loss of R waves in the anterior precordial leads. The loss of an R wave progression, sometimes called a **reverse R wave progression (RRWP)**, is suggestive of an anterior wall MI.

If the transition occurs early (i.e., before V3), it may be indicative of a posterior wall AMI, and the Paramedic may want to consider obtaining leads V7, V8, and V9 (these are discussed later). If the transient occurs later, after V4, it can be suggestive of an anterior wall MI. However, a late transition can also occur if the patient has a thick chest or has respiratory disease, particularly if there are small R waves in the right precordial leads. This may also be a normal variant in some women.

The isolated appearance of a RRWP should not be taken to mean that the patient is having an anterior wall MI. There are other causes of RRWP including a pre-existing left bundle branch block, dextrocardia, and Wolff–Parkinson–White (WPW) syndrome. Nevertheless, the presence of a reverse R wave progression, coupled with a good history for ACS and other 12-lead ECG changes in the anterior leads, is helpful in diagnosing an anterior wall MI.

STREET SMART

Reciprocal ST depression can be helpful in distinguishing infarction from the normal variants in African-American males who have ST elevations. This normal variant may be congenital and is a benign condition.

STREET SMART

Some Paramedics may use the term "poor R wave progression." The American Heart Association prefers the term "reverse R wave progression" instead.[32] It should be noted that improper lead placement can cause a reversed R wave progression.

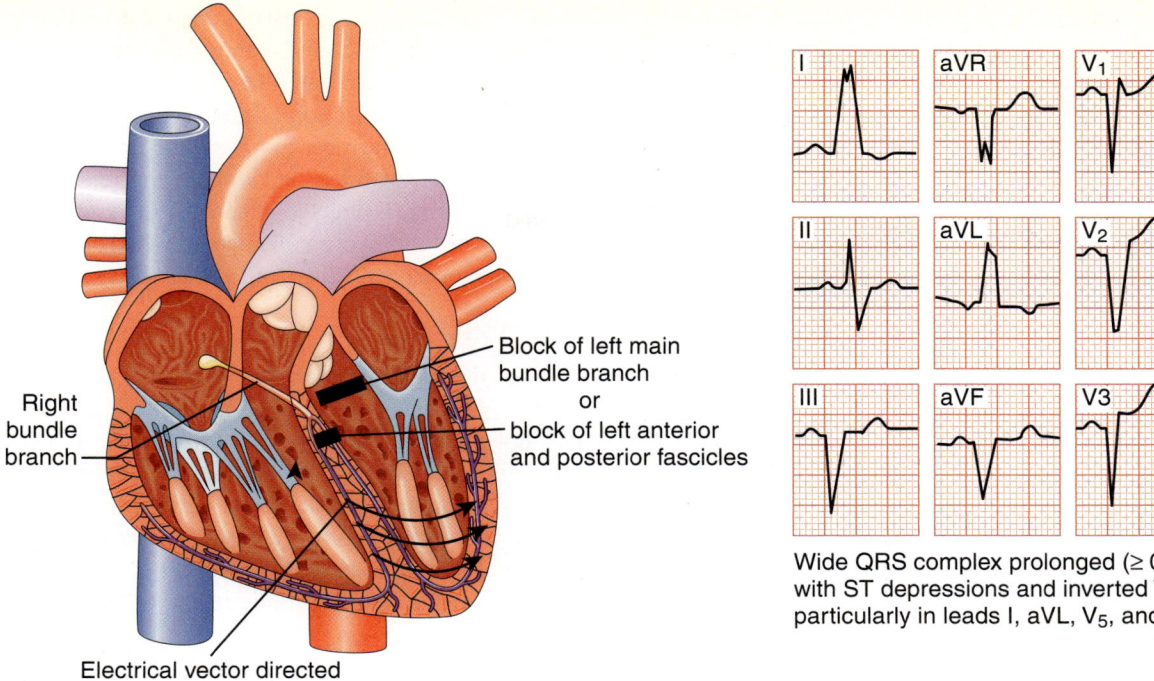

Wide QRS complex prolonged (≥ 0.12 second). with ST depressions and inverted T waves, particularly in leads I, aVL, V_5, and V_6

Right bundle branch

Block of left main bundle branch
or
block of left anterior and posterior fascicles

Electrical vector directed toward left ventricle as is normal, but delayed and prolonged

Figure 1-16 Left bundle branch block.

New Onset Left Bundle Branch Block

A left bundle branch block (LBBB) is a type of heart block (when the impulse fails to be conducted) that involves one or both the left fascicles of the left bundle (Figure 1-16). As a result, the ventricular wall of the affected side must be depolarized by a wave front from the opposite side. This delay in depolarization prolongs the QRS to greater than 0.14 seconds for a left bundle branch and a small narrow R wave (less than 0.04 seconds) in all leads. The Paramedic may also observe that the T wave is opposite in deflection to the QRS in all precordial leads, as well as a notching in the anterolateral leads.

The characteristic appearance of a notched QRS in V6 (i.e., RsR') is the result of the electrical impulse crossing the right bundle branch, depolarizing the right ventricle, then crossing the interventricular septum to depolarize the left ventricle.

A common cause of an LBBB is occlusion of either the left anterior descending (LAD) coronary artery or one of the septal perforators which branch from the LAD. These coronary arteries perfuse the septum and the bundle branches that lie within.

Because of the delayed repolarization, the ST segment of the septal leads will be elevated and the 12-lead ECG will have the appearance of an anterior wall MI (AWMI). However, there are a number of benign conditions, including advanced age and hypertension, that can also cause an LBBB.

In some cases, because of advanced atherosclerotic disease, the patient may experience a rate related bundle branch block. These blocks occur because the bundle branches are incapable of repolarizing, secondary to decreased perfusion,

at faster rates. Because of slower conduction there is reduced strength of contraction and, as a result, some patients may experience heart failure.

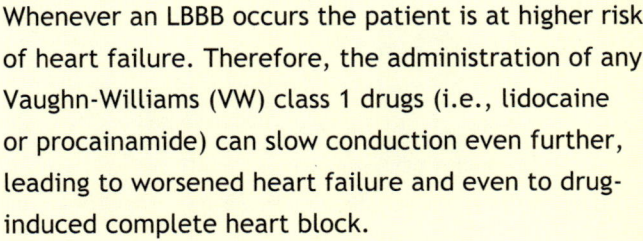

STREET SMART

Whenever an LBBB occurs the patient is at higher risk of heart failure. Therefore, the administration of any Vaughn-Williams (VW) class 1 drugs (i.e., lidocaine or procainamide) can slow conduction even further, leading to worsened heart failure and even to drug-induced complete heart block.

Typically, the altered electrical pathway associated with LBBB makes the ECG diagnosis of AMI complicated. Therefore, if a Paramedic observes an LBBB on initial 12-lead ECG, no further interpretation is possible because a diagnosis of AMI by ECG cannot be made with confidence. However, the presence of a new onset LBBB during the course of patient care is an ECG finding highly suggestive of an AMI.[33–35] The Paramedic should report the appearance of a new onset LBBB and, coupled with a patient history suggestive of ACS, have a high index of suspicion that the patient is having an AMI. Patients with a new onset LBBB have a worse prognosis for their AMI compared to those without the conduction delay. Because of the prolonged conduction, and the resultant decreased inotropy, a patient with an LBBB may experience as much as a 25% loss of cardiac output.[36] Paramedics should treat new onset LBBB more aggressively, with a keen eye on the development of heart failure.

Right Bundle Branch Block

A right bundle branch block (RBBB) is a type of heart block in which the impulse fails to be conducted down the right bundle of the bundle of His (Figure 1-17). In an RBBB, the impulse travels rapidly to depolarize the interventricular septum and down the left bundle branch to activate the left ventricle. When the right bundle branch is blocked, the impulse must cross the interventricular septum to activate the right ventricle. Because it takes more time to depolarize the entire ventricle, the QRS is greater than 0.12 seconds in width.

The ECG diagnosis of RBBB is also supported by a small terminal R wave in V1 and a slurring of the S wave in the lateral leads (i.e., leads I and V6). The T wave in V1 will also be in the opposite deflection of the QRS.

An RBBB is one of the most common defects in ventricular conduction. RBBB occurs often, and without apparent cause, in normal hearts. Treatment is directed at the cause of the conduction defect, which can include myocardial infarction (MI) or ischemia, heart failure, pulmonary embolism, or valvular disease.

Nondiagnostic Electrocardiogram

In some cases the patient may have a benign 12-lead ECG. However, the absence of patterns of ischemia on a 12-lead ECG does not preclude the diagnosis of an AMI. When the 12-lead ECG is nondiagnostic, the Paramedic should maintain a high index of suspicion based on the patient's clinical presentation and, more specifically, the history of present illness.

In some cases the diagnosis of AMI on 12-lead ECG is missed because of the low amplitude of the QRS. When the amplitude of the QRS is less than 5 mm in the standard limb leads (i.e., low amplitude QRS), an assessment of ST segment change is nearly impossible. Causes of low voltage, resulting in a low amplitude QRS, include pericardial effusions leading to constructive pericarditis, pleural effusions, and obesity.

Electrical Alternans

When every other ECG complex has alternating amplitude (i.e., the one QRS complex is smaller when compared to the next), then the patient may have **electrical alternans**.

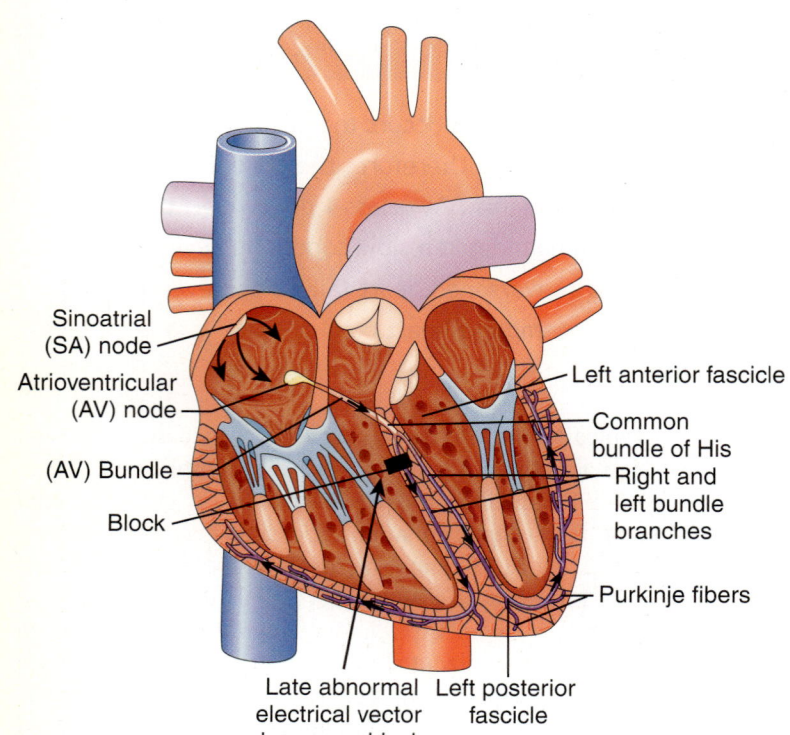

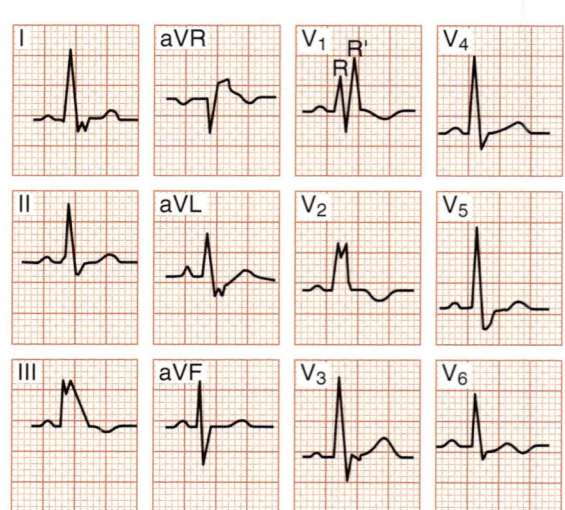

Total QRS complex prolonged (≥0.12 second). Terminal broad S wave in lead I. RSR' complex in lead V_1

Delmar/Cengage Learning

Figure 1-17 Right bundle branch block.

Electrical alternans is more frequently seen in the precordial leads and is a sign suggestive of pericardial effusion.

The alternating amplitude of the QRS is thought to be the result of the heart swinging, in a pendulum fashion, from the wave created in the pericardium as the heart beats within the accumulation of fluid.

Alternative Etiologies for Electrocardiogram Abnormalities

The Paramedic should keep an open mind when reading a 12-lead ECG for alternative causes of prolonged QT intervals, T wave abnormalities, and ST segment elevations. These aberrant changes do not typically mimic the pattern of ischemia but at a quick glance could mislead a Paramedic into thinking that there is a pattern of ischemia. Careful attention to the ECG for patterns of ischemia and a disciplined approach to interpretation will provide the Paramedic with the best results.

Prolonged QT Intervals

One of the first ECG changes which can occur as a result of AWMI can be a prolonged QT interval. However, there are a host of other etiologies for prolonged QT intervals as well. The majority of causes of acquired prolonged QT intervals involve electrolyte abnormalities (e.g., hypokalemia) and medications. Vaughn–Williams class I and III drugs are the leading offenders and have been repeatedly implicated as the cause of prolonged QT intervals. Other potential offenders include psychotropic medications, particularly tricyclic antidepressants and phenothiazines; antibiotics such as erythromycin; and toxins such as organophosphates.[37,38]

In some cases the cause of the prolonged QT interval is congenital. These patients may have presented in their youth as unexplained syncopal episodes. For this reason any patient, regardless of age, who has an unexplained syncope should be a candidate for a 12-lead ECG.

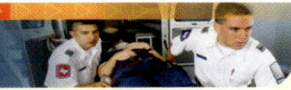

STREET SMART

One of the first ECG changes associated with hypothermia is a prolonged QT interval. The difficulty in obtaining a 12-lead ECG, because of the cold skin and resultant poor penetration of the electrode gel, makes this assessment problematic.

The length of the QT interval is inversely related to the patient's heart rate. Therefore, when calculating a patient's QT interval it must be corrected with the heart rate. Typically Paramedics and physicians use Bazett's formula to obtain the correct QT interval. Under emergency conditions the QTc (corrected QT) can be derived from information on the 12-lead ECG. Alternatively, the Paramedic can take the heart rate and, for every ten (10) beats above 70, subtract 0.02 seconds from 0.40 seconds, Likewise, for every ten (10) beats below 70, the Paramedic can add 0.02 seconds. Finally, many cardiac monitors will calculate the QTc, displaying this value on the 12-lead ECG. The Paramedic should also confirm the QTc by another method since the computer computation is inaccurate in some cases.

T Wave Abnormalities

Generally the T wave in a normal ECG is in the same deflection as the preceding QRS in the limb leads. The normal T wave is slightly asymmetrical, with the upstroke of the leading edge of the T wave being gentle compared to the downstroke. Any deviation from those conditions would be abnormal.

T wave abnormalities can include T wave inversion, flattened or low amplitude T waves, and peaked or hyperacute T waves. There are numerous causes for the T wave abnormalities that can be suggestive of a number of disorders (Table 1-5). With the exception of hyperkalemia, the isolated presence of a T wave abnormality is not diagnostic of any condition and requires further investigation.

Table 1-5 Potential Causes of T Wave Abnormalities

- CNS disorders
  - Cerebrovascular accident (CVA)
  - Subarachnoid hemorrhage
- Cardiac disease
  - Mitral valve prolapse
  - Myocarditis
  - Pericarditis
  - Ventricular hypertrophy
  - Conduction disorders
    - Bundle branch block
    - Ventricular pre-excitation
    - Post-ventricular tachycardia
- Electrolyte disorders
  - Hyperventilation
- Pulmonary conditions
  - Pulmonary embolism
  - Pneumothorax
- Gastrointestinal conditions
  - Acute pancreatitis
  - Acute cholecystitis
- Pharmacology
  - Digitalis
  - Antidysrhythmic agents
  - Alcohol
  - Cocaine

Hyperacute T Waves

Hyperacute T waves are defined as T waves greater than 5 mm in the limb leads and greater than 10 mm in the precordial leads. While a peaked T wave in contiguous leads is suggestive of ischemia, hyperacute T waves in all leads are highly suggestive of hyperkalemia. Hyperkalemia can be the result of renal failure or crush injury, or can be seen in cases of diabetic ketoacidosis (DKA).

Conversely, flattened T waves are suggestive of hypokalemia, a deficit in serum potassium that can be the result of potassium-wasting diuretics, such as Furosemide (Lasix®).

ST Segment Abnormalities

Although an ST segment depression is suggestive of ischemia when seen in select contiguous leads, when the ST segment depression is global, affecting all of the precordial leads, then the etiology of the ST segment depression is likely extracardiac (Table 1-6).

Medications, for example, can cause alterations in the ST segment. A classic cause of ST segment depression is digitalis. Digitalis alters ventricular depolarization, resulting in a "ladle" appearance of the ST segment (Figure 1-18).

Table 1-6 Three Possible Causes
of ST Segment Depression

- Hypokalemia
- Hypothermia
- Hypertrophy—ventricular

Other causes of ST segment depression include subarachnoid hemorrhage and hypokalemia. Hypokalemia, serum potassium less than 2.8, will produce ST segment depression in 80% of patients, along with flattened T waves (Figure 1-19).[39]

Similarly, ST segment elevation can be a normal variant, with some patients demonstrating a 1 to 2 mm ST segment rise, particularly if the ST segment has an upward concavity and/or a notch at the J point (Table 1-7). This finding is particularly common among African Americans and leaves the ST segment with an appearance of a fishhook.

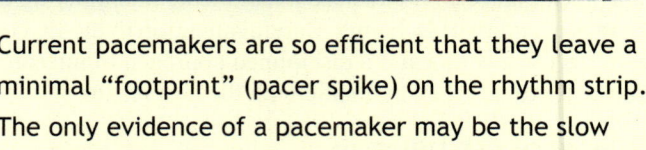

STREET SMART

Current pacemakers are so efficient that they leave a minimal "footprint" (pacer spike) on the rhythm strip. The only evidence of a pacemaker may be the slow and wide QRS as well as a slight ST segment elevation noted in the precordial leads.

Nonspecific ST Changes

In some instances the ST segment changes do not fit a pattern of ischemia nor are they contributory toward another diagnosis. In some cases the ST changes are transitory but not evolutionary. In those cases the Paramedic merely notes that the 12-lead ECG has **nonspecific ST changes**.

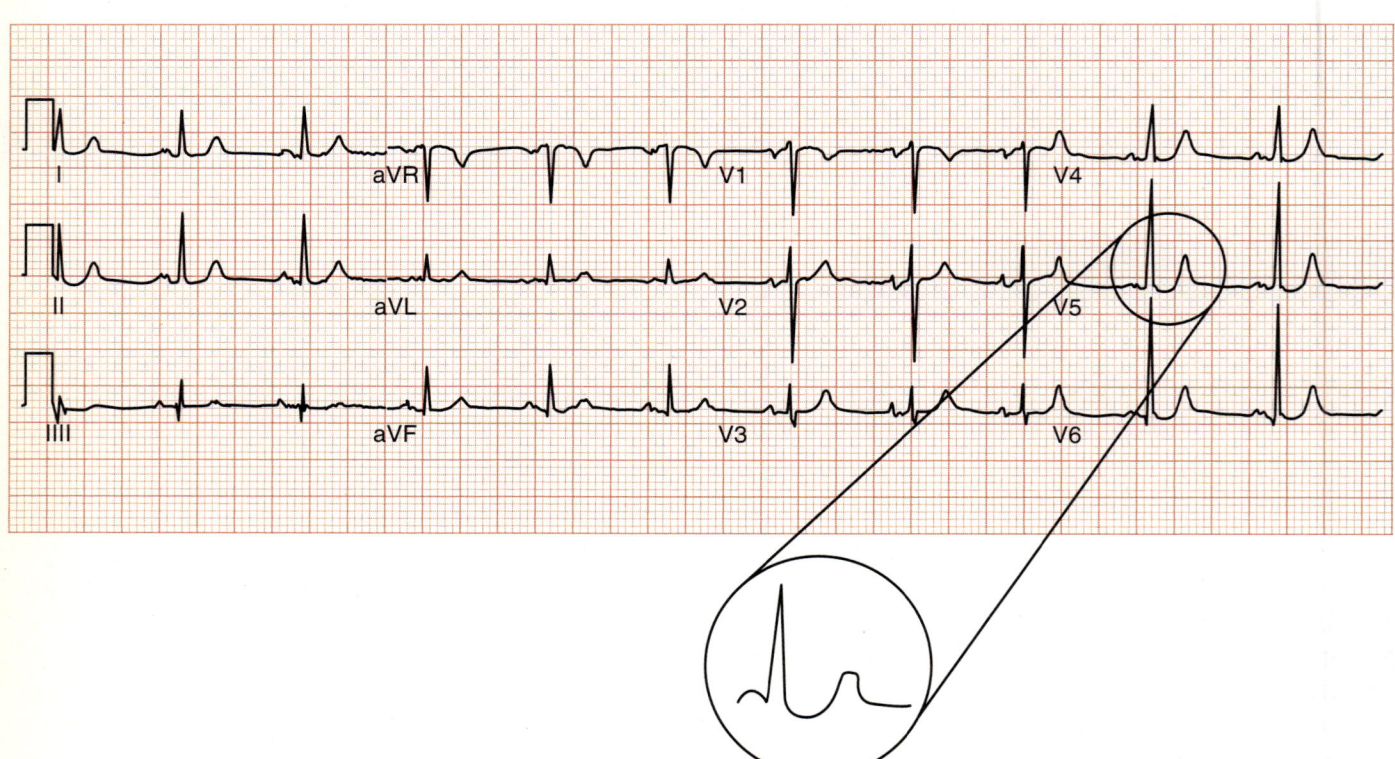

Figure 1-18 Digitalis effect on the ST segment.

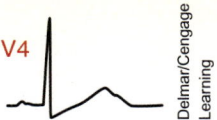
V4

Figure 1-19 Hypokalemia, a condition in which the patient's serum potassium is less than 2.8.

Table 1-7 Etiologies of Normal ST Segment Elevation

- Therapeutic digoxin
- Pre-excitation syndromes
  - WPW
  - LGL
- Early repolarization syndromes (congenital)
  - Brugada syndrome

There are a number of causes of nonspecific ST changes including improper lead contacts, electrolyte abnormalities, drug-induced changes, and hyperventilation. Even a drink of cold water can cause nonspecific ST changes.

Vasospastic Angina

One of the causes of transient patterns of myocardial ischemia is vasospasm. This vasospasm may be the result of many etiologies, including hyperventilation. These patients may present with symptoms consistent with acute coronary syndrome. Any 12-lead ECGs taken during this time will demonstrate ST segment elevations that seemingly disappear spontaneously. This condition is called variant or Prinzmetal's angina.

Approach to 12-Lead Electrocardiogram Interpretation

Several published approaches to the analysis and interpretation of the 12-lead ECG are available, and each of these methods has one common characteristic. Success in accurate 12-lead interpretations requires a disciplined approach to the analysis as well as the avoidance of any presumptions. Most Paramedics read a 12-lead ECG from left to right, starting at the left corner. The left corner provides information about calibration, speed, and diagnostic quality.

Calibration

The 12-lead ECG machine is a scientific instrument. As such, it needs to be calibrated to ensure its accuracy. Unlike the past, when Paramedics had to physically calibrate the ECG machine, current machines are self-calibrating (Figure 1-20). To demonstrate this internal calibration, the ECG machine marks the calibration as a squared off calibration mark at the beginning of the recording. Standard gain is 1 mv to 10 mm (10 small boxes) of amplitude.

Speed

The paper speed is critical for the analysis of the 12-lead ECG. The correct paper speed should be 25 mm/second. In some instances the Paramedic may have slowed the paper speed to better analyze slope characteristics; for example, the delta wave of WPW is sometimes difficult to discern when the paper speed is 25 mm/second. However, a slower, or faster, paper speed will impact on the measurement of intervals (i.e., PRI, QRS, and QT), leading to errors in interpretation.

Diagnostic Quality

The last information in the left lower corner of the 12-lead ECG is related to frequency response. When the ECG is used as a monitor for dysrhythmia, the machine reduces the frequency response (i.e., the sample from the signal) to 0.5 Hz and 20 to 50 Hz. This helps eliminate some of the artifact but also diminishes the quality of the ECG.

The 12-lead ECG must have a frequency response of 0.05 (not 0.5) Hz to 150 Hz. By "opening" the range, minor changes in the ECG are observable and the 12-lead ECG can be diagnostic. Unfortunately, the artifact and noise eliminated by the narrow sample supports the importance of proper skin preparation and proper electrode placement.

12-Lead Electrocardiogram Analysis

Having confirmed that the 12-lead is accurate (calibrated) and that the 12-lead ECG is diagnostic, the Paramedic can then proceed to analysis. There are several systems of analysis.[40,41] The P, Q, R, S, T method (described shortly) helps to ensure that no change or abnormality is left undetected. Regardless of the methodology of analysis, the Paramedic should always maintain a detailed approach to analysis and never rush to judgment over what appears to be obvious signs of ECG changes. The decision to label a 12-lead ECG as indicative of acute coronary syndrome must be coupled with the patient's clinical picture and the whole picture must be taken into consideration.

Every 12-lead ECG analysis starts with confirmation that the patient is not experiencing a dysrhythmia. The first mission of a Paramedic and emergency physician remains the treatment of dysrhythmia. This point is emphasized by the placement of a rhythm strip on the bottom of some 12-lead ECGs. Once the Paramedic has confirmed that the patient's rhythm is normal (i.e., there is a P wave associated with a QRS) and sinus in origin, then the Paramedic can proceed to the rest of the analysis.

Some Paramedics analyze the 12-lead ECG by proceeding in a left to right and top to bottom fashion. Other Paramedics, with a trained eye, look for Q waves in the leads that are associated with specific coronary arteries; for example, leads II, III, and aVF overlying the right coronary artery located in the inferior wall. Paramedics look for pathologic Q waves that are indicative of either an old myocardial infarction or a new myocardial infarction that is late in its evolution.

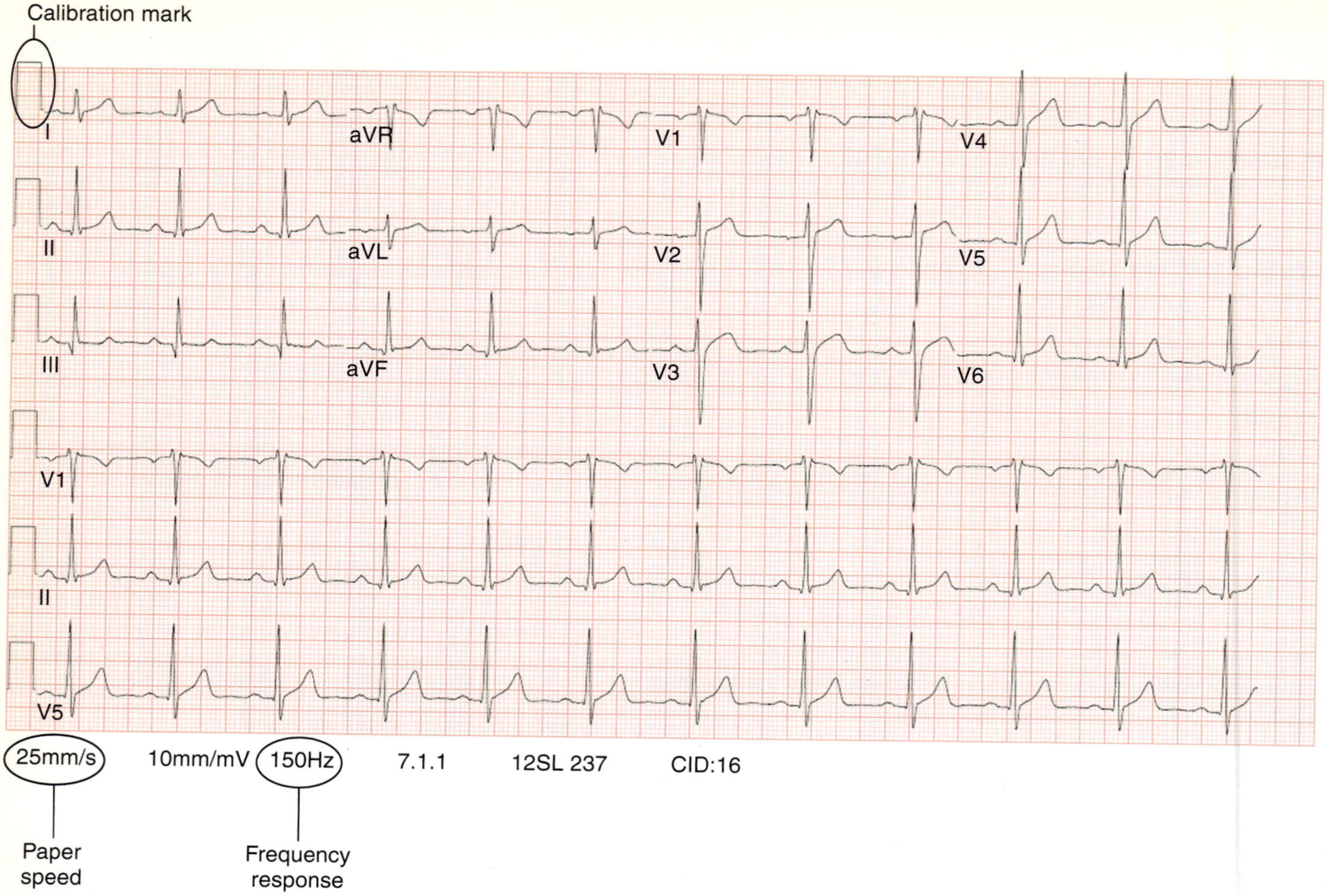

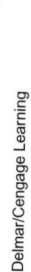

Calibration mark

I   aVR   V1   V4

II   aVL   V2   V5

III   aVF   V3   V6

V1

II

V5

(25mm/s)   10mm/mV   (150Hz)   7.1.1   12SL 237   CID:16

Paper speed   Frequency response

Delmar/Cengage Learning

Figure 1-20 ECG calibration mark, paper speed, and frequency response.

The latter finding, Q waves in a late evolving MI, have some implications for further complications.

Following a search for Q waves, the Paramedic should take a moment and look at the R wave progression. A reverse R wave progression is suggestive of anterior ischemia. Anterior wall MI (AWMI) can rapidly progress to either heart failure or sudden cardiac death. A RRWP can be likened to an early warning system, alerting the Paramedic to the possibility of sudden cardiac death before other ECG changes, such as ST segment elevation, occur.

Next the Paramedic should look for ST segment elevations and ST segment depressions, which are indicative of reciprocal changes. The importance of delaying to find ST segment elevations, suggestive of an ST elevation myocardial infarction (STEMI), is to reinforce the importance of a disciplined approach and to prevent the Paramedic from leaping to conclusions.

Finally, the Paramedic would turn to analysis of the T waves. While T waves are supportive of an argument for ACS, isolated T wave abnormalities may have no significance at all. Therefore, T wave changes should only be considered in the context of other ECG changes and the patient's history.

12-Lead Electrocardiogram Interpretation

Like the approach to a 12-lead ECG analysis, the approach to the 12-lead ECG interpretation must likewise be disciplined. First, the Paramedic should assemble the list of abnormalities (i.e., presence and location of Q waves, R wave progression, ST changes, and T wave abnormalities). Reflecting on these changes, the Paramedic should assess for lead groupings. Lead groupings are ECG changes in contiguous leads that are suggestive of involvement of a specific ventricular wall.

Armed with this information, the Paramedic can attempt to identify the culprit artery that is involved. Understanding coronary artery involvement can help the Paramedic predict the progression of the acute coronary event and prepare for these predictable events. For example, the right coronary artery (RCA) supplies the AV node in the vast majority of patients. ECG changes suggestive of an inferior wall myocardial infarction (IWMI) implicate the RCA and vice versa via the AV node ischemia. This AV node ischemia can manifest as type I heart block. The first indication of a type I heart block is a prolonged PR interval (PRI). Therefore, a Paramedic confronted with a possible IWMI would monitor the PRI in an IWMI for a possible heart block.

Finally, the Paramedic should consider the 12-lead ECG as a whole. ECG changes in adjoining walls may be suggestive of the extent and the evolution of the AMI. For example, ST changes and T wave abnormalities across all of the precordial leads, from V1 to V6, is suggestive of an extensive AMI. Such a pattern of ischemia could be suggestive of a left main coronary artery occlusion. The potential implications of left main coronary artery occlusion include acute pulmonary edema (backward failure), cardiogenic shock (forward failure), and sudden cardiac death (cardiac arrest).

A combination of Q waves, ST changes, and T wave abnormalities across one or more ventricular walls may be suggestive of an AMI later in its evolution. While every STEMI has the potential for reversal, the prognosis in a late evolution AMI is poorer and the morbidity higher.

Prognosis

In the event that the AV node is suffering from a lack of oxygenated blood, it will malfunction. The AV node is responsible for delaying the impulse and allowing the atria to contract and push blood into the ventricles. The node is also the electrical connection between the atria and the ventricles. The RCA serves the AV node in 90% of the population. If ischemic or injury patterns in the ECG leads which look at the area served by the RCA occur, the Paramedic can anticipate conduction abnormalities in the monitoring strip. The conduction abnormalities may lead to a decrease in coronary output sufficient to decrease preload and drop the blood pressure. Concurrently, blood may back up into the venous system, leading to distention in the neck veins. RCA occlusions are also associated with bradycardia.

With LAD occlusions, the conduction is affected at the bundle of His, making for more serious conduction abnormalities and unreliable escape mechanisms. The anterior wall is the largest portion of the left ventricle and is responsible for ejecting blood into the high pressure system. Damage to the anterior wall may impair the ability to eject the blood delivered to the left ventricle and create a backup of blood to the lungs. Anterior wall damage caused by occlusion of the LAD may lead to pump failure. Treatment options for anterior wall damage include anticipation of cardiogenic shock and anticipation of gross irritability of the muscle cells, leading to ventricular fibrillation.

Further 12-Lead Electrocardiogram Interpretation

As the heart's muscle depolarizes, the energy moves down the electrical pathway from the sinoatrial node (SA node) to the atrioventricular node (AV node) as a wave front. The electrical wave front then moves across the septum in a left to right fashion, then to the bundle branches, and finally the wave front radiates outward across the ventricular mass. Each of these electrical events can be recorded, over time, on an ECG. The graphic representation of these events is the traditional PQRS complexes seen on an ECG. However, there is another way to look at the electrical event. Instead of looking at depolarization in fragments of P, Q, R, and S, the Paramedic could look at the sum of these events. The sum of these electrical events would be the common direction of the electrical wave front, called the mean electrical **vector** (Figure 1-21).

To explain vectorography in another way, these electrical events could be likened to a battle front during a war. While an army may send out many patrols, some going in different directions, the army's main objective is to move the front forward. This common direction would be the army's vector. Similarly, although there may be minor deflections on the ECG, the major direction of the energy during depolarization is toward the apex of the heart. This common direction, or vector, of the energy of depolarization is called the heart's electrical **axis**. Any aberration from a normal electrical axis could be indicative of disease; this is explained in more detail shortly.

To help conceptualize the heart's normal axis, and to help determine if there is any axis deviation, an artificial construct called the **hexaxial reference system** (Figure 1-22) was created. To create the hexaxial system, the limb leads were drawn around the heart. Lead I, the lead that is horizontal

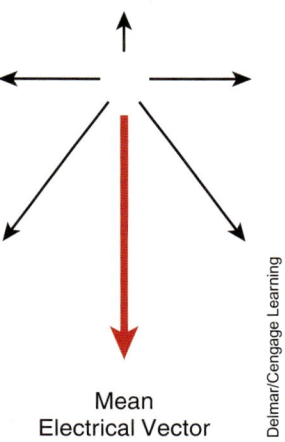

Mean
Electrical Vector

Figure 1-21 Electrical vector.

Delmar/Cengage Learning

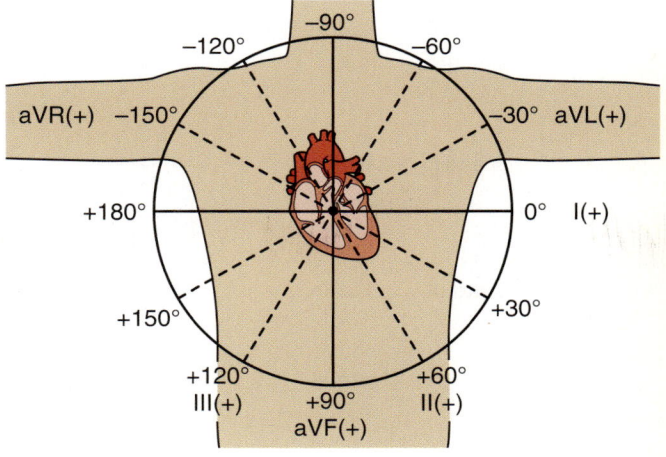

Figure 1-22 Hexaxial reference system.

Delmar/Cengage Learning

and on the right side, was assigned 0 degrees and the left side 180 degrees. Since the limb leads are part of Einthoven's triangle, an equilateral triangle, then Lead II would be at 60 degrees and negative 120 degrees and Lead III would be at 120 degrees and negative. The three axes are then all drawn into the middle of the heart and the three augmented leads overlaid with aVF at 90 degrees, aVL at negative 30 degrees, and aVR at 30 degrees and negative 150 degrees. The resulting construct shows the heart divided into equal 30 degree segments.

The traditional method of calculating the mean electrical axis was to find the most equiphasic lead of the frontal leads (I, II, III, aVR, aVL, and aVF); an equiphasic lead is a QRS complex where the R wave is equal in height to the depth of the S wave. An equiphasic wave would be neither going toward the vector nor away from it but would be perpendicular to it. The Paramedic would plot that lead on the hexaxial reference system, and the lead represented on the perpendicular spoke would be the heart's mean electrical axis in degrees (Figure 1-23). For example, if the equiphasic QRS was Lead I then the perpendicular axis would be 90 degrees.

This method of axis determination, while very accurate, is cumbersome in the field. An acceptable alternative is the Grant method. With the Grant method, the Paramedic would refer to Lead I and Lead II only (Figure 1-24). If both leads are upright, then there is a normal axis deviation. If Lead I is upright but Lead II is primarily downward in deflection,

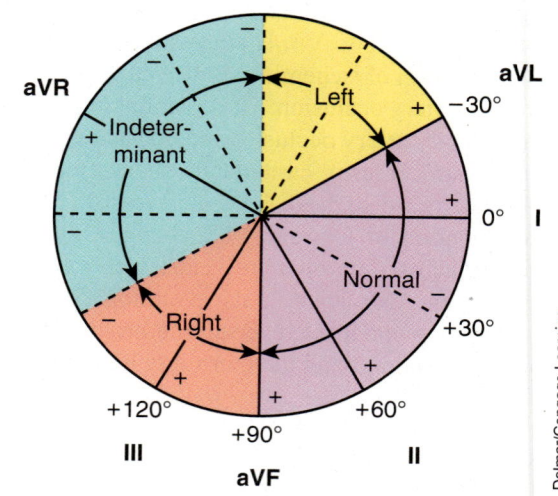

Figure 1-23 Axis determination using the hexaxial reference system.

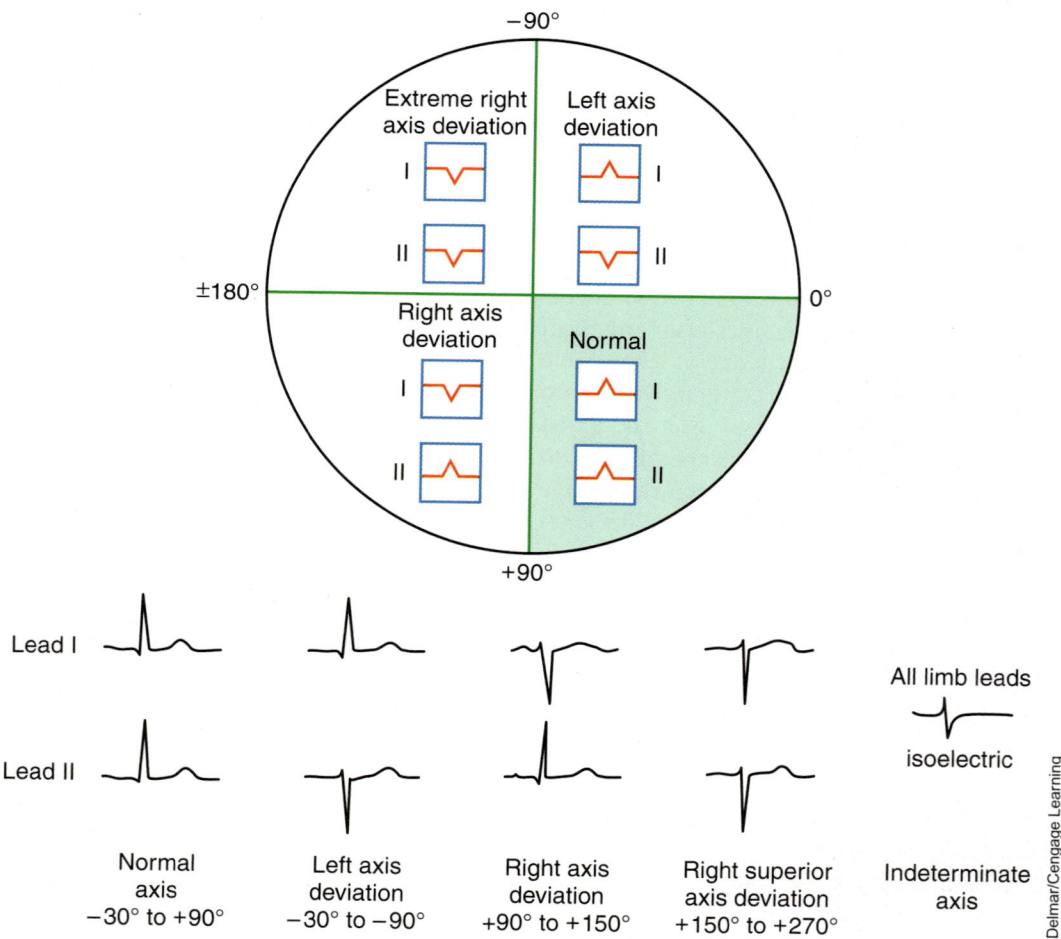

Figure 1-24 Determination of axis using Lead I and Lead II.

then a left axis deviation is assumed. Alternatively, if Lead I is primarily downward but the QRS in Lead II is upright, then it can be assumed it is a right axis deviation. If both Lead I and Lead II's QRS is negatively deflected, then the axis is called an extreme right axis deviation. This is nicknamed "no man's land" because it represents extreme abnormal depolarization.

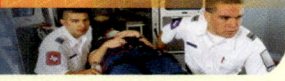

STREET SMART

Many 12-lead ECGs provide a reading of the axis, listed as P-R-T axes. The Paramedic need only read the R axis and compare it to the hexaxial reference to determine the axis.

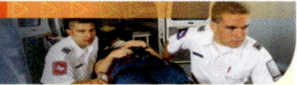

STREET SMART

To reduce confusion, some Paramedics use their thumbs to represent the QRS deflection, Lead I on the right hand and Lead II on the left hand. If Lead I is upright (i.e., the right thumb is up and the left thumb is down), then there is a left axis deviation. If both Lead I and Lead II are negative, then both thumbs are down.

Axis Deviation

Axis deviation occurs any time the heart's axis is not normal. Determining axis deviation is another means of observing many pathological conditions. Coupled with other physical findings, axis determination can help the Paramedic establish a diagnosis. For example, a right axis deviation, which is abnormal, can often suggest pulmonary pathologies such as pulmonary embolism and chronic obstructive pulmonary disease.

A slight left axis deviation, from 0 to (−) 40 degrees, may be physiologic and is seen in obese patients or women who are in their third trimester of pregnancy. A larger left axis deviation, from (−) 40 to (−) 90 degrees, is often associated with left ventricular hypertrophy, secondary to heart failure, inferior wall MI, or, in some cases, Wolff–Parkinson–White syndrome.

Of greater concern to the Paramedic is an extreme left axis deviation (>180 degrees) into "no man's land." While conditions such as congenital transposition of the great vessels and dextrocardia can produce this, in the normal heart extreme left axis deviation is suggestive of ventricular tachycardia

(VT). During ventricular tachycardia, the electrical source is in the ventricle and the wave front runs backward through the conduction system.

Differentiating Ventricular Tachycardia from Supraventricular Tachycardia with Aberrant Conduction

Paramedics (and other practitioners) often have difficulty determining whether a fast rhythm with a wide QRS complex is ventricular tachycardia (VT) or supraventricular tachycardia (SVT) with aberrant conduction. Some patients can tolerate a sustained monomorphic ventricular tachycardia for a prolonged period of time, despite opinion that patients cannot tolerate ventricular tachycardia (VT). Because the patient is tolerating what appears to be a wide complex tachycardia of unknown etiology, the assumption is it must be supraventricular tachycardia (SVT) with aberrant conduction; however, some patients do develop a rate-related bundle branch block (Table 1-8).

The determination is important as treatments for SVT, such as calcium channel blockers, can lead to rapid patient deterioration if the rhythm is actually VT. Instead of trialing a medication to "see if it works," at the risk of patient discomfort and wasted time, a 12-lead ECG can provide the necessary information.

Ventricular tachycardia occurs most often in patients with acute cardiac ischemia or those with a previous cardiac history. The Paramedic should first obtain a quick patient history, paying attention to anti-arrhythmic medications that indicate a previous history of cardiac dysrhythmia or medications that may predispose the patient to arrhythmias (pro-arrhythmic medications).

Table 1-8 Characteristics of Ventricular Tachycardia versus Supraventricular Tachycardia with Aberrancy

Ventricular Tachycardia	Supraventricular Tachycardia with Aberrancy
• History of ischemia	• Healthy individual
• Proarrythmic medications	• History of SVT
• Regular or irregular rhythm	• Regular or irregular rhythm
• Dissociated P wave activity	• P waves before each QRS
• Concordance in the chest leads	• R wave progression
• In V1 (MCL1), R wave, Rr', QR, RS	• In V1 (MCL1), rSR'
• In V6 (MCL6), rS, QS,QR	• In V6 (MCL6), qRs
• QRS duration of 0.16 sec or more	• QRS duration > 0.12 but < 0.16 sec
• Initial notching or slurring of QRS	• Absent or ending slurring of QRS
• Axis of −90 to −180	• Axis of −90 to +180

Alternatively, supraventricular tachycardias often occur in otherwise healthy individuals. Some of these patients may have a history of SVT or a diagnosis of WPW or Lown-Ganong-Levine (LGL) syndromes.

Next, the Paramedic should obtain a 12-lead ECG, paying particular attention to axis deviation and R wave progression. The first step is to determine if the rhythm is regular. Ventricular tachycardia is usually very regular. SVT with aberrancy is also usually regular unless the underlying cause is an atrial fibrillation with a rapid ventricular response. If the rhythm is atrial fibrillation, then the ventricular response will be irregularly irregular. While regularity will not help differentiate an interpretation of either VT or SVT, an irregularly irregular rhythm is suggestive of atrial fibrillation.

Next the Paramedic should examine the QRS morphology in V1. In ventricular tachycardia, the V1 lead will be an R wave where typically there is no R wave. Looking across the chest leads, the Paramedic may also observe an S wave where typically there is no S wave.

If fact, if all of the QRS complexes in the chest (leads V1 through V6) are in the same direction, a phenomenon called concordance, the ECG interpretation favors VT. The direction of the QRS (the polarity) can be either positive or negative but should be in the same direction.

Next, the Paramedic should look at Lead I and Lead II. If both leads are negative, or if the R vector on the 12-lead ECG reads between (−) 90 degrees and (−) 180 degrees (i.e., extreme left axis deviation), then the interpretation of VT is supported.

Finally, the Paramedic should observe the 12-lead ECG for the presence of P waves. Atrial depolarization still occurs in VT, independent of the ectopic ventricular pacemaker. Because of the independent atrial and ventricular activity (i.e., atrial–ventricular dissociation), P waves will randomly appear throughout the 12-lead ECG. P waves that appear regularly in front of a QRS suggest a supraventricular ectopic pacemaker.

Miscellaneous Effects on the Electrocardiogram

Electrolyte abnormalities, particularly potassium, can cause changes in the appearance of the 12-lead ECG. While the Paramedic does not usually have access to lab results, the patient's history may suggest the potential for electrolyte disturbances. For example, patients in end-stage renal disease may experience elevation of potassium levels while those patients receiving diuretics may have a decreased level of potassium unless they receive potassium supplementation.

A normal potassium level, between 3.5 mEq/L and 4.5 mEq/L, is important for optimum cardiac cell function. If the patient is hypokalemic (i.e., serum potassium less than 3.5 mEq/L), then the patient may be prone to decreased inotropy, leading to generalized weakness or malaise, and/or dysrhythmias such as atrial flutter and bradycardia.[42]

Causes of hypokalemia are numerous and include vomiting, aggressive gastric suctioning, diarrhea (secondary to infectious diseases), or abuse of potassium-wasting diuretics such as furosemide. With hypokalemia, the 12-lead ECG may show T wave flattening, ST segment depression, and/or U wave development; U waves are thought to be late after-depolarizations in the Purkinje fibers and may be an error of automaticity that gives rise to Torsade de pointes.

Hypokalemia is often associated with low magnesium levels or hypomagnesemia. Hypomagnesemia may predispose the patient to a form of polymorphic ventricular tachycardia called Torsade de pointes.[43]

Albuterol is a bronchodilator but it also drives potassium into the cells. Aggressive use of albuterol (i.e., stacked treatments) may cause changes in cellular uptake of potassium, putting the patient at risk for low potassium levels and dysrhythmias. Various ECG changes are associated with hypokalemia and hyperkalemia (Figure 1-25).

Perhaps more problematic for the Paramedic may be hyperkalemia, a serum potassium level above 4.5 mEq/L. One of the most common causes of hyperkalemia is kidney failure. Patients who are on kidney dialysis are at obvious risk of hyperkalemia prior to dialysis. Other at-risk patients include patients with diabetes who are experiencing diabetic ketoacidosis, patients with severe burns, patients with crush injury, and those patients with acute tubular necrosis secondary to shock.

The common ECG alterations seen in hyperkalemia are changes in the T wave.[44,45] At potassium levels greater than 4.5 mEq/L but less than 6.5 mEq/L, the T wave appears tall and peaked and is best seen in inferior leads (Lead II and Lead III). As the potassium level continues to climb toward 8 Eq/L, the QRS starts to widen and a left axis deviation may be appreciated. Finally, as the potassium level climbs above 8 mEq/L, the P waves all but disappear and the QRS starts to flatten into a sine wave configuration. At this time, the patient's cardiac output has dropped precipitously and the patient is at risk for ventricular fibrillation or asystole.

STREET SMART

Calcium is needed for regular cell function. Loss of calcium (serum calcium levels less than 8.5 mg/dL), also known as hypocalcemia, is rare. Typical causes of calcium disturbances are chronic diseases.

The effect of calcium is seen on the QT interval. Hypocalcemia causes a widened QT interval whereas an elevated serum calcium causes a short QT interval. To remember that calcium is related to QT, the Paramedic need only remember that QT interval is corrected for heart rate and recorded on the 12-lead ECG as such (i.e., QTc). The little c could represent calcium, to remind the Paramedic of other causes of prolonged/shortened QT intervals.

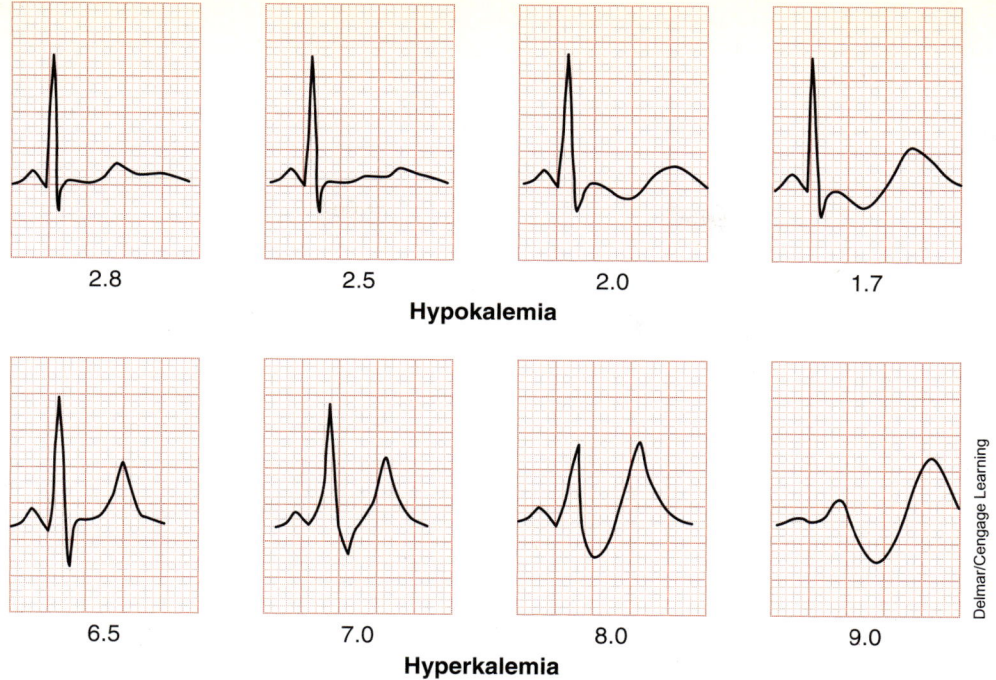

Figure 1-25 ECG changes associated with hypokalemia and hyperkalemia.

Arrhythmias caused by hyperkalemia are very difficult to treat with defibrillation or the usual emergency drugs without lowering the serum potassium level. Calcium chloride, calcium gluconate, or sodium bicarbonate—all competitive electrolytes—may be used to lower potassium levels. Alternatively, serial treatments with Albuterol may help to treat mild to moderate hyperkalemia. In severe cases, it may be necessary to administer 50% dextrose with short acting insulin. The insulin helps to drive both glucose and potassium into the cells.

Extracardiac Causes of Electrocardiogram Changes

Potentially devastating extracardiac pathologies, such as intracranial hemorrhage, hypothermia, and periocarditis, can also cause changes on the 12-lead ECG. While not pathognomonic for these pathologies, they are another sign to be added to the symptom complex for diagnosis.

An acute rise in intracranial pressure secondary to subarachnoid hemorrhage, intracerebral bleed, or an epidural bleed may lead to wide and deeply inverted T waves in the chest leads. Although the Paramedic's attention is likely focused on other, more urgent matters during one of these events, 12-lead ECG evidence, if obtained, may be useful at the emergency department.

Hypothermia affects all cellular functions and can also cause changes in the ECG. When a patient is hypothermic all of the interval durations (i.e., PR, QRS, and QT) lengthen and positive deflections at the J point, or point where the ventricular complex ends and the ST segment begins, become noticeable. These deflections are in the same direction (polarity) as the QRS and are termed "Osborn waves." They are also sometimes called the camel–hump sign. The Osborn wave can be seen in all leads, but is more prominent in the inferior limb leads. The size of the Osborn waves correlates directly with the degree of hypothermia.[46] Osborn waves are often difficult to discern because of artifact from muscle tremors (Figure 1-26), but are seen in 80% of patients with hypothermia (below 33°C/91.4°F).[47]

Finally, pericarditis, an inflammation of the pericardium, can cause chest pain and 12-lead ECG abnormalities. Initially the Paramedic may be led to believe that the chest pain is secondary to acute coronary syndrome. However, nitrates are not useful in treating the pain of pericarditis, so it is important for the Paramedic to seek historical clues to the diagnosis of pericarditis (i.e., fevers, etc.) as well as ECG evidence.

The inflammation that occurs between the sac surrounding the heart and the epicardium leads to swelling which puts some pressure on the myocardium. The myocardium cannot repolarize as it normally does due to the swelling, so there are T wave changes. The T will become pointed and tall, similar to a hyperacute T wave found in an MI. However, the changes tend to occur in all leads rather than within contiguous leads only, leading the Paramedic to suspect other causes for the chest pain, such as pericarditis.[48]

Evaluation

One of the advantages of the 12-lead ECG is its ability to predict the clinical progression of the patient's disease. For example, in the case of a patient with AWMI, the patient may

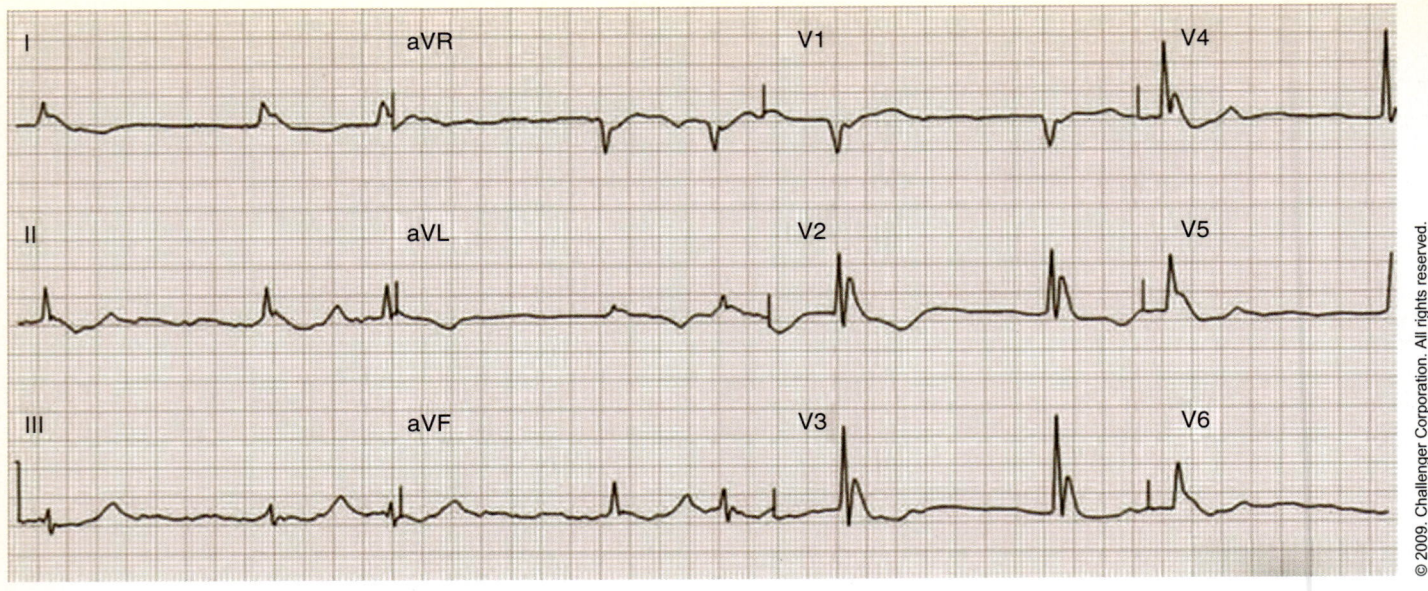

Figure 1-26 Osborn wave secondary to hypothermia.

eventually develop cardiogenic shock secondary to lost myocardial function. In this case, the patient may have an IWMI that could, predictably, either extend to the mitral valve, causing mitral valve regurgitation, or extend into the right ventricle. It is estimated that 50% of IWMI extend into the right ventricle, with a resultant loss of preload.

> ### STREET SMART
>
> The right ventricle essentially primes the pump (the left ventricle). Loss of right ventricular function, secondary to myocardial injury, can lead to profound hypotension. For this reason, some Paramedics perform a 15-lead ECG to identify right ventricular involvement before administering vasodilators such as nitroglycerin or morphine sulfate.

15-Lead Electrocardiogram

If the Paramedic suspects right ventricular involvement, an additional diagnostic test available for testing is the 15-lead ECG.[49] The electrode placement for a 15-lead ECG will place positive electrodes onto the right side of the chest and view the right ventricle (Figure 1-27).

Locations for these electrodes are the fifth right intercostal space at the midclavicular for V4R, fifth right intercostal space anterior axillary line, and fifth right intercostal space at midaxillary. The corresponding V4 to V6 wires from the left chest electrodes are switched over to the right electrodes and

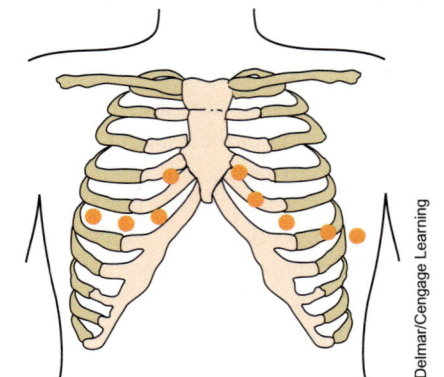

Figure 1-27 Lead placement for 15-lead ECG.

the ECG is rerecorded. The repeated ECG is marked **right chest leads** or V4R, V5R, and V6R.

Disposition

Although a 12-lead ECG is not a perfect tool, the combination of positive ST elevations on a 12-lead ECG with a patient history that is consistent for acute coronary syndrome should encourage the Paramedic to transport the patient to an interventional cardiac center, sometimes called an ST elevation MI (STEMI) center.

National standards have encouraged rapid intervention, less than 90 minutes, from arrival at the emergency department to balloon inflation in a cardiac catheterization lab for patients with a suspected STEMI.[50] Clearly the emphasis has been on rapid assessment and intervention in these cases. Paramedics can improve that efficiency by acquiring and analyzing prehospital 12-lead ECGs and making a rapid transport decision to a STEMI center.

The Paramedics had obtained an ECG right after placing Mrs. Swinter on oxygen. It showed ST elevation and hyperacute T waves in Leads II, III, and aVF. Mrs Swinter said her pain was gone but she complained of feeling very lightheaded and afraid. Repeat vital signs were obtained and rather than the 118/66 found earlier, she had a pressure of 80/48. She also had jugular venous distention while semi-sitting and clear lung sounds. One Paramedic continued with treatment while the other transmitted her ECG to a STEMI center.

Mrs. Swinter was taken to the local STEMI center. Later in the week, the Paramedics received a brief note from their medical director telling them that Mrs. Swinter underwent angioplasty with placement of a stent. Based in part on promptly obtaining an ECG and transmitting it to the center, Mrs. Swinter's door to balloon time was 59 minutes.

CRITICAL THINKING QUESTIONS

1. What is the significance of the ST changes in leads II, III, and AvF?
2. Why was the "door to balloon" (D2B) time so important?

CONCLUSION

The 12-lead ECG provides the Paramedic with a wealth of knowledge regarding the heart's electrical conduction system. As the Paramedic becomes more proficient with 12-lead ECG interpretation, this assessment tool becomes more useful in patient care.

KEY POINTS:

- Death from AMI remains a national health problem.

- Aggressive prehospital treatment including obtaining and interpreting a 12-lead ECG can favorably impact patient mortality and morbidity.

- Paramedics must have a higher index of suspicion with patient populations that may present with atypical cardiac symptoms.

- A regular ECG uses standard limb leads, augmented limb leads, and precordial leads.

- The regular ECG allows for views of the inferior, anterior, and lateral left ventricle, as well as combinations of these views.

- Accurate 12-lead ECG requires proper patient preparation including standardized electrode placement.

- A 12-lead ECG is printed in a standard configuration.

- Viewing specific combinations of leads, called contiguous leads, allows correlation to specific ventricular walls.

- Based upon coronary artery anatomy, ECG changes in contiguous leads permit estimating damage in specific arteries.

- Estimation of damage in specific arteries permits prognosis and planning.

- Understanding an acute myocardial infarction requires an understanding of penumbra.

- Additional ECG evidence, such as new onset left bundle branch block (LBBB) and reverse R wave progression (RRWP), are important in supporting the diagnosis of myocardial infarction.

- Some 12-lead ECGs do not show acute changes; therefore, the Paramedic should focus on treating the patient based on history.

- There are numerous extracardiac causes to ECG abnormalities.

- The 12-lead ECG interpretation takes a disciplined approach that gathers all the pertinent information to prevent premature interpretation.

- Based on the 12-lead ECG interpretation and the patient history, the Paramedic can make a field diagnosis.

- Additional information is also available from the 12-lead ECG that can lend insight into other health conditions.

- The 12-lead ECG can help differentiate ventricular tachycardia (VT) from supraventricular tachycardia (SVT).

- The addition of three right-sided leads can help identify right ventricular AMI.

- Early detection of MI, via 12-lead ECG, and rapid transportation to an interventional cardiac care center can lead to better patient outcomes.

REVIEW QUESTIONS:

1. Why is Paramedic use of 12-lead ECG the first step in a critical pathway for patients with acute coronary syndrome?

2. What are the key elements necessary for an accurate acquisition of a 12-lead ECG?

3. List the ECG abnormalities associated with an inferior wall MI, anterior wall MI, and lateral wall MI.

4. Which leads are affected on an ECG of a patient experiencing an inferolateral MI? An anteriolateral MI?

5. Where are leads placed for a right-sided ECG?

CASE STUDY QUESTIONS:

Please refer to the Case Study in this chapter, and answer the questions below:

1. What does the scene tell you about Mrs. Swinter's previous level of activity? Do you think her complaint is of an acute nature or chronic nature? Explain your answer.

2. Is Mrs. Swinter experiencing a STEMI? Defend your answer.

3. What is the relationship between the location of Mrs. Swinter's damaged myocardium and her resultant drop in blood pressure?

4. What is the national standard for STEMI management at the receiving hospital? What is the Paramedic involvement in this standard?

REFERENCES:

1. Brady WJ, Chan TC, et al. Electrocardiographic manifestations: patterns that confound the EKG diagnosis of acute myocardial infarction—left bundle branch block, ventricular paced rhythm, and left ventricular hypertrophy. *J Emerg Med*. 2000;18(1):71–78.

2. Nikus KC. Electrocardiography. *Timely Topics in Medicine: Cardiovasc Dis*. 2007;11:E29.

3. Alpert JS, Thygesen K. A new global definition of myocardial infarction for the 21st century. *Pol Arch Med Wewn*. 2007;117(11–12):485–486.

4. Canto JG, Goldberg RJ, et al. Symptom presentation of women with acute coronary syndromes: myth vs reality. *Arch Intern Med*. 2007;167(22):2405–2413.

5. Methot J, Hamelin BA, et al. Does hormonal status influence the clinical presentation of acute coronary syndromes in women? *J Women's Health (Larchmt)*. 2004;13(6):695–702.

6. Geddes JS (Editor). *The Management of the Acute Coronary Attack: The J. Frank Pantridge Festschrift*. London: Academic Pr.; 1986.

7. Purim-Shem-Tov YA, Rumoro DP, et al. Emergency department greeters reduce door-to-ECG time. *Crit Pathw Cardiol*. 2007;6(4):165–168.

8. Diercks DB, Kirk JD, et al. Door-to-ECG time in patients with chest pain presenting to the ED. *Am J Emerg Med*. 2006;24(1):1–7.

9. Cajavilca C, Varon J. Resuscitation great. Willem Einthoven: the development of the human electrocardiogram. *Resuscitation*. 2008;76(3):325–328.

10. Davis DP, Graydon C, et al. The positive predictive value of Paramedic versus emergency physician interpretation of the prehospital 12-lead electrocardiogram. *Prehosp Emerg Care*. 2007;11(4):399–402.

11. Garvey JL, MacLeod BA, et al. Pre-hospital 12-lead electrocardiography programs: a call for implementation by emergency medical services systems providing advanced life support—National Heart Attack Alert Program (NHAAP) Coordinating Committee; National Heart, Lung, and Blood Institute (NHLBI); National Institutes of Health. *J Am Coll Cardiol*. 2006;47(3):485–491.

12. Whitbread M, Leah V, et al. Recognition of ST elevation by Paramedics. *Emerg Med J*. 2002;19(1):66–67.

13. Greiff SJ. Taking it to the street: advanced monitoring and 12-lead EKGs in prehospital care. *Emerg Med Serv*. 1998;27(9):47–48, 54–55.

14. Patel SI, Souter MJ. Equipment-related electrocardiographic artifacts: causes, characteristics, consequences, and correction. *Anesthesiology*. 2008;108(1):138–148.

15. Wan SW, Nguyen HT. 50 Hz interference and noise in ECG recordings—a review. *Australas Phys Eng Sci Med*. 1994;17(3):108–115.

16. Davies A. Recognizing and reducing interference on 12-lead electrocardiograms. *Br J Nurs*. 2007;16(13):800–804.

17. Krucoff MW, Johanson P, et al. Clinical utility of serial and continuous ST-segment recovery assessment in patients with acute ST-elevation myocardial infarction: assessing the

dynamics of epicardial and myocardial reperfusion. *Circulation.* 2004;110(25):e533–e539.

18. Pope JH, Selker HP. Diagnosis of acute cardiac ischemia. *Emer Med Clin North Am.* 2003;21(1):27–59.

19. Madias JE. Comparability of the standing and supine standard electrocardiograms and standing, sitting, and supine stress electrocardiograms. *J Electrocardiol.* 2006;39(2):142–149.

20. Ferguson JD, Brady WJ, et al. The prehospital 12-lead electrocardiogram: impact on management of the out-of-hospital acute coronary syndrome patient. *Am J Emerg Med.* 2003;21(2):136–142.

21. Drew BJ, Krucoff MW. Multilead ST-segment monitoring in patients with acute coronary syndromes: a consensus statement for healthcare professionals. ST-Segment Monitoring Practice Guideline International Working Group. *Am J Crit Care.* 1999;8(6):372–386; quiz 387–388.

22. Morrison LJ, Brooks S, et al. Prehospital 12-lead electrocardiography impact on acute myocardial infarction treatment times and mortality: a systematic review. *Acad Emerg Med.* 2006;13(1):84–89.

23. Antzelevitch C. Cardiac repolarization. The long and short of it. *Europace.* 2005;7 Suppl 2:3–9.

24. Burke AP, Virmani R. Pathophysiology of acute myocardial infarction. *Med Clin North Am.* 2007;91(4):553–572; ix.

25. Herlitz J, Hansson E, et al. Predicting a life-threatening disease and death among ambulance-transported patients with chest pain or other symptoms raising suspicion of an acute coronary syndrome. *Am J Emerg Med.* 2002;20(7):588–594.

26. Peacock WF, Hollander JE, et al. Reperfusion strategies in the emergency treatment of ST-segment elevation myocardial infarction. *Am J Emerg Med.* 2007;25(3):353–366.

27. Shah SR, Hochberg CP, et al. Reperfusion strategies for ST-elevation myocardial infarction. *Curr Cardiol Rep.* 2007;9(4):281–288.

28. Ornato JP. Accelerating time to reperfusion in acute myocardial infarction: prehospital and emergency department strategies, systems of care, and pharmacologic interventions. *Rev Cardiovasc Med.* 2006;7 Suppl 4:S49–S60.

29. O'Connor R, Persse D, et al. Acute coronary syndrome: pharmacotherapy. *Prehosp Emerg Care.* 2001;5(1):58–64.

30. Magid DJ, Wang Y, et al. Relationship between time of day, day of week, timeliness of reperfusion, and in-hospital mortality for patients with acute ST-segment elevation myocardial infarction. *J Am Med Assoc.* 2005;294(7):803–812.

31. Eskola MJ, Nikus KC, et al. Value of the 12-lead electrocardiogram to define the level of obstruction in acute anterior wall myocardial infarction: correlation to coronary angiography and clinical outcome in the DANAMI-2 trial. *Int J Cardiol.* 2008.

32. Gami AS, Holly TA, et al. Electrocardiographic poor R-wave progression: analysis of multiple criteria reveals little usefulness. *Am Heart J.* 2004;148(1):80–85.

33. Kontos MC, McQueen RH, et al. Can myocardial infarction be rapidly identified in emergency department patients who have left bundle-branch block? *Ann Emerg Med.* 2001;37(5):431–438.

34. Miller WL, Sgura FA, et al. Characteristics of presenting electrocardiograms of acute myocardial infarction from a community-based population predict short- and long-term mortality. *Am J Cardiol.* 2001;87(9):1045–1050.

35. Brilakis ES, Wright RS, et al. Bundle branch block as a predictor of long-term survival after acute myocardial infarction. *Am J Cardiol.* 2001;88(3):205–209.

36. Spiers CM. Using the 12-lead ECG to diagnose acute myocardial infarction in the presence of left bundle branch block. *Accid Emerg Nurs.* 2007;15(1):56–61.

37. Cavero I, Mestre M, et al. Drugs that prolong QT interval as an unwanted effect: assessing their likelihood of inducing hazardous cardiac dysrhythmias. *Expert Opin Pharmacother.* 2000;1(5):947–973.

38. De Ponti F, Poluzzi E, et al. Safety of non-antiarrhythmic drugs that prolong the QT interval or induce torsade de pointes: an overview. *Drug Saf.* 2002;25(4):263–286.

39. Ballantyne F, 3rd, Vander Ark C. The difficult diagnosis of hypokalemia. *Am Fam Physician.* 1986;33(2):256–258.

40. Kligfield P, Gettes LS, et al. Recommendations for the standardization and interpretation of the electrocardiogram: part I: The electrocardiogram and its technology: a scientific statement from the American Heart Association Electrocardiography and Arrhythmias Committee, Council on Clinical Cardiology; the American College of Cardiology Foundation; and the Heart Rhythm Society: endorsed by the International Society for Computerized Electrocardiology. *Circulation.* 2007;115(10):1306–1324.

41. Dubin D. *Rapid Interpretation of EKG's, sixth edition.* C.O.V.E.R.; 2000.

42. Humphreys M. Potassium disturbances and associated electrocardiogram changes. *Emerg Nurse.* 2007;15(5):28–34.

43. Roden DM. A practical approach to torsade de pointes. *Clin Cardiol.* 1997;20(3):285–290.

44. Burger CM. Hyperkalemia. *Am J Nurs.* 2004;104(10):66–70.

45. Diercks DB, Shumaik GM, et al. Electrocardiographic manifestations: electrolyte abnormalities. *J Emerg Med.* 2004;27(2):153–160.

46. Aslam AF, Aslam AK, et al. Hypothermia: evaluation, electrocardiographic manifestations, and management. *Am J Med.* 2006;119(4):297–301.

47. Patel A, Getsos JP, et al. The Osborn wave of hypothermia in normothermic patients. *Clin Cardiol.* 1994;17(5):273–276.

48. Brady WJ, Perron AD, et al. Cause of ST segment abnormality in ED chest pain patients. *Am J Emerg Med.* 2001;19(1):25–28.

49. Somers MP, Brady WJ, et al. Additional electrocardiographic leads in the ED chest pain patient: right ventricular and posterior leads. *Am J Emerg Med.* 2003;21(7):563–573.

50. Fesmire FM, Brady WJ, et al. Clinical policy: indications for reperfusion therapy in emergency department patients with suspected acute myocardial infarction. American College of Emergency Physicians Clinical Policies Subcommittee (Writing Committee) on Reperfusion Therapy in Emergency Department Patients with Suspected Acute Myocardial Infarction. *Ann Emerg Med.* 2006;48(4):358–383.

CHAPTER 2

ACUTE CORONARY SYNDROME

KEY CONCEPTS:

Upon completion of this chapter, it is expected that the reader will understand these following concepts:

- That coronary heart disease is the number one killer of Americans of both genders
- How the anatomy and physiology of the heart are the key to cardiac conditions
- That chest pain or discomfort is the primary complaint of most persons experiencing an acute coronary event, although respiratory complaints, weakness, fatigue, or malaise may also be the presenting complaint
- How myocardial infarction is death of heart tissue; treatment varies for ST elevation MI compared with non-ST elevation MI
- How angina occurs when oxygen demand exceeds oxygen supply to the heart tissue
- The causes of pain: infections, damage to the pericardium, valve disorders, vessel disorders, or specific respiratory, musculoskeletal, or gastrointestinal disorders
- That initial treatments for acute coronary syndrome include oxygen, intravenous access, 12-lead ECG, and nitrates
- How the results of the 12-lead ECG help determine further treatment and destination

ANATOMY CONCEPTS:

Prior to reading this chapter the Paramedic student should be familiar with the following anatomy and physiology concepts:

- Valves and chambers of the heart
- Functions of the left and right ventricles
- Hemodynamic concepts
  - Preload
  - Cardiac output
  - Ejection fraction
  - Systemic vascular resistance
- Great vessels

CASE STUDY:

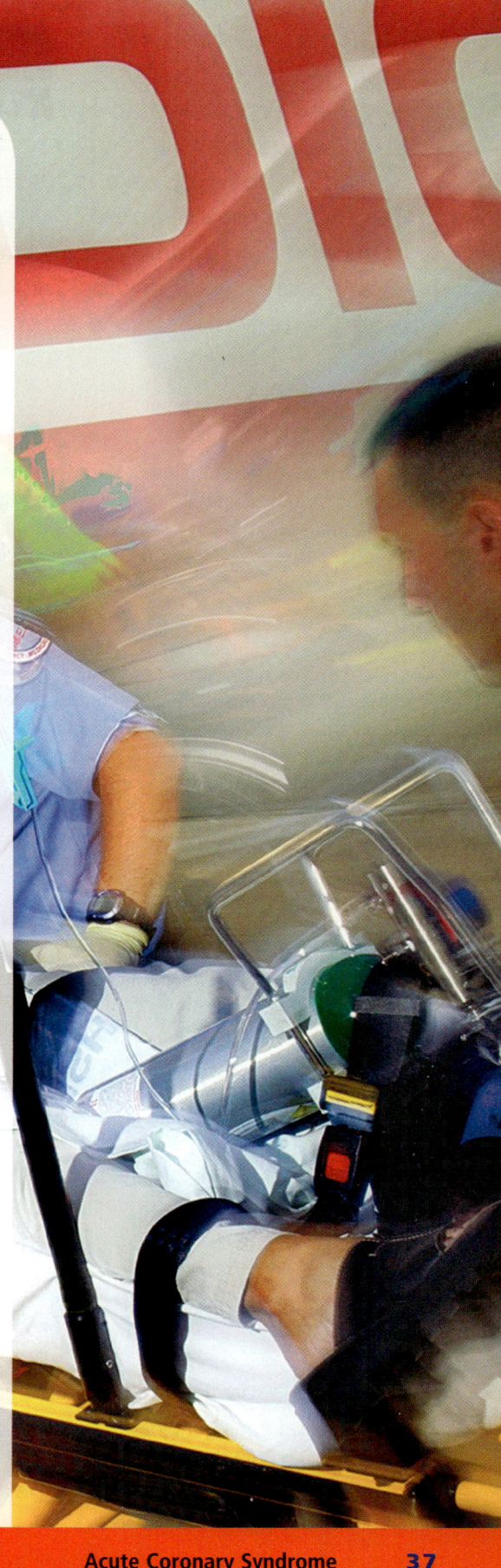

"County Paramedic 1, Conto Corners Rescue Squad, respond to 4351 Old Brick Church Road, for a 42-year-old male patient complaining of chest pain and trouble breathing."

The Paramedic starts the engine on his SUV Paramedic response vehicle and starts off for the scene. During the 10-minute drive, he hears the volunteer providers from the rescue squad come on the air acknowledging the call and then calling en route to the scene. During the drive, he considers the many possible conditions that can cause chest pain, reviewing the Continuing Medical Education (CME) lecture he attended at the state conference the week before.

CRITICAL THINKING QUESTIONS

1. What are some of the possible causes of cardiac-related chest pain?
2. How is trouble breathing related to chest pain?

OVERVIEW

An estimated 16 million people in the United States have some form of coronary heart disease.[1] In 2008, estimates indicated an additional 770,000 Americans would have a new **acute cardiac event (ACE)**, formerly called a "heart attack," and another 430,000 would have a recurrent ACE.

Coronary heart disease is responsible for one in every five deaths in the United States. Furthermore, approximately half of the men and almost two thirds of the women who die suddenly of an acute coronary event, or sudden cardiac death, will not have any warning symptoms. Patients who have a history of, or symptoms related to, coronary artery disease are among the more common reasons for patients to access EMS.

Chief Concern

There are many different causes of chest pain, some of which are cardiac in nature, and others that are not. Of those that are cardiac in nature, some are related to coronary heart disease while others are related to structural or electrical disorders of the heart.

Acute Coronary Syndrome

Acute coronary syndrome (ACS) is a generic term used to describe the symptom pattern related to coronary artery disease that, untreated, results in unstable angina and myocardial infarction (MI).[2–4] The most common symptom reported by patients with ACS is chest pain; however, there are many other complaints associated with ACS. Even the term "pain" may be misleading, as the patient may report the sensation as a pressure or ache rather than a pain, and deny pain when questioned by the Paramedic.

ACS typically presents with chest pain or pressure that is either substernal or left sided and can radiate to the left arm, shoulder, neck, or jaw. This pain is often associated with nausea, dyspnea, and diaphoresis. A patient may also complain of atypical descriptions of pain, including pressure, tightness, sharp pain, or pain that is only present in the arm, jaw, or neck. Some patients, especially those who are elderly or those who have diabetes, may only complain of shortness of breath, diaphoresis, or nausea rather than pain.[5] These atypical presentations, when linked with cardiac-related events, are often termed **angina equivalents**, meaning the patient will develop these complaints rather than pain with ACS events.

STREET SMART

Some patients with jaw pain may assume that they have a dental emergency and go to the dentist's office for relief of their symptoms.

Pathophysiology of Acute Coronary Syndrome

The most common pathophysiology of ACS involves gradual build-up over time of atherosclerotic plaque along the lumen of the coronary arteries. These plaque build up until an acute event occurs, at which point the plaque ruptures and a clot is formed at the site of the plaque. The clot, or thrombus, occludes the coronary artery, which produces a total or near total blockage of blood flow to the myocardium distal to the obstruction (Figure 2-1).

Pain occurs when the amount of blood flowing through the narrowed or blocked coronary artery is less than required to supply adequate oxygen to the myocardium. Acidic by-products build up which irritate the myocardium, causing pain and dysrhythmia.

Alternatively, an obstruction can be caused by an embolus. An embolus may form within the heart and then break off, only to float into the sinus of Valsalva and into the coronary arteries. This phenomenon must often occur during atrial fibrillation. During atrial fibrillation, the atriums quiver and blood becomes stagnant within pockets of the atria, and particularly within the valve's leaflets. Stagnant blood quickly congeals into a blood clot on the walls of the atria; these are called mural thrombi. When the heart's rhythm returns to normal (either naturally or because of electrical cardioversion, for example), the mural thrombi come off the walls of the atria and go on to occlude the coronary arteries.

A very small percentage of patients, approximately 1% to 2%, may have a rupture of an coronary artery aneurysm.[6] A coronary artery aneurysm is an out-pouching of the blood vessel wall and represents a weakness in the blood vessel. If this aneurysm ruptures, then the patient will bleed from the coronary artery into the pericardial sac and eventually develop a pericardial tamponade. There is little that a Paramedic can do for this condition in the field and it is presented only for the purpose of a complete discussion of the causes of coronary artery-induced chest pain.

Another mechanism of coronary artery occlusion is vasospasm. A number of etiologies can cause focal coronary

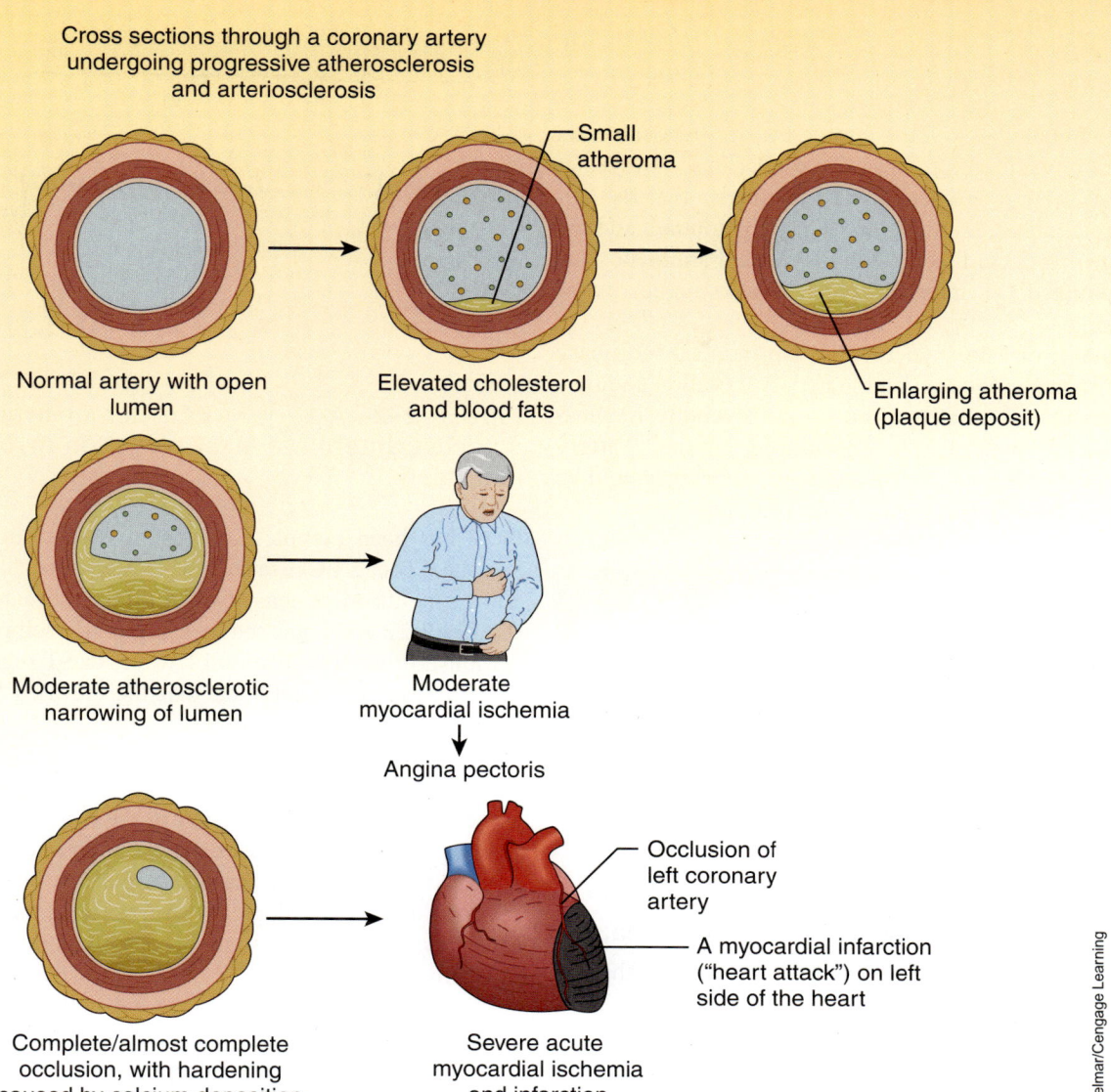

Figure 2-1 Arteriosclerotic build-up narrows the coronary artery, decreasing blood flow to the myocardium.

Cross sections through a coronary artery undergoing progressive atherosclerosis and arteriosclerosis

Small atheroma

Normal artery with open lumen

Elevated cholesterol and blood fats

Enlarging atheroma (plaque deposit)

Moderate atherosclerotic narrowing of lumen

Moderate myocardial ischemia

Angina pectoris

Occlusion of left coronary artery

A myocardial infarction ("heart attack") on left side of the heart

Complete/almost complete occlusion, with hardening caused by calcium deposition

Severe acute myocardial ischemia and infarction

Delmar/Cengage Learning

artery vasospasm including cocaine intoxication, calcium channel blockers, and atherosclerotic coronary artery disease.[7] The latter, atherosclerosis, prevents normal coronary artery vasoconstriction and vasodilation, leaving the artery prone to vasospasm.

Patients with a history of Raynaud's phenomenon, specifically those who smoke cigarettes and those that use cocaine, are at particular risk of coronary artery vasospasm. It should be noted that the patient with a coronary artery vasospasm may manifest all the same symptomology as a patient with a coronary artery occlusion, including transient ST segment elevation. Fortunately, coronary vasospasm responds well to the vasodilator nitroglycerin.

Typically the diagnosis of coronary artery vasospasm, also called Prinzmetal's angina, only occurs after a coronary artery angiography shows minor coronary artery disease or coronary arteries without a critical lesion; a critical atherosclerotic lesion occludes 70% of the coronary artery.

Hyperventilation Syndrome

Hyperventilation can lead to coronary artery spasm and chest pain.[8] There are a number of factors that are thought to contribute to hyperventilation syndrome including panic disorders, agoraphobia, and stimulants such as caffeine. These result in agitation, hyperpnea, and tachypnea, the cardinal signs of hyperventilation syndrome.

Patients with hyperventilation syndrome (HVS), also known as psychogenic dyspnea, markedly decrease their arterial pCO_2 levels, causing a leftward shift in the oxyhemoglobin curve and hypocalcemia. The latter, hypocalcemia, can lead to coronary artery vasospasm.

Other associated signs of hypocalcemia, secondary to hyperventilation, include a feeling of perioral numbness, the presence of cramps in the hand or carpopedal spasm, and muscle twitching. Another simple test for hypocalcemia secondary to hyperventilation is Chvostek's sign. Nerves at the angle of the jaw are sensitive to hypocalcemia. By tapping the facial nerve, the facial muscles will contract and the face will grimace. On the 12-lead ECG, the Paramedic may note a prolonged QT interval, which is also suggestive of hypocalcemia.

Treatment of the hyperventilation-induced coronary artery vasospasm is focused on the hyperventilation and may include the use of sedatives and/or antipsychotic medications. However, hyperventilation-induced coronary artery vasospasm can induce ischemia and these patients should be routinely treated with standard cardiac protocols.

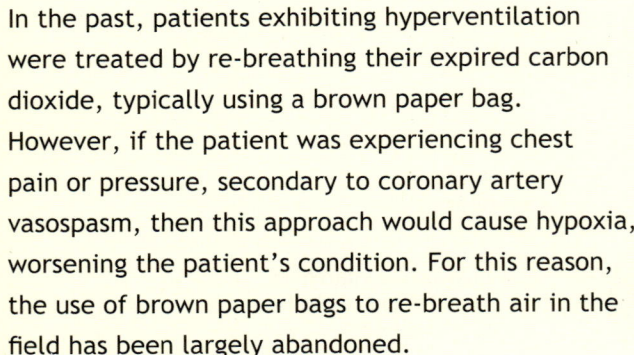

STREET SMART

In the past, patients exhibiting hyperventilation were treated by re-breathing their expired carbon dioxide, typically using a brown paper bag. However, if the patient was experiencing chest pain or pressure, secondary to coronary artery vasospasm, then this approach would cause hypoxia, worsening the patient's condition. For this reason, the use of brown paper bags to re-breath air in the field has been largely abandoned.

Myocardial Infarction

A myocardial infarction is death of myocardial muscle cells. This occurs acutely when an embolus or thrombus occludes a narrowed coronary artery, completely eliminating blood flow to a specific portion of the myocardium (see Figure 1-7 and Table 1-3). When this occurs, the coagulation cascade is initiated, causing propagation of the clot and ultimately completely occluding the coronary artery. These occlusions will manifest on the 12-lead ECG as patterns of ischemia.

ST Elevation Myocardial Infarction versus Non-ST Elevation Myocardial Infarction

Myocardial infarctions can be divided into ST elevation myocardial infarction (STEMI) and non-ST elevation myocardial infarction (NSTEMI). While there is myocardial damage in each type, the acute treatment (discussed later in this chapter) is different.

Approximately half of the patients who are having a myocardial infarction have an STEMI an their initial 12-lead ECG.[9] In an **ST elevation myocardial infarction (STEMI)**,

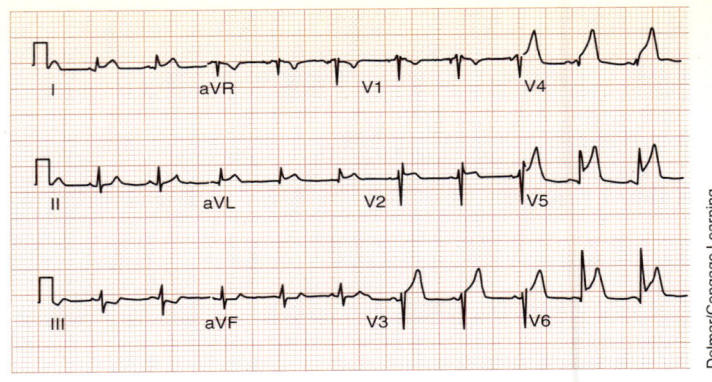

Figure 2-2 A 12-lead ECG demonstrating an acute anterolateral ST elevation myocardial infarction.

there has been complete occlusion of the coronary artery and the 12-lead ECG reveals at least 1 mm elevation of the ST segments in at least two contiguous anatomical leads (Figure 2-2). As discussed in Chapter 1, reciprocal changes demonstrating either inverted T waves or ST segment depression increase the likelihood that the elevated ST segments have been caused by an acute MI.

Initially, the myocardium is able to survive with minimal cell damage as the ECG undergoes the typical changes associated with the progression of the MI (see Figure 1-15). Eventually, the myocardial cells die and are unable to regenerate. At this point, the cardiac event has been present for several hours, pathologic Q waves have developed, and acute revascularization strategies are unlikely to salvage the myocardium.

Eventually the dead myocardial cells are replaced by collagen, a connective tissue, and a scar forms in the heart muscle. This scar is sometimes seen on later ECGs as smaller Q waves or persistent ST segment or T wave changes, indicating a past MI. Depending upon the amount of myocardial damage, the scar may affect the contractility of the heart muscle, reducing the ejection fraction.

Surrounding the damaged myocardium is an **ischemic penumbra** (see Figure 1-11) consisting of adjacent myocardium that is ischemic, but not yet dead. This nearly dead tissue can often be salvaged by aggressive treatment, limiting the morbidity of the cardiac event. It should be noted that the tissue in the ischemic penumbra can easily become permanently damaged, resulting in a larger area of infarct and increased morbidity and mortality without interventional cardiac catheterization.

In the case of ACS, the clot needs to be treated either mechanically or chemically in order to revascularize the myocardium, by opening up the blocked coronary artery, and reperfuse the myocardium.

Non-ST Elevation Myocardial Infarction

In a **non-ST elevation myocardial infarction (NSTEMI)** there is still permanent damage to myocardial cells; however, at the time of presentation, the 12-lead ECG does not demonstrate ST segment elevations. This may occur because the acute event is now several hours old and the 12-lead ECG has evolved past the acute injury pattern. This is sometimes seen in patients who have had intermittent severe symptoms over several hours. A non-ST elevation MI may also occur if there is less than a complete occlusion.

While the initial 12-lead ECG with pain may not demonstrate ST elevations, it is important to be aware that in patients who are diagnosed with a myocardial infarction, the 12-lead ECG is normal in only about 4% of patients.[9]

In these patients, the myocardial infarction is detected by measuring serum levels of troponin, CK-MB, and myoglobin enzymes. When myocardial cells die, the cell membrane breaks down and these three enzymes are released at different rates. While the myoglobin can be detected within two to three hours of the onset of the myocardial infarction, it is not as specific for myocardial infarction because it is present in skeletal muscle in addition to myocardial cells. CK-MB is a subtype of creatine kinase that is more specific for myocardial cells, but is still found to a small extent in skeletal muscle. The most specific enzyme for a myocardial infarction is troponin.[10,11] Troponin is essentially present only in myocardial cells and can be detected as early as six hours after the myocardial infarction. A non-ST elevation MI is diagnosed when the serum troponin is elevated above the threshold for MI, which may not happen for several hours.

Angina Pectoris

Angina pectoris is cardiac pain secondary to ischemia that occurs as a result of the narrowing of the coronary arteries. Angina is a condition in which the supply of oxygenated blood cannot meet the demand for oxygen by the myocardium, creating a demand and supply mismatch. While the body automatically regulates the diameter of the coronary arteries to maximize blood flow to keep up with the demand, the arteries become too narrow, because of atherosclerotic plaque, to provide sufficient blood flow. Angina is further subdivided into stable angina and unstable angina.

Stable angina occurs with exertion and goes away with rest. When the patient exerts himself past the point where coronary blood flow can supply enough oxygen, the patient will develop symptoms. Once the patient rests, the pain will often resolve within several minutes without any other intervention. Occasionally, the patient will take one of the prescribed sublingual nitroglycerin tablets and completely relieve the symptoms. The nitroglycerin works by dilating the coronary arteries, increasing blood flow to the myocardium.

In general, stable angina does not produce death of myocardial cells. However, over long periods of time, chronic myocardial ischemia can lead to weakening of the myocardium, decrease in ejection fraction, and dilation of the left ventricle. The 12-lead ECG in a patient who has stable angina is likely to be nondiagnostic.

In contrast, **unstable angina** may occur at rest and persist for a longer time period. Unstable angina tends to require repeated administration of nitroglycerin to relieve the symptoms. Unstable angina is also defined as angina which occurs with increasing frequency or requires more than the usual nitroglycerin to resolve symptoms.[12]

Unstable angina is also defined as new onset exertional chest pain or pre-infarction angina. Often, the patient's 12-lead ECG will show patterns of ischemia (Figure 2-3). The ECG signs of ischemia may resolve once the patient is pain free, providing further evidence of a cardiac origin for the symptoms as well as highlighting the patient as one with unstable angina. On the other hand, it may be difficult clinically to differentiate between a non-ST elevation myocardial infarction and unstable angina as the ECGs may be nondiagnostic in both cases. For this reason, any patient with unstable angina is assumed to be having an acute coronary event.

Angina can also occur as a result of coronary vasospasm. This variation of angina is called Prinzmetal's angina and

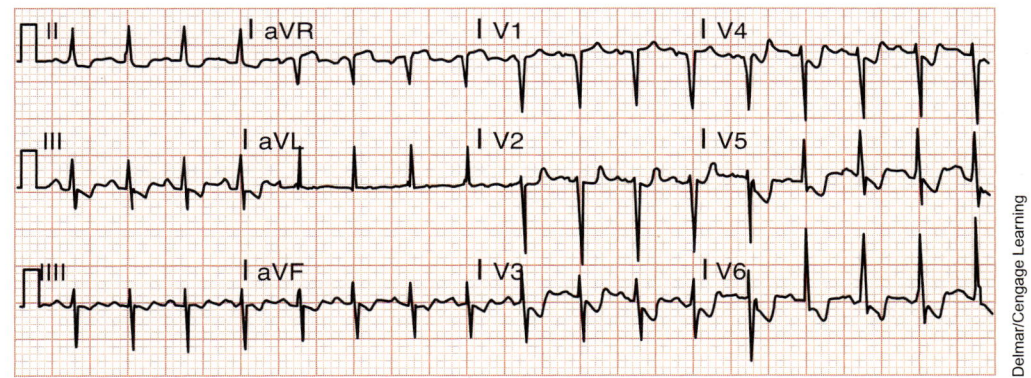

Figure 2-3 ECG findings that are suggestive of myocardial ischemia include T wave inversions or ST depressions greater than 1 mm in at least two anatomically contiguous ECG leads. This ECG is from a patient who has inferior wall ischemia.

occurs most of the time while the patient is at rest. Often, the patient has either minimal or no atherosclerotic build-up in the coronary arteries, as evidenced by cardiac catheterization. This form of angina is thought to be caused by spasm of the coronary arteries, often with an unknown cause, though smoking may be a risk factor. The ECG may either be non-diagnostic or show signs of ischemia. This is a relatively uncommon variation of angina.

Cocaine-Related Acute Coronary Syndrome

Cocaine use is a significant risk factor for an acute coronary syndrome. Cocaine is a sympathomimetic drug (adrenalin-like) which is often snorted, but it can be smoked or made into an injectable form that can be inserted into a vein. As a sympathomimetic drug, it produces vasospasm, an increase in heart rate, and a marked increase in blood pressure. These effects are increased when alcohol or cigarettes are used at the same time, which is often the case.

Cocaine does several things from a cardiovascular standpoint. Cocaine increases the myocardial oxygen demand by increasing heart rate as well as causing the heart to work harder against increased systemic vascular resistance. Cocaine produces vasospasm of the coronary arteries, which in turn limits myocardial blood flow and oxygen delivery. The reduction of blood flow is even greater in individuals who have coronary artery disease.

Finally, cocaine also encourages thrombus formation and accelerates the rate of arteriosclerotic plaque development, both of which set the cocaine user up for a myocardial infarction. Repeated hypertensive episodes which develop from cocaine use also increase the risk for thoracic aortic dissection, which the Paramedic should also consider when conducting a differential diagnosis of chest pain.[13,14]

Most of the time, chest pain related to cocaine use occurs within three hours after ingesting cocaine. The patient is most at risk for ACS within that first hour after ingestion at which time the sympathomimetic effects of cocaine are at their peak. In some individuals, the symptoms may not begin for 24 to 96 hours after the last use of cocaine. This is thought to be due to metabolites or breakdown products of cocaine that are active and produce vasospasm hours after the sympathomimetic surge subsides.[15] It is important to remember that cocaine also accelerates the development of arteriosclerosis; therefore, the cardiac complaint the patient is experiencing may be due to an embolic cause of coronary artery occlusion rather than vasospasm.

Cardiac Infections

Infections in and around the heart can cause both parietal and visceral pain. The group of cardiac-related infections includes infections of the pericardium, the myocardium, and the valve surfaces. Often these infections incite an inflammatory response; as a result fever, chills, and malaise are often associated with these infections.

Pericarditis

Pericarditis is an inflammation of the pericardium and can be caused by infections, malignancy, medications, systemic inflammatory conditions, renal failure, or can occur after a myocardial infarction.[16] Classically, pericarditis occurs within two weeks of a viral illness. In pericarditis, the pericardium becomes thickened and inflamed. The small amount of pericardial fluid that is normally present to allow the heart to slide easily within the pericardial sac is displaced and a significant amount of friction develops, producing pain. The somatic pain associated with pericarditis is often sharp and positional, improving when the patient leans forward and worsening when the patient lies back. The pain may radiate to the back between the shoulders or to the epigastrium, depending upon which sections of the pericardium are affected. Pericarditis may be associated with a fever less than 101°F.

The inflammatory process which occurs with pericarditis may also cause a pericardial effusion. A pericardial effusion is a collection of pericardial fluids around the heart. The volume in a pericardial effusion can become large, creating increased pressure in the pericardium, and affect the ventricle's ability to expand. The resultant pericardial tamponade can reduce blood outflow (Figure 2-4). The large pericardial effusion produces tamponade physiology and eventually causes hypotension.

Pericardial Effusion and Tamponade

A **pericardial effusion** is an increased amount of fluid or blood in the pericardial sac surrounding the heart. When an effusion becomes larger, it can develop into a pericardial tamponade. **Pericardial tamponade** occurs when the amount of pericardial fluid becomes large enough to interfere with ventricular

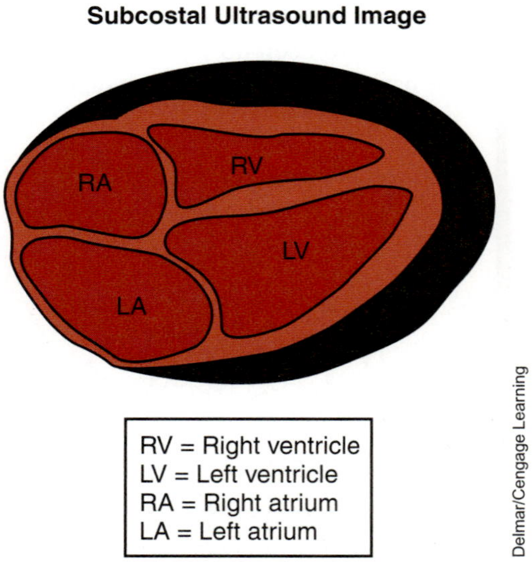

Subcostal Ultrasound Image

RV = Right ventricle
LV = Left ventricle
RA = Right atrium
LA = Left atrium

Delmar/Cengage Learning

Figure 2-4 A large pericardial effusion can develop, impeding the ventricle's ability to expand, therefore reducing blood output. This is called tamponade physiology.

filling, and thus impairs cardiac output. This can occur either medically or traumatically. The discussion of pericardial tamponade in this chapter will be limited to medical causes.

As previously discussed, acute pericarditis is one cause for a pericardial effusion. Other causes include renal failure, malignancy, infection, pulmonary disease, and rheumatologic disorders. Another cause is a dissection of the thoracic aorta that extends back to the root of the aorta where it meets the left ventricular outflow tract (Figure 2-5). At this point, the pericardium surrounds the vessel. A tear in the vessel that extends down toward the aortic valve may leak into the pericardium, producing a pericardial effusion that usually rapidly progresses to a pericardial tamponade.

Pericardial tamponade occurs when the pressure of the fluid in the pericardium impairs the ability of the ventricles to expand. If the pericardial fluid develops acutely, it takes a relatively small amount of fluid to produce tamponade because the pericardium does not have the ability to stretch quickly. If the pericardial fluid develops more slowly, a significant effusion can develop. Up to a liter of fluid may be present before the patient shows life-threatening signs of a pericardial tamponade.[17] This is because over time the pericardium has the ability to slowly stretch. However, even these patients will develop fatigue and dyspnea on exertion after a small fluid collection develops.

The classic presentation of the patient with pericardial tamponade is Beck's triad. Beck's triad consists of dropping systolic pressure, secondary to decreased ventricular filling; increased venous pressure, from backward failure; and distant heart sounds. Clinically the patient will present with hypotension, accompanied by a sustained tachycardia without exertion, marked jugular venous distention even while seated, and diminished heart sounds even over the point of maximal intensity (PMI) at the apex of the heart.

ECG findings in acute pericarditis may include diffuse ST segment elevations across multiple anatomic territories (Figure 2-6); in other words, ischemic patterns suggesting global ischemia. These ST elevations are the result of myocardial irritation and typically do not include V1. Another classic ECG finding in acute pericarditis is depression of the PR segment, commonly seen in the inferior leads, but which can

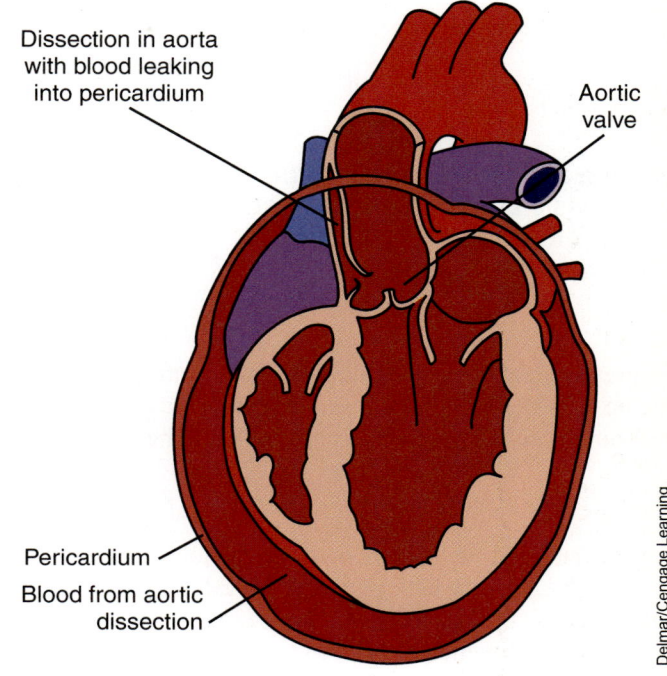

Dissection in aorta with blood leaking into pericardium

Aortic valve

Pericardium

Blood from aortic dissection

Figure 2-5 Acute pericardial tamponade caused by a thoracic aortic dissection that involves the aortic valve and aortic root.

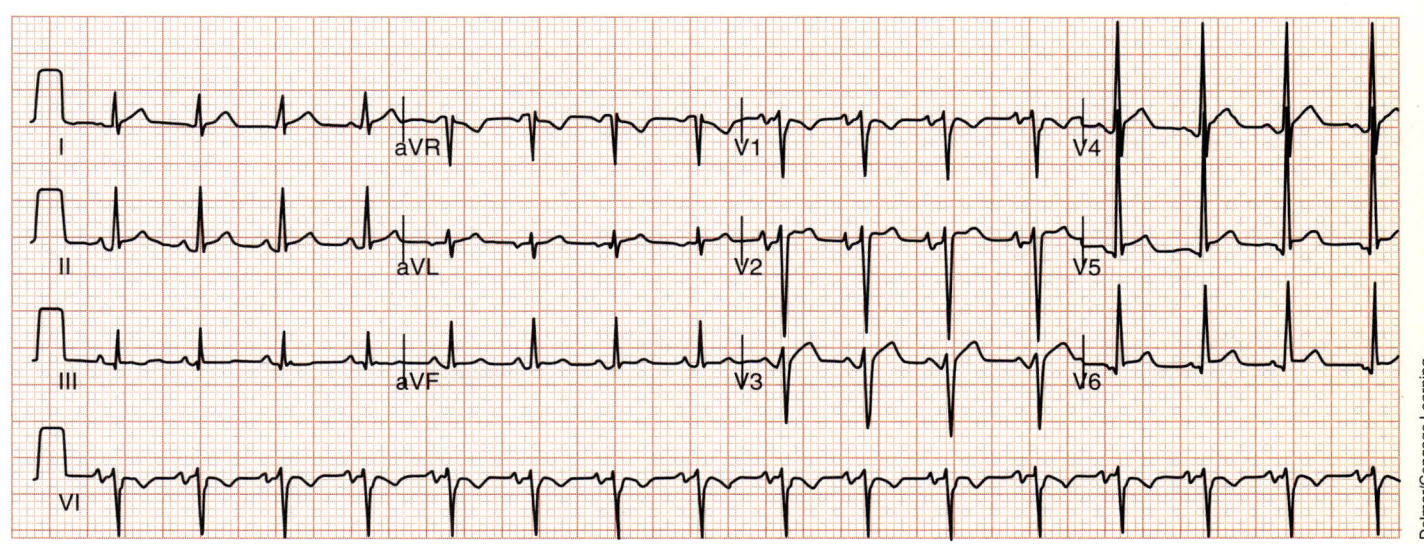

Figure 2-6 Diffuse ST elevations suggestive of acute pericarditis rather than an ST elevation myocardial infarction.

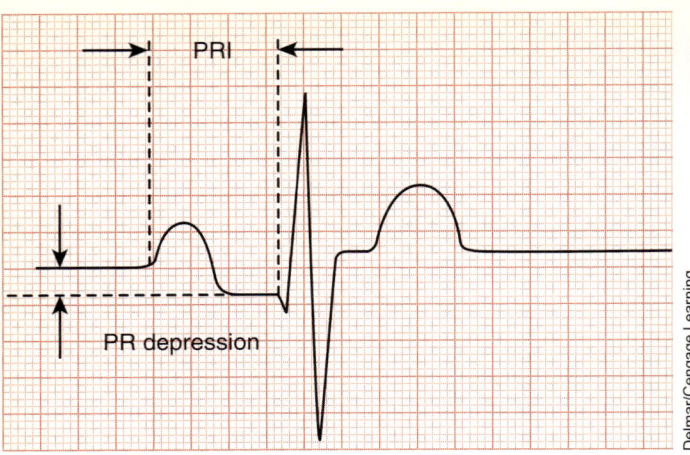

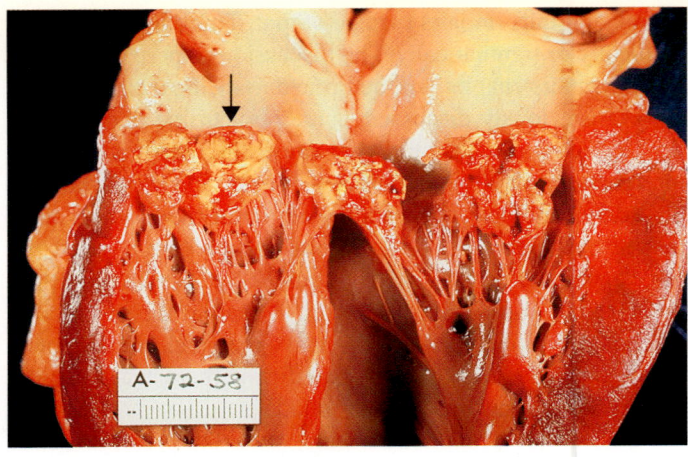

Figure 2-7 Depression of the PR segment is a classic ECG finding suggestive of acute pericarditis.

Figure 2-8 Infective endocarditis produced this vegetation on a valve.

be present in any lead (Figure 2-7). As a reminder, the Paramedic uses the T-P segment as the isoelectric baseline when measuring ST or PR segment changes from the baseline.

Endocarditis

Endocarditis is an infection of the endocardial, or inner, layer of the heart, which includes the valves' tissue and the inner surface of the chambers. Endocarditis may also affect artificial valves which have been implanted to replace a diseased valve.[18]

The endocardium receives its oxygen and nutrients directly from the blood circulating through the heart. Endocarditis occurs when bacteria gain access to the bloodstream and subsequently infect the endocardial tissue. Bacteria can gain access to the bloodstream either through spread of an infection elsewhere in the body or through instrumentation (i.e., surgery on areas of the body that contain normal amounts of bacteria). In certain patients, the American Heart Association and American Dental Association recommend taking antibiotics one hour prior to invasive procedures that may release bacteria into the bloodstream.[19] Intravenous drug users are also at risk for endocarditis from sharing needles, reusing needles, or practicing inadequate aseptic technique when injecting drugs.

Bacterial vegetations, pockets of pus, can develop on affected valves (Figure 2-8), pieces of which can become dislodged by constant valve movement and be propelled downstream, further spreading the infection or causing more serious problems. If the tricuspid or pulmonic valves develop a bacterial vegetation, an infective emboli can be released and can lodge in the lung, causing an infective pulmonary embolus. If the mitral or aortic valve develops a vegetation, the embolus can lodge in the smaller arteries supplying the gut or the lower legs, causing an acute arterial occlusion. Alternatively, the vegetation can travel to the brain and cause abscesses in the brain.

Due to the nature of the endocarditis, it may be difficult to identify that a patient has this condition. The diagnosis may not be definitively made without extensive hospital workup. However, it should be considered in the paramedical differential diagnosis in a patient with a fever, cardiac sounding chest pain, a loud new murmur, and those who use intravenous drugs of abuse. If the affected valve begins to leak, the patient may complain of dyspnea, hypoxia, and fatigue, secondary to pulmonary edema, due to the decreased forward blood flow through the pulmonary valve. Some patients may present in acute heart failure as described in Chapter 3.

Myocarditis

Myocarditis is an inflammation of the myocardial tissue. As with endocarditis and pericarditis, myocarditis can occur from an infectious cause—toxicity from both medications and environmental poisons—as well as rheumatological or autoimmune disorders. In severe cases, the inflammation that occurs within the heart can impede ventricular filling as well as myocardial contraction, leading to heart failure and death. More frequently, mild cases occur without significant symptoms.

The vast majority of specific causes of myocarditis are the result of viruses which attack the myocardium. As with endocarditis, it is often difficult to detect myocarditis clinically. Many of the signs and symptoms include constitutional symptoms and very little chest pain unless the pericardium becomes involved (pericarditis). If chest pain does occur it is often described as stabbing in nature.

Myocarditis is a significant cause of sudden death in younger populations. Myocarditis can also cause heart failure, in some cases requiring a heart transplant, in a young person.

Valve Disorders

Valve disorders can occur either acutely or as a slow and progressive process. Acute changes are more likely to produce severe signs and symptoms whereas the progressive conditions will either intermittently produce symptoms or may produce more severe symptoms if the patient cannot compensate for added stressors on the body.

Valve disorders can be divided into two categories. Disorders occur from scarring down of the valve, which limits valve opening and therefore provides significant resistance to forward blood flow, or valve incompetence, in which the valve cannot prevent backward flow of blood during ventricular contraction, thereby also limiting forward blood flow. The most common complaint in patients who have an acute valve problem is dyspnea due to either pulmonary congestion or lack of forward blood flow. A valve disorder should be considered when a patient presents with these symptoms and has a new murmur upon physical examination.

Valve Stenosis

Scarring of a cardiac valve is called **stenosis** and may occur for a variety of reasons. Endocarditis and rheumatic fever are the most common causes of valve stenosis. For the aortic valve, other common causes include calcium deposits at the aortic root or on the valve leaflets as well as congenital changes in the shape of the valve or number of leaflets.

If the mitral valve is affected, blood flow between the left atrium and the ventricle is restricted because of the increased resistance as the opening of the valve decreases. As a result, the pressure in the left atrium increases, which in turn increases the backward pressure in the pulmonary circulation. As the pressure in the pulmonary vessels increases, pulmonary edema develops and the patient begins to complain of dyspnea. **Hemoptysis**, or a cough producing either frank blood or bloody sputum, may occur if the smaller pulmonary venules rupture from the increased pulmonary vessel pressure. Mitral stenosis can exist for decades before the patient becomes symptomatic. Events which can cause an acute decompensation and heart failure include tachydysrhythmia (e.g., atrial fibrillation), exertion, anemia, pregnancy, and emotional upset.[20]

While mitral stenosis can be caused by the rupture of pulmonary venules, resulting in hemoptysis, it is relatively rare. When confronted with a patient with hemoptysis and chest pain, the Paramedic should first consider the possibility of tuberculosis and take appropriate precautions.

Alternatively, if the aortic valve becomes stenotic, the left ventricle needs to generate additional force to overcome the resistance of outflow from this valve. This increased work causes a dilation of the left ventricle and an increase in systemic blood pressure from the increased force of contraction. As with mitral stenosis, aortic stenosis develops gradually over time, sometimes taking two or three decades for the patient to become symptomatic. Most often, symptoms occur with exertion, in that the heart cannot keep up with the blood flow demand.

The classic symptom pattern for aortic stenosis includes dyspnea, chest pain, and syncope; however, this symptom pattern generally only occurs in the most severe cases of disease. With less severe disease, the patient may complain of dyspnea on exertion or paroxysmal nocturnal dyspnea, or dyspnea which wakes the patient from sleep. Approximately 25% of patients who have aortic stenosis develop sudden cardiac arrest from dysrhythmias.[21]

The murmur associated with aortic stenosis tends to be harsh and loud, and is heard best at the second intercostal space at the right sternal border with radiation of the sound into the right side of the neck. The murmur of aortic stenosis is the most frequently heard as a pathological systolic murmur.

In severe disease, the patient may require the elevated blood pressure just to have blood flow across the valve. In severely hypertensive patients with a loud harsh murmur in the second intercostal space at the right sternal border, the Paramedic should use caution in administering medications, such as nitroglycerin, that lower the blood pressure. These medications can cause a precipitous drop in blood pressure with resultant syncope.

Valve Regurgitation

Regurgitation of blood across the valve occurs when the valve is incompetent and cannot prevent the backward flow of blood. During ventricular contraction, the mitral valve prevents the backward flow of blood from the left ventricle into the left atrium. Loss of the mitral valve can result in backward failure and pulmonary edema.

Similarly, during ventricular relaxation, the aortic valve prevents the backward flow of systemic blood in the aorta from flowing back into the left ventricle. Loss of the aortic valve can result in decreased ejection fraction and systemic hypotension.

There are many causes of valvular destruction. Endocarditis may cause valve dysfunction due to direct damage to either of these valve's leaflets. The mitral valve can be damaged as a result of ischemia during a myocardial infarction of the inferior wall. During an IWMI, the papillary muscle—anchored in the inferior wall—ruptures, releasing the leaflets of the valve.

Similarly, the aortic valve can become dysfunctional if an aortic dissection involves the aortic root. As the dissection advances, the root of the aorta becomes disrupted, causing failure of the valve. When aortic regurgitation occurs acutely, the patient often complains of dyspnea, fatigue, and stabbing chest pain and has tachycardia, tachypnea, and rales on examination.

Tricuspid and Pulmonary Valves

The valves on the right side of the heart cause symptoms much less often than the valves on the left side of the heart (i.e., mitral and aortic valves). However, the tricuspid and pulmonic valves may also become stenotic from endocarditis. Regurgitation often occurs when the pulmonary vessel pressures are chronically or acutely increased.

The end result for the patient with either pulmonic or tricuspid regurgitation is that the patient will develop signs of right-sided heart failure, including increased jugular venous pressure, hepatic distention, abdominal tenderness, and peripheral edema.

Pulmonary Hypertension

The pulmonary system normally has a very low pressure, with a normal systolic pressure between 20 to 30 mmHg and normal diastolic pressure between 8 to 14 mmHg. On occasion patients may develop pulmonary hypertension. **Pulmonary hypertension** is defined as an elevated pressure in the pulmonary vascular system.[22] Pulmonary hypertension may develop gradually from a variety of causes including chronic obstructive pulmonary disease (COPD), stimulant use, liver disease, obstructive sleep apnea, chronic pulmonary embolism, and systemic collagen vascular disease.

Systemic collagen vascular disease causes the elastic fibers in the body to become stiff. When this occurs in the pulmonary vessels, the blood vessels are slightly narrower in diameter and the result is an increase in the blood pressure in the pulmonary vessels (i.e., pulmonary hypertension).

Obstructive sleep apnea can also cause pulmonary hypertension. Obstructive sleep apnea generally occurs in overweight individuals who intermittently obstruct their airway during the night as they sleep. These individuals become apneic for prolonged periods of time while sleeping, and then suddenly wake to clear the obstruction of their throat and restart breathing. Pulmonary hypertension develops over time as a result of the obstructions.

The use of stimulants, including cocaine, amphetamines, and some dietary aids, increases systemic blood pressure, including pressure in the pulmonary vessels. The long-term increases in blood pressure produce changes which make the vessels less elastic, and therefore produce chronically elevated blood pressures.

Some patients with liver disease develop portal hypertension, a condition in which the pressure of the blood flowing through the portal vein in the liver is elevated. A small percentage of patients with portal hypertension also have concomitant pulmonary hypertension.

Pulmonary hypertension can develop acutely if the pulmonary vessel pressure increases due to acute mitral valve regurgitation (e.g., during an IWMI). Pulmonary hypertension can also develop in patients with either mitral or aortic stenosis as a result of long-standing elevated pressures in the left side of the heart.

Pulmonary hypertension also develops when a large pulmonary embolism occludes the larger branches of the pulmonary arteries, obstructing flow through the lungs and increasing the pulmonary pressure.

At the extreme, right ventricular failure can occur, secondary to pulmonary hypertension, as the right ventricle attempts to overcome the pressure in the pulmonary vessels and move blood forward through the lungs to the left side of the heart. Patients with pulmonary hypertension, as with valvular disease, often initially complain of dyspnea on exertion and fatigue. Syncope, ischemic chest pain, and signs of right heart failure, including elevated jugular venous pressure and peripheral edema, will develop as the pulmonary hypertension worsens.

Noncardiac Causes of Chest Pain

There are many noncardiac causes of acute chest pain (Table 2-1). The Paramedic should also consider these conditions when assessing a patient complaining of chest pain and forming a differential diagnosis.

The Paramedic should always consider trauma, either present or in the recent past, especially if an accurate history is difficult to obtain. Most of these conditions are covered in depth in other chapters of this volume.

Dissection of the Thoracic Aorta

Dissection of the thoracic aorta is an uncommon condition that presents with sharp chest pain which, often, does not radiate, yet will migrate as the dissection extends. The dissection occurs when a small tear develops in the intimal layer of the aorta. The force of blood flowing over the tear causes an extension of the tear. As the tear extends, the intima and media layers separate and create a false lumen or pathway for blood to travel. This false lumen eventually occludes the true lumen and distal blood flow stops.

Table 2-1 Noncardiac Causes of Acute Nontraumatic Chest Pain

- Respiratory
  - Pulmonary embolism
  - Pneumonia/bronchitis
  - Spontaneous pneumothorax
  - Carcinoma (primary lung or metastatic from another location)
- Cardiovascular
  - Thoracic aortic dissection
- Musculoskeletal
  - Intercostal muscle strain
  - Pathological rib fracture
  - Thoracic vertebral fracture or degeneration
- Gastrointestinal
  - Gastroesophageal reflux (GERD)
  - Peptic ulcer disease
  - Hiatal hernia

If the dissection is confined to the intima, it can travel proximal to the aortic root and distal through the abdomen and into the iliac arteries. If the dissection involves the media layer, the aorta will rupture and the patient will expire from sudden acute exsanguination.

In some cases, the aortic dissection will extend upward and involve the aortic valve, causing acute systolic dysfunction and cardiogenic shock. In other cases, the dissection will block the opening of the coronary arteries, at the sinus of Valsalva, where they branch off from the aorta. The patient will then develop myocardial ischemia or infarction from the lack of blood flow. The dissection may also involve the arteries that branch off from the aorta, including one or both of the carotid arteries, and produce signs and symptoms consistent with an acute cerebrovascular accident (CVA).[23] The varying nature of this condition can make it difficult to identify patients who have a thoracic aortic dissection.

Patients who are at risk for aortic dissection include patients with a long-standing history of poorly controlled hypertension and smokers. This is also the same group of patients who are at risk for other cardiovascular events.

CASE STUDY (CONTINUED)

At the scene, the Paramedic is greeted by Mr. Wilson, who is sitting just inside the door, leaning forward, tightly holding his chest.

"Hello, I'm from County Paramedic. What can we do for you today, sir?"

"I'm having severe pain in the center of my chest!"

The Paramedic takes a history on Mr. Wilson and finds out this began about two hours ago and has progressively worsened. It is a pressure quality pain that does not radiate unless he exerts himself, and then the pain radiates to his left shoulder. He also complains of mild dyspnea and diaphoresis. The pain is non-migrating. He states he does not have a primary care physician, is a heavy smoker, and has never had any medical problems. He said in the past two weeks he has noticed that he is more fatigued with exertion; however, he feels that is due to working two jobs.

CRITICAL THINKING QUESTIONS

1. What are the important elements of the history that a Paramedic should obtain?
2. What is the symptom pattern for acute coronary syndrome?

History

The classic symptom pattern related to acute coronary syndrome consists of substernal chest pain, with or without radiation to the neck or left shoulder. However, the pain, or discomfort associated with acute coronary syndrome, can extend from the epigastrium to the jaw; hence, the saying "pain from the nose to the navel is cardiac until proven otherwise."

The Paramedic should be cautious about using the term "pain" or expecting the patient to use the word. It may be wiser to ask the patient if she is experiencing any "discomfort," then let the patient describe the discomfort. Often patients with acute coronary syndrome will complain of a vise-like pressure or epigastric discomfort rather than pain.

When considering symptoms related to acute coronary syndrome, most people think of chest pain. However, the specific complaint or symptoms can vary from patient to patient. Many patients will complain of nonclassic symptoms with their ACS.

Myocardial by Presentation

Patients whose AMI involves the anterior wall frequently complain of the classic symptom pattern associated with ACS: substernal chest pain with radiation into the jaw and/or shoulders. These patients often describe an intense pain or pressure that lasts longer than 15 minutes. Tachycardia and gross diaphoresis often accompany this patient presentation.

Patients whose AMI involves the inferior wall of the left ventricle are more likely to complain of epigastric discomfort and may even experience vomiting from the discomfort. Because the coronary artery that supplies the inferior wall of the left ventricle—the right coronary artery—also supplies the atrioventricular (AV) node, in 90% of the population these patients also may experience type I AV blocks and bradycardia secondary to AV node ischemia.

However, some 50% of IWMI are thought to display none of the previously listed symptoms. These patients have an atypical presentation of their ACS.

Atypical Presentations of Acute Coronary Syndrome

Some patients may provide a history indicating that, with their past myocardial infarction(s), the patient only experienced dyspnea or diaphoresis or that the pain was located in an atypical location. Women, especially those under 60 years old, often present with atypical symptoms which ultimately are from ACS.[24,25]

Elderly patients often do not complain of the typical chest pressure during their cardiac events. Instead, these patients complain of unexplained weakness, sudden diaphoresis, or an acute shortness of breath not related to exertion.[26,27]

Patients with a long history of diabetes also may not have pain during their ACS event. The elevated blood glucose over time affects the sensory nerve's ability to transmit information to the brain, called a neuropathy, thus blunting the sensation of pain. Often these patients will present with either respiratory complaints or complaints of weakness, fatigue, or malaise.

These patient populations who have an atypical presentation of acute coronary syndrome, such as women, elderly, and patients with diabetes, may be said to be experiencing a "silent" AMI (i.e., without the usual manifestations of chest pain). Approximately one quarter of all AMI are silent; therefore, Paramedics should have a higher index of suspicion regarding the possibility of ACS, especially when treating these patient populations.

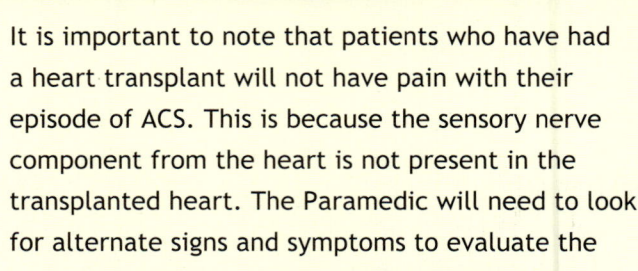

STREET SMART

It is important to note that patients who have had a heart transplant will not have pain with their episode of ACS. This is because the sensory nerve component from the heart is not present in the transplanted heart. The Paramedic will need to look for alternate signs and symptoms to evaluate the heart transplant patient for ACS, such as absence of bradycardia with vagal stimulation.

If the patient has had a past cardiac event, it is important to ask the patient to compare the current symptoms with the past events, and describe how they are different. Many of these patients may have had a stent placed in their coronary artery. A stent is a small scaffolding that holds the lumen of the coronary artery open. In some cases the stent becomes obstructed by a new coronary thrombus.

The OPQRST AS/PN mnemonic (Onset, Provocation, Quality of pain, Radiation, Severity, Timing, Associated Symptoms, Pertinent Negatives) will help the Paramedic elicit important information regarding ACS. An important and key piece of information that will affect emergency treatment is the time the pain began. As discussed later in this chapter, the time of onset combined with the ECG findings dramatically affects immediate treatment and may affect destination decisions.

Activity during onset of the pain, including exacerbating factors, may assist in narrowing the Paramedic's differential diagnosis. The quality of the pain can also be helpful in developing the paramedical diagnosis. It is also very important to consider atypical complaints in the specific groups listed previously.

The Paramedic should ask about the location of the pain or discomfort, about any radiation of the pain, whether the pain is intermittent or constant, and if there are factors, including position, which relieve or worsen the pain. A young patient who describes sharp midsternal chest pain that is worse lying back and is better leaning forward is more likely to have acute pericarditis than a patient who describes more classic ACS symptoms of crushing chest pressure that radiates to the left jaw and arm. A patient who describes the pain as a severe tearing pain that migrates may have a dissection of the thoracic aorta.

The Paramedic should assess the severity of the pain, either by using the 0 to 10 scale or by asking the patient to rate the pain as mild, moderate, or severe. Asking for associated symptoms (e.g., diaphoresis and dyspnea) may help narrow the Paramedic's differential diagnosis. Finally, the Paramedic should report the pertinent negative findings from the history (e.g., lack of dyspnea on exertion) in his documentation and report to the emergency physician.

The past medical history, family history, and social history are important in detecting risk factors that heighten the Paramedic's awareness of a cardiac cause for the patient's chief complaint. The most significant risk factor for cardiac disease is a past history of a myocardial infarction, angina, or a cardiac catheterization which demonstrates coronary artery disease (Figure 2-9).

Other risk factors include a patient with a past medical history of hypertension, high cholesterol (hypercholesterolemia), angina, and diabetes.[28,29] Patients with a past history of angina should be asked about their normal pattern of chest pain and if there has been a change in their pattern.

Crescendo angina is an increasing frequency of symptoms over time and may indicate progressive coronary artery disease. If the patient provides a history of peripheral vascular disease or stroke, the patient is likely to have undiagnosed coronary artery disease.

The Paramedic should ask the patient if he is aware if he has a heart murmur. While most murmurs are benign, the patient may relate a history of a murmur that is being followed by a physician, thereby indicating moderate valvular disease.

A history of pulmonary hypertension places the patient at greater risk for heart failure and valve disease. A surgical history of a past coronary angioplasty to open up an obstructed coronary artery, a coronary artery bypass graft (CABG) operation, and vascular procedures in the extremities for peripheral vascular disease all point to a history of coronary artery disease.

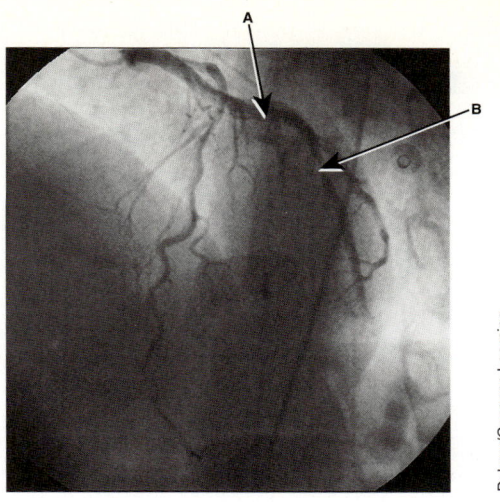

Delmar/Cengage Learning

Figure 2-9 An angiogram that demonstrates a coronary artery with a normal size lumen (a) and narrowing from coronary artery disease (b).

A history of smoking, cocaine use, or some other stimulant use also accelerates coronary artery disease. A family history of myocardial infarction prior to age 60 is a significant risk factor. A family history of sudden unexplained death in a young family member is also a risk factor, but is typically associated with dysrhythmias and not coronary artery disease. Finally, medications and herbal products the patient uses need to be reviewed for interactions with prehospital medications.

CASE STUDY (CONTINUED)

The basic life support (BLS) crew from the rescue squad arrives on scene and comes inside to assist in completing the physical examination. One of the EMTs had recently attended a 12-lead ECG training session and assists in placing the leads and acquiring a 12-lead ECG while the Paramedic performs a focused physical examination. Another EMT obtains a pulse of 100 regular and strong, a blood pressure of 180/96, a respiratory rate of 20 and labored, and a room air SaO_2 of 97%. On examination, Mr. Wilson is seated and in significant distress. Rales (crackles) are detected at both lung bases but no frank pulmonary edema is present. He has a normal jugular venous pressure and no murmurs on cardiac auscultation. Mr. Wilson's peripheral pulses are equal and there is no peripheral edema present. Mr. Wilson's skin is diaphoretic and his chest needs to be dried with a towel to allow the ECG leads to stick. The remainder of the exam is unremarkable.

CRITICAL THINKING QUESTIONS

1. What are the elements of the physical examination of a patient with suspected acute coronary syndrome?

2. Why is a 12-lead ECG a critical element in this examination?

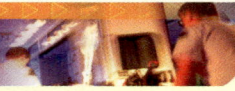
Examination

While the physical examination is important to detect decompensation, narrow down the Paramedic's diagnosis, and guide treatment, the 12-lead ECG is a vitally important early assessment tool. As we will discuss later in the Disposition section, the 12-lead ECG determines the appropriate hospital destination and the speed of treatment. An early 12-lead ECG obtained by EMS may also detect ST elevations that disappear with subsequent treatment (Figure 2-10a), identifying a high risk patient that is treated differently in the emergency department (ED) and hospital. Due to the significant differences in time to obtain treatment and choice of destination, the 12-lead ECG should be considered part of the primary assessment and rapidly obtained in all patients with suspected acute coronary syndrome (Figure 2-10b).

Serial ECGs should be considered if the patient becomes pain free during the Paramedic's contact with the patient (Figure 2-11a). Normalization of nonspecific changes (e.g., T wave flattening or nonsignificant ST segment depression) may frequently occur, identifying patients who are at a higher risk for progressing to a myocardial infarction (Figure 2-11b). If the patient develops another episode of

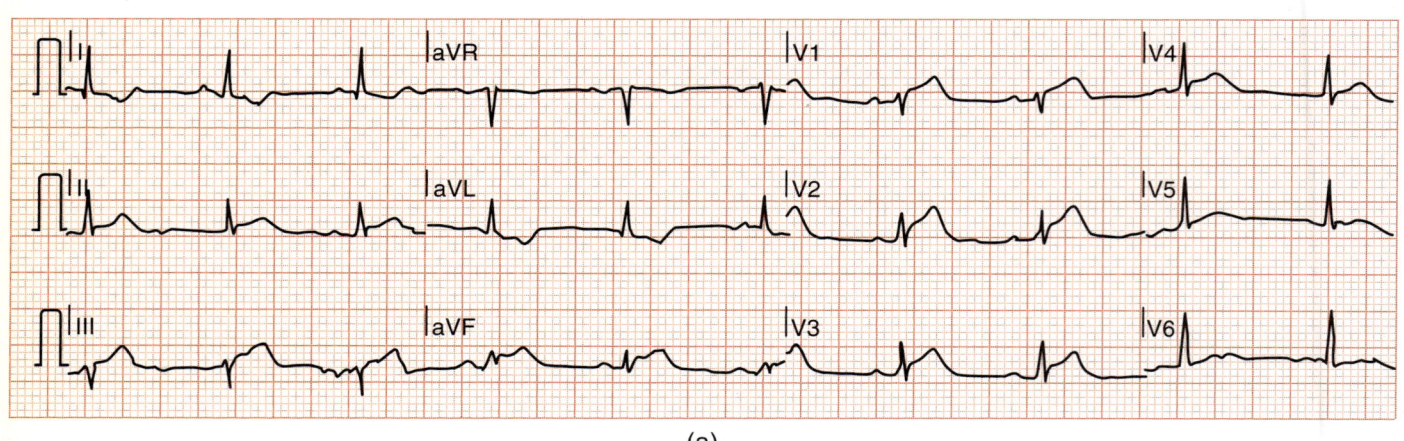

(a)

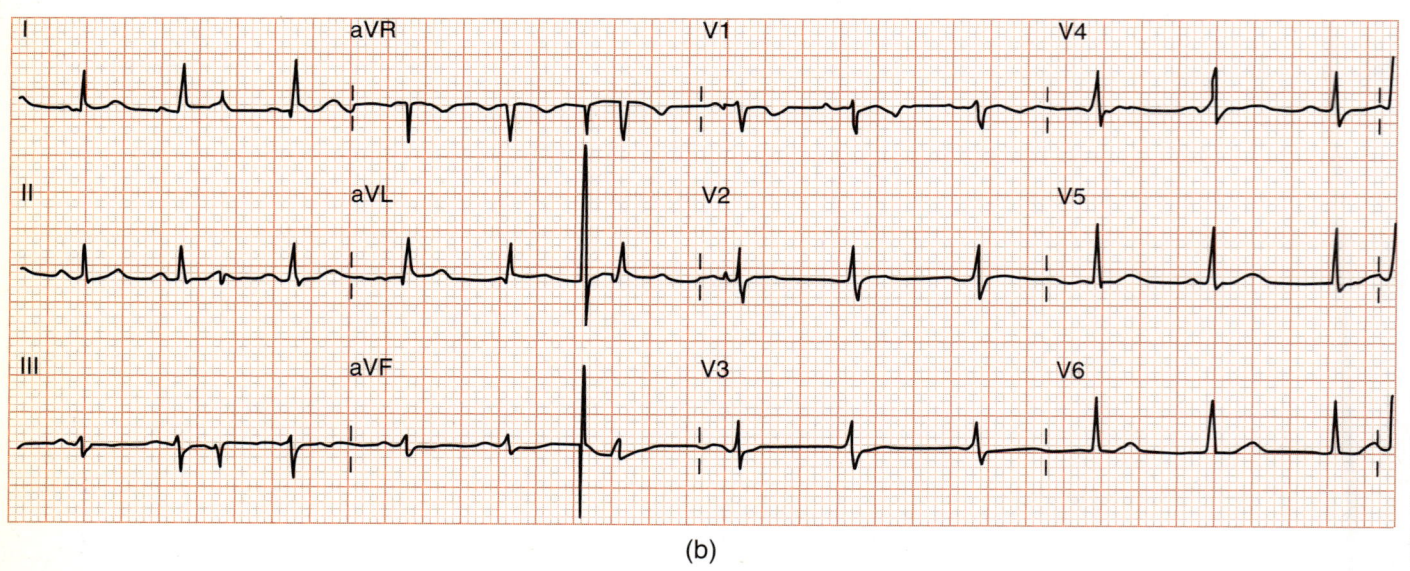

(b)

Delmar/Cengage Learning

Figure 2-10 A 56-year-old female patient who initially presented with an inferior wall ST elevation myocardial infarction (a) who became pain free after administration of oxygen. The ED ECG (b) shows normalization of the ST segments. This patient was admitted to the Coronary Care Unit and treated aggressively with anticoagulants.

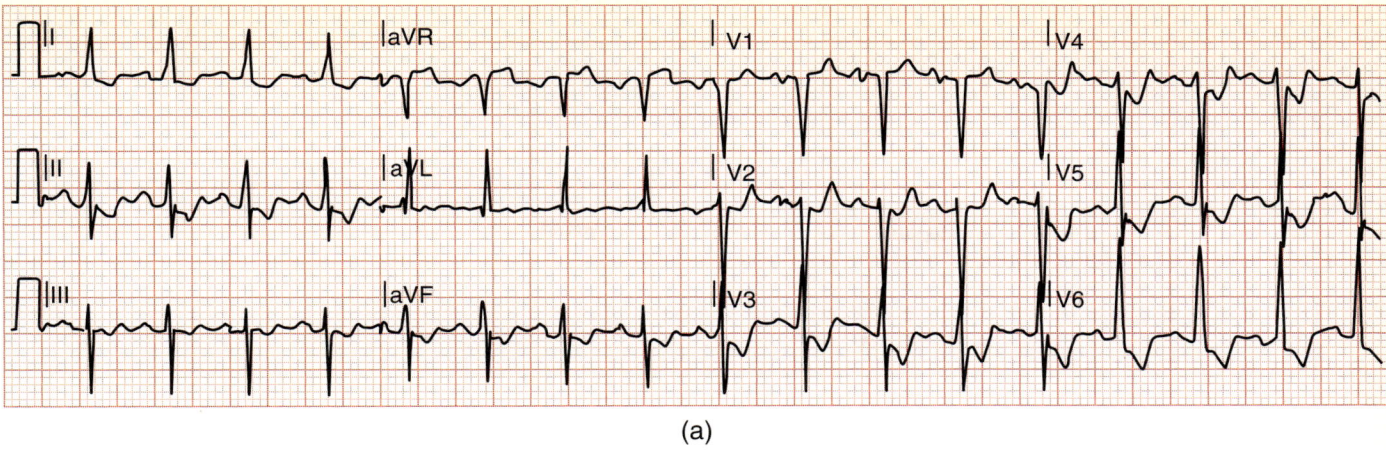

(a)

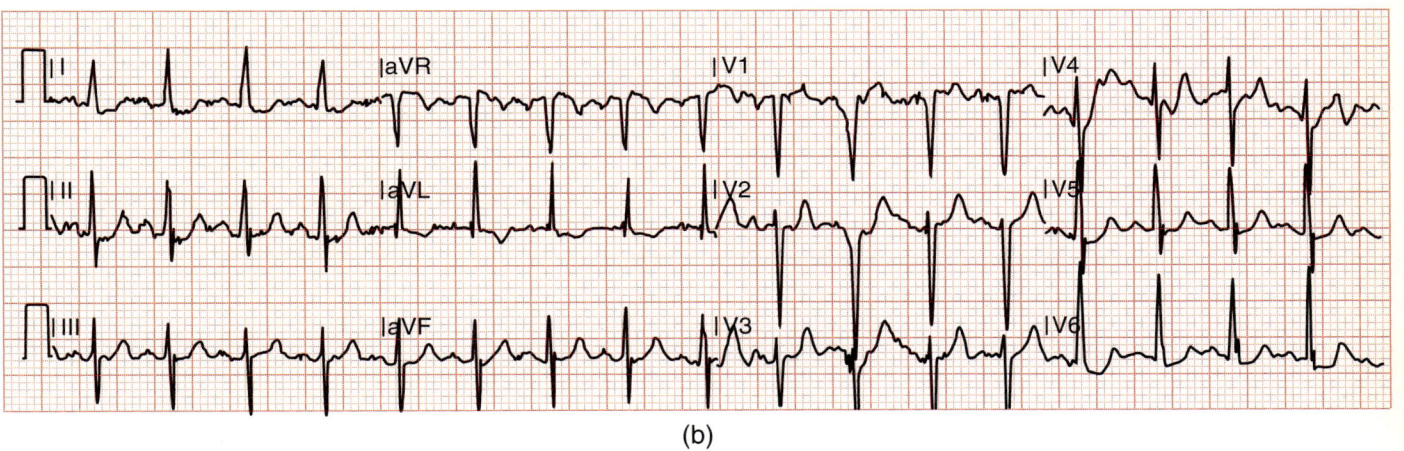

(b)

Figure 2-11 Normalization of nonspecific ST and T wave changes (a) once the patient is pain free (b) identifies high risk patients.

chest pain, the Paramedic should acquire another ECG and look for a return of the changes. If ECG changes occur with pain and resolve with rest, this indicates what is referred to as dynamic ECG changes.

If the patient presents with hypotension and an inferior wall acute STEMI, the Paramedic should acquire a right-sided ECG (see Chapter 1) to assess for a possible right ventricular posterior infarction.[30] The presence of an inferior or posterior wall MI will change the initial management of the patient.

Abnormal vital signs, including hypotension, unstable dysrhythmias, or airway, breathing, or circulation issues, must be immediately addressed by the Paramedic. Once these issues are addressed, the Paramedic can move on to the focused physical examination.

The focused examination includes assessment of the cardiovascular, respiratory, gastrointestinal, and neurologic systems as well as palpation of the thorax. Starting at the head, an increased jugular venous pressure may indicate right-sided heart failure from valve dysfunction, pulmonary hypertension, or a myocardial infarction which suddenly decreases the patient's ejection fraction. The Paramedic should auscultate the heart for murmurs that may be new or worse than baseline, indicating valve dysfunction. Auscultation of the lungs for signs of heart failure should also be performed (see Chapter 3 for a more complete discussion of heart failure). The peripheral pulses should also be assessed for equality and strength and the blood pressure should be checked in both upper extremities. Unequal pulses or a significant difference in systolic blood pressure may indicate aortic dissection as the cause of the patient's symptoms.

Next, the Paramedic should palpate the chest to assess for a thrill, the upward heave of the heart, indicating increased myocardial work, as well as tenderness over the bony structures. The Paramedic should remember that up to 25% of patients with confirmed myocardial infarctions have palpable chest wall tenderness.[31,32] Hepatojugular reflux, an increase in the jugular venous distention with the application of pressure over the right upper quadrant over the liver, may also indicate heart failure or pulmonary hypertension. A brief neurological examination will detect abnormalities that may be caused by a dissection of the thoracic aorta.

The EMT hands the ECG to the Paramedic to interpret. The ST segments in leads V2 through V4 are elevated 2 mm above the baseline. Leads II, III, and aVF demonstrate inverted T waves and 1 mm ST depressions. The Paramedic announces to the patient his suspicion, elevating the patient and the crew's awareness.

CRITICAL THINKING QUESTIONS

1. What is the significance of the elevated ST segment?
2. What diagnosis did the Paramedic announce to the patient?

Assessment

In this specific case, the 12-lead ECG confirms the presence of an acute STEMI. While in rare circumstances this may be due to dissection of the thoracic aorta, the vast majority of the time if ST elevations greater than 1 mm above the baseline are present in at least two anatomically contiguous leads and there are reciprocal changes in at least two anatomically contiguous leads, this is highly suggestive of a myocardial infarction in evolution.

However, in many patients who develop acute chest pain, the ECG is either nondiagnostic or there are contradictory ischemic changes present on the 12-lead ECG. If the patient presents with signs and symptoms suggestive of a cardiac origin for the chest pain, treat the patient as if she was having an acute coronary event. In this specific case, the patient's symptoms are more consistent with ACS than an aortic dissection.

Symptoms which may suggest a respiratory origin of the chest pain include a symptom pattern of sharp pain that changes during the respiratory cycle (often worse with deep inspiration); signs of respiratory infection, including fever and a productive cough; tachypnea; tachycardia; and hypoxia.

Symptoms suggesting a gastrointestinal cause include a symptom pattern that includes burning pain that begins in the epigastrium and radiates up the center of the chest to the back of the throat, a sour taste when waking after sleep, worsening symptoms at bed time, and symptoms worsened by certain foods.

As discussed earlier, symptoms suggesting acute pericarditis include pain that is often sharp and nonradiating that improves when the patient leans forward, worsens when the patient leans back, and is also suggested when the classic ECG findings are present.

The 12-lead ECG helps to divide the treatment of acute coronary syndrome into three categories: ST elevation MI (STEMI), nonspecific ischemic changes, and normal (Figure 2-12). For patients diagnosed with an STEMI, much of the literature supports either fibrinolytic therapy or percutaneous coronary angioplasty as first line in-hospital treatment. Destination decision will be discussed later in the chapter and often is specific to the region in which the Paramedic practices.

Patients who have been identified as having an acute STEMI should be questioned further to determine contraindications to fibrinolysis. Many systems have developed a checklist to expedite this process (Figure 2-13). Checklists allow the Paramedic to rapidly identify patients who have contraindications to STEMI treatments, which in turn may affect destination decision, emergency department treatment, and interfacility transfer.

Patients who have nondiagnostic ECGs or nonspecific ECG changes comprise the largest group encountered by Paramedics. The Paramedic should remember that these patients may still be having a myocardial infarction. Treatment of patients in this category includes the standard treatments for acute coronary syndrome in an effort to alleviate the patient's symptoms.

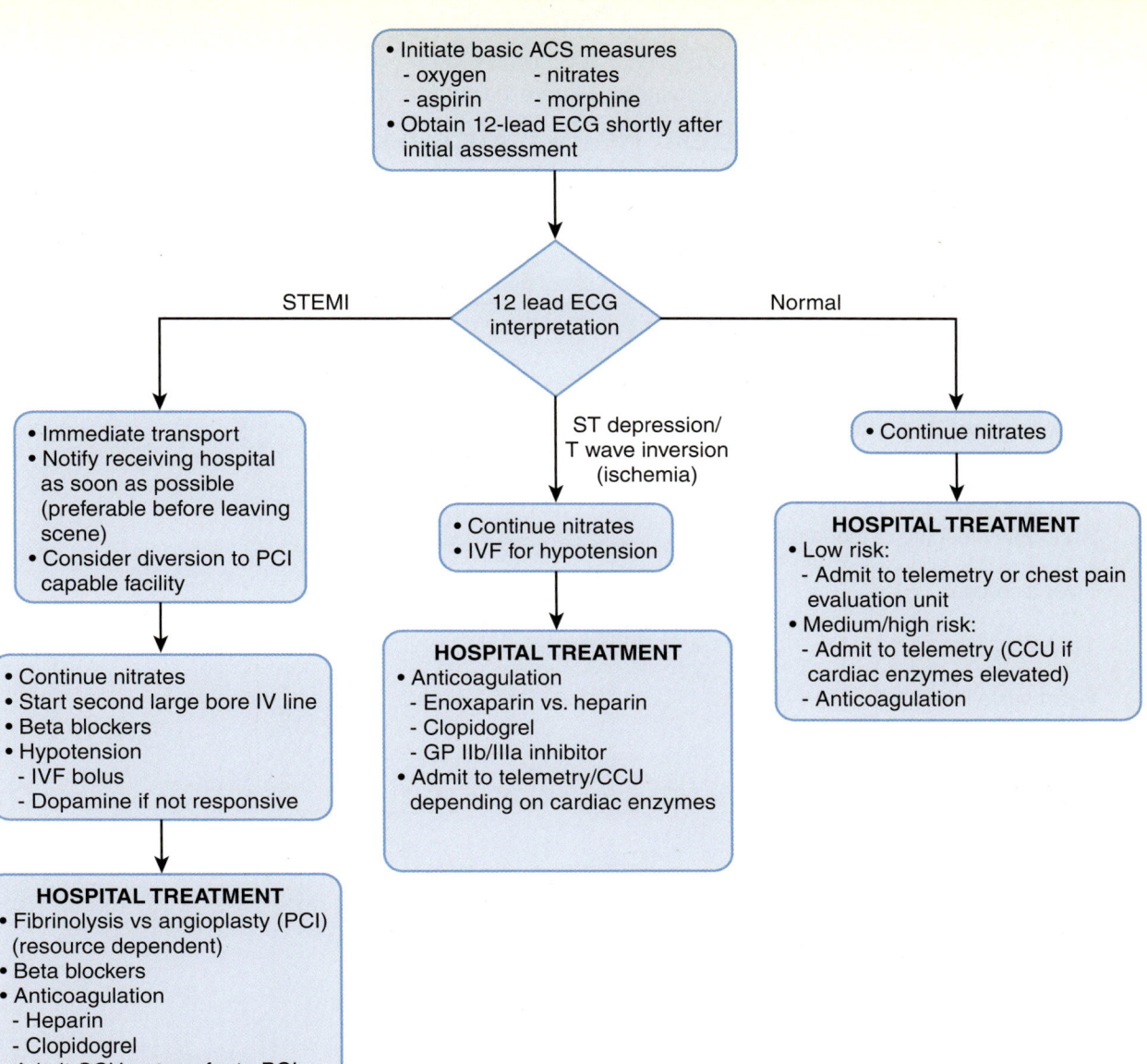

Figure 2-12 Treatment algorithm for acute coronary syndrome.

Delmar/Cengage Learning

This checklist should be completed where indicated in the *Chest Pain* protocol

CHEST PAIN CHECKLIST

Patient name: _____

Date: _____

Ambulance Co.: _____ Vehicle ID: _____

Time pain began: _____

Have you ever had or do you now have:	Yes	No
GI bleeding or peptic ulcer?	_____	_____
Abnormal bleeding or blood disease?	_____	_____
Liver disease?	_____	_____
Stroke?	_____	_____
Heart valve infection?	_____	_____
Cancer?	_____	_____
Diabetic eye disease?	_____	_____
Poorly controlled blood pressure?	_____	_____
Recent head injury, brain tumor, or aneurysm?	_____	_____

In the past two weeks, have you had:

	Yes	No
surgery?	_____	_____
major trauma or injury?	_____	_____
CPR?	_____	_____
Are you pregnant?	_____	_____
Are you currently taking blood thinners?	_____	_____
Ever receive any clot dissolving medication for a heart attack or stroke?	_____	_____
Recent angiogram or cardiac catheterization?	_____	_____ When? _____

EMT name: _____

Courtesy of Western Regional Emergency Medical Advisory Committee

Figure 2-13 A fibrinolytic checklist completed by the Paramedic expedites appropriate treatment for patients with an STEMI.

The Paramedic proceeds to administer routine care for patients with suspected acute coronary syndrome according to the algorithm provided by local medical control, understanding that treatment is part of a large national standard of care.

CRITICAL THINKING QUESTIONS

1. What is the national standard of care of patients with suspected acute coronary syndrome?
2. What are some of the patient-specific concerns and considerations that the Paramedic should consider when applying this plan of care that is intended to treat a broad patient population presenting with acute coronary syndrome?

Treatment

As with all patients, the Paramedic should rapidly address life-threatening conditions that affect the airway, breathing, or circulation. The Paramedic should then proceed with treatments. Standard treatment of acute coronary syndrome includes rapid 12-lead acquisition, administration of oxygen and aspirin, and sublingual or intravenous nitroglycerin. The mnemonic "MONA–B" (Morphine, Oxygen, Nitrates, Aspirin, and Beta/adrenergic blockers) is often used by Paramedics to remember the medications used to treat ACS, though they will not necessarily be administered in that order.

Oxygen

Oxygen is traditionally administered to patients with acute chest pain to improve oxygen delivery to the myocardium in hopes of decreasing ischemia. The goal of oxygen administration should be to maintain oxygen saturation greater than 90% in the normovolemic patient.

The choices of devices for oxygen administration should be guided by the patient's condition, pulse oximetry readings, and protocols. In some EMS systems Paramedics are allowed to administer low-flow oxygen, two to four liters, by nasal cannula, provided the patient has normal vital signs and is not hypoxic. However, if the patient is hypoxic, or there is any doubt about the patient's respiratory status (i.e., potential for pulmonary edema), then high-flow, high-concentration oxygen via nonrebreather mask should be administered.

If the patient states that the oxygen relieved the chest discomfort, then the patient may have had an episode of angina pectoris. While this result may encourage the patient to refuse further medical treatment, the Paramedic should recognize that this is a case of unstable angina and the patient should be convinced to seek medical evaluation.

Aspirin

Aspirin (acetylsalicylic acid or ASA) interferes with the platelets' ability to bind to one another through suppression of the production of thromboxanes, specifically thromboxane

A2. The resulting anticoagulant property is useful for treatment of an AMI. However, it should be noted that aspirin prevents platelets from binding and forming a larger platelet plug. Aspirin has little effect on pre-existing platelet plugs and thrombus that formed prior to administration of the aspirin.

Aspirin, from 162 mg to 324 mg, should be administered, preferably chewed, to patients with suspected ACS unless there is a contraindication. The most common contraindications to aspirin administration include an allergy to aspirin, which appears in about 5% of the population, or active upper gastrointestinal (GI) bleeding.[33] If GI bleeding is suspected, some patients have been prescribed 300 mg aspirin suppositories.

It has also been stated that between 5% and 10% of patients with asthma can experience aspirin-induced asthma attacks (AIA).[34] While the exact mechanism is unknown, aspirin may stimulate the body to produce leukotrienes, a potent bronchoconstrictor, which leads to the asthma attack.

Nitrates

Nitroglycerin, an organic nitrate, has been the mainstay of treatment of angina pectoris secondary to acute coronary artery disease for centuries. Nitroglycerin works when it is converted into nitric oxide (NO) in the body. NO is a potent smooth muscle relaxer.

Originally it was thought that nitroglycerin caused direct dilation of the coronary arteries via relaxation of the smooth muscle in the tunica media, but recent studies have suggested that atherosclerotic plaques limit the action of nitroglycerin on the coronary arteries. The greater benefit of nitroglycerin may be in the peripheral vasodilation that occurs. At lower doses nitroglycerin causes venous dilation and venous pooling, thus causing decreased venous return and subsequently decreased left ventricular end-diastolic pressure or preload. This decreased preload decreases the work of the heart.

At higher doses, such as those that Paramedics typically administer, nitroglycerin is an arterial vasodilator. Arterial dilatation, especially in the aorta, decreases systemic vascular resistance, also called afterload, that the pumping heart has to overcome for perfusion to occur. This afterload can be grossly estimated by Paramedics using the diastolic pressure in the blood pressure. However, the coronary arteries fill during diastole and depend on diastolic pressure to maintain coronary perfusion.

Nitroglycerin's onset of action is generally within one to three minutes and peaks at about five minutes; thereafter, its effects decline for about 25 minutes. Nitroglycerin can be rapidly absorbed by any mucous membrane, including the buccal pocket, but the rich venous plexus under the tongue, the sublingual area, is preferred.

Nitroglycerin is manufactured in several doses including 0.3 mg, 0.4 mg (1/150 grain or 400 mcg), and 0.6 mg and may be administered sublingually as either a pill or spray. If the pill form is used, then the Paramedic should be cautious about inadvertent exposure to the nitroglycerin by contact with the moisture in the palm of the hand and subsequent absorption. Nitroglycerin needs moisture to dissolve and be absorbed. If the patient's saliva is insufficient (for example, secondary to anticholinergic medications or tricyclic antidepressants), then the patient may use chewing gum to moisten the mouth.

Nitroglycerin is easily denatured by sunlight and moisture. Therefore, nitroglycerin pills should be stored in their original dark glass container with the cotton plug in place. Ideally, nitroglycerin should be stored at a controlled room temperature of 68°F to 77°F.

Nitroglycerin is capable of inducing hypotension and therefore should not be used in hypotensive patients. Patients receiving nitroglycerin should be seated, not standing, when the medication is administered in case there is a precipitous drop in blood pressure leading to syncope.

Patients should be advised that the administration of nitroglycerin may cause a headache and/or lightheadedness. Concurrent use of nitroglycerin and alcohol is more likely to cause hypotension.

Typically Paramedics administer up to three doses of 0.4 mg approximately every three to five minutes until the patient's chest pain is relieved, provided the patient's blood pressure remains greater than 90 to 100 mmHg systolic or drops no more than 30 mmHg below the patient's baseline systolic blood pressure. Caution is advised when administering nitroglycerin to patients with bradycardia (less than 50 bpm) or tachycardia (greater than 100 bpm). These heart rates may reflect conditions under which the heart cannot compensate if hypotension occurs.

Nitroglycerin should not be administered to patients who are allergic to organic nitrates or to those taking phosphodiesterase inhibitors (medications for erectile dysfunction). Coadministration of nitroglycerin with erectile dysfunction medications can cause an unsafe drop in blood pressure as these medications tend to potentiate the effects of nitroglycerin.

Patients who routinely take nitroglycerin, in one formulation or another, may develop a tolerance to nitroglycerin.

In those cases, larger doses may be necessary for angina pain relief. Otherwise, use of morphine sulfate should be considered.

Once the patient is pain free, transdermal nitroglycerin paste may be applied to maintain vessel dilation. An approximately one inch ribbon of transdermal nitroglycerin paste is squeezed out of the tube of paste onto an application paper. This paper is then applied to the patient and the time and dose noted.

STREET SMART

Nitroglycerin is a potent vasodilator, and nitroglycerin paste releases NO for an extended period of time. In many instances emergency physicians order intravenous nitroglycerin because it can be more carefully titrated. The combination of transdermal and intravenous nitroglycerin may cause an unsafe drop in blood pressure. Therefore, it is important to notify hospital staff when and where nitroglycerin paste has been applied.

Morphine Sulfate

If the patient's chest pain does not resolve with three doses of nitrates, morphine may be administered. Morphine has also been used for centuries for the treatment of ACS, in part because of its excellent safety profile. Morphine, like nitrates, is a potent vasodilator and is thought to have similar actions upon the heart's function as nitroglycerin.

Morphine sulfate, as a potent vasodilator, can cause hypotension. Therefore, the same recommendations and precautions provided for nitroglycerin administration are also indicated for morphine administration.

Typically the dose of morphine sulfate for the patient with ACS is 2 mg to 4 mg intravenously and then additional doses of 2 mg to 8 mg every 5 to 10 minutes, depending on the patient's response to the medication.

Morphine sulfate should also be considered if the patient is taking erectile dysfunction medications. The vasodilation caused by morphine is thought to be caused by the release of histamine, which creates a different action than that of nitroglycerin. Therefore, phosphodiesterase inhibitors will not potentiate the effects of the morphine sulfate like they would potentiate nitroglycerin.

Beta/Adrenergic Blockers

For patients who present with an STEMI, particularly an AWMI, a beta blocker is often given to help reduce the size of the infarction and reduce the risk of ventricular tachycardia or ventricular fibrillation.

The intravenous administration of a beta-1 selector adrenergic blocker, or beta blocker, helps to decrease the automaticity of the myocardium and thereby prevent tachycardia. Beta blockers also slow the heart rate, resulting in decreased myocardial oxygen demand (MvO_2).

Five milligrams of intravenous beta blockers are administered in three doses every five minutes or until the target heart rate of 60 to 90 bpm is obtained. Beta blockers should be administered cautiously, if at all, to patients with asthma as the medication may induce an asthma attack. Other contraindications to beta blocker administration include bradycardia, especially if induced by a second or third degree heart block, and hypotension, as represented by a systolic blood pressure less than 100 mmHg.

Anticoagulants

Some EMS systems may carry heparin, an intravenous anticoagulant that is administered to help reduce propagation of the clot in the coronary artery. A Paramedic involved in interfacility transports of patients with ACS will routinely encounter patients who have an intravenous heparin infusion.

CASE STUDY (CONTINUED)

Mr. Wilson is reassessed after nitrate administration. He has become pain free after three nitrates and morphine. The Paramedic applies an inch of nitropaste (approximately 1 gram). Mr. Wilson's blood pressure is 120/60 and his heart rate is 80. He receives metoprolol, an intravenous beta blocker, while the EMT acquires a second 12-lead ECG. The second ECG shows continued elevation of the ST segments in the anterior leads with reciprocal changes in the inferior leads.

CRITICAL THINKING QUESTIONS

1. What are some of the predictable complications associated with acute coronary syndrome?
2. What are some of the predictable complications associated with the treatments for acute coronary syndrome?

Evaluation

The Paramedic should be aware of several specific situations in which the standard treatment with nitroglycerin may require more careful consideration. Hypotension is a common side effect of nitroglycerin. In lower doses, nitroglycerin is a venodilator. However, in higher doses, such as the sublingual doses traditionally given every five minutes, it is a potent arteriodilator.

If the circulatory system dilates and the volume of blood in the system stays the same, the pressure within the system will decrease. This can be beneficial to assist in reducing myocardial work and oxygen demand, as well as limiting infarct size. However, hypotension will significantly decrease coronary blood flow and causes a risk of worsening the infarction. If the patient complains of worsening chest pain with the administration of nitroglycerin, then readministration of subsequent doses should be reconsidered. If the patient's systolic blood pressure drops below 100 mmHg, then nitroglycerin should be withheld.

Right Ventricular Myocardial Infarction

The right coronary artery provides blood to the infeior wall of the left ventricle. When it is occluded, the result is an inferior wall myocardial infarction (IWMI). The distal branch of the right coronary artery—the posterior descending coronary artery—provides blood to a portion of the right ventricle. Patients who present with an IWMI often have extension of ischemia into the right ventricle.

The right ventricle is responsible for left ventricular filling, called the preload. The preload of the left ventricle is determined by the force of contraction and blood volume from the right ventricle. If the right ventricular contractility is diminished, secondary to ischemia, and is unable to provide a sufficiently strong contraction, it will affect the volume of blood going to the left side of the heart. Then, if the patient is given the vasodilator nitroglycerin, further diminishing the venous preload, the patient's blood

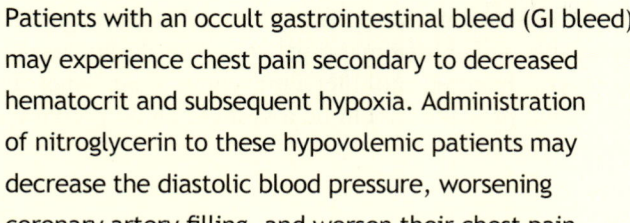

STREET SMART

Patients with an occult gastrointestinal bleed (GI bleed) may experience chest pain secondary to decreased hematocrit and subsequent hypoxia. Administration of nitroglycerin to these hypovolemic patients may decrease the diastolic blood pressure, worsening coronary artery filling, and worsen their chest pain.

pressure may drop significantly after the administration of nitroglycerin. If this occurs, the Paramedic should first lay the patient supine and monitor the patient's vital signs closely. The half-life of nitroglycerin is short, approximately five minutes, and the patient's blood pressure may return to more normal values within that time. While waiting for the return of the blood pressure, the Paramedic may want to consider establishing additional intravenous access and ensure adequate fluid resuscitation by administering normal saline fluid boluses and closely monitoring the patient's blood pressure.

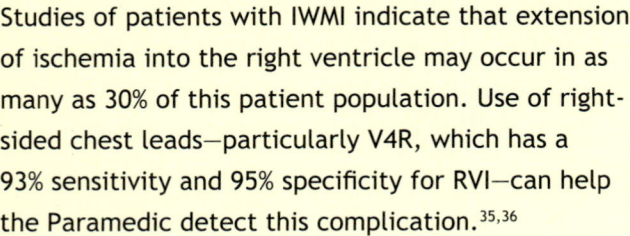

STREET SMART

Studies of patients with IWMI indicate that extension of ischemia into the right ventricle may occur in as many as 30% of this patient population. Use of right-sided chest leads—particularly V4R, which has a 93% sensitivity and 95% specificity for RVI—can help the Paramedic detect this complication.[35,36]

Right ventricular infarction is always suspected when the patient with an IWMI has hypotension in the absence of rales. With a loss of preload, secondary to right ventricular involvement, the clinical goal is to replace the preload. This is best accomplished by the administration of a minimum of 1 to 2 liters of isotonic solution over one to two hours. This initial volume loading may need to be either increased or vasopressors may need to be added, according to the patient's condition, in order to restore adequate coronary and cerebral perfusion. However, the key to long-term survival lies with early reperfusion of the occluded coronary artery through the use of either fibrinolytics or coronary angioplasty.

Mitral Regurgitation

Another predictable complication of an IWMI is extension of the ischemia along the inferior muscle bundle, or whorl, into the **papillary muscles**. These muscles secure the chordae tendineae (heart strings) that open the two leaflets of the mitral valve.

Under stress, the papillary muscles or the chordae tendineae can rupture and the mitral valve will experience a catastrophic failure. The resultant condition, ischemic mitral regurgitation, causes blood to flow backward into the lungs (acute pulmonary edema) as well as reduce forward flow out the aortic valve (acute hypotension) with every contraction of the heart.

With a patient mortality of approximately 80%, the Paramedic must assess and treat the patient quickly if the patient is expected to survive.[37] During ischemic mitral regurgitation, there is a dramatic drop in blood pressure, usually resulting in patient dizziness or syncope. This hypotension is accompanied by diffuse rales in all lung fields, associated with sudden hypoxia and a drop in the patient's oxygen saturation. There may also be marked jugular venous distention as a result of backward failure. Upon auscultation of the chest for rales, the Paramedic may also note a high-pitched pansystolic murmur that radiates to the left axilla.

The treatment in the prehospital setting is limited to treating the hypotension with volume loading and transporting the patient to a cardiac center where an intra-aortic balloon pump may be placed and other pharmacological therapies, such as nitroprusside, can be initiated.

Aortic Stenosis

Another special situation where caution should be observed when administering nitroglycerin involves a patient with aortic stenosis and hypertension. The hypertension is often required to overcome the decreased opening of the aortic valve secondary to stenosis. Nitroglycerin dilates the systemic veins and decreases the volume of blood returning to the heart. If this preload drops significantly, the patient loses forward blood flow and may become profoundly hypotensive. The result is a sudden drop in the pressure gradient needed to maintain forward blood flow and a dramatic drop in the cardiac output. Nitroglycerin should be used cautiously in these patients, and only once intravenous access is established and intravenous fluids can be administered to support the blood pressure.

The first-line treatment for hypotension is generally to administer fluid boluses to the patient to improve preload. The exception to that is for patients who are in cardiogenic shock, with acute pulmonary edema, heart failure, and myocardial infarction. These patients may require blood pressure support with a vasopressor. The vasopressor most often used is dopamine. These vasopressors contain a beta/adrenergic component which helps increase the force of contraction.

Alternative vasopressors, used more often in interfacility transfers, is phenylephrine or norepinephrine. Use of pure alpha adrenergic vasopressors (e.g., phenylephrine or norepinephrine) will increase systemic vascular resistance and increase myocardial workload without increasing the force of contraction. Vasopressors may also be required in hypotensive and symptomatic patients who do not respond to a several hundred milliliter intravenous fluid bolus. The target blood pressure should be a systolic blood pressure of at least 90 mmHg.

The Paramedic requests a helicopter for transport to the STEMI center. The trip by ground would take at least 60 minutes from this rural location; however, it will be significantly less time by air. The closest community hospital is 40 minutes away. He then calls the medical control line at Valley Regional, discusses Mr. Wilson's case with the ED physician, and requests activation of the cardiac catheterization team. The ECGs were transmitted to the STEMI center.

The crew loads Mr. Wilson into the ambulance and they travel down the road to the local fire department where a landing zone is being established behind the station. The helicopter arrives shortly after the ambulance arrives. Report was given and care transferred to the Paramedic and nurse from the helicopter crew. Five minutes later, the helicopter lifts off for the 10-minute flight to the STEMI center.

CRITICAL THINKING QUESTIONS

1. What is the most appropriate transport decision that will get the patient to definitive care?
2. What are the advantages of transporting a patient with suspected acute coronary syndrome to these hospitals, even if that means bypassing other hospitals in the process?

Disposition

The in-hospital treatment changes dramatically based upon the 12-lead ECG findings. The goal is to open up the occluded coronary artery as rapidly as possible. Both fibrinolysis and angioplasty achieve that objective; however, the literature suggests an approach based upon availability of these treatments as well as time from the onset of symptoms.[38]

Fibrinolysis works well early in the disease process when the clot in the occluded coronary artery (Figure 2-14a) has not solidified. As time passes, the clot is more difficult to dissolve by administering systemic fibrinolytic medications and may require mechanical revascularization by **angioplasty**, a procedure used to widen vessels narrowed by stenosis or occlusions (Figure 2-14b, c, and d). Angioplasty is also preferred if the patient is in cardiogenic shock or has contraindications to fibrinolysis (Table 2-2). Patients who have a history of renal failure typically are not able to receive the contrast dye that is injected into the coronary arteries to detect the blockage and confirm flow. They may need fibrinolysis at the ED to treat the acute ST elevation myocardial infarction.

The decision to preferentially transport a patient past a closer community hospital to a tertiary hospital that has been designated as an STEMI center or PCI center is largely a regional or local decision based upon resources and made by the medical oversight authority in conjunction with the hospitals in that region. Some systems have developed an automatic referral system between local EMS, community hospitals, and tertiary care PCI centers through collaboration of these different partners in patient care.[39] Other systems have instituted automatic activation of an aeromedical transport agency to meet the Paramedic transporting a patient to a distant community hospital to decrease overall medical contact to balloon times.[40] A system's medical oversight authority can make appropriate destination decisions for patients with an STEMI. There is an effort underway to include EMS contact time as an indication of overall system effectiveness and some systems have demonstrated the ability to decrease EMS contact to balloon times to below 90 minutes.[40] If in doubt, or if there is a specific situation where the choice of destination is not as clear, the Paramedic should not hesitate to consult on-line medical control to discuss the specific patient and situation.

Table 2-2 Comparison of Fibrinolysis to Primary Angioplasty

Fibrinolysis	Primary Angioplasty
• Fibrinolysis less than three hours from onset of pain	• Greater than three hours from onset of pain
• Contraindication to angioplasty	• Contraindications to fibrinolysis
• No contraindications to fibrinolysis	• Heart failure present at same time as MI

Note: If the time to reperfusion is less than three hours, there is no preference between treatments[39]

Comparison of fibrinolysis to primary angioplasty (adapted from: American Heart Association. Part 8: Stabilization of the patient with acute coronary syndrome, Circulation 2005;112:IV-89–IV-110)

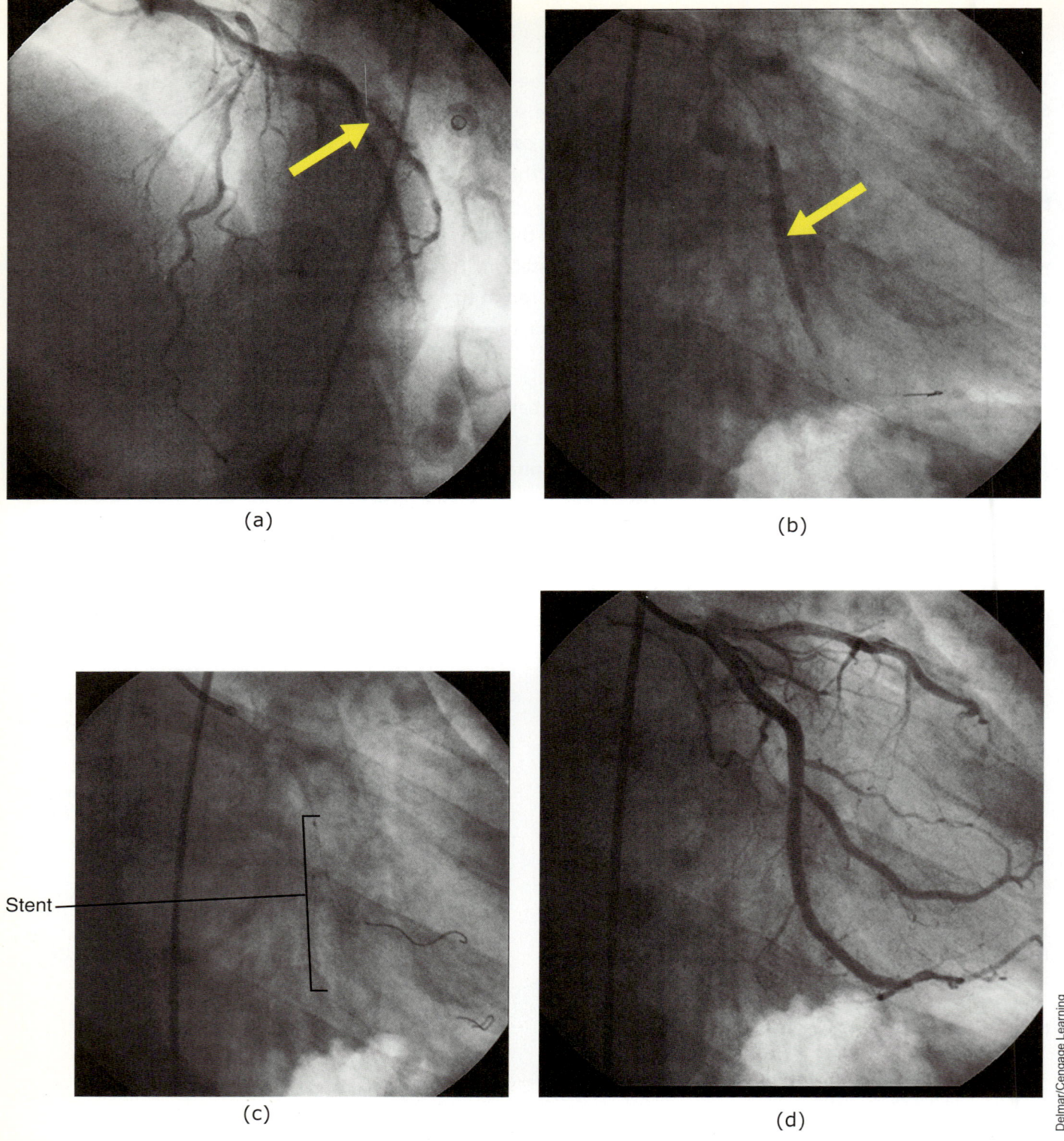

Figure 2-14 Primary angioplasty performed in a patient with an acute myocardial infarction. (a) The coronary occlusion is indicated by the arrow. (b) A wire is passed through the obstruction and a balloon is inflated to open the artery. (c) A metal stent is placed to keep the artery open. (d) The dye flows freely downstream after the obstruction is removed.

CONCLUSION

The American Heart Association has issued treatment standards which dictate that 90% of patients undergoing primary angioplasty for an STEMI should have a door-to-balloon time of less than 90 minutes. For patients receiving fibrinolysis as treatment for an STEMI, 90% of those patients should have a door-to-fibrinolysis time under 30 minutes.

For patients who have acute coronary syndrome that is not an STEMI, the patient should be transported to the nearest appropriate emergency department for evaluation and treatment. For patients who clearly have a valve rupture or aortic dissection, the patient should be transported to a facility with cardiothoracic surgery capability.

This condition is very difficult to definitively determine without ultrasound, X-ray, or CT scan confirmation. In addition, the decision to transport an unstable patient to a more distant center may not be appropriate for that specific patient. If in doubt, either transport the patient to the closest appropriate facility or consult on-line medical control to discuss that specific patient.

KEY POINTS:

- Calls for patients with a history or symptoms related to coronary heart disease are among the more common reasons for patients to access EMS.

- Acute coronary syndrome (ACS) is a generic term used to describe acute events related to coronary artery disease.

- Atherosclerotic build-up narrows the coronary arteries, decreasing blood flow to the myocardium.

- Chest pain is the most common ACS complaint; however, atypical signs/symptoms may present as ACS. These atypical presentations are often called anginal equivalents.

- A myocardial infarction is death and permanent damage of myocardial muscle cells.

- Myocardial infarctions are ST elevation myocardial infarction (STEMI) or non-ST elevation myocardial infarction (NSTEMI). The acute treatment of each is different.

- Surrounding the infarct is an ischemic penumbra. This nearly dead tissue can often be salvaged by aggressive treatment.

- As myocardial cells die, enzymes are released into the blood. The most specific enzyme for a myocardial infarction is troponin.

- Angina is a condition where the supply of oxygen cannot meet the demand for oxygen by the myocardium. Patterns include stable, unstable, and crescendo, a form of unstable angina.

- Cocaine increases myocardial oxygen demand by increasing heart rate and systemic vascular resistance. It produces vasospasm of the coronary arteries. It also encourages thrombus formation and accelerates the rate of atherosclerotic plaque development.

- Infections of the heart can affect the pericardium, the myocardium, or the endocardium and valves. All may produce acute coronary syndrome type complaints.

- Valves may become incompetent through narrowing or failure to close.

- Pulmonary hypertension is an elevated pressure in the pulmonary vascular system above the normal systolic pressure of 20 to 30 mmHg and normal diastolic pressure of 8 to 14 mmHg.

- Noncardiac causes of chest pain arising from trauma, or the respiratory, musculoskeletal, or gastrointestinal systems, should be considered in developing the paramedical diagnosis.

- The most significant risk factor for cardiac disease is a past history of a myocardial infarction, angina, or a cardiac catheterization that demonstrates coronary artery disease. Other risk factors include a past medical history of hypertension, high cholesterol, angina, and diabetes.

- The 12-lead ECG determines the appropriate hospital destination and the speed of treatment.

- Paramedics address life-threatening conditions that affect the airway, breathing, or circulation and then provide the standard treatment for acute coronary syndromes including rapid 12-lead acquisition and the administration of aspirin, nitroglycerine, and oxygen. This treatment also includes continuous rhythm monitoring.

- Nitroglycerine should be used carefully or avoided in patients with inferior or posterior wall MI right ventricular involvement, aortic stenosis with hypertension, or when the patient has used medications for erectile dysfunction within the past 24 to 48 hours.

- Anticoagulants or antiplatelets should be used cautiously in patients with risk of bleeding.

- Patients with STEMIs should be transported to a facility capable of providing fibrinolysis and angioplasty if possible. Beta blockade and anticoagulation may be started prior to arrival at the facility.

- Patients without STEMIs may be transported to a community hospital. Call medical control for advice.

REVIEW QUESTIONS:

1. What are anginal equivalents?
2. What differentiates angina from myocardial infarct?
3. What is the goal of aggressive treatment in the face of an acute myocardial infarction?
4. How does the use of cocaine increase the risk for an acute coronary event?
5. Name noncardiac causes of chest pain that should be considered in the paramedical differential diagnoses.
6. Which wave(s) on the 12-lead determine destination hospital and speed of treatments?
7. Which class of medications causes a clot to break apart or "dissolve"?

CASE STUDY QUESTIONS:

Please refer to the Case Study in this chapter, and answer the questions below:

1. What is the most common clue to Mr. Wilson's diagnosis of acute coronary syndrome?
2. In assessing Mr. Wilson's history, which medications/drug use would have caused the Paramedic to alter his plan of nitrates and beta blockade?
3. What would be the purpose of administering aspirin to Mr. Wilson?
4. How does the Paramedic contribute to a reduced door-to-balloon time?

REFERENCES:

1. American Heart Association. Heart disease and stroke statistics: 2008 update at a glance. Available at: **http://www.americanheart .org/downloadable/heart/1200082005246HS_Stats%202008 .final.pdf.** Accessed April 15, 2008.
2. White HD, Chew DP. Acute myocardial infarction. *Lancet.* 2008;372(9638):570–584.
3. Brogan GX, Jr. Bench to bedside: pathophysiology of acute coronary syndromes and implications for therapy. *Acad Emerg Med.* 2002;9(10):1029–1044.
4. Hoekstra JW, Pollack CV, Jr., et al. Improving the care of patients with non-ST-elevation acute coronary syndromes in the

emergency department: the CRUSADE initiative. *Acad Emerg Med.* 2002;9(11):1146–1155.

5. Gupta M, Tabas JA, et al. Presenting complaint among patients with myocardial infarction who present to an urban, public hospital emergency department. *Ann Emerg Med.* 2002;40(2):180–186.

6. Pahlavan PS, Niroomand F. Coronary artery aneurysm: a review. *Clin Cardiol.* 2006;29(10):439–443.

7. Yasue H, Nakagawa H, et al. Coronary artery spasm—clinical features, diagnosis, pathogenesis, and treatment. *J Cardiol.* 2008;51(1):2–17.

8. Nakao K, Ohgushi M, et al. Hyperventilation as a specific test for diagnosis of coronary artery spasm. *Am J Cardiol.* 1997;80(5):545–549.

9. Hollander JE. Acute coronary syndromes: acute myocardial infarction and unstable angina. In: Tintinalli JE, Kelen GD, Stapcsynski JS. *Emergency Medicine, a Comprehensive Study Guide,* sixth edition. American College of Emergency Physicians; 2004:343–352.

10. Tucker JF, Collins RA, et al. Early diagnostic efficiency of cardiac troponin I and troponin T for acute myocardial infarction. *Acad Emerg Med.* 1997;4(1):13–21.

11. Gupta S, Alagona P, Jr. Troponins: not always a myocardial infarction. *Am J Med.* 2008;121(9):e25, author reply e29.

12. Wong CK, White HD. Implications of the new definition of myocardial infarction. *Postgrad Med J.* 2005:81(959):552–555.

13. Hsue PY, Salinas CL, et al. Acute aortic dissection related to crack cocaine. *Circulation.* 2002;105(13):1592–1595.

14. Gadaleta D, Hall MH, et al. Cocaine-induced acute aortic dissection. *Chest.* 1989;96(5):1203–1205.

15. McCord J, Jneid H, Hollander JE, et al. Management of cocaine associated chest pain and myocardial infarction. *Circulation.* April 2008;117:1897–1907.

16. Spangler S, MD. Acute pericarditis. Available at: **http://www .emedicine.com/med/TOPIC1781.HTM.** Accessed January 2009.

17. Karam N, Patel P, et al. Diagnosis and management of chronic pericardial effusions. *Am J Med Sci.* 2001;322(2):79–87.

18. Habib G, Thuny F, et al. Prosthetic valve endocarditis: current approach and therapeutic options. *Prog Cardiovasc Dis.* 2008;50(4):274–281.

19. American Heart Association. Endocarditis prophylaxis information. Available at: **http://www.americanheart.org/ presenter.jhtml?identifier=11086.** Accessed April 17, 2008.

20. Cline DM. Valvular emergencies. In: *Emergency Medicine, a Comprehensive Study Guide,* sixth edition. American College of Emergency Physicians; 2004:373–378.

21. Baumgartner H. Aortic stenosis: medical and surgical management. *Heart.* 2005;91(11):1483–1488.

22. Michelakis ED, Wilkins MR, et al. Emerging concepts and translational priorities in pulmonary arterial hypertension. *Circulation.* 2008;118(14):1486–1495.

23. Gaul C, Dietrich W, et al. Neurological symptoms in aortic dissection: a challenge for neurologists. *Cerebrovasc Dis.* 2008;26(1):1–8.

24. McSweeney JC, Cody M, et al. Women's early warning symptoms of acute myocardial infarction. *Circulation.* 2003;108(21):2619–2623.

25. McSweeney JC, Crane PB. Challenging the rules: women's prodromal and acute symptoms of myocardial infarction. *Res Nurs Health.* 2000;23(2):135–146.

26. Hwang SY, Ryan C, et al. The influence of age on acute myocardial infarction symptoms and patient delay in seeking treatment. *Prog Cardiovasc Nurs.* 2006;21(1):20–27.

27. Rich MW. Epidemiology, clinical features, and prognosis of acute myocardial infarction in the elderly. *Am J Geriatr Cardiol.* 2006;15(1):7–11; quiz 12.

28. Smith SC, Jr. Current and future directions of cardiovascular risk prediction. *Am J Cardiol.* 2006;97(2A):28A–32A.

29. Han JH, Miller KF, et al. Factors affecting cardiac catheterization rates in elders with acute coronary syndromes. *Acad Emerg Med.* 2007;14(3): 228–233.

30. Fijewski TR, Pollack ML, et al. Electrocardiographic manifestations: right ventricular infarction. *J Emerg Med.* 2002;22(2):189–194.

31. Husser D, Bollmann A, et al. Evaluation of noncardiac chest pain: diagnostic approach, coping strategies and quality of life. *Eur J Pain.* 2006;10(1):51–55.

32. How J, Volz G, et al. The causes of musculoskeletal chest pain in patients admitted to hospital with suspected myocardial infarction. *Eur J Intern Med.* 2005;16(6):432–436.

33. Ng W, Wong WM, et al. Incidence and predictors of upper gastrointestinal bleeding in patients receiving low-dose aspirin for secondary prevention of cardiovascular events in patients with coronary artery disease. *World J Gastroenterol.* 2006;12(18):2923–2927.

34. Kim SH, Park HS. Pathogenesis of nonsteroidal antiinflammato drug-induced asthma. *Curr Opin Allergy Clin Immunol.* 2006;6(1):17–22.

35. Tragardh E, Claesson M, et al. Detection of acute myocardial infarction using the 12-lead ECG plus inverted leads versus t 16-lead ECG (with additional posterior and right-sided chest electrodes). *Clin Physiol Funct Imaging.* 2007;27(6):368–3

36. Zalenski RJ, Cooke D, et al. Assessing the diagnostic value ECG containing leads V4R, V8, and V9: the 15-lead ECG. *Emerg Med.* 1993;22(5):786–793.

37. Russo A, Suri RM, et al. Clinical outcome after surgical correction of mitral regurgitation due to papillary muscle rupture. *Circulation.* 2008;118(15):1528–1534.

38. American Heart Association. Part 8: stabilization of the with acute coronary syndromes. *Circulation.* 2005;112: IV-89–IV-110.

39. Rokos IC, Larson DM, Henry TD, et al. Rationale for establishing regional ST elevation myocardial infarctio receiving center networks. *Am Heart J.* 2006;152:661–

40. Hyde RJ, Kociszewski C, Thomas SH, Wedel SK, Bre Prehospital STEMI diagnosis and early helicopter dis to expedite interfacility transfer reduces time to reper *Prehosp Emerg Care.* 2008;12(1):107.

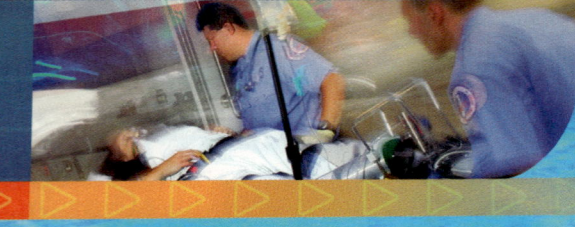

CHAPTER 3

HEART FAILURE

KEY CONCEPTS:

Upon completion of this chapter, it is expected that the reader will understand these following concepts:

- The effects of heart failure on patient and society
- Methods to identify, assess, and manage a patient who is experiencing an acute medical emergency due to heart failure or device failure
- Technologic advances such as LVAD, IABP, bi-level, and CPAP

ANATOMY CONCEPTS:

Prior to reading this chapter the Paramedic student should be familiar with the following anatomy and physiology concepts:

- Hemodynamic concepts
- Autonomic nervous system control
- Neurotransmitter effects
- Renin-angiotensin-aldosterone mechanism
- Heart sounds

The call came in the same as any other routine call, "Medic 7, respond to 14 Bowie Lane, the Smith residence, for a female who is weak and short of breath." As the Paramedics head for the ambulance, they discuss how this residence sounds familiar. "Wasn't that address where we intubated that lady last week?"

CRITICAL THINKING QUESTIONS

1. What are some of the possible causes of cardiac-related shortness of breath?

2. How is trouble breathing related to chest pain?

OVERVIEW

Cardiac disease has been a major focus of the health industry for years. Through aggressive public education and improved treatment modalities in both the in-hospital and out-of-hospital environments, a decline has been seen in the mortality of cardiovascular disease. Patients are now surviving once fatal cardiac events only to live with a damaged heart, one that may be unable to act as a pump, as it was originally designed.

Heart failure has become the only cardiovascular disease that is increasing in prevalence in the United States. It affects 10 patients out of every 1,000 after the age of 65 and cost the United States $27.9 billion in 2005.[1] The American Heart Association estimates that there are 5,000,000 people living with heart failure in the United States and there are approximately 550,000 new diagnoses every year. Of those, 80%—over 1 million—of all patient admissions over the age of 63 will be hospitalized, and nearly 55,000 will die. Risk factors to heart failure are similar to those of acute coronary syndrome (ACS) and include **ischemia** (insufficient supply of blood to an organ), hypertension, alcohol abuse, smoking, and infections of the heart and valves.[1]

Chief Concern

Heart failure is a multisystem disorder whereby abnormalities in the cardiovascular and renal systems cause a state of low **cardiac output** (blood pumped from the heart) and eventually lead to the development of impaired cardiac function. This impaired function prevents the heart from meeting the body's metabolic demands. Essentially, the pump's effectiveness is impaired due to any number of structural or functional causes. This, in turn, decreases the amount of blood pumped forward through the circulatory system. The body's compensatory mechanisms activate but yet are unable to meet the body's demands, thus starving the cells of oxygen and nutrients, thereby worsening the condition (Figure 3-1).

Although heart failure may be thought of as a chronic condition, it may also present as an acute emergency as well. It can result from *any* structural or functional disorder in the body that impairs the heart's filling or pumping action such as volume overload, excessive **vascular resistance** (that which must be overcome to push blood through the circulatory system), and/or ventricular **dysfunction** (difficult or abnormal function).

This means that not only are there cardiac factors within the heart, or **intrinsic**, dysfunctions that cause heart failure as well as an abnormal load on the left ventricle, but also **extrinsic** factors (those not from within the heart) as well.

Pathophysiology of Heart Failure

The effects of heart failure generally begin to appear when there is a dysfunction in myocardial **contractility** (the capability of muscle cells to shrink or contract), preload, and/or afterload. Patients will often complain of **dyspnea** (difficulty in breathing) as a result of impaired forward blood flow, backward failure, and **pulmonary edema** (an accumulation of fluids in interstitial spaces of the lungs).

General Development of Heart Failure

As the body senses a decrease in cardiac output or oxygen delivery, the compensatory mechanisms activate, redistributing blood flow to the core and vital organs through **shunting** (diverting flow from one area to another) and increasing

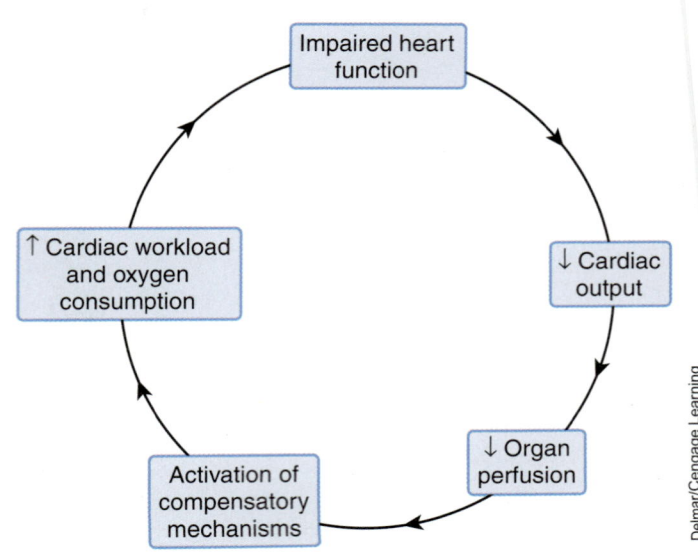

Figure 3-1 The cycle of heart failure.

cardiac output (CO) by increasing stroke volume (SV) and/or heart rate (HR):

$$\uparrow SV \times \uparrow HR = \uparrow CO.$$

The compensatory response by the sympathetic nervous system and the renin-angiotensin-aldosterone system (RAAS) are the body's most important responses, but they are only meant to be temporary. Prolonged activation of the sympathetic nervous system or activation in the presence of another disease state, such as with an acute myocardial infarction (AMI), may lead to long-term consequences such as heart failure.

Autonomic Nervous System Response

The sympathetic nervous system is immediately activated when the baroreceptors in the carotids and the aorta recognize a state of low pressure, sensing a drop in cardiac output. The adrenal gland releases the catecholamine, norepinephrine, and epinephrine to increase cardiac output by increasing stroke volume and heart rate.[2]

Norepinephrine binds with alpha 1 receptors, causing vasoconstriction of the smooth muscle in the peripheral systemic arterioles. This shunts needed blood to the core and vital organs at the cost of increased afterload.

Norepinephrine also binds with beta 1 sites within the heart to increase **chronotropy** (rate) while having little to no effect on **inotropy** (force). However, as the afterload increases, secondary to the effects of norepinephrine upon the alpha 1 receptors, so does the need for increased contractile force of the left ventricle to overcome the increased resistance and pressure within the aorta.

Epinephrine, the other rescue hormone, has both positive inotropic and chronotropic effects but little *direct* effect on blood pressure. Indirectly epinephrine increases blood pressure by increasing cardiac output ($\uparrow BP = \uparrow CO \times$ Systemic Vascular Resistance). As cardiac output increases, so too will the blood return to the heart and thusly preload.

Both epinephrine and norepinephrine work to improve the performance of the heart by maintaining the **mean arterial pressure (MAP)**, the average blood pressure during a cardiac cycle, which in turn maintains the net blood pressure to the brain, or **cerebral perfusion pressure (CPP)** (CPP = MAP − ICP). However, these adjustments come at the price of increasing the myocardial workload and oxygen demand.

Normally the heart spends one third of its time in systole and two thirds of its time resting in diastole, when the coronary arteries fill. As the heart rate increases to compensate, the diastolic and, thus, the coronary artery filling time decrease. This can lead to angina and myocardial ischemia. With prolonged myocardial ischemia, eventually heart failure follows. Thus, both of these catecholamines are contributing factors to the development of heart failure. However, they are continually released by the sympathetic nervous system as long as cardiac output is low and the heart fails in meeting the body's metabolic demands (i.e., perfusion).

Activation of the Renin-Angiotensin-Aldosterone System

The renin-angiotensin-aldosterone system (RAAS) is activated through either sustained stimulation of the sympathetic nervous system or at times when there is a decrease in renal perfusion pressure. Activation of the RAAS not only increases the release of norepinephrine but also promotes a greater preload and afterload through increasing venous and arterial tone (Figure 3-2).

The RAAS increases the concentration of angiotensin II, a potent vasoconstrictor, by increasing the amount of angiotensin I that is converted with the angiotensin-converting enzyme (ACE). This causes profound vasoconstriction in the renal and systemic circulation by releasing additional amounts of norepinephrine. Damage to the myocardium occurs as angiotensin II increases permeability of the coronary arteries, allowing growth factors, which cause necrosis, into the interstitium (the space between the myocardial cells). Angiotensin II not only stimulates the release of norepinephrine but aldosterone as well. Aldosterone causes the kidneys to reabsorb sodium and water from urine produced by the kidneys, increasing the intravascular volume while at the same time causing an increase in the excretion of potassium and the development of **hypokalemia** (a low serum potassium level).[3]

Renin, as with aldosterone, aids in the reabsorption of sodium and water, increasing the intravascular volume. With an acute drop in cardiac output, this is a beneficial response. However, if there is a continued state of decreased cardiac output, this continued reabsorption could be a contributory factor to systemic fluid overload.

The Paramedic must remember that this is typically a gradual response and that oftentimes acute pulmonary edema is not the result of fluid overload but more often the misdistribution of fluid in the body.

Other Hormonal Responses

Natriuretic peptides are also released in response to volume expansion and pressure overload. They act as a physiological antagonist to angiotensin II. The atrial natriuretic peptides (ANP) are released from the atria in response to stretching whereas brain natriuretic peptides (BNP) are released from the ventricles.[4,5] Paramedics may often see BNP levels being referred to with patients in heart failure as it confirms ventricular engorgement and increased strain on the ventricles.

In response to raising ANP and BNP hormone levels, the **antidiuretic hormone (ADH)**, also known as vasopressin, is released by the posterior pituitary and assists in increasing the intravascular volume by acting upon the smooth muscle of the arterioles and kidney tubules. This constricts blood vessels while also stimulating the reabsorption of water.

Endothelin, released by the endothelial cells, is another hormone that is a potent vasoconstrictor, especially in the renal vasculature. There it promotes sodium retention, contributes to peripheral vasoconstriction, and may have adverse effects

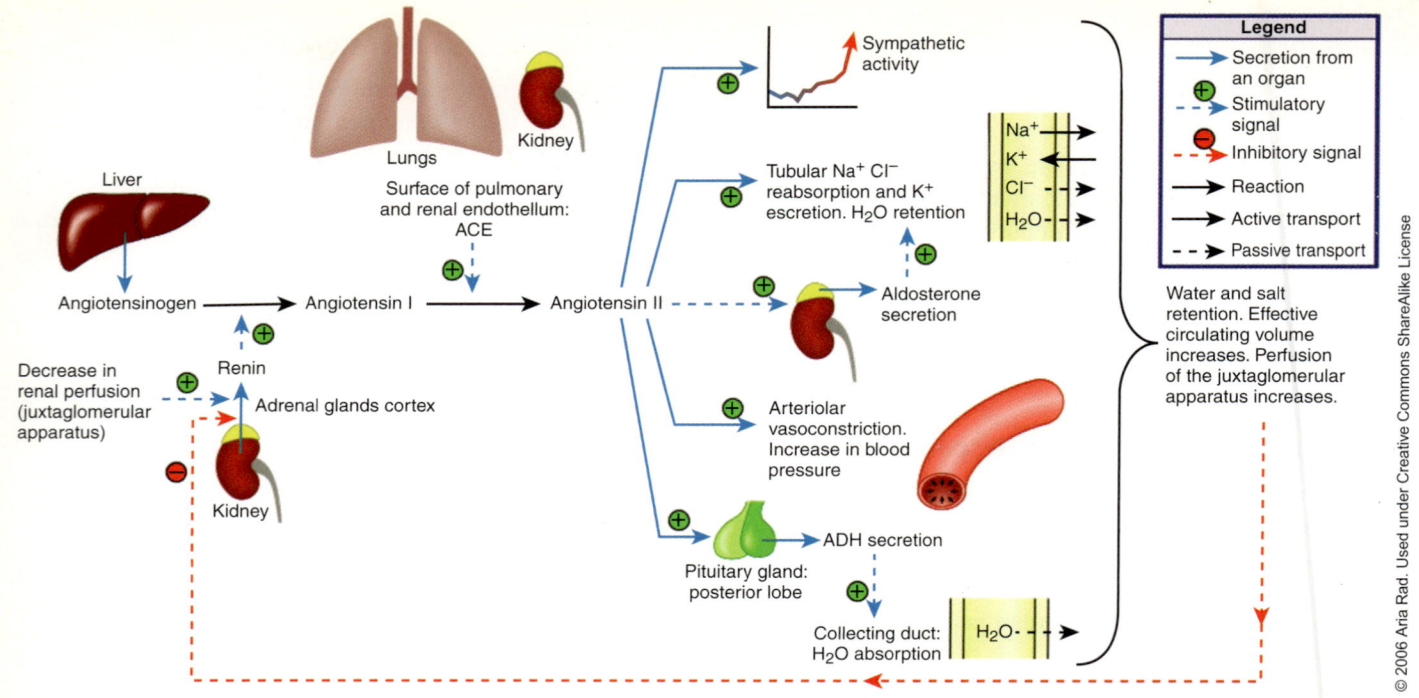

Figure 3-2 Activation of the RAAS.

upon ventricular remodeling (adaptations) by promoting myocardial hypertrophy.

Ventricular Remodeling

When an injury occurs, or when the heart is required to work harder, there are numerous changes that happen within it to allow the heart to adapt to its new environment. These changes, termed **ventricular remodeling**, develop over time as a result of an increased hemodynamic load and/or neurohormonal activation. Causes are numerous, but they are grouped as physiological (as with a well-conditioned athlete) or pathological (as would occur from myocardial damage post AMI (see Table 3-1).

In the case of an AMI, the process begins within hours of ischemia and continues to progress until the heart fails, the severity of which is dependent upon additional neurohormonal activation.

During an acute coronary event the myocardial (heart muscle) cells become necrotic and the affected ventricular wall becomes akinetic (loss of function). Over time necrotic tissue is absorbed and scar tissue replaces it.

As pressure overload remains in the ventricle, the infarcted area expands, forming an aneurysm. The ventricle then dilates and begins to reshape itself. These changes alter the heart in size and shape, making it less elliptical and more spherical.

As ventricular mass, composition, and volume change, cardiac function changes as well. The amount of functional change is dependent upon the percentage of the ventricle wall that is damaged. The larger the infarction, the greater the dilation, and the greater the change in the ventricle and its functional capacity. This causes a decrease in **ejection fraction** (the percentage of blood expelled by the heart with each contraction) and cardiac output (Figure 3-3).

Ventricular Hypertrophy

Ventricular hypertrophy, ventricular muscle enlargement, is the heart's adaptive response to stress. It allows the heart to compensate by enabling the ventricles to enhance their pumping capacity by increasing their mass. Benign

Table 3-1 Conditions That Cause Remodeling

- Acute myocardial infarction
- Pressure load
- Aortic stenosis
- Hypertension
- Inflammatory heart muscle disease
- Idiopathic dilated cardiomyopathy or volume overload
- Ventricular regurgitation
- Compensatory change due to functional change of the heart
  - Athletes

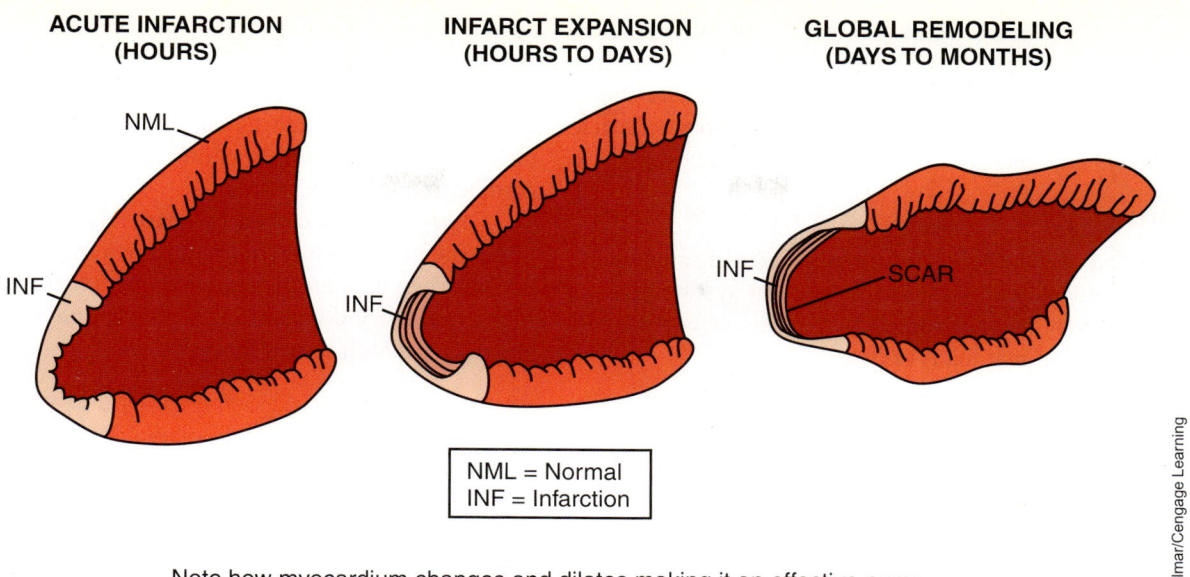

ACUTE INFARCTION (HOURS)

NML

INF

INFARCT EXPANSION (HOURS TO DAYS)

INF

GLOBAL REMODELING (DAYS TO MONTHS)

INF

SCAR

NML = Normal
INF = Infarction

Delmar/Cengage Learning

Note how myocardium changes and dilates making it an effective pump

Figure 3-3 Ventricular remodeling after an AMI.

ventricular hypertrophy may be the result of physiological stress (i.e., exercise) allowing the ventricle to pump a greater volume of blood. This characteristic is fully reversible and often seen in well-conditioned athletes. It may also be a result of a pathological stress, as with chronic hypertension, and allows the heart to maintain a normal stroke volume in the presence of an increased systemic vascular resistance (i.e., afterload). Although initially pathological hypertrophy may be beneficial, it will lead to functional demise and ultimately heart failure.

The good way to introduce the concepts of ventricular hypertrophy is by looking at what occurs during aerobic exercise. As athletes condition their bodies, making them work harder, one is able to see how their muscles increase in size. This is especially noticeable in runners who develop strong legs or body builders who develop large biceps. The bodies of these types of athletes have an increased need for skeletal and myocardial oxygen, glucose, and removal of waste by-products.

To accomplish this, there is an increase in blood return to the heart, creating a volume overload. This volume overload increases the stretch of the ventricle and subsequently the contraction (Frank-Starling Law).[3] The heart responds to this increased workload by allowing the ventricle to dilate by adding new muscle filaments in series to those already existing. This allows for greater expansion of the ventricle and thus a greater volume of blood. As the ventricle dilates, support is required. Therefore, the myocardium generally responds by increasing the thickness of the ventricular wall (i.e., hypertrophy).

Alternatively, if the heart is constantly exposed to increased systemic vascular resistance (chronic hypertension), the thickness of the ventricular wall undergoes hypertrophy. To maintain stroke volume against an increased systemic vascular resistance (i.e., afterload), the ventricle is required to generate forces greater than the pressures resisting its output. Increased ventricular muscle mass helps maintain this

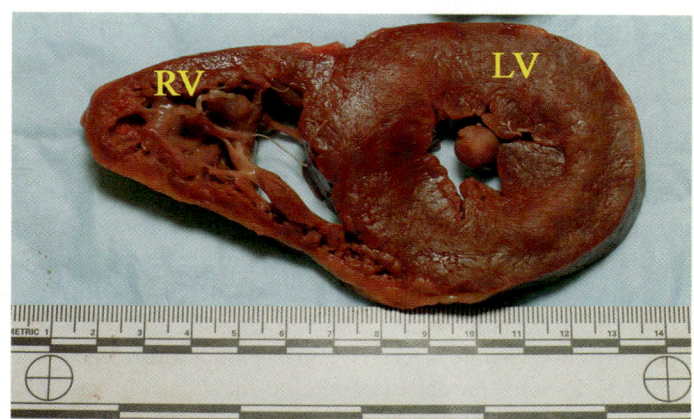

RV

LV

Delmar/Cengage Learning

Figure 3-4 Left and right ventricular hypertrophy.

cardiac output. However, the advantage of ventricular hypertrophy eventually reaches its limits. The ventricular walls become stiff and rigid, secondary to ventricular hypertrophy; this can be compared to becoming "muscle bound" when weight lifting. With decreasing ventricular wall compliance the ventricles do not fill as effectively. Without ventricular filling, the atrial "kick" that occurs (i.e., augmented end-diastolic ventricular filling) does not take advantage of Starling's law. As a result of the decreasing ventricular filling, there is less cardiac output. This syndrome is referred to as **diastolic dysfunction** (Figure 3-4).

Continued Progression of Ventricular Remodeling

As blood flow to the area diminishes, the tissue becomes necrotic. As a result, apoptosis (progressive cell death) occurs and causes progressive ventricular dysfunction, a process that is not fully understood. Fibrosis begins and eventually collagen accumulates in the cardiac interstitium. An increase in chamber size occurs while decreasing the compliance, or ability to stretch to fill with blood. To help compensate, norepinephrine, angiotensin, and endothelian are released. However, because of this neurohormonal response cardiac function begins to deteriorate (i.e., heart failure).

Causative Factors of Heart Failure

As mentioned earlier, heart failure may occur through acute or chronic changes within the cardiovascular system. Causes are many but may be categorized as intrinsic causes (abnormal ventricular volume load) or extrinsic causes.

Intrinsic Causes

Intrinsic myocardial damage occurs when there is a direct injury to the myocardium. Although the causes of intrinsic myocardial damage are numerous, approximately 30% are caused by ischemia and infarction due to coronary artery disease. Other causes include infections such as myocarditis, toxicity from alcohol abuse and other cardiotoxic substances, metabolic insults from diseases like hyperthyroidism, and cardiomyopathy where the heart mass has become excessively large in response to any of these or other chronic conditions (Table 3-2).

Abnormal Volume Load on the Left Ventricle

Factors that may create an abnormally high volume load on the left ventricle include fluid retention (e.g., from an excessive intake of sodium) or fluid overload (e.g., when a renal failure patient misses dialysis and is not secreting urine). These expand the intravascular volume, increasing the preload to the heart.

Another cause of an abnormal load occurs when there is excessive vascular resistance or a chronic pressure overload, as with systemic arterial hypertension, requiring the left ventricle to work harder to overcome the systemic vascular resistance (Table 3-3).

Extrinsic Causes

Oftentimes there are causes of heart failure that occur from forces from outside the heart and are fully reversible if caught and treated early. For example, pericardial restrictive diseases, such as pericarditis and cardiac tamponade, do not allow the heart to expand as it normally would. This decreases the cardiac output and leads to heart failure.

Tachycardias, such as supraventricular and ventricular tachycardias, diminish diastolic filling times. As a result, cardiac output drops.

Other extrinsic causes of heart failure can be classified under the rubric of high output failures. A high output failure occurs when the heart is unable to meet the body's unusually high circulatory demands, as with hyperthyroidism, chronic anemia, or a high fever (Table 3-4).

Pathophysiology Summary

The amount of dysfunction that occurs in the ventricles is dependent upon two factors: the degree of neurohormonal activation and the extent of hemodynamic changes as a result of increased volume load. As cardiac output falls, neurohormonal activation responds accordingly through the primary release of norepinephrine and angiotensin II, which are both major components of the progression of heart failure. If sustained, they cause physical and functional changes to the heart.[6]

The Frank-Starling Law states that the greater the stretch, the greater the contraction. Just like overinflating a balloon too many times weakens the balloon, the ventricle walls eventually become overstretched and weakened. This stretching causes excessive myocardial dilation that eventually diminishes contractility and stroke volume and subsequently diminishes the ejection fraction.

With a greater amount of blood remaining in the ventricle, hydrostatic pressure increases, leading to venous congestion in the tissues and organs located before the affected ventricle. As cardiac output diminishes, the body increases the heart rate to compensate, decreasing coronary filling times and leading to hypoxia and ischemia. This constant work by the heart causes it to enlarge, or hypertrophy, thus increasing its oxygen demand. This action is affected by the decreased coronary filling times.

Remodeling, including hypertrophy, initially begins as an adaptive process. These changes initially may be beneficial, allowing the heart to maintain a forward flow of blood in the face of an increased afterload. As with any compensatory mechanism, a short-term solution becomes counterproductive if prolonged, and instead becomes a contributory factor in the development of heart failure. Once this compensatory mechanism becomes counterproductive, decompensation is noted and cardiac output drops, thus reactivating the aforementioned neurohormonal compensatory mechanisms (in particular the renin-angiotensin-aldosterone system).

Table 3-2 Intrinsic Causes of Heart Failure

- Coronary artery disease
- Myocarditis
- Toxicity from substance abuse
- Metabolic insults
- Cardiomyopathy

Table 3-3 Causes of Abnormal Ventricular Load

- Fluid retention due to sodium consumption
- Fluid overload due to decreased urine output
- Excessive systemic vascular resistance

Table 3-4 Extrinsic Causes of Heart Failure

- Pericarditis
- Cardiac tamponade
- Tachycardias
- Heart unable to meet the circulatory demands

Upon arriving outside of the home, it hits them. "Oh, not Mabel!" they both exclaim as they look at each other, for Mabel's past medical history is notorious for cardiorespiratory problems including heart failure and chronic obstructive pulmonary disease (COPD). The last time she went in, she ended up admitted with pneumonia.

The crew grabs their first-in bag that has their BLS and ALS airway equipment, as well as their oxygen, their drug bag, the cardiac monitor, and a stair-chair as they head up the steep stairs leading to Mabel's apartment. As they ascend the stairwell, they discuss Mabel's medication list, recalling that she takes furosemide, albuterol, and nitroglycerin.

As they walk through the door, they see Mabel where they usually find her: sitting upright in her recliner and in obvious distress. They ask what seems to be the matter. Mabel, sounding very tired, manages to get up enough energy to say, "I . . . can't . . . catch . . . my . . . breath." Is it her COPD or maybe pneumonia again?

CRITICAL THINKING QUESTIONS

1. What are the important elements of the history that a Paramedic should obtain?
2. What is the symptom pattern for suspected congestive heart failure?

History

It is not often that an EMS call comes across as heart failure; instead, it is usually for complaints or symptoms that are associated with the disease, such as trouble breathing. Oftentimes patients with heart failure will present with a history of fatigue or general malaise, acute respiratory distress, syncope secondary to hypotension, or any combination thereof (Figure 3-5). The Paramedic must remember that heart failure is a complex multisystem syndrome that may develop from an acute insult or through chronic activation of the compensatory mechanisms and remodeling.

Although there are numerous disease processes (Table 3-5) that may stem from these complaints, they can be classified as a result of acute respiratory distress or syncope. The Paramedic must be diligent in obtaining a complete and thorough history to narrow the list while developing the field diagnosis.

History of Present Illness— Acute Respiratory Distress

Patients may experience acute respiratory distress because of any number of reasons. Patients with chronic illnesses such as COPD, asthma, or even heart failure will often be aware of, and even educated about, their disease, simplifying the job of gathering a patient history.

On the opposite side, patients experiencing an acute illness such as anaphylaxis or heart failure due to an AMI may be a little more difficult. To aid in the assessment of the patient in acute respiratory distress, the Paramedic can utilize the HAPISOCS mnemonic (Table 3-6).

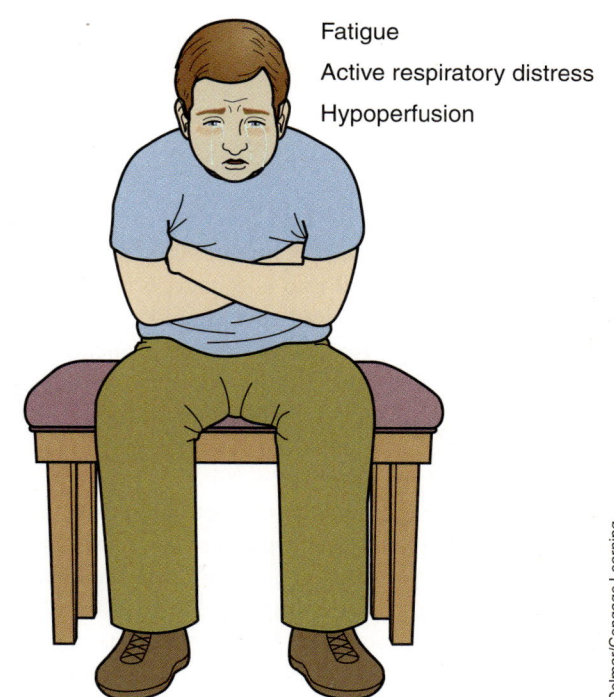

Fatigue
Active respiratory distress
Hypoperfusion

Figure 3-5 Common presentations of heart failure patients.

Delmar/Cengage Learning

Table 3-5 Differential Diagnoses

- Acute respiratory distress
  - Pulmonary embolus
  - Pneumonia
  - Anaphylaxis
  - Aspiration
  - Heart failure
  - Pneumothorax
- Syncope
  - AMI
  - Heart failure
  - Sepsis syndrome
  - Hypovolemia
  - Hemorrhage
  - Cardiac tamponade
  - Tension pneumothorax

Table 3-6 HAPISOCS

H	History of pulmonary disease
A	Activity at onset of SOB
P	Pain on inspiration
I	Infectious signs
S	Smoker
O	Orthopnea
C	Cough and sputum
S	Supplemental questions

History of Pulmonary Disease

There are both pulmonary and nonpulmonary causes for dyspnea. Heart failure may fall into both categories and should be assessed as such. The Paramedic should ask the patient if he or she has a history of COPD, asthma, pneumonia, or heart failure. Wheezing does not only occur in patients with COPD or asthma but in anaphylaxis and heart failure as well. **Cardiac asthma** occurs when fluid accumulates in the lungs, causing bronchoconstriction.[7,8]

A pulmonary embolism can restrict blood flow through the lungs, leading to increased pulmonary vascular resistance, or pulmonary hypertension. In turn, this leads to right ventricular failure and diminished left ventricular filling, leading to left ventricular failure. Patients with clotting problems may be aware of, and prone to, pulmonary embolisms. Knowing this information early in the assessment will help the Paramedic later when forming his field diagnosis.

Activity at Onset of Shortness of Breath

Acute disease states that occur during rest may progress rapidly. A patient complaining of sudden onset of dyspnea while resting may deteriorate more quickly and require more assertive airway management when compared to the patient that has had a gradual worsening over a period of time. Heart failure patients may experience rapid onset of respiratory distress as a result of acute pulmonary edema (APE) from acute left ventricular dysfunction or they may have more of a gradual onset from general fluid overload.

Patients with heart failure are often fatigued, having **dyspnea on exertion (DOE)**, and tend to be more sedentary, similar to those with COPD. They may complain that their shortness of breath worsens with climbing stairs or with simple movement around the house. DOE is defined as just that and is a result of the patient's heart being unable to meet the body's metabolic and oxygen demands either as a result of impaired cardiac output or a diffusion problem at the alveoli. These symptoms typically subside when the patient rests and their severity may be dependent upon the progression of their disease.

The onset of these conditions typically occurs at rest or possibly even during sleep, causing patients to awake short of breath (SOB). These patients are experiencing **paroxysmal nocturnal dyspnea (PND)** as a result of being in a supine position, causing an increase in the return of fluid to the lungs.

Since fatigue and DOE are common symptoms of the patient in heart failure, acute onsets during activity may lead the Paramedic to believe that the SOB may be a result of another disease process such as an AMI with APE. Determining the activity at the onset is important and allows the Paramedic to eliminate disease processes that do not fit the patient history.

Pain on Inspiration

Patients with heart failure typically do not have pain on inspiration although they may have cardiac chest pain. Trauma, cardiac infections, pleurisy, and costochondritis may all present with pain.

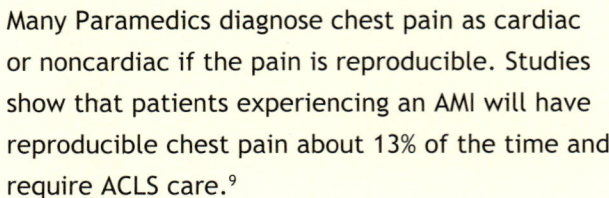

STREET SMART

Many Paramedics diagnose chest pain as cardiac or noncardiac if the pain is reproducible. Studies show that patients experiencing an AMI will have reproducible chest pain about 13% of the time and require ACLS care.[9]

Infectious Signs

Every Paramedic has asked himself or herself, "Is it pneumonia or heart failure?" Both may present similarly but oftentimes a decision comes down to if the patient has been experiencing any signs of infection. Patients presenting with night sweats, chills, fever, and productive cough of yellow or greenish sputum, may lead the Paramedic toward a field diagnosis of pneumonia.

As with the previous diagnosis, the differentiation was important because the treatments for pneumonia and heart failure are sometimes contradictory. For example, Paramedics usually give fluid to the pneumonia patient, whereas they take it away from the heart failure patient. Giving an incorrect treatment to the wrong patient would have grave consequences. Recent trends in the initial treatment of heart failure have eliminated this confusion and will be addressed later in this chapter.

Smoker

Nicotine causes a release of catecholamines and therefore increases heart rate, blood pressure, venous constriction, cardiac workload, and oxygen demand. All of these are causative factors of heart failure. Patients who smoke over 20 pack-years begin to develop clinical signs of disease and are at the greatest risk for acute coronary syndromes and stroke. One pack year equals smoking an average of one pack of cigarettes a day for a year or a similar combination of smoking and years.

This does not mean that a nonsmoker will not develop heart failure, only that it is more likely to occur in a smoker. In addition, a 20 pack-years smoker whose ventilation and oxygenation is already compromised may not tolerate APE or hypoxia for extended periods.

Orthopnea

Like a patient with PND, when a patient with heart failure lies down fluid returns to the pulmonary capillaries, decreasing the patient's ability to diffuse gasses. This is known as **orthopnea**. These patients will feel better sitting up (Figure 3-6). This allows the fluid to settle into the lower lobes of the lungs, allowing for oxygenation of the upper, nonobscured lung fields.

These patients will often sleep with their heads propped up to facilitate breathing. The Paramedic should consider asking the patient how many pillows she sleeps with and if that number has increased recently. An increased pillow count will help to demonstrate the progression of the illness. Orthopnea in some patients is so severe that they need to sleep sitting up in a recliner chair.

Cough and Sputum

Determine if the patient has a cough, the cough's duration, and if it is productive. Heart failure patients may start out with a dry cough but, as pulmonary vascular congestion worsens and the hydrostatic pressures increase due to left ventricular dysfunction, red blood cells and fluid are forced into the alveoli from the capillaries. This is what gives the classic sign often associated with acute pulmonary edema—pink-frothy sputum.

There are other causes of this as well, for the pink-frothy sputum is only a sign that there is an air-blood mix in the alveoli. It may be a result of trauma or other diseases, such as tuberculosis.

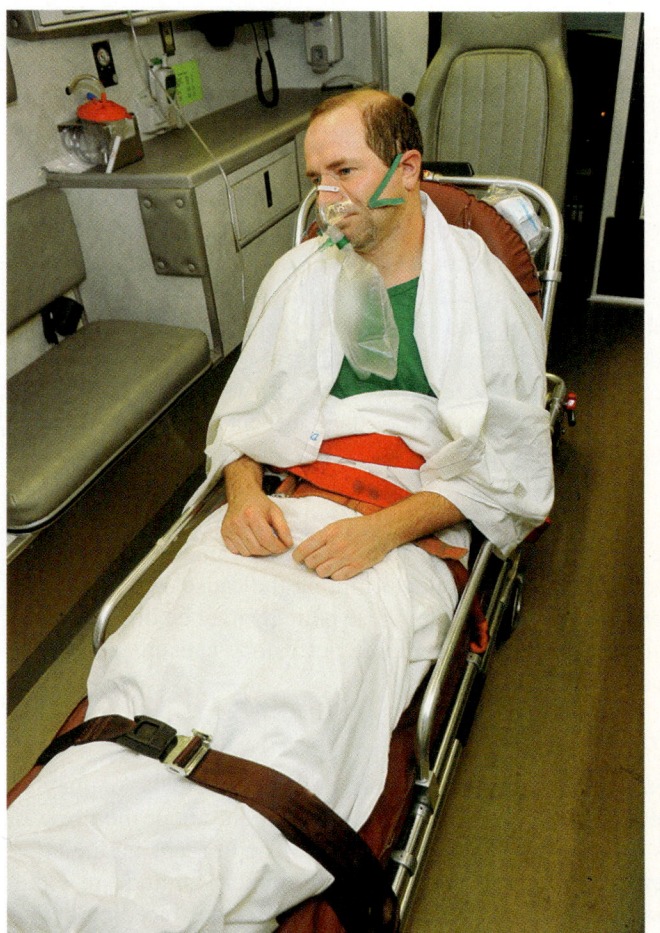

Figure 3-6 Patient positioning.

Supplemental Questions

To assist in determining disease progression, the Paramedic should inquire if the patient's dyspnea has been constant, worsening, or even subsiding since its onset. There are times that the patient may have experienced similar episodes. If so, the Paramedic should ask how long ago the episode occurred, if the patient was hospitalized, what the patient did to help the condition, and if the patient knows what exacerbated it. The answers to these questions will then lead to the next line of questioning.

The Paramedic should have the patient rate her dyspnea from 0 to 10, making 0 no trouble breathing and 10 the worst trouble she has ever experienced. This will allow the Paramedic to form a comparison of previous episodes and to evaluate their treatment. The Paramedic should ask the patient if she has ever been intubated or on a non-invasive ventilation device, such as continuous positive airway pressure (CPAP) or bi-level positive airway pressure (BiPAP). If so, this indicates the patient is at high risk of respiratory failure and the Paramedic should plan accordingly. Some patients who have had a good experience with CPAP or BiPAP in relieving their dyspnea may know they need non-invasive ventilation and ask for it.

History of Present Illness—Syncope

Heart failure may also present as syncope, with or without APE. As the Paramedic works toward developing his field diagnosis, he must keep in mind that the syncope may actually be a result of the heart's inability to fill and expel its contents. In other words, the syncope may be due to a decrease in the patient's ejection fraction as with left ventricular dysfunction due to an AMI, cardiac tamponade, or tension pneumothorax.

Syncope may also be a result of hypovolemia, uncontrolled bleeding, and other causes of shock. These lead to a decrease in preload while increasing the amount of blood remaining in the system, preventing forward flow. This causes the circulation to become stagnant, increasing hydrostatic pressure at the capillary level, which leads to APE.

Patients suffering from syncope will generally have complaints or symptoms based upon the underlying cause. Using the mnemonic OPQRST will help the Paramedic organize her interview and assist in determining the cause of the syncope. Obtaining a history from these patients may be difficult since syncope may affect cerebral perfusion, causing an altered level of consciousness.

Onset/Activity

Syncope may occur suddenly and unexpectedly, or may be preceded by dizziness. Asking the patient about the onset of his symptoms may assist the Paramedic in focusing the interview. Causes of hypovolemia are numerous, and are either traumatic or nontraumatic in nature. Besides bleeding, hypovolemia may occur due to an illness that causes uncontrolled vomiting and diarrhea, both of which may develop over days.

Provocation/Palliation

The Paramedic should determine what makes the patient's symptoms, if any, worse and better. A patient with a history of angina, stable or unstable, may state that generally the pain goes away with rest, but not so with an AMI.

Quality

The patient in heart failure due to an AMI may complain of heaviness or pain in her chest. However, the Paramedic should remember that this is not always the case. The Paramedic should have the patient explain, in her own words, how she feels. Remember that patients experiencing acute respiratory distress may ignore the chest pain. Patients experiencing asthma or exacerbation (worsening) of their COPD may complain of tightness in their chest as well. Some may even describe it as a belt being tightened around their chest.

Region/Radiation

Before asking the patient where the pain goes, it is best for the Paramedic to ask him where it starts. The Paramedic should have the patient point, with one finger, to the area where the pain originates, keeping in mind that with sudden severe dyspnea the patient may ignore or be unable to recognize his chest pain. Patients experiencing a pulmonary embolism, pericarditis, or trauma are often able to do this. However, patients experiencing an AMI or another condition that causes hypoxia to the heart muscle may complain of a more generalized pain or pressure, and may be unable to point to just one area. These patients may experience radiation into their neck, jaw, shoulder, or back. However, if their dyspnea is severe, these associated symptoms may be ignored.

Reoccurrence

The progression of the illness is important. Asking the patient if her symptoms have been constant or coming and going since their onset can be beneficial for the Paramedic. A majority of the differential diagnoses will be constant, but those of hypovolemia and sepsis may have symptoms that have occurred, changing intensity, over a period.

Severity

If the patient is having pain, have him rate it on the 0 to 10 scale. Ask him what the pain is currently, what it was at onset, and, if he has self-medicated, what the pain was afterwards.

Not all patients will have pain to rate. Pressure, dyspnea, and dizziness are just a few symptoms that patients present with that will allow for the use of this scale and may help the Paramedic see the disease's progression and intensity, especially when compared to previous episodes. If the patient is unable to give a numerical value, the Paramedic may ask the patient to rate his pain by using descriptions like mild, moderate, or severe.

Time

This may have already been ascertained earlier in the patient interview, but asking the patient what time, or how long ago, her complaint began allows the Paramedic to establish a timeline.

Heart failure patients may have been experiencing symptoms for years, but generally only call when there is an acute change. It is important to keep the patient focused on her immediate complaint early in the assessment. However, one should never ignore past complaints of worsening fatigue, DOE, or orthopnea, as these may help the Paramedic build a field diagnosis of heart failure.

Associated Signs/Symptoms and Pertinent Negatives

Besides increased fatigue, there are several other signs and symptoms that a patient may have heart failure. Since heart failure involves the renal system, there is no surprise that the kidneys are affected. Heart failure patients may have decreased urine output as the body retains sodium and water in an attempt to increase the intravascular volume. This may also be a sign of severe hemodynamic compromise as the blood is being shunted away from the kidneys to perfuse other organs (prerenal acute renal failure).

Patients who are hemodynamically stable may have an increase in urine production, especially at night. Nocturia occurs when the patient is lying down and fluid returns to the kidneys, similar to PND. To assess the patient's output, the Paramedic should inquire about the amount, color, smell, and frequency of urination.

Another area to assess is in regard to weight gain. Patients with chronic heart failure weigh themselves daily and an increase in weight may signify fluid retention and potentially fluid overload. Patients may also complain of nausea and vomiting. As the sympathetic nervous system activates, blood flow to the digestive tract decreases, slowing peristalsis. This causes a backup of bile and fluids into the stomach.

Allergies

Obtaining a list of the patient's allergies is crucial. The Paramedic should not only ask the patient about hypersensitivity to medications but also allergies to foods and latex as well. Patients allergic to sulfa drugs are particularly of interest in that these patients may develop an allergic reaction to furosemide or hydrochlorothiazide, even though the risk is very low.

If the patient does state he has an allergy to a medication, the Paramedic should inquire as to what occurs if he is given that medication. Many patients may misinterpret the side effects of a drug as an allergic reaction; for example, getting a headache from nitroglycerin.

Medications

Patient's experiencing an acute onset of heart failure may have a limited medication history. However, patients with chronic heart failure will often be on numerous medications that assist in diuresis, adjust preload and afterload, and increase contractility. The Paramedic should also inquire as to the use of nonprescribed, over-the-counter, and so-called natural medications.

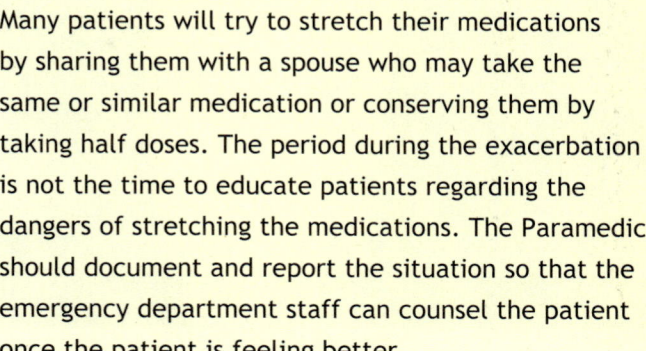

PROFESSIONAL PARAMEDIC

Many patients will try to stretch their medications by sharing them with a spouse who may take the same or similar medication or conserving them by taking half doses. The period during the exacerbation is not the time to educate patients regarding the dangers of stretching the medications. The Paramedic should document and report the situation so that the emergency department staff can counsel the patient once the patient is feeling better.

Nitrates

Nitrates are often prescribed to patients who have a history of angina, but they may also be given to patients with chronic heart failure. Nitroglycerin causes **vasodilatation** (widening of blood vessels), which decreases preload and alleviates some of the heart's workload as a result of increased venous return. This often causes the symptoms of dyspnea on exertion and orthopnea.

Patients who have been prescribed nitroglycerin are told to take it anytime that they experience chest pain or pressure, and possibly dyspnea if they have heart failure. The problem arises if the patient is experiencing a right ventricular wall infarct or is hypovolemic. Nitrates can drop the blood pressure due to the decreased preload. Right ventricular infarcts commonly cause inferior wall ST elevations or elevations in the V3R and V4R leads on a right-sided ECG.

Nitroglycerin Patches

Upon encountering a patient who is hypotensive, in heart failure, and has been prescribed nitrates, the Paramedic should always assess the patient from head to toe in search of a nitroglycerin patch. These may be flesh-colored or even clear and are commonly found on the arms, chest, or back, although other areas are also possible locations (Figure 3-7). Upon finding one, removal with gloved hands and further assessment is warranted. There have been times a patch is placed on a patient without removing the other, so the idea of multiple patches should not be overlooked.

Angiotensin-Converting Enzyme Inhibitors

A classification of drug that is becoming more prevalent in the management of heart failure is angiotensin-converting enzyme (ACE) inhibitors. They are designed to block the

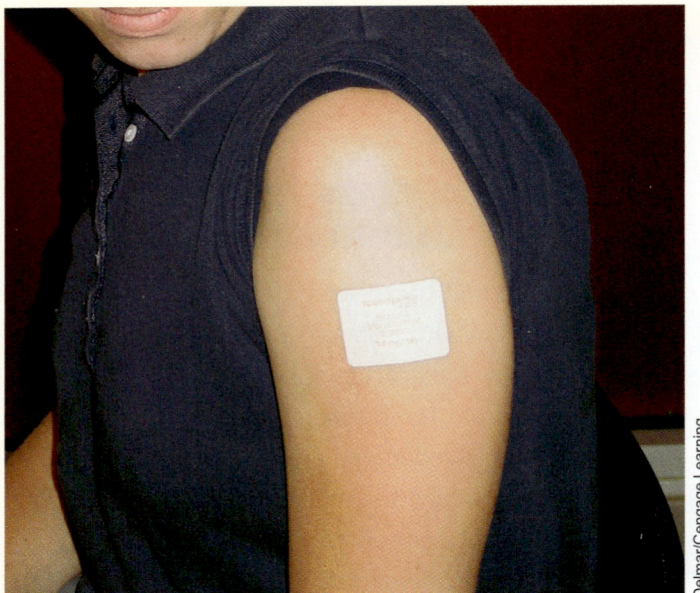

Figure 3-7 Nitroglycerin patches.

Glomerulus Proximal tubule Distal tubule
Bowman's capsule
Cortex
H_2O
Outer medulla
Descending limb
Inner medulla
Loop of Henle
H_2O ← Cl⁻ / Na⁺ H_2O →
H_2O ← Cl⁻ / Na⁺
Cl⁻ / Na⁺
Ascending limb
H_2O ← NaCl
NaCl
NaCl
Collecting duct
Urea ← H_2O →
Urea ← H_2O →
Urea ←
H_2O →
Urine

Delmar/Cengage Learning

Figure 3-8 Diuretics and the loop of Henle.

effects of the renin-angiotensin-aldosterone system through interfering with the conversion of angiotensin I into angiotensin II. Therefore, ACE inhibitors decrease water and sodium retention, afterload, and blood pressure.

ACE inhibitors do have their share of side effects. A patient may present with a persistent, dry, nonproductive cough that is common and not dangerous. Generally, the cough is not associated with position or time of day and stops once the ACE inhibitor therapy ceases.

Diuretics

There are different reasons for a patient to develop a state of expanded intravascular volume, ranging from sodium and water retention to excessive sodium intake. As the fluid levels increase, so does the hydrostatic pressure. This forces fluid into the interstitial space, a process called "third spacing."

Diuretics, most commonly furosemide, cause the patient to lose fluid through diuresis by decreasing the absorption of sodium in the loop of Henle. As sodium is expelled, so too is water (Figure 3-8).

The therapeutic levels of furosemide differ from patient to patient. The Paramedic should obtain how many milligrams per dose the patient receives as well as the patient's total daily dose.

This information may be used as a starting point for emergency diuretic treatment. However, the use of furosemide as the first-line agent in acute pulmonary edema is rapidly declining.

Spironolactone is a potassium-sparing, commonly prescribed diuretic whose mechanism of action is not widely understood. Theoretically, it is an antagonist to aldosterone, competing for receptor sites in the distal renal tubule, and allows the excretion of sodium and chloride while preserving

potassium. Spironolactone is not a powerful diuretic, so it is often prescribed in conjunction with ACE inhibitors, digoxin, and other diuretics.

Other diuretics that the patient may be taking include the thiazides, such as hydrochlorothiazide. Hydrochlorothiazide works by interfering with the absorption of sodium in the distal renal tubules. Therefore, sodium, potassium, chloride, bicarbonates, and water are excreted. Common side effects of thiazides include hypoglycemia and hypokalemia.[10]

Digoxin

Digoxin, a cardiac glycoside, is a positive inotrope that increases the force and velocity of the contraction of the ventricles while decreasing the velocity of conduction through the AV node.

Although digoxin has been used for centuries for heart failure, there is little evidence that it improves mortality. Its primary use is to alleviate the symptoms associated with heart failure. Although digoxin is a relatively safe drug, sufficient blood levels are a requirement for its use due to a narrower therapeutic index than possessed by many other drugs. Patients who have high digoxin levels may experience anorexia, nausea, vomiting, diarrhea, and visual disturbances (such as a green–yellow halo around lights), along with ECG changes including bradycardia and a ladle-shaped ST segment.

Beta Blockers

A primary causative factor in the progression of heart failure is the compensatory mechanisms of the sympathetic nervous system. Norepinephrine increases rate and contractility through stimulating the beta 1 receptor sites. Beta blockers prevent this.

A patient receiving beta blocker therapy should *never* be suddenly taken off them. The sudden cessation may in fact cause a rebound tachycardia that may be fatal to the patient.

Past Medical History

Obtaining the medical history of a patient in heart failure is important not only because it helps the Paramedic focus the patient's attention, but also because it may lead the Paramedic to causative as well as comorbid factors that cause rapid deterioration or limited ability to compensate.

These comorbid factors include a history of acute myocardial infarction, cardiac infections, trauma, atrial fibrillation, or any other injury that decreases the preload (Table 3-7).

The Paramedic should also ascertain if the patient has a pacemaker and/or defibrillator implanted. If the patient has a defibrillator, the Paramedic should inquire if it has discharged and, if so, how many times.

If the patient were to present with an arrhythmia such as bradycardia or tachycardia, the Paramedic may consider the heart failure to be due to pacemaker failure. Patients with such devices implanted will have a card that will tell the healthcare provider the kind of device implanted, such as an atrial, ventricular, AV sequential, or demand pacemaker.

Conditions Leading to Heart Failure

Hypertension increases the amount of pressure that the left ventricle must exert to open the aortic semilunar valve and overcome the pressure within the aorta. This constant workload creates the hypertrophic ventricle and sets into motion the process of remodeling as previously described.

Table 3-7 Comorbid Factors Causing Possible Rapid Deterioration

- AMI
- Cardiac infections
- Trauma
- Atrial fibrillation
- Any disease/injury that decreases preload

Diabetes mellitus is a major causative factor for numerous diseases, including heart failure. It causes microvascular disease that decreases tissue perfusion, which leads to hypoxia and ischemia in many organs including the kidneys. This ischemia in the kidney leads to renal dysfunction that results in fluid overload and hypertension. Diabetes also results in macrovascular disease that leads to coronary artery disease and peripheral vascular disease, both of which may lead to heart failure.

Damage to heart valves can also lead to heart failure. The heart valves are made of endocardial tissue and therefore any dysfunction of the endocardium will affect the valves. Typically, acquired valvular disease may be due to inflammatory diseases such as rheumatic fever and endocarditis. Damage occurs leading to stenosis, preventing forward flow. This leads to hypertrophy. Regurgitation allows blood to leak back into the atrium, thereby causing the heart to work harder to maintain cardiac output. This leads to hypertrophy and, eventually, a decreased ejection fraction and failure (Figure 3-9). Complete failure of a valve is also possible, due to either disease or trauma, rendering the pumping action of the ventricle ineffective. This failure will present with sudden onset of symptoms if severe enough.

Cardiomyopathy is a general term that describes any functional or structural disease of the myocardium as a result of hypertrophy, dilation, rigidity of the walls, or constriction of the ventricles (Figure 3-10). Causes of cardiomyopathy may include exposure to infectious disease or toxins (such as alcohol or smoking), systemic connective tissue disease, or nutritional deficiencies. The resulting ventricular alteration impairs the heart's ability to act as an effective pump, thereby decreasing cardiac output and starting the compensatory mechanisms down the path into heart failure.

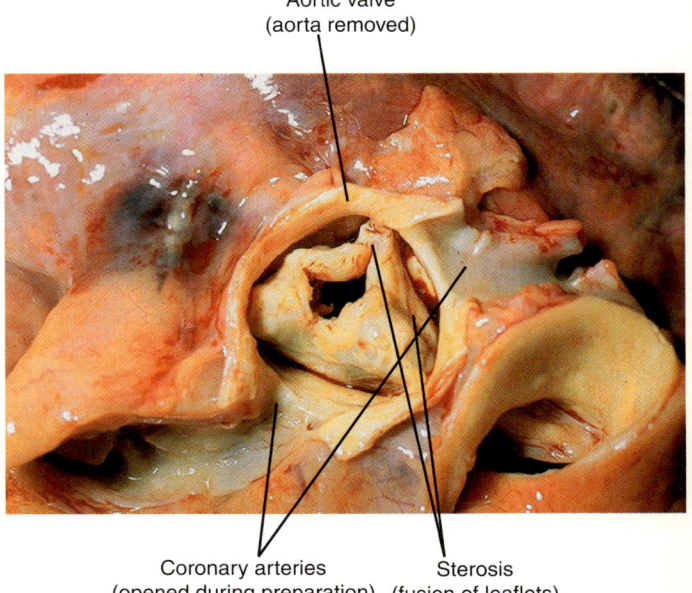

Aortic valve
(aorta removed)

Coronary arteries
(opened during preparation)

Sterosis
(fusion of leaflets)

CDC/ Dr. Edwin P. Ewing, Jr.

Figure 3-9 Valvular stenosis.

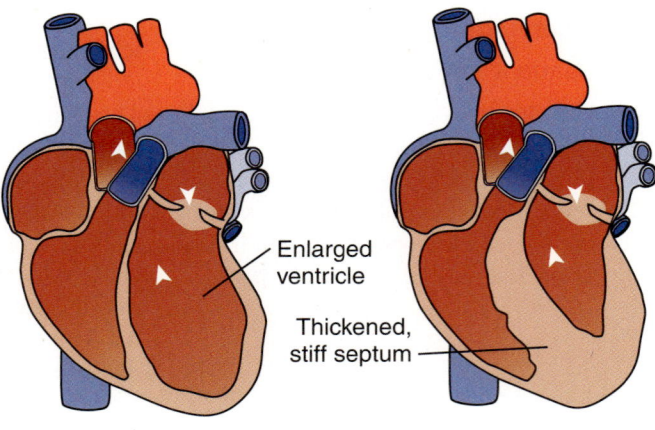

Cardiomyopathy

A condition in which a ventricle has become enlarged, thickened, and/or stiffened. As a result, the heart's ability to pump is reduced. Two types of cardiomyopathy include:

Normal

Dilated cardiomyopathy

Hypertrophic cardiomyopathy

Healthy septum

Healthy left ventricle

Enlarged ventricle

Thickened, stiff septum

Delmar/Cengage Learning

A healthy left ventricle pumps enough oxygenated blood to meet the body's needs.

An enlarged, weakened left ventricle struggles to pump enough blood to meet the body's needs.

Left ventricle cannot fully relax between heartbeats, resulting in less blood flow.

Figure 3-10 Cardiomyopathy.

Sexually transmitted diseases may also lead to heart failure. It is estimated that from 20% to as many as 70% of patients with acquired immunodeficiency syndrome (AIDS) have cardiac disease caused by the inflammatory response, drugs, and malignancies such as Kaposi sarcoma. Only about 10% of those patients with HIV have clinical manifestations resulting in left ventricular heart failure. These are usually due to ventricular dilation and dysfunction.

Obesity is another contributor to heart failure, as obese patients often develop left ventricular hypertrophy. To meet the increased demand on the heart from being overweight, the myocardium must increase in mass to perfuse the tissue and meet the increased oxygen demand.

These are only a few of the causative factors leading to heart failure. In fact, any disease that increases the workload of the heart or causes structural or functional damage can lead the heart into failure (Table 3-8).

Substance Use and Abuse

Patients who routinely use alcohol and illicit drugs, cocaine in particular, are at risk for heart failure. These drugs increase the heart's workload and oxygen demand, leading to the progression of heart failure.

Psychosocial

The Paramedic should obtain a psychosocial history as well. Elderly patients, for example, may forget to fill prescriptions or take their medication as prescribed. When a patient does not take her medications as prescribed, the levels fall below the therapeutic index, become ineffective, and the patient begins to develop symptoms of disease progression.

Table 3-8 Various Causes of Heart Failure

- Hypertension
- Diabetes
- Dyslipidemia
- Valvular heart disease
- Coronary or peripheral heart disease
- Myopathy
- Rheumatic fever
- Viral myocarditis
- Mediastinal irradiation
- Sleep disorders
- Exposure to toxic agents
- Collagen vascular disease
- Current or past alcohol consumption
- Smoking
- Sexually transmitted diseases
- Thyroid disorder
- Obesity

For example, a patient who fails to take her ACE inhibitor may develop uncontrolled hypertension, or a patient who fails to take his beta blocker may develop tachydysrhythmias, both of which may lead to heart failure and pulmonary edema. Many elderly patients utilize a daily medication dispenser. The Paramedic should check to see if the medications are emptied out of the days that have gone past. If a medication is in the current day's chamber, try asking the patient when she takes her medications, since some patients may take them later in the day. Unfilled prescriptions may be a little more difficult to determine; however, an astute observer may notice unfilled prescriptions in various places including on the refrigerator, kitchen table, or nightstands.

Last Oral Intake

Many patients with a previous diagnosis of heart failure keep track of their fluid intake and output (I/O) as well as their sodium consumption. The Paramedic should ask the patient when and what he last ate, as well as his fluid intake in terms of what, when, and how much.

CASE STUDY (CONTINUED)

Mabel is pale, maybe even a little cyanotic, and does not acknowledge their presence, nor does she look at them as they enter. Looking around the room, there are numerous prescription pill bottles on the kitchen table and a large pile of dirty dishes in the sink, some with rotting food. The house, which is usually very neat and clean, appears very disheveled and dirty. Mabel looks to have gained some weight and her ankles seem larger than normal. There are rales (crackles) in her lung bases and some wheezing in the apical aspects.

CRITICAL THINKING QUESTIONS

1. What are the elements of the physical examination of a patient with suspected congestive heart failure?
2. Why is an environmental assessment helpful?

Examination

Since the list of differential diagnoses is lengthy, and many of the conditions have similar presentations to that of heart failure, the Paramedic needs to be an astute observer when it comes to the assessment. A determination of heart failure generally occurs once several pre-established criteria are met during the patient assessment (Table 3-9).

The following assessment focuses upon findings specific to heart failure and its associated differential diagnosis. The Paramedic should still perform a thorough assessment on each patient.

Scene Survey

Chronic heart failure patients whose symptoms are not managed often have fatigue and dyspnea on exertion. These symptoms may prevent the patient from caring for his home. The Paramedic should look for clues that the patient may be unable to care for himself and may have little help in doing so.

Initial Assessment

First, the general impression of the heart failure patient is critical. The Paramedic must utilize the time taken to walk up to the patient to determine her stability. The Paramedic is not

Table 3-9 Framingham Criteria for the Determination of Heart Failure

- Major criteria (Figure 3-11)
  - Paroxysmal nocturnal dyspnea (PND)
  - Elevated jugular venous pressure (JVP)
  - Rales (fine crackles)
  - Cardiomegaly
  - Acute pulmonary edema
  - S3 gallop
  - Increased venous pressure
- Minor criteria
  - Extremity edema
  - Night cough
  - Dyspnea on exertion (DOE)
  - Hepatomegaly
  - Pleural effusions
  - Vital capacity reduced by 1/3 normal
  - Tachycardic (>120 bpm)

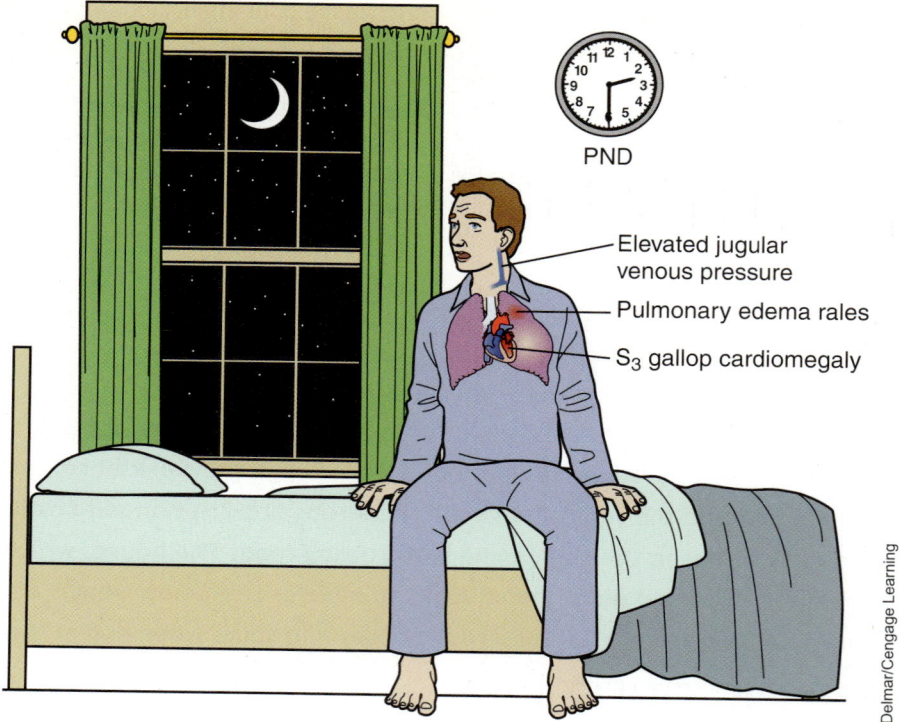

PND

Elevated jugular
venous pressure

Pulmonary edema rales

S₃ gallop cardiomegaly

Delmar/Cengage Learning

Figure 3-11 A patient meeting the Framingham major criteria for heart failure.

only evaluating the patient's level of consciousness, but her respiratory status as well.

Patients in heart failure may already be in respiratory distress. Therefore, the Paramedic must recognize this immediately since this distress may quickly develop into respiratory failure. Patients in respiratory distress have an increased breathing effort that may include nasal flaring, pursed lips, broken speech, retractions, tripod positioning, and audible adventitious breath sounds. However, they are compensating, getting the exchange of gasses that they need, and may be alert, looking around, sitting up, and talking (Table 3-10).

As the Paramedic forms his general patient impression, he will also determine the nature of illness (NOI). A patient grabbing or rubbing her chest while grimacing may be having chest pain, whereas a patient sitting upright in a tripod position is most likely having trouble breathing.

The patient's mental status demonstrates the patient's perfusion, oxygenation, and ventilation status as it shows that blood, oxygen, and sugar are getting to the brain and carbon dioxide is being removed. A patient in heart failure may exhibit signs of impairment in these processes, such as having an altered mental status as a result of acute respiratory distress or syncope. Typically, mental status changes of the patient in acute respiratory distress manifest themselves as apprehension, anxiety, confusion, or, in severe cases, head bobbing. All these lead to unconsciousness as the patient becomes fatigued, hypoxic, and hypercarbic. Although these may be signs of syncope as well, signs tend to lead more toward a decreased level of consciousness, as the brain is not perfused.

Table 3-10 Comparison between Respiratory Distress and Failure

	Respiratory Distress (compensating)	Respiratory Failure (not compensating)
Appearance	Alert	Altered mental status
	Interacts	Limited or no interaction
	Good muscle tone	Poor muscle tone
Work of Breathing	Increased (flaring, retractions, tripod)	Increased or decreased
Skin	Pink	Cyanotic/pale

Airway

Starting the assessment of a patient in heart failure with the ABCs (airway, breathing, circulation) is important since this disease may alter all three. In cases of severe APE, the patient may have pink or white frothy sputum that may develop within seconds. This sudden onset is often referred to as flash pulmonary edema. Any patient with an altered level of consciousness should be assessed for his ability to maintain his airway and given suction as needed.

Breathing

The Paramedic should assess the patient more thoroughly for signs of severe respiratory distress. These patients are leading to respiratory failure and may present with severe dyspnea, tachypnea, and inspiratory retractions in both the intercostal and supraclavicular regions.

Pulmonary edema is a key finding suggestive of backward heart failure. When listening to the lungs of a patient suspected of being in heart failure, the Paramedic should always listen carefully to the dependent areas.

The first change in breath sounds during pulmonary edema is actually an absence of breath sounds. As the pulmonary venous system distends, it compresses the adjunct airways, thereby diminishing air movement. These diminished breath sounds are difficult to ascertain without a baseline to compare them against. This fact stresses the importance of serial assessments.

The Paramedic may also encounter a patient who is wheezing. Wheezing signifies a narrowing of the lower airways and is typically heard upon exhalation as the patient tries to force air out. However, in severe cases, the wheezing may be both inspiratory and expiratory. Patients in heart failure may present with wheezing—known as cardiac asthma—as fluid begins to build up in the lungs, narrowing the passageways. In contrast, true asthma is an inflammatory process that causes the narrowing. Pneumonia patients and those with COPD may have wheezing as well. The wheezing in heart failure, COPD, asthma, and anaphylaxis is generally bilateral, whereas the wheezing in pneumonia is often localized.

Finally, the Paramedic may appreciate fine crackles, or rales. **Rales** are soft, short, high-pitched sounds usually heard in the late-inspiratory phase in the lower, or dependent, lung fields. They signify opening of the small airways and alveoli against fluid. Rales are generally bilateral and usually found in the dependent fields, as the fluid spreads out if the patient is seated. In severe cases, fine rales may be heard higher in the lung fields and may signify a serious condition.

Circulation

The Paramedic should start by assessing the presence, strength, regularity, and estimated rate of peripheral pulses. Weak or nonexistent peripheral pulses with tachycardia are signs of shock as the blood is being shunted to vital organs.

Patients with an irregular pulse may lead the Paramedic to think atrial fibrillation, which is common with heart failure patients, or premature ventricular contractions, which may occur with hypoxia. These signs may be present in any of the aforementioned conditions as each can cause hypoxia and shock.

The skin of a patient in heart failure will depend upon the major contributing factor to the illness. Skin color is important—hypoxia will lead to cyanosis (blue-tinted), shock will be pale, and cardiac insufficiency will be ashen, or gray. Skin temperature is also used to evaluate perfusion status. As a patient goes into shock, the body shunts blood away from the skin, making it cold. However, if in a cold environment, the body will do the same to preserve body heat. As with color and temperature, the condition of the body will also indicate the patient's perfusion status (i.e., is the patient's skin wet or dry?). However, this is not always easy to tell in a hot environment or if the patient was active prior to onset. The Paramedic should touch the patient with a gloved hand, then rub her fingers together. If she senses a greasy feeling, the wetness is sweat (diaphoresis). As blood is shunted away, the oil glands in the skin release their contents.

Focused Physical Exam

The focused physical exam supplements both the initial exam and the history. It allows the Paramedic to confirm his field diagnosis so he can work toward a plan of treatment. The focused physical examination of the patient with suspected heart failure should be completed in a head-to-toe fashion.

Head, Eyes, Ears, Nose, and Throat

Starting at the eyes, the Paramedic should assess the patient's conjunctiva (lining membrane of the eyelids). The conjunctiva is an excellent area to assess the patient's perfusion and oxygenation status, and is an ideal evaluation area for patients with dark complexions. Pale conjunctivas indicate a state of poor perfusion, as can occur with heart failure. Cyanosis demonstrates hypoxia and may be associated with many of the disease processes including heart failure.

Next, the Paramedic should evaluate the patient's oral cavity and mouth. She should look at the mucous membranes for similar findings as appeared at the conjunctiva. The Paramedic should also attend to how the patient speaks. If the patient stops speaking every couple of words to catch his breath, this is a sign of increasing dyspnea, especially if the patient is at rest. The Paramedic may describe this condition as *x* (number) word dyspnea. The patient's lips will also provide clues. Circumoral cyanosis is central cyanosis and a sign of hypoxia.

Jugular Venous Distention

With a patient supine at a 45-degree angle, the Paramedic should assess for jugular venous distention (JVD), an outward manifestation of jugular venous pressure. Jugular venous pressure has a direct correlation to right atrial pressure. If the jugular veins are engorged, it is a sign of increased right atrial pressure, suggestive of increased venous volume secondary to venous pooling.

Chest

Assessment of the chest is imperative in the patient experiencing dyspnea, chest pain, altered mental status, or any vague complaints such as fatigue. The Paramedic should take a "look, listen, then feel" approach to the assessment of the chest.

Heart failure will present with breath sounds that are similar bilaterally. Breath sounds heard in the patient experiencing heart failure may range from clear fields to extensive rales heard throughout all lung fields, which are representative of fulminate pulmonary edema.

Wheezing is another possible breath sound but it is important to reiterate the fact that not all wheezing is due to bronchoconstriction from asthma. It can also occur when airways are narrowed from an accumulation of fluid.

The Paramedic should look for accessory muscle use along with retractions in the subcostal, intercostal, or supraclavicular areas. Patients with a history of COPD may have well-defined (hypertrophied) accessory muscles from years of struggling to breathe. A prolonged expiratory phase is significant for air trapping, which is common with COPD and asthma.

While listening to the lungs, the Paramedic should assess for the transmission of sound as the patient speaks. The Paramedic should have the patient say, "Boy-oh-boy" and listen for how clearly it sounds. Normally speech is muffled when assessing the lungs; however, if one hears it clearly then this may signify that there is fluid from heart failure or consolidation from pneumonia.

The Paramedic should then place her hands on the patient's back and have him say, "Boy oh boy" as she feels for vibrations. With the exception of the second intercostal space on the right side and between the scapulas—areas both close to the bronchial bifurcation—little vibration should be felt.

Presence of a vibration may indicate consolidation of fluids as can occur with pneumonia. Percussion of the chest wall may be resonant; a dull thud would mean consolidation and possibly pneumonia.

Heart Sounds

One of the early signs of heart failure is a split heart sound. Normally the heart sounds, appreciated at the point of maximal intensity (PMI) at the fifth intercostal space at the midclavicular line, is the "lub–dub," of S1 and S2. Patients in heart failure may have a third sound, S3, having a cadence like "Ken-tuc-ky," signifying the split of S2 into two sounds. The S2 sound normally indicates the closure of the semilunar valves. Normally the two ventricles beat synchronously, thus creating one sound. However, when the heart is stressed, the left ventricle contraction is slower than the right ventricle. As a result, the second heart sound, S2, is split into S2 and S3. This splitting of the second heart sound is suggestive of a heart going into failure. In fact, 70% of patients over the age of 40 with an ejection fraction less than 30% will have this extra sound, known as an **S3 gallop** as the result of ventricular overdistention.[11]

Abdomen

As edema develops, the patient may develop fluid in the peritoneal cavity. The Paramedic should assess for **ascites**, serous fluid in the peritoneal cavity, by having one person press down firmly on the midline of the patient's abdomen while the Paramedic presses on one side of the abdomen, feeling for a wave transmission on the other side. If this wave is noted, the patient has ascites, which may indicate heart failure. The Paramedic should assess the upper right quadrant, feeling for the lower margin of the liver as well as tenderness. If noted, the liver is considered to be enlarged (hepatomegaly). This may be a sign of venous engorgement from heart failure or may indicate liver disease such as with cirrhosis.

Extremities

The Paramedic should take note of any nonpitting, hard, or pitting edema. If an impression is left, the Paramedic may make a measurement as to the severity of the edema. However, this may not always be feasible, so documenting a good description of the edema indicating its depth, how far up the leg it appears, and how long it remains depressed may be more beneficial. With heart failure, both extremities will have edema. A deep vein thrombosis (DVT) will generally only have edema of one extremity. The Paramedic should also note any weeping or redness to the extremity, for this may be a sign of **cellulitis** (skin infection). The Paramedic should remember that just because the patient does not have pitting edema, it does not mean that he does not have heart failure. Left ventricular failure, especially due to an acute cause (e.g., an acute MI), does not generally present with pedal edema.

Posterior

A patient who is lying in bed, such as in a nursing home, may not have pedal edema but will have edema in other dependent areas. Sacral edema is common in these patients and may be assessed in a similar manner.

Vital Signs

The signs and symptoms of heart failure, whether acute or chronic, manifest as a result of the catecholamine released by the sympathetic nervous system. The vital signs the Paramedic obtains should reflect this; otherwise, the Paramedic should look for other causes of the patient's complaint or consider that the patient is decompensating.

Blood Pressure, Pulse, and Respirations

Due to an increase in the sympathetic nervous system and the subsequent vasoconstriction, the blood pressure increases. However, in the case of APE, significantly high blood pressure may be the cause as it increases the hydrostatic pressure of the capillaries in the lungs. A low blood pressure demonstrates poor cardiac output and may be a grave sign in the patient in heart failure. The Paramedic must recognize an at-risk patient early by calculating the MAP, especially as she is giving medications that lower the blood pressure. As the MAP becomes closer to 60, there is less chance of perfusing vital organs such as the brain and kidneys. A patient with a MAP of 30 or below can be classified as being in decompensated shock.

The pulse will typically be fast due to the catecholamine release. However, in some cases it may be weak due to the decreased cardiac output. Patients on beta blockers may not be tachycardic due to the blockade of norepinephrine, causing a relative bradycardia and not allowing the compensatory mechanisms to work.

The Paramedic should assess for a **paradoxical pulse** (one that decreases during inhalation) by feeling for a weakening of the patient's radial pulse during inspiration. A more accurate measurement is made by taking the patient's blood pressure and noting a drop in the systolic pressure greater than 10 mmHg. This shows an abnormally increased pressure within the thoracic cavity and may be a result of asthma, COPD, pulmonary embolism, pneumothorax and tension pneumothorax, and anaphylaxis. However, a drop of less than 10 mmHg is normal; a patient in cardiogenic shock may also present with such a pulse.

As the oxygen levels in the blood decrease and the carbon dioxide levels increase, or as the patient becomes acidotic, the body compensates by increasing the respiratory rate. Patients in heart failure may have tachypnea with labored respirations as the airflow obstruction increases and the patient increases the use of accessory muscles. Slowing respirations, or **bradypnea**, is a sign of respiratory failure and impending respiratory arrest.

Pulse Oximetry (SaO$_2$)

Although pulse oximetry has become a common assessment tool in EMS, it may not be useful when used intermittently. It is best used in a continuous manner and by determining the patient's room air SaO$_2$ before oxygen administration. Although a room air SaO$_2$ less than 94% is abnormal, a SaO$_2$ less than 90% is indicative of hypoxemia.[12]

These readings may be misleading or even normal if the patient does not present with APE. A patient with a low saturation (< 94%) without APE suggests that a pulmonary disease may be complicating the heart failure. COPD patients, or those with other chronic pulmonary diseases, may live with a low SaO$_2$ and are usually the contributing factors to hypoxemia in heart failure. A falling SaO$_2$, despite treatment,

is a dire sign. The Paramedic must be able to recognize that the patient is in respiratory failure with impending respiratory arrest.

End-Tidal Carbon-Dioxide Measurement (EtCO$_2$)

Only recently has EtCO$_2$ monitoring become an important factor in patient assessment. Generally EtCO$_2$ monitoring is thought of as a way to verify placement of an endotracheal tube. However, as EtCO$_2$ monitoring becomes more widely accepted, it is able to give the Paramedic information about the patient's hemodynamic and respiratory status. For example, a patient with syncope will have little blood return to the lungs; therefore, EtCO$_2$ will be low. A high EtCO$_2$ in a well-perfused patient indicates **hypercarbia** (too much carbon dioxide in the blood) and may alert the Paramedic to impending respiratory failure, allowing her to prepare accordingly.

Cardiac Rhythms

Any patient complaining of dyspnea, chest pain, fatigue, or any other symptom that has been discussed in this chapter needs to have a 12-lead ECG performed to assess for ischemic heart disease, a major cause of acute heart failure. Patients with chronic heart failure should also receive assessment via 12-lead ECG, as ventricular dysrhythmias are common findings and may be directly related to mortality. It has been estimated that patients with heart failure have premature ventricular contraction (PVCs) approximately 78% of the time and periods of nonsustained ventricular tachycardia 43% of the time.[13]

Dysrhythmias in the patient with heart failure may be a result of the medication the patient is on, the disease process itself, or a combination of the two. Common ECG findings in the heart failure patient may include a significant U wave and flattened T waves as the result of diuretic-induced hypokalemia (low potassium in the blood). In this case, digitalis may cause a scooping, or sagging, ST segment and a prolonged PR interval.

Ventricular hypertrophy (Figure 3-12), a consequence of chronic heart failure, is evident on the ECG with greater-than-normal amplitude for the leads that are over that particular ventricle. Right ventricular hypertrophy (RVH) is seen in V1 with a tall R wave, right axis deviation, and many times T wave inversion. The R wave in V1 represents depolarization of the right ventricle that, in the case of RVH, is enlarged. Commonly RVH is caused by diseases that strain the right ventricle like COPD or any other chronic lung disease. With this increase in pressure that the right ventricle must pump against, a right ventricle strain pattern may be seen as ST depression and T wave inversion in leads V1 and V2. **Right atrial enlargement (RAE)**, an increase in the size of the right atrium, commonly accompanies RVH as evident by tall (≥ 2.3 mmHg) and peaked P waves in leads II and/or V1 (Figure 3-13).

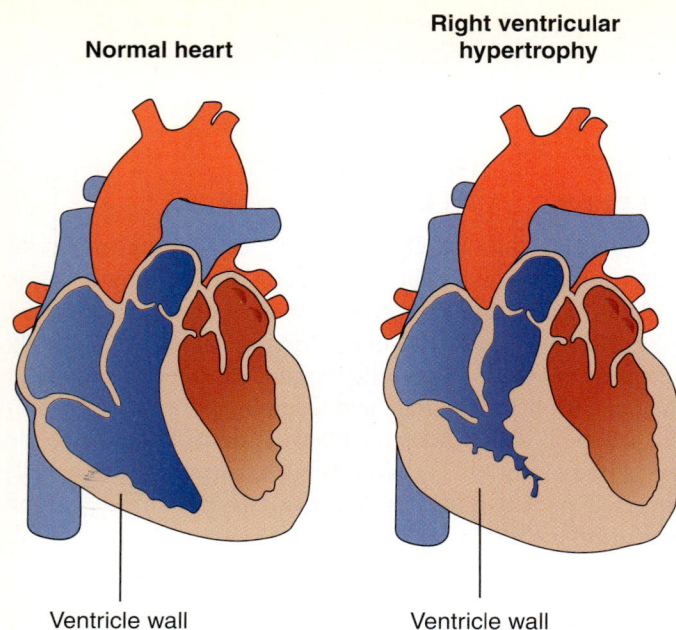

Normal heart

Right ventricular hypertrophy

Ventricle wall

Ventricle wall

Figure 3-12 Right ventricular hypertrophy.

Left ventricular hypertrophy (LVH), an increase in the muscle mass of the left ventricle, develops from increased resistance that the left ventricle must contract against to expel its contents, such as with hypertension. On the ECG, LVH may produce or even hide ST elevation and depression, and have tall, inverted T waves; this essentially includes all of the changes that the Paramedic uses to assess for ACS (Figure 3-14). The indication of LVH occurs by using one of three methods to look at the amplitudes of the R wave and, in one case, the S wave. One criterion used to determine the presence of LVH is if the sum of the height of the S wave in V1 and the taller of the two R waves in V3 or V6 is equal to or greater than 33 mm. The second is if the R wave in aVL is equal to or greater than 11 mm. The final criterion is if the R wave in V3 or V6 is equal to or greater than 27 mm. LVH may show a strain pattern as well, involving ST depression and T wave inversion in leads I, aVL, V3, and V6—the left-sided leads. Left atrial enlargement (LAE) may also accompany LVH, but most commonly because of mitral valve disease. LAE is present if the P wave is notched with 0.04 second between peaks in Lead II, the P wave starts above the isoelectric line then dips down and is ≥1 mm deep and ≥1 mm wide in V1, or if the P wave is ≥0.11 seconds wide in any lead.

Both severe tachycardias and bradycardias impede the forward flow of blood. Tachycardias do not allow the left ventricle to fill, thereby causing pulmonary edema, whereas bradycardias create a poor cardiac output. The Paramedic must be diligent in his assessment. Before he determines the treatment, the Paramedic must determine the underlying cause of the patient's dysrhythmia. The Paramedic should consider any of the aforementioned causes as well as hypoxia, which is an easy correction. Review of Chapter 2 will assist in differentiating these various causes.

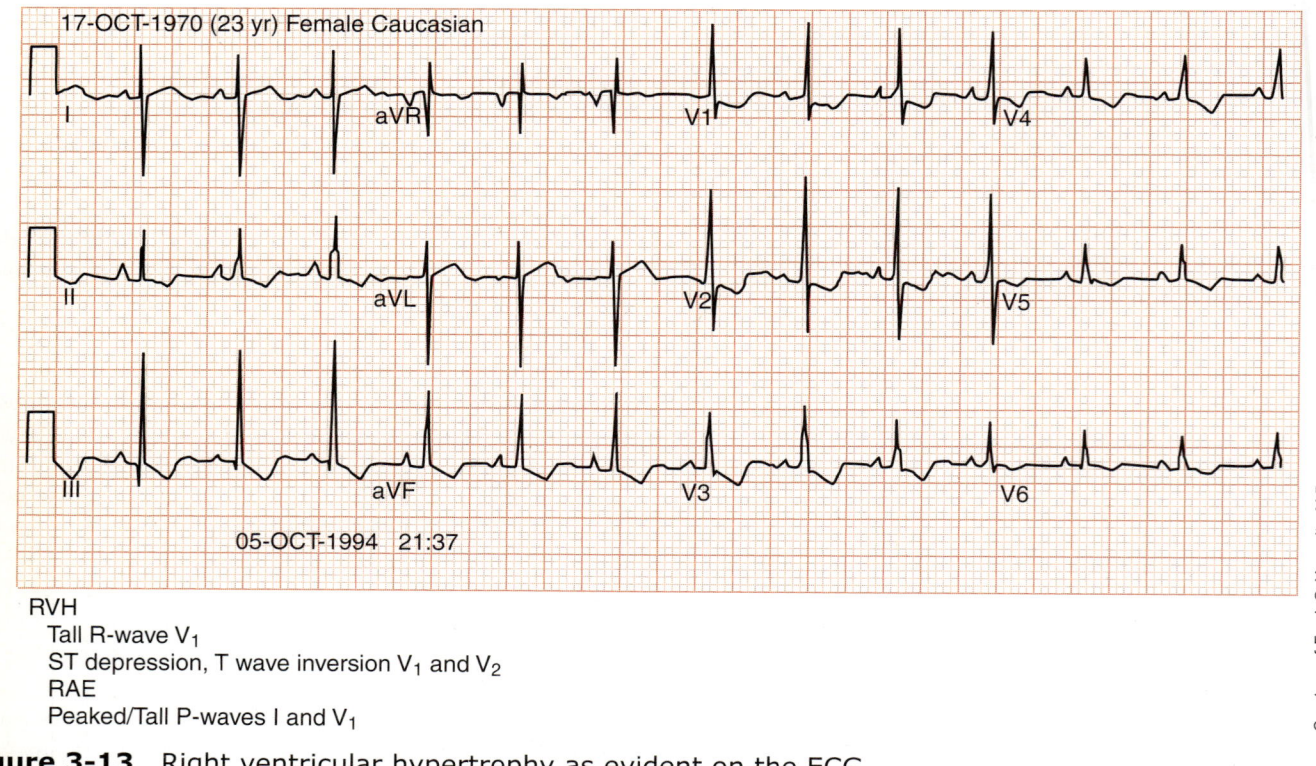

17-OCT-1970 (23 yr) Female Caucasian

I   aVR   V1   V4

II   aVL   V2   V5

III   aVF   V3   V6

05-OCT-1994   21:37

RVH
 Tall R-wave V$_1$
 ST depression, T wave inversion V$_1$ and V$_2$
 RAE
 Peaked/Tall P-waves I and V$_1$

Figure 3-13 Right ventricular hypertrophy as evident on the ECG.

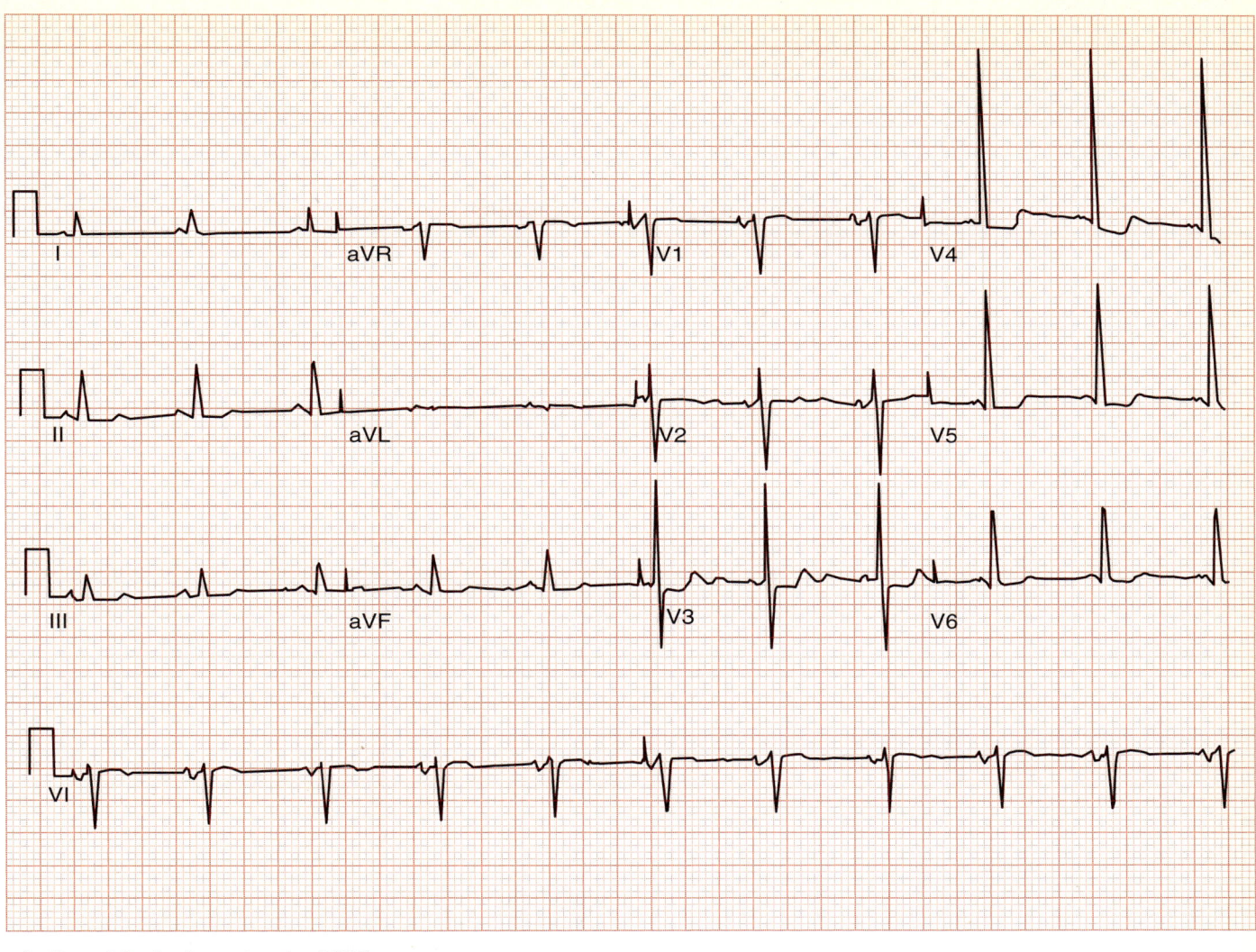

Left ventricular hypertrophy (LVH)

There are many different criteria for LVH.

- Sokolow + Lyon *(Am Heart J, 1949;37:161)*
  - S V1 + R V5 or V6 > 35 mm
- Cornell criteria *(Circulation, 1987;3: 565–72)*
  - SV3 + R avl > 28 mm in men
  - SV3 + R avl > 20 mm in women
- Framingham criteria *(Circluation, 1990; 81:815–820)*
  - R avl > 11 mm, R V4–6 > 25mm
  - S V1-3 > 25 mm, S V1 or V2 +
  - R V5 or V6 > 35 mm, R I + S III > 25 mm
- Romhilt + Estes *(AM Heart J, 1986:75:752–58)*
  - Point score system

Left atrial abnormality (dilatation or hypertrophy)

- M shaped P wave in lead II
- Prominent terminal negative component
  to P wave in lead V1 (shown here)

Figure 3-14   Left ventricular hypertrophy as evident on the ECG.

The Paramedics decide that Mabel appears to be in heart failure but are not sure of the type of heart failure that she is suffering. Although Mabel has signs of right-sided heart failure, the pulmonary edema is evidence that Mabel is in left-sided heart failure as well.

CRITICAL THINKING QUESTIONS

1. What is the symptom pattern for right-sided heart failure? Left-sided heart failure?
2. What factors complicate the diagnosis of suspected heart failure?

Assessment

Heart failure is a generalized term to define the heart's inability to meet the body's demands. Although classifying heart failure is not always necessary or possible to do in late stages, it may be helpful early in describing symptoms, discovering the causes, and proposing treatment.

Systolic versus Diastolic Heart Failure

Systolic dysfunction (low cardiac output) occurs when the impaired ventricle is unable to overcome the pressure in the receiving artery to expel its contents. These patients will present with signs of inadequate cardiac output that include weakness, fatigue, and reduced exercise intolerance. In severe cases, like with an AMI, the patient may present with signs of syncope.

Diastolic dysfunction impairs the heart's ability to relax and fill normally. Any injury or illness that elevates filling pressures may impede this process and are able to cause diastolic failure (high filling pressures). Constrictive pericarditis along with hypertensive and hypertrophic cardiomyopathy increase resistance to the ventricular inflow as well as reduce the capacity of the ventricle, thus decreasing the amount of blood the ventricle can receive and expel during systole. Acute myocardial ischemia and hypertrophic cardiomyopathy may impair ventricular relaxation, decreasing filling time and thus stroke volume. Myocardial fibrosis and infiltration cause the heart to dilate, creating chronic ischemia and restrictive cardiomyopathy. Oftentimes both diastolic and systolic heart dysfunction coexists.

High Output versus Low Output Heart Failure

High output heart failure leads to both peripheral edema and pulmonary congestion simultaneously because of elevated diastolic pressures and circulatory overload. These patients have an above normal cardiac output because of high contractility. If left untreated, systolic dysfunction occurs, the symptoms progress, and the cardiac output returns to normal levels or even lower. Eventually these patients develop the classic signs of heart failure. The causes of high output heart failure include hyperthyroidism, anemia, pregnancy, and arteriovenous fistulas (an abnormal connection between an artery and vein).

Low output heart failure is the more typical type of failure that the Paramedic may encounter and involves any state that decreases the cardiac output. It generally occurs secondary to ischemic heart disease, hypertension, dilated cardiomyopathy, valvular and pericardial disease, or any condition that impedes the forward flow of blood.

Acute versus Chronic Heart Failure

Acute heart failure develops abruptly, usually secondary to an illness or injury. The prototype is the normally healthy person who develops a massive myocardial infarction or acute heart valve rupture. The sudden reduction in cardiac output may cause syncope accompanied by acute pulmonary edema and left ventricular dysfunction.

Chronic heart failure occurs as the result of dilated cardiomyopathy and a general deterioration of cardiac function, which covers most of the patients with heart failure. Their physical presentation of peripheral edema and the other classic signs of heart failure are a result of fluid retention and the continued compensatory mechanisms of the neuroendocrine system.

Right-Sided versus Left-Sided Heart Failure

Although it is not completely true that one ventricle may fail without affecting the other, this is the most common way that providers classify heart failure, through describing the symptoms that the patient presents with.

An easy way to remember right versus left heart failure is that the signs and symptoms will relate to the structures before the dysfunctional ventricle. In the presence of chronic heart failure, patients will generally tend to develop biventricular heart failure.

Failure of the Right Ventricle

As the right ventricle fails as a forward pump, venous congestion develops, increasing the systemic blood pressure. As venous return diminishes the right atrium distends, neck veins engorge, the liver becomes congested, and peripheral signs (Table 3-11) of heart failure become evident. This occurs because the right ventricle is unable to keep up with venous return. Stroke volume decreases because of the lower preload (decreased return). Right atrial pressures then increase as well, affecting the pressure within the vena cavae and the rest of the venous system. As these pressures increase, so do the hydrostatic pressures in the periphery, forcing a fluid shift from the vascular system into the interstitial space. This causes the peripheral edema.

The causes of right ventricular heart failure are many. However, the most common cause of right-sided heart failure is left-sided failure. As the pressure in the pulmonary circulation is impeded, the pumping ability of the right ventricle decreases, causing it to create higher pressures to expel the blood. Other causes of right-sided heart failure include isolated right ventricular infarct as seen on V4R in the presence of an IWMI, infarct of the right atrium, valvular disruptions or infections such as with pulmonic stenosis, large pulmonary emboli, chronic hypertension, COPD, and cor pulmonale.

Patients will generally present with compensatory tachycardia from the neuroendocrine system as well as with venous congestion as noted by JVD and organ engorgement. Fluid accumulation may occur in dependent areas such as pedal or pedal aspects of the patient or in serous cavities like the abdomen, pleural space, and pericardium.

Failure of the Left Ventricle

Left ventricular heart failure may occur as a result of the heart being mechanically overloaded, as with aortic stenosis, or being weakened such as post-AMI. Whatever the cause, when the ventricle loses its ability to contract, it loses its

Table 3-11 The Peripheral Signs and Symptoms of Right-Sided Heart Failure

- Peripheral edema
- Ascites
- Nocturia
- JVP
- Hepatomegaly
- Right ventricular heave
- Abdominal tenderness

Table 3-12 The Pulmonary Signs of Left-Sided Heart Failure

- Dyspnea
- Orthopnea
- Rales (crackles)
- DOE
- Nocturnal cough
- PND

ability to pump blood to the body. As the forward flow is impeded, blood begins backing up, starting in the left ventricle, and progressing backward into the lungs. This causes increased pressure within the capillaries, causing fluid to leak out, and causing pulmonary edema. As the forward flow from the left ventricle slows, so does the flow throughout the remainder of the system, thus causing right failure and peripheral edema.

These patients will present with pulmonary symptoms (Table 3-12) and, if in the presence of right-sided heart failure, the peripheral signs as well. These patients may also have fatigue, cool extremities, diaphoresis, and in late stages confusion and memory impairment. Patients with decompensated left-sided heart failure may have a displaced apical beat typically to the left side because of **cardiomegaly** (enlarged heart). They may also have a pathologic S3 gallop as well as an S4 heart tone. Percussion will be dull and **tactile fremitus**, vibrations felt on the chest wall when the patient speaks, will be present.

Backward versus Forward Heart Failure

Backward heart failure is when the pressure develops in the vascular system before the ventricle increases. The ventricle is unable to expel its contents or fails to fill normally. Pressures within the atrium and venous system rise. The retention of sodium and water further increase the pressures within the systemic veins and capillaries, forcing fluid into the interstitial spaces. Left ventricular failure results in decreased cardiac output and causes an increase of the blood volume in the pulmonary vascular beds. This blood remains there as it is not able to empty into the overdistended and weakened left ventricle. The lung then has a greater perfusion when compared to ventilation, causing a V/Q mismatch.

Forward heart failure occurs when there is an inadequate discharge of blood into the arterial system, also known as decreased cardiac output. As perfusion to the renal system diminishes, it responds by activating the RAAS, reabsorbing sodium, and retaining water. Patients will present with fatigue, weakness, decreased urine production, and possibly hypotension and shock.

The Paramedics place Mabel on high-flow, high-concentration oxygen while sitting her up into a semi-Fowler's position. Mabel receives one sublingual nitroglycerin. Remembering their Paramedic class, the Paramedics recall that furosemide and morphine were part of the treatment for heart failure. They had, however, attended a cardiac symposium at the hospital last week and discuss that neither of those two drugs were talked about. In fact, they recall that the treatment of heart failure has changed drastically from the original class.

CRITICAL THINKING QUESTIONS

1. What is the typical treatment plan for patients with suspected heart failure?
2. What are some of the patient-specific concerns and considerations that the Paramedic should consider when applying this treatment plan that is intended to treat a broad patient population presenting with heart failure?

Treatment

As heart failure has shown an increase in prevalence, so too has the understanding of this multisystem disease. In recent years, the management of heart failure has undergone many changes, some requiring a new outlook on the previous treatment. Remembering that heart failure may present as acute respiratory distress and/or syncope, the goals of management are to improve both.

In the presence of acute respiratory distress because of cardiogenic pulmonary edema, the primary goal is to restore the balance of oxygen supply with that of oxygen demand by increasing diffusion within the alveoli, increasing cardiac output by improving the heart's pumping action, reducing the body's need for oxygen, decreasing the sum pressures, and decreasing sodium retention.

With the patient in a state of syncope (lack of awareness of one's surroundings), the Paramedic must base the management upon the cause by asking if this is a (1) rate problem, (2) pump problem, (3) volume problem, or (4) vascular resistance problem. The treatment for each may be different, so the patient's history, examination, and assessment will assist in this.

The toolbox that the Paramedic has for the treatment can be diverse. No matter how many of these treatments the Paramedic has access to, they should be methodical and thoughtful in their process. The Paramedic should not "throw everything" at the patient, but rather have a process whereby she gives a treatment and then assesses its effectiveness in relation to alleviating the patient's symptoms. This then assures that the patient receives the least invasive measures first, reserving the more invasive and potentially hazardous treatments for last.

Oxygenation and Ventilation

The most important treatment the Paramedic can give to any patient is ensuring both oxygenation and ventilation. To help balance oxygen supply and demand, the Paramedic should place the patient at rest by sitting him up into a high-Fowler's position with legs dependent. This will increase the lung volume and vital capacity while decreasing the work of breathing and venous return to the heart.

There may come a time when the Paramedic encounters a patient who is hypotensive and has pulmonary edema. Sitting this patient up will improve his ability to breathe while sacrificing cerebral perfusion, causing ischemia. However, lying this patient down will essentially drown him. These are patients that will require positive pressure ventilation via endotracheal tube with positive end expiratory pressure (PEEP) or **continuous positive airway pressure (CPAP)** (a method that maintains airway pressure above atmospheric pressure throughout the respiratory cycle) to ensure oxygenation occurs.[14–16] Once one of these treatments is applied, the Paramedic may then lay the patient down some. Using mean arterial pressure (MAP) may help the Paramedic determine the appropriate height for the patient.

Generally, these patients are hypoxic because of a ventilation/perfusion (V/Q) mismatch. This hypoxia causes pulmonary vasoconstriction and hypertension. Since the administration of oxygen will reverse this process, all patients should receive oxygen.

Typically the use of the nonrebreather mask in these patients is warranted. However, if the oxygen saturation levels are above 94% a nasal cannula may be chosen instead as long as the saturation levels are measured continuously, the patient does not have physical exam findings of severe respiratory distress, and it is acceptable per local protocol.

Non-Invasive Pressure Support Ventilation

Non-invasive pressure support ventilation is quickly becoming a standard in the treatment of patients with APE and many other respiratory diseases like COPD. There are two types of non-invasive pressure support ventilation: continuous

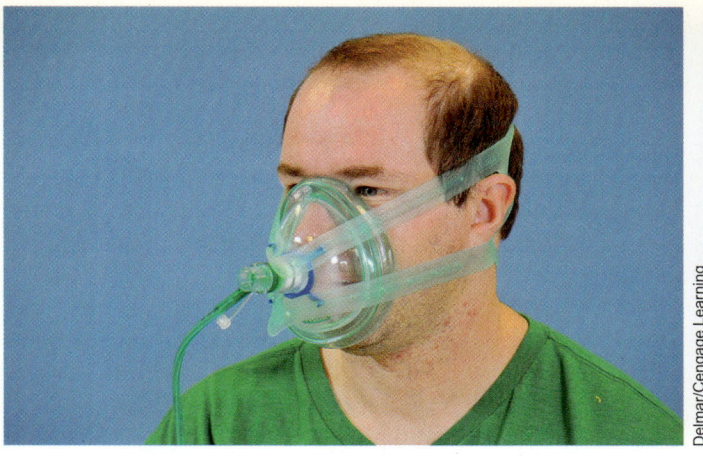

Figure 3-15 Non-invasive pressure support ventilation.

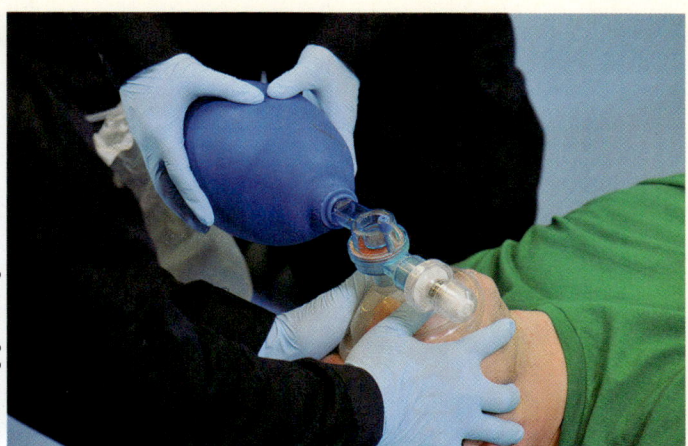

Figure 3-16 BVM with PEEP.

positive airway pressure (CPAP) and bi-level positive airway pressure (Bi-PAP). CPAP is the most common device found in EMS (Figure 3-15). It provides a constant pressure during both inspiration and expiration, whereas **bi-level positive airway pressure (Bi-PAP)** provides a lower pressure during expiration as compared to inspiration. Both require that the patient have spontaneous respirations, be conscious, and be able to maintain her own airway.

The concept behind non-invasive pressure support ventilation is that the positive pressure keeps the smaller airways open to enhance gas exchange. It increases alveolar pressures by keeping them open. It also increases thoracic cavity pressure, including the area around the left ventricle, making it easier to move blood into the system circulation. This "splinting open of the airway" from the positive pressure also significantly decreases the patient's work of breathing as the airways do not have to be reopened with every inhalation. Not only does non-invasive pressure support ventilation decrease the rate of endotracheal intubation by 30% to 90%, but it is the only heart failure treatment that, when initiated early, has shown to improve patient mortality.

For systems that do not use CPAP or Bi-PAP, the Paramedic may use a bag-valve-mask device to create a pseudo–non-invasive pressure support ventilation. The Paramedic will apply a PEEP valve to the exhalation port (Figure 3-16) of the bag-valve-mask assembly and ventilate the patient. This will take some coordination between the patient and Paramedic, but may eliminate the need to intubate the patient.

Tracheal Intubation

Although there is no contraindication to intubation, the Paramedic must weigh the consequences, specifically the weaning process of older adults from the ventilator. This may be very difficult to do with this patient population. However, if the patient requires invasive airway management due to apnea, prolonged transport, fluids in the airway, or if, despite treatment, the patient is becoming fatigued and respiratory failure is imminent, intubation is an option.

Typically, these patients will be conscious enough that the Paramedic will not be able to perform a standard endotracheal intubation. Therefore, the Paramedic must choose nasotracheal intubation or medication-facilitated intubation. Nasotracheal intubation is a standard method of securing an airway. However, the consequences (i.e., hemorrhage) may cause the Paramedic to defer this procedure.

Rapid sequence induction (RSI) intubation is a procedure for sedating and paralyzing a patient for intubation. Once accomplished, this may also help to decrease oxygen consumption. If the patient is to remain in a constant state of paralysis, the Paramedic needs to be sure the patient remains sedated. Otherwise, the oxygen consumption increases as the patient becomes conscious in this state of paralysis.

Facilitated intubation using medications such as morphine and diazepam to create a state of respiratory depression has many complications and, in some medical circles, is falling out of favor. The initial medications used for traditional RSI are short acting, whereas morphine and diazepam are longer acting and may induce hypotension. Morphine also has a negative impact on the heart that includes the release of catecholamines, an effect that could be detrimental to the failing heart. Once the patient has been intubated, the application of PEEP will perform much in the same way as CPAP does upon expiration.

Some emergency medicine physicians would state that giving a patient in heart failure beta 2 agonists would be detrimental to the patient as it increases the patient's heart rate and myocardial oxygen demand (MvO_2). Although this would not be the first treatment given, administering albuterol will improve oxygenation by dilating the constricted airways.

Intravascular Access

Obtaining intravascular access early in the patient with heart failure is important in that it not only provides a route to administer medications, but it also allows for the administration of fluid. Fluid boluses should be given to any patient that is showing signs of syncope, even if the patient has "wet" lung sounds. Most likely the pulmonary edema is a result of the decreased cardiac output due to an inferior wall MI, severe dehydration, or any other condition that causes hypovolemia. The pulmonary edema present in these patients is not a result of fluid overload but misdistribution of that fluid into the lungs and interstitial spaces by any of the aforementioned mechanisms. By providing fluid, the Paramedic is increasing the preload that increases stroke volume and, thus, cardiac output. This then in turn improves perfusion to the kidneys, allowing the patient to diuresis any extra vascular fluid.

Pharmacological Treatment

The focus of pharmacological treatment of the patient in heart failure is goal directed toward three problem areas: preload, afterload, and cardiac output. The end result of the treatment of heart failure is to improve cardiac output while controlling the rate and preventing an increased workload on the heart (Table 3-13).

Decreasing Preload

Decreasing the preload is the principal goal in the management of a patient in heart failure. This occurs by increasing the venous capacitance through vasodilatation and by eliminating fluid through diuresis.

Nitroglycerin

Nitroglycerin is the best and safest drug to use to decrease preload. It has limited adverse effects as well as a very short half-life, so if the patient's blood pressure drops the negative effects of the nitroglycerin will be brief.

Nitroglycerin should be used with caution, however, if the patient is hypotensive, has valvular heart disease, or suffers from an inferior wall MI with suspected right ventricular involvement.

Nitroglycerin is absolutely contraindicated if the patient has taken phosphodiesterase enzyme inhibitors (PDE$_3$), erectile dysfunction medications, within the previous 24 hours, as they will cause a state of severe hypotension that is often unresponsive to standard treatment.

Nitroglycerin is supplied sublingually by tablet or spray as well as topically. In the patient with heart failure, the topical method is not recommended because of the erratic absorption rate, especially if the patient is diaphoretic.

The Paramedic should administer 0.4 mg (400-mcg) of sublingual nitroglycerin every three minutes as long as the blood pressure remains above 100 mmHg systolic. Administration via the sublingual route allows 73% of the nitroglycerin to be absorbed. Therefore, of the 400-mcg tablet, the patient receives only 300-mcg over three minutes or 60 mcg/min (300 mcg divided by 3 minutes).[17]

Although only a few EMS systems carry IV nitroglycerin, every Paramedic that performs interfacility transport will encounter it. This is the best form of the drug to use, as it allows for immediate and 100% absorption while being easily titrated. The administration of IV nitroglycerin is more appropriate in the treatment of heart failure as compared to patients with ACS and demonstrates many benefits when higher dosing is used. Recommended dosing of IV nitroglycerin of a patient in heart failure should be set at least 100 mcg/min. In some cases, administering boluses at 300 to 600 mcg/min may be beneficial as well. Patients receiving these high doses of IV nitroglycerin have done well, decreasing the incidence

Table 3-13 Emergency Medications Used in the Treatment of Heart Failure

	Goal	Mechanism	Medication	Notes
Improve Oxygenation	Increase alveolar surface area and time for gas exchange	Pushing fluid out and keeping alveoli open Delay exhalation	CPAP/PEEP	The only treatment that has shown to be beneficial
Decrease Preload	Increase venous capacitance	Vasodilate	Nitroglycerin	Watch for IWMI Quick relief Also decreases afterload
	Increase fluid elimination	Increase diuresis	Furosemide	CAUTION If kidneys are not perfusing, will have delayed onset If not fluid overloaded, will lead to dehydration and hypokalemia
Decrease Afterload	Decrease systemic vascular resistance	Stop conversion of angiotensin I into angiotensin II	Captopril	Also reduces preload

of endotracheal intubation and length of stay. It has also resulted in faster resolution of pulmonary edema.[17]

Furosemide

Another method of decreasing preload is by decreasing the fluid within the venous container by diuresis. By administering a diuretic such as furosemide (a potassium-wasting loop diuretic), the venous volume is diminished.

For years furosemide has been the first-line drug for patients in heart failure, removing the extra fluid from the system. However, literature shows that the onset of diuresis is delayed, often up to 90 minutes post-administration. This delayed diuresis occurs with patients who have severe APE because the decreased perfusion to the kidneys allows for very little diuresis.

In most cases of heart failure, the patient is not fluid overloaded, but rather the body's fluids are maldistributed as a result of failing circulation. Administrations of furosemide to a patient without fluid overload, or to a patient not in heart failure (such as a patient with sepsis or pneumonia), may cause harmful side effects. These may include marked dehydration, electrolyte disturbances that may cause dysrhythmias, and a drop in cardiac output and stroke volume. For these reasons, furosemide has become a third-line drug after nitroglycerin and ACE inhibitors and may fall completely out of favor for the treatment of acute pulmonary edema. Furosemide may still play a role in exacerbations of chronic heart failure, however, in cases where the patient is clinically fluid overloaded.

Once reduction of the preload and afterload occurs, administration of furosemide has almost immediate effects because of increased perfusion of the kidneys.

Morphine Sulfate

For years morphine was the third drug of choice in heart failure. However, many clinicians increasingly feel that the use of it in the treatment of heart failure is not only inappropriate but also dangerous. There is no sound evidence that morphine helps, and there is mounting evidence through the Acute Decompensated Heart Failure National Registry (ADHERE) that the administration of morphine increases mortality, ICU admissions, rate of endotracheal intubation and mechanical ventilation, and hospital stays.[18] The administration of morphine was thought to cause vasodilatation, thereby decreasing preload through a release of histamine. However, this release also causes a release of catecholamines. This sudden venous dilation then causes an increase in heart rate and oxygen demand, two effects that can both worsen a patient's condition.

Another use of morphine was to reduce anxiety. For patients who are anxious, administration of a benzodiazepine would be more beneficial in treating anxiety with fewer side effects than using morphine.[17]

Decreasing Afterload

Decreasing the afterload is another step in pharmacologically treating a patient in heart failure. By decreasing afterload, cardiac output increases as the pressure by which the left ventricle pumps against is decreased. Some of the medications used to decrease afterload also simultaneously reduce preload.

Angiotensin-Converting Enzyme (ACE) Inhibitors

Angiotensin-converting enzyme (ACE) inhibitors are the treatment of choice when it comes to a patient in heart failure, especially if the patient is in renal failure or fluid overloaded. Typically, the use of ACE inhibitors has been with patients in chronic heart failure, but their use in acute situations is gaining popularity. In fact, they may be used in place of nitroglycerin when nitroglycerine is contraindicated.

There are two formulations and doses for ACE inhibitors. Enalaprilat (IV form of enalapril) is a single dose of 1.23 mg given IV, and captopril is a dose of 12.5 mg given sublingually. Both formulations cause a rapid reduction in afterload, as well as preload, by decreasing blood pressure, dilating the arterial system, improving cardiac output, and reducing volume by the excretion of sodium.

ACE inhibitors should be used with caution in patients with aortic stenosis, renal failure, or those who are hypotensive. ACE inhibitors should never be used in the patient who has experienced angioedema secondary to ACE inhibitors. Otherwise, they are very safe and hemodynamically stable drugs that have been shown to decrease hospital stays and rates of intubation.

Other Medications to Reduce Afterload

Nitroglycerin at lower doses decreases preload through venodilation. However, in high doses, nitroglycerine causes arterial dilation, reducing afterload. When given in combination with an ACE inhibitor, the resultant effects are greater than either drug given independently. Nitroprusside is another medication that reduces afterload by decreasing systemic vascular resistance. Generally, the use of nitroprusside is limited as it requires hemodynamic monitoring and it is extremely sensitive to light (it requires a foil covering), which causes logistical issues that make its prehospital use rare.

Drugs used to block the compensatory mechanisms of heart failure are also in use. They inhibit the effects of the neuroendocrine system by either blocking **beta receptors** (beta blockers) or blocking the conversion of angiotensin I into angiotensin II. Angiotensin II receptor blockers (ARBs) are increasing in their popularity as they block the effects of the RAAS system.

Beta blockers are not recommended in acute heart failure as it can drop the patient's blood pressure. Beta blockers tend to be used later after the acute event has improved to help reduce the remodeling that occurs in heart failure.

Inotropic Support

Some patients may not tolerate preload or afterload reduction, as with a patient in cardiogenic shock, and therefore may require inotropic support to maintain their blood pressure. Unfortunately, there is a high mortality rate as these medications are asking an already sick heart to work harder. Positive inotropics include catecholamines and phosphodiesterase inhibitors. **Intra-aortic balloon pumps** are also used in patients with cardiogenic shock to support the blood pressure and may be encountered during interfacility critical care transport.

Catecholamines, such as dopamine and dobutamine, provide temporary improvement of left ventricular function. Unfortunately, these medications cause tachycardias and increase myocardial ischemia as oxygen demand increases, although dobutamine does not cause the same release of endogenous norepinephrine as dopamine and therefore there is less tachycardia. Even though they appear to work initially, they do not improve the mortality rate. Oftentimes, patients with heart failure may be prescribed beta blockers that would suppress the inotropic agents. Essentially, they do not work in the end.

Treatment Summary

When dealing with a patient in heart failure and complaining of chest pain, the Paramedic must ask himself if the failure, combined with the body's compensatory mechanisms, is causing the chest pain or if the failure is due to an acute injury to the myocardium, causing left ventricular dysfunction. Chest pain is representative of cardiac ischemia. Hypoxia is a common cause and may be easily correctable in the patient with heart failure. The Paramedic should initially focus on improving myocardial oxygenation while decreasing myocardial workload through the administration of high-flow, high-concentration oxygen and nitrates. However, administration of thrombolytics to a patient suffering ischemia due to hypoxia who does not have a clot could be detrimental.

CASE STUDY (CONTINUED)

About five minutes into the transport, Mabel's work of breathing is diminished. This change isn't good, though, as Mabel's head bobs and she stops responding.

CRITICAL THINKING QUESTIONS

1. What are some of the predictable complications associated with acute coronary syndrome?
2. What are some of the predictable complications associated with the treatments for acute coronary syndrome?

Evaluation

Once treatment has begun, the Paramedic needs to continually reassess the patient and his response to treatment. The Paramedic should take vital signs every five minutes and consider serial 12-lead ECGs whenever a patient presents with a change. Be aware that a patient in heart failure may develop respiratory failure and/or cardiogenic shock.

Respiratory Failure

In ill patients, ventilatory oxygen consumption may increase upward of 20%. This then increases the patient's work of breathing and, if not corrected, fatigue sets in. The patient's ventilatory status declines and the patient becomes hypoxic and hypercarbic with respiratory acidosis soon to follow. These patients begin to develop an altered level of consciousness with the hallmark head bob, a slowing respiratory rate, and decreased work of breathing in the late stages. Alveoli begin to collapse, except in the apices, during exhalation. Pulmonary edema washes out the surfactant, increasing surface tension of the alveoli and requiring a considerable effort to reopen.

Breathing against resistance, such as with pursed lips or nasal intermittent positive pressure ventilation (NIPPV), prevents the collapse of the alveoli. The work of breathing decreases, relieving respiratory muscle fatigue and doubling the time that gas is exchanged. It also increases alveolar pressures and stops the movement of fluid into the alveoli.

Cardiogenic Shock

Cardiogenic shock, hypoperfusion attributed to the heart, is the most extreme form of pump failure. The left ventricular dysfunction is so great that it is unable to meet the body's metabolic demands, exhausting the compensatory mechanisms. Hypotension worsens the condition by decreasing coronary artery perfusion. This, in turn, suppresses cardiac performance, resulting in total pump failure.

Generally, cardiogenic shock is the result of extensive myocardial damage from a left ventricular infarct, diffuse ischemia, or decompensated heart failure. Hypoxia occurs as a result of V/Q mismatch that occurs early on in shock and decreases contractility. In late shock, the heart failure worsens, becoming irreversible due to the low state of perfusion.

Table 3-14 Triad of Cardiogenic Shock[11]

- Pump failure
- Pulmonary edema
- Hypotension

This continued state of hypoxia leads to anaerobic metabolism and respiratory acidosis as well as metabolic acidosis. In turn, renal perfusion decreases even more. Myocardial ischemia begins to develop, if it has not already, as the atrial pressures fall further, compromising contractility.

To determine if the patient is in cardiogenic shock, the Paramedic should assess for the presence of pump failure, pulmonary edema, and hypotension (Table 3-14). These patients will have a systolic blood pressure less than 80 to 90 mmHg and may have a drop of 30 to 60 points from baseline.

Evidence that blood is being shunted to the core is evident by peripheral vasoconstriction through cool, diaphoretic, and dusky/ashen skin. Cerebral hypoxia may present as restlessness, apprehension, confusion, apathy, lethargy, or even coma. Signs of left-sided heart failure may also be present. In addition, the patient may have compensatory tachycardia. The Paramedic should correct dysrhythmias first, for they may be the cause of failure.

Management of the patient in cardiogenic shock involves rapid transport in a supine position while maintaining the ABCs. The Paramedic should establish an IV and administer fluid boluses if the lungs are clear to maintain a MAP of at least 60 mmHg to perfuse the brain. If fluid is not effective, then the administration of vasopressors such as dopamine is warranted.

Stressors of Transport

Sometimes in EMS, the thought of "getting them there fast" is not always the best thing for the patient. The Paramedic also needs to consider that the emergency transport of the patient will have an impact upon the patient's condition and that temperature changes, noise, vibration, fatigue, and gravitational forces will all affect the patient as well, possibly in a negative way through activation of the neuroendocrine system.

For this reason, performing a complete assessment in the residence is beneficial. Once the patient is in the ambulance and transport has begun, there will be a catecholamine release causing changes to the patient's condition. If the heart failure is a result of an AMI, and the Paramedic is not careful, these stressors will further worsen the condition, as they increase the oxygen demand from the heart and may cause secondary infarcts.

The Paramedic and the driver should discuss the transport mode and route of travel before the transport begins. The driver needs to be aware as to how fast they stop, start, and take turns. They should also pick the smoothest route that has the fewest turns. The use of red light and sirens during transport has been under scrutiny for several years, with some studies showing that it may save, at best, 30 to 40 seconds. The Paramedic must weigh the costs versus the benefits to the patient when using red light and sirens.

CASE STUDY CONCLUSION

After placing Mabel on CPAP, her condition begins to improve. Mabel is transported to the regional medical center that specializes in cardiology. There they diagnose Mabel with class IV heart failure and schedule her for surgery to have a left ventricular assist device (LVAD) implanted.

CRITICAL THINKING QUESTIONS

1. What is the most appropriate transport decision that will get the patient to definitive care?
2. What are the advantages of transporting a patient with suspected heart failure to these hospitals, even if that means bypassing other hospitals in the process?

Disposition

The destination hospital may be one of the most important decisions that a Paramedic makes in relation to the patient's treatment. If the patient is experiencing signs and symptoms consistent with ACS or if the patient's 12-lead ECG demonstrates an STEMI, then transport to a hospital with interventional cardiology that performs cardiac catheterization and cardiac surgery is crucial. If the transport time is greater than 30 minutes, the Paramedic may consider air medical transport. Transportation to these specialty centers may allow placement of devices such as implanted pacemaker/defibrillators to prevent harmful dysrhythmias or other devices to improve cardiac output.

Mechanical Circulatory Support

As more patients are diagnosed with heart failure, the Paramedic may encounter more medical devices either in the interfacility transport environment or at the patient's home. The Paramedic should have a basic understanding of these devices.

Ventricular Assist Devices

Ventricular assist devices are implanted "mechanical hearts" that perform the duties of the dysfunctional ventricle and are generally reserved for patients who have end-stage heart failure and are awaiting transplant.[19]

Ventricular assist devices consist of an intake tube, a pump, and an output tube that are implanted and have an external power source, emergency battery backup, computer controller, and in some cases a hand pump. They are classified as left ventricular (LVAD), right ventricular (RVAD), or biventricular (BiVAD). Ventricular assist devices work by diverting blood from the dysfunctional ventricle into an artificial pump that then returns to the adjoining vasculature. For example, a left ventricular assist device diverts blood from the left ventricle into the pump and returns the blood into the aorta (Figure 3-17).

VADs are becoming increasingly prevalent, as studies have shown recovery of the myocardium with their use. Many patients are going home with these devices, so the chances of the Paramedic encountering such a device is increasing. However, their use should not be a surprise as hospitals are charged with educating not only the families, who are the best resource, but the community and EMS personnel as well. Most likely EMS will arrive when the pump has failed. If this occurs, the patient will present with signs of inadequate perfusion. If a hand pump is available, the Paramedic should attempt to use that first, assessing for improvement in patient status. If the patient is in cardiac arrest, chest compressions are not contraindicated but should only be attempted *after* trying to use the hand pump.

There are numerous VADs on the market with different operating and care instructions, and new ones now in development. In-depth care of the patient with a VAD, as well as all the different types of alarms and conditions possible, is beyond the scope of this chapter.

Intra-Aortic Balloon Pumps (IABP)

Placement of an intra-aortic balloon pump (IABP) occurs when all other measures have failed to increase the cardiac output and the patient develops cardiogenic shock. This involves placing a balloon in the aorta that inflates during diastole, increasing perfusion to the coronary arteries and myocardium. During systole, the balloon deflates, decreasing the afterload on the left ventricle. The goal of IABP treatment is to increase myocardial oxygen supply and cardiac output while decreasing myocardial oxygen demand.

Although the Paramedic will not encounter a patient with an IABP at home, she may be involved in transporting a patient with one. This is an involved process as the IABP connects to a large external console that includes the power supply, inflation control, monitor, and gas cylinder. The Paramedic will typically never have to transport these devices alone, since the sending facility generally has a team responsible for the IABP that will accompany the Paramedic (Figure 3-18).

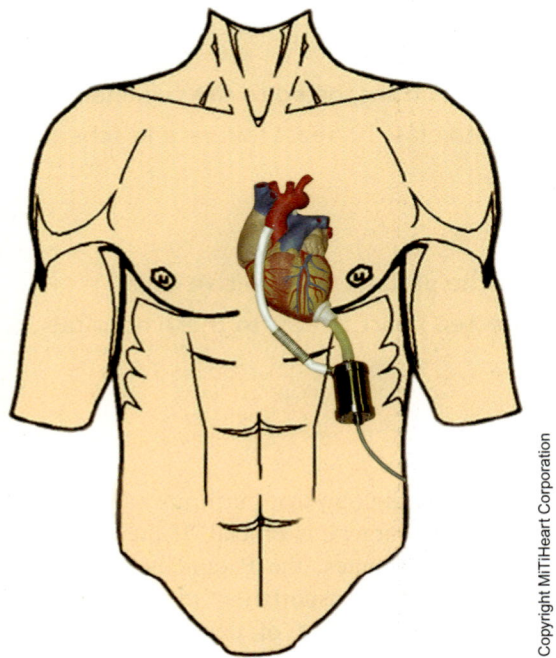

Figure 3-17 Left ventricular assist device (LVAD).

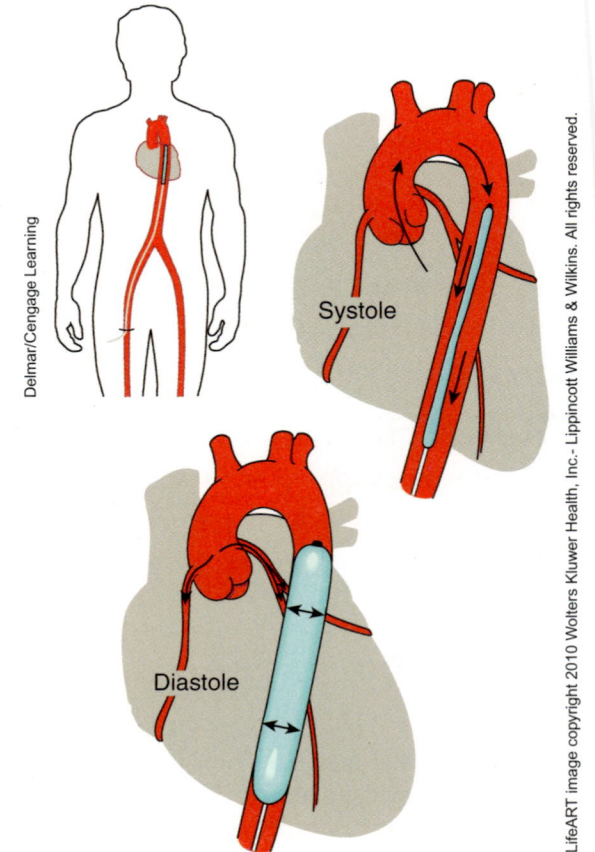

Systole

Diastole

Figure 3-18 Intra-aortic balloon pump (IABP).

CONCLUSION

Because heart failure involves many different systems and may be a result of any number of causes, the Paramedic must be diligent in obtaining an accurate history and performing a detailed assessment. The Paramedic must then take a look at the various differential diagnoses and determine if the patient fits the criteria of heart failure.

Studies have shown that the misdiagnosis of heart failure is common (18% to 42%) and that inappropriate treatment may be harmful.[17,18] Studies have also shown that 23% of the patients given furosemide developed significant electrolyte imbalances and hypotension requiring fluid boluses.[18] Treatment with both furosemide and morphine found a 22% mortality rate where nitroglycerin alone had only a 2% rate.

While it may be difficult to differentiate between heart failure, COPD/asthma, and pneumonia, standardized treatment with bronchodilators, nitroglycerin, and NIPPV while avoiding morphine and furosemide is typically the standard of care.[17,18]

The treatment of heart failure should focus on improving oxygenation through NIPPV while reducing preload and afterload with nitroglycerin and ACE inhibitors. The Paramedic needs to constantly reassess the patient and assess how the treatment has affected her, both positive and negative effects, as he transports her to an appropriate facility.

KEY POINTS:

- Heart failure is the only cardiovascular disease increasing in prevalence in the United States.

- Heart failure is the ineffectiveness of the pump which may have many etiologies and is considered multisystem in nature.

- Heart failure may present as a chronic condition or an acute condition.

- Patients in heart failure usually call EMS due to dyspnea.

- Whenever the body senses a decrease in oxygen, compensatory mechanisms are activated.

- The heart normally spends one third of its time in systole and two thirds in diastole. An increasing heart rate decreases coronary artery filling time.

- Activation of the renin-angiotensin-aldosterone system by the autonomic nervous system leads to increased preload and afterload.

- Pulmonary edema is less likely caused by fluid overload than by inappropriately distributed fluid.

- The heart changes its size and shape to meet demands placed upon it. The term for these changes is "remodeling."

- Ventricular hypertrophy is an increase in muscle mass caused by increased demands.

- Initially hypertrophy of the left ventricle assists in pumping capability but continued hypertrophy and the left ventricle becomes stiff and rigid.

- Intrinsic myocardial damage results from direct injury to the myocardium.

- Extrinsic causes result from forces outside of the heart.

- The extent of failure results from the amount of activation of the sympathetic nervous system and the hemodynamic changes caused by excessive fluid.

- Patients in heart failure often present in respiratory distress.

- In addition to signs of respiratory distress, the patient may show signs of decreased urine output, nocturia, and weight gain.

- Medications used by patients for control of their heart failure include:
  - Nitrates
  - ACE inhibitors
  - Diuretics
  - Digoxin
  - Beta blockers

- Many comorbid factors can lead to or exacerbate heart failure.

- Once the initial assessment has been completed, assessment must include multiple body systems, since heart failure is a multisystem disorder.

- Pulse oximetry is best used as a continuous device to monitor trends.

- Dysrhythmias in heart failure may result from medications used to control the heart failure, the disease process, or a combination of the two.

- As the heart is a multichamber device which pumps to low and high pressure systems, heart failure has been classified in multiple ways:
  - Systolic versus diastolic failure
  - High output versus low output
  - Acute versus chronic
  - Right side versus left side
  - Backward versus forward

- Emergent interventions for heart failure concentrate upon oxygenation and hemodynamic changes:
  - CPAP or Bi-PAP
  - Decrease preload
  - Decrease afterload

- In-hospital treatments may also include use of an intra-aortic balloon pump and left ventricular assist device.

- A triad of abnormalities are seen in cardiogenic shock:
  - Pump failure
  - Pulmonary edema
  - Hypotension

- Ventricular assist devices are similar to a mechanical heart.

- Intra-aortic balloon pumps increase coronary blood flow by inflating during diastole and decreasing afterload by rapid deflation at the beginning of systole.

REVIEW QUESTIONS:

1. How does the autonomic nervous system affect heart failure?
2. Compare the amount of time that the heart normally spends in diastole with the amount of time it spends in systole. How does an increase in heart rate affect this?
3. Name at least three of the following:
   - Intrinsic causes of heart failure
   - Extrinsic causes of heart failure
   - Abnormal volume load on the left ventricle
4. Name the two factors responsible for the degree of dysfunction in the left ventricle.
5. Describe the focused assessment that should be performed for a patient with heart failure.
6. Name the five classifications of heart failure.
7. Name the triad of abnormalities seen in cardiogenic shock.

CASE STUDY QUESTIONS:

Please refer to the Case Study in this chapter, and answer the questions below:

1. What initial differential diagnoses do you have for weakness and shortness of breath?

2. What is the significance of the patient's weight gain and swollen ankles? If these are the only signs, what type of failure is the patient likely in? What type of failure is present if there are rales and wheezing?

3. Which medications or interventions decrease preload? Which decrease afterload?

4. How does NIPPV decrease the work of breathing?

REFERENCES:

1. Hunt SA, et al. ACC/AHA 2005 guidelines update for the diagnosis and management of chronic heart failure in the adult. *Circulation.* 2005;112:1825–1852. Available at: **http://circ.ahajournals.org**. Accessed June 16, 2007.

2. Tintinalli J, et.al. *Emergency Medicine.* New York: McGraw-Hill, Medical Pub. Division; 2004.

3. Pikilidou MI, Lasaridis AN, et al. Blood pressure and serum potassium levels in hypertensive patients receiving or not receiving antihypertensive treatment. *Clin Exp Hypertens.* 2007;29(8):363–373.

4. Peacock WF, Mueller C, et al. Emergency department perspectives on B-type natriuretic peptide utility. *Congest Heart Fail.* 2008;14(4 Suppl 1):17–20.

5. Chung T, Sindone A, et al. Influence of history of heart failure on diagnostic performance and utility of B-type natriuretic peptide testing for acute dyspnea in the emergency department. *Am Heart J.* 2006;132(3):949–953.

6. Shiels HA, White E. The Frank-Starling mechanism in vertebrate cardiac myocytes. *J Exp Biol.* 2008;211(Pt 13):2003–2013.

7. No author listed. Cardiac asthma. *Lancet.* 1990;335(8691):693–694.

8. Jorge S, Becquemin MH, et al. Cardiac asthma in elderly patients: incidence, clinical presentation and outcome. *BMC Cardiovasc Disord.* 2007;7:16.

9. Aufderheide T, Brady W, Gibler W. Acute ischemic coronary syndromes. In: Marx JA, Hockenberger RS, Walls RM, eds. *Rosen's Emergency Medicine: Concepts and Clinical Practice* (Vol. 2), third edition. St. Louis: Mosby; 2002:1017.

10. Shorr RI, Ray WA, et al. Antihypertensives and the risk of serious hypoglycemia in older persons using insulin or sulfonylureas. *JAMA.* 1997;278(1):40–43.

11. Mattera CJ. Heart failure and pulmonary edema: understanding and correcting problems with the body's amazing pump. *J Emerg Med Serv.* 2000;23(3):36–47.

12. Hess D. Detection and monitoring of hypoxemia and oxygen therapy. *Respir Care.* 2000;43(1):63–80; discussion 80–83.

13. Ballew CC, Reigle J. Mechanisms and management of ventricular dysrhythmias in heart failure. *AACN Clinical Issues: Advanced Practice in Acute and Critical Care.* 1998;9(2):208–224.

14. Levitt MA. A prospective, randomized trial of BiPAP in severe acute congestive heart failure. *J Emerg Med.* 2001;21(4):363–369.

15. Philip-Joet FF, Paganelli FF, et al. Hemodynamic effects of bilevel nasal positive airway pressure ventilation in patients with heart failure. *Respiration.* 1999;66(2):136–143.

16. Craven RA, Singletary N, et al. Use of bilevel positive airway pressure in out-of-hospital patients. *Acad Emerg Med.* 2000;7(9):1063–1068.

17. Mattu A. (Speaker). *Cardiac Update* (Audio podcast EM2321). San Francisco: Audio Digest Emergency Medicine; 2006;23(21).

18. Peacock WF, Hollander JE, et al. Morphine and outcomes in acute decompensated heart failure: an ADHERE analysis. *Emerg Med J.* 2008;23(4):203–209.

19. Aggarwal S, Slaughter MS. Acute myocardial infarction complicated by cardiogenic shock: role of mechanical circulatory support. *Expert Rev Cardiovasc Ther.* 2008;6(9):1223–1233.

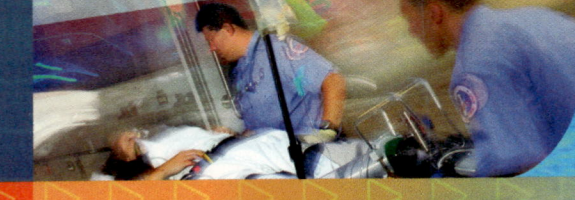

CHAPTER 4

ERRORS OF AUTOMATICITY

KEY CONCEPTS:

Upon completion of this chapter, it is expected that the reader will understand these following concepts:

- Automaticity as an etiology of dysrhythmia
- The ability to identify, given an ECG strip in either Lead II or MCL1, dysrhythmias caused by a change in automaticity
- The treatments for dysrhythmias caused by an error of automaticity

ANATOMY CONCEPTS:

Prior to reading this chapter the Paramedic student should be familiar with the following anatomy and physiology concepts:

- Cardiac conduction
- Myocardial cell electrophysiology
- Electrolyte balance

The Paramedics are called to a local factory for a 52-year-old male who is complaining of weakness, some dizziness and a "fluttering" in his chest. The foreman says that Aaron, one of his best machine operators, came to work today looking "green" around the edges and now is hunched over at his machine. During the walk back to the patient, both Paramedics talk about causes of weakness coupled with dizziness.

CRITICAL THINKING QUESTIONS

1. What is the implication of "fluttering" in the chest and what are some of the possible causes of cardiac-related weakness and dizziness?

2. How is weakness related to his fluttering in the chest?

OVERVIEW

A dysrhythmia, an irregular cardiac rhythm, occurs whenever the rhythm is not a sinus rhythm. Dysrhythmia can be either a rhythm with a rapid rate, called a **tachydysrhythmia**, or a rhythm with a slower rate, called a **bradydysrhythmia**.

In the past, these dysrhythmia were defined by ECG characteristics. However, as the science of medicine has advanced, via electrophysiology mapping of the heart, the origins of these dysrhythmias have been identified and an improved system of dysrhythmia classification was devised upon these findings.

The origin of a dysrhythmia, **arrhythmogenesis**, can be caused by either an **error in automaticity**, a disorder of impulse formation, or by an **error of conduction**, in which an impulse takes an altered pathway through the heart (Table 4-1). While it is difficult to accurately determine the cause of dysrhythmia in the field, generalizations made about a common dysrhythmia can provide clues to the dysrhythmia's effect on cardiac output and help drive decisions as to which treatments would be most effective to terminating the dysrhythmia.

Chief Concern

The chief concern of weakness and dizziness can be precipitated by a varied number of disorders in the body. It is important for the Paramedic to consider the possibility that a dysrhythmia can decrease cardiac output, resulting in decreased blood flow to the brain or cerebral perfusion. Dysrhythmia can alter the hemodynamics of the heart and may lead to a significant decline in cerebral blood flow, even in otherwise healthy individuals.[1]

Dysrhythmia caused by a change in automaticity—either an increase in automaticity or a decrease in automaticity—may lead to a faster or slower heart rate than can be tolerated by the patient, resulting in a number of symptoms including lightheadedness, syncope, chest pain, and shortness of breath.

Normal Automaticity

Normally the sinoatrial (SA) node is the primary pacemaker of the heart, at a rate of 60 to 100 bpm, and the atrioventricular (AV) node is the latent or backup pacemaker, at a rate of 40 to 60 bpm. Under normal conditions, the sinus node has the fastest automaticity and thus its rate of depolarization controls the rate and rhythm of the heart. This concept is called **dominance**, where the fastest pacemaker assumes control of the rate of depolarization of the atrium and ventricles. These areas beat as one in synchrony, a concept called **syncytium**.

Table 4-1   Chart of Dysrhythymias by Origin

	Abnormalities in Conduction	Abnormalities in Automaticity
Bradyarrhythmias	**Conduction Block**	**Decreased Automaticity**
	SA block	Sinus bradycardia
	AV block	Wandering atrial pacemaker
	Bundle branch block	
Tachyarrhythmias	**Re-entry {Short RP Interval}**	**Increased/Abnormal Automaticity {Long RP Interval}**
	Atrial flutter	Sinus tachycardia
	AV nodal re-entry tachycardia (AVNRT)	Atrial fibrillation
	Wolff–Parkinson–White	Focal atrial tachycardia
	AV re-entrant tachycardia (AVRT)	Accelerated junctional tachycardia
	Ventricular tachycardia	Multifocal atrial tachycardia
		Junctional ectopic tachycardia

The sinoatrial node is faster because it has an increased slope in phase four of the action potential: the repolarization phase. The slope of phase four readily responds to chemical changes on the cell membrane caused by the autonomic nervous system. These biochemical changes either accelerate or inhibit the SA node, allowing the SA node to change the heart rate according to conditions.[2]

Errors in Automaticity

However, any of the heart's pacer cells or conduction cells can be affected by chemical changes—such as hypoxia, acidosis, and hyperkalemia, for example—that lead to errors in automaticity (Table 4-2). Therefore, any chemical changes in the sinus node, along the internodal conducting tracts, AV junctional tissue, bundle of His, right or left bundle branches, and the Purkinje fibers, or out in the myocardium can result in dysrhythmia due to an error in automaticity.

Accelerated Automaticity

Factors that can accelerate the heart's automaticity include medications, hypoxia, ischemia, and stimulation of the autonomic nervous system. Stimulation of the sympathetic branch of the autonomic nervous system—from fear, pain, or medications such as beta agonists, for example—will cause an increase in the slope of phase four, effectively increasing the spontaneous conduction of the myocardium. This is called **accelerated automaticity**. Conversely, depression of the parasympathetic branch (i.e., the vagus nerve) with medications such as atropine, a parasympathetic antagonist, will allow the sympathetic nervous system to predominate and thus increase automaticity.

Fibers of both the sympathetic and parasympathetic branches serve the atrial tissue from the sinus node and down to the level of the AV node. The ventricular tissue is served by sympathetic fibers only. Therefore, parasympathetic antagonists, such as atropine, are ineffective when the error of automaticity arises from the ventricles.[3]

Additionally, any increase in the body's metabolic needs from fever, work, or exercise will stimulate the sympathetic branch and can cause an increase in the heart rate. That rate increase is limited by the pacing and/or conducting tissues' ability to form impulses.

Ischemia-Induced Increased Automaticity

Myocardial ischemia can also cause increases in cellular automaticity. The myocardial ischemia can be due to a local thromboembolic event in the coronary arteries or from global hypoxia from a pulmonary embolism. As a result of ischemia, cellular membranes can no longer maintain the ion gradients necessary, resulting in varying repolarization rates and subsequent spontaneous depolarizations.

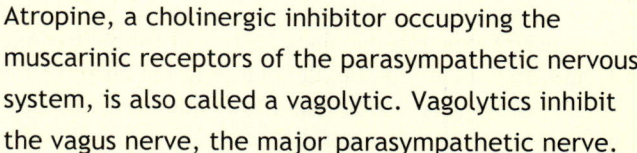

STREET SMART

Atropine, a cholinergic inhibitor occupying the muscarinic receptors of the parasympathetic nervous system, is also called a vagolytic. Vagolytics inhibit the vagus nerve, the major parasympathetic nerve.

Regular Narrow Complex Tachycardia

The initial approach to dysrhythmia analysis is to ascertain if the rhythm is regular or irregular. Irregular rhythms, by their nature, signify dysrhythmia, regardless if the rate is within the normal range. Therefore, the assessment of dysrhythmia can be done with a simple pulse check. This immediately puts the Paramedic on alert that there is a potential cardiac problem.

The next step is to determine if the QRS complex is wide or narrow. A wide complex QRS is more ominous and suggests a ventricular origin for the rhythm. Ventricular dysrhythmias need immediate attention and may require rapid intervention.

Table 4-2 Rhythms Attributed to an Error in Automaticity

- Increased automaticity
  - Narrow QRS complex
    - Regular rhythm
      - Sinus tachycardia (ST)
      - Focal atrial tachycardia (FAT)
      - Accelerated junctional rhythm (AJR)
      - Junctional ectopic tachycardia (JET)
    - Irregular rhythm
      - Multifocal atrial tachycardia (MAT)
      - Atrial fibrillation (AF)
  - Wide QRS complex
    - Regular rhythm
      - Accelerated ventricular rhythm (AVR)
- Ectopic beats
  - Supraventricular ectopic beats
    - Premature atrial complex (PAC)
    - Premature junctional complex (PJC)
  - Ventricular ectopic beats
    - Premature ventricular complex (VPB)
- Decreased automaticity
  - Narrow QRS complex
    - Regular rhythm
      - Sinus pause
      - Sinus bradycardia (SB)

The first set of dysrhythmias due to errors of automaticity is the regular narrow complex tachycardia, then the irregular narrow complex tachycardia, then the wide complex tachycardia. Following the tachycardias will be errors of automaticity that lead to bradycardia. The last set of dysrhythmias discussed are not abnormal rhythms, as rhythms are the regular recurrent beating of the heart, but rather irregular beats, called ectopic beats, that interfere with the underlying rhythm.

Many of the regular narrow complex tachycardias are due to either excessive sympathetic stimulation (by such sympathomimetic drugs as cocaine or medications such as epinephrine, for example), digitalis toxicity, or both.

Sinus Tachycardia

The pacemaker in a sinus tachycardia is the sinus node. When the sinus rhythm exceeds 100 beats per minute, it is called a **sinus tachycardia**. Sinus tachycardia rarely causes a rhythm problem for most patients and it may be considered benign (although troublesome to the patient). The appearance of sinus tachycardia may indicate the use of stimulants like caffeine. Sinus tachycardia is a normal response to a wide range of activities, including exercise, in most people.

Conversely, sinus tachycardia may be a sign of a pathological process. For example, ischemia of the SA node can cause sinus tachycardia. In approximately 55% of people, the sinus node gets its blood from a coronary artery that branches from the right coronary artery, and in the remaining 45% the blood comes from the left circumflex. Ischemia, as a result of occlusion of these coronary arteries, can cause a tachycardia to ensue.[4]

Similarly, the SA node is very sensitive to chemical, pressure, and temperature changes within the body, and constantly adjusts rates to meet various conditions and the body's needs (Table 4-3). Hyperthermia, acidosis, and hypovolemia can also cause a sinus tachycardia.

Impulses formed in the sinus node will follow the internodal and Bachmann bundle, depolarizing the atria. Following the delay at the AV node that allows augmentation of the diastolic volume in the ventricles, the impulse will follow the conduction pathways down the bundle of His and bundle branches to ultimately depolarize the ventricles.

Dysautonomia, a disorder of the autonomic nervous system which enhances sinus automaticity, can cause a patient's heart rate to be abnormally high, even at rest, and cause the patient's heart rate to increase with the slightest provocation.

One condition that is the result of dysautonomia is the **syndrome of inappropriate sinus tachycardia (SITS)**. SITS is most often seen in younger women and has no apparent stimulus (i.e., no physiological etiology such as hypoxia, hypoglycemia, hypovolemia, etc.) to explain the sudden increase in heart rate to 140 to 150 bpm. The mechanism is thought to be hypersensitivity of the SA node. The patient often presents with palpitations, dyspnea, dizziness, and syncope.

Table 4-3 Increased Automaticity—Sinus Node

- Physiologic
  - Pain
  - Anxiety
  - Exercise
- Pathologic
  - Hypoxia
  - Hypoglycemia
  - Hypovolemia
- Pharmacologic
  - Beta/adrenergic agonists
    - Albuterol
    - Dopamine
    - Epinephrine
    - Methylxanthine
      - Caffeine
  - Increased serotonin levels
    - Antidepressants
    - Selective serotonin reuptake inhibitors (SSRI)
  - Sympathomimetics
    - Cocaine
    - Methamphetamine

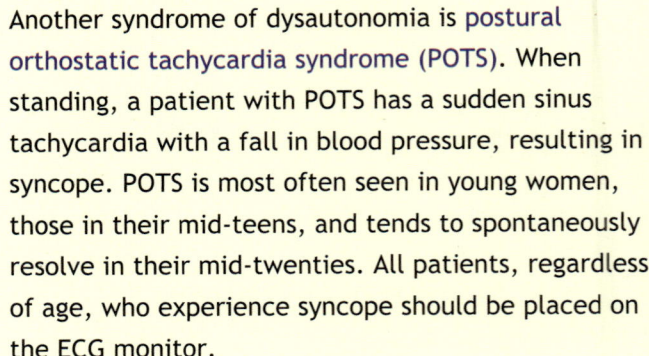

STREET SMART

Another syndrome of dysautonomia is postural orthostatic tachycardia syndrome (POTS). When standing, a patient with POTS has a sudden sinus tachycardia with a fall in blood pressure, resulting in syncope. POTS is most often seen in young women, those in their mid-teens, and tends to spontaneously resolve in their mid-twenties. All patients, regardless of age, who experience syncope should be placed on the ECG monitor.

Focal Atrial Tachycardia

Focal atrial tachycardia, sometimes called ectopic atrial tachycardia, is the result of an enhanced automaticity in the atrium, usually near the pulmonary veins proximal to the atrial septum, that creates very fast heart rates. The ectopic foci fires at rates typically around 150 bpm with a range of 100 to 250 bpm. However, unlike atrial flutter, these automatic atrial tachycardias have a 1:1 conduction rate through the AV node. Thus, heart rates of greater than 200 beats per minute are possible.

A focal atrial tachycardia may occur during periods of increased sympathetic stimulation, such as hypoxia, hypoglycemia, exercise, when taking sympathomimetics such as xanthines (coffee, theophylline) or cocaine, or even when ingesting alcohol.[5] Digitalis has been implicated as the cause of some focal atrial tachycardias.

The elderly may occasionally experience paroxysmal atrial tachycardia, a burst of 100 to 150 bpm that lasts for only minutes and then spontaneously subsides. Depending on the patient's cardiovascular health, he or she may be asymptomatic, may only be aware of palpitations, or may experience syncope.

Focal atrial tachycardia can be difficult to distinguish from sinus tachycardia, particularly if the heart's rate is between 100 and 120 bpm. The only distinguishing characteristic may be the shortened PR interval. Also characteristic of atrial tachycardia is the warm-up phenomena, where the heart rate gradually speeds up and then slowly terminates. Focal atrial tachycardia has been implicated as a cause of atrial fibrillation, another rhythm arising from an error of automaticity.

Wandering Atrial Pacemaker

A **wandering atrial pacemaker (WAP)** is thought to be akin to a multifocal atrial tachycardia, without the tachycardia. It appears that ectopic foci within the atria start to compete with the SA node in a subtle manner whereby some sinus impulses may create depolarization and others do not.

A wandering atrial pacemaker has been observed in some patients while they sleep, particularly if the patients have obstructive lung disease. In other cases, a wandering atrial pacemaker is thought to occur because of structural damage to the atria or as a result of the effects of medications such as digitalis.

A wandering atrial pacemaker has three or more morphologically different P waves and an irregular PR interval, representing the shifting pacemakers and a heart rate less than 100 bpm. As a result, the rhythm is irregularly irregular and may be mistaken for slow atrial fibrillation. However, atrial fibrillation does not have any P waves.

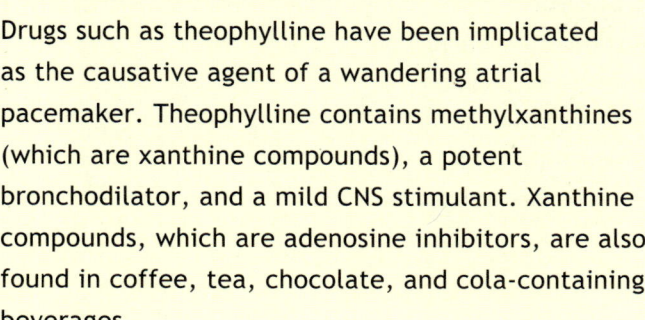

STREET SMART

Drugs such as theophylline have been implicated as the causative agent of a wandering atrial pacemaker. Theophylline contains methylxanthines (which are xanthine compounds), a potent bronchodilator, and a mild CNS stimulant. Xanthine compounds, which are adenosine inhibitors, are also found in coffee, tea, chocolate, and cola-containing beverages.

Accelerated Junctional Rhythm

An **accelerated junctional rhythm** is any junctional rhythm faster than the inherent automaticity of the AV node (i.e., faster than 60 bpm). A junctional tachycardia is a junctional rhythm that is faster than 100 bpm. An accelerated junctional rhythm is the result of the AV node spontaneously depolarizing faster than the SA node, and thus gaining dominance.

Two common causes of an accelerated junctional rhythm are ischemia, typically due to an occlusion of the right coronary artery that supplies blood to the AV node, and digitalis toxicity. Hemodynamically speaking, an accelerated junctional rhythm is generally well-tolerated by the patient who is not aware of its presence.

Junctional Ectopic Tachycardia (JET)

Junctional ectopic tachycardia (JET) is a rare dysrhythmia thought to be due to increased automaticity of an ectopic focus, probably outside of the AV node and near the bundle of His. Junctional ectopic tachycardia has been noted following valvular surgery, after IWMI, during active endocarditis secondary to rheumatic fever, and with digitalis toxicity.

Junctional ectopic tachycardia is not typically triggered by a premature atrial complex and is not responsive to adenosine, making it difficult to treat. Amiodarone may be used to control ventricular response if adenosine is unsuccessful in converting the rhythm.

Irregular Narrow Complex Rhythms

An irregular narrow complex tachydysrhythmia is either atrial fibrillation with a rapid ventricular response or an atrial flutter with a varying conduction ratio. In the first case, atrial fibrillation with a rapid ventricular response, the rhythm is irregularly irregular and can even be detected in the patient's pulse. In the second case, atrial flutter with a varying conduction ratio, the rhythm is regularly irregular, meaning that a pattern of grouped beats, such as a burst of beats, can be felt in the patient's pulse.

Multifocal Atrial Tachycardia

At least two ectopic atrial foci are needed to create **multifocal atrial tachycardia (MAT)**. The resultant rhythm appears like ectopic atrial tachycardia. However, as a result of the competing ectopic foci, the rhythm is irregular.

This rhythm is often experienced by patients with exacerbation of their chronic lung disease. Chronic obstructive lung diseases, such as emphysema, create pulmonary hypertension, which leads to right ventricular strain and right ventricular hypertrophy.[6] As a result of the hypertrophy, remodeling of the right ventricle occurs and gives rise to increased atrial automaticity.

Sudden hypoxia can initiate multifocal atrial tachycardia. The Paramedic must assess for signs of hypoxia and increased work of breathing, while placing the patient in a position so as to maximize the patient's lung expansion while decreasing the work of breathing. Adequate ventilation alone may lead to a conversion of the rhythm before any medications are given.

Other conditions implicated in MAT include heart failure, particularly with pulmonary edema; sepsis, particularly with adult respiratory distress syndrome; and methylxanthine overdose. Methylxanthine is found in caffeine and theophylline.

Atrial Fibrillation (AF)

Atrial fibrillation (AF) is a common ECG dysrhythmia affecting some two million Americans, a far greater percentage than any other dysrhythmia. In addition, the incidence of atrial fibrillation increases with age, from 0.5% for the fifth decade to 8.8% of the population in the eighth decade, with an average of 5% of patients over the age 65 experiencing atrial fibrillation.[7]

The causes of atrial fibrillation and atrial flutter are numerous, including thyrotoxicosis (i.e., symptomatic hyperthyroidism), electrolyte abnormalities (such as hypocalcemia), and even acute alcohol intoxication. Atrial fibrillation is also thought to occur in cardiac conditions (including acute myocardial infarction and pericarditis) and pulmonary diseases (such as pulmonary embolism).

Atrial fibrillation can be divided into three classifications, according to presentation: uncontrolled atrial fibrillation, paroxysmal atrial fibrillation, and persistent atrial fibrillation. By definition, uncontrolled atrial fibrillation is an atrial fibrillation with a rapid ventricular response (greater than 100 bpm). The first manifestation of atrial fibrillation can be an uncontrolled atrial fibrillation that makes the patient symptomatic. Alternatively, uncontrolled atrial fibrillation can be the result of inadequate medication (e.g., secondary to noncompliance).

Patients can also experience paroxysmal atrial fibrillation as a result of any number of temporary or potentially reversible conditions (Table 4-4). These patients become symptomatic secondary to the atrial fibrillation, then the atrial fibrillation spontaneously resolves. These are cases where the atrial fibrillation is thought to be due to an error in automaticity. In some cases, these episodes of atrial fibrillation are so short lived that the Paramedic's ECG may be the only evidence of paroxysmal atrial fibrillation.

Patients with persistent atrial fibrillation often do not use medication, either because the atrial fibrillation is resistant to medications or the side effects of the medications make taking the medications undesirable. In addition, some patients can tolerate the atrial fibrillation and do not need medication. There are a number of complications that can occur as a result of persistent atrial fibrillation, including dilated cardiomyopathy with concomitant remodeling of the heart. However, the single largest danger of atrial fibrillation may be in the development of strokes, discussed in more detail under the Treatment section.

Atrial fibrillation and atrial flutter can also have another common etiology: a re-entry phenomena, or error of conduction, discussed in Chapter 5 regarding tachycardia.

During atrial fibrillation, irregular waves of depolarization rain down on the AV node. The AV node propagates those waves at an irregular rate, according to its ability to accept another depolarization. As a result, the ECG rhythm becomes irregularly irregular, a hallmark of atrial fibrillation.

During atrial fibrillation, the atria are never depolarized as a unit, since multiple impulses depolarize small areas. Without atrial contraction, the heart loses the "atrial kick," or augmented end-diastolic ventricular filling, that increases the cardiac output by 30%. Thus, there is a substantial loss of cardiac output.[8,9] To maintain the cardiac output in the face of dropping stroke volume, the heart increases its rate: $CO = HR \times SV$.

Table 4-4 Conditions Causing Atrial Fibrillation

- Uncontrolled hypertension
- Hypothermia
- Heart disease
- Mitral valve disease
- Atrial ischemia
- Atrial fibrosis
- Inflammatory diseases
- Pericarditis
- Amyloidosis
- Intoxications
- Caffeine
- Alcohol (Holiday Heart)
- Endocrine disorders
- Pheochromocytoma
- Hyperthyroidism
- Pulmonary hypertension
- Pulmonary embolism
- Surgery
- Heart transplant

Digitalis Toxicity

A drug used for the control of atrial fibrillation is digitalis, though its use has started to decline in favor of alternative therapies such as atrial pacemakers. Digitalis, an old world medicine, is a cardioglycoside that provides a positive inotropic effect to the heart as well as a negative chronotropic effect.[10] It exerts its effects by binding to the sodium–potassium pump and increasing the intracellular sodium and calcium. The increased sodium and calcium increases the slope of phase four, slowing conduction, and allowing for a longer contraction.

Digitalis, through its effects on calcium, also affects the SA and AV node. These pacemakers are sensitive to changes in calcium levels. As a result of the increased intracellular calcium, digitalis slows the SA node and has a vagal effect on the AV node, both slowing the rate of conduction. This is a negative chronotropic effect.

There are a number of causes of digitalis toxicity. The most obvious would be an overdose—intentional or accidental—secondary to errors in administration or prescription. Taking twice the dose can lead to minor toxic effects. A more likely cause of digitalis toxicity is electrolyte imbalance. Digitalis affects intracellular concentrations of sodium and calcium. Therefore, any abnormalities in the sodium–potassium balance and/or calcium levels could lead to a form of pseudotoxicity.

Hypokalemia (low potassium levels) can intensify effects of digitalis upon the sodium–potassium pump, resulting in toxic effects. Causes of hypokalemia include use of common potassium-wasting diuretics (such as furosemide) or diarrheal losses. Similarly, low calcium levels (hypocalcemia) can also lead to digitalis toxicity. As the kidneys control electrolyte balance, any renal dysfunction, perhaps secondary to forward heart failure (i.e., cardiogenic shock), could lead to digitalis toxicity.

Cardiotherapeutic medications can also exacerbate digitalis toxicity. Drugs within the Vaughn–Williams classification I (sodium channel blockers, such as procainamide), classification II (beta/adrenergic blockers), or classification IV (calcium channel blockers, such as diltiazem or verapamil) can aggravate digitalis toxicity. Amiodarone, which has effects on sodium, potassium, and calcium channels, is used to treat patients with atrial fibrillation but also can exacerbate digitalis toxicity.

Since digitalis affects intracellular sodium and calcium levels, it can affect nervous tissue as well as muscle tissue. Systemic effects of digitalis toxicity upon the central nervous system include lethargy, headaches, visual changes, and even hallucinations. A classic sign of digitalis toxicity is impact on the optic nerve. The patient who is digitalis toxic will visualize yellow–green halos around lights as well as decreased visual acuity.[11] The latter may cause the patient to seek assistance from an optometrist.

One of the more troubling effects of digitalis toxicity is nausea, vomiting, and diarrhea, with concurrent abdominal pain. Vomiting and diarrhea can lead to digitalis toxicity; likewise, digitalis toxicity can lead to vomiting and diarrhea (Figure 4-1). In some cases, the impetus for digitalis toxicity is a minor stomach virus, which causes vomiting and/or diarrhea, leading to digitalis toxicity and more vomiting and diarrhea, and so on, and so on, and so on.

Since digitalis can affect both the conduction system and the myocardium directly, it can cause errors of automaticity and errors of conduction. It can also cause almost any dysrhythmia except sinus tachycardia and atrial fibrillation with a rapid ventricular response. Through a combination of increased automaticity and depressed conduction, digitalis toxicity can cause paroxysmal atrial tachycardia, multifocal atrial tachycardia, sinus bradycardia, and ventricular ectopy.

Regular Wide Complex Tachycardia

Under normal circumstances, a wide complex tachycardia would be cause for concern. However, the accelerated idioventricular rhythm is a transitional rhythm toward sinus rhythm. Strictly speaking, an accelerated idioventricular rhythm is not a tachycardia; however, it is relatively tachycardic compared with the normal idioventricular rate of 20 to 40 beats per minute.

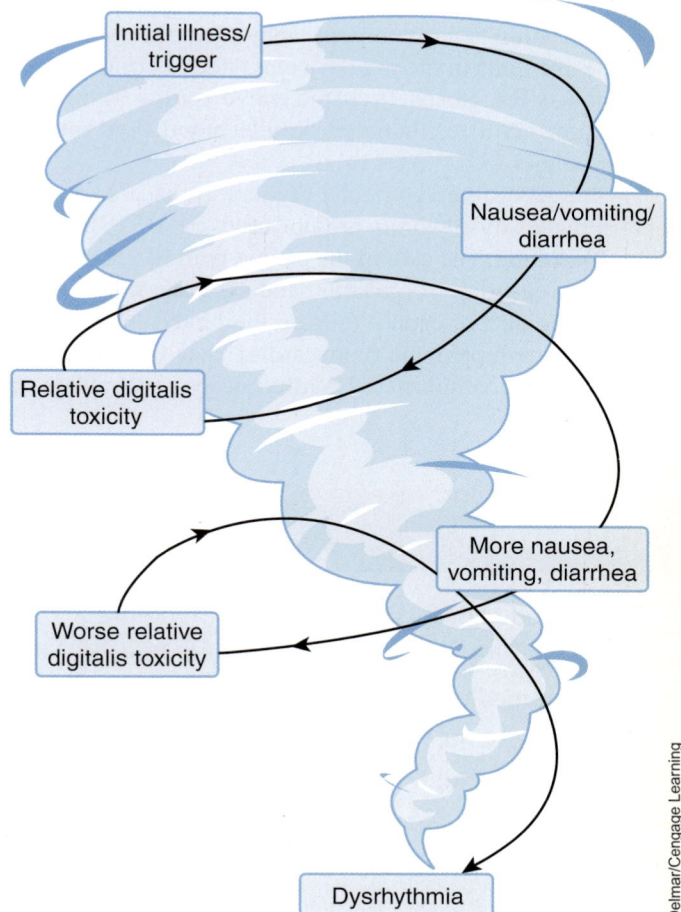

Figure 4-1 Cycle of digitalis toxicity.

Accelerated Idioventricular Rhythm

Accelerated idioventricular rhythms (AIVR) are the result of enhanced automaticity of the bundle of His–Purkinje fibers, which occur under certain metabolic conditions. In the prehospital setting, this rhythm is generally caused by increased vagal tone that depresses both the SA node and the AV node. Combined with enhanced automaticity of the escape rhythm (an idioventricular rhythm), the result is an accelerated idioventricular rhythm.

Conditions that support an AIVR include IWMI, especially with treatment of bradycardia with epinephrine or dopamine drips; digitalis toxicity; or electrolyte imbalances, most notably hypokalemia.

The ventricular response rate in AIVR may be regular and the onset gradual (i.e., nonparoxysmal or maybe irregular), as the SA node periodically assumes dominance for a period of time. The ectopic ventricular foci then assume dominance. As a result, fusion beats may occur. A fusion beat is the combination of atrial depolarization, initiated by the SA node, and ventricular depolarization, initiated by the ventricular foci. It appears like a premature ventricular complex with a P wave preceding the complex.

Patients with AIVR may experience hypotension, secondary to the loss of "atrial kick" (end-diastolic ventricular augmentation by atrial contraction) as a result of AV dissociation. The Paramedic may also observe cannon waves (pulsations in the jugular veins) due to atrial contraction against the closed tricuspid valve during ventricular contraction, with resultant retrograde blood flow into the jugular veins.

While AIVR is a ventricular rhythm, the usual treatments for ventricular dysrhythmia are not used, as AIVR is generally self-limiting. The care of the patient with AIVR is largely supportive, ensuring oxygenation and adequate fluid resuscitation. If the patient cannot tolerate the bradycardia (i.e., he suffers from symptomatic bradycardia), then 0.5 to 1 mg of atropine can be administered intravenously to stimulate the SA node.

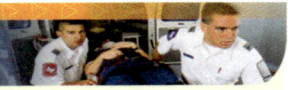

STREET SMART

Accelerated idioventricular rhythms (AIVR) are a sign of reperfusion following fibrinolytic therapy. Some Paramedics may witness AIVR as they transport patients from outlying hospitals, where they were treated with fibrinolytics, to cardiac centers for percutaneous transluminal coronary angioplasty (PTCA).

Ectopy

Myocardial cells have the property of automaticity, or more correctly autorhythmicity. Autorhythmicity is an ability to spontaneously depolarize in a rhythmic fashion according to the degree of ion gradient across the cell membranes. Abnormal automaticity occurs in the myocardium, away from the conductive tissue, when myocardial cells are irritable. Sources of irritability that can trigger abnormal automaticity include hypoxia, ischemia, or hyperkalemia, to name a few. An area of irritability that causes an abnormal spontaneous depolarization is called an **ectopic focus**.[12] (Some define an ectopic focus as any pacemaker other than the SA node.)

If the ectopic focus depolarizes before the SA node depolarizes, then this premature pacemaker will depolarize the remainder of the myocardium. Premature ectopy can originate in the atriums, in the junctional tissue, or in the ventricular myocardium. Premature complexes, which occur earlier than expected, are not a rhythm; instead, they are an interruption in a rhythm. The premature complex interrupts the underlying rhythm, making it irregular.

The relationship of the premature complex to the preceding complex is called its **coupling interval**. When a fixed coupling interval between the premature beat and the preceding normal one is observed, then a re-entry mechanism is suspected (an error of conduction). If the coupling interval is variable, it suggests an independent ectopic focus.

The premature beat will usually depolarize surrounding tissue. If this depolarization reaches the SA node, the entire sinus node rhythm will be reset. The underlying rhythm will begin from the premature beat. The R-R-R—which includes a normal beat, the premature beat, and another normal beat—will be shorter than one containing three normal beats. This describes a **noncompensatory pause**.

If the premature depolarization does not reach the SA node, then the underlying rhythm is not changed since the SA node is not reset. The R-R-R sequence that contains a normal beat, the premature beat, and another normal beat will equal the same time frame as the R-R-R of three normal beats. This defines a **compensatory pause**.

Premature beats may occur repetitively. If every other complex is premature, the sequence is termed **bigeminy** (Figure 4-2). Every third complex as a premature beat is called **trigeminy** (Figure 4-3) and every fourth is called **quadrageminy**.

Premature beats may also arise from different foci. When premature beats present with different morphologies, or shapes, they are called **multifocal** (Figure 4-4), since a presumption is made that they arise from different foci. If there is identical morphology for all of the premature beats, they are termed **unifocal** (Figure 4-5).

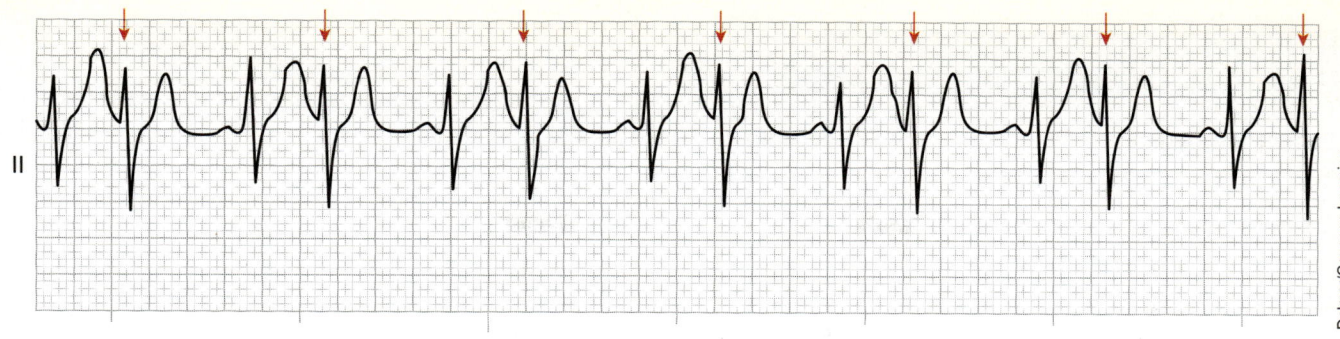

Figure 4-2 Sinus rhythm with atrial bigeminy.

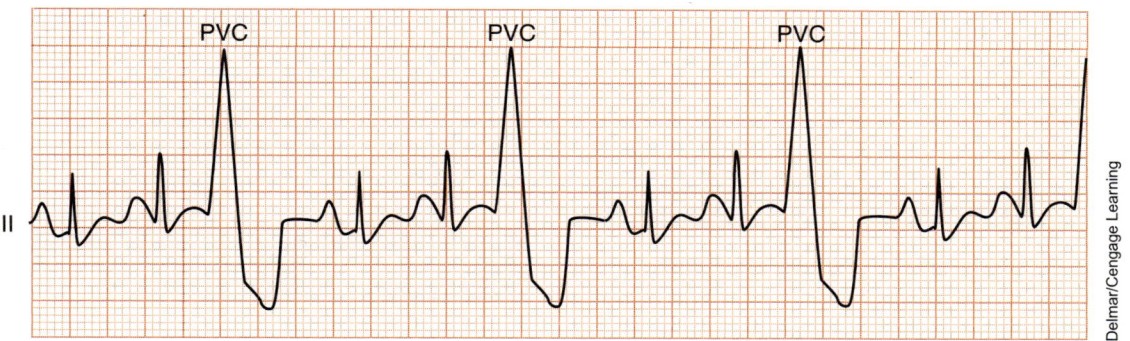

Figure 4-3 Sinus rhythm with ventricular trigeminy.

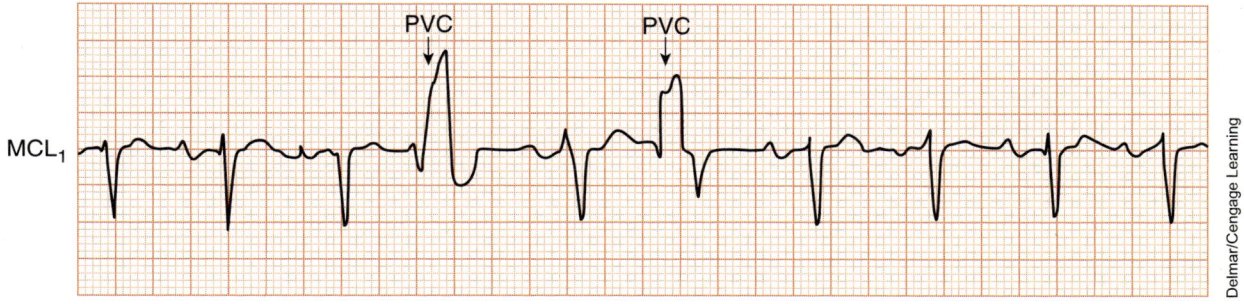

Figure 4-4 Sinus rhythm with multifocal PVC.

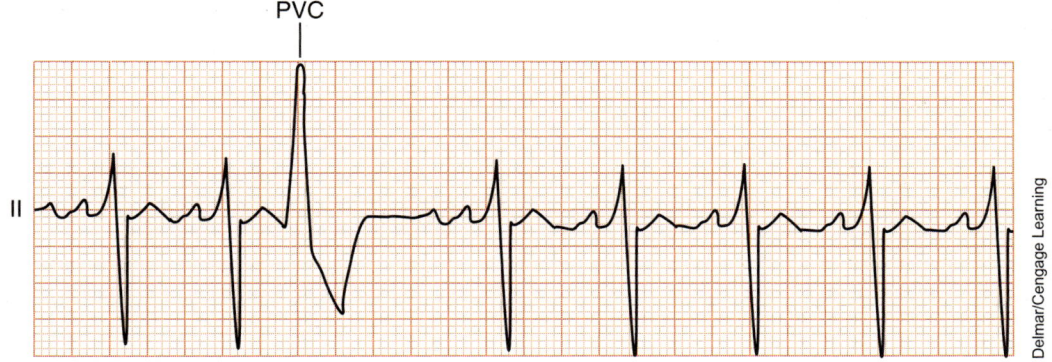

Figure 4-5 Sinus rhythm with unifocal PVC.

Standardized Rhythm Descriptions

While ectopic beats should be viewed with concern, the underlying rhythm is of greater importance. For example, although a premature beat (such as a late beat) may indicate increased cellular automaticity secondary to hypoxia and a potential life threat, an escape beat, as might be seen in a profound bradycardia, may be life-saving. Therefore, whenever a Paramedic describes a rhythm, the description always starts with the primary underlying rhythm and the ectopic beats are described as secondary modifiers. For example, the description of this rhythm (Figure 4-6) would be a sinus rhythm with a premature junctional complex.

Premature Atrial Complexes

A **premature atrial complex (PAC)** (Figure 4-7) is the result of an early depolarization of an irritable ectopic foci in the atria. PACs are common in the healthy patient population and may signify emotional stress or use of common substances such as alcohol, caffeine, or tobacco. Occasionally the patient will describe a feeling that her heart "skipped" a beat.

When they occur in a patient with a history of cardiac or pulmonary disease, these complexes may indicate a worsening of the patient's condition. The Paramedic should observe the frequency of the PACs while investigating the underlying etiology. A patient with frequent PACs, who has a history of heart or pulmonary disease, may be at risk for atrial fibrillation.

Some PACs occur when the ventricle is in a refractory period and are unable to be conducted down the bundle of His. These PACs are called nonconducted PACs. **Nonconducted PACs** (Figure 4-8) are recognizable by the pause that is created following the QRS, as the PAC interrupts the sinus rhythm, and by the peaked T wave. The P wave is in the T wave.

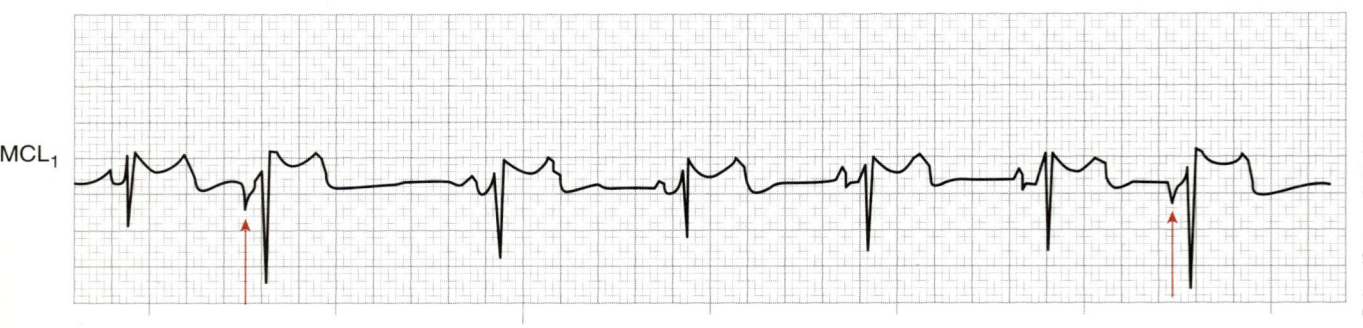

Figure 4-6 Sinus rhythm with PJC.

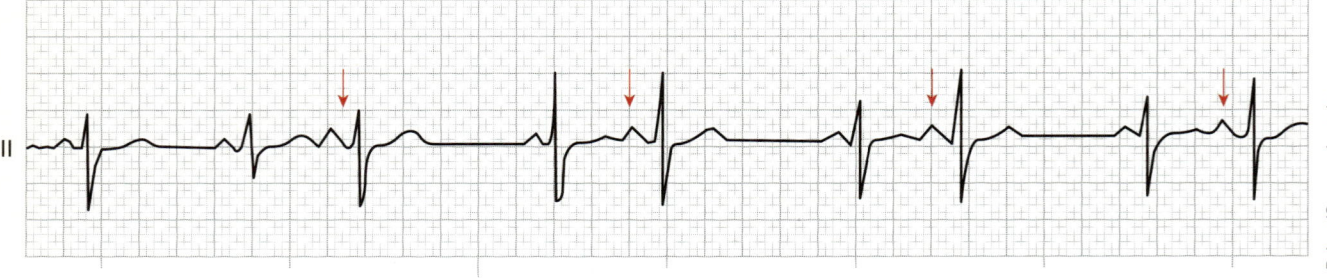

Figure 4-7 Premature atrial contraction.

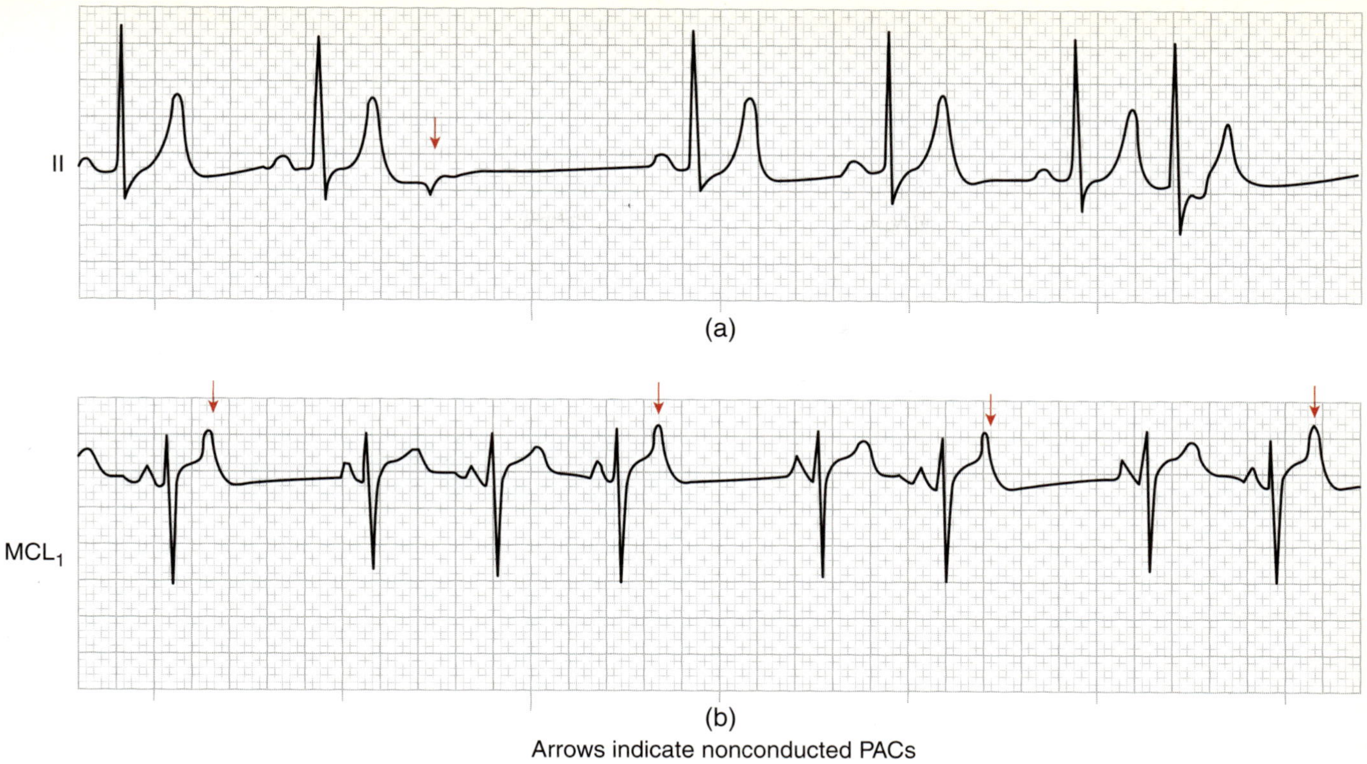

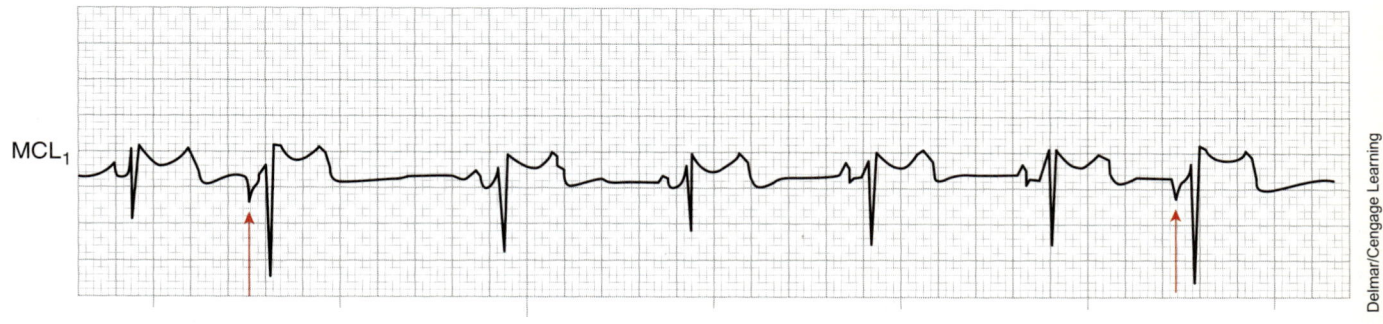

Figure 4-8 (a) shows ECG lead II with an arrow indicating a nonconducted PAC.

Figure 4-8 (b) shows ECG lead MCL₁ with arrows indicating nonconducted PACs.

(a)

(b)

Arrows indicate nonconducted PACs

Delmar/Cengage Learning

Figure 4-8   Sinus rhythm with a nonconducted PAC.

Delmar/Cengage Learning

Figure 4-9   Sinus rhythm with premature junctional complex.

Premature Junctional Complex

A **premature junctional complex (PJC)** (Figure 4-9) arises from either just above, within, or just below the junctional tissue. As a result, the impulse continues down the bundle of His, producing a narrow QRS complex. However, depending on the origin of the PJC, there may be an inverted P wave, secondary to retrograde conduction of the atria, that precedes the QRS complex; a P wave that is not visible, because it is obscured by the QRS complex; or a P wave that immediately follows the QRS in the ST segment. PJCs typically have a noncompensatory pause because of the retrograde conduction of the impulse through the atrium.

PJCs are the result of errors of automaticity and therefore usually do not have a fixed coupling distance, further supporting the assumption that PJC is an error of automaticity.

PJC may occur in response to stress, stimulants such as caffeine or nicotine, or worsening of pulmonary *or* heart disease.

Ventricular Premature Beat

A **ventricular premature beat (VPB)**, also known as a **premature ventricular complex (PVC)**, is an early beat that originates in the ventricles. PVCs can be divided into two classifications: benign and malignant (Table 4-5). Some patients have benign PVCs that are caused by a number of stimulants, such as caffeine, cocaine, and cold remedy formulations containing pseudoephedrine. Other PVCs are more likely to precipitate a potentially life-threatening dysrhythmia, either ventricular tachycardia or ventricular fibrillation, and may be especially evident in the face of known cardiac disease.

Like other dysrhythmias, such as atrial fibrillation, premature ventricular complex can be due to either a re-entry phenomena, making it an error of conduction, or an error of automaticity. The former, the error of conduction, has a tendency to establish a re-entry circuit that can cause a ventricular tachycardia. The latter, the error of automaticity, is secondary to local ischemia, electrolyte imbalances, and increased sympathetic tone in the ventricles. These factors lead to the development of one or more ectopic foci that can generate PVCs.

PVCs should not be confused with ventricular escape beats. PVCs may indicate an active pathologic process, which can deteriorate into ventricular fibrillation and sudden cardiac death.[13–15] Ventricular escape beats occur because of the failure of higher pacemakers in the SA and AV node and help sustain the heart until the primary or secondary pacemakers can resume dominance.

Table 4-5 Causes of PVC

- Systemic
  - Hypoxemia
  - Acidosis
    - Diabetic ketoacidosis
    - Acute renal failure
- Electrolyte imbalances
  - Hyperkalemia
  - Hypomagnesemia
- Cardiac disease
  - Ischemic heart disease
    - Acute coronary syndrome
  - Valvular disease
    - Mitral valve prolapse
    - Aortic regurgitation
  - Cardiomyopathy
- Medications
  - Digitalis
  - Methylxanthine
    - Theophylline
  - Psychiatric medications
    - Antipsychotic medication
    - Tricyclic antidepressants
  - Antidysrhythmics
    - Vaughn–Williams Class I
- Lidocaine
- Quinidine
- Stimulants
  - Caffeine
  - Cocaine
  - Ephedrine
  - Pseudoephedrine

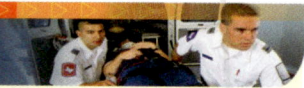

STREET SMART

Some Paramedics and physicians refer to premature ventricular contractions (PVC) as extrasystoles or ventricular premature beats (VPB). These various names all represent the same entity, the ventricular ectopic beat.

Forms of Premature Ventricular Complex

PVCs originating from a single ectopic focus will be uniform in shape, or morphology, and are called **unifocal PVCs** (Figure 4-10). These wide and bizarre QRS complexes may occur rarely (i.e., less than 6 minutes), may occur as frequently as every other complex (i.e., bigeminy) (Figure 4-11), on every third complex (i.e., trigeminy), or on every fourth complex (i.e., quadrageminy).

Unifocal PVCs sometimes appear two in a row and are called **couplets**. These couplets are not as ominous as bigeminy because of a phenomena called R on T. With R on T phenomena, the QRS complex of the PVC falls on the T wave of the previous complex, whether it's normal or ventricular. The T wave of the ECG represents the period of repolarization. During the first half of the T wave, the ventricles are unable to sustain a depolarization. This is called the **absolute refractory period**. During the second half of the T wave, some ventricles are able to sustain a depolarization. This period is referred to as the **vulnerable period** or the **relative refractory period**

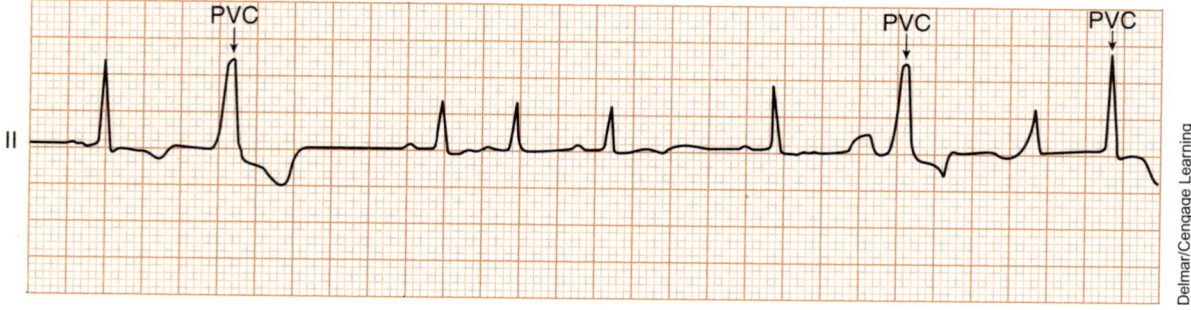

Figure 4-10 Unifocal PVC.

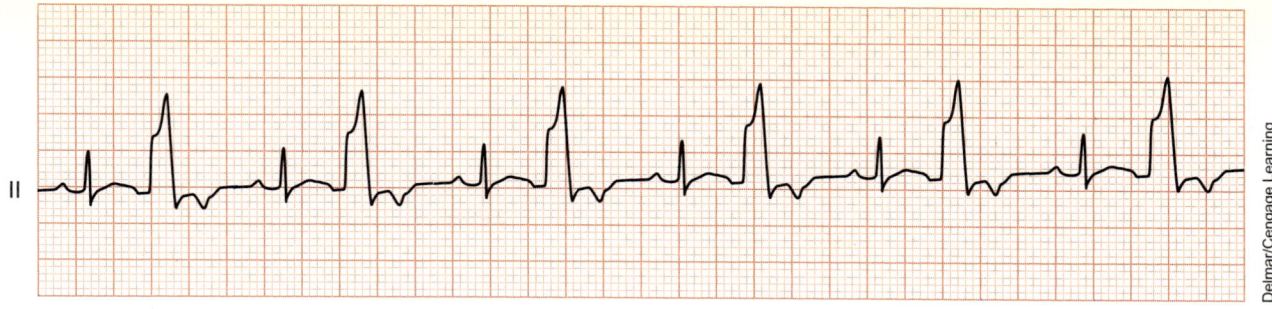

Figure 4-11 PVC in bigeminy.

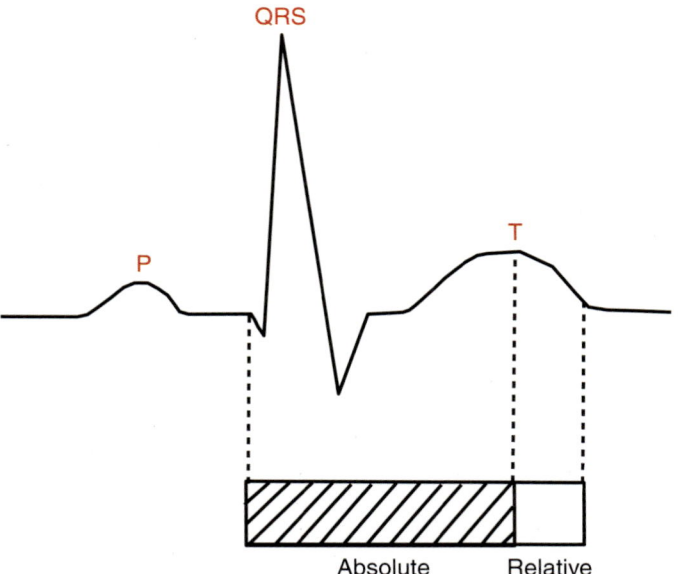

Figure 4-12 Refractory periods.

(Figure 4-12). If a stimulus strikes the ventricles during the vulnerable period, then a chaotic and disorganized depolarization can occur and ventricular fibrillation ensues.

When PVCs occur more than two at a time, but are not sustained and self-terminate after a few beats, they are called **salvos** or **runs of ventricular tachycardia**. Like couplets, runs of VT risk R on T phenomena (Figure 4-13).

Lown's Criteria

At one time PVCs were treated aggressively, using lidocaine, according to a prognostic criteria called Lown's criteria (Table 4-6). This practice stopped when it was discovered that lidocaine offered no survival advantage over nontreatment and, in some instances, the lidocaine was proarrhythmic. While there has been some discussion about the utility of Lown's criteria for prognosis, it is valuable to Paramedics as an illustration of potentially dangerous PVC, especially if the patient is experiencing an acute coronary event.

Decreased Automaticity

Decreased automaticity can be caused by either decreased sympathetic stimulation or excess parasympathetic tone. Causes of increased parasympathetic tone include vagal stimulation from head to toe, increased intraocular pressure, stimulation of the carotid sinus (e.g., by wearing a necktie that is too tight), brushing the teeth (for patients with carotid sinus hypersensitivity), abdominal distention secondary to small bowel obstruction, performing a Valsalva maneuver while bearing down to defecate, and micturition from an overdistended bladder, to name just a few.

Ischemia-Induced Decreased Automaticity

Ischemia can also cause decreases in automaticity. As a result of ischemia, cellular membranes can no longer maintain the ion gradients necessary, resulting in prolonged repolarization and subsequent bradycardia. A major cause of coronary ischemia is ruptured plaques formed during arteriosclerosis. If one of these ruptured plaques subsequently creates a thrombus, blocking a coronary artery, then myocardial ischemia can occur downstream.

The right coronary artery, found in the inferior wall, supplies blood to the AV node in the majority (over 90%) of patients. When a plaque ruptures, causing ischemia to the AV node, the AV node can become depressed. As a result, the patient will initially experience a prolonged PR interval, followed by bradycardia and subsequent heart block as the ischemia progresses.

Table 4-6 Modified Lown's Criteria—Pathological PVC

0. Low risk
○ No VPB
○ Rare unifocal VPB (<30 VPB/hr)
1. Immediate risk
○ Frequent VPB (>30 VPB/hr)
2. High risk
○ Multifocal VPB
○ Repetitive VPB
○ Couplets
○ Salvos
○ R on T phenomena

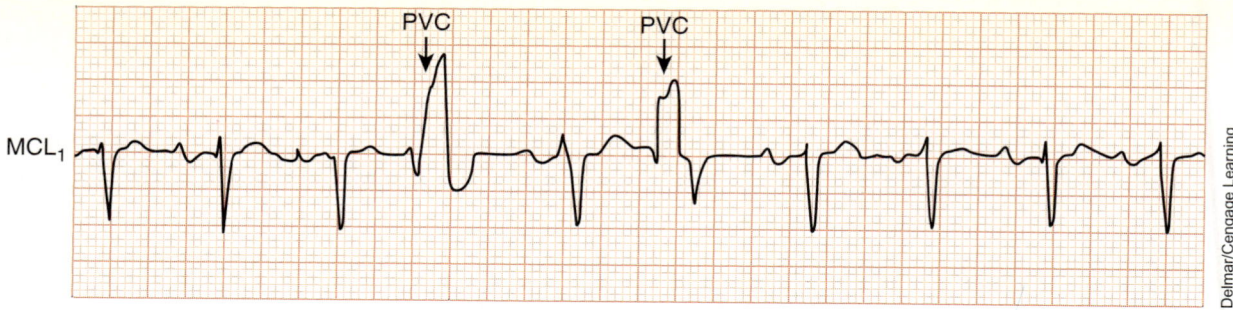

Figure 4-13 Multifocal PVC.

Similarly, the left circumflex coronary artery, found on the septal wall, supplies blood to the SA node. When a plaque ruptures, causing ischemia to the SA node, there is a decrease in the automaticity to the sinus node. As a result, the patient will experience bradycardia and possibly even syncope.

Sinus Pause/Arrest

When the SA node is temporarily suppressed, there may be a pause in the sinus rhythm. Since the only representation of sinus node activity on the ECG is the P wave that represents atrial depolarization, it is difficult to distinguish if a sinus pause is due to an error of automaticity (i.e., the sinus node failed to initiate an impulse) or an error in conduction, because of a block of the sinus impulse.

The etiology of a sinus pause/arrest may be due to increased vagal tone, suppressing the SA node, or hypoxia of the SA node, secondary to ischemia from occlusion of either the right coronary artery or the circumflex artery, or from the effects of medications such as beta/adrenergic blockers, calcium channel blockers, or digitalis. Regardless, a sinus pause is only significant if the patient becomes symptomatic. Further discussion of sinus pause/sinus block is found in Chapter 6 on errors of conduction: bradycardia.

Stokes–Adams Attacks

A **Stokes–Adams attack** is characterized by a sudden loss of consciousness, without warning, while seated or standing, which may be followed by a convulsion. A Stokes–Adams attack is thought to occur because of ventricular asystole, such as what occurs in a prolonged sinus arrest.

A Stokes–Adams attack is typically preceded by a momentary paleness, and flushing immediately afterward. Any convulsive activity, probably secondary to cerebral hypoxia, is short-lived (15 to 20 seconds), and the patient awakens without the typical postictal symptoms associated with epilepsy. The patient's pulse is often bradycardic following the syncope.

However, there are other potential causes of this cardiogenic syncope including vasovagal syncope or simple faint, orthostatic syncope and carotid sinus hypersensitivity, as well as bradydysrhythmia. In every case, a person who experiences syncope, whether seated or standing, should be placed on an ECG monitor.

Sinus Bradycardia

By definition, **sinus bradycardia** is a slow sinus rhythm, with a heart rate less than 60 beats per minute. Sinus bradycardia occurs regularly during the course of a person's day, while he sleeps or while he rests. Sinus bradycardia may also be the resting heart rate of conditioned athletes.

Sinus bradycardia can also be a warning sign of more serious conditions including IWMI, increased intracranial pressure, exposure to toxins, and certain electrolyte disorders, as well as medication effects. Sinus bradycardia is the result of increased parasympathetic stimulation, vagal tone, or sinus node dysfunction. The latter, sinus node dysfunction, as manifest in sick sinus syndrome, is discussed in Chapter 6 on errors of conduction: bradycardia.

The plant nurse states that Aaron's medical information card says that he has no allergies and that he takes Lisinopril® for his high blood pressure. The foreman tells the Paramedic that, to his knowledge, Aaron doesn't drink alcoholic beverages, he avoids caffeine, and he quit smoking about 15 years ago. Aaron says that he ate a light lunch because he "just wasn't up to eating." He does admit to a "sour stomach" over the past two weeks and has been taking antacids. He denies any exposures to toxins or poisons. Other than not feeling well, he denies any specific stressors.

CRITICAL THINKING QUESTIONS

1. What are the important elements of the history that a Paramedic should obtain?
2. What is the symptom pattern for someone with a suspected bradydysrhythmia? Tachydysrhythmia?

History

The general impression of a patient with weakness and dizziness can vary from one of serious illness to mild discomfort. The source of this complaint can arise from metabolic or neurological origins, or may be a cardiac event. Noncardiac origins of a concern of weakness and dizziness will be covered in later chapters. Nevertheless, the Paramedic must also keep those other potential etiologies in mind and be prepared to either redirect the examination or to entertain multiple pathologies (for example, new onset atrial fibrillation leading to stroke).

After completing an initial survey and treating any life threats, the Paramedic should try to obtain a succinct history of the present illness, using an OPQRST mnemonic (Onset, Provocation, Quality of pain, Radiation, Severity, Timing, focusing on the cardiac in this case) and a past medical history using the SAMPLE mnemonic (Symptoms, Allergies, Medications, Past medical history, Last meal or drink, and Events preceding the incident).

The Paramedic's history taking should focus on the hemodynamic effects of the dysrhythmia. The correlation that is being made is that decreased cardiac output, secondary to either profound bradycardia or tachycardia, has led to cerebral hypoperfusion. The patient should be asked about the precise time of onset and whether it was gradual or sudden. The patient should also be asked if she was standing or seated and experienced any syncope, especially while seated. If so, that should be thoroughly investigated.

Often patients with a dysrhythmia experience chest pressure or angina. The Paramedic should obtain a complete heart history, using the OPQRST mnemonic, if the patient has these complaints.

Dysrhythmia can lead to forward heart failure, as manifest by the symptoms weak and dizzy or syncope. Similarly, dysrhythmia can lead to backward failure including pulmonary edema.[16-18] The patient should be asked if she is experiencing any shortness of breath or has noticed any peripheral swelling (edema) recently.

Some patients with a tachydysrhythmia, and even some with bradycardia secondary to heart block, will experience palpitations, an awareness of one's heart beating, and may describe this as "skipped beats," "heart in the throat," "fluttering in the chest," and "heart flip flopping." These symptoms may be accompanied by feelings of anxiety or fright. The patient should be reassured that these are normal symptoms associated with an abnormal cardiac rhythm and that the symptoms will disappear when the dysrhythmia is treated.

The Paramedic should obtain an accurate medication record and focus on changes in medications. Often medications, or changes in doses of medications, can be the source of cardiac dysrhythmia (Table 4-7). For example, tricyclic antidepressants can affect the QT interval, prolonging it and leading to depressed myocardial function.[19-22]

Table 4-7 Potentially Cardiotoxic Substances

- Medications
  - Calcium channel blocker overdose
  - Beta/adrenergic blocker overdose
  - Tricyclic antidepressant overdose
  - Chemotherapy
  - Digitalis toxicity
- Illicit Drug—Sympathomimetics
  - Cocaine
  - Methamphetamine
- Other
  - Snake venom

The Paramedic should also decide if the weakness and dizziness may have caused stimulation or inhibition of the autonomic nervous system. Metabolic disorders such as hypoglycemia can stimulate the autonomic nervous system, leading to tachycardia and exacerbating underlying cardiac conditions. The Paramedic should also look for exposure to potentially cardiotoxic poisons.

CASE STUDY (CONTINUED)

During the initial exam, Aaron had a very slow radial pulse. His skin was cool and moist. After ensuring good oxygenation and IV access, the monitoring leads were applied and showed a sinus bradycardia of 42. Aaron states that he is not an athlete and does not participate in any athletic sport. The 12-lead ECG obtained immediately after the monitoring strip was obtained showed greater than 2 mm depression in leads II, III, and aVF.

CRITICAL THINKING QUESTIONS

1. What are the elements of the physical examination of a patient with disorder of rhythm?
2. Why is a 12-lead ECG a critical element in this examination?

Examination

The quick check of circulation performed during the initial assessment will alert the Paramedic to a rate that is too fast or too slow. Most adults will tolerate a fast rate up to 150 bpm or a slow rate of 50 bpm for short periods of time without significant hemodynamic compromise. However, older adults may have significant complaints related to a decrease in cardiac output at rates of 120 to 130 bpm.

The Paramedic should obtain a blood glucose reading and a full set of vital signs, including a systolic over diastolic blood pressure reading, to identify early hypoperfusion. The hemodynamic implications of tachydysrhythmia or bradydysrhythmia may require fast and decisive action.

Although urgency of the situation, in high priority cases, may dictate quick action, the Paramedic should, minimally, perform a cardiovascular examination. This cardiovascular examination should include an assessment for central cyanosis, jugular venous distention, breath sounds at apices and base, heart sounds (one should be particularly attentive to murmurs and a ventricular gallop), hepatojugular reflex, abdominal tenderness, and peripheral dependent edema.

Time should be taken to carefully assess the pulse. An irregular pulse with bounding pulses may indicate ventricular premature beats, whereas an irregularly irregular pulse may indicate atrial fibrillation. A central pulse should be compared to the peripheral pulse to ascertain any pulse deficit; a pulse deficit of > 20 bpm is significant. This advanced assessment can be performed while basic life support treatments (such as high-flow, high-concentration oxygen) are offered, blood sugar tests are performed, and a set of vital signs is obtained.

Electrocardiograph Analysis

Key to the clinical decision making for the patient with suspected tachydysrhythmia is the ECG. A monitoring ECG strip, and possibly a 12-lead ECG, should be the next priority. The patient's heart rate is helpful in determining the lead selection. If the patient's heart rate is tachycardic, > 120 bpm, then the Paramedic may want to choose the MCL1 ECG lead. This lead leaves the patient's chest (i.e., the defibrillation platform) open for pacer/defibrillator pads or paddles if synchronized cardioversion is needed.

12-Lead Electrocardiograph

Errors of automaticity, either bradycardia or tachycardia, can either be the cause of myocardial ischemia or the result of myocardial ischemia. Therefore, a 12-lead ECG should be quickly obtained, provided the patient's condition does not require immediate intervention to prevent sudden cardiac death. The information on the 12-lead ECG, such as PR interval and QT length, can be invaluable in the rhythm strip analysis.

Increased Automaticity

The rhythms that are the result of increased automaticity of the heart and that can cause a tachydysrhythmia can be categorized as narrow–regular, narrow–irregular, wide–regular, and wide–irregular, and include ectopic atrial tachycardia, accelerated junctional rhythm, junctional ectopic tachycardia, multifocal atrial tachycardia, and accelerated ventricular rhythm.

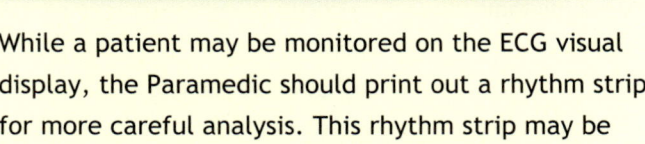

STREET SMART

While a patient may be monitored on the ECG visual display, the Paramedic should print out a rhythm strip for more careful analysis. This rhythm strip may be the only documentation of the rhythm and, as such, is invaluable to cardiologists at the hospital.

Sinus Tachycardia

Sinus tachycardia (Table 4-8 and Figure 4-14) has all of the same ECG characteristics as a sinus rhythm except the rate. The rate can range from 100 to 220 bpm minus the patient's age, although most patients cannot sustain a heart rate above 120 bpm without becoming symptomatic.

Focal Atrial Tachycardia

Differences between focal atrial tachycardia (Table 4-9 and Figure 4-15) and normal sinus rhythm are found in the heart rate and morphology of the P wave. Focal atrial tachycardia results from the fast firing of atrial tissue rather than from the SA node. Some atrial tachycardias (e.g., paroxysmal atrial tachycardia) utilize a re-entry circuit; this dysrhythmia is discussed in Chapter 5 on errors of conduction: tachycardia.

However, for focal atrial tachycardia, the key is the increased automaticity of an ectopic focus.

Wandering Atrial Pacemaker

In a wandering atrial pacemaker (WAP) (Table 4-10), the pacer site shifts between the sinus node and other ectopic atrial sites. In general, atrial and ventricular depolarization occurs normally, although some atrial depolarization may occur earlier depending upon the actual location of the ectopic focus. The primary differences between this rhythm and normal sinus rhythm are in the shape of the P wave and the PR interval, which will both change as the site shifts from the ectopic site to the sinus node.

Irregular Narrow Complex Tachycardia

The two irregular narrow complex tachycardias are atrial fibrillation and atrial flutter. These two tachydysrhythmias are grouped together because the treatments are the same and the associated complications of treatment can be the same as well.

Atrial Fibrillation/Flutter (AFF) with Rapid Ventricular Response (RVR)

The signs and symptoms of atrial fibrillation (Table 4-11 and Figure 4-16) revolve around the subtle loss of cardiac output. Initially the patient may complain of sudden unexplained weakness, shortness of breath, and even chest discomfort, particularly during exertion. For the patient in atrial fibrillation with a rapid ventricular response (Figure 4-17), cardiac output may be sufficient at

Table 4-8 Sinus Tachycardia

Ventricular Rhythm	
Rhythm	Regular
Rate	Greater than 100 bpm
Width QRS	Less than 0.12 seconds
Atrial Rhythm	
Rhythm	Regular
Rate	Same as ventricular rate
Shape of P wave	Rounded and upright Lead II
Atrial rate	Same as ventricular
PR interval	0.12 to 0.20 seconds
AV relationship	1 P wave for every QRS

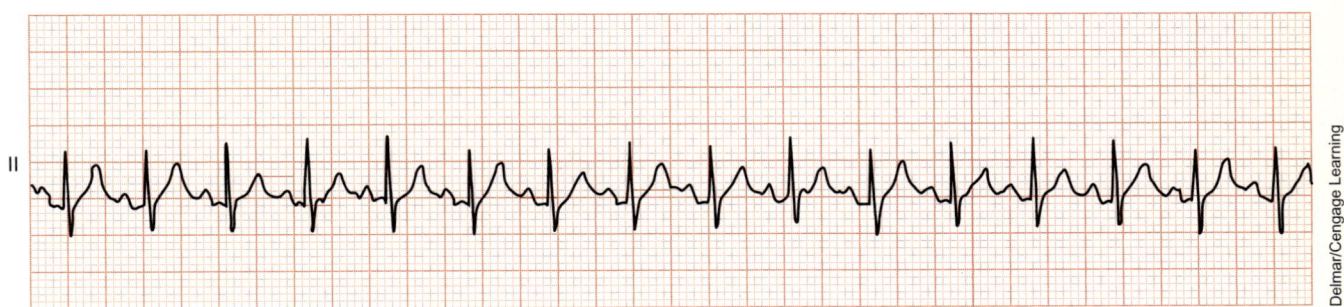

Figure 4-14 Sinus tachycardia.

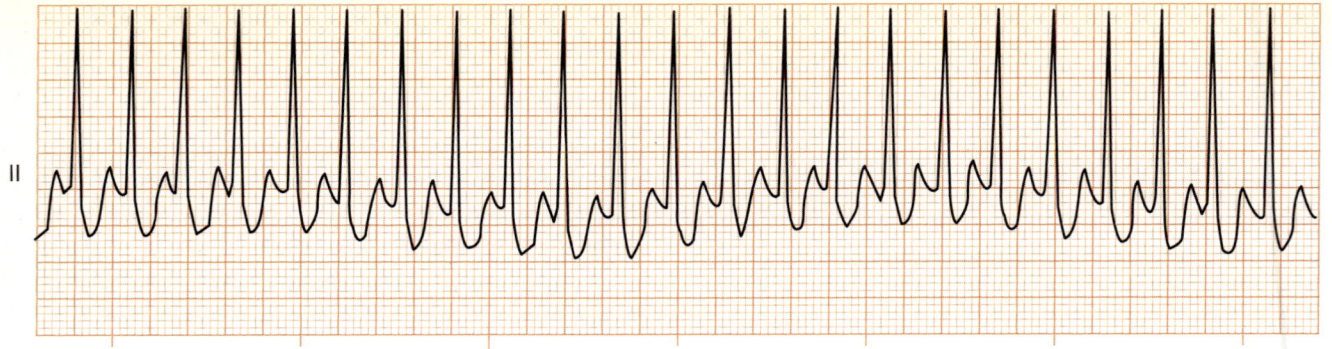

Figure 4-15 Focal atrial tachycardia.

Table 4-9 Focal Atrial Tachycardia

Ventricular Rhythm	
Rhythm	Regular
Rate	Greater than 100 bpm, generally greater than 150 bpm
Width QRS	Less than 0.12 seconds
Atrial Rhythm	
Rhythm	Regular
Rate	Same as ventricular rate
Shape of P wave	Ectopic P wave, peaked
Atrial rate	Same as ventricular
PR interval	Less than 0.12 seconds
AV relationship	1 P wave for every QRS

Table 4-10 Wandering Atrial Pacemaker

Ventricular Rhythm	
Rhythm	Irregular
Rate	60 to 100 bpm
Width QRS	Less than 0.12 seconds
Atrial Rhythm	
Rhythm	Regular
Rate	Same as ventricular rate
Shape of P wave	Grossly irregular
Atrial rate	Same as ventricular
PR interval	Varies
AV relationship	1 P wave for every QRS

rest. However, any increase in physical or metabolic activities can lead to decompensation. If the average ventricular rate exceeds 150 bpm (in the elderly, the rate at which signs and symptoms develop may be much lower), chest pain may develop secondary to inadequate ventricular filling times and decreased coronary perfusion. New onset atrial fibrillation rates usually are uncontrolled, sometimes averaging 150 beats per minute or faster.

As a result of the irregular filling of the ventricles, the patient's pulses may also be irregular. In some cases, the pulse will be intermittently weak, strong, or absent, depending on the degree of augmentation of the end-diastolic filling. The last finding, absent pulses, is characteristic of atrial fibrillation. While the cardiac output is strong enough to create a central pulse, it is not strong enough to create a peripheral pulse. Therefore, there is a difference between central pulses, or complexes observed on the ECG monitor, and the peripheral pulse (e.g., a radial pulse). This difference is called a **pulse deficit**. Any time there is a pulse deficit of greater than 20 bpm, it is considered significant and should be treated.

Patients with atrial fibrillation are particularly prone to backward heart failure, as venous congestion occurs as a result of incomplete ventricular filling. The Paramedic should assess for signs of cardiac failure. Pulmonary edema should be assessed by listening to the lung sounds for rales and wheezes. The Paramedic should note if there is jugular venous distention with the patient

sitting at a 45-degree angle and assess the patient for a hepatojugular reflex.[23] Finally, the Paramedic should assess for abdominal tenderness, swelling, and the dependent areas for edema.

Ashman's Phenomenon

At first glance a wide complex beat occurring in atrial fibrillation may be thought to be a ventricular premature beat. However, upon closer examination it will be discovered that these wide complex beats are supraventricular beats that are aberrantly conducted. These short bursts of abnormally conducted supraventricular impulses seen in atrial fibrillation are called **Ashman's phenomenon** (Figure 4-18).[24] Ashman's phenomenon occurs because the ventricles are not completely repolarized, thus allowing one branch of the bundle branches to be depolarized. Retrograde depolarization depolarizes the remainder later, resulting in a widened QRS complex. Clues to Ashman's phenomena include a short R to R interval before the aberrantly conducted beat, then a long R to R interval following the aberrantly conducted beat. Another clue to Ashman's phenomenon is a QRS pattern of rsR in V1 or MCL1.

Chronic/Persistent Atrial Fibrillation

In chronic or persistent atrial fibrillation, multiple impulses complete multiple circles within the atria, and these impulses bombard the AV node repeatedly. The result is that the AV produces irregularly spaced ventricular responses. Each impulse

Table 4-11 Atrial Fibrillation

Ventricular Rhythm	
Regularity	Irregularly irregular (without pattern)
Rate	Controlled >100, uncontrolled >100 complexes per minute
Width of QRS	0.04 to 0.12 seconds
Atrial Rhythm	
Regularity	None
Rate	None
Shape of P wave	None, fine fibrillatory "f" waves
PR interval	None
AV relationship	None
{Insert rhythm strip here}	

that tries to reach the ventricles depolarizes a portion of the AV node, increasing the difficulty that subsequent impulses will get through. The irregular response is due to this competition from multiple atrial impulses trying to get through the AV node.

Accelerated Junctional Rhythm

In this rhythm, junctional tissue initiates impulses at a rate greater than its intrinsic rate of 40 to 60 bpm (Table 4-12 and Figure 4-19). Depending on exactly where in the junction this initiation takes place, a P wave may occur before the QRS with a shorter-than-normal PRI. This may occur simultaneously with the QRS complex and thus not be evident on the rhythm strip. It may also occur after the QRS as an inverted P, representing the reverse or **retrograde conduction** of the stimulus backward through the atrium. If the junctional impulse then causes the atrial tissue to be depolarized after ventricular depolarization, retrograde depolarization has occurred and the P wave is found after the QRS complex.

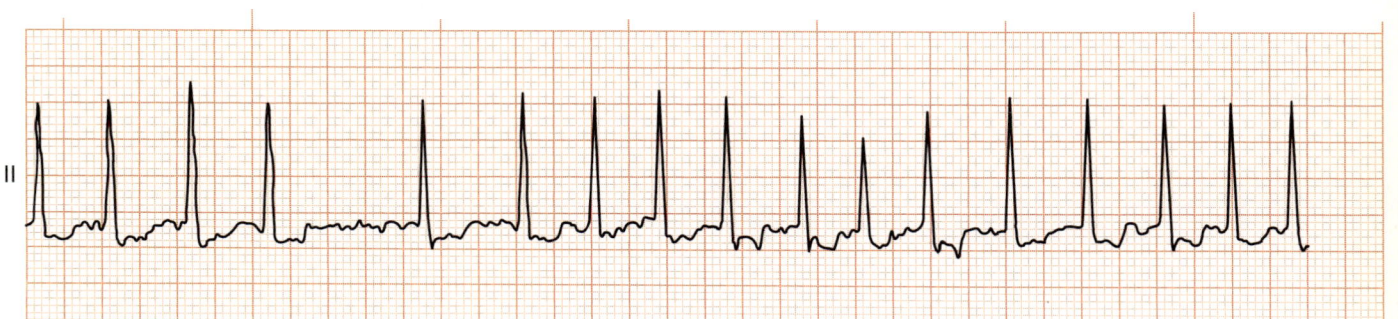

Figure 4-16 Atrial fibrillation.

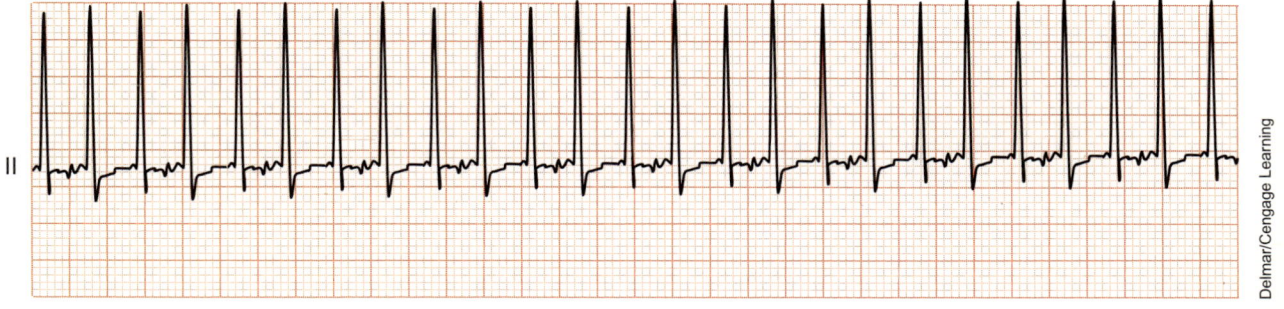

Figure 4-17 Atrial fibrillation with a rapid ventricular response.

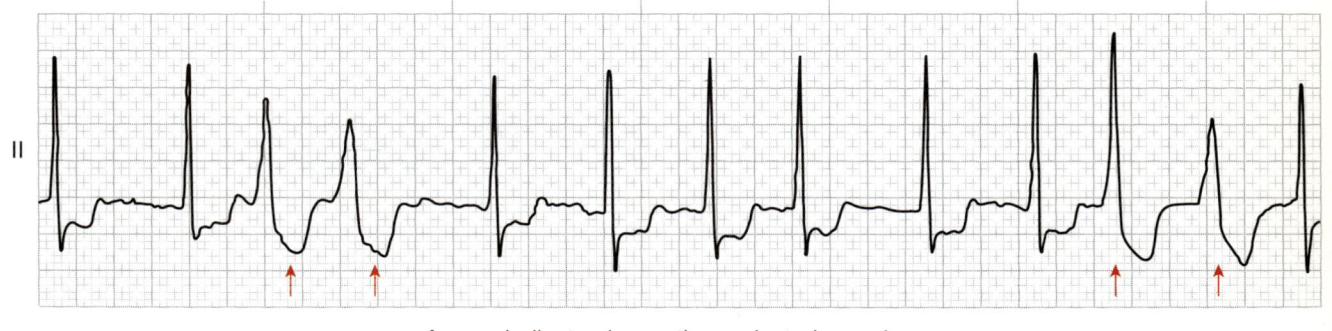

Arrows indicate aberrantly conducted complexes

Figure 4-18 Atrial fibrillation with Ashman's phenomenon.

Table 4-12	Accelerated Junctional Rhythm		Table 4-13	Junctional Ectopic Tachycardia
Ventricular Rhythm			**Ventricular Rhythm**	
Rhythm	Regular		Rhythm	Regular
Rate	60 to 100 bpm		Rate	100 to 180 bpm
Width QRS	Less than 0.12 seconds		Width QRS	Less than 0.12 seconds
Atrial Rhythm			**Atrial Rhythm**	
Rhythm	Irregular		Rhythm	Irregular
Rate	Same as ventricular rate, when P wave visible		Rate	Same as ventricular rate, when P wave visible
Shape of P wave	Rounded and upright Lead II		Shape of P wave	Rounded and upright Lead I
Atrial rate	Same as ventricular		Atrial rate	Same as ventricular
PR interval	Less than 0.12 seconds for P waves before the QRS		PR interval	Less than 0.12 seconds for P waves before the QRS
AV relationship	1 P wave for every QRS		AV relationship	1 P wave for every QRS

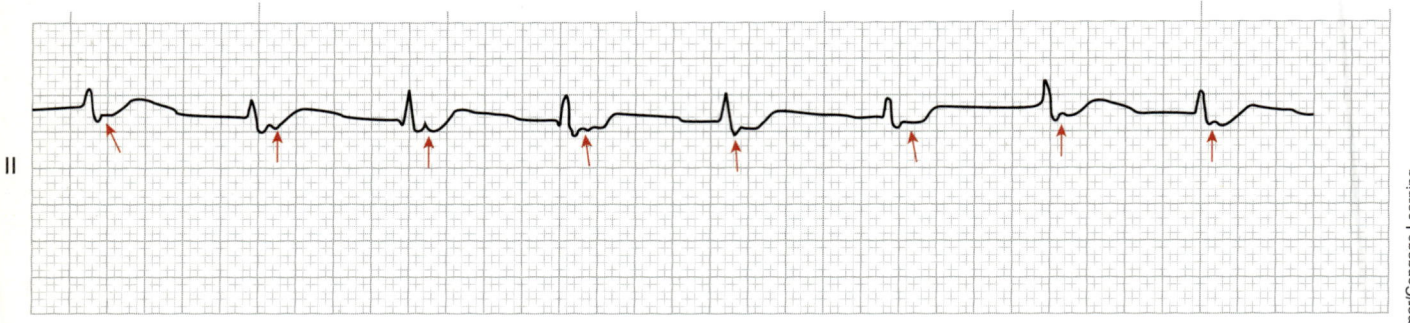

Retrograde P waves indicated by arrows

Delmar/Cengage Learning

Figure 4-19 Accelerated junctional rhythm.

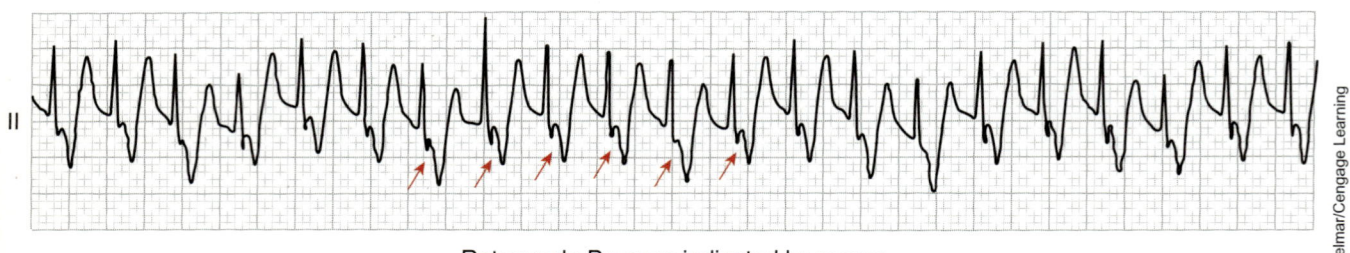

Retrograde P waves indicated by arrows

Delmar/Cengage Learning

Figure 4-20 Junctional ectopic tachycardia.

Junctional Ectopic Tachycardia

Junctional ectopic tachycardia (JET) (Table 4-13 and Figure 4-20) is the result of an ectopic focus either near the AV node or adjunct to the bundle of His. The QRS is the same as the preceding sinus rhythm with a 1:1 retrograde conduction up the atria (i.e., ventricular atria (VA) conduction), causing an inverted P wave that appears before the QRS, buried in the QRS, or immediately following the QRS.

Junctional ectopic tachycardia can have a tendency to change rates quickly, even from R to R. As a result of the changing rates (which result in an irregular rhythm) and the appearance and disappearance of the P wave, JET may be confused with multifocal atrial tachycardia, discussed shortly. Fortunately, both rhythms are errors of automaticity and can be similarly treated.

STREET SMART

Junctional ectopic tachycardia (JET) may occur during an acute myocardial infarction, particularly in IWMI. It is prudent to obtain a 12-lead ECG on any patient presenting with a junctional ectopic tachycardia.

Narrow QRS with an Irregular Rhythm

An irregular rhythm suggests multiple foci for the tachycardia. The only narrow QRS complex tachycardia that is irregular is multifocal atrial tachycardia.

Accelerated Idioventricular Rhythm (AIVR)

AIVR (Table 4-14 and Figure 4-21) originates in the ventricles rather than from above the ventricles as the supraventricular rhythms do. Any atrial activity that is occurring is independent of the ventricles or may be hidden in the QRS complex.

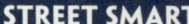
Premature Atrial Complex

A premature atrial complex (PAC) (Figure 4-22) is a beat initiated in ectopic atrial tissue that occurs before an expected complex. A PAC occurs within a rhythm; for example, the patient has a sinus rhythm with PACs. The P wave that occurs with the early complex is abnormal in its appearance. Additionally, the PR interval that occurs with the early complex may be different than that of the underlying rhythm.

Premature Junctional Complex

A premature junctional complex (PJC) (Figure 4-23) is similar to a PAC in that it occurs within a rhythm and interrupts the rhythm. Because the ectopic focus is within junctional tissue, the QRS generally has the same morphology as the preceding normal beat. If the focus is near the AV junction, a P wave may occur before the QRS complex. It will have a shortened PRI and will likely be of a different polarity and morphology than the sinus P waves. Depolarization of the atria can also occur after the QRS complex. This is termed a retrograde P wave.

Table 4-14 Accelerated Idioventricular Rhythm (AIVR)

Ventricular Rhythm	
Rhythm	Regular
Rate: ventricular	40 to 100 bpm
Width of QRS	Greater than 0.12 seconds
Atrial Rhythm	
Rhythm	Regular
Rate	60 to 100 bpm
Shape of P wave	Normal, rounded and upright in Lead II
PR interval	None
AV relationship	None

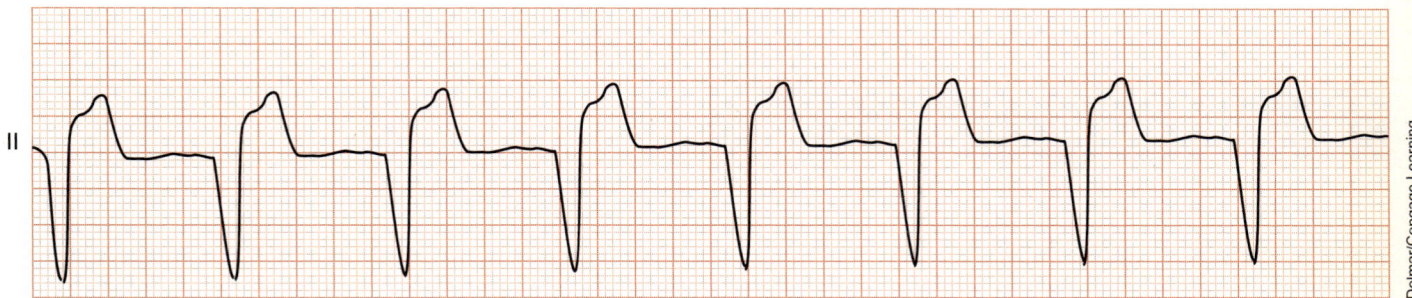

Delmar/Cengage Learning

Figure 4-21 Accelerated idioventricular rhythm (AIVR).

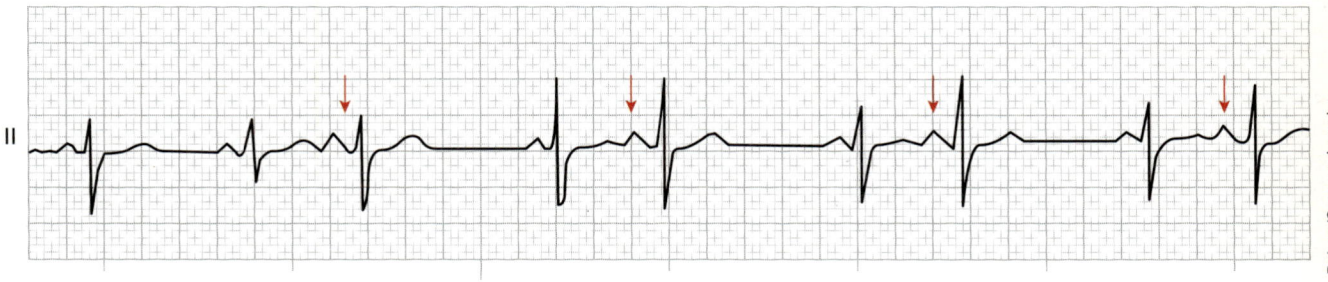

Delmar/Cengage Learning

Figure 4-22 Premature atrial complex.

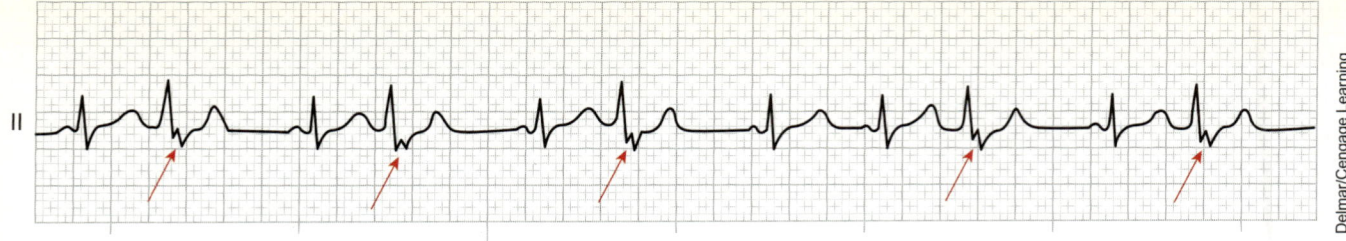

P waves indicated by arrows

Figure 4-23 Premature junctional complex.

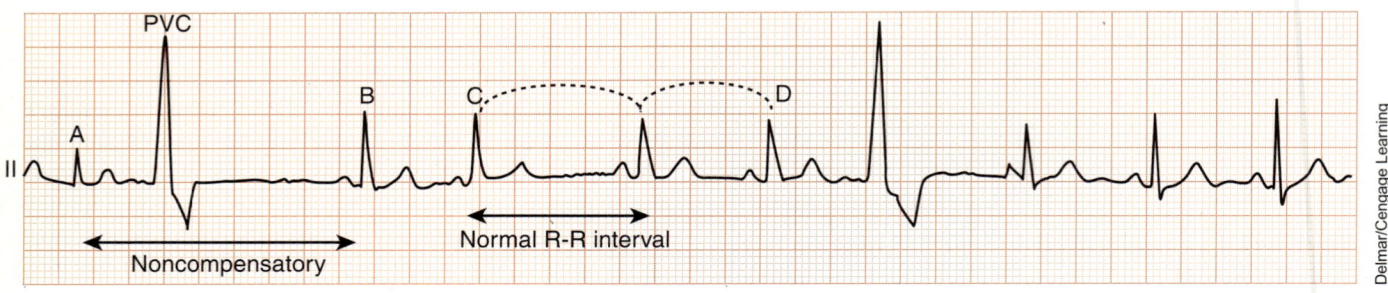

Figure 4-24 Premature ventricular beat showing the compensatory pause.

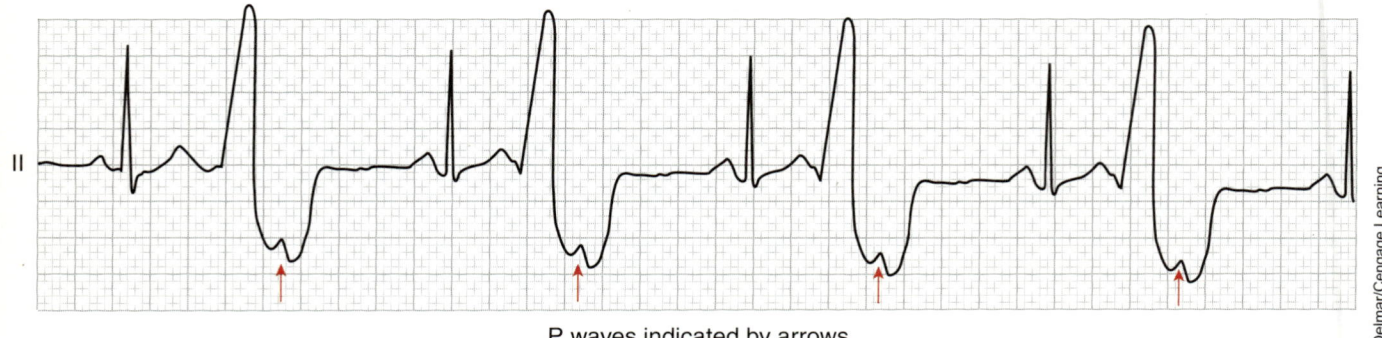

P waves indicated by arrows

Figure 4-25 Sinus rhythm with R on T phenomenon.

Premature Ventricular Complex

Premature ventricular complexes (PVC) have wide and bizarre QRS complexes that generally have a T wave in the opposite direction of the preceding T wave. While atrial activity may occur, it is generally obscured by the PVC QRS complex. There is generally a compensatory pause following a PVC before the next beat (Figure 4-24). This compensatory pause permits augmented ventricular filling

and a bounding pulse that follows. PVCs may occur very early in the cycle, actually impinging on the preceding T wave. This creates the R on T phenomenon discussed earlier (Figure 4-25).

Decreased Automaticity

The primary cause of decreased automaticity is increased parasympathetic stimulation. This parasympathetic stimulation has its greatest effects on the atria.

Sinus Pause/Arrest

A **sinus pause** (Table 4-15 and Figure 4-26) is identifiable not only by the loss of rhythm in a sinus rhythm, as manifest by a single irregular R to R ratio, but sometimes by the escape beat that tends to intercede between the sinus rhythm. A sinus pause, often termed a sinus arrest, occurs when the sinus node fails to initiate an impulse due to a change in automaticity. When the SA node resumes initiating impulses, a

Table 4-15 Sinus Pause/Arrest

Ventricular Rhythm	
Rhythm	Irregular
Rate	Greater than 100 bpm
Width QRS	Less than 0.12 seconds
Atrial Rhythm	
Rhythm	Irregular
Rate	Same as ventricular rate
Shape of P wave	Rounded and upright Lead II
Atrial rate	Same as ventricular
PR interval	0.12 to 0.20 seconds
AV relationship	1 P wave for every QRS

Table 4-16 Sinus Bradycardia

Ventricular Rhythm	
Rhythm	Regular
Rate	Less than 60 bpm
Width QRS	Less than 0.12 seconds
Atrial Rhythm	
Rhythm	Regular
Rate	Same as ventricular rate
Shape of P wave	Rounded and upright Lead II
Atrial rate	Same as ventricular
PR interval	0.12 to 0.20 seconds
AV relationship	1 P wave for every QRS

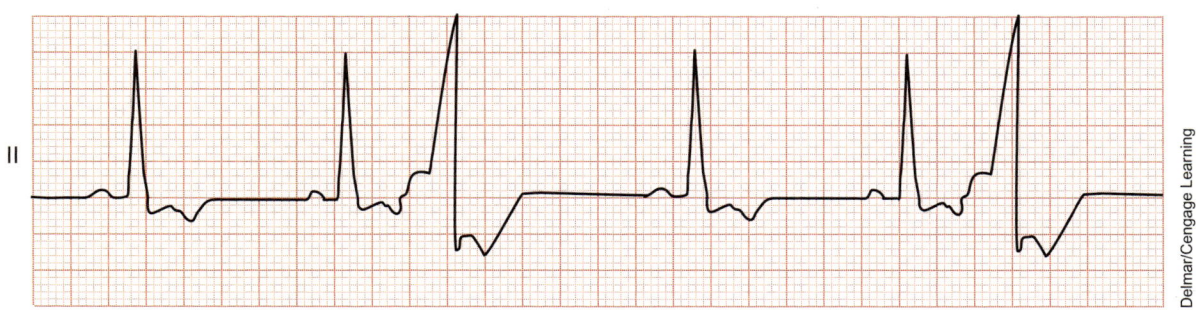

Figure 4-26 Sinus pause with ventricular escape beats.

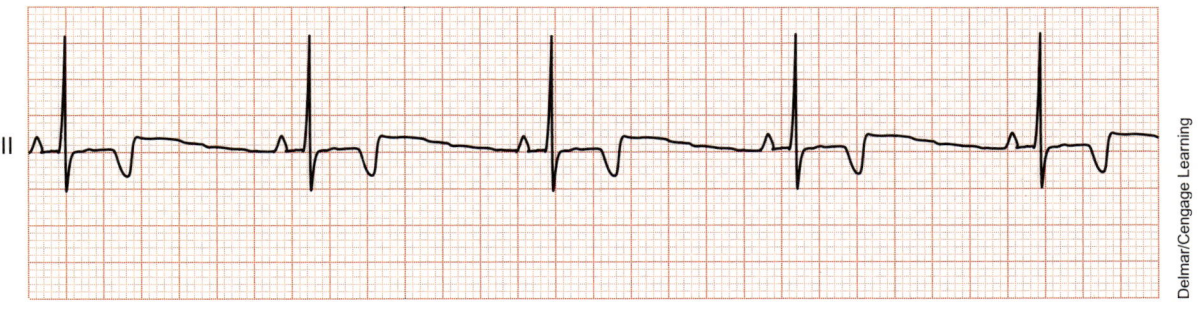

Figure 4-27 Sinus bradycardia.

noticeable break in the rhythm has occurred. The defining difference is in the sinus rhythm, which exhibits periods of rhythm coupled with pauses. In other words, the rhythm is regularly irregular.

Sinus Bradycardia

Just as in sinus tachycardia, the pacemaker site for sinus bradycardia (Table 4-16 and Figure 4-27) is in the sinus node. Atrial and ventricular depolarization occurs normally. The defining difference is in the rate, which is less than 60 beats per minute.

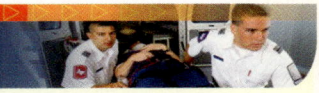

STREET SMART

The heart rate slows normally during relaxation and sleep. Well-conditioned athletes may develop slow heart rates that produce strong effective ventricular contractions. Many patients take medications (especially beta and calcium channel blockers and digoxin) that slow the heart rate below 60 bpm.

Aaron does not feel that his problems warrant medical attention and that he would rather go home from work to get some rest. The Paramedic makes the decision that Aaron should be encouraged to seek medical attention and enlists the assistance of the foreman and the nurse to help convince Aaron of that recommendation.

CRITICAL THINKING QUESTIONS

1. What is the significance of the bradycardia?
2. What information should be provided to Aaron so that he can make an informed decision?

Assessment

All supraventricular tachycardia have a short PR interval. This makes distinguishing tachydysrhythmias due to errors of conduction from the tachydysrhythmias due to errors of automaticity difficult. The differential diagnosis between the tachydysrhythmia from errors of conduction and errors of automaticity does not focus on the PR interval, but rather on the refractory period (RP). The refractory period is that time from the beginning of the QRS complex to the end of the T wave and represents the time of repolarization.

In those tachydysrhythmias due to an error of conduction, discussed in the next chapter, the RP is shorter than the PR interval (RP<PR) secondary to the use of accessory pathways. Tachydysrhythmias due to errors of conduction should be treated aggressively because they tend to lead to

cardiovascular collapse. These cases can be some of the most challenging for a Paramedic because the medications usually used to treat them cause peripheral vasodilation, creating hypotension, which is added to the tachycardia-induced hypotension.

In those tachydysrhythmias due to errors of automaticity, the refractory period is longer than the PR interval (RP>PR). Tachydysrhythmias are usually due to secondary or extracardiac causes, such as sympathomimetic stimulation. Rather than treat the consequence of these extracardiac causes, it is more effective to treat the causes to terminate the dysrhythmia; in many cases, the rhythm self-terminates without any further intervention from the Paramedic. When the cause cannot be effectively treated in the field, then the plan of treatment includes supportive care and medications to control the rate.

After the Paramedic's explanation, Aaron consents to treatment provided his wife is called by the Paramedic. Aaron didn't want his wife to be unduly concerned and thought the Paramedic's explanation would ally her fears.

CRITICAL THINKING QUESTIONS

1. What is the national standard of care for patients with bradydysrhythmia? Tachydysrhythmia?
2. What are some of the patient-specific concerns and considerations the Paramedic should consider when applying this plan of care that is intended to treat a broad patient population presenting with an error of automaticity?

Treatment

Based on the clinical information obtained during the history and physical, the Paramedic has to make a decision regarding whether the patient is stable or unstable (Table 4-17). The goal of Paramedic cardiac care is to maintain perfusion

to the vital organs: heart, lungs, and brain. Therefore, a patient who does not perfuse to these end organs is, by definition, unstable. Signs and symptoms of hypoperfusion of the lungs include shortness of breath and hypoxia. Signs and symptoms of hypoperfusion of the heart include chest pain and hypotension, and signs and symptoms of hypoperfusion

Table 4-17 Unstable Criteria—Vital Organs

- Brain: Altered mental status
  - Signs
    - Syncope
  - Symptoms
    - Confusion
- Lungs: Hypoxia
  - Signs
    - Pulmonary edema
  - Symptoms
    - Shortness of breath
- Heart: Myocardial hypoperfusion
  - Signs
    - Hypotension
  - Symptoms
    - Chest pain

to the brain include dizziness, syncope, and altered mental status.

When there is evidence of hypoperfusion of the vital organs, secondary to dysrhythmia, the Paramedic should take measures to convert the rhythm, or control its effects, that have the least potential for harm to the patient.

If the patient is unstable, and has a tachydysrhythmia, then elective synchronized cardioversion (discussed at the end of the chapter) may be necessary. The decision to provide direct current (DC) countershock to a beating heart should not be taken lightly, since one of the potential outcomes of DC countershock is asystole.

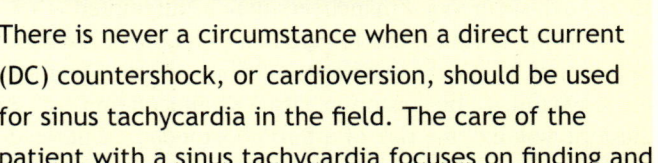

STREET SMART

None of the signs and symptoms of instability can be taken individually. Instead, the entire symptom complex should be appraised as one and, in light of the patient's clinical condition, a determination of stable versus unstable should be made.

Wide versus Narrow Complex Tachycardia

Next, the Paramedic needs to ascertain if the tachydysrhythmia is a wide complex tachycardia or a narrow complex tachycardia. A wide complex tachycardia is more ominous, as it is suggestive of ventricular tachycardia, and can quickly deteriorate into a ventricular fibrillation/flutter. A narrow complex tachycardia is more likely to be tolerated by the patient and amenable to pharmacological intervention.

Wide Complex Tachycardia

Accelerated idioventricular rhythm (AIVR) is a wide complex tachycardia that owes its origins to an error of automaticity. AIVR is generally a life-saving rhythm that only occurs during increased vagal tone, IWMI, digitalis toxicity, or electrolyte imbalance. Therefore, treatment focuses on supportive care.

Narrow Complex Tachycardia

While sinus tachycardia is a narrow complex tachycardia that arises from an error of automaticity, the approach to sinus tachycardia is different than the approach to the other tachy-dysrhythmias that arise from errors of automaticity. The treatment of sinus tachycardia focuses on treating the underlying cause of the tachycardia.

STREET SMART

There is never a circumstance when a direct current (DC) countershock, or cardioversion, should be used for sinus tachycardia in the field. The care of the patient with a sinus tachycardia focuses on finding and treating the cause of the sinus tachycardia.

After performing an examination and providing supportive care, such as oxygen, intravenous access, and an ECG monitor, the Paramedic should proceed with treating the patient with a regular narrow complex tachycardia.

While vagal maneuvers and administration of adenosine, described more fully in the next chapter, may provide some insight into the exact nature of the dysrhythmia, they are seldom effective therapies. These approaches produce AV slowing but do not affect the ectopic focus. Rather, the treatment for tachydysrhythmias that originate from errors of automaticity should focus on controlling the rate, rather than converting the rhythm in the field. Drugs that are effective at rate control are the calcium channel blockers, such as diltiazem, and the beta/adrenergic blockers.

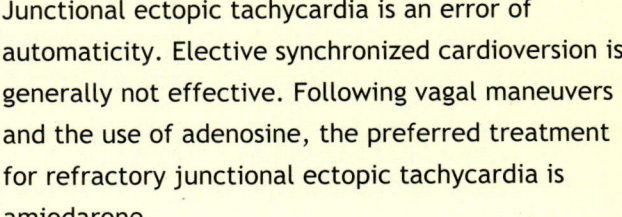

STREET SMART

Junctional ectopic tachycardia is an error of automaticity. Elective synchronized cardioversion is generally not effective. Following vagal maneuvers and the use of adenosine, the preferred treatment for refractory junctional ectopic tachycardia is amiodarone.

Irregular Narrow Complex Tachycardia

An irregular narrow complex tachycardia can be atrial fibrillation with a rapid ventricular response (AF-RVR), a flutter with variable conduction, or a MAT. A MAT might be suspected in this case because the patient is on digitalis and has had vomiting and diarrhea, which tends to cause digitalis toxicity, and MAT is a dysrhythmia commonly seen in digitalis toxicity.

While it can be difficult to discern a MAT from atrial fibrillation with a rapid ventricular response, particularly if the heart rate is above 150 bpm, both rhythms are errors of automaticity and the treatments are similar.

Pharmacological Intervention

Atrial fibrillation (AF) with a rapid ventricular response (RVR) can cause an irregular narrow complex tachycardia. In some cases, it is difficult to distinguish if the rhythm is regular or irregular when the R to R interval is extremely short. In those cases, either a 12-lead ECG may be obtained to help with the ECG analysis or vagal maneuvers may be attempted.

The therapeutic goal for atrial fibrillation in the field is rate control. While the restoration of sinus rhythm can improve hemodynamics, by restoring atrial augmentation of end-diastolic volume, the risk of a thromboembolic event, leading to stroke, outweighs its usefulness.[25,26] It should be noted that approximately 50% of patients with new onset atrial fibrillation will spontaneously convert to sinus rhythm, without pharmacological intervention, in the first 24 to 48 hours. This lends importance to transporting the patient to the hospital for anticoagulation.[27] Drugs that have been shown to convert atrial fibrillation to sinus rhythm include procainamide and amiodarone and thus should be avoided in the field unless the patient is hemodynamically unstable secondary to the tachycardia. Furthermore, patients who receive procainamide for treatment of atrial fibrillation are at greater risk for torsades de pointes (TDP).

In some cases, the rate can be lowered, and the blood pressure improved, by a modest fluid bolus provided the patient is not in pulmonary edema. An increased preload, from the fluid bolus, increases stroke volume. This, in turn, slows the heart rate while maintaining cardiac output (HR × SV = CO). Agents used for pharmacological control of ventricular response in atrial fibrillation are intravenous calcium channel blockers, such as diltiazem, and the beta/adrenergic blockers,

such as metoprolol. The former, diltiazem, was effective in slowing the ventricular response rate during AF, within four minutes, in 94% of patients in one study. The latter, metoprolol, is also effective in controlling heart rates. While adenosine reduces AV node conduction, its short time of action makes it ineffective in the treatment of atrial fibrillation.

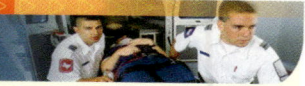

STREET SMART

It is best to avoid adenosine in patients with a history of pre-excitation syndromes, such as Wolff-Parkinson-White. The reduction of the AV node conduction only stimulates the accessory pathway, leading to runaway tachycardia with rates as high as 300 bpm.

Treatment of Digitalis Toxicity

Initially, the treatment of digitalis toxicity is largely supportive: oxygen for hypoxia and tachycardia-induced increases in mVO_2, and fluid bolus for hypotension. The definitive treatment for digitalis is correction of the underlying electrolyte imbalance and/or administration of digoxin-specific antibody fragments (Digibind) that bind to the digitalis.[28,29]

If the patient is experiencing either profound sinus bradycardia or AV block, then atropine may be necessary to overcome the vagal stimulation. If the patient is experiencing atrial tachydysrhythmia, then a beta/adrenergic blocker can be used to slow the rapid ventricular response. If the patient is experiencing ventricular tachycardia, then lidocaine would be the drug of choice. Lidocaine (VW1B), a weak sodium channel blocker, shortens the action potential and is more effective. As procainamide (VW1A) is contraindicated in AV blocks and digitalis toxicity tends to create an AV block, procainamide is therefore contraindicated in digitalis toxicity.

An alternative drug therapy, if the first-line antidysrhythmics are ineffective, is magnesium. As the body loses potassium, it also loses magnesium. Since hypokalemia is a cause of digitalis toxicity, it follows that the patient may also have hypomagnesemia. Magnesium is an important cofactor used by the sodium–potassium pump; administration of magnesium acts as an indirect antagonist to the digitalis.

CASE STUDY (CONTINUED)

Aaron's heart rate picks up and the Paramedic notes that he appears to be in atrial fibrillation. The Paramedic immediately restarts his assessment, starting with the primary assessment, and considers his treatment options.

CRITICAL THINKING QUESTIONS

1. What are some of the predictable complications associated with error of automaticity?
2. What are some of the predictable complications associated with the treatments for atrial fibrillation?

Evaluation

If the atrial fibrillation is thought to be less than 48 hours, and the patient is hemodynamically unstable, then the Paramedic can proceed with the administration of amiodarone 150 mg over 10 minutes.

If the amiodarone is ineffective, or the patient is decompensating rapidly, it may be necessary to cardiovert the ventricular tachycardia. Cardioversion is hazardous and the patient may convert to ventricular fibrillation or intractable asystole. Furthermore, cardioversion may release mural thrombi and cause a stroke, discussed shortly.[30] Some experts suggest that energies as low as 10 to 25 joules is sufficient, although current American Heart Association recommendations suggest starting at 50 to 100 joules. A more complete description of cardioversion and how to perform the procedure are contained in Chapter 5.

STREET SMART

In the case where digitalis toxicity has led to profound bradycardia that causes hemodynamic compromise, then pacing is indicated. However, there is a higher rate of complications, as high as 36%, with pacing dysrhythmia induced by digitalis toxicity. Therefore, pacing should be reserved for hemodynamically unstable patients who are unresponsive to medications such as atropine.

Atrial Fibrillation and Stroke

When the atria are in fibrillation, blood flow in portions of the atria—particularly near the valves—slows. This stagnant blood has a tendency to form clots on the walls of the atria. These clots are called mural thrombi. If the atria starts to rhythmically contract, these mural thrombi break off the atrial walls and float upstream to the brain. Subsequently, the patient experiences a stroke.

For this reason, the goal of prehospital care is to control the rate, not to convert the rhythm. The rhythm may be converted in the hospital at a later date, after the patient has been anti-coagulated.

STREET SMART

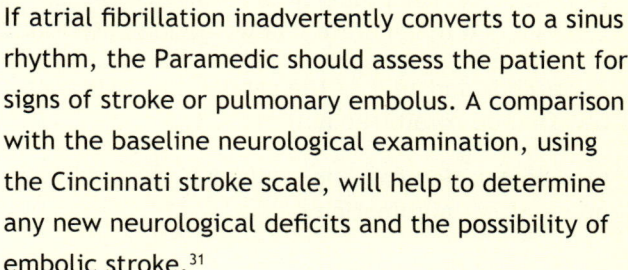

If atrial fibrillation inadvertently converts to a sinus rhythm, the Paramedic should assess the patient for signs of stroke or pulmonary embolus. A comparison with the baseline neurological examination, using the Cincinnati stroke scale, will help to determine any new neurological deficits and the possibility of embolic stroke.[31]

CASE STUDY CONCLUSION

The Paramedics found that Aaron had UA/NSTEMI (unstable angina non-ST elevation myocardial infarction) affecting the area surrounding the sinus node. He was transported to the heart center at the local hospital, which was capable of immediately treating the cause of the bradycardia plus the other signs and symptoms.

CRITICAL THINKING QUESTIONS

1. What is the most appropriate transport decision that will get the patient to definitive care?
2. What are the advantages of transporting a patient with suspected disorder of automaticity to these hospitals, even if that means bypassing other hospitals in the process?

Disposition

Dysrhythmia, whether tachydysrhythmia or bradydysrhythmia, due to errors of automaticity represent a separate class of dysrhythmia and require a different approach to treatment both in the field and in the hospital. Many of these dysrhythmias will need a catheter ablation. A catheter ablation is a procedure that delivers energy, usually radio waves, to areas of the myocardium suspected of harboring an ectopic foci, burning out the area, and effectively terminating the ectopy. The patient with a suspected error of automaticity should be transported to a cardiac center with capabilities to perform a catheter ablation in an electrophysiology lab.

CONCLUSION

Patients who develop disorders related to errors of automaticity may present with subtle complaints that initially may not appear to be cardiac in nature. These conditions can indicate a more serious underlying pathophysiology, especially when the onset is acute or the first episode. Paramedics are often the first medical professionals to detect and treat these rhythms.

KEY POINTS:

- Dysrhythmia may be caused by a change in automaticity, the property of cardiac cells that allows a cell to generate its own action potential.

- Pacer cells and cells of the conduction system can be affected by altered automaticity.

- Increases or decreases in the body's metabolic needs affect automaticity.

- Stimulation or inhibition of the autonomic nervous system can affect automaticity.

- Rhythms caused by an increase in automaticity are:
  - Sinus tachycardia
  - Atrial tachycardia
  - Wandering atrial pacemaker
  - Multifocal atrial tachycardia
  - Accelerated junctional rhythm

  - Premature atrial complex
  - Premature junctional complex
  - Premature ventricular complex
  - Accelerated ventricular rhythm

- Rhythms caused by an decrease in automaticity are:
  - Sinus bradycardia
  - Sinus pause
  - Sick sinus syndrome (tachy-brady syndrome)

- Treatment for an increase in automaticity is to remove the cause. If the rhythm is causing hemodynamic compromise, then vagal maneuvers, medications, or electrical interventions are indicated.

- Treatments for a decrease in automaticity are to find and remove the cause. Medications may be indicated. Pacing is rarely indicated.

REVIEW QUESTIONS:

1. How does a change in automaticity cause a rhythm disturbance?
2. List causes of changes to automaticity.
3. What classes of medications decrease automaticity?
4. What classes of medications increase automaticity?

CASE STUDY QUESTIONS:

Please refer to the Case Study in this chapter, and answer the questions below:

1. How does ischemia in the inferior leads cause a sinus bradycardia?
2. Explain the rationale for choosing to pace Aaron in the face of his ischemia.
3. How is the mechanism of dopamine or epinephrine different from that of atropine?

REFERENCES:

1. Walsh CA. Syncope and sudden death in the adolescent. *Adolesc Med.* 2001;12(1):105–132.

2. Baruscotti M, Robinson RB. Electrophysiology and pacemaker function of the developing sinoatrial node. *Am J Physiol Heart Circ Physiol.* 2007;293(5):H2613–H2623.

3. Gill MA, Miscia VF, et al. The treatment of common cardiac arrhythmias. *J Am Pharm Assoc.* 1976;16(1):20–29.

4. Vassallo JA, Cassidy D, et al. Relation of late potentials to site of origin of ventricular tachycardia associated with coronary heart disease. *Am J Cardiol.* 1985;55(8):985–989.

5. Patel A, Markowitz SM. Atrial tachycardia: mechanisms and management. *Expert Rev Cardiovas Ther.* 2008;6(6):811–822.

6. Scher DL, Arsura EL. Multifocal atrial tachycardia: mechanisms, clinical correlates, and treatment. *Am Heart J.* 1989;118(3):574–580.

7. Lazar, J, MD, MPH. Atrial fibrillation. Available at: http://www.emedicine.com/EMERG/topic46.htm. Accessed April 23, 2008.

8. Crijns HJ, Van den Berg MP, et al. Management of atrial fibrillation in the setting of heart failure. *Eur Heart J.* 1997;18 Suppl C:C45–C49.

9. Boriani G, Biffi M, et al. Rate control in atrial fibrillation: choice of treatment and assessment of efficacy. *Drugs.* 2003;63(14):1489–1509.

10. Ramlakhan SL, Fletcher AK. It could have happened to Van Gogh: a case of fatal purple foxglove poisoning and review of the literature. *Eur J Emerg Med.* 2007;14(6):356–359.

11. Rietbrock N, Alken RG. Color vision deficiencies: a common sign of intoxication in chronically digoxin-treated patients. *J Cardiovasc Pharmacol.* 1980;2(1):93–99.

12. de Bakker JM, Ho SY, et al. Basic and clinical electrophysiology of pulmonary vein ectopy. *Cardiovasc Res.* 2002;54(2):287–294.

13. Albert NM. Ventricular dysrhythmias in heart failure. *J Cardiovasc Nurs.* 2004;19(6 Suppl):S11–S26.

14. Abbott AV. Diagnostic approach to palpitations. *Am Fam Physician.* 2005;71(4):743–750.

15. Alexander ME, Berul CI. Ventricular arrhythmias: when to worry. *Pediatr Cardiol.* 2000;21(6):532–541.

16. Gowda RM, Misra D, et al. Acute pulmonary edema after cardioversion of cardiac arrhythmias. *Int J Cardiol.* 2003;92(2-3):271–274.

17. Khan IA. Atrial stunning: basics and clinical considerations. *Int J Cardiol.* 2003;92(2-3):113–128.

18. Frishman WH, Del Vecchio A, et al. Cardiovascular manifestations of substance abuse: part 2: alcohol, amphetamines, heroin, cannabis, and caffeine. *Heart Dis.* 2003;5(4):253–271.

19. Sala M, Coppa F, et al. Antidepressants: their effects on cardiac channels, QT prolongation and torsade de pointes. *Curr Opin Investig Drugs.* 2006;7(3):256–263.

20. Allen LaPointe NM, Curtis LH, et al. Frequency of high-risk use of QT-prolonging medications. *Pharmacoepidemiol Drug Saf.* 2006;15(6):361–368.

21. Olsen KM. Pharmacologic agents associated with QT interval prolongation. *J Fam Pract.* 2005;Suppl:S8–S14.

22. Goodnick PJ, Jerry J, et al. Psychotropic drugs and the ECG: focus on the QTc interval. *Expert Opin Pharmacother.* 2002;3(5):479–498.

23. Marantz PR, Kaplan MC, et al. Clinical diagnosis of congestive heart failure in patients with acute dyspnea. *Chest.* 1990;97(4):776–781.

24. Smith DC. Ashman's phenomenon—a source of nonsustained wide complex tachycardia. *J Emerg Med.* 1993;11(1):98.

25. Crijns HJ. Rate versus rhythm control in patients with atrial fibrillation: what the trials really say. *Drugs.* 2005;65(12):1651–1667.

26. Saxonhouse SJ, Curtis AB. Risks and benefits of rate control versus maintenance of sinus rhythm. *Am J Cardiol.* 2003;91(6A):27D–32D.

27. Boriani G, Diemberger I, et al. Pharmacological cardioversion of atrial fibrillation: current management and treatment options. *Drugs.* 2004;64(24):2741–2762.

28. Bateman DN. Digoxin-specific antibody fragments: how much and when? *Toxicol Rev.* 2004;23(3):135–143.

29. Ramlakhan SL, Fletcher AK. It could have happened to Van Gogh: a case of fatal purple foxglove poisoning and review of the literature. *Eur J Emerg Med.* 2007;14(6):356–359.

30. Sherman DG. Stroke prevention in atrial fibrillation: pharmacological rate versus rhythm control. *Stroke.* 2007;38(2 Suppl):615–617.

31. Kothari RU, Pancioli A, et al. Cincinnati Prehospital Stroke Scale: reproducibility and validity. *Ann Emerg Med.* 1999;33(4):373–378.

CHAPTER 5

ERRORS OF CONDUCTION: TACHYCARDIA

KEY CONCEPTS:

Upon completion of this chapter, it is expected that the reader will understand these following concepts:

- Effects on the cardiac output equation and coronary filling time from heart rates that are too fast
- Re-entry, either as a macrocircuit or microcircuit, and how it is the most likely cause of tachycardic errors of conduction
- Mechanical, pharmacological, or electrical treatment options

ANATOMY CONCEPTS:

Prior to reading this chapter the Paramedic student should be familiar with the following anatomy and physiology concepts:

- Cardiac conduction system
- Electrophysiology

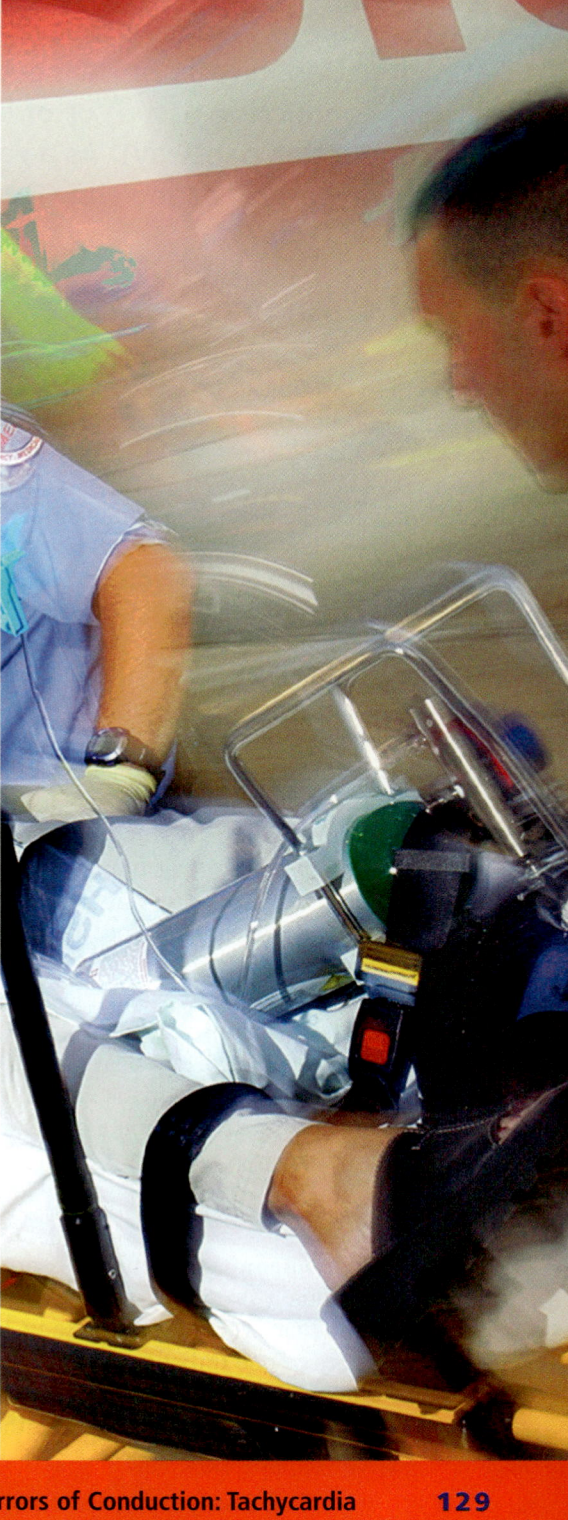

CASE STUDY:

Paramedics are called to the local diner for a 24-year-old female patient who feels faint. Upon arrival, Kaylie, the short order cook, is seated on a stool in the kitchen. She is tachypneic and appears anxious. The waitress says that Kaylie was managing the dinner crowd alone when suddenly she complained of feeling faint. She looked pale, so the waitress had her sit down and then called EMS. Kaylie states that she feels weak and slightly dizzy. She also says it feels as if her heart is going to beat right out of her chest.

CRITICAL THINKING QUESTIONS

1. What are some of the possible causes of Kaylie's palpitations?
2. How can the palpitations and the dizziness be related?

OVERVIEW

Electrocardiograms were originally grouped in order of similar characteristics (e.g., narrow complex tachycardia and wide complex bradycardia). However, as our understanding of the mechanisms of these dysrhythmia increased, with the advent of electrophysiologic mapping of the heart, it become apparent that there were two primary mechanisms for dysrhythmia: (1) errors of automaticity (i.e., problems with impulse formation, discussed in the previous chapter) and (2) errors in conduction.

The second mechanism for the development of dysrhythmia, errors of conduction, is a disorder of impulse propagation through the conduction system. These errors of conduction may be of the re-entry type (in which an impulse continues to circle around conducting tissue) or of a block (in which the impulse does not continue along the conducting pathway). As a result of errors of conduction, the heart rate can go too fast (tachycardia) or too slow (bradycardia), with devastating effects on hemodynamics.

Chief Concern

The crux issue with errors of conduction is the heart rate that is either too fast (generally greater than 150 bpm) or too slow (less than 50 bpm). Although heart rates that are too fast or too slow affect the equation for cardiac output (Cardiac Output = Stroke Volume × Heart Rate, or CO = SV × HR) in different ways, the outcome is quite similar. Heart rates that are too fast or too slow ultimately affect cardiac output. Blood flow to the body and brain is reduced, leaving the patient with complaints of weakness and dizziness. Older patients, or those with comorbidities, may also complain of chest pain and shortness of breath due to these rate abnormalities.

The pathologic mechanism for a too fast heart rate is thought to be due to a re-entry phenomena. These phenomena, described shortly, permit tachycardias in excess of 150 bpm. Most patients cannot sustain a heart rate above 150 bpm for long without becoming symptomatic. When the heart races, the period of diastole in cardiac cycle, which is normally two-thirds of the cardiac cycle, is reduced to 50% or less. During the diastolic period, the coronary arteries fill. Therefore, the result of sustained tachycardia is diminished coronary artery filling just when the heart is working the hardest (i.e., there is a mismatch between the coronary artery filling and the demand of the heart for oxygenated blood). Without the needed oxygen that is normally supplied during diastole, the heart starts to become ischemic and the patient becomes symptomatic.

Re-Entry Phenomena

Re-entry phenomena is the return passage of a depolarization wave through a structure, such as the AV node, that has passed through that structure once already. It utilizes a circuit that depolarizes in one direction while allowing the impulse to return via another direction. When the impulse reaches the starting point, it finds the first arm of the circuit ready to accept the impulse again and the circuit persists. If conditions are right, then the depolarization wave will persist in retrograde fashion and create an antidromic circus movement.

A re-entry circuit can depolarize the entire myocardium rapidly and repeatedly, establishing a re-entry tachycardia, or it can depolarize small segments of myocardium, creating either an atrial or ventricular fibrillation (Figure 5-1).

Causes of Re-Entry Phenomena

There are thought to be many causes of re-entry; however, three conditions must exist in order for a re-entry circuit to occur. First, there must be an available circuit. This pathway for conduction of an impulse should be a circular depolarization wave. It can be a large, or **macrocircuit**, such as may exist between the atria and ventricles, through the AV node. It can also be an alternate bundle of conduction tissue, a congenital

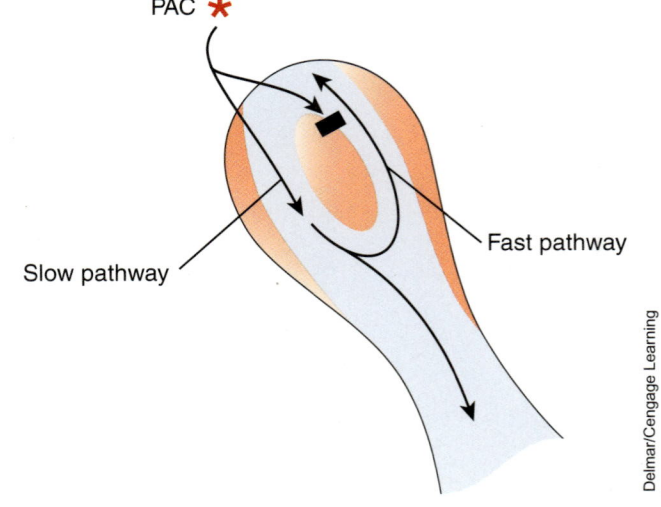

PAC

Slow pathway

Fast pathway

Delmar/Cengage Learning

Figure 5-1 Re-entry phenomena.

conductive pathway. Alternatively, it can be a small **microcircuit** that exists within either the atrium or the ventricles.

Second, there must be a pathway for impulse, or a difference in the refractory periods of one part of the circuit and another part. One arm of the circuit, sometimes referred to as the alpha pathway, must be slower than the other arm of the circuit, sometimes referred to as the beta pathway. The difference in the speeds of depolarization and repolarization allow the impulse to continually find cells ready to accept the impulse and depolarize again.

Third, the alpha circuit must have slowed conduction so that the impulse never catches up with itself. This slowed conduction can be due to acidosis, hypoxia, or ischemia, or it can be the result of medications such as tricyclic antidepressants.

If any of the three conditions fails to exist, the circuit is extinguished and the dysrhythmia ends. Treatments are directed toward eliminating the circuit through such techniques as radio ablation (use of radio energy to destroy tissue in an electrophysiology lab) or neutralizing one part of the circuit, making the refractory periods equal (i.e., electrical cardioversion/defibrillation). Other techniques include using medications that slow conduction so much that the impulses fail to move forward or speeding up conduction so the impulse overtakes itself and self-extinguishes. Many dysrhythmias can be attributed to an error of conduction (Table 5-1).

Table 5-1 Rhythms Usually Attributed to an Error in Conduction

- Macrocircuit
  - Atrial tachydysrhythmia
    - Paroxysmal atrial tachycardia
    - Atrial flutter
  - AV tachydysrhythmia
    - Re-entrant tachycardia (AVRT)
    - AV nodal re-entrant tachycardia (AVNRT)
      - Pre-excitation disorders
        - Wolff–Parkinson–White
        - Long–Ganong–Levine
    - Junctional tachycardia
  - Ventricular tachydysrhythmia
    - Ventricular tachycardia
      - Monomorphic
      - Polymorphic
    - Ventricular flutter
- Microcircuit
  - Atrial fibrillation*
  - Ventricular fibrillation

Note: *One theory suggests that atrial fibrillation is an error of conduction, whereas others attribute atrial fibrillation to an error of automaticity.

Supraventricular Tachycardia

All tachycardias that originate above the ventricles are called **supraventricular tachycardias (SVT)** (Table 5-2). These designations have a certain utility when trying to treat unstable patients under emergent conditions. However, since specific types of SVT respond more favorably to specific medications, distinguishing the different types of SVT is helpful in choosing the most effective medication.

SA Node Re-Entry Tachycardia

Sinoatrial node re-entry tachycardia is a relatively rare tachydysrhythmia that results from a re-entry circuit around the SA node. All of the morphological features of the ECG, P wave, and QRS, as well as the intervals and interval relationships in SA node re-entry tachycardia, are the same as sinus tachycardia. The only feature that should cause alarm in the Paramedic is the sudden and abrupt sinus tachycardia without plausible explanation; typically sinus tachycardia starts gradually then slows gradually. SA node re-entry tachycardia can also be initiated by ectopic beats, such as a premature atrial complex. Patients with SA node re-entry tachycardia can complain of palpitations and become extremely diaphoretic. While supportive care is generally all that is needed, the use of vagal maneuvers may terminate this tachydysrhythmia.

Atrial Flutter

Atrial flutter is a re-entry phenomena that occurs in the atria. This re-entry phenomena can result in either atrial fibrillation or atrial flutter.[1-3] The difference in the two rhythms is the size of the circuit; atrial flutter has a slightly larger or macrocircuit and atrial fibrillation has a microcircuit. Because of the common etiology, atrial flutter can break down and convert into an atrial fibrillation and then revert back into atrial flutter again.

Table 5-2 Supraventricular Rhythms— Errors of Conduction

- Regular narrow complex tachycardia
  - Sinus node
    - SA nodal re-entry tachycardia (SANRT)
  - Atria
    - Atrial flutter*
    - Paroxysmal atrial tachycardia (PAT)
  - AV node
    - AV nodal re-entry tachycardia (AVNRT)
    - Re-entrant tachycardia (AVRT)
      - Pre-excitation syndromes
        - Wolff–Parkinson–White (WPW)
        - Long–Ganong–Levine (LGL)
  - Junctional tachycardia

Note: *A flutter can be irregular depending on AV node block.

Atrial flutter caused by re-entry phenomena are referred to as type I atrial flutter. Atrial flutter can also be caused by an ectopic foci, creating an error of automaticity. This variety of atrial flutter, called type II atrial flutter, is less common than type I atrial flutter. Type I atrial flutter tends to be regular, with atrial rates of between 250 and 350 beats per minute and a regular ventricular response, secondary to the AV block, which is described shortly. Type II atrial flutter can be more irregular, because of its ectopic origins, and can sustain atrial depolarization of greater than 350 beats per minute.

The atrial response in atrial flutter can be between 250 to 350 beats per minute. The AV node cannot sustain repeated depolarizations and repolarizations at these rates and subsequently an AV block is created. While a 2:1 AV block is commonly seen in atrial flutter it is possible to have 4:1 and less commonly 3:1 or 5:1 AV blocks. At atrial rates greater than 350 (i.e., type II atrial flutter), the AV block becomes variable and the protection offered to the ventricles by the AV block is gone.

Patients with a history of heart failure, valvular disease (particularly the tricuspid valve), or pulmonary diseases (such as pulmonary embolism or chronic obstructive pulmonary disease) are prone to atrial flutter. Men are more prone to atrial flutter than woman by an almost 2 to 1 ratio. In addition, the prevalence of atrial flutter increases with age. The complications of atrial flutter include syncope and congestive heart failure, secondary to loss of atrial kick and subsequent decreased cardiac output.

Paroxysmal Atrial Tachycardia

Like the other dysrhythmias that arise from errors of conduction, **paroxysmal atrial tachycardia** arises from a microreentry circuit located in the atria wall and creates a sustained tachycardia. Usually paroxysmal atrial tachycardia is triggered by a premature atrial contraction and can sustain heart rates of more than 200 beats per minute. At heart rates this fast, the patient is usually acutely aware of his racing heart (an effect called palpitations) and may become lightheaded and experience syncope. Some patients, particularly those who have experienced PAT previously, will perform self-vagal maneuvers to terminate the tachydysrhythmia.

A/V Nodal Re-Entry Tachycardia (Intranodal)

The most common supraventricular tachycardia may be the A/V nodal re-entry tachycardia, seen in approximately 60% of SVT. A/V nodal re-entry tachycardia is thought to be triggered by a premature complex, such as a premature atrial complex (PAC) or a ventricular premature complex (VPC). Certain types of A/V nodal re-entry tachycardias occur in young adults who have no evidence of heart disease. There is greater prevalence of A/V nodal re-entry tachycardias in women than men.

A/V nodal re-entry tachycardia should not be confused with multifocal atrial tachycardia (MAT). MAT has an irregular heartbeat caused by an error of automaticity (e.g., created by digitalis toxicity). In contrast, A/V nodal re-entry tachycardia is usually a regular rhythm caused by an error of conduction. A/V nodal re-entry tachycardia is also not a pre-excitation syndrome, which is described shortly. These pre-excitation syndromes, such as Wolff–Parkinson–White syndrome, usually have specific ECG evidence of accessory pathways. In addition, A/V nodal re-entry tachycardia is not atrial fibrillation. Atrial fibrillation, discussed later, also has specific ECG findings and is an irregularly irregular rhythm.

A/V nodal re-entry tachycardia typically has an abrupt beginning (in some cases patients can provide an exact time of onset to the minute) and may last for seconds, minutes, and, rarely, days. A/V nodal re-entry tachycardia then ends as abruptly as it began. Generally patients tolerate the momentary burst of tachycardia, unless they have pre-existing coronary artery disease or other structural heart diseases (such as mitral regurgitation).

Functionally, but not anatomically, the AV node of the heart in these patients is divided into two branches. Conduction normally occurs over both of these branches simultaneously. The tachycardia of A/V nodal re-entry tachycardia is the result of re-entry phenomena in which either one of the two branches of the AV node conducts the impulse forward (**anterograde**) and then the other branch conducts the impulse backward (**retrograde**), called **orthodromic** tachycardia. The reverse can also occur, in which one branch of the AV node conducts the impulse forward and the other branch of the AV node conducts it backward (called **antidromic** tachycardia).

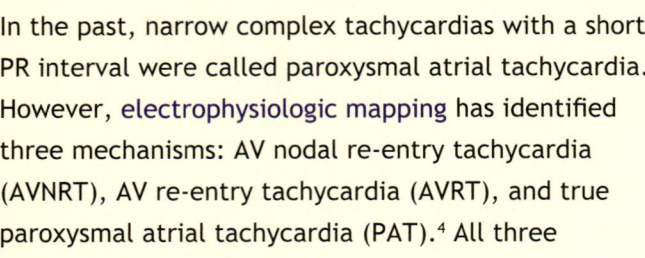

STREET SMART

In the past, narrow complex tachycardias with a short PR interval were called paroxysmal atrial tachycardia. However, electrophysiologic mapping has identified three mechanisms: AV nodal re-entry tachycardia (AVNRT), AV re-entry tachycardia (AVRT), and true paroxysmal atrial tachycardia (PAT).[4] All three tachydysrhythmias are errors of conduction.

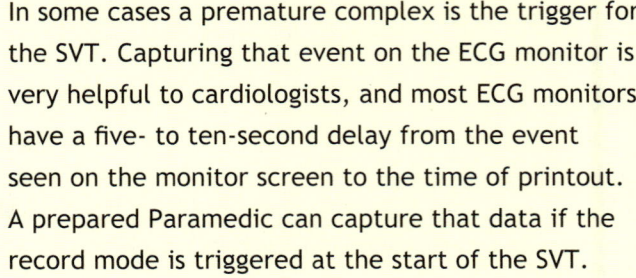

STREET SMART

In some cases a premature complex is the trigger for the SVT. Capturing that event on the ECG monitor is very helpful to cardiologists, and most ECG monitors have a five- to ten-second delay from the event seen on the monitor screen to the time of printout. A prepared Paramedic can capture that data if the record mode is triggered at the start of the SVT.

Precipitating factors that can cause A/V nodal re-entry tachycardia include fatigue, stress, and anxiety; all are factors that influence the autonomic nervous system. The increased heart rate causes a variety of physical signs and symptoms which may include weakness associated with dizziness and near syncope. The effects are real, debilitating, and can be very frightening.

A/V Re-Entry Tachycardia (Extranodal)

A/V re-entry tachycardia (AVRT) occurs when the early or premature activation of the ventricles, through the use of a congenital accessory tract that goes around the AV node, allows a circus movement to occur. These AVRT are loosely grouped as **pre-excitation disorders**. Pre-excitation disorders are not rhythms in and of themselves, but rather are the manifestation of a pre-existing cardiac anomaly that results in AVRT. An AVRT is due specifically because of congenital pathways, such as a bundle of Kent or a James Bundle. Several forms of pre-excitation disorders exist, including **Wolfe–Parkinson–White syndrome (WPW)**, the best known pre-excitation disorder, and **Lown–Ganong–Levine (LGL) syndrome**, that use the congenital accessory pathway that bypasses the AV node.

Pre-excitation disorders rely on these congenital accessory pathways for the re-entry circuit. When the depolarization wave passes down the conduction system, some of the depolarization wave passes down the accessory pathway, bypassing the AV node, and then circles back. Typically, the tissue is in a state of repolarization and the cells are refractory to further depolarization. However, if conditions are correct then a circus movement can occur and a tachycardia ensues. These re-entry rhythms can allow for very rapid ventricular responses.

Some older patients may know that they have a pre-excitation disorder, secondary to previous episodes of palpitations. Younger patients may not know that they have a pre-excitation disorder until they experience their first episode of tachycardia. Patients with a diagnosis of Wolff–Parkinson–White (WPW) syndrome have an accessory pathway, called the bundle of Kent, that bypasses the AV node to connect the atria and ventricles.[5–7] This pathway is normally weak. However, when the patient experiences a tachycardia, for whatever reason, the primary pathway fatigues. The two pathways then become equal, electrophysiologically speaking, and an antidromic circus movement can occur. Other examples of pre-excitation syndrome include Long–Ganong–Levine (LGL) syndrome; patients diagnosed with LGL have a bundle of tissues called the Lewis bundle that serves as an accessory pathway. WPW is more common than LGL.

All pre-excitation disorders produce a tachycardia with a slightly widened QRS complex and a shortened PR interval of less than 0.12 seconds. A distinguishing characteristic of WPW is the **delta wave**, a slurring of the upstroke of the R wave that broadens the QRS slightly. WPW can also be distinguished by a number of minor changes in the precordial leads that distinguish WPW into types A, B, and C.

Junctional Tachycardia

The pacemaker site for junctional tachycardia is adjacent and inferior to the AV node. The mechanism may involve an accessory pathway around the AV node or a small area completely within the AV junction that allows a circular motion. Infants and young children often display junctional tachycardia rhythms; however, as they grow older they tend to lose the tissue necessary for this rhythm to continue. Some children will display a junctional tachycardia immediately after cardiac surgery which resolves during the recovery period.

Emergency treatment during a junctional tachycardia is aimed toward maintaining an adequate cardiac output. In junctional tachycardia, the atria do not contract in synchrony with the ventricles. An analogy can be made to atrial fibrillation. Atrial contribution of blood to the stroke volume is lost (i.e., the atrial kick), and cardiac output subsequently decreases.[8]

Wide Complex Tachycardia of Unknown Origin

The ventricles can also produce a re-entry circuit like atrial fibrillation and atrial flutter called ventricular tachycardia, ventricular flutter, and ventricular fibrillation. The last, ventricular fibrillation, is particularly worrisome and is discussed, in detail, in Chapter 7 on cardiac resuscitation. These re-entry rhythms can all produce a wide complex tachycardia of unknown origin, which can be divided into those that are regular and those that are irregular. Those wide complex tachycardias that are regular include monomorphic ventricular tachycardia, ventricular flutter, and supraventricular tachycardia with aberrant conduction secondary to pre-excitation disorder. The irregular wide complex tachycardias include polymorphic ventricular tachycardia and torsades de pointes.

Monomorphic Ventricular Tachycardia

Like all tachycardia **monomorphic tachycardia** can be tolerated for a short period of time before the patient becomes symptomatic. The amount of time it can be tolerated depends on the patient. The mechanism of decompensation is similar to the mechanism of decompensation that occurs with supraventricular tachycardia, which was described earlier. The heart races and diminishes coronary artery filling at a time when the heart's demand for oxygen is the greatest. Therefore, the quick identification and treatment of ventricular tachycardia is essential.

The typical origin of ventricular tachycardia is associated with ischemia; however, there are other etiologies of ventricular tachycardia including prolonged QT syndromes; medications that prolong the QT interval; valvular disease, such as mitral valve prolapse; and other causes of electrical instability.[9,10] Extracardiac causes of ventricular tachycardia can include medications such as digitalis, sympathomimetics (such as cocaine), and conditions such as sarcoidosis. Sarcoidosis is an immune system disorder that can affect all organs of the body and lead to associated symptoms of fatigue, shortness of breath, and cutaneous lesions called erythema nodosum (an inflammation of adipose in the flesh).

Cardiac causes of ventricular tachycardia usually involve coronary artery insufficiency secondary to atherosclerosis or sudden coronary occlusion secondary to thrombus, embolus, aneurysm, or vasospasm. All of these conditions cause ischemia, which in turn leads to an irritation of the myocardium and creation of an ectopic pacemaker.

Since an ectopic pacemaker in the ventricles can take dominance over the natural pacemakers, and the ventricular depolarization renders the AV node refractory to further depolarization, atrial–ventricular dissociation is one of the hallmarks of ventricular tachycardia. During an episode of ventricular tachycardia, atrial depolarization continues to occur, represented by P waves, but the depolarization is not conducted into the ventricles. Ventricles continue to depolarize according to the rate of the ectopic foci; by definition, this is atrial–ventricular dissociation. Therefore, as a result of AV dissociation, augmentation of the end-diastolic volume is lost. Also, as a result of the tachycardia, the time for ventricular filling is shortened. The cumulative result of these two events is to markedly diminish the cardiac output, leading to systemic hypoperfusion and its sequella.

Ventricular Flutter

Ventricular flutter is often grouped together with ventricular tachycardia, and may be considered a form of extreme ventricular tachycardia. The difference between ventricular tachycardia, which can be tolerated for a limited time, and ventricular flutter, which cannot be tolerated, is the rate. While ventricular tachycardia can be rapid with rates ranging from 120 beats per minute to over 150 beats per minute, ventricular flutter is said to occur when the monitor complexes exceed 200 complexes per minute.

At this fast rate there is little time for ventricular filling. The result is a dramatic decrease in blood pressure and coronary artery perfusion. Without coronary artery perfusion the myocardium becomes ischemic and the patient's rhythm generally deteriorates into ventricular fibrillation.[11] The utility of knowing ventricular flutter is understanding the implications of a cardiac rhythm over 200 complexes per minute and the impending deterioration into ventricular fibrillation and sudden cardiac death.

Irregular Beats

On occasion, an atrial depolarization occurs during an episode of ventricular tachycardia at a time when both the AV node and then the ventricle can conduct it. As a result of this normal conduction, a normal narrow complex appears. These beats are referred to as capture beats and generally have a shorter RR interval than the RR interval of the ventricular tachycardia.

Similarly, the atrial depolarization can occur at the precise moment of ventricular depolarization and is manifest by a normal P wave and PR interval with a wide QRS complex. These beats are called fusion beats; in these cases, the RR interval is unchanged.

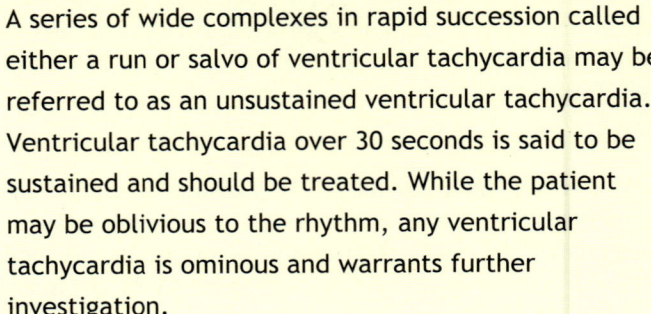

Polymorphic Ventricular Tachycardia

Another ventricular tachydysrhythmia is **polymorphic ventricular tachycardia**. The term "polymorphic" is given to this rhythm because there are at least two different morphologies, or shapes, of the QRS complex. Polymorphic ventricular tachycardia has a ventricular rate of over 150 bpm. This rhythm is the result of a delay in phase three of the action potential. During phase three the calcium channels close while the potassium channels remain open. This prolonged phase three results in hyperpolarization of the cell, which results in the creation of an ectopic pacemaker that triggers the ventricular tachycardia.

Electrolyte imbalances that predispose a patient to polymorphic ventricular tachycardia include hypokalemia and, particularly, **hypomagnesemia** (low serum magnesium levels). Hypomagnesemia occurs in patients with alcoholism, probably as a result of a combination of a poor diet and diarrhea as well as the use of diuretics (such as loop diuretics or thiazides). Certain antibiotics, such as the mycins and the aminoglycosides, interfere with the reabsorption of magnesium in kidneys. Symptoms associated with hypomagnesemia include weakness, muscle cramps, and prolonged QT intervals on the ECG.

Drugs that block the potassium channels, such as class III antidysrhythmics including amiodarone, delay the phase three repolarization, increasing the effective refractory period and terminating any re-entry circuits by eliminating susceptible myocardium.

When polymorphic ventricular tachycardia is preceded by a rhythm with a prolonged QT interval, either congenital or medication induced, it is called torsades de pointes. Torsades de pointes, French for "twisting of the point," appears to wax and wane along the isoelectric line. Medications implicated as causative agents of Torsades de pointes include the mycin antibiotics such as erythromycin, the antipsychotic drug haloperidol, methadone, and class 1c anti-arrhythmics, such as procainamide. Patients with Torsades de pointes have otherwise structurally sound hearts and appear healthy. Death in these patients appears to occur for no apparent reason. A variety of prescribed medications can lead to a prolongation of the QT interval of the ECG (Table 5-3).

Table 5-3 Partial List of Common Medications That Prolong QT Intervals

- Vaughn–Williams classification
  - 1A
    - Procainamide
    - Quinidine
- Organophosphates
- Antibiotics
  - Erythromycin
  - Clindamycin
  - Chloroquine
- Antifungals
  - Ketoconazole
- Antipsychotropics
  - Haloperidol
  - Phenothiazines
- Antidepressants
  - Tricyclic
  - Tetracyclic
- Citrate
  - Massive blood transfusions

Congenital Long QT Syndromes

One form of polymorphic ventricular tachycardia that is characterized by QT prolongation (QTc > 0.47 seconds) and T wave abnormalities is **Romano–Ward syndrome** **(RWS)**. Romano–Ward syndrome is a genetic abnormality that causes the heart rhythm to degenerate into Torsades de pointes (TdP).[12,13] Patients with Romano–Ward syndrome often present with syncope during exercise or during times of high emotion. They are also more prone to torsades de pointes when their serum potassium is low.

Similarly, some other unfortunate individuals are born with **exercise–induced polymorphic ventricular tachycardia**. This ventricular tachycardia is thought to be induced by epinephrine, a catecholamine. Typically this condition manifests in childhood, usually by a syncopal episode during play that is followed by a spontaneous recovery. However, in some cases the ventricular tachycardia progresses to ventricular fibrillation and sudden cardiac death. In many cases, the family has a history of premature death and/or has positive genetic testing for these conditions. The drug of choice to treat both of these cases, if the patient is stable, is a beta/adrenergic blocker.

CULTURAL/REGIONAL DIFFERENCES

Male adolescents were thought to be at greater risk of sudden cardiac death when compared to the same aged females. However, research published in 2006 shows there was no significant difference in risk for life-threatening events between males and females aged 13 to 20.

CASE STUDY (CONTINUED)

Kaylie's concern began about 15 minutes ago. She denies substernal pain but does complain of a "quivering" in her chest and a nagging sense of pressure. Aside from asthma, which she says she manages well and has not had an attack in months, she is healthy. Kaylie does admit to a lot of stress with a full-time job and demanding school schedule. She drinks six to seven cups of coffee daily, often after work, so she can get her homework done for her night classes. She admits that all that coffee keeps her up and that she does not sleep well.

CRITICAL THINKING QUESTIONS

1. What are the important elements of the history that a Paramedic should obtain?
2. What is the symptom pattern associated with a tachydysrhythmia?

History

The history of the patient with a tachycardia focuses on the precipitating factors and temporal events surrounding the episode of tachycardia. Starting with broad questions and narrowing the questions down to specifics, the Paramedic should inquire about time of onset, specifically what activity the patient was doing at the time of the episode. The OPQRST mnemonic (onset, provocation, quality of pain, radiation, severity, timing) is a useful tool for questioning. In addition, pertinent negative symptoms (i.e., loss of consciousness, chest pain, shortness of breath, and abdominal pain) can help the Paramedic assess the severity of the episode.

There is a common symptom complex that occurs in all patients with a tachycardia, regardless of the origin of the dysrhythmia. All tachycardias can markedly diminish cardiac output with resultant hypoperfusion of the end organs. The symptoms associated with these tachycardias are the result of that hypoperfusion. For example, hypoperfusion of the brain can lead to a sense of anxiety and even a sense of doom (i.e., a premonition of an impending disaster). Some patients complain of lightheadedness, particularly upon standing, and some even experience syncope.

The result of coronary hypoperfusion includes symptoms of neck or chest discomfort. In some cases, the patient may sense her heart beating faster within her chest, in an attempt to make up for the lost atrial kick. This abnormal awareness of one's heart beating in her chest is called a **palpitation**.

Many events can precipitate a tachycardia, including overexertion or use of stimulants (such as caffeine) or sympathomimetics (such as cocaine or methamphetamine). Certain disease states can also cause the patient to experience tachycardia. These diseases typically make the patient hypermetabolic. Conditions that make a patient hypermetabolic include hyperthyroidism, epinephrine-secreting tumor of the adrenal gland called a pheochromocytoma, and other hypermetabolic syndromes.

Some tachycardias, especially atrial fibrillation, are triggered by dehydration. As part of a hydration history, the Paramedic should ask about any recent infections that include vomiting or diarrhea. The Paramedic should also tactfully inquire about alcohol use. Alcohol is a known diuretic and

Table 5-4 Symptom Pattern of Tachydysrhythmia

- Heart
  - Palpitations—96%
  - Chest and/or neck discomfort—35%
- Lungs
  - Dyspnea—47%
- Brain
  - Dizziness—75%
  - Syncope—20%
- Other
  - Unexplained fatigue—23%
  - Unexplained diaphoresis—17%
  - Nausea—13%

excessive alcohol use may have been the predicating event (Table 5-4). The Paramedic should take the patient's symptom complex and compare it to the symptom pattern of tachydysrhythmia to form a paramedical diagnosis.

The etiology of some tachydysrhythmias is genetic, while the etiology of some others is medication related. A careful past medical history may reveal a history of the same tachydysrhythmias. If the patient has a history of tachydysrhythmias, the Paramedic should inquire about pharmacologic interventions used in the past or an electrical therapy including cardioversion and/or ablation. The co-existence of coronary artery disease is ominous, so the Paramedic should carefully explore the history of such cardiac disease.

CASE STUDY (CONTINUED)

Kaylie says that the oxygen that the EMT gave her is helping but that she continues to feel the chest pressure and palpitations. With those words the Paramedic asks to see the rhythm strip and inquires about Kaylie's vital signs.

CRITICAL THINKING QUESTIONS

1. What are the elements of the physical examination of a patient with suspected tachydysrhythmia?
2. Why is a 12-lead ECG a critical element in this examination?

Examination

Although the physical examination of the patient with a tachydysrhythmia focuses on the primary assessment, the Paramedic should also take a moment to perform a cardiovascular examination for life threats, vital signs, and the ECG. Persistent tachycardia can lead to heart failure, so the Paramedic should examine the patient for signs of heart failure including jugular venous distention, pulmonary edema,

ventricular gallop, hepatic–jugular reflex, abdominal tenderness, and dependent peripheral edema.

A patient with a tachydysrhythmia will have a heart rate greater than 100 bpm, but it is sustained tachycardia above 150 bpm that is problematic. At rates over 150 bpm the heart has insufficient time for ventricular filling, resulting in decreased cardiac output. A heart rate of over 150 bpm also creates a shortened diastolic period. During the diastolic period the coronary arteries fill. As a result of the tachycardia, there is decreased coronary artery filling and subsequent myocardial ischemia. Patients with a pre-existing history of poor left ventricular function (e.g., those with a previous acute myocardial infarction) may become grossly symptomatic at lower heart rates and will manifest signs of heart failure earlier.

However, if time permits, the Paramedic should attempt to obtain as much diagnostic information as possible. A 12-lead ECG, combined with clinical information, may help the Paramedic determine if the tachydysrhythmia is an error of conduction or an error of automaticity. This diagnostic information can help the Paramedic determine the most appropriate treatment pathway. Further information can be obtained from vagal maneuvers and/or the use of adenosine.

Vagal Maneuver

The heart's rate is usually kept in check by the parasympathetic nervous system, specifically the vagus nerve. During periods of tachydysrhythmia the vagal control of the heart can be exaggerated by performing **vagal maneuvers** (methods used to evaluate and treat cardiac arrhythmias and conduction abnormalities). In some instances the vagal maneuver is therapeutic, converting the rhythm back to normal. However, in most cases it is simply diagnostic.

There are several methods of eliciting a vagal response including facial immersion in ice water, used for pediatrics, the Valsalva maneuver; and carotid sinus massage.[14] The last, carotid sinus massage (CSM) or carotid sinus pressure (CSP), are to be avoided in the field. Patients with a history of **hypercholesterolemia** (a presence of an abnormal amount of cholesterol in the blood) who are at risk for arteriosclerosis, or those with a history of thrombus formation, are at risk for stroke if CSM is performed.

The preferred method of vagal stimulation in the field is the Valsalva maneuver. The **Valsalva maneuver** increases the intrathoracic pressure and thereby compresses the great vessels and the heart. As a result of this compression, there is a decrease in venous return to the heart, along with a decrease in ventricular filling. The combination of reduced filling and preload causes a drop in cardiac output (the inverse of the Frank–Starling law). When the patient breathes, the aortic pressure is increased, cardiac output increases, and the baroreceptors in the aorta reflexively signal the heart to slow through the vagus nerve.

To perform the Valsalva maneuver, the patient is instructed to take a deep breath and then hold his breath while either trying to blow out or by bearing down, as if to have a bowel movement, and then hold that way for 20 to 30 seconds. Children can be encouraged to forcefully blow through a straw for 20 seconds.

Typically the Valsalva maneuver is only used for narrow complex tachycardia, though it can be helpful in distinguishing SVT with aberrancy from ventricular tachycardia. If the tachydysrhythmia is supraventricular, the rhythm tends to stop abruptly, then paroxysmally return. If the rhythm is a sinus tachycardia the rate tends to slow gradually, then the heart gradually increases the rate again. If the rhythm is atrial fibrillation, the Paramedic may witness a slowing of the ventricular rate, which makes the fibrillatory "f" waves more prominent. Finally, ventricular tachycardia does not respond to vagal maneuvers as a rule.

While the use of vagal maneuvers can be helpful, the ECG is the primary diagnostic tool for distinguishing tachydysrhythmias. The following sections review those rhythms that can cause tachycardia.

Atrial Flutter

Atrial flutter is an uncommon rhythm that may be found in patients with ischemic heart disease or valvular disorders. The rhythm is unstable, reverting back to sinus rhythm or progressing to atrial fibrillation (Table 5-5). The pacemaker site is in the atrium. A single impulse completes a circle within the atrial tissue and creates the characteristic sawtooth F waves, which are best seen in Lead II. In type I, or typical atrial flutter, these F waves are inverted in Lead II secondary to the counterclockwise depolarization wave that traverses the re-entry circuit.

The AV node is usually able to prevent most of the circular activity from reaching the ventricles (i.e., AV block). With an atrial rate of 225 to 350, this block serves to protect the ventricles. Untreated or new onset atrial flutter usually presents with two flutter waves for each QRS complex with an effective ventricular rate of 150 times per minute (i.e., 2:1 AV block) (Figures 5-2 and 5-3).

Paroxysmal Atrial Tachycardia

Differences between paroxysmal atrial tachycardia and normal sinus rhythm are found in the heart rate and morphology of the P wave (Table 5-6). Focal atrial tachycardia results from the fast firing of atrial tissue rather than from the SA node. Although some atrial tachycardias utilize a re-entry circuit, for others the key is the increased automaticity of an ectopic focus. Some atrial tachycardia may be initiated by a premature beat, such as a PAC (Figure 5-4).

Table 5-5 Atrial Flutter

Ventricular Rhythm	
Regularity	May be either regular or slightly irregular
Rate	Usually 50 to 60, 75 to 80, 100 to 120, 150 complexes per minute
Width of QRS	Usually 0.04 to 0.12 seconds
Atrial Rhythm	
Regularity	Regular
Rate	300 to 400 waves
Shape of P wave	Sharp pointed "F" waves
PR interval	None
AV relationship	2–3–4 F waves per QRS

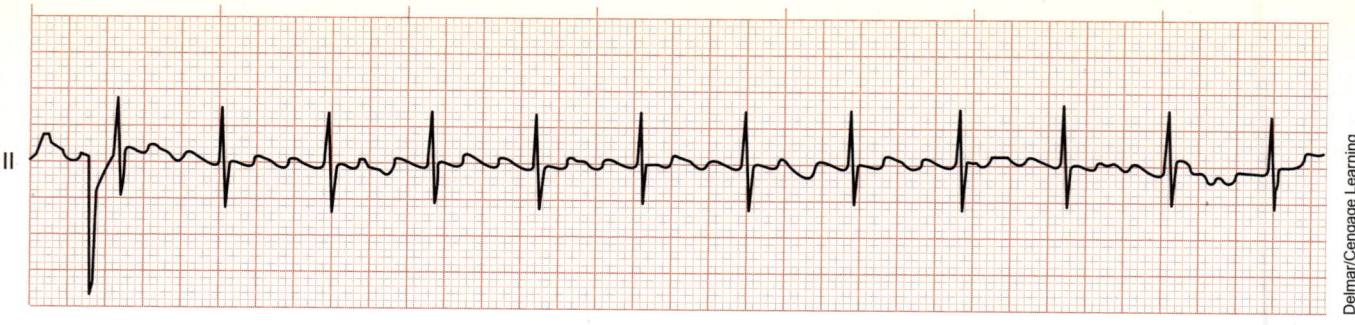

Figure 5-2   Atrial flutter.

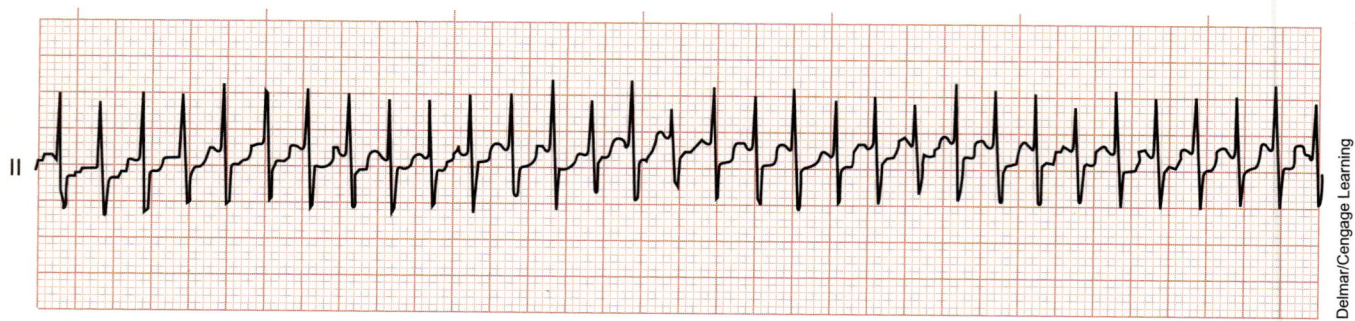

Figure 5-3   Atrial flutter with 1:1 conduction.

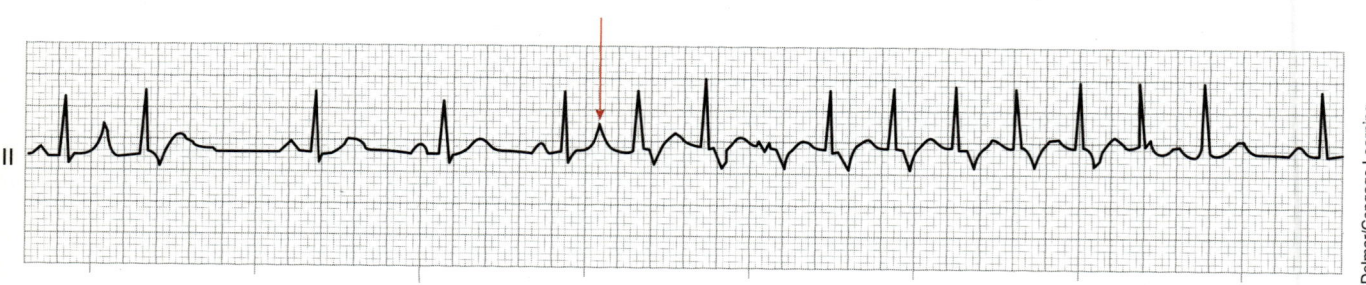

Figure 5-4   Paroxysmal atrial tachycardia initiated by a premature atrial complex.

Table 5-6   Paroxysmal Atrial Tachycardia

Ventricular Rhythm	
Rhythm	Regular
Rate	Normal with bursts greater than 150 bpm
Width QRS	Less than 0.12 seconds
Atrial Rhythm	
Rhythm	Regular
Rate	Same as ventricular rate
Shape of P wave	Ectopic P wave, peaked
Atrial rate	Same as ventricular
PR interval	Less than 0.12 seconds
AV relationship	1 P wave for every QRS

A/V Nodal Re-Entry Tachycardia

A/V nodal re-entry tachycardia is a fast rhythm initiated above the level of the ventricles (Table 5-7). The rapid rates associated with AVNRT decrease filling time and therefore lead to decreased cardiac output. Additionally, the fast rate increases the heart's need for oxygen. Patient complaints reflect this imbalance between the heart's needs and the supply. Common signs and symptoms associated with SVT include palpitations, lightheadedness or dizziness, change in level of consciousness, chest pain, or shortness of breath (Figure 5-5).

AV Re-Entry Tachycardia

The key identifying feature of a pre-excitation syndrome is the shortened PR interval, which is owed to an accessory pathway that accelerates conduction into the ventricles.

Table 5-7 A/V Nodal Re-entry Tachycardia (AVNRT)

Ventricular Rhythm	
Regularity	Regular
Rate	Greater than 150 complexes per minute
Width of QRS	Usually 0.04 to 0.12 seconds
Atrial Rhythm	
Regularity	Regular; if visible—usually buried in QRS
Rate	Varies
Shape of P wave	Upright and rounded in Lead II
PR interval	Less than 0.12 seconds; if visible
	PR interval shortens at onset of AVNRT
	PR interval lengthens at termination of AVNRT
AV relationship	1 P wave per QRS

Table 5-8 AV Re-entry Tachycardia (Wolff–Parkinson–White Syndrome)

Ventricular Rhythm	
Regularity	Regular
Rate	Greater than 100 complexes per minute
Width of QRS	Usually > 0.12 seconds; delta wave evident
Atrial Rhythm	
Regularity	Regular
Rate	Same as ventricular
Shape of P wave	Upright if before QRS, buried in QRS, or inverted following rhythm
PR interval	Less than 0.12 seconds
AV relationship	1 P wave per QRS

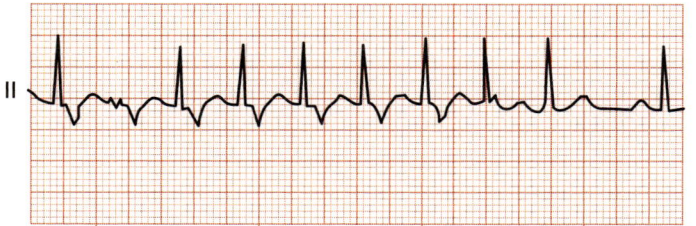

Figure 5-5 A/V nodal re-entry tachycardia.

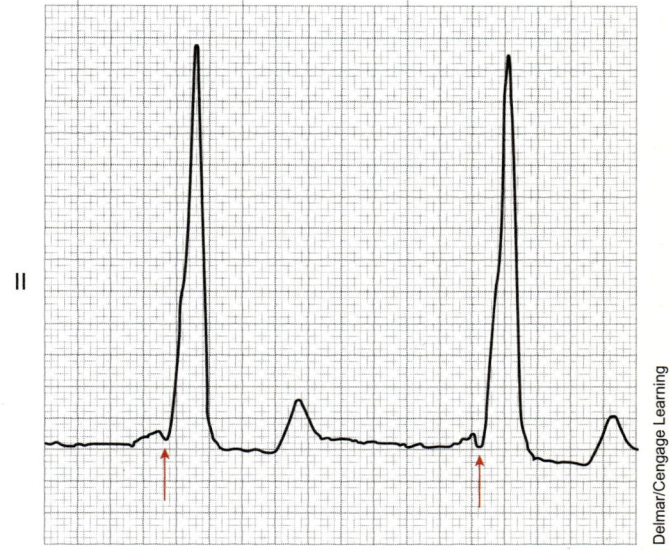

Figure 5-6 Delta wave associated with Wolff–Parkinson–White syndrome.

The QRS widens in some patients during their tachycardia. The widened QRS occurs because the changes of aging do not permit the bundle branches to sustain the rhythm. As a result, the patient experiences a "rate related bundle branch block" (type II first degree block) that quickly resolves when the tachycardia resolves and the QRS becomes narrow again.

However, patients with these syndromes—such as Wolff–Parkinson–White (WPW) (Table 5-8), types A and B (Figure 5-6), and Long–Ganong–Levine (Figure 5-7)—are prone to atrial dysrhythmias such as atrial fibrillation/flutter. However, the greatest danger of these short PR interval disorders is the rapid tachydysrhythmia, with rates exceeding 170 bpm.

WPW has a shortened PR interval and a distorted QRS complex. The additional pathway, the bundle of Kent, produces a delta wave on the ECG.

Junctional Tachycardia

Junctional tachycardia is sometimes confused with sinus tachycardia or atrial flutter (Table 5-9). In a junctional tachycardia, the P waves may be found inverted, as a result of retrograde depolarization, in front of the QRS complex. In addition, the PR interval is shorter. In atrial flutter, very pointed F waves, not P waves, are seen in Lead II. If the ventricular rate slows at all, additional pointed F waves (the flutter waves) can occur approximately 300 times a minute (Figure 5-8).

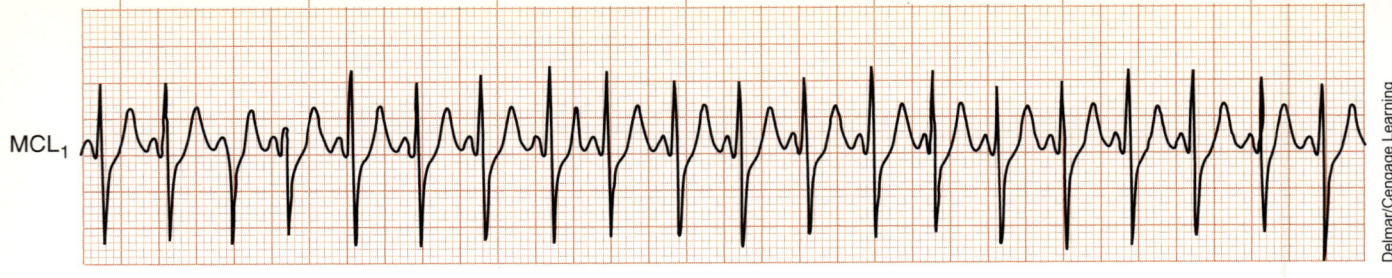

Figure 5-7 Long–Ganong–Levine syndrome.

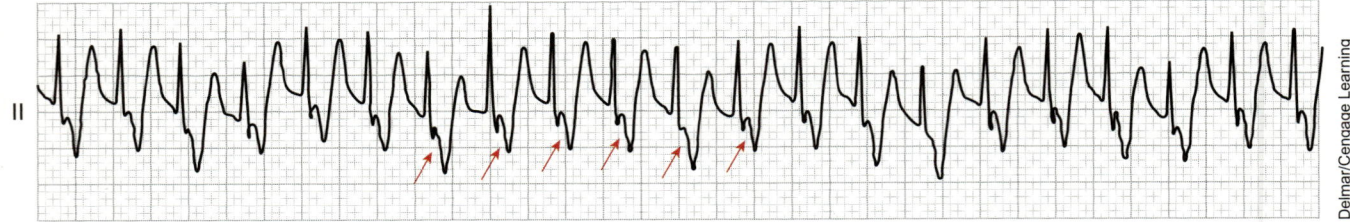

P waves noted by arrows

Figure 5-8 Junctional tachycardia.

Table 5-9 Junctional Tachycardia

Ventricular Rhythm	
Regularity	Regular
Rate	Greater than 100 complexes per minute
Width of QRS	Usually 0.04 to 0.12 seconds
Atrial Rhythm	
Regularity	Regular
Rate	Same as ventricular
Shape of P wave	Upright if before QRS, buried in QRS, or inverted following rhythm
PR interval	Less than 0.12 seconds if preceding QRS; otherwise none
AV relationship	1 per QRS if visible

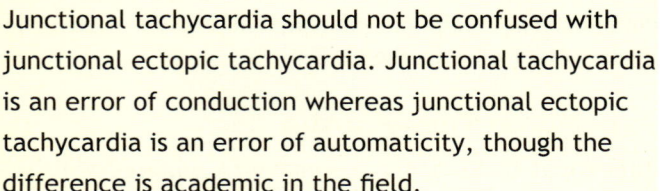

STREET SMART

Junctional tachycardia should not be confused with junctional ectopic tachycardia. Junctional tachycardia is an error of conduction whereas junctional ectopic tachycardia is an error of automaticity, though the difference is academic in the field.

Ambulatory Electrocardiography Monitoring

Some patients with paroxysmal tachycardia, particularly those that are symptomatic, will be placed on ambulatory monitors. In honor of the inventor of long duration, ambulatory monitoring, the procedure is usually called **Holter monitoring**. Holter monitors consist of a recorder capable of recording two or three ECG leads simultaneously for rate, rhythm, and rhythm disturbances.[15,16] Current recorders utilize frequencies in the 0.05 to 150 Hz range and are capable of analyzing ST segment variations and the QT interval. Most recorders have an event marker that allows the patient to instruct the Holter monitor to record and identify the timing of a particular symptom. Patients must also complete a diary as part of the monitoring procedure.

Ambulatory Holter monitoring is usually conducted for 24 to 48 hours. However, newer, longer duration, infrequent event monitors may be used for weeks. These long duration Holter monitors require activation by the patient when the event is recognized and the information is sent by telephone for possible identification of immediate threats and management. Regardless of the duration of the monitoring, the device is returned to a central location for complete analysis.

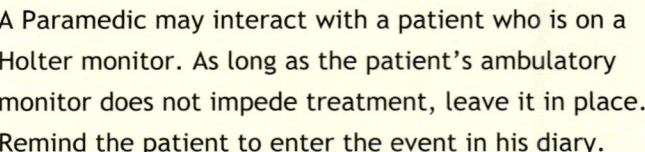

STREET SMART

A Paramedic may interact with a patient who is on a Holter monitor. As long as the patient's ambulatory monitor does not impede treatment, leave it in place. Remind the patient to enter the event in his diary.

Wide Complex Tachycardia

By definition, any QRS complex greater than 0.12 seconds is wide. The wide complex tachycardias of unknown origin are typically either one of two ventricular rhythms (monomorphic ventricular tachycardia or polymorphic tachycardia) or one of two supraventricular rhythms (supraventricular tachycardia with aberrant conduction or supraventricular tachycardia with excitation pathways).

Ventricular Tachycardia (VT)

The pacemaker site for ventricular tachycardia is located in the ventricles within a small re-entry circuit, allowing the impulse to circle just within the ventricles. Treatment varies for ventricular tachycardia, generally depending on the presence of pulses and specifically on the stability of the patient. If there are pulses present, observe for changes in mental status, alterations in skin condition, temperature and color, or complaints of chest pressure or dyspnea. These are signs and symptoms suggestive of impending instability (Table 5-10 and Figure 5-9). Unstable ventricular tachycardia can be terminated by antidysrhythmic medications or electricity.

Ventricular Flutter

The mechanism for ventricular flutter is the same re-entry circuit that causes ventricular tachycardia. Like atrial flutter, it is often associated with deterioration of the rhythm to ventricular fibrillation. Ventricular flutter is monomorphic and can be thought of as a rapid ventricular tachycardia (Table 5-11 and Figure 5-10). Fortunately, ventricular flutter responds to the same treatment as ventricular tachycardia.

Table 5-10 Monomorphic Ventricular Tachycardia

Ventricular Rhythm	
Regularity	Regular
Rate	Greater than 100 complexes per minute; usually 150 to 200 complexes per minute
Width of QRS	Usually > 0.12 seconds
Atrial Rhythm	
Regularity	Regular
Rate	Varies
Shape of P wave	Upright and rounded in Lead II
PR interval	None
A/V relationship	None: A/V disassociation

Table 5-11 Ventricular Flutter

Ventricular Rhythm	
Regularity	Regular
Rate	Greater than 200 complexes per minute
Width of QRS	Usually > 0.12 seconds
Atrial Rhythm	
Regularity	Regular
Rate	Not discernable
Shape of P wave	Not visible
PR interval	None
A/V relationship	None; A/V dissociation

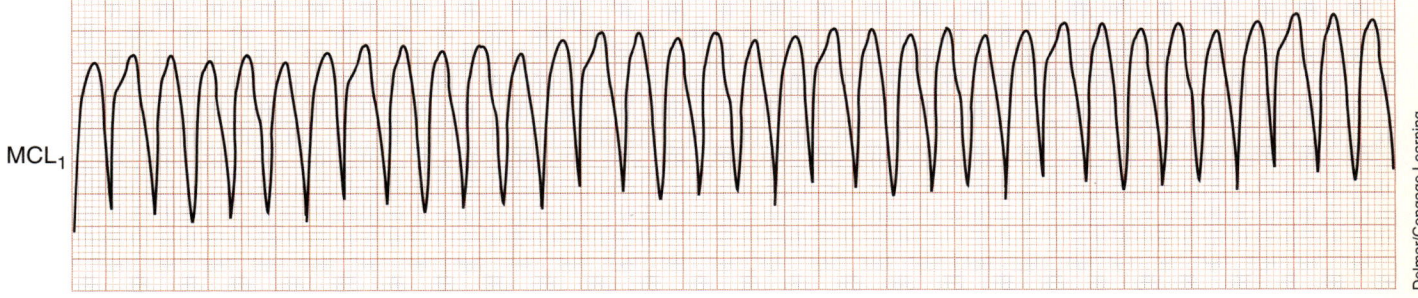

MCL$_1$

Delmar/Cengage Learning

Figure 5-9 Monomorphic ventricular tachycardia.

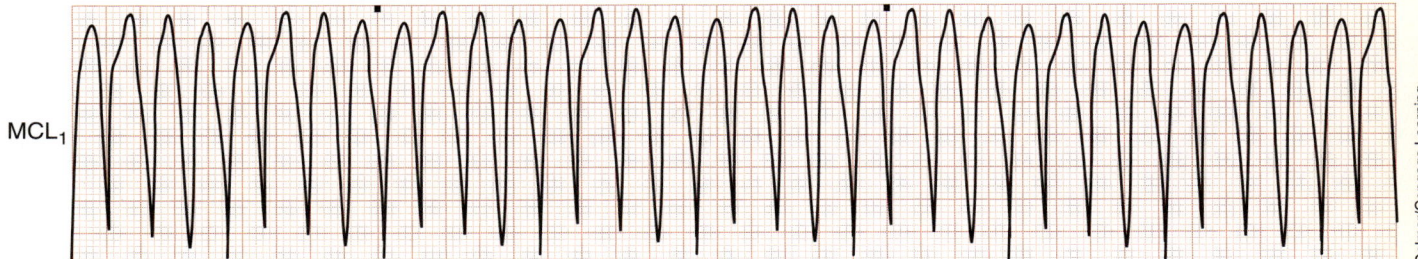

MCL$_1$

Delmar/Cengage Learning

Figure 5-10 Ventricular flutter.

Polymorphic Ventricular Tachycardia

Polymorphic ventricular tachycardia is associated with a long QT interval, which is often a result of hypomagnesemia (Table 5-12 and Figure 5-11). Polymorphic ventricular tachycardia can be paroxysmal. Between runs of the ventricular tachycardia the Paramedic should ascertain if there is a prolonged QT interval; this information can be most easily obtained by a 12-lead ECG. Although there can be pulses with this rhythm, cardiac output is likely to be impaired secondary to decreased ventricular filling. If a prolonged QT interval or the characteristic waxing and waning of the ECG over the isoelectric line is observed, or there is a history suggestive of hypomagnesemia, then the dysrhythmic of choice is magnesium.

Torsades de Pointes

Torsades de pointes (TdP), a subset of polymorphic ventricular tachycardia, occurs with patients who either have congenital prolonged QT syndromes, or who have a drug-induced QT interval prolongation. The distinguishing characteristics of torsades de pointes are the morphological features of the QRS. There is a waxing and waning of the QRS along the isoelectric line. Starting with a small wave, called the node, the waves become larger, then smaller again. Each of these units is called a spindle. At the termination of the spindle, the deflection of the QRS changes from positive to negative, or negative to positive as the case may be.

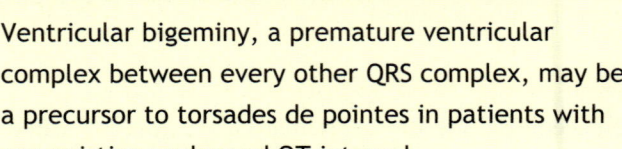

Aberrancy

Normally the QRS of a supraventricular tachycardia is narrow, less than 0.12 seconds. However, as the rate of depolarization increases, conductive tissue (particularly the right bundle branch) becomes fatigued and unable to accept another impulse. The fatigued bundle branch acts essentially as a block, forcing conduction of the impulse to bypass the conductive pathway and go from cell to cell across the right ventricle. This cell-to-cell conduction around the conductive pathway is called **aberrant conduction**. Aberrant conduction in the right ventricle results in a widened QRS complex on the ECG and a characteristic right bundle branch block.

The Paramedic can detect a right bundle branch block (RBBB) by looking at either MCL1 on the monitor or at V1 on the 12-lead ECG (Figure 5-12). The QRS complex of a RBBB will typically have an rSR configuration and the second R wave will be taller (Figure 5-13).

Aberrant Supraventricular Tachycardia versus Ventricular Tachycardia

Differentiating the abnormal or aberrant conduction of SVT, which causes a wide complex tachycardia, from ventricular tachycardia can be challenging. Since treatments vary for these rhythms, and the treatment of one rhythm with the other rhythm's medications can be devastating, it is important for the Paramedic to search for clues revealing the presence of each.

When confronted with wide complex tachycardia of unknown origin, the Paramedic's first instinct is to suspect ventricular tachycardia, because of its ominous implications. The Paramedic then begins to ascertain if the patient is stable or unstable. If the patient is unstable, regardless of the rhythm, then cardioversion (discussed shortly) is in order.

Table 5-12 Polymorphic Ventricular Tachycardia

Ventricular Rhythm	
Regularity	Irregular
Rate	Greater than 100 complexes per minute; usually > 150 complexes per minute
Width of QRS	Usually > 0.12 seconds
Atrial Rhythm	
Regularity	Regular; if visible
Rate	Varies
Shape of P wave	Upright and rounded in Lead II
A/V relationship	None: A/V disassociation

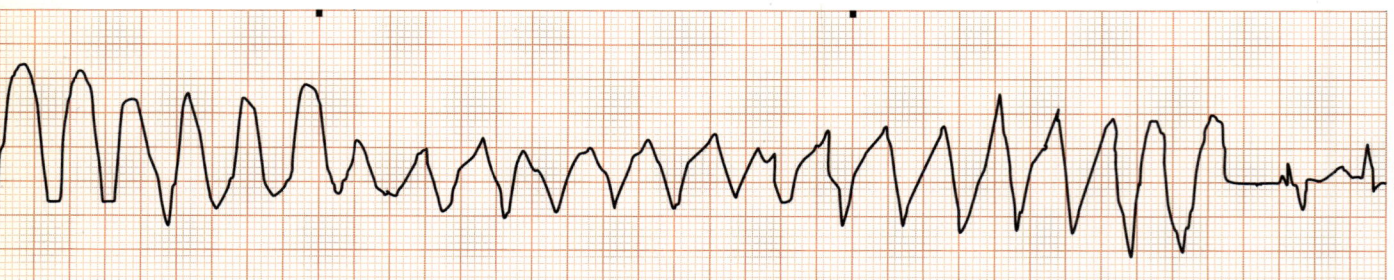

Figure 5-11 Polymorphic ventricular tachycardia.

Delmar/Cengage Learning

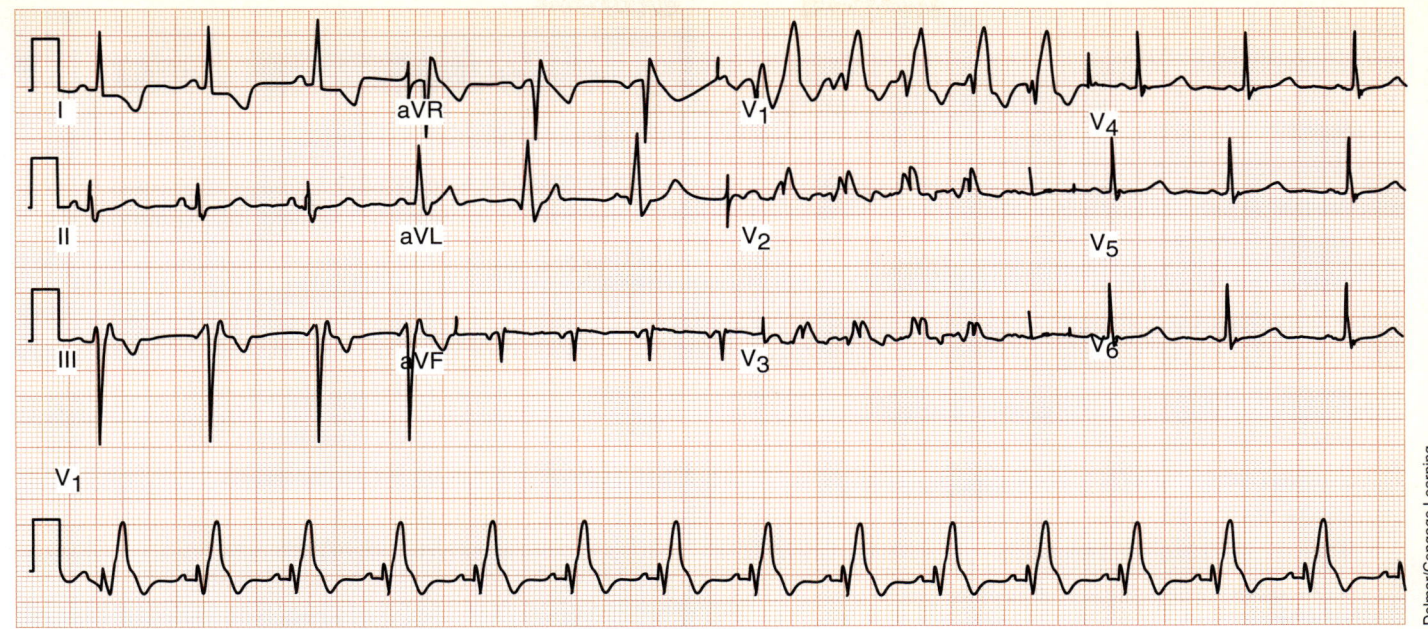

Figure 5-12 Right bundle branch block.

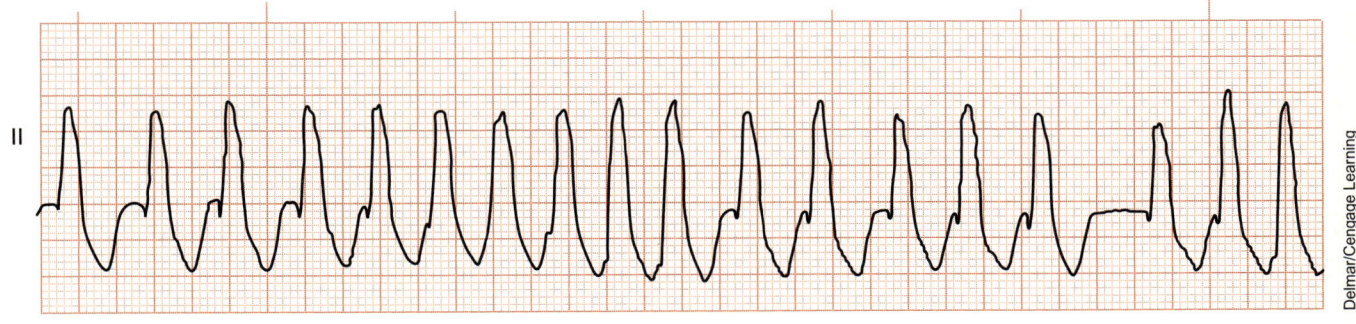

Figure 5-13 Atrial fibrillation with right bundle branch block.

However, if the patient is stable (i.e., without hemodynamic compromise) and can tolerate further investigation (and perhaps a pharmacological approach to management of the dysrhythmia), then the Paramedic should obtain a 12-lead ECG immediately.

Distinguishing ventricular tachycardia from supraventricular tachycardia with aberrancy is the primary concern. Treating a borderline wide QRS tachycardia that is thought to be a supraventricular tachycardia with adenosine, diltiazem, or verapamil not only delays the appropriate treatment of ventricular tachycardia but risks ventricular fibrillation. A 12-lead ECG can be very helpful in making this distinction.

An analysis of the 12-lead ECG will first show a common deflection across the precordial leads. The R wave progression in a normal rhythm (i.e., supraventricular) would be primarily negative in V1 and positive in V6. However, since the pacemaker in ventricular tachycardia is in the ventricles, the deflection of the R waves is all in the same direction, or in **concordance** across the precordial leads.

Next, the Paramedic should ascertain the axis deviation. Ventricular tachycardia has an extreme axis deviation, with a QRS axis of (−) 30 degrees to (−) 180 degrees (i.e., extreme left axis deviation). However, there are numerous causes of left axis deviation.

Therefore, the Paramedic should either closely examine the 12-lead ECG for atrial activity, or perform a vagal maneuver in an attempt to slow the ventricular response (Table 5-13 and Figure 5-14). Visible P waves, denoting atrial activity, will not have any association with the QRS complexes in ventricular tachycardia (A/V dissociation). Furthermore, the ventricular response will not be affected by the vagal maneuver.

However, when in doubt the Paramedic should assume ventricular tachycardia over supraventricular tachycardia. Ventricular tachycardia accounts for greater than 80% of wide complex tachycardia and over 95% of wide complex tachycardia in patients with a history of acute coronary syndrome.

Table 5-13 Differentiating Wide Complex Tachycardia

- Characteristics favoring supraventricular tachycardia with aberrancy
  - Triphasic morphology in V1 and V6
  - V1 rSR'
  - V6 QRS
  - Associated atrial activity
    - Vagal maneuvers
  - QRS axis of −30 to +90 degrees
  - Previous diagnosis of aberrancy
- Characteristics favoring ventricular tachycardia
  - Single R wave or QR, RS, or Rsr' in V1
  - rS, QS, or QR in V6
  - QRS axis of −30 to −180 degrees (extreme left deviation)
  - Concordance across the precordial leads
  - Atrial ventricular dissociation QRS greater than 0.16 seconds

Rate Related Bundle Branch Block

The impulses from above the ventricle speed up until one bundle branch (usually the right) remains refractory longer. Although the impulse will traverse the nonrefractory bundle, aberrant conduction (as a wide QRS) will show on the tracing. The rate at which the aberrancy develops is called the **critical rate**. If the rate decelerates, it must drop below the critical rate before normal conduction resumes.

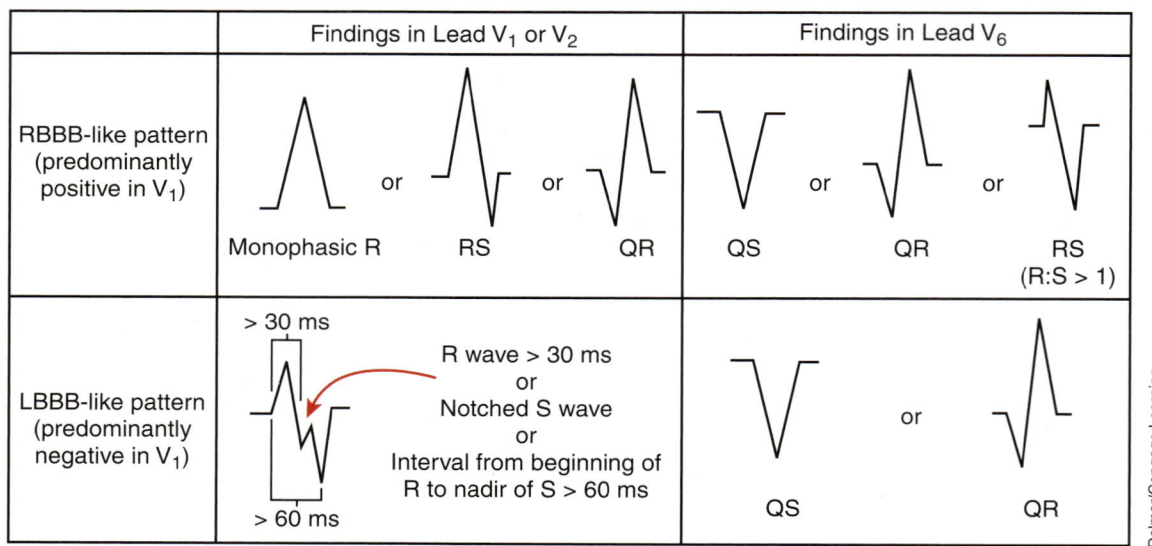

Figure 5-14 Brugada criteria.

CASE STUDY (CONTINUED)

As the Paramedic suspected, Kaylie has a tachydysrhythmia. The Paramedic advises Kaylie that her heart is racing and that there are medications available to treat her condition.

CRITICAL THINKING QUESTIONS

1. Hemodynamically speaking, what is the significance of a tachydysrhythmia?
2. What diagnosis did the Paramedic announce to the patient?

Assessment

The patient's presentation of a sudden onset narrow complex tachycardia, in the face of autonomic nervous system stimulation, is suggestive of A/V nodal re-entry tachycardia. The hypotension associated is likely induced by the tachycardia.

If the patient is grossly symptomatic and unstable, then the Paramedic needs to intervene.

AV nodal re-entry tachycardia can be difficult to treat. The patient is in imminent cardiovascular collapse secondary to the tachycardia-induced hypotension and the medications used to treat the dysrhythmia tend to cause hypotension.

CASE STUDY (CONTINUED)

Kaylie did not have a change in rhythm after the vagal maneuver so she was given adenosine. Following a 6 mg dose of adenosine, Kaylie converted to a sinus tachycardia at 110. She said she felt much better and would like to return to work. While the Paramedic advises Kaylie against a return to work before he performs a complete workup, Kaylie says she feels terrible. Her monitor is now showing a wide complex tachycardia at 200.

Since the leads are still in place from the 12-lead ECG, the Paramedic's partner obtains a 12-lead tracing which shows an average QRS axis of +45 degrees, no acute ST-T wave changes, good R wave progression through the V leads, rSR' in V1 lead, and initial deflection in V1 is the same as on the earlier ECG.

CRITICAL THINKING QUESTIONS

1. What is the national standard of care of patients with suspected tachydysrhythmia?
2. Why did Kaylie suddenly decompensate?

Treatment

As previously discussed, there are three conditions necessary for a re-entry tachycardia to exist. If any of the conditions is removed, the dysrhythmia is eliminated. Therefore, treatments are directed toward correcting one or more of the sustaining conditions.

First, a re-entry circuit must be available. It can be a macrocircuit, such as may exist between the atria and ventricles through the AV node and an alternate bundle of conduction tissue, or a microcircuit that exists within the atriums or ventricles. In an emergency, when the patient is unstable, the re-entry circuit is eliminated by electrical therapies, such as cardioversion. Cardioversion, discussed shortly, depolarizes all of the myocardium, allowing the primary pacemakers to dominant the rhythm.

Medications that affect the cell membrane potential can also be used to slow either the alpha or beta pathway of the re-entry circuit.

Vascular Access

The foundation of pharmacological intervention is intravenous access. This fact lends importance to the Paramedic obtaining intravenous access as soon as reasonably practical. While central venous access may be desirable, particularly in administering medications like adenosine that have an extremely short half-life, the time needed to obtain such access generally makes it prohibitive in the field. However, if the patient already has an established central access—for example, via peripherally inserted central venous catheter (PICC)—and medical control permits Paramedics to access these lines, then central venous access should be considered.

The newest form of intravenous access in adults is intraosseous (IO). IO allows near central venous access and is generally a dependable form of intravenous access. The decision to use IO should be based on careful consideration of the patient's status and the need for immediate access. For example, a trial of medications via an intraosseous access may be preferable to a failed intravenous attempt and elective cardioversion.

Pharmacological Intervention for Symptomatic Tachycardia

The general intelligence for medical interventions is to choose the most effective therapy that is least invasive. For patients with tachycardia, the order of treatment starts with vagal maneuvers, proceeds to medications, and ends with electrical therapy. The key is matching the patient's condition, and the urgency of intervention, to the treatment modalities (Table 5-14). This critical decision is based upon many factors including the patient assessment findings, the ECG analysis, the Paramedic's skills, and the patient's stability.

Table 5-14 Treatment Algorithm for Tachydysrhythmia

Stable				Unstable
Wide Complex		Narrow Complex		
Regular	Irregular	Regular	Irregular	Cardioversion
Amiodarone	Amiodarone	Vagal maneuver	Calcium channel blocker	
Lidocaine	Magnesium	Adenosine	Beta blocker	
Procainamide	Cardioversion			
Cardioversion				

Stable versus Unstable

As discussed in the previous chapter, the treatment of tachydysrhythmia first focuses on whether the patient is stable or unstable. This concern is more urgent for the patient with a tachydysrhythmia owed to an error of conduction. This class of dysrhythmia tends to cause more hemodynamic compromise and patients suffering from this class tend to be more symptomatic. Classic signs of instability include altered mental status, shortness of breath, and chest pain.

A pharmacological trial of medications is acceptable before more invasive therapies (such as cardioversion) are used, provided the patient is stable enough to tolerate the delays inherent in a pharmacological approach.[17]

Paramedics have an advantage in the treatment of these patients as they often can multitask (i.e., start intravenous access, draw up medications while obtaining an ECG), using team members for various tasks. This efficiency is borne of practice and drill.

Wide versus Narrow Complex Tachycardia

Next, the Paramedic needs to ascertain if the tachydysrhythmia is a wide complex tachycardia or a narrow complex tachycardia. A wide complex tachycardia is more ominous, as it suggests ventricular tachycardia, and can quickly deteriorate into a ventricular flutter/fibrillation.

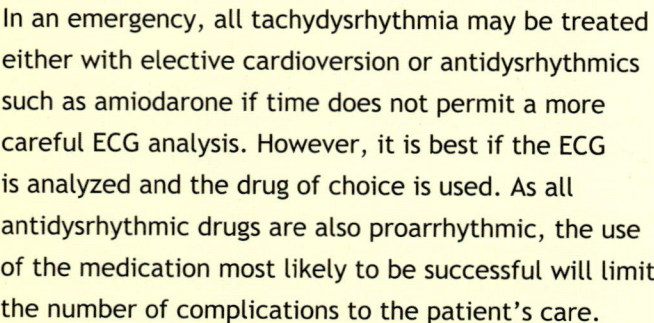

STREET SMART

In an emergency, all tachydysrhythmia may be treated either with elective cardioversion or antidysrhythmics such as amiodarone if time does not permit a more careful ECG analysis. However, it is best if the ECG is analyzed and the drug of choice is used. As all antidysrhythmic drugs are also proarrhythmic, the use of the medication most likely to be successful will limit the number of complications to the patient's care.

Pharmacological Intervention— Wide Complex Tachycardia

A regular wide QRS tachycardia is most likely ventricular tachycardia, although the rhythm could be a supraventricular tachycardia with aberrancy or a pre-excitation tachycardia such as Wolff–Parkinson–White. There are three mainstays to treat regular wide complex tachycardia: amiodarone, lidocaine, and procainamide.

Amiodarone

The antidysrhythmic amiodarone has several effects on the action potential, affecting sodium, potassium, and calcium channels as well as beta/adrenergic receptors. As a result of these multiple actions, amiodarone effectively treats several tachydysrhythmias including monomorphic ventricular tachycardia, atrial fibrillation with aberrancy, and atrial fibrillation with Wolff–Parkinson–White syndrome. In fact, amiodarone is an effective medication for any wide complex tachycardia of unknown origin.

The usual dose of amiodarone is 150 mg administered over 10 minutes, either in normal saline solution (NSS) or dextrose 5% in water (D_5W). The Paramedic should administer amiodarone carefully, continuously monitoring for signs of hypotension and/or bradycardia induced by the medication.

After the initial bolus of amiodarone is complete, it may be necessary for the Paramedic to administer additional boluses of amiodarone, at doses of 150 mg over 10 minutes each, until the tachydysrhythmia is suppressed or to a maximum of 2.2 grams in 24 hours. Once the tachydysrhythmia is abated, then an amiodarone infusion of 1 mg per minute should be administered for the first six hours and 0.5 mg per minute thereafter.

Lidocaine

Lidocaine may be one of the oldest medications used for the treatment of wide complex tachycardia, even though the drug of choice for the treatment of wide complex tachycardia is amiodarone.[18] Lidocaine can be effective in treating monomorphic ventricular tachycardia as well as polymorphic ventricular tachycardia with a normal QT interval.

The dose of lidocaine is usually 0.5 to 0.75 mg per kg intravenous bolus. Lidocaine bolus can be repeated every five to ten minutes until it reaches either a maximum of

3 mg per kg or dysrhythmia suppression. It is important to follow the initial dose of lidocaine with a bolus of one-half of the initial dose approximately 10 to 15 minutes after the initial dose. This prevents breakthrough tachydysrhythmias during the chemical hiatus.

Once the dysrhythmia is suppressed, the Paramedic should begin a lidocaine drip of between 1 to 4 mg per minute (typically 2 mg per minute). The lidocaine infusion should be incrementally increased as a repeat bolus of lidocaine is administered to treat "breakthrough" dysrhythmia (Table 5-15).

The therapeutic plasma level for lidocaine is approximately 1.5 to 5.0 micrograms per mL. Levels above 6 micrograms per mL can become toxic. This toxicity is particularly problematic for the patient with liver disease or heart failure who has trouble clearing the medication from the bloodstream. The Paramedic should observe for signs of toxicity, such as slurred speech, muscle twitching, and seizures, especially in these populations.

Procainamide

Procainamide hydrochloride, like amiodarone, is effective in ventricular tachycardia, pre-excitation tachycardia, and supraventricular tachycardia with aberrancy, making it desirable in treating wide complex tachycardia of unknown origin. Because procainamide slows conduction, it effectively controls the rate of AV node conduction in atrial flutter and atrial fibrillation as well. Procainamide may also be superior to lidocaine in the treatment of monomorphic ventricular tachycardia.

However, the difficulty encountered when using procainamide is its lengthy administration time. To administer procainamide, the Paramedic must first calculate the total dose at 17 mg per kilogram. The medication then must be administered at a maximum of 20 mg per minute. Therefore, administering the maximum dose of procainamide to a 220-pound male (100 kg) at 20 mg per minute would take almost an hour and a half (85 minutes).

Unfortunately, increasing the rate of administration to greater than 20 mg per minute can lead to hypotension. If hypotension occurs, then the infusion should be slowed and the blood pressure rechecked in 10 minutes. If the patient remains hypotensive despite the slowed infusion, then the medication

infusion should be stopped. Paramedics may also note a reflexive tachycardia, warning the Paramedic that the patient's blood pressure has decreased as a result of the cardiotoxic anticholinergic effects of procainamide upon the AV node.

Procainamide also has several caveats that further complicate its administration. Because procainamide is a Vaughn–Williams class IA medication, its use affects the action potential, lengthening the QT interval. Administration must be stopped if the QRS widens by 50%. For this reason, procainamide should not be administered to patients with a prolonged QT interval, since inadvertent administration could lead to polymorphic ventricular tachycardia. If procainamide is inadvertently bolused (i.e., too rapid intravenous infusion), ventricular asystole can occur (Table 5-16).

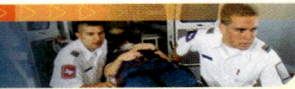

STREET SMART

Some Paramedics perform serial 12-lead ECG to monitor the QRS width and the QT interval. The 12-lead ECG monitors are very accurate at measuring these intervals.

Procainamide must be cautiously administered to patients with bronchospastic disease, such as asthma, who may have a hypersensitivity to the medication.[19] Similarly, procainamide must be cautiously administered to patients with heart failure, liver failure, or renal failure. These conditions may lead to a possible accumulation of the drug and subsequent toxicity.

Careful analysis of the ECG to eliminate the possibility of heart block must also be undertaken before the administration of procainamide. Procainamide administration, especially in larger doses, can lead to or aggravate a pre-existing heart block.

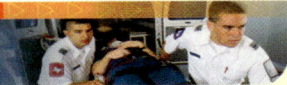

STREET SMART

Because of the anticholinergic properties of procainamide, co-administration of neuromuscular blockade may result in a prolonged paralysis of the patient.

Table 5-15 Lidocaine Infusion

Standard Concentration:	1 gram in 250 cc or 2 gm in 500 cc—Concentration 4 mg per cc.	
Standard Drip Set:	60 drops per cc	
Bolus	**Infusion**	**Drip Rate**
0.5 to 0.75 mg	1 mg/min	15 drops per minute
1 to 1.5 mg	2 mg/min	30 drops per minute
2 to 2.5 mg	3 mg/min	45 drops per minute
2.5 to 3 mg	4 mg/min	60 drops per minute

Table 5-16 Indications for Termination of Procainamide Administration

- Maximum dose of 17 mg per kilogram administered
- Hypotension occurs; first slow the infusion then stop if hypotension remains unresolved
- 50% increase in the width of the QRS complex
- Cessation of dysrhythmia; start an infusion of 1 to 4 mg per minute

Pharmacological Intervention— Irregular Wide Complex Tachycardia

Typically ventricular tachycardia is a regular rhythm stimulated by a re-entry circuit within the ventricles. If the Paramedic observes an irregular wide complex tachycardia of unknown origin, other possibilities should be considered including atrial fibrillation with aberrancy, atrial fibrillation with pre-excitation (such as WPW), and polymorphic ventricular tachycardia, including Torsades de pointes (TdP). In these cases, amiodarone is the drug of choice. The Paramedic should avoid the use of adenosine or calcium channel blockers, as these medications are ineffective and can cause a paradoxical rise in the heart rate and a potentially lethal tachydysrhythmia.

Amiodarone

Amiodarone is the drug of choice in these cases as it can treat ventricular tachydysrhythmias as well as atrial tachydysrhythmias.[20] If the rhythm is atrial fibrillation, either with aberrancy or with pre-excitation, amiodarone will control the rate of AV node conduction and ventricular depolarization. Amiodarone should be administered as previously discussed.

Magnesium

Magnesium is the drug of choice for any polymorphic ventricular tachycardia (PVT) with a prolonged QT interval. When confronted with a PVT, the Paramedic should first stop any medications, such as procainamide, that may be inducing the PVT. Next, the Paramedic should prepare to administer magnesium while considering potential causes of electrolyte imbalances (e.g., vomiting and diarrhea), as well as any toxicology (e.g., tricyclic antidepressants).

The dose of magnesium for PVT is 1 to 2 grams over 10 minutes or more, up to 60 minutes. This may be administered over 1 to 2 minutes in patients with cardiac arrest. Ensuing patient hypotension usually controls the rate of infusion and therefore the rate can be very patient dependent. If the rhythm is resistant to conversion with magnesium, it may be possible that the tachydysrhythmias may not be a prolonged QT PVT and would be more responsive to amiodarone instead.

STREET SMART

If profound hypotension and/or asystole occurs during magnesium administration, calcium gluconate (10 to 20 mL of 10% solution) may be administered. Calcium gluconate is the antidote for iatrogenic hypermagnesemia.

Overdrive Pacing

In some instances, polymorphic ventricular tachycardia is resistant to pharmacological therapies. In those cases, the Paramedic may consider the use of **overdrive pacing**. Based on the concept of dominance, the Paramedic attempts to gain control of the tachydysrhythmia by increasing the rate of a transcutaneous pacer (TCP) until the TCP takes control and then gradually slows the rhythm to a tolerable range.[21] The process of transcutaneous pacing is described in Chapter 6 on the errors of conduction: bradycardia. The only difference between TCP on a patient with bradycardia and a patient with tachycardia is the rate of the pacer.

Pharmacological Intervention— Regular Narrow Complex Tachycardia

A regular tachycardia with a narrow QRS that is not a sinus tachycardia most likely involves an error in conduction (i.e., a re-entry circuit). If that is the case, then the Paramedic should initially attempt a vagal maneuver, like a Valsalva maneuver, before using a medication. It has been estimated that the Valsalva maneuver effectively converts 20% to 25% of AVNRT.

Sinus Tachycardia

The clinical goal of the therapeutic intervention is to return the patient to a normal sinus rhythm. Therefore, it would be inappropriate to administer antidysrhythmic medication if the patient is already in a sinus rhythm, albeit a sinus tachycardia. However, several tachydysrhythmias are difficult to discern from sinus tachycardia. Subtle ECG findings, such as a shortened PR interval, may be the only difference between an AVNRT and ST. Careful attention to these subtle differences can have a significant impact on the patient's outcome. One clinical clue is the heart rate. Rarely does a patient have a sustained sinus tachycardia greater than 150 bpm. ECGs with a rate less than 150 bpm should be more carefully examined. If sinus tachycardia is suspected, the Paramedic should focus on ascertaining the underlying etiology (e.g., fever, anemia, and/or hypofusion) and treat these disorders accordingly.

Adenosine

If a vagal maneuver is not effective in terminating the tachydysrhythmias, then the Paramedic should consider using adenosine next. Adenosine is an ultra short-acting endogenous nucleoside that slows conduction through the AV node, effectively eliminating one pathway in the re-entry circuit. The result is that, when the next impulse fires, it essentially depolarizes the entire myocardium and effectively terminates any re-entry pathways.

Adenosine leaves the circulation, via cellular uptake, where it is deaminated by the enzyme adenosine deaminase into inosine. Inosine can be further degraded by xanthine compounds. Methylxanthine compounds are found in coffee, tea, and the respiratory drug theophylline. Those patients who have these methylxanthine compounds circulating in the blood will require higher doses of adenosine or will be resistive to the effects of adenosine.

Adenosine can also stimulate bronchoconstriction in susceptible individuals. Therefore, adenosine should be avoided in patients with a history of reactive airway disease (including asthma) and given cautiously to those with obstructive airway disease (such as emphysema).

Adenosine is an ultra short-acting medication, with a half-life of less than 10 seconds, and thus requires the closest venous access to the heart and a rapid intravenous administration, often coupled with a simultaneous bolus of 20 mL of solution and elevation of the limb. The initial dose is usually 6 mg with repeat doses of 12 mg given in two to three minutes for a total dose of 30 mg of adenosine.

Studies have shown that 60% of patients with SVT convert with 6 mg adenosine rapid intravenous bolus.[21–24] If the patient does not convert with 6 mg, the Paramedic should reconsider the venous access (the method of administration) and ascertain from the patient if he has been drinking coffee or using the medication theophylline. Over 90% of patients with an SVT convert with a subsequent 12 mg rapid intravenous bolus.

Since adenosine slows, or stops, conduction in the AV node, it should not be used in patients with high-degree AV blocks (e.g., AV block type II, second degree, or any third degree block). Similarly, if sick sinus syndrome or bradycardia–tachycardia syndrome, indicating sinus node disease, is suspected, then adenosine should be avoided.

Similarly, adenosine will provide increased AV block in atrial fibrillation/flutter, revealing the underlying f waves or F waves. However, adenosine seldom converts either atrial fibrillation or atrial flutter into a sinus rhythm.

Prolonged asystole, but rarely ventricular fibrillation, has been reported with the administration of adenosine. This tends to occur especially if the patient is either on digitalis or a calcium channel blocker. For this reason, the Paramedic should be prepared to provide cardiac resuscitation, including CPR, intubation, and transcutaneous pacing.

Approximately 18% of patients will experience facial flushing, while a much smaller percentage will experience headaches (2%), chest pressure (7%), and shortness of breath (12%). Immediately following cardioversion with adenosine, the Paramedic may note premature complexes—both atrial and ventricular—as well as AV nodal block. These dysrhythmias are common (appearing in up to 55% of patients) and are transitory in nature, lasting only a few minutes. As such, they do not require immediate treatment.

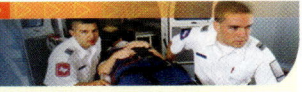

STREET SMART

Adenosine may not terminate errors of automaticity, such as new onset atrial fibrillation or multifocal atrial tachycardia, but it may induce a temporary A/V block. Following the chemical induction of the A/V block by adenosine, the Paramedic should focus on the first complex that follows to help clarify the rhythm.

Calcium Channel Blockers

If the adenosine is not effective in terminating a regular narrow complex tachycardia, the Paramedic should consider using a calcium channel blocker. The AV node is particularly sensitive to calcium, and calcium channel blockers can slow the conduction within the AV node, thereby slowing the rate of impulses conducted to the ventricles. This slowed rate is often all that is necessary to interrupt the re-entry circuit and restore normal conductive pathways.

Diltiazem and verapamil are two calcium channel blockers that are effective in terminating regular narrow complex tachycardias. The first dose of diltiazem is 0.25 mg per kg. If needed, a second dose of 0.35 mg per kg may be administered. The usual initial dose is therefore 20 to 25 mg IV injected over two minutes. Diltiazem converts greater than 75% of patients with PSVT.

An alternative calcium channel blocker is verapamil. Although 5 mg of verapamil is the standard dose used for tachydysrhythmias, many Paramedics divide the dose into two 2.5 mg doses, each administered over two minutes. A divided dose allows the Paramedic to reassess the patient, with attention to hypotension, before administering the second dose, and potentially withholding the second dose if it is contraindicated. The 5 mg doses of verapamil can be repeated every 15 to 30 minutes to a maximum of 20 mg or until termination of the dysrhythmia. Alternatively, some Paramedics infuse the verapamil via 50 cc of 0.9% saline solution.

Verapamil should be administered cautiously to patients with a history of heart failure.[25,26] Verapamil inhibits the influx of calcium in vascular smooth muscle, found in the tunica media of blood vessels, resulting in systemic vasodilation. Systemic vasodilation, in turn, leads to venous pooling, reduced preload, and diminished cardiac output manifested as hypotension.

Some Paramedics have resorted to pretreatment with either 1 g of calcium gluconate or 10 mL of 10% calcium chloride solution, administered over three to five minutes, to prevent hypotension in this susceptible population. Calcium given during the pretreatment occupies the calcium channels, thereby preventing the calcium channel blocker from working. This creates a competitive inhibition. However, the calcium infusion does not interfere with verapamil's effects on the AV node, which is a conductive tissue.

All calcium channel blockers should be given cautiously if the patient is on beta/adrenergic blocker medications, or if a beta/adrenergic blocker has been given. The combination of a beta/adrenergic blocker, affecting the ventricles, and a calcium channel blocking agent, affecting the AV node, leaves the patient predisposed to high degree AV block and/or profound bradycardia. The same precautions should be observed with digitalis, as digitalis has effects on both the AV node and the ventricles.

Diltiazem has a lesser tendency to cause hypotension; for example, hypotension (systolic < 90 mmHg) occurred in only 18% of patients in one study. Therefore, diltiazem is generally considered preferable in the treatment of supraventricular tachycardia. While pretreatment with calcium salts is an option, studies are inconclusive whether this pretreatment is advantageous for diltiazem.

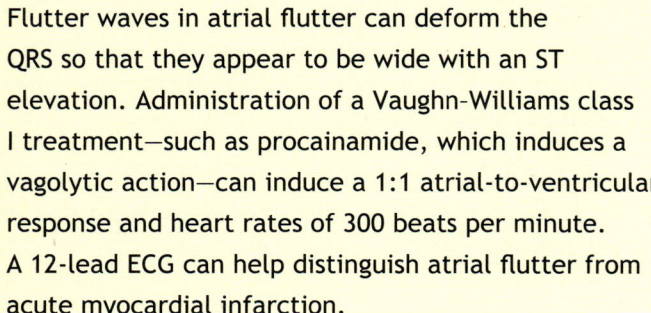

STREET SMART

Flutter waves in atrial flutter can deform the QRS so that they appear to be wide with an ST elevation. Administration of a Vaughn-Williams class I treatment—such as procainamide, which induces a vagolytic action—can induce a 1:1 atrial-to-ventricular response and heart rates of 300 beats per minute. A 12-lead ECG can help distinguish atrial flutter from acute myocardial infarction.

Beta/Adrenergic Blockers

Beta/adrenergic blocking agents have an antidysrhythmic effect that is cardioprotective to patients with acute coronary syndrome. Considered a third line drug for the treatment of AVRNT, this class of drugs works directly on the ventricles to both prevent tachycardia and treat SVT.

Metoprolol, a selective beta 1 adrenergic blocker, is typically given in 5 mg doses, administered over five minutes, with a repeat dose of 5 mg every 10 minutes to a maximum of 15 mg.

Propranolol is an alternative beta/adrenergic blocker that is less selective for beta 1 receptors. As a result, propranolol can cause bronchospasms in patients with asthma or emphysema and therefore should not be given to these patients. The treatments for these respiratory diseases are sympathomimetics that produce tachycardia and would be counterproductive. Propranolol is usually given as 0.1 mg per kg in three doses, each one given over three minutes or as an infusion of 1 mg per minute.

Common side effects reported with beta/adrenergic blockers include heart blocks and bradycardia as well as hypotension. Patients given a beta/adrenergic blocker may be prone to postural hypotension and syncope. For this reason, patients receiving these drugs must be supine and on the ECG monitor.

STREET SMART

Some patients experience atrial flutter as a part of their hyperthyroidism (thyrotoxicosis-induced atrial flutter). Thyrotoxicosis increases the sympathetic tone and therefore the atrial flutter of these patients will respond more favorably to beta/adrenergic blockers.

Amiodarone

Amiodarone has effects on the sodium (Na^+) channels, potassium (K^+) channels, calcium (Ca^{++}), and beta/adrenergic receptors. Having the action of several of the medications just discussed, amiodarone is an acceptable alternative, especially if the adenosine and calcium channel blockers were unsuccessful against AVRNT.

Atrial Fibrillation and AV Re-Entry Tachycardia

When atrial fibrillation occurs in patients with pre-existing AV re-entry tachycardia (AVRT), such as WPW, extremely fast heart rates can occur. As there are two existing conductive pathways, and atrial impulses at a rate of 250 to 300 per minute are running down these two pathways, the ventricles can be besieged with impulse after impulse and sustain heart rates over 250 bpm. This can lead to myocardial fatigue, irritability, and even ventricular fibrillation.

Administration of calcium channel blockers to this vulnerable group only encourages conduction via the accessory pathway, bypassing the AV node, and increases the risk of ventricular fibrillation and sudden cardiac death. For this reason, calcium channel blockers should not be administered to patients with atrial fibrillation who have AVRT such as WPW or LGL. Instead, the Paramedic should consider the use of either amiodarone or procainamide.

CASE STUDY (CONTINUED)

Kaylie begins complaining of chest pain and some difficulty breathing. The Paramedics prepare her for electrical cardioversion by administering a benzodiazepine for sedation.

CRITICAL THINKING QUESTIONS

1. What are some of the predictable complications associated with a sustained wide complex tachycardia?
2. What are some of the predictable complications associated with the treatments for sustained wide complex tachycardia?

Evaluation

A patient is unstable when the tachydysrhythmia causes decreased cerebral perfusion (as manifest by an altered mental status), decreased coronary perfusion (as manifest by chest pain), decreased pulmonary perfusion (as manifest by shortness of breath), systemic hypoperfusion (as manifest by hypotension), and other signs of shock. These potentially life-threatening conditions require immediate action to terminate the tachydysrhythmia. The most effective treatment is synchronized cardioversion.

Electrical Cardioversion

Cardioversion is defined as changing the heart's rhythm. It can be accomplished by mechanical means such as vagal maneuvers or a blow to the chest (precordial thump); through pharmacological methods after administration of dysrhythmia medication (pharmacological cardioversion); or, in the most common usage, with a timed DC countershock (electrical cardioversion).

If time permits, then a trial of intravenous medications can be attempted. However, if unsuccessful, or if the patient becomes grossly symptomatic, then the Paramedic must be prepared to deliver a synchronized cardioversion.

By electrically depolarizing (i.e., "stunning") the entire myocardium, cardioversion removes two of the necessary components for a re-entry rhythm: a different refractory period and slowed conduction in one of the arms of the re-entry circuit. However, if the energy is delivered at the period of time in the cardiac cycle called the relative refractory period (the latter half of the T wave), there is a chance that the patient's rhythm can convert to ventricular fibrillation (the R on T phenomena). Delivering an electrical countershock at a specific time within the cardiac cycle, outside of the vulnerable period, via a timed or synchronized countershock eliminates the likelihood of unintentionally initiating a ventricular fibrillation.

Synchronized cardioversion is a medical procedure that has potential for serious complications, including death. The patient must be properly informed about the procedure—and consent obtained, if possible—prior to synchronized cardioversion. Cardioversion should be avoided if the patient has a tachydysrhythmia as a consequence of digitalis toxicity. Cardioversion under those circumstances can lead to refractory ventricular tachycardia, ventricular fibrillation, or intractable asystole. If cardioversion must be performed, then the lowest possible energy setting (usually 50 joules) should be used.[27]

If time permits, and the patient consents, the patient should be sedated prior to synchronized cardioversion. The drug of choice when performing this is benzodiazepines such as diazepam or midazolam. Benzodiazepines have several desirable qualities including anxiolysis and amnesic properties. It is also a smooth muscle relaxer.

The Paramedic should place the leads on the patient in a way that provides a clear electrocardiogram without interfering with the defibrillation platform. Usually MCL1 is the best lead. After ensuring a good quality monitoring lead, the Paramedic should place the defibrillation/pacer pads over the upper right chest wall and the lower left rib cage. Care should be taken to avoid jewelry, medication patches, or vascular access devices. If necessary, the Paramedic should dry the skin with a gauze pad or towel before applying the defibrillation/pacer pads.

Next, the Paramedic should turn on the synchronization mode. The ECG monitor should start to mark, or flag, the R waves of the QRS. The Paramedic should check to ensure that the ECG flags identify the R wave. If the R waves are not flagged, then the Paramedic should consider changing the lead to a more favorable lead.

With the R waves flagged, the Paramedic should select the correct energy level for the rhythm. For regular narrow complex tachycardias, 100 joules or a biphasic equivalent is used, with escalating doses of 50 to 100 joules for successive synchronized cardioversion until successful. For regular wide complex tachycardias, 100 to 200 joules or the biphasic equivalent is used, with escalating doses of 100 joules to a maximum of 360 joules, or the biphasic equivalent.

After ensuring that the sedation administered has taken effect, the Paramedic should charge the ECG monitor. First, to ensure the safety of all team members, the Paramedic should announce that a shock will be given at the end of a count of three. After visually sweeping the patient from head to toe to check for any possible physical contact by members of the team, the Paramedic should press the record button (a continuous ECG strip should be recorded during the cardioversion). Then the Paramedic should press and hold the shock button. Since the device is set to deliver the shock on the R wave, it may take a moment before the discharge occurs. Prematurely releasing the shock button will only delay the cardioversion. If paddles are used, the paddles should be kept in contact with the patient and the shock button should stay depressed until the charge is delivered.

After the countershock is delivered, the Paramedic should stop the ECG recording and re-evaluate the patient's status. If the rhythm persists, it will be necessary for the Paramedic to reset the synchronization mode on some ECG monitor/defibrillators; however, some newer model ECG monitor/defibrillators do not need to be reset. It is the Paramedic's responsibility to know the operations of the ECG monitor/defibrillator in her system.

Some current and older model ECG monitor/defibrillators automatically default to unsynchronized mode after the shock is delivered in the event the patient converts to ventricular fibrillation, allowing immediate defibrillation. If the patient should revert to ventricular tachycardia, without pulses, or ventricular fibrillation, then immediate unsynchronized cardioversion at 360 joules, or the biphasic equivalent, should be used immediately. As most ECG monitor/defibrillators automatically default to the defibrillation mode after discharge, there should be a minimal delay (less than 10 seconds) in delivering an unsynchronized cardioversion or defibrillation (**Skill 5-1**).

For a step-by-step demonstration of Elective Synchronized Cardioversion, please refer to Skill 5-1 on pages 153–154

Cardioversion and Atrial Fibrillation

Elective cardioversion of the patient with atrial fibrillation/flutter (AFF) and a rapid ventricular response (RVR) should be avoided unless absolutely necessary. The risk of stroke from thromboembolism released during the cardioversion is high and the potential benefits are limited. If the patient is unstable, then the patient can be electively cardioverted at 100 joules monophasic or 75 joules biphasic. However, lower energies, such as 50 joules, can be effective in atrial flutter.

Failed Cardioversion

Cardioversion works best when the tachydysrhythmia is the result of an error of conduction. If the cardioversion failed, then the mechanism for the tachydysrhythmia may be an error of automaticity. Tachydysrhythmias, such as junctional ectopic tachycardia (JET) and multifocal atrial tachycardia (MAT), both caused by errors of automaticity, will be resistant to cardioversion. Occasionally there may be a paradoxical increase in the tachycardia. Under those conditions, the Paramedic should return to pharmacological treatments and/or focus on methods of rate control, such as fluid bolus.

CASE STUDY CONCLUSION

Kaylie converted to a sinus tachycardia following a synchronized DC shock of 100 joules. She was transported to the cardiac center and received diltiazem. Two weeks later, as the Paramedics were getting lunch, they saw Kaylie at the diner. She thanked them for their help and let them know that she was scheduled for electrophysiology studies to determine the cause of her issue and find the best ongoing treatments.

CRITICAL THINKING QUESTIONS

1. What is the most appropriate transport decision that will get the patient to definitive care?
2. What are some of the transportation considerations?

Disposition

Patients with tachydysrhythmia need to be transported to the hospital for further medical treatment including antidysrhythmic drugs and/or anticoagulation. As many of these patients will be followed up by a cardiologist, it is helpful to transport these patients to a cardiac center, particularly one with an electrophysiology lab and/or an interventional cardiology suite.

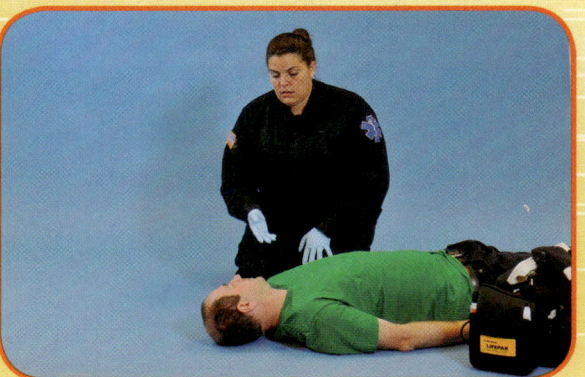

1 Explain the procedure to the patient.

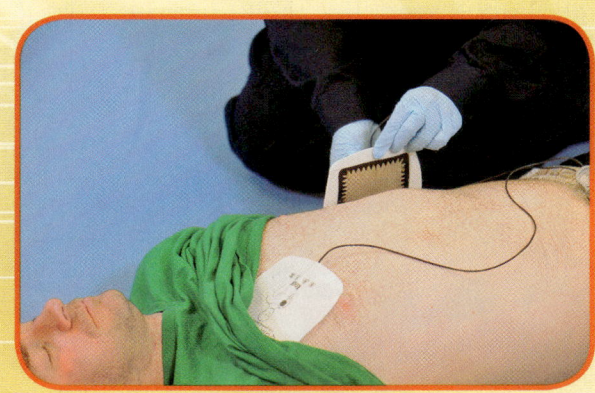

2 Adequately sedate the patient.

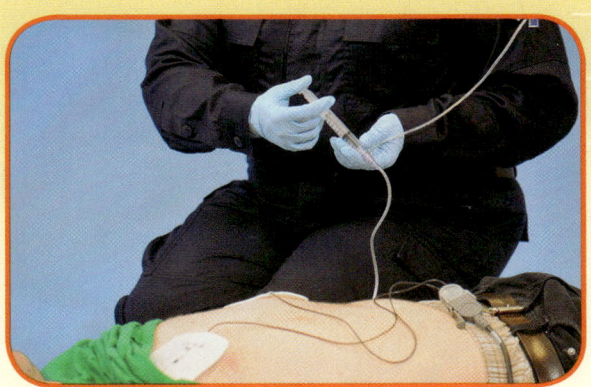

3 Place pads on the patient in an anterior–posterior position.

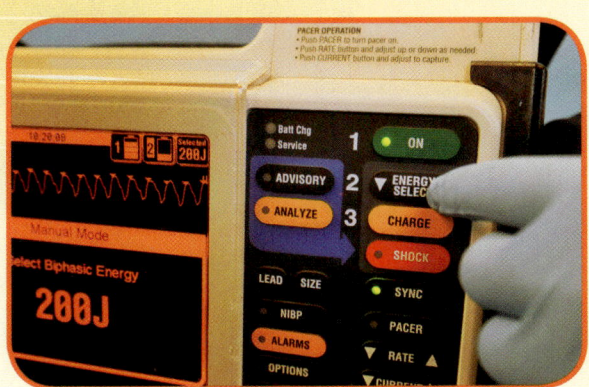

4 Select the energy setting.

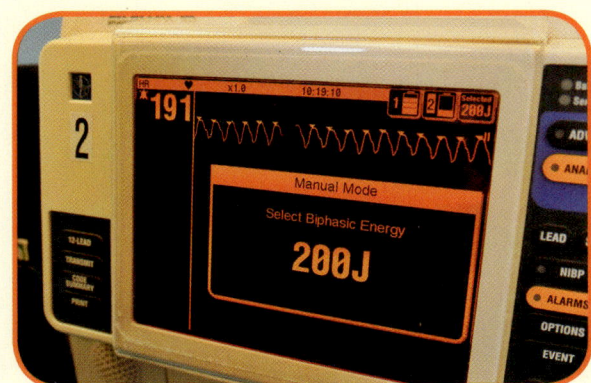

5 Confirm synchronization.

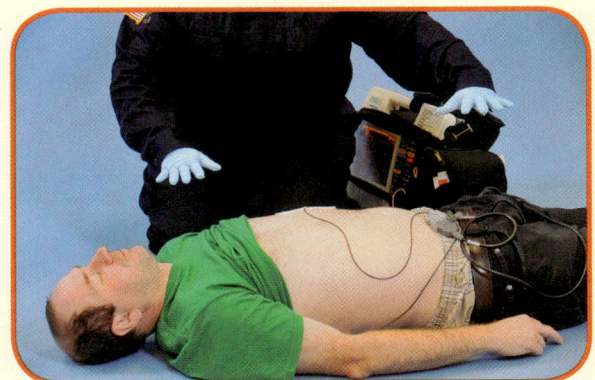

6 Signal all clear.

Delmar/Cengage Learning

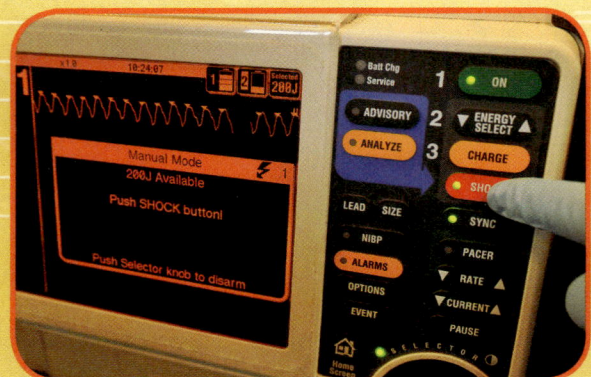

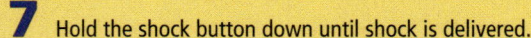

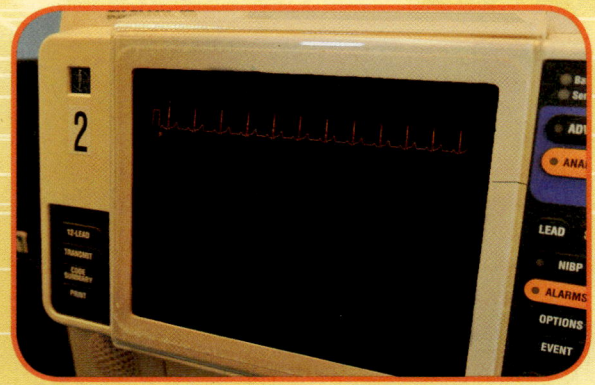

7 Hold the shock button down until shock is delivered.

8 Reassess for conversion.

Delmar/Cengage Learning

CONCLUSION

Errors of conduction that cause tachydysrhythmias may produce subtle patient complaints. The astute Paramedic will pick up on these complaints and look for the possibility of a tachydysrhythmia as the source of the complaint.

KEY POINTS:

- Two mechanisms exist for dysrhythmia formations: errors of automaticity and errors of conduction.

- The equation for cardiac output is cardiac output equals stroke volume multiplied by heart rate.

- Re-entry is the passage of a depolarization wave through a structure that it has just passed through.

- Three conditions must exist in order for re-entry to occur:
  - Available circuit
  - Pathway for impulse
  - Slowed conduction

- Circuits can be macrocircuits, as exist between atria and ventricles, or microcircuits, as within the atria or ventricle.

- Supraventricular dysrhythmias caused by an error of conduction (tachycardic) and originating in each region are:
  - SA node
    - SA nodal re-entry tachycardia
  - Atria
    - Atrial flutter
    - Paroxysmal atrial tachycardia
  - AV node
    - AV nodal re-entry tachycardia
    - Re-entrant tachycardia
  - Pre-excitation syndromes
    - Wolff-Parkinson-White
    - Long-Ganong-Levine
  - Junction
    - Junctional tachycardia

- Wide complex tachycardias
  - Monomorphic ventricular tachycardia
  - Ventricular flutter
  - Irregular beats
  - Polymorphic ventricular tachycardia

- Long QT intervals may predispose to a specific type of polymorphic ventricular tachycardia called torsades de pointes.

- Significant history includes precipitating factors.

- Tachydysrhythmias may place the patient at risk for heart failure.

- Vagal maneuvers include facial immersion in iced water, the Valsalva maneuver, and carotid sinus massage.

- Ventricular tachycardia differs from SVT in axis and R wave progression.

- The rate at which aberrancy develops is called the critical rate.

- Treatment of tachydysrhythmias first focuses on whether the patient is stable or unstable.

- Amiodarone affects sodium, calcium, potassium channels, and beta receptors.

- Lidocaine can lead to toxicity which shows as lateralizing CNS effects.

- Procainamide should be discontinued if the QRS widens by 50% of original, hypotension ensures, 17 mg per kilogram has been given, or the dysrhythmia terminates.

- Overdrive pacing is an attempt to dominate the dysrhythmia by pacing at a rate faster than the dysrhythmia and gradually slowing the pacemaker down.

- Sinus tachycardia is treated by determining its cause, such as fever or pain, and addressing that issue.

- Calcium channel blockers are usually effective in treating narrow complex tachycardias. Verapamil can lead to greater hypotension than diltiazem.

- Electrical cardioversion should be avoided in patients with digoxin toxicity for fear of inducing ventricular tachycardia or fibrillation which is not amenable to electrical interventions or placing the patient into asystole.

- Cardioversion is an electrical intervention that may place the patient and practitioner at risk. Obtain consent if possible. Strict safety should be followed. The procedure hurts, so the Paramedic should consider sedation if time permits.

REVIEW QUESTIONS:

1. How do dysrhythmias caused by errors of automaticity differ from those caused by errors of conduction?

2. How does an increase in heart rate affect diastolic filling time?

3. Describe myocardial oxygen demand during a period of sustained tachycardia.

4. Describe the difference between a macrocircuit and a microcircuit.

5. Which vagal maneuver is preferred in the field? Why?

6. How does R wave progression differ in ventricular tachycardia from supraventricular tachycardia with aberrancy?

7. What phases of the action potential are affected by amiodarone?

CASE STUDY QUESTIONS:

Please refer to the Case Study in this chapter, and answer the questions below:

1. Using the cardiac output equation, explain why Kaylie feels weak and dizzy.

2. What components of Kaylie's history point toward a cardiac rhythm disturbance?

3. Explain the mechanism of vagal maneuvers upon heart rhythm.

4. How is adenosine administered?

5. What is the significance of the following finding: average QRS axis of +45 degrees, no acute ST-T wave changes, good R wave progression through the V leads, rSR' in V1 lead, initial deflection in V1 is the same as on the earlier ECG?

6. What findings suggest that Kaylie has become unstable?

7. What is the mechanism of action for diltiazem?

8. Would you have tried to slow down Kaylie's rhythm of sinus tachycardia? Why or why not?

REFERENCES:

1. I've heard the terms "atrial flutter" and "atrial fibrillation" used interchangeably when describing certain heart-rhythm disorders, but I thought atrial flutter was a less-serious condition. Can you elaborate? *Heart Advis.* 2008;11(7):12.

2. Patel A, Markowitz SM. Atrial tachycardia: mechanisms and management. *Expert Rev Cardiovasc Ther.* 2008;6(6):811–822.

3. Andrew P, Montenero AS. Atrial flutter: a focus on treatment options for a common supraventricular tachyarrhythmia. *J Cardiovasc Med (Hagerstown).* 2007;8(8):558–667.

4. Bulava A, Peichl P, et al. Atrioventricular nodal reentrant tachycardia: anatomical and electrophysiological considerations. *Ital Heart J.* 2003;4(3):163–172.

5. Sethi KK, Dhall A, et al. WPW and preexcitation syndromes. *J Assoc Physicians India.* 2007;55 Suppl:10–15.

6. Fengler BT, Brady WJ, et al. Atrial fibrillation in the Wolff–Parkinson–White syndrome: ECG recognition and treatment in the ED. *Am J Emerg Med.* 2007;25(5):576–583.

7. Luedtke SA, Kuhn RJ, et al. Pharmacologic management of supraventricular tachycardias in children. Part 1: Wolff–Parkinson–White and atrioventricular nodal reentry. *Ann Pharmacother.* 1997;31(10):1227–1243.

8. Alpert JS, Petersen P, et al. Atrial fibrillation: natural history, complications, and management. *Ann Rev Med.* 1988; 39:41–52.

9. Ernoehazy W, Jr, MD. Ventricular tachycardia. Available at: **http://www.emedicine.com/emerg/topic634.htm**. Accessed March 17, 2008.

10. Nabar A, Nathani PJ. Ventricular tachycardia: tricks and traps. *J Assoc Physicians India*. 2007;55 Suppl:39–42.

11. Luqman N, Sung RJ, et al. Myocardial ischemia and ventricular fibrillation: pathophysiology and clinical implications. *Int J Cardiol*. 2007;119(3):283–290.

12. Morita H, Wu J, et al. The QT syndromes: long and short. *Lancet*. 2008;372(9640):750–763.

13. Chiang CE. Congenital and acquired long QT syndrome. Current concepts and management. *Cardiol Rev*. 2004;12(4):222–234.

14. Olshansky B. Atrioventricular nodal reentry tachycardia. Available at: **http://emedicine.medscape.com/article/160215-overview**. Accessed November 20, 2009.

15. Abbott AV. Diagnostic approach to palpitations. *Am Fam Physician*. 2005;71(4):743–750.

16. Thakor NV. From Holter monitors to automatic defibrillators: developments in ambulatory arrhythmia monitoring. *IEEE Trans Biomed Eng*. 1984;31(12):770–778.

17. Innes JA. Review article: adenosine use in the emergency department. *Emerg Med Australas*. 2008;20(3):209–215.

18. October TW, Schleien CL, et al. Increasing amiodarone use in cardiopulmonary resuscitation: an analysis of the National Registry of Cardiopulmonary Resuscitation. *Crit Care Med*. 2008;36(1):126–130.

19. Vargaftig B, Coignet JL. A critical evaluation of three methods for the study of adrenergic beta-blocking and anti-arrhythmic agents. *Eur J Pharmacol*. 1969;6(1):49–55.

20. Vassallo P, Trohman RG. Prescribing amiodarone: an evidence-based review of clinical indications. *JAMA*. 2007;298(11):1312–1322.

21. Israel CW, Gronefeld G, et al. Suppression of atrial tachyarrhythmias by pacing. *J Cardiovasc Electrophysiol*. 2002;13(1 Suppl):S31–S39.

22. Luber S, Brady WJ, et al. Paroxysmal supraventricular tachycardia: outcome after ED care. *Am J Emerg Med*. 2001;19(1):40–42.

23. Melio FR, Mallon WK, et al. Successful conversion of unstable supraventricular tachycardia to sinus rhythm with adenosine. *Ann Emerg Med*. 1993;22(4):709–713.

24. Gausche M, Persse DE, et al. Adenosine for the prehospital treatment of paroxysmal supraventricular tachycardia. *Ann Emerg Med*. 1994;24(2):183–189.

25. Holdgate A, Foo A. Adenosine versus intravenous calcium channel antagonists for the treatment of supraventricular tachycardia in adults. *Cochrane Database Syst Rev*. 2006;(4):CD005154.

26. Bailey DG, Dresser GK. Interactions between grapefruit juice and cardiovascular drugs. *Am J Cardiovasc Drugs*. 2004;4(5):281–297.

27. Ewy GA. The optimal technique for electrical cardioversion of atrial fibrillation. *Clin Cardiol*. 1994;17(2):79–84.

CHAPTER 6

ERRORS OF CONDUCTION: BRADYCARDIA

KEY CONCEPTS:

Upon completion of this chapter, it is expected that the reader will understand these following concepts:

- Re-entry as an etiology for dysrhythmias
- Conduction abnormalities as an etiology for dysrhythmias
- Given an ECG strip in either Lead II or MCL1, identification of dysrhythmias caused by re-entry or conduction abnormalities

ANATOMY CONCEPTS:

Prior to reading this chapter the Paramedic student should be familiar with the following anatomy and physiology concepts:

- Cardiac conduction system
- Electrophysiology

Just before breakfast, the Paramedics are dispatched to the Farmer's Market on West Street and Haven Boulevard for a 55-year-old man who has passed out. Dispatch reports that he is now conscious and breathing. While en route, the Paramedics discuss likely causes for this event. It was very early in the season, and there wasn't a lot of activity at the Farmer's Market as yet. The weather was pleasant—neither too hot nor too cold. Pesticides weren't in use.

When they turn the corner of West Street they see a small knot of people at the market's entrance and hear a man yelling, "Why did you call an ambulance? I'm fine!" Getting out of the rig, the Paramedics push through to a man seated on a display bench. He appears pale but his voice is booming. "Hello, we are from the ambulance service," they say. "Can we help you?"

Mr. Tedesco tells them that he is a local farmer, born in Italy, and used to taking care of himself. He doesn't know why anyone bothered the ambulance service just because he got a little weak. "It's just hard work," he says, "Nothing to worry about."

CRITICAL THINKING QUESTIONS

1. What are some of the possible causes of cardiac-related syncope?
2. Why is the cause of the fall more important than the fall?

OVERVIEW

Syncope, the sudden loss of consciousness followed by a fall, is one of the more frequent reasons for an EMS call. There are many causes of syncope, from the benign to the potentially lethal. The Paramedic must determine which syncope episodes are deadly and which are harmless. The differentiation of these etiologies is one of the most complex diagnostic challenges that a Paramedic will face.

Chief Concern

The brief sudden loss of consciousness and postural tone is called **syncope**. Unlike convulsions, which have a prolonged postictal period, syncope has an almost spontaneous revival. However, like the convulsion, syncope represents a disturbance in brain function. In the case of syncope, the disturbance of brain function can be the result of hypoperfusion.

Several cardiac mechanisms can be responsible for the sudden loss of blood pressure and subsequent cerebral hypoperfusion, including ventricular diastolic disorders, dysrhythmia, and outflow obstructions.[1] Ventricular diastolic disorders are conditions that prevent ventricular filling during diastole and include tension pneumothorax and cardiac tamponade. These conditions generally develop gradually, albeit in a short period of time, and do not tend to produce the rapid loss of consciousness seen in syncope.

However, orthostatic or postural hypotension, due to loss of compensatory mechanisms that ensure ventricular filling, can produce syncope. Orthostatic hypotension is defined as an excessive loss of blood pressure, generally greater than 20 mmHg systolic, when standing.[2] Symptoms accompanying orthostatic hypotension include lightheadedness, dizziness, and blurred vision for a few moments before the patient collapses. In some instances, the patient is aware of the impending fall and takes self-protective measures. These measures may be evidenced by abrasions and contusions to the patient's forearms, elbows, and knees.

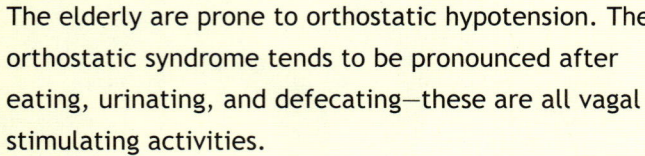

Barriers to cardiac output, called outflow obstructions, can cause a sudden loss of blood pressure. Although there are many causes of outflow obstruction, such as aortic stenosis and intracardiac tumors (**myxoma**), the classic outflow obstruction that causes syncope is the pulmonary embolism.

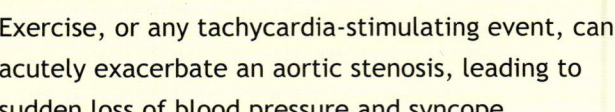

A principal cause of cardiogenic syncope is dysrhythmia. Either a tachydysrhythmia or a bradydysrhythmia can lead to insufficient cardiac output and subsequently cause syncope. Tachydysrhythmias have a rate that is too fast for adequate ventricular filling. In contrast, bradydysrhythmias have a rate that is too slow for adequate ventricular emptying. Generally, any heart rate over 150 beats per minute or less than 50 beats per minute can be problematic; however, in some instances it is not the rate but the drop in rate that becomes problematic. The addition of any outflow obstructions, such as aortic stenosis, only compounds the problem.

This chapter focuses on bradydysrhythmias that can cause syncope. These bradydysrhythmias can be broken down into causes and conditions of profound sinus bradycardia, such as sick sinus syndrome, and atrioventricular heart block or A/V blocks. The key to understanding cardiogenic syncope is recognition that the underlying disorder, and not the syncope itself, is the potentially life-threatening condition.

Sinus Bradycardia

Bradycardia can occur as a result of age-related changes in the conduction system (i.e., fibrosis and calcification) and/or because of medications such as digitalis, beta/adrenergic blockers, and calcium channel blockers. However, sudden drops in heart rate, resulting in syncope, are often due to hypersensitive carotid sinus syndrome, neurocardiogenic syncope, or sick sinus syndrome.

Hypersensitive carotid sinus syndrome (i.e., **shaver's syndrome**) is syncope caused by an exaggerated reflex response to carotid sinus stimulation.[3] When the carotid sinus, located proximal to the angle of the jaw, is stimulated (e.g., via direct pressure by a too-tight necktie) there are two effects. The first is an increase in parasympathetic tone. An increase in parasympathetic tone leads to a slowed heart rate, via vagal stimulation, which is manifest on the ECG as sinus arrest or AV block with subsequent asystole for as much as three seconds. This increased parasympathetic effect is termed the cardioinhibitory effect. Second, stimulation of the carotid sense leads to a decrease of sympathetic tone. The sympathetic nervous system maintains peripheral vascular tone and a loss of sympathetic stimulation causes vasodilation, significant venous pooling, and subsequent hypotension. This effect is called the **vasodepressor effect**.

Although they have a similar mechanism (an abnormal neural reflex) and a similar outcome (syncope), neurocardiogenic syncope does not involve the carotid sinus. **Neurocardiogenic syncope** (i.e., vasovagal syncope) is caused by cardioinhibitory and vasodepressor effects on the body. Like hypersensitive carotid sinus syndrome, they also cause syncope.[4–6] Neurocardiogenic syncope can be triggered by pain (such as when an IV is started), by stress, or even by the anxiety of being in a crowded place. It has been suggested that 10% to 40% of episodes of adult syncope may be attributed to neurocardiogenic syncope. Many of these patients initially present with nausea and diaphoresis just prior to the syncope; however, this is not always true for the elderly. Fortunately, neurocardiogenic syncope is self-limited and the patient recovers with sequela.

STREET SMART

Following heart transplant, bradydysrhythmia may occur in as many as 23% of the patient population. The initial presentation of these patients may be syncope induced by the bradydysrhythmia.

Sick Sinus Syndrome

Sick sinus syndrome, a condition that can cause a profound bradycardia, may be the result of natural fibrosis of the SA node that occurs with aging, or pathological conditions such as acute myocardial infarction and subsequent ischemia of the SA node.[7,8] Sick sinus syndrome may also be caused by Lyme disease or infiltrative diseases, such as **amyloidosis**, which damages the atrial muscle. Certain antidysrhythmia medications have been implicated in sick sinus syndrome, specifically procainamide, verapamil, diltiazem, and amiodarone.

Regardless of the etiology, the sum result is the same. The patient experiences a marked bradycardia, typically less than 40 bpm, and has a syncopal episode. Upon arrival at the patient's side, the ECG may show a sinus rhythm and even a sinus tachycardia in some cases, leading to some confusion about the origins of the syncope. Patients with sick sinus syndrome may also complain of lightheadedness prior to the event and dyspnea, angina, and/or palpitations.

Although the disease is called sick sinus syndrome, the pathology can also affect the AV node. Eventually, patients with sick sinus syndrome, particularly those with multiple episodes of syncope, are treated with a pacemaker.

Conduction Blocks

In the past the diagnosis of heart block was based on either change in pulses or changes in the ECG. However, a better understanding of the pathological origin of these heart blocks has led to a modified identification schema that relies on coronary artery involvement and the changes of ischemia.

SA Node Blocks

The SA node, like the AV node, receives its blood supply from the coronary arteries. If there is an interruption in blood flow, then the SA node may fail. As a result of the ischemia the SA may fail to fire, leading to an error of automaticity called sinus arrest, or the impulse may be blocked, resulting in an error of conduction.

A/V Blocks

A/V heart blocks were frequently classified by degrees only. A first degree block meant added delay at the AV junction shown by an elongated PR interval. Second degree blocks demonstrated occasional nonconduction of sinus impulses through the AV node with pauses felt in the pulse and an absence of a QRS complex on the ECG. Third degree blocks demonstrated a complete atrial ventricular dissociation in which sinus impulses were formed but did not initiate ventricular activity and either junctional or ventricular escape rhythms occurred. This classification system did not include information on the likely cause of the block or its location.

The division of the heart between the atria and the ventricles is at the crux (Latin Cross) of the heart. Within the crux (Figure 6-1) is a strip of conductive tissue connecting the atria and the ventricle that contains the AV node, junctional tissue, and the bundle of His. This conductive tissue is critical to the establishment of systole, the contraction of the heart. The upper portion, containing the AV node, receives its blood supply from the right coronary artery (RCA) in 90% of patients; in the remaining 10%, blood comes from the left coronary artery. This 10% of patients is referred to as left dominant. The lower portion of the conduction system, including the bundle of His and the bundle branches, receives its blood supply from the left coronary artery. Therefore, any vascular occlusive event involving either coronary artery will subsequently cause injury to the associated conductive pathway.

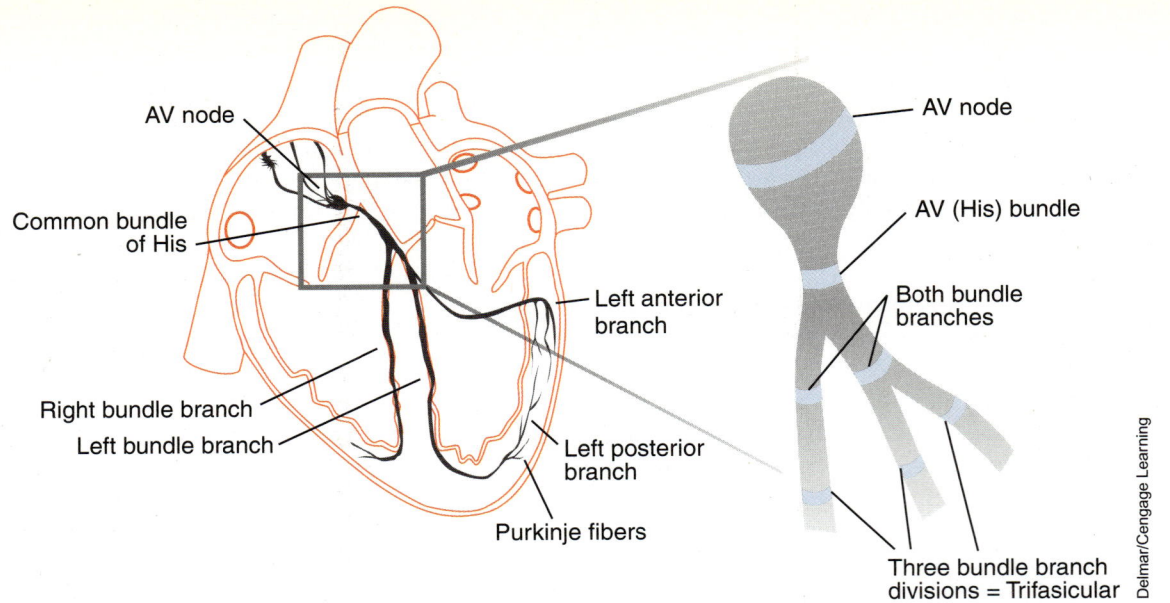

Figure 6-1 AV conduction at the heart's crux.

The proper term is A/V block, not AV block. The term AV supposes a block at the AV node, whereas A/V means atria–ventricle and could mean a block anywhere along the conduction pathway from the AV node to the junction to the bundle of His and includes the bundle branches.

Heart Blocks and Penumbra

The severity of the injury to the conductive pathway can be predicted based on the progression of cellular damage. As cells experience hypoxia the cells are, at first, ischemic. As the hypoxia continues the cells become injured. If the hypoxia persists, then the cells die and infarct. If the cells are conductive cells, then the ischemic progression will also affect these cells in a similarly predictable fashion. These changes result in the two types and three degrees of heart block (Table 6-1).

Type I Heart Blocks (Supranodal Block)

A/V heart blocks are divided into type I and type II. The first classification of heart blocks (type I) affect the AV node. Vasculo-occlusive events in the right coronary artery, involving the inferior wall and the AV node, can lead to type I heart blocks. The AV node can also be affected by other factors, including extreme vagal stimulation (see hypersensitive

Table 6-1 Causes of A/V Heart Blocks

- Acute coronary event
  - Right coronary artery
    - Supranodal
  - Left coronary artery
    - Infranodal
- Medications
  - V–W class I (sodium channel blockers)
    - Procainamide
  - V–W class II (beta blockers)
    - Metoprolol
  - V–W class IV (calcium channel blockers)
    - Verapamil
  - V–W class V (Other)
    - Digitalis
- Infections
  - Diphtheria
  - Rheumatic fever
  - Lyme disease
- Infiltration
  - Syphilis
  - Scleroderma
  - Sarcoidosis
- Aging
  - Idiopathic fibrosis

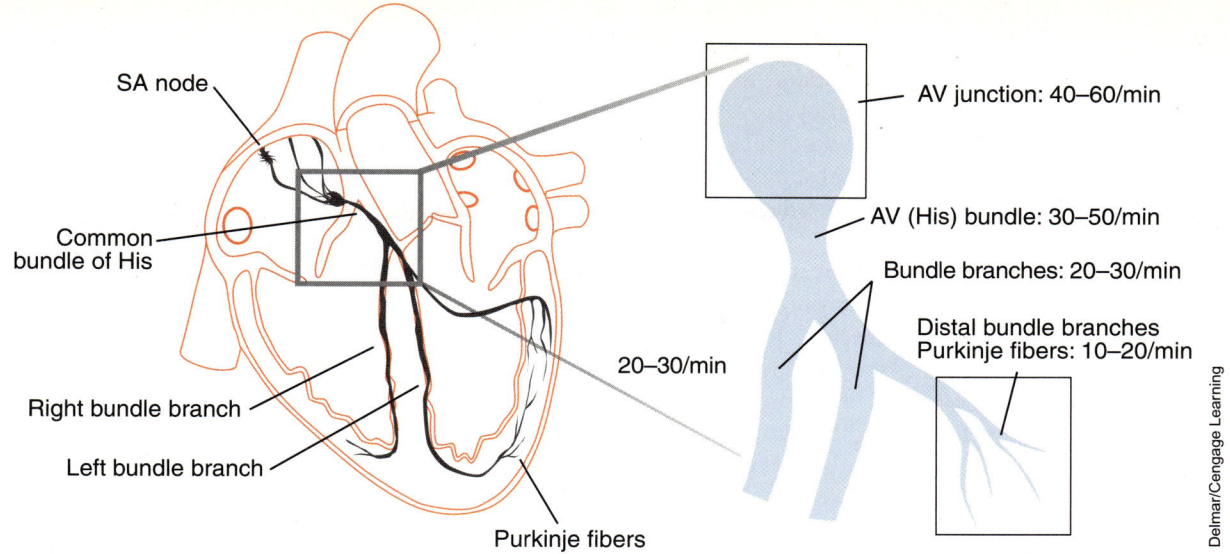

Figure 6-2 Intrinsic heart rates at the heart's crux.

carotid syndrome), digitalis toxicity (see Chapter 4 on errors of automaticity), and changes of old age (i.e., fibrosis and calcification of the AV node).

Type II Heart Block (Infranodal Block)

The other heart block is called a type II heart block. A type II heart block, like a type I heart block, can be either benign (as a result of fibrotic changes of aging) or pathological. A pathological type II heart block can occur because of a vasoocclusive event in the left coronary artery that supplies blood to the septum. The resultant hypoxia causes an infranodal conduction delay. Because the heart block occurs below the AV node, and therefore the escape rhythm would be ventricular, there

is a high mortality associated with type II heart blocks that progress to a complete heart block.[9]

Dangers of Heart Blocks

Unabated, heart blocks deteriorate into complete heart blocks. Depending on the level of the block, the subsequent escape rhythm may, or may not, be sufficient for the patient's needs. For example, a supranodal heart block that progresses to a complete heart block will have a junctional escape rhythm at a rate of 40 to 60 beats per minute, whereas an infranodal heart block that progresses to a complete heart block may have an idioventricular escape rhythm at a rate of 20 to 30 beats per minute or profound bradycardia that is incompatible with life (Figure 6-2).

CASE STUDY (CONTINUED)

Mr. Tedesco agrees to let the Paramedics examine him after they assure him that he isn't taking them away from any customers who really need them. During the interview, he tells them that 8 years ago, he had a "spell" in which he had gotten really weak. Neighbors thought that he had been exposed to pesticides. The doctor thought otherwise and Mr. Tedesco got a pacemaker implanted in his chest.

CRITICAL THINKING QUESTIONS

1. What are the important elements of the history that a Paramedic should obtain, especially in light of the fact that Mr. Tedesco has not seen a physician in a number of years?
2. What questions should the Paramedic ask about events that occurred before the syncope?

History

Most patients are asymptomatic from their heart block unless there is a high degree of block or a complete heart block. Patients with a high degree of block, or complete heart block, may complain of symptoms associated with a loss of cardiac

output, including lightheadedness and dizziness. Any patient who experiences syncope and has severe bradycardia (less than 50 beats per minute) should be suspected of having a high degree of heart block or possibly even a complete heart block. Patients with ischemia-induced heart block will have the traditional signs of an acute coronary event including chest pain/pressure, shortness of breath, or heart failure as well.

A careful medication history is important. Many medications, particularly those in the Vaughn–Williams classification, can cause bradycardia. Of particular concern are the beta/adrenergic blockers and digitalis. These drugs can also have direct effects on the ventricular mass, decreasing contractility and diminishing blood pressure.

Although it would seem that the heart is controlled by the autonomic nervous system, the endocrine system also exerts influence on cardiac function. Low levels of thyroid hormones lead to bradycardia. Patients with hypothyroidism, or those who have not been compliant with their thyroid hormone replacement therapy, may experience symptomatic bradycardia. A hypothermic patient may present with a bradycardia and treatment is focused on warming the patient.

Finally, the Paramedic should inquire if the patient has a pacemaker. Pacemakers are inserted into patients for a variety of reasons and on occasion these pacemakers fail. Without a properly functioning pacemaker, the patient's underlying, or native, rhythm will become evident.

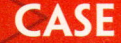

STREET SMART

Patients on beta/adrenergic blockers will not be able to mount a compensatory tachycardia to offset the negative inotropic effect of the medications. Therefore, these patients can present with bradycardia and hypotension.

CASE STUDY (CONTINUED)

Immediately the Paramedics seize on the fact that Mr. Tedesco's pulse is slow and irregular and the patient is placed on the ECG monitor. After the history fails to reveal any untoward effects of medications, as well as indicating Mr. Tedesco doesn't take any medicine nor have any symptoms consistent with acute coronary syndrome, the Paramedic still insists on obtaining a 12-lead ECG.

CRITICAL THINKING QUESTIONS

1. What are the elements of the physical examination of a patient with suspected syncope secondary to bradycardia?
2. Why is a 12-lead ECG a critical element in this examination?

Examination

The presence of bradycardia should alert the Paramedic to the potential for a heart block.[10] A regular pulse, within the normal limits, suggests that the patient may have a first degree heart block. A slowed and irregular pulse may suggest that the patient has a second degree heart block, secondary to dropped beats. A bradycardia may indicate that the patient has either a high degree block or a complete heart block with an escape rhythm. A bradycardia is usually associated with

STREET SMART

Second degree heart blocks tend to drop beats in a pattern that can be detected in the pulse and is described as regularly irregular. This pattern differs from that of atrial fibrillation, where the pulse is irregularly irregular.

the signs of poor perfusion, such as lethargy, chest pain, shortness of breath, and hypotension.

ECG Findings

Any patient with the aforementioned symptom complex (i.e., chest pain, shortness of breath, etc.) should be placed on the cardiac monitor and assessed for heart block. Traditionally Lead II is the lead of choice for detecting heart blocks.

A patient may have no outward manifestations of an A/V heart block if the cause is benign. These heart blocks are only detected during routine cardiac monitoring.

Sinus Disorders

The SA node, like the AV node, receives blood from the coronary arteries. If a coronary artery is occluded, ischemic changes occur that may lead to a sinus block. A sinus disorder occurs when the impulse is either blocked in the atria, making it an error of conduction, or the SA node fails to fire, making it an error of automaticity. In both cases there is a dropped beat with no preceding P wave.

As the SA node does not produce a wave on the ECG, it is necessary to analyze the P to P interval to ascertain if either a sinus block or a sinus arrest occurred. If the P to P interval during the dropped beat is a multiple of the previous P to P (i.e., the dropped beat does not change the rhythm), then it is a sinus block (Table 6-2), which is an error of conduction (Figure 6-3). If the P to P interval during the dropped beat is not a multiple of the previous P to P intervals (i.e., the dropped beat changes the rhythm), then it is a sinus arrest (Figure 6-4). Sinus arrest, along with Stokes–Adams attacks, are discussed in Chapter 4 on errors of automaticity.

When the SA node ceases to fire entirely (e.g., because SA node is infarcted), then no P waves will be visible and a lower escape pacemaker will assume dominance, typically the AV node. This rhythm would be called a junctional escape rhythm. In those cases, the QRS complex will remain narrow and no P waves are visible.[11] Sinus disorders—both sinus arrest and sinus block—can occur with inferior wall MI, posterior wall MI, and digitalis toxicity. SA blocks are only treated if the patient becomes symptomatic.

Sinus Rhythm with Type I A/V Heart Block

A type I first degree heart block can either be benign, as a result of fibrotic changes associated with old age, or pathological, as a result of an acute coronary event. When an acute coronary event occurs in the right coronary artery, the AV node starts to malfunction. Initially the patient will experience a vagally induced bradycardia as a result of the hypoxia. This bradycardia would seem to be incongruent with a patient experiencing epigastric discomfort and/or nausea. As the cellular damage progresses, the AV node depolarization (represented by the PR interval) slows and the PR interval starts to lengthen.

The exact PR interval is less important than the amount of change observed over the course of the Paramedic/patient interaction. A PR interval measuring 0.24 seconds and

Table 6-2 Sinus Block

Ventricular Rhythm	
Regularity	Regular except for pauses
Rate	Normocardia to bradycardia
Width of QRS	Usually 0.04 to 0.12 seconds
Atrial Rhythm	
Regularity	Regular
Rate	Normocardia
Shape of P wave	Rounded and upright in Lead II
PR interval	0.12 to 0.20 seconds
A/V relationship	1 P wave for each QRS; pause without P wave or QRS

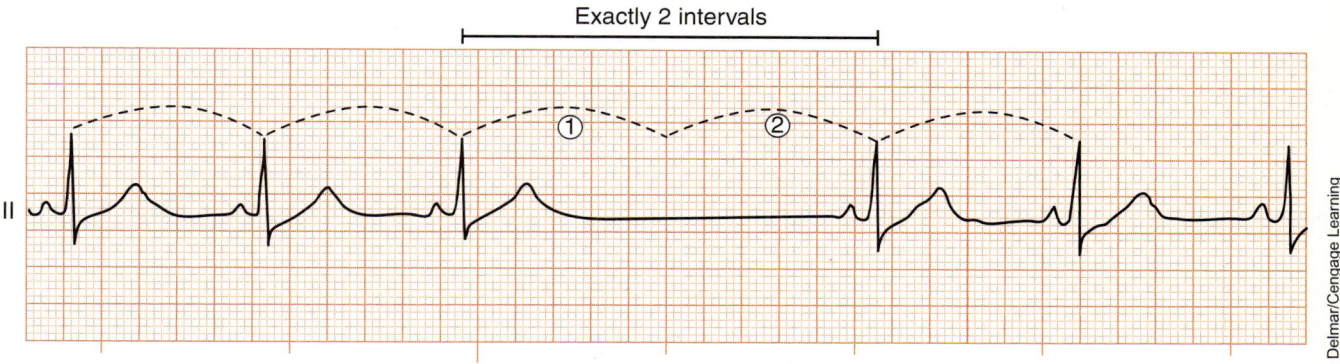

Figure 6-3 Sinus block.

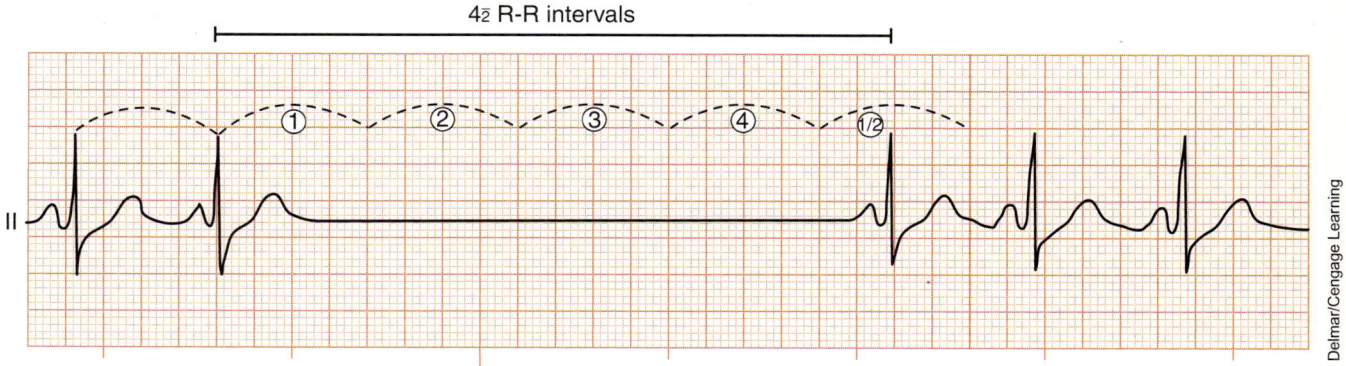

Figure 6-4 Sinus arrest.

remaining unchanged is less likely to indicate an acute problem than is a PRI that began at 0.12 seconds and has lengthened to 0.24 seconds during the transport time. The change in the PRI should be an indication of ischemia.

Sinus Rhythm with Type I Block—First Degree Block

The first dysrhythmia associated with a **type I first degree heart block** is usually sinus bradycardia. Cellular hypoxia, in the AV node, does not allow the pacemaker cells to depolarize and repolarize as quickly as normal, resulting in bradycardia.

STREET SMART

Increased vagal tone, secondary to vagal stimulation, may produce a transient type I first degree A/V heart block. When the heart rate returns to normal, the PR interval shortens and the A/V block disappears.

Eventually the hypoxic AV node develops ischemia that progresses to a type I first degree heart block (Table 6-3 and Figure 6-5).

Sinus Rhythm with Type I Block—Second Degree Block

As the cellular damage progresses, the AV node starts to become ischemic. These changes (increased AV node refractoriness) are evidenced by a lengthening PR interval until the impulse is blocked by a refractory AV node, represented on the ECG as a dropped beat. This pattern of lengthening PR intervals and then a dropped beat is called a **type I second degree block** or **Wenckebach's phenomena**.[12]

Early in the development of a sinus rhythm with a type I second degree block, the patient may sense the dropped beat as a palpitation (Table 6-4). As the frequency of dropped beats occurs, the patient's cardiac output may fall as well as the blood pressure (Figures 6-6 and 6-7). When the number of blocked beats becomes so high that the patient experiences a bradycardia, then the heart is said to have a high degree of block.

Table 6-3 Sinus Rhythm with Type I Block—First Degree Block

Ventricular Rhythm	
Regularity	Regular except for pauses
Rate	Normocardiac
Width of QRS	Usually 0.04 to 0.12 seconds
Atrial Rhythm	
Regularity	Regular
Rate	Normocardiac
Shape of P wave	Rounded and upright in Lead II before QRS
PR interval	Greater than 0.20 seconds
A/V relationship	1 P wave for each QRS

Table 6-4 Sinus Rhythm with Type I Block—Second Degree Block

Ventricular Rhythm	
Regularity	Regularly irregular
Rate	Normocardiac
Width of QRS	Usually 0.04 to 0.12 seconds
Atrial Rhythm	
Regularity	Regular
Rate	Normocardiac
Shape of P wave	Rounded and upright in Lead II before QRS
PR interval	Greater than 0.20 seconds; lengthens with each QRS until dropped QRS complex
A/V relationship	1 P wave for each QRS; except dropped QRS complex

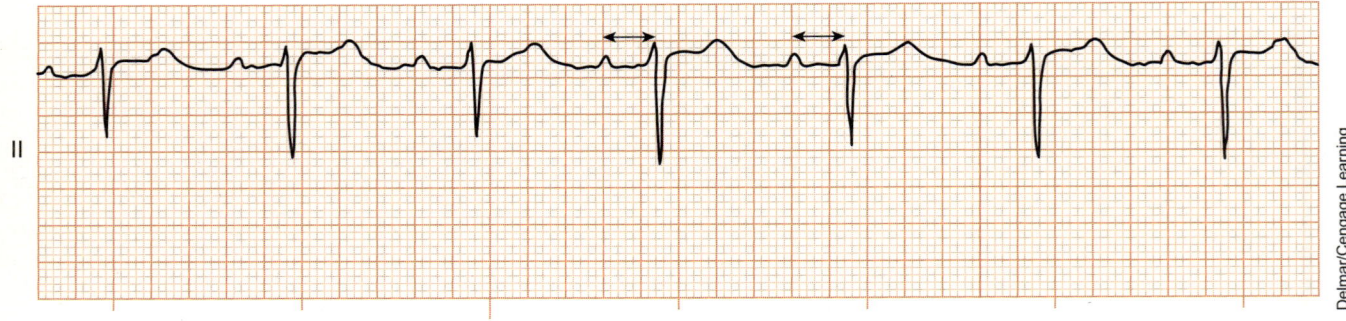

Figure 6-5 Sinus rhythm with type I first degree A/V block.

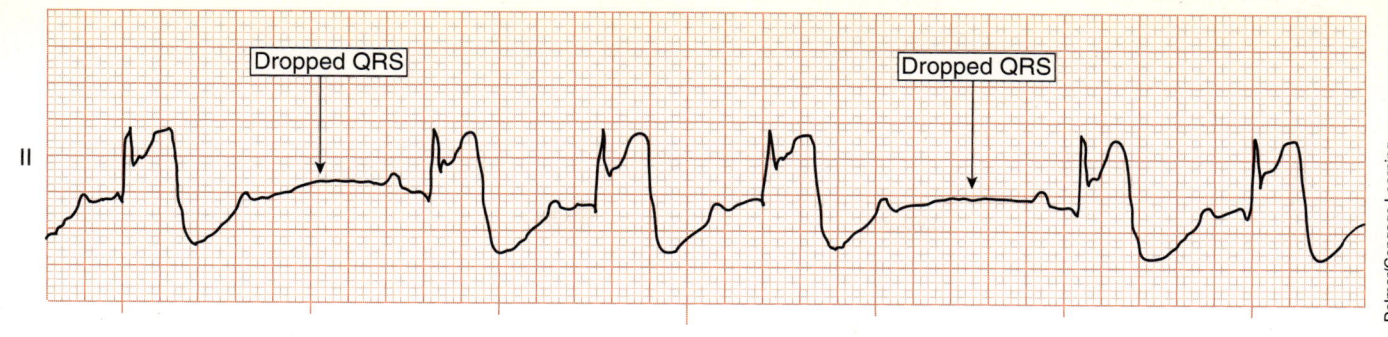

Figure 6-6 Sinus rhythm with type I second degree A/V block (Wenckebach's phenomena).

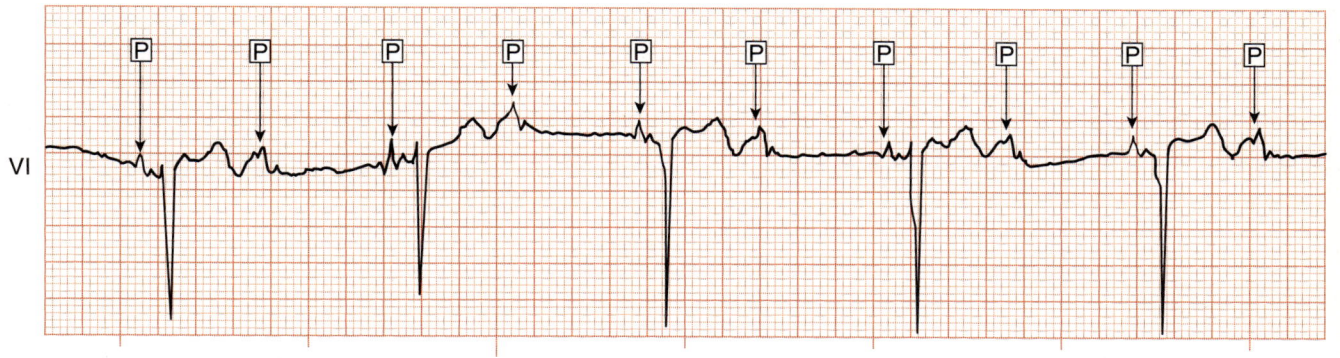

Figure 6-7 Sinus rhythm with type I second degree A/V block—high degree block.

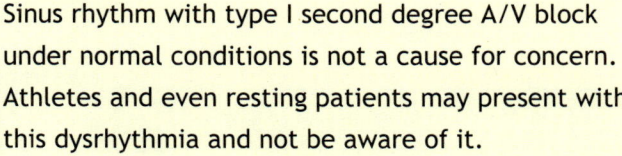
Sinus Rhythm with Type I—Third Degree Block

In the end, the injured AV node starts to infarct and a sinus rhythm **type I third degree block** occurs. The necrotic tissue of the infarcted AV node is unable to propagate the impulse to ventricles, establishing a complete heart block. The next pacemaker immediately inferior to the AV node is within the junction and a junctional escape rhythm ensues (Table 6-5 and Figure 6-8). However, the SA node continues to depolarize the atria, creating a P wave. However, these two activities—the sinus rhythm and the junctional escape rhythm—are disconnected (a state called A/V dissociation).

Type II Block

Type II heart blocks are infranodal blocks that involve the bundle of His and the bundle branches. Type II heart blocks can also occur as a result of an acute coronary event. The appearance of type II blocks should alert the Paramedic to the possibility of an anterior wall MI (AWMI). AWMI comes with attendant risks for forward failure and subsequent hypotension.

Sinus Rhythm with Type II—First Degree Block

When the left coronary artery becomes occluded, the septal wall (and specifically, the bundle of His and/or the bundle branches) start to become ischemic. That ischemia could affect only one branch of the bundle branch, creating an intraventricular conduction delay (QRS greater than 0.12 seconds but less than 0.16), or the ischemia could affect two fascicles of the left bundle or one fascicle of the left bundle and the right bundle, resulting in a **type II first degree block** (i.e., **bundle branch block**) (Table 6-6 and Figure 6-9).

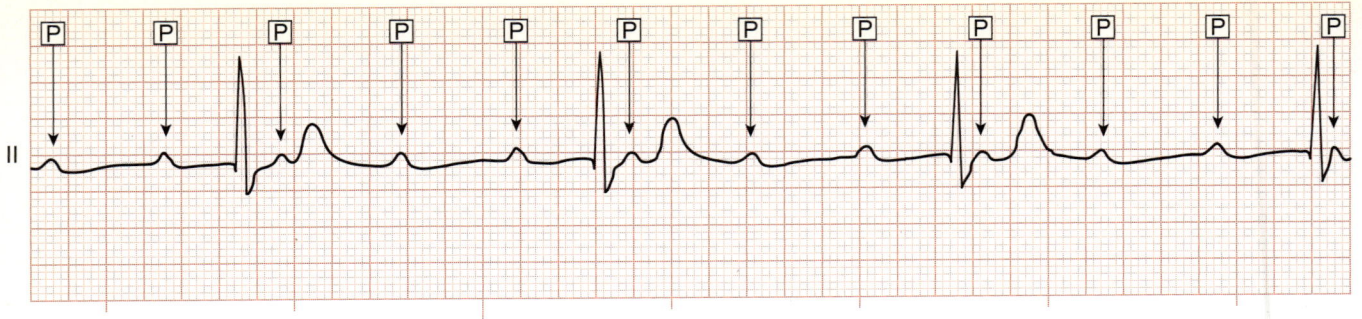

Figure 6-8 Sinus rhythm with type I third degree A/V block.

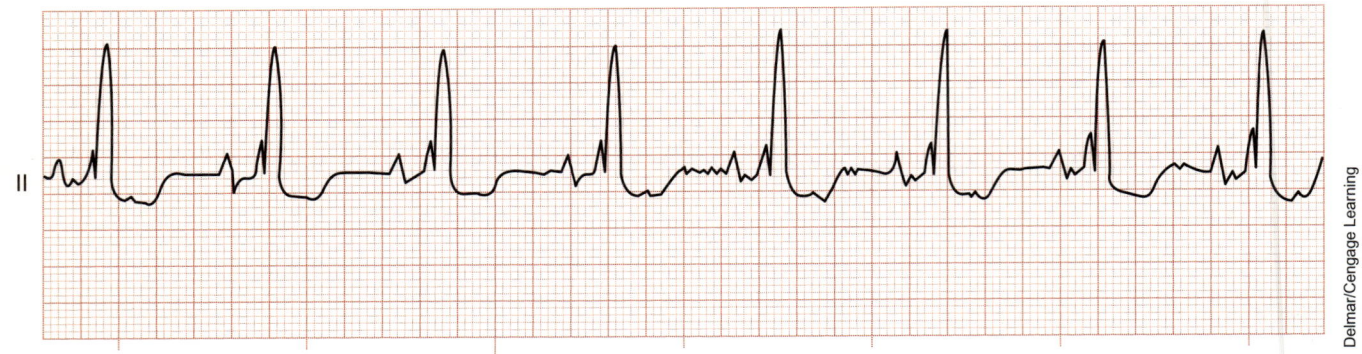

Figure 6-9 Sinus rhythm with type II first degree A/V block, also known as a bundle branch block.

Table 6-5 Sinus Rhythm with Type I Block—Third Degree Block with Junctional Escape Rhythm

Ventricular Rhythm	
Regularity	Regular
Rate	Bradycardia; 40 to 60 complexes per minute
Width of QRS	Usually 0.04 to 0.12 seconds
Atrial Rhythm	
Regularity	Regular
Rate	Normocardiac
Shape of P wave	Rounded and upright in Lead II before QRS
PR interval	None
A/V relationship	None; A/V dissociation

Table 6-6 Sinus Rhythm with Type II Block—First Degree Block

Ventricular Rhythm	
Regularity	Regular
Rate	Normocardia; 40 to 60 complexes per minute
Width of QRS	Greater than 0.12 seconds
Atrial Rhythm	
Regularity	Regular
Rate	Normocardiac
Shape of P wave	Rounded and upright in Lead II before QRS
PR interval	Greater than 0.20 seconds
A/V relationship	1 P wave for each QRS complex

Sinus Rhythm with Type II—Second Degree Block

As the hypoxia continues, and the ischemia worsens within the bundle of His, the patient may start to experience dropped beats. Unlike type I dropped beats, **type II second degree block**, also known as a classic block, gives no indication of an impending dropped beat (Table 6-7 and Figure 6-10). However, like a type I second degree block, if the number of dropped beats is so high that the patient experiences a bradycardia, then the block is referred to as a high degree block.

STREET SMART

While type I second degree blocks can be benign and self-resolving, type II second degree blocks tend to progress to complete heart blocks and potentially deadly idioventricular rhythms.

Sinus Rhythm with Type II—Third Degree Block

Eventually, as the bundle branches infarct, all communication between the atria and the ventricles is lost. As the break in the conduction system occurs below the AV node, the resulting escape rhythm is ventricular (Table 6-8 and Figure 6-11). The ventricular pacemakers are unreliable and the resulting profound bradycardia can convert to ventricular fibrillation or asystole. An overview of all these blocks in a matrix that is attributed to coronary artery involvement (Table 6-9) can be helpful for a Paramedic.

Heart Transplantation

Patients with conduction abnormalities include those patients with cardiac transplantation. The first human-to-human transplant occurred in 1967 in Cape Town, South Africa. The recipient lived 18 days. Since then, cardiac transplantation has extended patients' lives from days into decades.[13]

Patients with end-stage cardiac failure are registered with the United Network for Organ Sharing. Approximately 3,500 transplants occur annually, with the number being held down by the unavailability of donor hearts. While awaiting a

Table 6-7 Sinus Rhythm with Type II Block—Second Degree Block (Classic)

Ventricular Rhythm	
Regularity	Regularly irregular
Rate	Normocardia; 40 to 60 complexes per minute
Width of QRS	Greater than 0.12 seconds
Atrial Rhythm	
Regularity	Regular
Rate	Normocardiac
Shape of P wave	Rounded and upright in Lead II before QRS
PR interval	Greater than 0.20 seconds; constant
A/V relationship	1 P wave for each QRS complex; except dropped beat

Table 6-8 Sinus Rhythm with Type II Block—Third Degree Block—Idioventricular Escape Rhythm

Ventricular Rhythm	
Regularity	Regular
Rate	Bradycardia; 20 to 40 complexes per minute
Width of QRS	Greater than 0.12 seconds
Atrial Rhythm	
Regularity	Regular
Rate	Normocardiac
Shape of P wave	Rounded and upright in Lead II
PR interval	None
A/V relationship	None; A/V dissociation

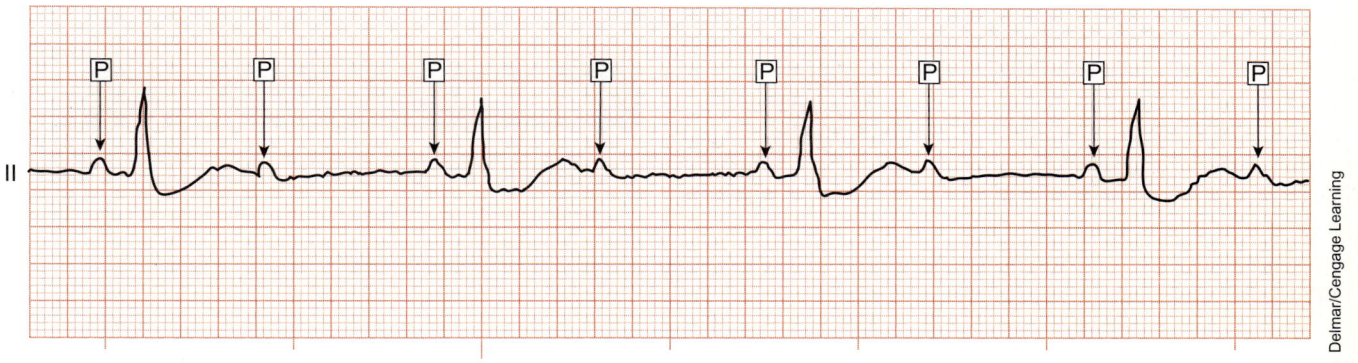

Figure 6-10 Sinus rhythm with type II second degree A/V block—high degree of block.

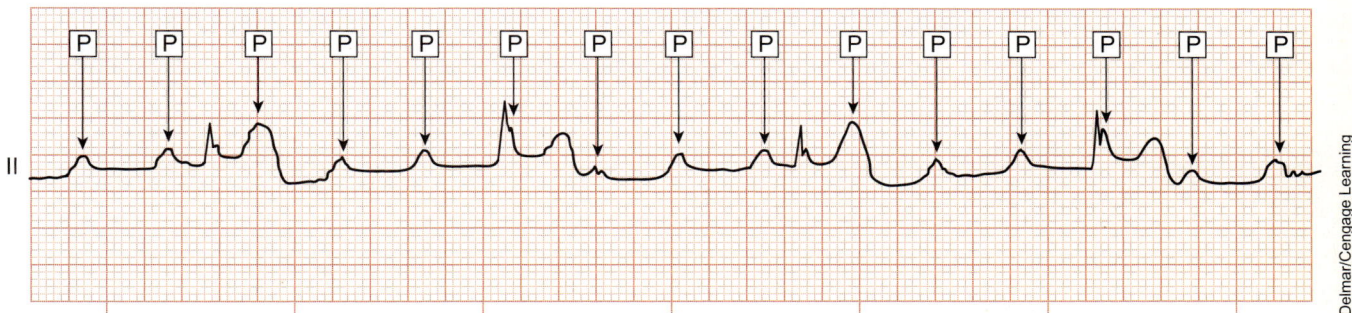

Figure 6-11 Sinus rhythm with type II third degree A/V block.

Table 6-9 Heart Blocks by Coronary Perfusion

Pathological	Type I Right Coronary Artery Inferior Wall MI	Type II Left Coronary Artery Anterior Wall MI
Sinus Rhythm with:		
First degree block		
Ventricular rhythm	Regular	Regular
PR interval	Widened	Normal
AV association	1:1	1:1
Old terminology		Bundle branch block
Second degree block		
Ventricular rhythm	Irregular	Irregular
PR interval	Extending	Constant
AV association	# P wave > # QRS	# P wave > # QRS
Old terminology	Wenckeback/Mobitz type I	Classic heart block/Mobitz type II
Third degree block		
Ventricular rhythm	Regular	Regular
PR interval	None	None
AV association	None	None
Escape rhythm	Junctional	Ventricular
Rate	40 to 60 per minute	20 to 40 per minute
Old terminology	Complete heart block	Complete heart block

donor heart, many patients are assisted by a left ventricular assist device (LVAD) or an artificial heart.

The most common procedure for transplantation is to remove the native heart at the mid-atrial level and replace it with the donor heart. The great vessels of the recipient are preserved as are the valves of the donor heart. This procedure leaves the patient at risk for conduction abnormalities including atrial dysrhythmia and atrioventricular nodal blocks. A newer procedure reconstructs the great vessels and grafts the entire donor heart into place. There are less conduction disturbances with this procedure as the entire right atrium along with the SA node and internodal pathways are preserved. The procedure takes longer to perform and thus places the patient at risk for decreased blood flow and ischemic events during the surgery.

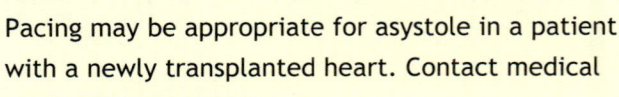

STREET SMART

Pacing may be appropriate for asystole in a patient with a newly transplanted heart. Contact medical control for consultation.

CASE STUDY (CONTINUED)

The 12-lead ECG reveals a heart block-induced bradycardia in Mr. Tedesco. With that knowledge, the Paramedic tries to convince Mr. Tedesco that he should seek medical attention sooner rather than later. Fortunately for the Paramedic, Mrs. Tedesco shows up on scene and is able to convince her reluctant husband to go to the hospital.

CRITICAL THINKING QUESTIONS

1. What is the significance of the 12-lead ECG to the diagnosis of bradycardia-induced syncope?
2. What elements of the history, coupled with a knowledge of cardiology, should the Paramedic use to formulate his argument that Mr. Tedesco needed further medical attention?

Assessment

Regardless of the etiology of the bradycardia, decisions about patient treatment are predicated on whether the patient is symptomatic or asymptomatic. Signs of hemodynamic instability, as manifest by signs of hypoperfusion, include dizziness or syncope, chest discomfort, and shortness of breath. If the patient manifests signs of hypoperfusion, then treatment in the field is warranted.

CASE STUDY (CONTINUED)

Bolstered by the support of Mrs. Tedesco, the Paramedic lays out the treatment plan to Mr. Tedesco. At first Mr. Tedesco is resistant but agrees to receive treatment provided his wife can accompany him to the hospital.

CRITICAL THINKING QUESTIONS

1. What is the standard of care for patients with bradycardia?
2. What are some of the patient-specific concerns and considerations that the Paramedic should consider when applying this plan of care that is intended to treat a broad patient population presenting with bradycardia?

Treatment

The Paramedic treating a patient with suspected symptomatic sinus bradycardia will first focus on finding and treating the underlying cause (Table 6-10). Causes of symptomatic bradycardia are numerous and require the Paramedic keep an open mind to extracardiac causes as well as cardiac causes. If the patient is symptomatic then treatment with atropine, a parasympathetic blocker, may be needed.

The treatment of symptomatic bradycardia of A/V heart blocks is somewhat dependent on the type of A/V block. Type I A/V blocks are generally benign and only require the Paramedic to monitor the patient's condition. If the patient is symptomatic, then the Paramedic should administer 0.5 to 1 mg atropine, every three to five minutes as needed, to a maximum dose of 3 mg. As the patient's tolerance to atropine may vary, it is prudent to start the patient at the lowest dose of atropine (0.5 mg). Caution is advised with smaller doses of atropine. Small doses of atropine, less than 0.5 mg, or atropine given too slowly may cause a paradoxical drop in heart rate.[14]

Type II A/V heart blocks, or infranodal heart blocks, tend to be more problematic and patients with them tend to be more symptomatic. In those cases, the Paramedic should consider transcutaneous pacing. While the Paramedic can attempt a trial of atropine to see if the patient's heart is responsive, atropine is only effective on the parasympathetic nervous system. Unfortunately, the parasympathetic innervations end at approximately the AV node.

Table 6-10 Potential Causes of Symptomatic Sinus Bradycardia

- Parasympathetic stimulation
  - Persistent vomiting
    - Infection
    - Toxins
  - Small bowel obstruction
- Medications
  - Beta/adrenergic blocker overdose
  - Calcium channel blocker overdose
- Hypothermia
- Increased intracranial pressure
  - Trauma brain injury
  - Intracerebral hemorrhage
  - Stroke
- Pain

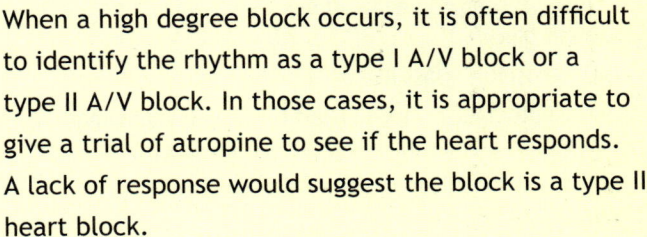

STREET SMART

When a high degree block occurs, it is often difficult to identify the rhythm as a type I A/V block or a type II A/V block. In those cases, it is appropriate to give a trial of atropine to see if the heart responds. A lack of response would suggest the block is a type II heart block.

Transcutaneous Pacing

In 1981, Dr. Zoll introduced a **transcutaneous external pacemaker (TEP)** that had a longer pulse duration (40 milliseconds) and a larger electrode (surface area 80 square centimeters). These features reduced the current needed for effective pacing and increased patient comfort, making TCP practical for use in the field. In the interim, TCP has become the standard of care for treating patients with severe symptomatic bradycardia (Table 6-11).

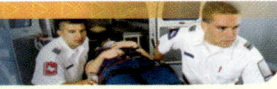

STREET SMART

The American Heart Association has stated that transcutaneous pacing should not be used in cases of asystole or pulseless electrical activity. However, some physicians think that transcutaneous pacing of primary asystole (asystole preceded by an error of conduction, such as A/V block) may be life-saving. TCP in those limited cases should be used only with medical consultation.[15,16]

TCP is particularly useful in heart blocks with severe bradycardia. Type I A/V heart blocks infrequently convert to high degree blocks or complete heart block. Even in those instances, the patient tolerates the junctional escape rhythm. A junctional escape rhythm has an intrinsic heart rate of 40 to 60 beats per minute.

Table 6-11 Indications for Transcutaneous Pacing

- Useful—class I
  - Symptomatic complete heart block
    - Unresponsive to medications
    - Suspected acute myocardial infarction
  - Symptomatic bradycardia
    - Type I second degree heart block
    - Type II second degree heart block
  - Type II second degree heart block with cardiac concerns
  - Type I second degree heart block with type II first degree heart block
- May be useful—class II
  - Asymptomatic complete heart block with ventricular response greater than 40 beats per minute
  - Type I second degree with cardiac concerns
- Not useful—class III
  - Type I first degree heart block
  - Type I second degree heart block (Wenckebach's phenomena)
  - Type II first degree heart block (BBB)

Note: Modified from the American Heart Association's recommendations.

More problematic is the patient with a type II second degree heart block. Approximately one third of patients with type II second degree heart blocks will progress to third degree or complete heart block and an idioventricular escape rhythm (the intrinsic heart rate of an idioventricular escape rhythm is 20 to 40 beats per minute). Seldom can a patient tolerate a heart rate of 20 to 40 bpm for any period of time without experiencing ischemia and deterioration into ventricular fibrillation or asystole. Studies have suggested that delays in pacing high degree heart blocks or idioventricular rhythms can lead to poorer survival rates.[17–19]

The heart is paced during transcutaneous pacing (TCP), sometimes called transcutaneous external pacing (TEP), by placing pacing pads (large cutaneous electrodes) on the patient. An electrical current, created by a pulse generator, then passes through the intact chest and depolarizes the heart in a rhythmic manner, resulting in cardiac pacing.

External cardiac pacing has two modes. The first mode is fixed or **asynchronous mode**. Fixed mode pacers pace the heart regardless of any underlying rhythm. Fixed mode is effective when the heart is in asystole but can be dangerous if the patient still has a native underlying rhythm. If the patient has a native rhythm, the pacer may inadvertently pace during the relative refractory period and cause ventricular fibrillation (R on T phenomena).

For this reason, most pacers are set in the synchronous or demand mode. In the demand mode, the pacer circuit senses the QRS and inhibits, or blanks, the pacemaker from discharging for about 100 milliseconds, in order to prevent R on T phenomena. If no QRS complexes are sensed, then the pacemaker reverts to fixed mode.

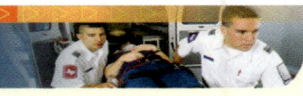

STREET SMART

While there is a theoretical chance that the R on T could produce ventricular fibrillation, this risk is probably greater with synchronized cardioversion than pacing. The energy to cause ventricular fibrillation in the heart is approximately 12 times the energy needed to pace the heart.

Procedure for External Pacing

Once the decision has been made to pace a patient, the preparation can be remembered using an ABCDE approach. The A stands for **A**irway management. The analgesics and sedatives used during pacing are respiratory depressants, and as such it may be necessary for the Paramedic to protect the airway.

Next, the Paramedic needs to prepare for ventilation (the B, for **B**reathing, in the mnemonic). Inadvertent phrenic nerve stimulation may lead to diaphragmatic exhaustion and the patient's ventilation will need support until the diaphragm recovers.

As there is always a risk of cardiovascular collapse, particularly in patients with severe bradycardia and with the attendant risk of R on T phenomena during pacing, intravenous access to support the Circulation (C) is vital.

As pacing can be an uncomfortable procedure, many Paramedics offer their patients sedation and/or analgesia prior to pacing (Drug). The drug of choice for sedation is diazepam, with a dose of 5 to 10 mg administered approximately one to five minutes before the pacing begins. Diazepam has two desirable qualities that make it ideal during external cardiac pacing: (1) Diazepam is a smooth muscle relaxer and, as such, quiets the muscular contracts of the chest, which are a source of discomfort for some patients, and (2) diazepam also has amnesic qualities.

Finally the Paramedic should obtain Expressed consent (E) in the steps in the procedure to the patient (Table 6-12). The Paramedic should advise the patient that the procedure is necessary to prevent further deterioration and that the patient may improve with pacing. The greatest concern the patient may have is pain. The Paramedic should alleviate the patient's concern by explaining that analgesia will be available and that the diazepam should lessen the muscular contractions. The Paramedic should also explain to the patient that the patient's heart rhythm may deteriorate with pacing but that antidysrhythmia medications are readily available. Finally, the Paramedic should advise the patient that transcutaneous pacing is only temporary and that either a temporary transvenous pacemaker or a permanent implanted pacemaker will be available at the hospital.

With the patient's consent, the Paramedic can proceed to placing the pacer pads on the patient. However, before placing the pacer pads, the Paramedic should adjust the lead placement to provide an optimal QRS. In many cases this lead is Lead II and the electrodes will be placed proximal to the pacer pads.

The preferred placement for pacer pads is anterior–posterior. With anterior–posterior placement, the positive pole is placed at the posterior chest slightly inferior to the scapulas and lateral of the spine on the left side. The negative pole is placed at the apex of the heart and proximal to the sternum border, effectively sandwiching the heart between the pads.

Alternatively, the Paramedic may choose an anterior–anterior placement. As many pacer pads are dual service (pacing and defibrillation), Paramedics often prefer to place the patient in the anterior–anterior placement. In this placement, the negative pole is placed in the right upper chest (proximal angle of Louis) and the positive pole is placed at the apex of the heart (fifth intercostal space, midclavicular line, similar to Lead II). While this placement has advantages for the Paramedic, it tends to cause greater pectoral muscle contraction and patient discomfort. If the patient cannot tolerate the anterior–anterior placement of the pacer pads, despite adequate analgesia, then the Paramedic should consider changing the pacer pads to the anterior–posterior placement.

With the pacer pads in place and attached to the pacing cables, the pacemaker is adjusted. The pacemaker is usually set at a rate between 60 and 80 beats per minute. Most Paramedics tend to start lower, at 60 bpm, and adjust the rate to minimize patient discomfort while improving the patient's symptoms and maintaining adequate cardiac output.

With the target heart rate set, the Paramedic starts the energy setting at zero milliamps (mA) and incrementally advances the energy, usually in 20 mA increments, until pacing is achieved. If the patient is in cardiac arrest, the pacemaker is used at the maximum energy setting.

Pacing started early has the greatest potential for successful capture. The incidence of capture can be as great as 90% if pacing is begun early and TCP has been used for over 100 hours with success (**Skill 6-1**).

For a step-by-step demonstration of Transcutaneous Pacing, please refer to Skill 6-1 on pages 180–181.

STREET SMART

If the patient is still experiencing pain despite adequate analgesia, the Paramedic may want to consider moving the positive electrode to the V6 placement (i.e., anterior-lateral position). This may create less pectoral contraction.

Capture

There are two forms of capture: electrical and mechanical. **Electrical capture** occurs when the pacer spike, a sharp vertical line on the ECG, is immediately followed by a QRS. The assumption is that the ventricular depolarization was caused by the pacemaker. If the capture is intermittent (i.e., some QRS are preceded by a pacer spike and some are not), then the energy setting needs to continue to be increased until 100% capture is achieved or the combined native QRS and pacemaker–induced QRS reach the targeted heart rate.

Once electrical capture is achieved, it is common practice to decrease the energy setting in increments of 5 mA while continuing to maintain capture. This ensures the minimum energy needed for capture is used. Alternatively, some Paramedics increase the energy to 10% more than is minimal for capture to ensure consistent pacing.

Table 6-12   Steps in Pacing Procedure

A	Airway	Advanced airway management
B	Breathing	Ventilatory management
C	Circulation	Venous access
D	Drugs	Analgesics and/or sedatives
E	Expressed consent	Procedural permission

Next, the Paramedic assesses the patient for **mechanical capture**. The focus of pacing is to produce palpable pulses. However, these pulses tend to be weaker because the pacer simultaneously paces the atria and the ventricles. This results in loss of the atrial kick and augmented end-diastolic ventricular filling. Starting at the radial pulse (a distal pulse is preferable to prevent confusion between pulses and muscle tremors from pacing), the Paramedic assesses for rate and quality. The patient's pulse should match the rate of the pacer.

If there is evidence of mechanical capture, the Paramedic should assess the patient for blood pressure and other signs of improved perfusion. If the patient remains hypotensive it may be necessary to increase the rate of the pacemaker to a maximum of 80 beats per minute, ever mindful that an increased heart rate can increase ischemia in an injured heart.

Special Case: Overdrive Pacing

Using the principle of dominance, transcutaneous pacemakers are used to terminate drug resistant supraventricular and ventricular tachycardias. The procedure for **overdrive pacing**, sometimes called **burst suppression**, is typical with the exception that the pacemaker is set at a rate higher than the underlying tachycardia. Once the pacemaker has obtained capture, and thus has established dominance as the primary pacemaker, the external pacemaker is slowed to a tolerable heart rate. While this technique can be effective, the accompanying chest discomfort may make it impractical for some patients.

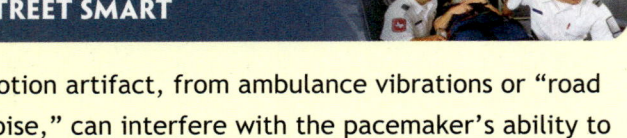

STREET SMART

Motion artifact, from ambulance vibrations or "road noise," can interfere with the pacemaker's ability to sense the QRS complex, forcing the pacemaker into fixed mode, and risking R on T phenomena. Movement of the ECG electrodes to optimize the QRS can prevent this problem.

CASE STUDY (CONTINUED)

While the Paramedic talks to Mr. Tedesco, an EMT applies oxygen, obtains vital signs, obtains a rhythm strip, and applies the 12-lead ECG electrodes. He apologizes for talking to the Paramedic while Mr. Tedesco was finishing his story and gives the vital signs as pulse 38 and regular, respirations 16 and labored, BP 104/60, pulse oximetry 97% on room air and 100% on oxygen.

The Paramedic notes that the rhythm strip shows type II third degree block with slowed ventricular response matching the patient's radial pulse. There is no evidence of pacemaker activity, which is a cause for concern.

CRITICAL THINKING QUESTIONS

1. What are some of the predictable complications associated with an implanted pacemaker?
2. What are some of the predictable complications associated with the prehospital treatments for pacemaker failure?

Evaluation

Permanent internal or implanted pacemakers, like their cousins the transcutaneous external pacemakers, deliver energy to the heart in order to either provide a rhythm (fixed mode) or to augment the heart's own rhythm (demand mode).

Approximately one million patients have permanent implanted pacemakers for a variety of indications including complete heart block, sinus node dysfunction such as sick sinus syndrome, Stokes–Adams syndrome, and atrial fibrillation.

The first pacemakers were ventricular pacemakers that were placed in cases when patients had degenerative changes—such as fibrosis of the AV node, the bundle of His, and the bundle branches—that caused bradycardia.

These pacemakers were followed up with dual chambered pacemakers. By synchronous pacing of the atria, then the ventricles, the patient was able to use the atrial kick to augment cardiac output, naturally.

The latest generation of pacemakers consists of **atrial pacemakers**. The first atrial pacemakers were placed in patients with atrial fibrillation. These pacemakers were placed either because the patient failed to respond to medications or ablation, or because they were preferred to medications or ablation.

Although type I first degree A/V block is normally benign, in some instances the advantage of augmented end-diastolic ventricular filling is lost with delayed atrial contraction. Atrial pacing returns the patient's atrial kick and improves cardiac output in patients with borderline heart function.

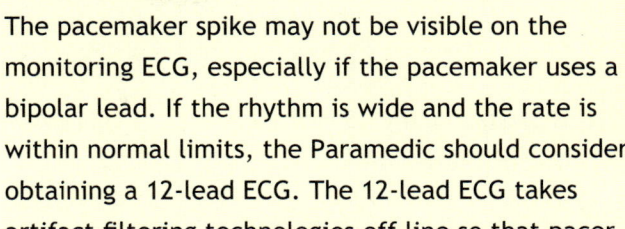
An internal pacemaker consists of a pulse generator, an electronic circuit board with resistors and capacitors, a microprocessor, and a Reed switch. The entire apparatus is contained in a hermetically sealed stainless steel case that is placed in a muscular "pocket" constructed by the cardiothoracic surgeon.

The pulse generator produces a three to four microjoule "pulse" that is stored in capacitors until it is permitted, by the microprocessor, to be transmitted to the heart via implanted electrodes. These electrodes are electrically isolated from the heart by diodes which permit electrical current to flow in one direction. The presence of diodes prevents the energy of defibrillation from entering the pacemaker assembly.

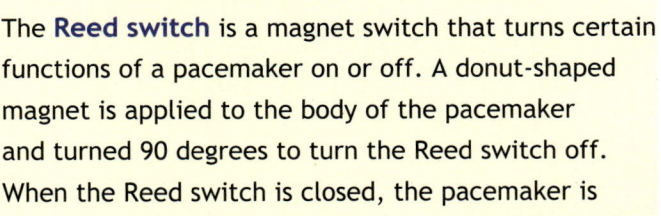
The pacemaker's microprocessor has three circuits. One circuit senses the patient's intrinsic heart rhythm. Another circuit contains the criteria for pacing, and is referred to as the pulse maker. The last circuit is the fail-safe. The fail-safe circuit is a redundant circuit that also contains the criteria needed for pacing. The pulse maker and the fail-safe circuits must agree before the pacemaker will discharge.

The heart of the pacemaker may be the leads. These leads conduct the pulse to the heart and must endure 30 million impulses a year. While these leads are conducting a pulse, they are also flexing every time the heart beats and thus are prone to breakage.

Leads can be either unipolar or bipolar and are placed into the myocardium by active fixation via a corkscrew or tines. Original pacemakers had unipolar leads that passed the current back to the pulse generator through the body and, as a result, created

a large spike on the ECG. Current pacemakers may use a bipolar lead, or coaxial lead, that returns the energy to the pacemaker via the lead. Thus, the result is a small pacer spike on the ECG.

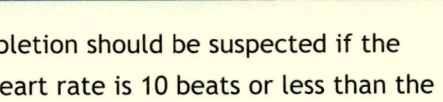
The second weak point in a pacemaker may be its power source. Original internal pacemakers used mercury–zinc batteries. These batteries created hydrogen gas and were prone to self-discharge and internal short circuits. The next generation of pacemaker batteries was made from lithium (Li). Lithium batteries can provide energy for a decade.

Currently the majority of internal pacemakers use lithium batteries because they have a predictable power curve that permits the microprocessor to "step up" the charge in order to maintain a constant output.

While scientists have experimented with nuclear batteries, which could last 20 years, there is increasing interest in biological batteries. Biological batteries derive their energy from the body, and thus last the patient's lifetime.

Over 100 models of pacemakers are currently available, and they can be grossly categorized as ventricular pacemakers, atrial pacemakers, and **dual chamber pacemakers**, which are pacemakers that fire to contract both the atria and ventricles. The current NASPE/BPEG Generic Pacemaker Code, 2000, for classifying pacemakers includes the chamber paced, the chamber sensed, the response to sensing, the rate modulation, and the site for pacing (Table 6-13).

Many patients carry a card with them that contains the previously listed code and the identification of their pacemaker. Paramedics tend to focus on the first three places as these represent the information needed to assess the patient.

For example, a VVI pacer would both pace and sense the ventricles but would be inhibited from discharge by ventricular

Table 6-13 The NASPE/BPEG Generic (NBG) Pacemaker Code (Revised 2000)[21]

Position	I	II	III	IV	V
Category	Chamber(s) Paced	Chamber(s) Sensed	Response to Sensing	Rate Modulation	Multisite Pacing
	O = None	O = None	O = None	O = None	O = None
	A = Atrium	A = Atrium	T = Triggered	R = Rate modulation	A = Atrium
	V = Ventricle	V = Ventricle	I = Inhibited		V = Ventricle
	D = Dual (A+V)	D = Dual (A+V)	D = Dual (T+I)		D = Dual (A+V)
Mfr Designation Only	S = Single (A or V)	S = Single (A or V)			

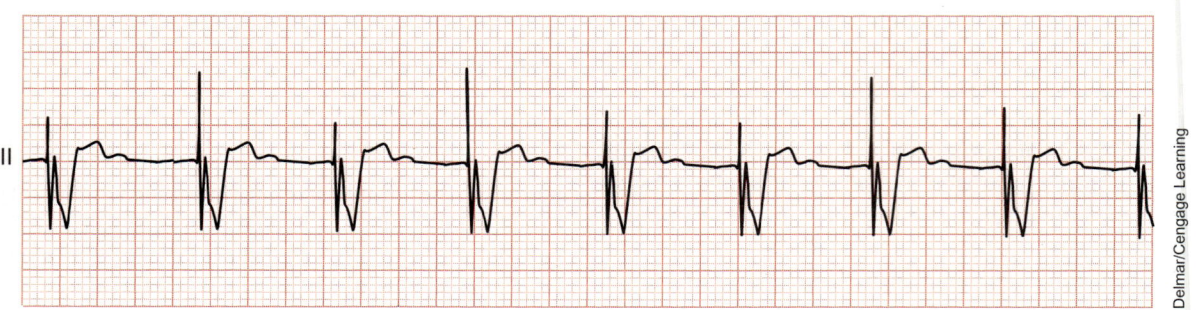

Delmar/Cengage Learning

Figure 6-12   Ventricular pacer with capture.

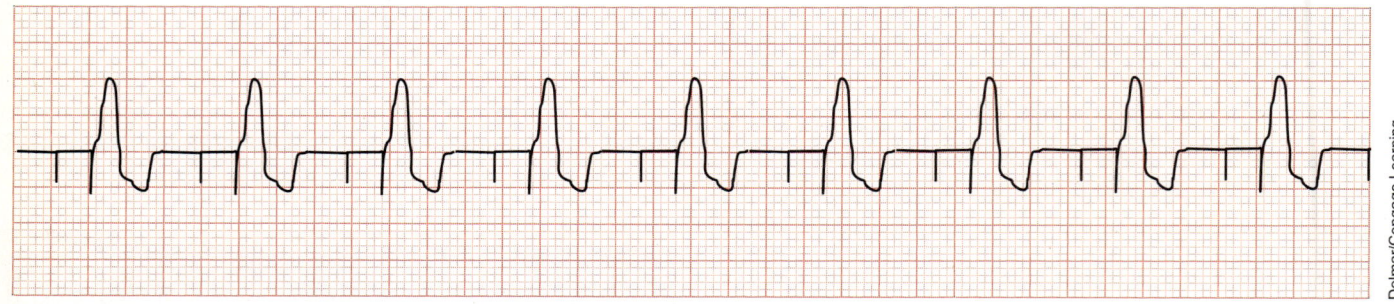

Delmar/Cengage Learning

Figure 6-13   Dual chambered pacemaker with capture.

complexes (i.e., a native beat). The fixed or demand trans-cutaneous pacemaker is a VOO pacemaker according to the code. The DDD pacemaker most closely replicates the natural conduction of the heart through pacing and sensing both chambers (Figures 6-12 and 6-13).

> ▷ ▷ ▷ ▷ ▷ ▷ ▷ ▷ ▷ ▷ ▷ ▷ ▷ ▷
>
> **STREET SMART**
>
> Approximately 97% of all pacemakers placed in the United States are rate responsive pacemakers. These pacemakers sense when the patient is exercising and trigger accelerations in pacing rate to meet metabolic demands.

Pacemaker Syndrome

When the ventricles alone are paced there is a loss of atrioventricular synchrony. As a result of A/V dysynchrony there are a number of physiologic impacts that create **pacemaker syndrome**.

First, there is a loss of the atrial kick, with a loss of up to 50% of the cardiac output.[22,23] This is accompanied by **cannon A waves**, pulsations in the neck and chest as the atria contract against the closed AV valves and pulsations flow backward. There is also increased atrial back pressure, leading to pulmonary hypertension and venous congestion.

Pacemaker syndrome is thought to occur in as many as 18% of patients with a pacemaker (16% in the first year post-implantation). Consequences of pacemaker syndrome include the development of atrial fibrillation (and its attendant risk of stroke) and heart failure.

Patients with pacemaker syndrome may complain of dizziness or confusion (secondary to cerebral hypoperfusion), shortness of breath and paroxysmal nocturnal dyspnea (secondary to backward heart failure), and fatigue or general malaise as a result of forward heart failure.

Patients with pacemaker syndrome will present with signs of shock, varying pulse pressures on palpation (the rhythm remains regular), and jugular venous distention with visible cannon waves from retrograde blood flow.

Although ventricular pacemakers (VVI or VOO) may cause pacemaker syndrome, dual chamber pacemaker malfunction, specifically interference with noise or battery depletion, can also cause pacemaker syndrome.

Pacemaker Malfunction

It is estimated that up to 6% of implanted pacemakers malfunction annually. These malfunctions include failure to discharge (18%), failure to capture (18%), and the clear majority that fail to sense (57%).[24] Patients with malfunctioning pacemakers will present with syncope, palpitations, and bradycardia (the original symptoms that necessitated the implanted pacemaker). Any patient with an implanted pacemaker who complains of weakness and dizziness, syncope, or chest pain should be assessed and transported for pacemaker malfunction.

The Paramedic should first obtain the most recent programmed mode, if possible. The information is available on the patient's pocket card and will tell the Paramedic the normal programmed rate as well as the type of pacemaker. The Paramedic should also obtain the date when the pacemaker was inserted (pacemaker batteries last about 8 to 10 years). Finally, the Paramedic should ask the patient to provide her resting heart rate.

Next, the Paramedic should obtain an ECG, preferably in Lead II, and assess the underlying or native rhythm.

If pacemaker spikes are visible, the Paramedic should ascertain if the pacemaker is atrial, ventricular, or both.

Next, the Paramedic should assess for capture. Normally there is a 1:1 relationship between each pacer spike and either the P wave or the QRS. Any relationship that is not 1:1 may indicate either a failure to sense or a failure to capture.

Undersensing, or failure to sense, is when the pacemaker fails to sense the underlying or native rhythm. Undersensing is detected when the pacer spike is inappropriately placed within or immediately following a P wave or a QRS complex. Undersensing (Figure 6-14) may be due to faulty connection, lead failure (for example, an insulation break), or improper lead position (i.e., the lead migrated within the chamber). Undersensing can also be the result of electrolyte abnormalities, such as hyperkalemia, or a post-defibrillation side effect. Regardless of the etiology, the pacemaker needs to be assessed and perhaps replaced.

Failure to capture (i.e., loss of capture) occurs when the pacemaker discharges, as evidenced by a pacer spike on the ECG. However, a QRS complex does not follow. Reasons for failure to capture include impending battery depletion, lead displacement, and conditions within the myocardium that increase the capture threshold such as medications and electrolyte abnormalities (Figure 6-15).

An acute myocardial infarction, which increases the capture threshold, may cause loss of capture.[25] Therefore, patients with pacemaker malfunction should be assessed for both typical and atypical signs of acute coronary syndrome.

Oversensing occurs when the pacemaker picks up artifact (termed noise) and the inhibition prevents the pacemaker from

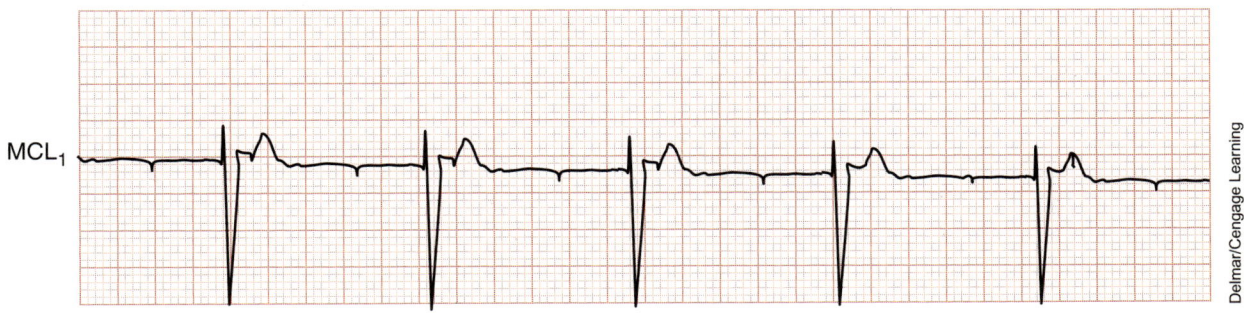

Figure 6-14 Failure to sense or capture.

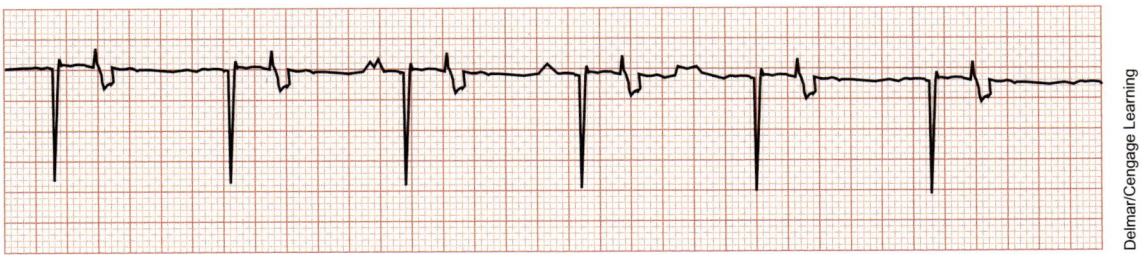

Figure 6-15 Complete heart block with ventricular escape rhythm and ventricular pacemaker with failure to capture.

pacing. Common sources of noise include hyperacute T waves, which may be secondary to ischemia or hyperkalemia, and shivering from hypothermia. The pacer sensing both the QRS complex and the T wave is inhibited and fails to pace (Figure 6-16).

If the patient is profoundly bradycardic, but still conscious, then the patient should be encouraged to perform cough CPR (described shortly) until the transcutaneous pacemaker can be applied. A patient's forceful coughing every second may generate enough energy (approximately 25 joules) to stimulate the heart to maintain cardiac output. Systolic pressures as great as 130 mmHg have been measured with cough CPR and patients have maintained consciousness for as long as 90 seconds.[26,27] The key to effective cough CPR is that it must begin immediately when the patient starts to lose consciousness.

Whenever bradycardia causes unconsciousness, chest compressions should be initiated, regardless of the underlying rhythm. Although CPR can generate systolic pressures of 60 mmHg, minimally sufficient for cerebral perfusion, percussion pacing may be more productive.

Percussion pacing is performed by applying sharp blows to the chest, in the same manner as a precordial thump but with one-quarter the force. Each blow to the sternum can produce between 0.04 to 1.5 joules of energy.[28,29] As the heart is contracting more naturally, twice the cardiac output is obtained than is possible with CPR. There have been documented cases where percussion pacing was able to sustain a patient for over 60 minutes.

The alternative to electrical pacing (via transcutaneous pacing) and manual pacing (with percussion pacing) is **chemical pacing** with either dopamine or epinephrine.

A dopamine infusion at 2 to 10 micrograms per kilogram per minute can stimulate the beta receptors and cause a satisfactory heart rate. If a dopamine infusion is not successful, then an epinephrine infusion can be instituted at 2 to 10 micrograms per minute (note that an epinephrine drip is not weight dependent).

In some instances, it may be beneficial to continue the dopamine infusion at higher levels to maintain its vasopressor effects while infusing the epinephrine to maintain the heart rate. Epinephrine and dopamine, both sympathomimetics, are compatible and can be infused together through the same intravenous access.

Special Case of Overdose

If the source of the bradycardia is a suspected beta/adrenergic blocker overdose, then an infusion of glucagon may be in order. In those cases 3 mg of glucagon should be administered intravenously followed by an infusion of 3 mg of glucagon per hour.

Implantable Cardioverter–Defibrillators

Implantable cardioverter–defibrillators (ICD) could be thought of as the next generation of pacemakers. An ICD detects and terminates potentially lethal tachydysrhythmia. This highly effective device is used to abort supraventricular tachycardia, ventricular tachycardia, and ventricular fibrillation by the delivery of a low energy countershock. Like the pacemaker, the ICD has an energy generator, a microprocessor, and ventricular leads. Formerly, the ICD had to

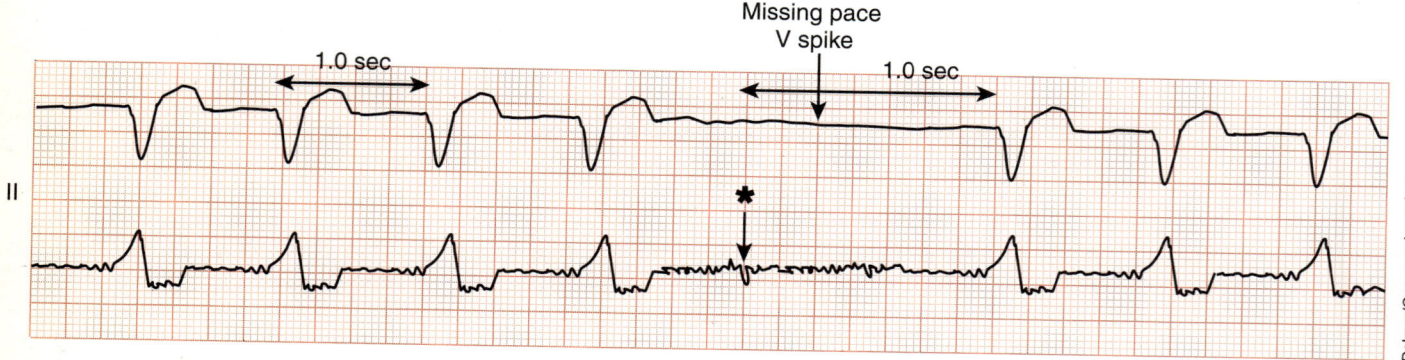

Figure 6-16 Oversensing.

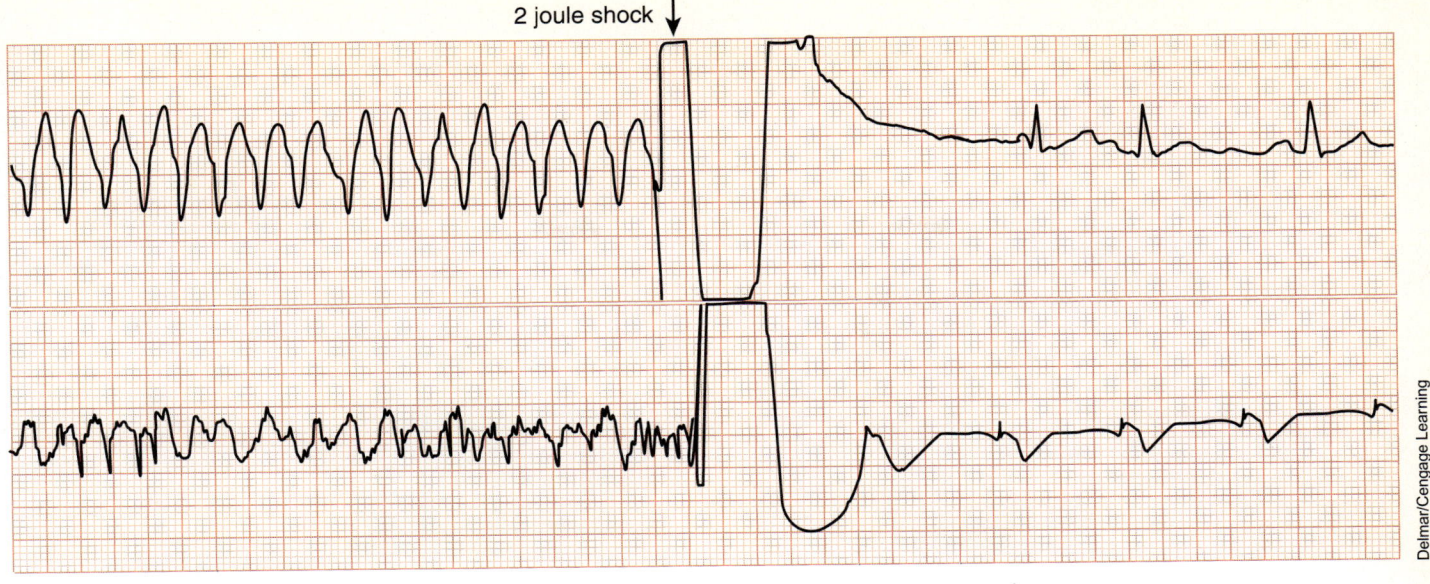

2 joule shock ↓

Figure 6-17 Functioning ICD.

be implanted in the abdomen (the battery made it too large to place elsewhere). However, current models of ICD can be placed in the same location as a pacemaker.

When the ICD senses a ventricular tachycardia, or supraventricular tachycardia, the ICD delivers a series of stacked countershocks, ranging from 0.1 joules to 30 joules, to the heart until the tachydysrhythmia resolves (Figure 6-17).

In some cases, the ICD does not function effectively. In those cases, the Paramedic should resort to standard transthoracic defibrillation or synchronized countershock, as the rhythm dictates. Persons performing CPR should not be concerned about the ICD.[30,31] Even if the ICD discharges, the rescuer will only feel a harmless low energy shock, described by some as a tingling sensation.

CASE STUDY CONCLUSION

Mr. Tedesco is transported to the cardiac center to meet with his cardiologist. The Paramedic muses that he can predict the future and Mr. Tedesco will be having surgery. Mr. Tedesco nods in agreement and says, "I guess it is time for my warranty checkup."

CRITICAL THINKING QUESTIONS

1. What is the most appropriate transport decision that will get the patient to definitive care?
2. What are the advantages of transporting a patient with suspected pacemaker failure to these hospitals, even if that means bypassing other hospitals in the process?

Disposition

Patients suffering from bradycardia secondary to A/V block, an error of conduction, should be transported to a cardiac center when possible. However, most emergency departments are capable of establishing a temporary transvenous pacemaker until the patient is stable enough for transport to a cardiac center for permanent pacemaker placement.

Documentation

The Paramedic should document a complete pacemaker history, including the date of insertion as well as the programmed rate. The patient care report should also indicate the percentage of the time that the patient's pacemaker was pacing. This can be calculated by comparing the number of paced beats in a six-second strip to the total number of beats in the six-second strip. For example, suppose there are five paced beats in a six-second strip with 10 total beats. The comparison is 5/10 and the pacemaker is pacing the patient 50% of the time.

If transcutaneous pacing was used, then the Paramedic should document an assessment of electrical and mechanical capture as evidenced by a rhythm strip and matching pulse rate. The Paramedic should also document the paced rate and the energy used in milliamps.

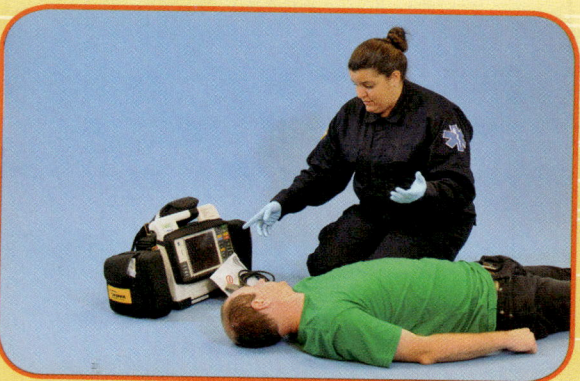

1 While setting up the equipment, explain the procedure to the patient. Consider analgesia and/or sedation.

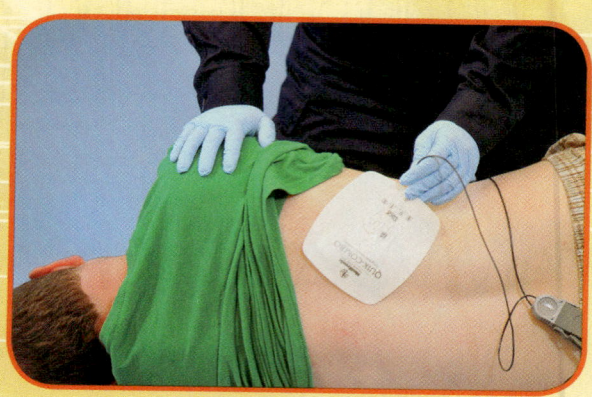

2 Apply pads to the chest/back and anterior–posterior (AP) position.

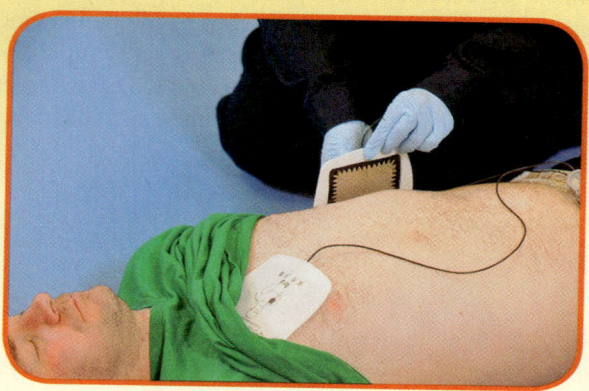

3 If an AP position is not possible, place the pads in an anterior–anterior (AA) position.

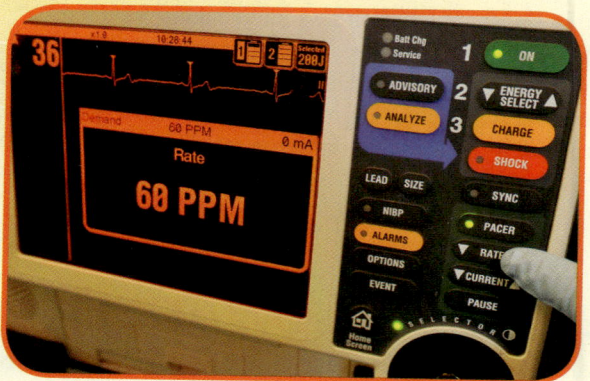

4 Set the rate dial to 60 and the milliamp dial to 0. Turn the pacer on.

Delmar/Cengage Learning

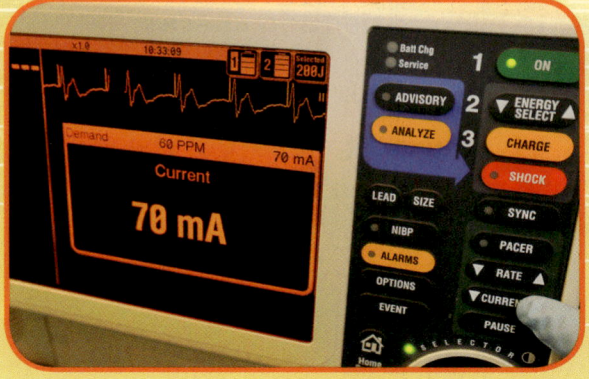

5 Increase the milliamp until electrical capture is obtained on the monitor. Use the lowest energy setting required for capture.

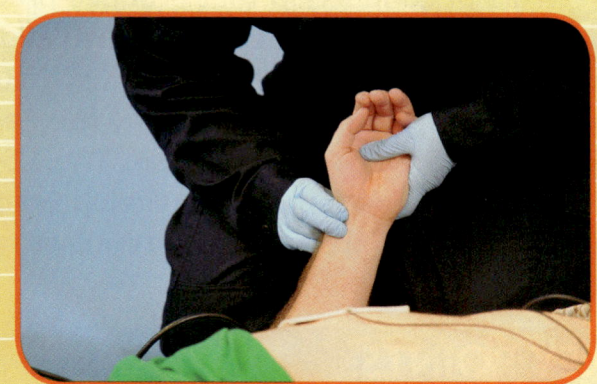

6 Palpate the pulse to confirm mechanical capture.

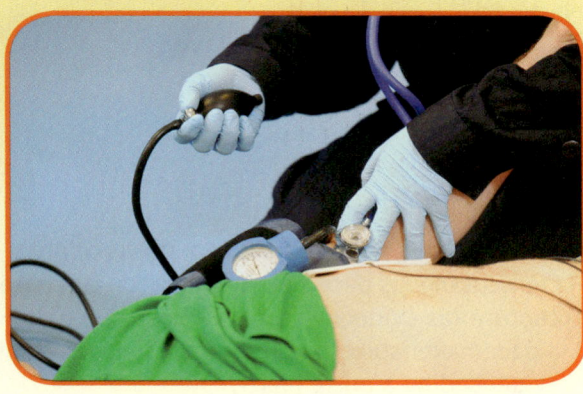

7 Reassess the patient's vital signs, mental status, and need for analgesia or sedation.

Delmar/Cengage Learning

CONCLUSION

Errors of conduction that produce bradydysrhythmias can present subtly with a range between feeling fatigued all the way to hypotension and altered mental status. Provided the blood pressure is normal or elevated, the patient only requires close monitoring by the Paramedic and transport to the hospital to address the underlying cause. The 12-lead ECG is an important part of the assessment of patients who develop bradydysrhythmias, as one of the causes is a myocardial infarction which requires rapid intervention.

KEY POINTS:

- Syncope represents a disturbance in brain function due to hypoperfusion. It has a spontaneous revival.

- Ventricular diastolic disorders, outflow obstructions, and dysrhythmias can cause cerebral hypoperfusion, although not all cause syncope.

- Syncope is not the life threat; rather, its underlying cause is the life threat.

- Bradydysrhythmias originating in the sinus node likely to cause syncope are:
  - Sinus bradycardia
    - Caused by hypersensitive carotid sinus syndrome, a vasovagal response, or sick sinus syndrome
  - Sinus block
  - Sinus arrest

- A/V blocks likely to cause syncope include those that result in an escape pacemaker that does not meet the body's needs.
  - Type II blocks
    - First degree
    - Second degree
    - Third degree
  - Type I blocks are usually not a cause for concern.

- Heart transplantation can cause conduction disturbances:
  - One type of procedure preserves the atria, valves, and great vessels but severs the conduction system.
  - Another type of procedure grafts the entire heart onto the great vessels and is less likely to cause conduction disturbances.

- Treatment for bradycardiac rhythms depends on the cause and location of the disturbance.
  - Sinus bradycardia
    - Atropine
    - Find cause
  - Type I A/V blocks
    - Atropine
  - Type II A/V blocks
    - Trial atropine
    - Pacemaker

- To assess the effectiveness of a newly applied transcutaneous pacemaker, check for electrical capture (as evidenced by a widened QRS following a pacemaker spike) and the mechanical capture (as evidenced by a pulse beat).

- Implanted pacemakers may pace the atria, the ventricles, or both.

- Modes may be fixed or asynchronous (in which the pacer disregards the activity of the underlying rhythm or demand) or synchronous (in which the pacemaker senses underlying electrical activity and does not discharge within a specified timeframe after the heart's own activity).

- Atrial pacemakers or dual chamber pacemakers preserve the atrial contribution to blood flow.

- Overdrive pacing uses the concept of the dominant rhythm being the faster rhythm to take control of a tachydysrhythmia and then slowing the pacemaker rate down.

- An implanted pacemaker contains a pulse generator, an electronic circuit board, a microprocessor, and a Reed switch.

- Areas likely to malfunction in an implanted pacemaker include the leads (wires) and the battery.

- Pacemaker syndrome results from asynchrony between the atria and ventricles:
  - Loss of atrial blood contribution to cardiac output

  - Backward pulse wave as the atria contract against closed valves
  - Pulmonary hypertension
  - Venous congestion

- Pacemaker malfunction includes:
  - Failure to discharge
  - Failure to capture
  - Failure to sense

- In addition to electrical pacing, a patient may be paced by percussion or through use of chemicals.

REVIEW QUESTIONS:

1. What types of dysrhythmias can cause syncope?
2. Explain the differences between hypersensitive carotid sinus syndrome and a vasovagal response.
3. Why are type II blocks of greater concern than type I blocks?
4. List the steps for applying a transcutaneous pacemaker. How are the settings assessed? What is the difference between electrical and mechanical capture?
5. Which pacemaker mode is most likely to result in ventricular fibrillation? Explain your answer.
6. What is the benefit of an atrial or dual chamber pacemaker to an active patient?
7. Using the NASPE/BPEG generic pacemaker code, describe a pacemaker that paces the ventricles, senses the ventricles, prevents firing if the patient's own beat is detected, doesn't allow for rate modulation, and doesn't have multisite pacing.

CASE STUDY QUESTIONS:

Please refer to the Case Study in this chapter, and answer the questions below:

1. What are some of the likely causes for syncope? What is the likely explanation for Mr. Tedesco being awake by the time friends were able to call for an ambulance?
2. Explain the relationship between type II third degree block and the patient's previous anterolateral MI.
3. Could the Paramedics have used their transcutaneous pacemaker if Mr. Tedesco's condition had required it? Explain your answer.

REFERENCES:

1. Thijs RD, Wieling W, et al. Defining and classifying syncope. *Clin Auton Res.* 2004;14 Suppl 1:4–8.

2. Roberts J. *Clinical Procedures in Emergency Medicine.* St. Louis: Saunders; 2003.

3. Kerr SR, Pearce MS, et al. Carotid sinus hypersensitivity in asymptomatic older persons: implications for diagnosis of syncope and falls. *Arch Intern Med.* 2006;166(5):515–520.

4. Medow MS, Stewart JM, et al. Pathophysiology, diagnosis, and treatment of orthostatic hypotension and vasovagal syncope. *Cardiol Rev.* 2008;16(1):4–20.

5. Vaddadi G, Lambert E, et al. Postural syncope: mechanisms and management. *Med J Aust.* 2007;187(5):299–304.

6. Bibb MH. Neurocardiogenic syncope. *N Engl J Med.* 1998;339(25):1857.

7. Roberts-Thomson KC, Sanders P, et al. Sinus node disease: an idiopathic right atrial myopathy. *Trends Cardiovasc Med.* 2007;17(6):211–214.

8. Gaffney BJ, Wasserman AG, et al. Sick sinus syndrome: mechanisms and management. *Cardiovasc Clin.* 1980;11(1):7–25.

9. Silverman ME, Upshaw CB, Jr., et al. Woldemar Mobitz and his 1924 classification of second-degree atrioventricular block. *Circulation.* 2004;110(9):1162–1167.

10. Fowler RL. The new ABCs of AV block. A revised classification to remove the mental block from recognizing AV block. *JEMS.* 2002;27(2):24–34.

11. Ufberg JW, Clark JS. Bradydysrhythmias and atrioventricular conduction blocks. *Emerg Med Clin North Am.* 2006;24(1):1–9, v.

12. Mendoza-Davila N, Varon J. Karel Wenckebach: The story behind the block. *Resuscitation.* 2008; (79): 189–192.

13. Marais M. *Heart Transplant: The Story of Barnard and the Ultimate in Cardiac Surgery.* Voortrekkerpers 1968.

14. Das G. Therapeutic review. Cardiac effects of atropine in man: an update. *Int J Clin Pharmacol Ther Toxicol.* 1989;27(10):473–477.

15. Sherbino J, Verbeek PR, et al. Prehospital transcutaneous cardiac pacing for symptomatic bradycardia or bradyasystolic cardiac arrest: a systematic review. *Resuscitation.* 2006;70(2):193–200.

16. Cummins RO, Graves JR, et al. Out-of-hospital transcutaneous pacing by emergency medical technicians in patients with asystolic cardiac arrest. *N Engl J Med.* 1993;328(19):1377–1382.

17. Bocka JJ. External transcutaneous pacemakers. *Ann Emerg Med.* 1989;18(12):1280–1286.

18. Syverud S. Cardiac pacing. *Emerg Med Clin North Am.* 1988;6(2):197–215.

19. Sliz NB, Jr., Johns, JA. Cardiac pacing in infants and children. *Cardiol Rev.* 2000;8(4):223–239.

20. Pinski SL. Emergencies related to implantable cardioverter-defibrillators. *Crit Care Med.* 2000;28(10 Suppl):N174–N180.

21. Bernstein AD, Daubert J-C, Fletcher RD, Hayes DL, Lüderitz B, Reynolds DW, Schoenfeld MH, Sutton R. The revised NASPE/BPEG generic code for antibradycardia, adaptive-rate, and multisite pacing. *PACE 2000.* 2000;25:260–264.

22. Alpert JS, Petersen P, et al. Atrial fibrillation: natural history, complications, and management. *Ann Rev Med.* 1988;39:41–52.

23. Crijns HJ, Van den Berg MP, et al. Management of atrial fibrillation in the setting of heart failure. *Eur Heart J.* 1997;18 Suppl C:C45–C49.

24. Woodruff J, Prudente LA. Update on implantable pacemakers. *J Cardiovasc Nurs.* 2005;20(4):261–268; quiz 269–270.

25. Erdinler I, Akyol A, et al. Long-term follow-up of pacemakers with an autocapture pacing system. *Jpn Heart J.* 2002;43(6):631–641.

26. Rieser MJ. The use of cough-CPR in patients with acute myocardial infarction. *J Emerg Med.* 1992;10(3):291–293.

27. Schultz DD, Olivas GS. The use of cough cardiopulmonary resuscitation in clinical practice. *Heart Lung.* 1986;15(3):273–282.

28. Amir O, Schliamser JE, et al. Ineffectiveness of precordial thump for cardioversion of malignant ventricular tachyarrhythmias. *Pacing Clin Electrophysiol.* 2007;30(2):153–156.

29. Cavalli A. Commotio cordis: a precordial thump? *Heart.* 1999;82(4):534.

30. Sowell LV, Sears SF, Jr., et al. Anxiety and marital adjustment in patients with implantable cardioverter defibrillator and their spouses. *J Cardiopulm Rehabil Prev.* 2007;27(1):46–49.

31. Luyster FS, Hughes JW, et al. Resource loss predicts depression and anxiety among patients treated with an implantable cardioverter defibrillator. *Psychosom Med.* 2006;68(5):794–800.

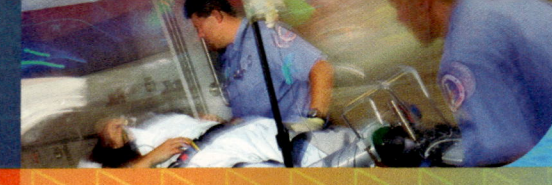

CHAPTER 7

CARDIAC RESUSCITATION

KEY CONCEPTS:

Upon completion of this chapter, it is expected that the reader will understand these following concepts:

- The four identifiable factors that lead to cardiac arrest
- Why resuscitation is only given to those with a reasonable expectation of survival
- Importance of finding and honoring a valid patient DNR order
- Ways teamwork is essential to perform a well-conducted resuscitation

ANATOMY CONCEPTS:

Prior to reading this chapter the Paramedic student should be familiar with the following anatomy and physiology concepts:

- Coronary artery distribution
- Electrophysiology
- Perfusion states

The EMS call came in the middle of the night stating a 50-year-old man had collapsed and wasn't breathing. His wife, a critical care nurse, was performing CPR. Dispatch reports that an ambulance was dispatched to the scene as well.

CRITICAL THINKING QUESTIONS

1. What are some of the possible causes of sudden cardiac death?
2. What importance, if any, is there that the wife has started CPR?

OVERVIEW

Out-of-hospital cardiac arrest occurs over 165,000 times a year, or in approximately 0.5 persons per 1,000 population. This all-too-common occurrence is the leading cause of death in the United States.[1,2] Of these out-of-hospital arrests, approximately 60% will be treated by EMTs or Paramedics.

In 20% to 40% of these sudden cardiac arrests (SCA), the first recorded ECG rhythm will either show ventricular fibrillation or ventricular tachycardia. In some cases, the timely delivery of defibrillation by the Paramedic can convert ventricular fibrillation/tachycardia into a perfusing rhythm. The key to successfully accomplishing this feat is the rapid delivery of energy at the right moment. Time is of the essence. As time elapses, the window of opportunity for successful defibrillation closes. Each second of inaction increases the likelihood of death. Paramedics, together with other members of the emergency medical team and the lay public, need to rapidly assess and confirm cardiac arrest in patients. EMS members must then proceed to treat the arrest with a combination of basic life support, as the foundation, and advanced life support.

Chief Concern

When a Paramedic encounters a patient who appears to be in cardiac arrest, but his medical history is unknown, acute coronary syndrome (ACS) might be suspected, since that is one of the more likely etiologies of cardiac arrest. However, the Paramedic must maintain an open mind as to other possibilities. Through a process of careful patient assessment, the Paramedic may find a readily correctable condition, treat that cause, and potentially cause a return of spontaneous circulation.

Factors Leading to Cardiac Arrest

There are four identifiable factors which can lead to cardiac arrest and can be traced following the circulatory pathway: decreased preload, decreased contractility, errors of automaticity, and increased afterload. This mechanistic approach encourages a process of deductive reasoning.

Decreased Preload

The first factor, **decreased preload**, can be the result of either hypovolemia or an obstruction to venous blood flow (preload is the sum of venous return). In the case of hypovolemia, there are a number of potential causes including absolute volume loss, via internal or external hemorrhage, and relative volume loss, such as occurs in anaphylaxis or septic shock (Table 7-1). In absolute volume loss, the treatment is aggressive fluid resuscitation that creates a functional blood volume. In relative volume loss, the treatment involves the use of potent vasoconstrictors such as epinephrine.

Table 7-1 Decreased Preload Leading to Cardiac Arrest

- Absolute volume loss
  - Hemorrhage
    - Internal
      - Gastrointestinal bleeding
    - External
      - Trauma
- Relative volume loss
  - Anaphylaxis
  - Systemic inflammatory response syndrome
    - Septic shock

Decreased Myocardial Contractility

The next factor, **decreased contractility** of the heart, involves those causes that exist outside of the heart. Contractility refers to the force of ventricular ejection of blood. Common extracardiac conditions that can cause decreased contractility include hypoxia, acidosis, and hypothermia. Hypoxia can be the culmination of problems of oxygenation, ventilation, and/or respiration. By providing a patent airway that is properly ventilated with a bag–mask assembly, using high-flow, high-concentration oxygen, the Paramedic can reduce or eliminate the patient's hypoxia.

The second problem, **acidosis**, is often a complication that accompanies all causes of cardiac arrest. Typically, acidosis following cardiac arrest is initially caused by an accumulation of respiratory acids (carbon dioxide).[3] This respiratory acidosis is best reversed by proper bag–mask assembly ventilation at a rate of approximately six to eight breaths per minute. While initial end-tidal carbon dioxide (EtCO$_2$) readings may be elevated greater than 45 mmHg, carefully controlled ventilation will cause the EtCO$_2$ to drop consistently and dependably in most cases.

Hypothermia is a special case. When patients suffer from severe hypothermia, Paramedics typically only deliver one defibrillation and withhold medications until the patient receives active internal rewarming. The Paramedic should remember the old adage, "The patient is not dead until he is warm and dead." Numerous causes of decreased myocardial contractility, singularly or combined, can lead to cardiac arrest (Table 7-2).

Errors of Automaticity

Errors of automaticity generally involve some biochemical derangement at the cellular level within the myocardium. While localized ischemia secondary to an acute coronary event is a likely cause of the irritability, other potential causes—such as electrolyte imbalances or drug impairment—are possible as well.

Since the heart muscle depends on sodium, potassium, calcium, and magnesium to properly function, an excess or deficit of any of these substances can lead to errors of automaticity and myocardial irritability (Table 7-3).[3,4] Of the four key electrolytes, a shift in potassium levels may be most problematic since elevated levels of potassium (i.e., hyperkalemia) can lead directly to ventricular fibrillation.[5]

Hyperkalemia

Hyperkalemia may occur in patients in end-stage renal disease, diabetic ketoacidosis, and Addison's disease. Addison's disease affects the adrenal glands. The adrenals glands secrete mineralocorticoids, such as aldosterone, which control electrolyte levels, such as those for potassium. An Addisonian crisis, or adrenal crisis, can lead to hyperkalemia and sudden cardiac death.

Hyperkalemia can also be caused by medication interference with urinary clearance. Medications implicated in hyperkalemia include angiotensin-converting enzyme (ACE) inhibitors; certain non-steroidal anti-inflammatory drugs (NSAIDs), such as celecoxib (Celebrex®); and potassium supplements.

Whatever the cause of the hyperkalemia, it must be treated promptly in a patient suffering from cardiac arrest. The drug of choice used in suspected hyperkalemic arrest is 10 mL of 10% solution calcium chloride (CaCl) over 10 minutes. CaCl is a competitive electrolyte that effectively neutralizes the effects of the elevated potassium in as little as one to three minutes.[6] If 10 mL of CaCl is not available, or is ineffective, then the Paramedic should administer 1 milliequivalent (mEq) per kilogram of sodium bicarbonate (NaHCO$_3$) instead. NaHCO$_3$ redistributes the electrolytes and drives potassium back into the cell. However, it can take as long as 10 minutes for the NaHCO$_3$ to take effect, which is why CaCl is the drug of choice in a cardiac arrest situation.[7]

Table 7-2 Decreased Myocardial Contractility Leading to Cardiac Arrest

- Hypoxia
  - Oxygen poor environment
  - Airway obstruction
    - Upper airway
      - Foreign body
    - Lower airway
      - Status asthmaticus
  - Insufficient ventilation
    - Medical
      - Neuromuscular paralysis
        - Botulism
    - Trauma
      - Pneumothorax
      - Flail ribs
  - Insufficient respiration
    - Cardiogenic pulmonary edema
    - Noncardiogenic pulmonary edema
  - Insufficient circulation
    - Acute coronary syndrome
    - Hypovolemia
      - Hemorrhage
  - Problems with cellular respiration
    - Carbon monoxide poisoning
    - Cyanide poisoning
- Acidosis
  - Diabetic ketoacidosis
- Hypothermia

Table 7-3 Errors of Automaticity

- Acute coronary ischemia
- Electrolyte imbalance
  - Hyperkalemia
    - Renal disease
    - Addison's disease
    - Diabetic ketoacidosis
  - Hypomagnesemia
  - Hypocalcemia
- Cardiotoxic medications
  - Tricyclic antidepressants
  - Beta/adrenergic blockers
  - Calcium channel blockers

When calcium chloride and sodium bicarbonate mix they form sodium chloride (common table salt) and calcium bicarbonate (chalk). To prevent this precipitant from forming, the Paramedic should perform a vigorous flush with a bolus of 20 mL of normal saline (0.9% NaCl) solution after every administration.

Table 7-4 Increased Afterload Leading to Cardiac Arrest

- Aortic aneurysm
- Pulmonary embolism

Cardiotoxic Medications

Although any medication, if given in a large enough dose, can cause death, certain medications are particularly problematic. These **cardiotoxic medications** can kill a patient with a dose as little as one pill. Naturally, these medications are a cause of great concern to Paramedics.

For example, some of the psychotic medications, such as the tricyclic antidepressants (TCA), affect the myocardium directly and cause a prolongation of the QT interval.[8] When confronted with a potential TCA overdose, and after establishing standard advanced cardiac life support, the Paramedic should consider administration of 1 mEq per kilogram body weight of sodium bicarbonate ($NaHCO_3$) intravenously.[9,10] If the $NaHCO_3$ is not effective, then the Paramedic may want to consider magnesium sulfate ($MgSO_4$). Magnesium is effective in the treatment of torsades de pointes (TdP), a polymorphic ventricular tachycardia seen with prolonged QT syndromes (Figure 7-1).[11] The dose of magnesium sulfate is usually 1 to 2 grams administered intravenously over five minutes during cardiac arrest.

An issue that may be more problematic—and more common—than TCA overdoses is overdoses of antihypertensive medications including calcium channel blockers and beta/adrenergic blockers. These two blockers affect the myocardial tissue directly, at the cellular level, and impair the myocardial cell function. The result of the overdose of these two medications is a profound drop in blood pressure secondary to pump failure.

Following a fluid bolus, the patient may need large amounts of intravenous glucagon (between 3 and 10 milligrams) and/or high dose epinephrine (0.2 mg/kg).[12,13] Glucagon works by bypassing the traditional metabolic pathways and increasing blood pressure through an alternative means. High dose epinephrine competes with the medication at the receptor. If both of these pharmacological methods fail, it may be necessary to pace the heart via transcutaneous pacing.

Increased Afterload

The final contributing factor to cardiac arrest is increased afterload. **Afterload** is the systemic vascular resistance, an alpha-adrenergic mediated vasoconstriction, that opposes outflow of blood from the heart to the lungs and systemic organs. An acute thrombosis at an aortic aneurysm, blocking caudal blood flow, can markedly increase the resistance to outflow from the left ventricle, causing increased afterload. Similarly, a pulmonary embolism (PE) can block the pulmonary artery and markedly increase the resistance to outflow from the right side of the heart. In both cases, the sudden increase in afterload overwhelms the heart's capacity to overcome the obstruction and blood flow stops (Table 7-4).

Cardiac Mnemonics

A number of mnemonics have been developed to help Paramedics and others remember some of the more common contributing causes of cardiac arrest. One of these is ITCH PAD (**I**nfarction, **T**ension pneumothorax, **C**ardiac tamponade, **H**emorrhage, **P**ulmonary embolism, **A**cidosis,

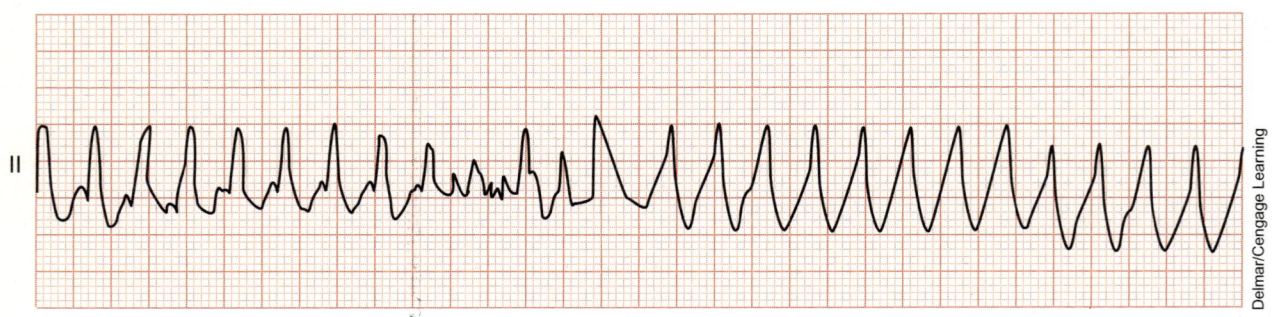

Figure 7-1 Torsades de pointes.

Delmar/Cengage Learning

and **D**rugs). Another mnemonic used to remember these causes is THE HAT (**T**ension pneumothorax, **H**ypovolemia, **E**mbolism (pulmonary), **H**ypothermia, **A**cidosis, **T**amponade (cardiac)).

However, the most commonly used mnemonic is probably the American Heart Association's five H's and five T's (**H**ypoxia, **H**ypovolemia, **H**ypothermia, **H**yper/hypokalemia, **H**ydrogen ion excess (acidosis), **T**oxins, **T**amponade (cardiac), **T**ension pneumothorax, **T**hrombosis (pulmonary), and **T**rauma) (Table 7-5).[14]

Even though all of these mnemonics are helpful, most Paramedics commit one to rote memory for use during a high stress cardiac arrest. Each of these causes of cardiac arrest can be summed up simply as problems of the pipes, pump, or the fluid. If the patient does not respond to standard advanced cardiac life support, the Paramedic can draw on her knowledge of these differential diagnoses to treat the patient and to produce a better outcome.

Table 7-5 Differential Diagnosis— Cardiac Mnemonics

ITCH PAD		Five H Five T		THE HAT	
I	Infarction	H	Hypoxia	T	Tension pneumothorax
T	Tension pneumothorax	H	Hypovolemia		
		H	Hypothermia	H	Hypoxia/ hypovolemia
C	Cardiac tamponade	H	Hyper/ hypokalemia		
				E	Embolism
H	Hemorrhage	H	Hydrogen ion excess	H	Hypothermia
P	Pulmonary embolism	T	Tablets/toxins	A	Acidosis
A	Acidosis	T	Tamponade (cardiac)	T	Thrombosis/ tamponade (cardiac)
D	Drugs	T	Tension pneumothorax		
		T	Thrombosis (pulmonary/ coronary)		
		T	Trauma		

CASE STUDY (CONTINUED)

When the Paramedics arrive, they find an obese male on the ground outside the residence. An EMT is performing CPR and an AED is in evidence. Report from the EMT who is in charge is that the man complained of chest pain and feeling hot. He went outside the residence to cool off. His wife followed him and was able to break his fall to the ground. She called 9-1-1 and then began CPR with both ventilations and compressions.

CRITICAL THINKING QUESTIONS

1. What are the elements that make performing a resuscitation reasonable? Unreasonable?
2. Why is the patient's history important?

Algorithmic Approach to Cardiac Arrest Management

Upon arrival at the scene of a possible cardiac arrest, the Paramedic should establish one of three antecedent conditions before starting or continuing the resuscitation. This determination will subsequently impact the course of treatment.

Realistic Chance of Survival

The first question the Paramedic should ask is whether the resuscitation is reasonable. In other words, "Is there a realistic chance of survival?" A patient with obvious signs of death is not a candidate for resuscitation. Some examples of obvious death include decapitation, incineration, decomposition, and mortal wounds (Table 7-6). The term "mortal wounds" may be a matter of interpretation. Wounds that were formerly thought to be mortal such as hemicorporectomy (amputation at the torso) are now considered survivable with modern surgery. However, it is generally agreed that the presence

of gray matter outside of the patient's cranium is a sign of mortal injury.

To the layperson, signs of death include an unresponsive patient whose eyes may be open, unblinking, and lackluster

Table 7-6 Signs of Obvious Death

- Mortal wounds
  - Decapitation
  - Incineration
  - Decomposition
  - Massive head injury
- Traditional signs of death
  - Rigor mortis
  - Algor mortis
  - Liver mortis

with skin that is pale and waxen in appearance. The layperson may also notice that the patient's sphincters have opened, allowing urine or stool to pass. On occasion, tinkling sounds can be heard by bystanders. These are not normal bowel sounds but instead are the sound of fluids within the body settling.

The more ominous signs of death are referred to as the three mortis: algor mortis, rigor mortis, and livor mortis.[15] The latter, livor mortis, may be the most obvious. **Livor mortis** is the pooling of blood in dependent portions of the body, leaving a reddish–blue discoloration on the body's underside. This is called **dependent lividity**.

However, caution is advised when deciding that these purplish patches are livor mortis. In cases of end-stage sepsis, the integrity of blood vessels is lost and blood collects under the skin in a condition called **purpura**. Along with the purpura, the patient with end-stage sepsis may be unconscious, hypotensive, and without palpable pulses, as well as cool to the touch. These signs are suggestive of death. However, closer examination reveals that the patient is actually in a coma. Furthermore, purpura occurs on all bodily surfaces, not just the dependent surfaces.

STREET SMART

When a patient is rolled over (e.g., so the Paramedic can examine for signs of death), the dependent lividity is on the upper surface, and this may appear similar to purpura. However, closer examination will reveal blanched pressure points where the body originally laid. The Paramedic should document in the patient care report the exact position in which the body was originally found as well as if the body was moved to examine for signs of death.

Next, the Paramedic may note algor mortis. **Algor mortis** is the natural cooling of the deceased body to the ambient temperature. Normally, the body cools at about 1°F per hour for the first 24 hours after death. However, if the patient is covered (e.g., with blankets) then the cooling process slows. Under these conditions, a patient who expired several hours ago may still feel warm to the touch.

Finally, the Paramedic may note rigor mortis, which is considered the classic sign of death. **Rigor mortis** is stiffening of muscles, which makes the body feel rigid. Rigor mortis is the result of biochemical changes within the muscle. Typically, the shorter muscles, such as those found in the jaw, stiffen first, followed by the larger muscles.

Again, caution is advised regarding making an assumption of death based on algor and rigor mortis. A patient with severe hypothermia may be both stiff and cold as a result of the effects of the cold upon the body. Furthermore, these patients will be unconscious, without readily palpable pulses. Although an ECG recording will show a flatline, it may be because the electrode gel has not melted to form a conductive pathway. For these reasons, no patient is dead until he is warm and dead.

Clinical Signs of Death

Most standard CPR classes teach that the traditional signs of death (the classic triad of signs) are unresponsiveness, apnea, and pulselessness. The Paramedic uses these signs as the basis for deciding whether or not to start CPR, although they are insufficient reasons to withhold CPR.

Following a quick check for unresponsiveness, breathlessness, and pulselessness, the Paramedic should consider using a look, listen, and feel approach for assessing signs of death. For example, the Paramedic should look for pupillary response. The pupils are a muscular sphincter; like all of the body's sphincters that relax at death, the pupils also relax, becoming dilated and unresponsive to even the brightest light.

While assessing the pupils, the Paramedic may elect to assess for corneal reflexes.[16] The corneal reflex is one of the last body reflexes remaining before death occurs. Using a sterile gauze pad, the Paramedic gently touches the globe of the patient's eye. If the reflex is intact, then the patient will involuntarily blink.

Moving to the chest, the Paramedic should auscultate for heart sounds at the apex of the heart for approximately 30 seconds to one minute (extreme bradycardia may not be appreciated in less time). The apex of the heart, or the point of maximal intensity (PMI), is typically found at the fifth intercostal space at the midclavicular line.

At this point, Paramedics traditionally place the ECG electrodes on the patient's chest. Modified chest leads (MCL) may be used for this task. MCL offer the Paramedic the opportunity to ascertain if there is any hope for ventricular activity.

Finally, the Paramedic should consider attempting a jaw thrust. As rigor mortis sets into short muscles first, the jaw should be rigid and difficult to elevate with manual pressure. The combination of these signs—absence of papillary and corneal reflexes, absence of heart activity, and the onset of rigor mortis, plus the traditional triad of signs—may be sufficient to convince the Paramedic to not initiate resuscitation.[17]

Do Not Attempt Resuscitation

The Paramedic may be bound by a medical order for "Do Not Attempt Resuscitation" (DNAR) under certain conditions. If a DNAR or a similar legally executed document is present, then the Paramedic should not attempt resuscitation.

If cardiopulmonary resuscitation (CPR) is already in progress, either by civilians or the Paramedic himself before the DNAR was produced, then the Paramedic should consider contacting medical control for guidance. While contacting medical control, the Paramedic should continue CPR until medical control orders termination of resuscitation.

Cardiopulmonary Resuscitation in Progress

When interfacing with civilians doing CPR in the field, the Paramedic should determine the adequacy of their CPR technique. First, the Paramedic should assess for the CPR compression rate and depth. Using the heel of one hand over the lower half of the sternum, between the nipples, the compressor should be compressing at a depth of 1 1/2 inches to 2 inches at a rate of approximately 100 compressions a minute in an adult.[14]

The Paramedic should make special note of the compression rate. Several studies have shown that the true compression rate is often less than predicted even when performed by trained healthcare providers who are being coached. The proper rate and depth of cardiac compression is important to maintaining minimally sufficient coronary perfusion pressures. If the rate and/or depth of compression is inadequate due to rescuer exhaustion or poor technique, then the Paramedic should replace the compressor at the end of the compression cycle.

In some cases, the civilian may have been directed to do compression-only CPR. In studies comparing conventional CPR (i.e., CPR with mouth-to-mouth ventilation) against compression-only CPR, there was no statistical benefit shown as to the use of mouth-to-mouth ventilation while performing CPR. Furthermore, although there have been no reported cases of HIV transmission with conventional CPR, there have been reported cases of tuberculosis and herpes simplex transmission. Studies have shown that the lay public, and even CPR instructors, are reluctant to perform mouth-to-mouth ventilation on strangers. Therefore, when comparing a possible risk of disease transmission, no matter how remote, with the potential benefit of performing mouth-to-mouth ventilation (practically none), it may be a reason to perform compression-only CPR.

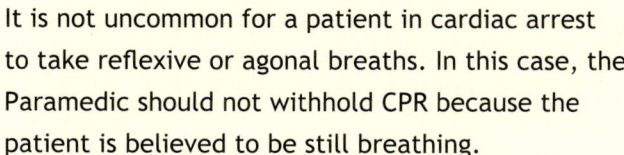

STREET SMART

It is not uncommon for a patient in cardiac arrest to take reflexive or agonal breaths. In this case, the Paramedic should not withhold CPR because the patient is believed to be still breathing.

The Paramedic should switch the patient over to ventilation with a bag–mask assembly as soon as possible if a civilian is performing mouth-to-mouth ventilation. While the oxygen provided by mouth-to-mouth ventilation is adequate (approximately 17% in exhaled air), the problem may be the carbon dioxide in the expired air (approximately 3.5% to 4%). This carbon dioxide is added to the carbon dioxide in the patient's lungs, increasing respiratory acid in the process. Even ventilation with ambient air, which contains one-third of 1%, is superior to ventilating the patient with exhaled air.

The Paramedic should establish, as accurately as possible from witnesses and rescuers, certain information from the scene: when the patient was found, whether the patient's collapse was witnessed, whether an automated external defibrillator (AED) was used, and when CPR was started. For example, if the AED's advisory message requested delivery of a shock, then the patient was likely in either ventricular fibrillation or ventricular tachycardia. This is suggestive of a recent collapse and may indicate a better chance of a successful patient resuscitation.[18–20]

While assuming responsibility for CPR, the Paramedic should apply the pads, or use paddles in quick–look function, to determine the patient's rhythm. One of three rhythms may be present. The desired rhythm would be ventricular fibrillation/tachycardia. This rhythm is amenable to defibrillation, which should be performed immediately following two minutes of CPR.

Alternatively, the patient may present in asystole, as represented by a flatline on the ECG monitor. Asystole is an ominous finding for the Paramedic, who would undoubtedly rather find the cardiac arrested patient in ventricular fibrillation. Therefore, asystole should be confirmed in two perpendicular leads in an attempt to find ventricular fibrillation. The initial rhythm should be confirmed by pads/paddles. The pad/paddle placement provides a view of the inferior wall in Lead II. The perpendicular view from Lead II is the anterior wall, which contains the majority of the myocardial mass. The best view of the anterior wall is in MCL1.

The patient may also present with an organized nonperfusing rhythm called **pulseless electrical activity (PEA)**, formerly called electromechanical dissociation (EMD). The key finding in PEA is a loss of a palpable carotid pulse. However, it is difficult to palpate a carotid pulse in an arrested patient. Severe peripheral disease, weakened cardiac contractions, acidosis, and hypovolemia can individually, or in combination, cause carotid pulses to be unpalpable despite the fact that a central pulse actually exists.

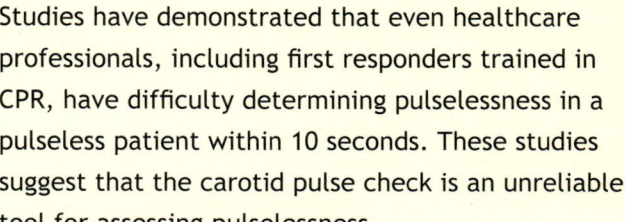

STREET SMART

Studies have demonstrated that even healthcare professionals, including first responders trained in CPR, have difficulty determining pulselessness in a pulseless patient within 10 seconds. These studies suggest that the carotid pulse check is an unreliable tool for assessing pulselessness.

When confronted with PEA, the Paramedic should continue CPR while trying to discover its source using any one of the mnemonic tools discussed earlier. Some common traits to all PEA, regardless of the etiology, is severe hypoxia and acidosis resulting in global ischemia.[21,22] The focus of advanced life support for PEA, a potentially survivable rhythm, should be on resolving the hypoxia and reversing the acidosis.

▶ CASE STUDY (CONTINUED)

The ambulance crew assesses the wife's compressions and find them to be adequate, so they allow her to continue while they set up the AED. The first rhythm is shockable and a Paramedic delivers a single shock. The ambulance crew then assumes responsibility for CPR. Two minutes are just about up and responsibility for the call is transferred to the Paramedic. The AED switches to the manual monitor/defibrillator and the Paramedic confirms ventricular fibrillation. The patient remains pulseless.

CRITICAL THINKING QUESTIONS

1. As the team leader, what factors should the Paramedic consider in order to ensure the greatest chance of success?
2. What are the qualities of a good team leader?

Teamwork in Resuscitation

The ECG finding of ventricular fibrillation is a rhythm of hope. Aggressive advanced life support can help convert an uncoordinated ventricular mass into a beating synchrony that produces a pulse and cause the **return of spontaneous circulation (ROSC)**. The key to a successful resuscitation of ventricular fibrillation is an effective defibrillation. A successful defibrillation results in asystole, quieting the chaotic cellular depolarizations. Ultimately, however, it is the return of an organized rhythm, by dominance of the SA node, coaxed by CPR, which causes the return of spontaneous circulation.

Resuscitations, almost by nature, are chaotic scenes initially. However, with leadership and teamwork the team can quickly coalesce into a functional unit. When starting resuscitation, the Paramedic should consider calling for additional responders early in the process so fresh responders will be available to help with CPR.

The Paramedic should also consider contacting medical control early on. Some systems have medical directors in the field that will respond to and assist with resuscitation. While the approach to performing a resuscitation is standardized (algorithmic), the success of a resuscitation may hinge on identifying and reversing the underlying cause of the arrest.

Teamwork

Cardiac resuscitation is first and foremost a team effort. It takes a large number of dedicated providers working at their tasks, in a seamless and integrated fashion, for a resuscitation to be successful. Furthermore, the team must have a team leader. The most successful resuscitations, regardless of the patient outcome, are run by informed team leaders who know how to delegate and communicate well.

In many instances the team leader, by design or default, is the Paramedic. The Paramedic's first objective as team leader is to remain focused on basic life support. While the complicated skills of advanced airway management and medication administration may seem important, studies indicate that continuous CPR, especially compressions and defibrillation, offer the patient the best hope for survival.

A good team leader is a good delegator. During cardiac arrest resuscitation a number of roles must be fulfilled. Often one person has multiple roles that, during the course of resuscitation, will change. The team leader must delegate responsibilities to avoid confusion, error, and duplication. Some teams who work together regularly—who have reassigned roles and have practiced their duties—will need a minimum of direction. Conversely, a team made up of responders from multiple emergency service agencies, with various levels of training and experience, may need more delegation and directed instruction in order to be an effective team.

The team leader also needs to be a good communicator. The team leader may need to clearly state the roles and responsibilities of the various team members. For example, if someone is assigned to perform cardiac compressions, the team leader might offer a short instruction to "push hard, push fast." These simple instructions help team members remember their skills during a stressful situation.

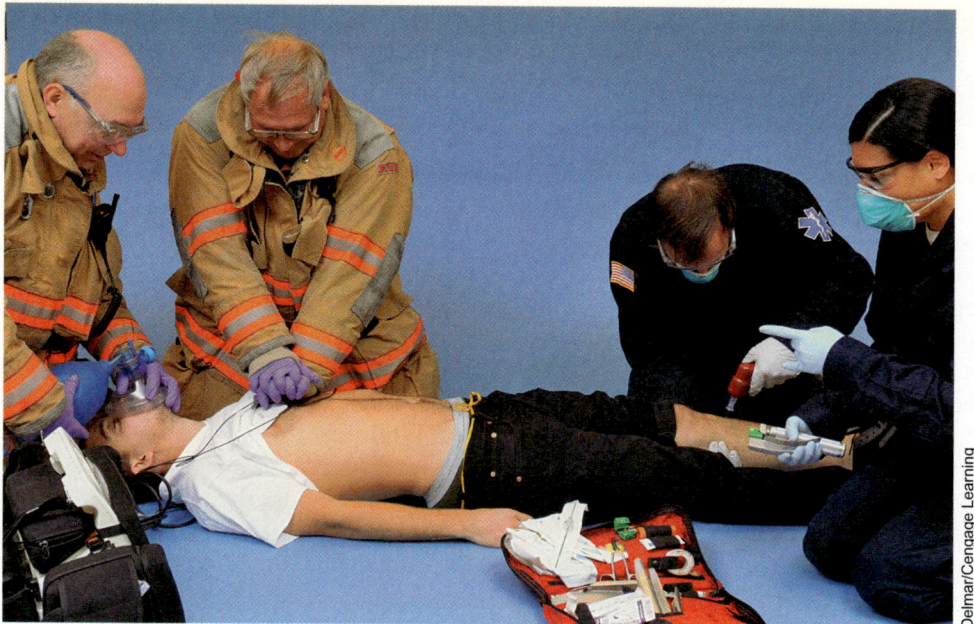

Figure 7-2 A team leader managing a cardiac arrest.

If possible, the team leader should take a hand's off approach. This allows the team leader the opportunity to survey the scene and to get a more global assessment. For example, the team leader may see that the compressor is tiring while another responder is idle and suggest that they switch.

Finally, the team leader generally interprets and announces the rhythm. This provides the team with a sense of direction and redirects them to the appropriate algorithm when the rhythm changes. The team leader should verbalize the observations and offer the team members opportunities for input should a problem arise (Figure 7-2).

The team leader should offer to review the care provided at the end of the resuscitation. These "**debriefings**" are important from both a performance improvement perspective and also from a psychological perspective.

In addition, the Paramedic should not forget about the patient's family while on scene. Although the resuscitation may seem routine, especially if the Paramedic rehearsed the resuscitation during simulations, a cardiac arrest of a loved one is a life-changing event for the family. While hospital providers sometimes debate if family members should be allowed to witness the resuscitation, Paramedics regularly experience the presence of family at the scene of the cardiac arrest. The Paramedic might consider assigning one team member to assist the family. This team member would be responsible for explaining, in lay terms, the resuscitation activities and effects.

CASE STUDY (CONTINUED)

The Paramedics deliver a single 200-joule biphasic defibrillation to the patient and immediately resume CPR. After two minutes the ECG monitor shows no change in the rhythm, so they deliver another defibrillation and resume CPR. The Paramedic completes a quick assessment to ensure that the patient's airway is open, ventilations are adequate, and supplemental oxygen is being given. The Paramedic also reviews compression depth and rate to make sure they are correct.

CRITICAL THINKING QUESTIONS

1. What is the difference between biphasic and monophasic defibrillation?
2. Why is it important to assess, and then reassess, the performance of proper CPR?

Basic Life Support for Cardiac Arrest

Airway

The resuscitation of the patient in cardiac arrest starts with the "ABCDs." Assuming that CPR is still in progress, the Paramedic would proceed to ensure that the airway is open and will remain open. The mantra "open, assess, suction, secure" reminds the Paramedic of the steps of basic airway management.

If trauma is suspected then a jaw thrust may be necessary. If the airway cannot be maintained with a jaw thrust, then the Paramedic may need to perform a two-handed triple airway maneuver (head-tilt, chin-lift with jaw thrust) until the airway opens enough to allow proper ventilation.

It is not uncommon for a patient who has received mouth-to-mouth ventilation to experience gastric distention and regurgitation. The Paramedic must clear the airway to prevent aspiration. Although aspiration can have long-term implications, such as aspiration pneumonia, at this point aspiration can prevent ventilation, leading to worsening hypoxia and acidosis.[23]

The Paramedic should assess the patient's airway for any obstructions. If an obstruction is visible, then she should perform a finger sweep using either a pair of fingers in a scoop-like fashion, with an oral airway wedged sideways between the teeth as a bite block, or by using a second oral airway as a scoop.

The Paramedic should then be prepared to suction the patient's oral cavity to the level of the hypopharynx. When doing this, it may be necessary to turn the patient's head to the side to allow fluids to pool in the buccal pocket. The final step in the process is to place the oropharyngeal airway into place and proceed to ventilation.

STREET SMART

Some Paramedics will also place a nasopharyngeal airway in the cardiac-arrested patient to increase the available airway space for ventilation.

Breathing

The presence of respiratory gasses (carbon dioxide) and subsequent acidosis has a profound impact on myocardial cell function. For this reason, careful ventilation is imperative. The Paramedic should ventilate at approximately five to six breaths per minute while maintaining compressions at a rate of at least 100 per minute.

Danger of Hyperventilation

Inadvertent hyperventilation is a danger in every cardiac arrest. Competing attentions can allow the person ventilating the patient to be distracted and to lose focus. Therefore, efforts should be taken to avoid hyperventilation.

Aggressive overventilation can cause respiratory alkalosis with resultant systemic vasoconstriction. In turn, vasoconstriction of cerebral arteries can lead to pancerebral anoxia and ischemia. In addition, vasoconstriction of coronary arteries can lead to decreased coronary artery perfusion and global myocardial hypoxia and ischemia.

Hyperventilation also causes air trapping within the chest, leading to an increase in the intrathoracic pressure. The complication of increased intrathoracic pressure is in low flow states, the pressure within the chest is higher than the pressure in the vena cava, limiting or ceasing blood return to the heart. If blood does not return to the heart, it cannot be expelled from the ventricle, ultimately decreasing systemic blood pressure.

While use of an automatic transport ventilator (ATV) during resuscitation might help ensure more even tidal volumes and a regular rhythm of ventilation, the timing of compressions to ventilations makes their use impractical. Instead, the Paramedic should emphasize the importance of proper ventilation and closely monitor the situation.

Effective Ventilation

An essential element of effective ventilation is a good mask seal, since loss of mask seal can result in loss of up to 50% of the ventilation volume. This results in erratic ventilation volumes and, more importantly, diminished exhalation of carbon dioxide. To maintain a good mask seal, the Paramedic should use a two-handed mask seal technique on the mask, pulling the patient's face up to the mask, when ventilating.[24]

During cardiac arrest, several factors combine to make ventilation more difficult and gastric insufflations more likely. Since air takes the path of least resistance, any decrease in pulmonary compliance, increase in airway resistance, or loss of esophageal sphincter tone will promote gastric insufflations and gastric distention. In turn, these will further decrease pulmonary compliance.

The lungs are intended to suspend in the chest cavity, allowing the abdomen to fall away, and improving lung compliance (the ease of ventilation). Whenever a patient lies supine, such as during a cardiac arrest, the lungs lose some compliance. This loss of compliance is increased if the patient is obese or pregnant. The enlarged abdomen in these patient populations pushes upward against the diaphragm and decreases the expansion of the lungs.

STREET SMART

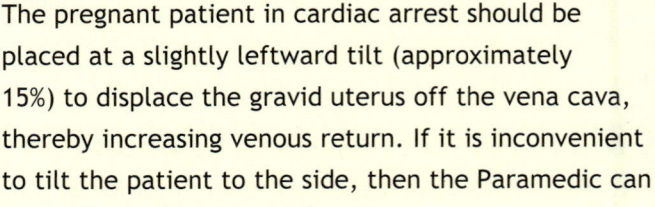

The pregnant patient in cardiac arrest should be placed at a slightly leftward tilt (approximately 15%) to displace the gravid uterus off the vena cava, thereby increasing venous return. If it is inconvenient to tilt the patient to the side, then the Paramedic can manually displace the abdomen.

Increased airway resistance will also hinder ventilation. Patients with chronic obstructive airway diseases—such as emphysema, asthma, or any condition that causes decreased airway diameter—will require increased airway pressure (force of ventilation) in order to overcome the airway resistance. This increased airway pressure against airway resistance can result in a backward airway pressure, causing air to spill into the esophagus.

Another area to consider that may help prevent gastric insufflations is the upper esophageal sphincter (UES) located between the esophagus and the pharynx. The opening and closing of the UES is caused by contraction of the cricopharyngeus and the superior and inferior hyoid muscles, which in turn are controlled by branches of the glossopharyngeal and vagal nerve. It takes as little as twenty (20) cm H_2O pressure to overcome the UES thereby allowing air into the esophagus. During a cardiac arrest, when muscle tone and nerve control may be lost, it may take less pressure to overcome the resistance of the UES.

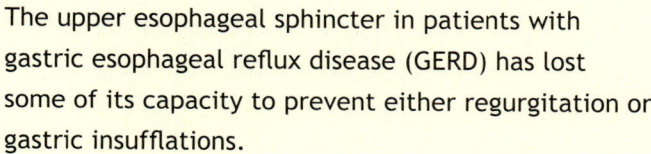

Pulmonary aspiration of gastric contents during resuscitation has been estimated to occur in between 10% and 35% of resuscitations. Paramedics can institute a two-prong approach to prevent this complication, by use of smaller ventilation volumes and the application of cricoid pressure, in the field. [25,26]

First, from the moment that the mask is applied to the arrested patient's face, the Paramedic should apply cricoid pressure to the patient's trachea. The application of cricoid pressure helps to prevent gastric insufflations by creating an artificial esophageal valve that augments the effectiveness of the upper esophageal sphincter.

Next, when ventilating the unintubated patient in cardiac arrest, the Paramedic should use approximately 500 mL, instead of the previously recommended 800 mL. This smaller volume can be obtained by either one-handed compression of the adult bag–mask assembly (typically about 1,700 mL volume, though volumes vary by manufacturer), or two-handed compression of a pediatric (child) bag–mask assembly (500 mL volume). The smaller volumes are intended to decrease peak airway pressures and avoid gastric insufflations.

Although the importance of ventilation has been emphasized, recent evidence supports the importance of compressions even more strongly. Compressions should be interrupted only minimally during CPR of the nonintubated patient and never interrupted during CPR of the intubated patient.

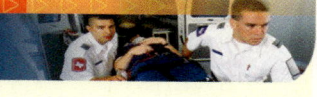

Circulation

In the past, defibrillation was attempted immediately upon arriving at the patient's side, regardless of the time since arrest (down time). It is now understood that the heart may not be ready to accept defibrillation at that time. Premature defibrillations are unsuccessful and may cause myocardial tissue damage.

When the heart initially goes into ventricular fibrillation, the wavelets are coarse (coarse ventricular fibrillation), indicating that the needed substrates (such as oxygen) are still present and that the heart may be responsive to defibrillation. However, as time elapses the activity of the myocardial cells weakens, as evidenced by smaller wavelets on the ECG monitor (fine fibrillation or asystole). When this happens, the heart can no longer produce a unified synchronized contraction despite defibrillation.

CPR must be performed to return the heart to a state of readiness. CPR, particularly chest compressions, helps to improve coronary artery perfusion, circulate oxygen to the myocardium, and eliminate by-products of anaerobic respiration (such as acid) that inhibit the cell's normal function.

Therefore, if the arrest is unwitnessed, CPR should be performed before defibrillation is attempted in an effort to return the heart to a state of readiness for defibrillation. [27] During a cardiac arrest, attention should be given to maintaining good compressions.

While the importance of exact hand placement during CPR has been de-emphasized (the dominant hand is simply placed on the center of the chest), the importance of depth, decompression, and the "duty cycle" has been re-emphasized.

During resuscitation the Paramedic should strive to see that the chest compression is at least 1 1/2 inches deep in an adult. However, studies have suggested that some patients may benefit from compressions that are 3 to 4 inches deep. Perhaps of greater importance than compression depth is rescuer fatigue. External cardiac compression is hard work and tired compressors cannot maintain a good and consistent depth of compression. Compressors should be switched frequently, perhaps as often as every five cycles, to ensure the delivery of hard and fast compressions.

Rotating compressors frequently will also prevent the rescuer from "resting on the chest" and causing incomplete chest recoil. Incomplete chest recoil prevents venous return, through increased intrathoracic pressure, and subsequently diminishes both coronary and cerebral perfusion.

Finally, the Paramedic should closely monitor the duty cycles during CPR. The "**duty cycle**" is the time spent in compression and decompression during each set of external cardiac massage. During the compression, phase blood is ejected from the heart into the systemic circulation, and specifically into the carotid arteries. During the decompression phase, the venous return to the heart fills the ventricles and the coronary arteries.

Normally, the heart spends one-third of the cardiac cycle in systole and two-thirds of the cardiac cycle in diastole. During diastole, the coronary arteries fill. During a cardiac arrest it is optimal if the duty cycle (i.e., compression and decompression) is approximately 50/50, more closely mimicking the natural percentage of the cardiac cycle. The 50/50 duty cycle can improve pulmonary, coronary, and cerebral perfusion.

Cardiopulmonary Resuscitation Assist Devices

Several CPR assist devices are available which compress the chest in a rhythmic fashion. The first of these devices is the inflatable circumferential chest vest. The vest is alternately inflated, like a blood pressure cuff, then deflated, in the process increasing and then decreasing intrathoracic pressure. The CPR vest is based upon the thoracic pump theory of CPR.

Similar to the vest device is the circumferential chest band. This device uses a pneumatic thoracic strap and also depends on the thoracic pump theory of CPR. Like the vest CPR device, it permits the Paramedic to perform other advanced life support skills while compressions are in progress.

The last device (one of the first CPR assist devices to appear on the market) is the piston device. This mechanical device more closely mimics manual external chest compressions using a piston plunger.

All of these devices are designed to ensure adequate and consistent depth of compression at the proper rate using a 50/50 duty cycle. These devices eliminate the issue of rescuer fatigue and errors as long as the Paramedic properly positions them. One of the major advantages of these CPR adjuncts is that they can release or replace one or more rescuers on the scene of a cardiac arrest, freeing them for other duties or to rest.

Precordial Thump

In the past, the precordial thump was considered an acceptable means of converting ventricular fibrillation, and was particularly effective in converting pulseless ventricular tachycardia to a perfusing rhythm. However, it recently has come under closer scrutiny. A precordial thump is most effective if delivered immediately after the patient develops ventricular fibrillation.[28] However, it rapidly loses its effectiveness as time passes. Currently, delivering one pericordial thump is acceptable when an ECG-monitored patient is observed to convert into either ventricular fibrillation or pulseless ventricular tachycardia.

To deliver a precordial thump, the Paramedic positions the fleshy ulnar prominence of the hand directly over the mid-sternum at about 10 to 12 inches (25 to 30 cm) and strikes a single sharp blow to the precordium. The delivery of the precordial thump is thought to produce from 2 to 5 joules of energy.[28]

It should be emphasized that the successful conversion with the precordial thump is limited and should not delay the use of a defibrillator. In addition, the use of the precordial thump does have its risks. While successful cardioversion from ventricular fibrillation to sinus rhythm can occur through use of a precordial thump, a precordial thump can also cause the patient's rhythm to deteriorate into other lethal rhythms, such as asystole. Therefore, the precordial thump should only be used on pulseless patients.[29]

STREET SMART

Paramedics may witness ventricular fibrillation in a conscious patient. If this occurs, the patient should be encouraged to cough. The rapid rise and fall of the intrathoracic pressure simulates CPR. This procedure, called "cough CPR," can allow the patient to maintain consciousness for up to 90 seconds, providing the Paramedic time to place defibrillation pads and defibrillate the patient.[30]

Defibrillation

Ventricular fibrillation is the chaotic and asynchronous firing of multiple irritable ectopic foci. Using the analogy of a stone and a lake, one can understand the mechanism of fibrillation. When one stone is thrown into a lake, one set of waves radiates outward across the lake's surface. Similar to a stone thrown into a lake, when the sinoatrial (SA) node fires then a wave of depolarization cascades down the person's heart. However, when a fist full of stones is thrown into a lake a series of waves is created. The waves collide into one another forming wavelets. In some instances, these colliding waves cancel each other out while in other cases the waves combine to form a larger wave, but under no circumstances is one wave dominant. Initially the wavelets are larger, and coarse, but over time they dissipate (similar to fine fibrillation) until the lake surface is quiet (similar to asystole).

The proverbial fist full of stones in the heart is the multiple irritable ectopic foci. These foci can be the result of local injury and ischemia from coronary artery occlusion or can be the result of global ischemia induced by some extracardiac event. Whatever the cause, these foci fire randomly and the result is ventricular fibrillation.

The treatment of ventricular fibrillation revolves around resolving whatever mechanisms cause ventricular irritability. At the onset it may be sufficient to defibrillate the heart in ventricular fibrillation; that would be like throwing a large rock into the lake, overwhelming all of the minor wavelets with one large wave.

However, as time passes the heart is not amenable to defibrillation and must be prepared before the defibrillation is delivered. To prepare the heart for defibrillation, the Paramedic should perform, at a minimum, two minutes of CPR. CPR helps to restore coronary artery perfusion, which in turn washes out metabolic acids created by ischemic tissue as well as delivers oxygen to the ischemic heart.

When the heart is ready—either when the patient is witnessed to go into ventricular fibrillation/pulseless ventricular tachycardia (VF/VT) or after two minutes (or five cycles) of CPR—a defibrillation (also called a countershock) should be delivered. The Paramedic should place either a pad or paddle of 12 cm diameter at the apex of the heart at the fifth intercostal space on the left side at the midclavicular line and the other pad or paddle at the fourth intercostal space at the right sternal border. A monophasic countershock of 360 joules or the approximately 200 j biphasic equivalent should then be administered.[14]

Current pacemakers are shielded to prevent harm to the pacemaker and the patient due to defibrillation. Nonetheless, if a pacemaker is noted in the upper right chest wall, then the defibrillation pads or paddles should be offset approximately 1 inch (2.5 cm) from the device as a precaution.

Monophasic versus Biphasic Defibrillation

Since Kouwenhouven demonstrated that an electrical shock could convert ventricular fibrillation into a perfusing rhythm, if delivered in a timely manner, defibrillation has been the standard of care for ventricular fibrillation.

Early defibrillators produced a direct current electrical energy pulse that delivered the energy in one direction down the heart (i.e., from the base of the heart to the apex). These defibrillators, pioneered by the cardiologist Bernard Lown, would deliver a high energy "spark" of 100 to 200 joules to the heart in approximately five milliseconds. This pulse was represented by a square sinusoidal wave on an oscilloscope and was later called a Lown waveform.

However, the human heart's electrical system is bidirectional. The depolarization wave for the upper portion of the heart travels down the heart from the SA node to the bundle of His. The depolarization wave for the bottom portion of the heart travels up the heart from the bundle branches and up the Purkinje fibers in a bottom-to-top manner.

Theoretically, delivering part of the defibrillation down the conduction system, then reversing the energy, would more naturally follow the heart's conductive pathway and allow for more complete depolarization of all of the myocardium. This defibrillation is called **biphasic defibrillation** and is seen on the oscilloscope as biphasic truncated waveform (BTE).[31] The advantage of biphasic waveforms over monophasic waveforms is that it takes less energy (115 joules biphasic defibrillation is equivalent to 200 joules monophasic defibrillation) and subsequently causes less injury of the myocardium from the electrical shock.[32]

Early defibrillation was performed in a series of "stacked" shocks designed to overcome **transthoracic impedance**, the electrical resistance of the chest wall to the passage of electricity. Many factors influence transthoracic impedance including the anatomy of the chest, volume of air in the lungs, the patient's muscle mass, and the gel on the defibrillation paddles (as well as their placement).

Modern biphasic defibrillators pass a "test" current through the chest wall to measure the transthoracic impedance. The energy to be delivered is then adjusted automatically in order to ensure the delivery of an optimal amount of energy with the first countershock. This minimizes the interruption of CPR while maximizing efficiency of defibrillation.

After two minutes, or five cycles, of CPR in the unwitnessed arrest, the patient in ventricular fibrillation should be defibrillated once. A single countershock at maximal energy provides the greatest opportunity for conversion of the rhythm while minimizing the interruption of compressions.

If defibrillation paddles are used, then a conductive medium (e.g., defibrillation gel) needs to be applied, usually a 1 inch ribbon that is then smeared over the surface of the paddles by pressing the paddles together and rotating them one against the other. It is important to ensure complete coverage of the paddles' surface without excess defibrillation gel coming in contacting with the Paramedic.

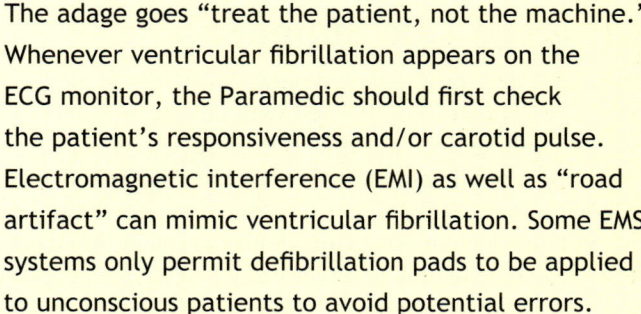

With the defibrillation pads in place, or defibrillator paddles on the chest and 25 pounds of force applied to the surface, the defibrillator is charged.[33] While the defibrillator is charging, the Paramedic should ensure that no one is in contact with the patient. If the patient is intubated, then the bag–mask assembly should be detached from the endotracheal tube and set at the patient's head.

With a focus on safety, the Paramedic should loudly announce "Stand clear!" repeatedly while visually scanning the patient from head to toe and back again. Some Paramedics actually wave a hand over the top of the patient to ensure that all persons have stepped back.

After the countershock has been delivered, cardiac compressions should resume immediately. Even if an organized rhythm appears, it is seldom a perfusing rhythm. CPR should be continued for two minutes, or five cycles. This maintains cerebral, pulmonary, and coronary perfusion while the heart recovers.

Some high-risk cardiac patients have an **automatic implanted cardiovertor–defibrillator (AICD)** placed inside the body which is designed to defibrillate the patient if she has a tachyarrhythmia or ventricular fibrillation. These devices are extremely effective. However, under certain circumstances (lead fracture, battery depletion, etc.) they may fail. If the patient has an AICD, the Paramedic should wait approximately 30 to 60 seconds after the AICD delivers its last countershock before manually delivering another defibrillation.

CPR can be performed without risk even if the AICD discharges. While the Paramedic can feel the countershock from the AICD, it is only approximately 2 joules, which is not uncomfortable or dangerous. In addition, it is possible to deactivate an AICD by use of a donut magnet that is placed over the upper right quadrant of the pulse generator.

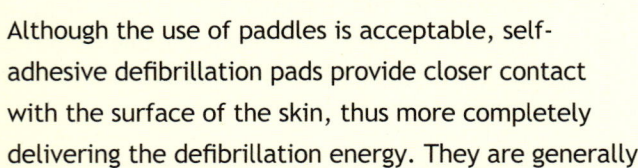

STREET SMART

Although the use of paddles is acceptable, self-adhesive defibrillation pads provide closer contact with the surface of the skin, thus more completely delivering the defibrillation energy. They are generally considered safer than standard defibrillation paddles.

Advanced Life Support

While CPR is in progress, and between rounds of defibrillation, the Paramedic can proceed with advanced life support (ALS) modalities such as intubation, intravenous access, and medication administration. It should be noted that the importance of these ALS modalities has been downgraded in favor of continuous compressions and defibrillation during cardiac arrest. They should only be attempted when sufficient personnel are on scene to ensure continuous CPR and defibrillation while ALS is being attempted.

Advanced Airway Devices

The decision to insert an advanced airway device, such as an endotracheal tube, should be based on assessment of basic airway management. If the patient's airway is being maintained by basic airway maneuvers, such as an oral airway, and ventilation is satisfactory, then endotracheal intubation could be deferred in favor of not interrupting compressions for intubation.

However, if the airway is not being maintained adequately with basic life support measures, then the Paramedic may elect to intubate. Reasons to consider intubation include airway control to prevent aspiration secondary to regurgitation resulting from gastric insufflations or to release personnel to other important tasks when there are a limited number of providers.

Following the endotracheal intubation the Paramedic should take steps to verify proper placement of the endotracheal tube in the trachea. After directly visualizing the endotracheal tube pass through the glottic opening and past the vocal cords, the Paramedic should attach the bag–mask assembly and observe for bilateral chest rise. Next, the Paramedic should use the stethoscope to auscultate the abdomen and chest. There should be an absence of sounds in the epigastrium and equal breath sounds in the chest. Finally, the Paramedic should consider the use of continuous end-tidal capnography to ensure continued placement of the endotracheal tube in the trachea.

The Paramedic should not hyperventilate the patient while performing these various verifications. Hyperventilation can have a deleterious effect on the patient. With the endotracheal tube secured with a commercial device, the Paramedic can maintain ventilations at a rate of six to eight ventilations a minute. If the airway is secured, it is not necessary to interrupt compressions to ventilate the patient. Continuous compressions at 100 compressions per minute should thus be maintained.

Alternative Advanced Airways

Under some circumstances it may be desirable to have the Paramedic use an alternative advanced airway device, such as the King® Tube or the Combitube®. In the hands of an expert user, placement of one of these supraglottic airways can be accomplished much faster than endotracheal intubation with less disruption of chest compressions. Inexperienced providers, or experienced providers with limited intubation practice, should consider these devices rather than risk an accidental—and potentially fatal—esophageal intubation. However, the decision to use any advanced airway device is dependent on

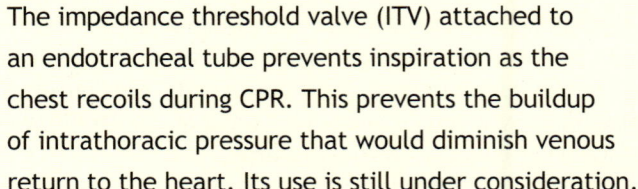

STREET SMART

The impedance threshold valve (ITV) attached to an endotracheal tube prevents inspiration as the chest recoils during CPR. This prevents the buildup of intrathoracic pressure that would diminish venous return to the heart. Its use is still under consideration.

the circumstances of the particular cardiac arrest and the competence of the Paramedic with those devices while at the same time keeping the patient's best interests foremost in mind.

Circulation Access

Circulatory access must be obtained in order to administer antidysrhythmic medications. Several options exist to gain this access including traditional intravenous access and the newer intraosseous access. Controversy exists whether intraosseous versus intravenous access is faster. During a cardiac arrest, the Paramedic should perform a rapid assessment to determine which means of access is quickest under the circumstances.

Although intravenous access can be obtained in the most convenient location, the majority of Paramedics prefer to access the venous system via either the veins in the antecubital space or the external jugular vein. A large bore (greater than 18 gauge) intravenous catheter can be placed in these locations.

Often the antecubital space is the site of choice in the field because it can be accessed while compressions and ventilations are ongoing. Once venous access has been obtained, then Paramedics typically maintain a continuous infusion of isotonic solutions, such as isotonic saline solution. Patients with suspected hypovolemia should receive volume loading.

Many Paramedics are choosing intraosseous access for medication administration during cardiac arrest. Intraosseous access is easier and faster to obtain when the patient is in cardiovascular collapse. Therefore, intraosseous medication administration is a safe and effective means of delivering the medications without interrupting resuscitation efforts.[34,35] With the fluid to be infused in a pressure bag to help maintain site patency, drug distribution through the noncollapsible venous plexus within the bone's marrow is almost as rapid as medications administered via a central line. Furthermore, the drug clearance in the bone marrow is so rapid that incompatible drugs may be given without an intervening fluid bolus.

Sites for intraosseous infusion are numerous and include both proximal tibia, distal femurs, and the humeral head. While the sternum is a viable site, compression during resuscitation makes it impractical.

Although it is permissible to administer medications down the endotracheal tube, this practice has several drawbacks. These include lower blood concentrations of medications and overall poorer survival rates. If intraosseous and intravenous access is not possible, then the Paramedic should use the endotracheal tube as the route of last resort.

The cardiac arrest medications that can be administered via an endotracheal tube can be remembered by the mnemonic NAVEL (**N**axolone, **A**tropine, **V**asopressin, **E**pinephrine, and **L**idocaine). The endotracheal dose of epinephrine is 2 to 2.5 mg and the endotracheal dose of atropine is thought to be 2 to 3 mg. The drug vasopressin has also been added to the list of drugs that can be given via the endotracheal tube. All drugs administered via the endotracheal tube should have a minimal volume of 10 cc and be aerosolized, with two or three ventilations, when possible to ensure the widest dispersion of the drug across the lung fields.

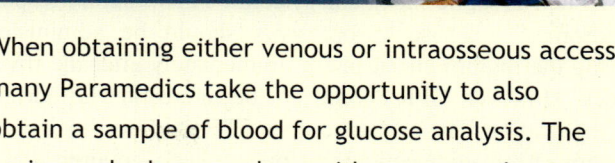
Advanced Cardiac Life Support (ACLS) Drugs

The use of medications in a cardiac arrest is less guided by science and more guided by expert judgment and conjecture. The general consensus has been that the first medications administered in a cardiac arrest should be vasopressors, followed by antidysrhythmics and other medications.

Vasopressors are thought to increase systemic vascular resistance (i.e., afterload) through vasoconstriction mediated by alpha receptors in the sympathetic nervous system. This increases the aortic diastolic pressure and thereby increases coronary artery filling. Improved coronary artery perfusion is thought to improve oxygenation of ischemic myocardial tissue as well as eliminate acid from the tissues. Vasopressors are also thought to improve the heart's contractility. In addition, vasopressors are thought to stimulate spontaneous contractions within the myocardium and pacemaker cells as well.

The vasopressor of choice for pulseless rhythms is epinephrine.[36–38] Epinephrine is administered in a 1 mg bolus followed by a 20 cc isotonic solution bolus, elevation of the limb (if possible), and a minimum of one minute of cardiac compressions. This procedure (bolus–bolus–limb lift–compressions) shows the greatest promise of distributing the drug from the periphery to the central circulation and onto the heart.

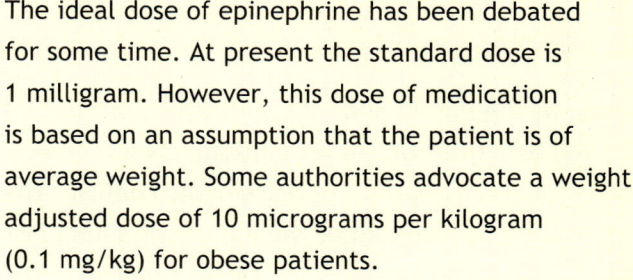
An alternative to epinephrine is the drug vasopressin, which can be given as either the first or second vasopressor. The dose of vasopressin (40 units) is administered either intravenously or via the intraosseous route and is a potent vasoconstrictor,

raising the peripheral vascular resistance. Vasopressin may be more effective than epinephrine in special cardiac arrest situations such as septic shock and systemic inflammatory response syndrome.[39–41] These vasopressors should be administered during the rhythm check phase, immediately after the rhythm check. However, CPR should not be interrupted to administer medication. The sequence goes CPR–countershock–CPR–rhythm check with concurrent pulse check–countershock as needed–CPR again for two minutes or five cycles. Epinephrine administration may be repeated every three to five minutes.[14]

Pulse checks should only occur during rhythm checks and only if an organized rhythm is observed. The pulse check should be brief (less than 10 seconds) and CPR resumed immediately regardless of the presence of a pulse. This is more fully discussed in the postresuscitative care section that follows.

Antidysrhythmics

The next classification of drugs administered is the antidysrhythmics. During a cardiac arrest the Paramedic's choice of antidysrhythmics should be the drug that will provide the patient with the most likely benefit. For example, if the patient's rhythm is polymorphic ventricular tachycardia then magnesium (discussed shortly) may be the drug of choice.

If the cause of the cardiac arrest is unknown and assumed to be sudden cardiac death, then the drug of choice is amiodarone. In the past lidocaine would have been the drug of choice. However, head-to-head studies have shown that, in a cardiac arrest situation, amiodarone is the superior choice and is more likely to cause conversion of ventricular fibrillation with defibrillation.[42–45]

The dose of amiodarone is 300 mg rapid bolus followed by a bolus of isotonic solution, elevation of the limb, and CPR during a cardiac arrest. Amiodarone 150 mg may be repeated in three to five minutes, if necessary, or an alternative antidysrhythmic, such as lidocaine, can be chosen.

Lidocaine, a traditional antidysrhythmic used for decades in cardiac arrest, is a weight-based medication. The dose of lidocaine is 1 to 1.5 mg per kg given rapid bolus via either intravenous or intraosseous, followed by a bolus of isotonic solution, elevation of the limb, and CPR. Like amiodarone,

the repeat dose is one-half the original dose. Lidocaine can then be repeated again, for a total dose of 3 mg per kg.

An old antidysrhythmic that is still used in some limited circumstances is procainamide. Procainamide lengthens the QT interval and should be used with caution if amiodarone has been used. Procainamide is administered via an infusion at 20 mg per minute, which can be raised to 50 mg per minute during a cardiac arrest. Like lidocaine, the dose of procainamide is weight dependent; the dose of procainamide is 17 mg per kg. The time for administration is a function of the total dose of the drug and the flow rate, making its use in a cardiac resuscitation cumbersome.

If hypomagesemia is suspected, or the patient is in torsades de pointes, then magnesium is the drug of choice. Magnesium is administered as a single dose of 1 to 2 grams and infused via either intravenous or intraosseous means over 5 to 20 minutes. Magnesium may also be useful in patients who are toxic on digitalis and experiencing life-threatening dysrhythmias.

Consideration of Other Possibilities

If the patient is unresponsive to initial resuscitative efforts, then the Paramedic should consider other etiologies for the cardiac arrest, some of which were discussed at the beginning of the chapter. These noncardiac etiologies may be amenable to other "nonstandard" therapies.

STREET SMART

If hyperkalemia, an elevated potassium level, is suspected, as in pre-dialysis end-stage renal failure or diabetic ketoacidosis, or calcium channel overdose is suspected, then 8 to 16 mg/kg of 10% calcium chloride solution can be used in a cardiac arrest. Otherwise, calcium chloride should not be used routinely in cardiac arrest management.

CASE STUDY (CONTINUED)

As soon as the Paramedics obtain intravenous access they administer a single milligram of epinephrine, followed by a flush of saline solution. They then resume CPR. At the end of two minutes of CPR, the ECG monitor shows asystole. The Paramedic confirms the asystole in a noncontiguous lead and then has the EMT resume CPR. Subsequently, the Paramedics administer 1 milligram of atropine intravenously and discuss the likely cause of the cardiac arrest based on the initial history.

CRITICAL THINKING QUESTIONS

1. Why is asystole confirmed in two leads?
2. What are some of the possible causes of asystole?

Evaluation

A successful defibrillation, by definition, results in a brief period of asystole. By quieting the waters (i.e., depolarizing all ectopic foci) and then performing cardiac compressions, the intention is that the SA node will resume dominance and there will be a return of spontaneous circulation. However, in some instances this does not happen and the Paramedic must take more dramatic action to restart the heart.

Asystole

When asystole appears on the ECG monitor, the Paramedic must first ensure that the patient is asystolic. Although the patient may appear to be in asystole in the monitoring lead, it is possible that the patient is still in ventricular fibrillation which is not visible in that lead. In order to ensure that the entire myocardium is in asystole, the ECG should be confirmed in two perpendicular leads (leads that look across both planes of the heart). Therefore, if the patient is monitored (for example, through the defibrillation pads) and the pads are conventionally placed in Lead II, then the perpendicular lead would be MCL1. These leads provide an opportunity to view both the inferior and anterior walls of the left ventricle, or the perpendicular planes.

Once asystole is confirmed in two leads, the Paramedic should immediately resume CPR and consider administering epinephrine (1 mg of a 1:10,000 concentration either IV/IO/ET) every three to five minutes and atropine (1.0 mg IV/IO/ET) every three to five minutes, for a total dose of 3 mg. At the same time, the Paramedic should continue searching for potentially reversible causes.[14]

Acidosis occurring during a cardiac arrest may be counterproductive and is best treated with careful ventilation and the use of sodium bicarbonate ($NaHCO_3$) to reverse the condition. $NaHCO_3$ administration creates an alkalosis which impacts the oxyhemoglobin curve and prevents the release of oxygen from hemoglobin. $NaHCO_3$ also inactivates epinephrine. Therefore, sodium bicarbonate use should be limited to known pre-existing metabolic acidosis, such as seen with diabetic ketoacidosis, hyperkalemia, and as seen in end-stage renal disease patients predialysis, as well as overdoses of aspirin and tricyclic antidepressants.[46,47] The dose of $NaHCO_3$ used in those cases is 1 mEq per kg.

Pulseless Electrical Activity

Pulseless electrical activity (PEA) is a catch all term for a number of rhythms including idioventricular or agonal rhythms, ventricular escape rhythms, bradyasystolic rhythms, and pseudomechanical dissociation (EMD). The common thread in all of these rhythms is that the patient remains pulseless. However, pulselessness is a function, in part, of the Paramedic's ability to palpate a pulse. If the patient's blood pressure is extremely low, then a pulse may not be palpable. However, even unpalpable pulses are insufficient for cerebral perfusion. Therefore, CPR is indicated for patients in PEA.

The goal in the treatment of PEA is to create a pulse. Until a pulse has returned it is imperative that continuous cardiac compressions continue throughout the resuscitation. A pulse is a sign of adequate cardiac output, determined by the formula stroke volume times heart rate equals the cardiac output ($SV \times HR = CO$). Therefore, to increase cardiac output the Paramedic should focus on increasing stroke volume or heart rate.

Epinephrine, which increases the force and rate of contraction (positive inotropic and chronotropic medication), is the first medication administered in treating PEA. The dose of epinephrine is 1 mg rapid intravenous bolus followed by a bolus of isotonic solution, elevation of the extremity, and a minimum of one minute of CPR.

Next, the Paramedic should turn to increasing the stroke volume. The easiest means to accomplish this is use of a fluid bolus. A fluid bolus increases the venous return, which in turn increases the end-diastolic volume or preload. The greater the end-diastolic volume, the greater the force of contraction of the heart (according to the Frank–Starling law).

If the patient's rhythm is bradycardiac, then the heart rate must be increased. This is the other portion of the formula. A bradycardia in PEA may be due to excessive parasympathetic stimulation secondary to ischemia, specifically of the AV node, or drug effect. Atropine is the drug of choice to overcome this parasympathetic effect. Atropine sulfate at a dose of 0.5 to 1 mg is administered in rapid intravenous bolus and doses of atropine are added until either the patient's heart rate is greater than 50 bpm or a maximum of 3 mg of atropine has been administered. While giving the combination of fluid boluses and epinephrine and atropine, the Paramedic should continue to look for potentially reversible causes of cardiac arrest.

Continuous monitoring of end-tidal CO_2 ($EtCO_2$) may help guide the Paramedic's decision making regarding termination versus continued resuscitation. $EtCO_2$ levels have been positively correlated with cardiac output and coronary artery perfusion, and have also been linked to successful cardiac arrest resuscitation.[48]

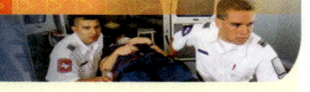

STREET SMART

In the past, transcutaneous pacing of asystolic rhythms was acceptable. However, recent research indicates that patient survival does not improve with pacing. Therefore, transcutaneous or external pacing of asystole is not recommended for routine cardiac arrest situations.

Obtaining a pulse during CPR is difficult at best. Traditionally, pulses are attempted at the femoral artery, the furthest point from where CPR is performed. However, the femoral artery is proximal to the femoral vein, which emanates from the inferior vena cava. As the vena cava has no valves, any compressions will create a backward pressure wave down the vena cava and into the femoral vein, giving the illusion that an arterial pulse is present even if one is not.

Disposition

The main therapeutic goal of resuscitation is a return of spontaneous circulation. Beyond return of spontaneous circulation, another therapeutic goal of resuscitation is the establishment of adequate cerebral and coronary perfusion pressure. The presence of a rhythm, even a normal sinus rhythm, is not sufficient to establish return of spontaneous circulation.

The first evidence of a perfusing rhythm often is not a palpable pulse but rather an increase in the end-tidal carbon dioxide ($EtCO_2$) level. As pulmonary perfusion increases, the $EtCO_2$ will gradually climb toward near normal levels (greater than 25 mmHg).

Similarly, a positive pulse reading on a pulse oximeter, particularly a second generation pulse oximeter, is another indicator of the return of perfusing rhythm. Often a pulse oximeter will register a faint pulse, with a pulsatile display, before a pulse can be palpated.

Finally, the gold standard used to establish return of spontaneous circulation is a palpable pulse, preferably the carotid pulse. When witnessing a potentially perfusing rhythm on the ECG monitor, such as a narrow complex tachycardia, the Paramedic should attempt to palpate a carotid pulse. Palpation of the carotid pulse should not take more than 10 seconds, and then should immediately be followed by CPR, even if pulses are detected.

Once return of spontaneous circulation is obtained, it must be maintained. To start, the Paramedic should perform a "reverse CPR check." After confirming a carotid pulse, the Paramedic could consider obtaining a radial pulse and/or blood pressure. As a result of epinephrine administration, as well as other actions, the patient can have a tachydysrhythmia. These dysrhythmias usually resolve with time and do not require further medication and/or cardioversion.

Patients with a return of spontaneous circulation are hemodynamically unstable, with their vital signs fluctuating moment to moment for a period of time. The Paramedic should closely monitor the ECG, pulse, and blood pressure every five minutes. Hypotension, secondary to myocardial dysfunction, low cardiac output, and/or acidosis-induced hypotension, may need fluid resuscitation and/or vasopressor support using dopamine.

Some medical directors support the use of antidysrhythmic medications immediately following return of spontaneous circulation. The current state of evidence is unclear as to whether antidysrhythmic medication is helpful in the postresuscitative phase. However, the current practice in many systems is to start a prophylactic infusion of the last effective antidysrhythmia medication.[49] Alternatively, some medical directors support the administration of beta blockers for their cardioprotective effects, provided there are no contraindications.

Next, the Paramedic would assess the patient's respiratory status. Often, these patients have apnea and require ventilation, either manual or (preferably) mechanical. Whether manual or mechanical ventilation is used, caution is advised to avoid hypocapnea (low carbon dioxide levels). Hyperventilation that leads to hypocapnea causes cerebral vasoconstriction and can induce pancerebral hypoxia.[50,51] This pancerebral hypoxia can worsen the neurological outcome for the patient. Therefore, the rate of ventilation should be aimed at creating a $EtCO_2$ of 35 to 45 mmHg.

Thereafter, the Paramedic should assess the patient's level of consciousness. In many cases, the patient will remain comatose. However, if the patient arouses it may be necessary to sedate the patient in order to properly ventilate him and to maintain a normal $EtCO_2$.

A meaningful neurological survival is based, in part, on maintaining an adequate cerebral perfusion pressure. Cerebral perfusion pressure is a function of the mean arterial pressure minus the intracranial pressure (CPP = MAP − ICP). As many patients with return of spontaneous circulation experience some cerebral edema, raising the ICP, the Paramedic should try to maintain a mean arterial pressure at or above 60 mmHg. The MAP can be obtained by non-invasive blood pressure (NIBP) monitoring in the field. If NIBP is not available, then a systolic pressure of 90 to 100 mmHg is the therapeutic goal.

Any increase in ICP can have profound effects upon the patient's neurological recovery. Prior to instrumentation of the throat, deep endotracheal suctioning, or any vagal stimulating event, the patient should be premedicated with 1 mg/kg of lidocaine to prevent elevations in the ICP. Although there is no evidence to support the use of prophylactic anticonvulsants, witnessed seizures should be treated immediately with diazepam or a similar rapid acting anticonvulsant to minimize the increase in ICP.

During cerebral insult, hypothermia can be protective, but hyperthermia can be deadly to the brain. Every increase of 1°F above normal increases the brain's metabolic demand by 13% to 15%, increases the intracranial pressure, and impacts on the oxyhemoglobin curve at a time when the brain needs a decrease in metabolic demand. If the patient is hyperthermic, the Paramedic should use cooling techniques to lower the body temperature to normal, and do so while avoiding shivering. Shivering increases heat production and the body's temperature.

The greatest danger to return of spontaneous circulation may be hypoxia and acidosis. After ensuring a patent airway and oxygenation with ventilation, the Paramedic should assess for acidosis via the $EtCO_2$. An elevated $EtCO_2$ indicates acidosis. Acidosis affects the oxyhemoglobin curve and can negatively impact on the patient's oxygenation. Typically, the patient's acidosis will abate with adequate ventilation. The administration of sodium bicarbonate is usually not necessary.

Besides adequate cerebral perfusion and oxygen, the brain requires glucose. The patient should be maintained as normoglycemic and hypoglycemia should be treated immediately with 50% dextrose intravenously. It should be noted that the traditional signs and symptoms of hypoglycemia may not be present as the patient recovers and the Paramedic should routinely obtain blood glucose in these patients.

Although little treatment can be provided for hyperglycemia in the field, it should be reported to the accepting physician at the emergency department. There are reports of poor survival and worsened neurological outcome in patients with return of spontaneous circulation and hyperglycemia.

Therapeutic Hypothermia

There is a current trend toward treating patients with return of spontaneous circulation with hypothermia. This hypothermia is more than permissive hypothermia, or natural cooling, but instead is actively induced **therapeutic hypothermia**.

Patients with return of spontaneous circulation who are subsequently cooled, either during resuscitation or after return of spontaneous circulation, have shown an improved neurological outcome.[52, 53] This may be because hypothermia reduces cerebral oxygen consumption approximately 6% for every degree in temperature drop. It has also been postulated that hypothermia may decrease reperfusion injury by limiting free radical production and/or preventing calcium shifts.

Therapeutic hypothermia is not without risks. Complications such as dysrhythmia and/or coagulopathy may occur. In addition, therapeutic hypothermia is generally limited to those patients without head injury, cerebral vascular accident, or opiate overdose.

To induce therapeutic hypothermia, the Paramedic should apply ice packs to the pulse points, such as the neck and groin and infuse 30 mL/kg (maximum of 2 liters) of cooled saline (4°C) over 30 minutes. The extended infusion time is intended to prevent pulmonary edema, a complication of too rapid infusion of cool saline. These techniques are used until the body's temperature is between 32°C and 34°C (90°F to 93°F). It is imperative that, once the therapeutic hypothermic goal is attained, the hospital can continue to maintain the temperature using cooling blankets and cool infusions. Some systems divert patients in this situation to a hospital that can continue the cooling process for 12 – 24 hours and the slow rewarm needed after. These hospitals preferably can perform emergent angioplasty as well, since it is assumed a coronary thrombus caused the cardiac arrest.

A 12-lead ECG should be performed as soon as possible after return of circulation to identify patients who have an ST-elevation MI. These patients would benefit from transport to a hospital capable of performing an emergent angioplasty, which may stabilize the heart by restoring blood flow to the myocardium.

Termination in the Field

Termination in the field is a point of contention for some EMS systems. Early Paramedics in Seattle, Washington, and Milwaukee, Wisconsin, pioneered termination of resuscitation in the field after seeing the dangers of transporting hopeless cases. Some of the hazards identified include continued bloodborne pathogens exposure, especially to hollow bore needles in a moving ambulance, and injuries associated with lifting and moving these patients. Further dangers exist for the citizens on public roadways from speeding ambulances using lights and siren as well as the substantial expense to the family for the emergency department's resuscitation efforts.

The medical literature supports the termination of adult resuscitation, and the American College of Emergency Physicians agrees in its policy statement to terminate resuscitation if further efforts would be futile and provided certain conditions are met. Specifically, the patient must be asystolic or in pulseless electrical activity at a rate less than 60 bpm. In addition, a trial of advanced cardiac life support must have been unsuccessful (i.e., the patient is unresponsive to standard medical treatment).[54] The trial of advanced cardiac life support typically includes CPR with defibrillation and advanced life support treatment modalities such as advanced airway management, venous access, medication administration, and possibly external pacing.

A termination in the field protocol for futile resuscitation is thought to reduce the number of patients transported to the hospital, in cardiac arrest, by approximately 65%. This would be expected to save hospitals and EMS systems tens of thousands of dollars, allowing them to stretch their limited resources.

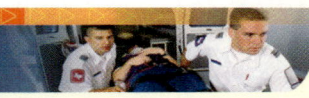

STREET SMART

Some studies have shown that patients in cardiac arrest with an $EtCO_2$ less than 10 mmHg after 20 to 30 minutes of appropriate advanced cardiac life support care do not survive. The use of $EtCO_2$ could be included in the criteria for termination of resuscitation protocols.

Despite performing high-quality CPR, the addition of advanced modalities such as intubation, and timely medication administration, the patient does not regain pulses. The Paramedic places a call to the County Medical Director and receives an order to terminate the resuscitation. The Paramedics prepare to talk with the man's wife and teenage children about the decision to terminate resuscitation.

CRITICAL THINKING QUESTIONS

1. Under what conditions should resuscitation be terminated?
2. What are the elements of a notification of death?

Notification

The decision to terminate resuscitation is accompanied by the need to notify the family. The decision to terminate resuscitation is predicated on three factors. The first factor is the family's wishes. If the family has been properly prepared, they are more likely to accept the decision. Proper preparation is a process that will be discussed shortly. The next factor is the Paramedic's ability to provide grief counseling. Preparation for grief counseling is a function of education and is a learned skill.

Finally, the Paramedic must be aware of the conditions necessary to terminate resuscitation, possibly including notification of medical control. The medical director and EMS administrators should develop a protocol which clearly describes the antecedent conditions, without room for ambiguity, and procedures for notifying the coroner/medical examiner and/or law enforcement. The protocol should include a mechanism for quality review for assurance of compliance with the protocol as well as guidelines for documentation for termination of resuscitation. It may be advisable that the protocol also include guidelines for care of the deceased which take into account cultural traditions and taboos.

Cherri D. Hobgood, MD, and Debbie Weir, MSW, have created a mnemonic, GRIEV_ING, for medical residents that is also useful for Paramedics who are tasked with death notification following termination of resuscitation (Table 7-7).

Before proceeding with a notification, the Paramedic should find an appropriate location. The setting for a notification is important; even though notifications can be made while the resuscitation is ongoing, the message is often lost as the family member focuses on the resuscitation. The best place for a notification is a place like a dining room, where there are chairs available. The Paramedic should try to avoid giving the news in the kitchen, since family members who have trouble accepting the patient's death may find an outlet by directing anger at the rescuers. A kitchen has many potential weapons.

The Paramedic should arrange to have chairs available so that family members can sit. Providing a box of tissues is also helpful. Grief reactions are very personal and providing a private place allows the family to grieve without concern for embarrassment.

The first letter in the GRIEV_ING mnemonic (G) stands for **G**athering the family together. The Paramedic should make every effort to deliver the same message to as many of the family members as possible. Although it may be important to call others first, there is typically little time on scene to assemble a large extended family. In those cases, the key individual who will relay the information to others should be identified. This person may be the oldest, youngest, male, or female, depending upon the family and cultural considerations.

While gathering the family, the Paramedic should consider calling for additional **R**esources (R), such as the fire service clergy. Often clergy are trained in death notification. It can be very helpful for the Paramedic to witness several notifications, in case a situation arises in which the clergy is unavailable. It is also helpful if the clergy is willing to stand by, observe, and offer instruction and correction while a Paramedic performs a notification.

Table 7-7   GRIEV_ING

G	Gather
R	Resources
I	Identify
E	Educate
V	Verify
_	Space
I	Inquire
N	Nut and bolts
G	Give

CULTURAL/REGIONAL DIFFERENCES

If English is not the family's primary language, it may be helpful for the Paramedic to have an interpreter available to avoid confusion in communications. Similarly, if the family is religious, it may be helpful to have the clergy available as well to lend guidance.

At this point, the Paramedic is ready to make contact with the family. Positioning is important: The Paramedic should take a position of about four feet away from the family, remaining at eye level and face to face with them. The Paramedic should then start the conversation, making a polite introduction Identifying (I) himself or herself by name, title, and position (e.g., Paramedic Smith, crew leader). One effective tool some Paramedics use is to ask the family to start with their recollection of events.

While avoiding the use of medical jargon, the Paramedic can pick up the story where the family called Emergency services and impart the severity of the situation (Educate). Using the patient's name, the Paramedic should paint a picture of the gravity of the situation and use the words "dead" or "died," avoiding euphemisms such as "passed away." It is best to keep the message simple. Providing unnecessary detail before announcing the death can raise false hopes and cause extreme anxiety in family members.

CULTURAL/REGIONAL DIFFERENCES

European cultures tend to believe a person is being honest when the two parties look at each other "eye to eye." However, some cultures feel eye to eye contact is threatening and inappropriate. The Paramedic should be aware of any cultural norms.

Next, the Paramedic should repeat the statement that the patient has died and ask if the family members understand. It is important to Verify (V) that the family understands what has been said.

At this point, it is wise to give the family members a little space (_) to let them absorb what they have been told. Often Paramedics feel anxiety at this emotional moment and feel compelled to say something. Tolerating silence is an important skill for a Paramedic to learn.

The family's initial response has been described as a "psychic pain spike." Although it lasts only a brief period of time (usually 5 to 15 minutes), it does occur. During this period, the family cannot make decisions. However, once this period of acute grief has ended, the family members may progress through other reactions: denial, anger, and/or guilt.

CULTURAL/REGIONAL DIFFERENCES

In some instances, a Paramedic may feel it necessary to offer a shoulder, or to put his arm around the family. While touching is OK, it should be carefully considered. The Paramedic should proceed only when it appears the family will accept the gesture.

When the moment has passed, the Paramedic should Inquire (I) if there are any questions. It is permissible for the Paramedic to express genuine concern with statements like "I am sorry for your loss" or "This must be very difficult for you."

Sometimes there are accusations of negligence or statements made about what should have been done. Although difficult to accept, Paramedics must see these as expressions of grief and not as personal attacks. Eventually the anger will dissipate, allowing the family to move on with the grieving process. These earlier statements of concern by the Paramedic do not make any implications about the care provided and are not an acceptance of responsibility for any alleged errors having been made.

The "Nuts and Bolts" (N) refer to the process of viewing the body. Many family members would like to take one last moment with the deceased patient. Although many jurisdictions have specific regulations regarding handling of the deceased, it is generally acceptable for the Paramedic to cap intravenous lines and then cover over the site with a bandage; to cover the body, leaving the arms exposed, and leaving electrodes in place; and to remove the adaptor from an endotracheal tube, while leaving the endotracheal tube in place. Paramedics are well advised to contact the local coroner/medical examiner for specific details and/or to follow written protocols. These regulations are provided to protect the patient and to assist with any investigations.

CULTURAL/REGIONAL DIFFERENCES

Some cultures have specific death rituals. Providing that these rituals do not violate local regulation, the Paramedic should facilitate the performance of these rituals by the family.

Once the patient's body is prepared, the family should be allowed into the room. At the same time, responders should quietly and reverently leave the room. It is helpful to have several providers remain with the family in case there are questions and to help if another medical emergency arises.

As a last act before the funeral director/medical examiner/coroner takes responsibility for the body, the Paramedic should Give (G) the family a telephone number or contact information in case there are questions later, like "Did he suffer?" Some Paramedics have a preprinted business card with all of the applicable information readily available to give to families.

CONCLUSION

Cardiac resuscitation seems somewhat mundane to some Paramedics who simply "follow the arrest protocol." Yet, every cardiac resuscitation provides the Paramedic with a unique opportunity to apply critical thinking to a situation. Using the problem-solving techniques described throughout this chapter, the Paramedic can search out the potentially reversible cause of cardiac arrest. Therein lies the opportunity to save a life.

KEY POINTS:

- Acute coronary syndrome is often cited as a likely cause of cardiac arrest.

- Four factors lead to cardiac arrest regardless of etiology.
  - Decreased preload
  - Decreased contractility
  - Errors of automaticity
  - Increased afterload

- The Paramedic should establish whether any of three historical conditions exist before starting or continuing resuscitation.
  - Is there reasonable hope of survival?
  - Are there clinical signs of death?
  - Does a valid DNR exist?

- Clinical signs of death include dependent lividity, body cooling, and stiffness.

- The signs of unresponsiveness, apnea, and pulselessness serve as the basis to start CPR but not as the basis for discontinuing CPR.

- Once CPR has begun, the Paramedic should contact medical control for an order to discontinue resuscitation.

- The Paramedic should assess the adequacy of bystander CPR:
  - Compression depth
  - Rate

- Agonal respirations do not signify an adequate respiratory effort.

- The Paramedic is responsible for taking over CPR from bystander CPR or arranging for continuation as needed.

- Rhythms come in many forms:
  - Shockable rhythms
    - Ventricular tachycardia
    - Ventricular fibrillation
  - Nonshockable rhythms
    - Asystole
    - Pulseless electrical activity

- Resuscitation is a team effort.

- The team leader delegates tasks.

- The team leader communicates with the team to both give and receive information.

- The team leader is responsible for determining and announcing the rhythm.

- Resuscitation begins with ABCD:
  - Airway
    - Open
    - Assess
    - Suction
    - Secure
  - Breathing
    - Normal ventilation; avoid hyperventilation
    - Cricoid pressure
  - Circulation
    - Compressions
      - 2 minutes of compressions
      - 1 1/2 inches in depth
      - Hard and fast
    - CPR assist devices
    - Vest
    - Chest band
    - Piston device
      - Correct placement

- Defibrillation
  - Preparation of the myocardium with oxygen and acid washout
- Monophasic defibrillators deliver energy in a single direction. If pads are properly applied, they are from base to apex.
- Biphasic defibrillators deliver energy down the conduction system and then reverse to allow flow back up the conduction system.
- The Paramedic controlling the defibrillator is responsible for electrical safety by ensuring that all persons, including the operator, are not in contact with the patient.
- Newer devices such as pacers and implanted cardiodefibrillators have been electrically isolated so they are not damaged by defibrillation energy. Prudence suggests that the pads be placed at least 1 inch away from the devices.
- The Paramedic should wait approximately 60 seconds after the implanted cardiodefibrillator has delivered a shock before initiating an external shock.
- Advanced life support modalities such as IV access and intubation should be completed only when there are sufficient personnel to deliver adequate CPR.
- An advanced airway is necessary only when basic airway interventions are not maintaining the airway.
- Alternative advanced airways should be available in case intubation is not successful.
- Intraosseous access is a fast alternative route for resuscitation medications.

- Endotracheal administration of drugs should occur only after IV or IO access has been attempted.
- The acceptable drugs for ET administration are lidocaine, epinephrine, atropine, vasopressin, and naloxone. Each drug should be administered in 10 mL of fluid.
- Cardiac resuscitation drugs and dosages are:
  - Vasopressors
    - Epinephrine (1 mg)
    - Vasopressin (40 units)
  - Antidysrhythmics
    - Amiodarone (300 mg followed in 10 minutes by 150 mg)
    - Lidocaine (1 to 1.5 mg/kg up to 3 mg/kg)
    - Procainamide (20 mg/minute until hypotension ensues, QRS widens by 50% of original, 17 mg/kg have been given, or dysrhythmia terminates)
    - Magnesium (1 to 2 grams over 5 to 20 minutes)
- Treatment of asystole and pulseless electrical activity includes epinephrine or atropine (if the pulseless electrical activity is bradycardiac and treating the cause of the event).
- Return of spontaneous pulses is the goal of resuscitation, although the patient remains at risk of a re-arrest.
  - Monitor $EtCO_2$
  - Pulse oximetry
  - Vital signs
- Therapeutic hypothermia reduces cerebral oxygen consumption.
- A patient's family must be notified of termination of resuscitative efforts.

REVIEW QUESTIONS:

1. What etiologies cause cardiac arrest?
2. List three signs that serve as the basis for determining whether to initiate CPR.
3. Describe ABCD as applied to cardiac resuscitation.
4. In the case of defibrillation, who is responsible for safety?
5. What is the correct procedure for manually defibrillating someone with an implanted cardiodefibrillator?
6. What are likely causes of asystole and pulseless electrical activity rhythms?
7. How would the Paramedic assist in therapeutic hypothermia?

CASE STUDY QUESTIONS:

Please refer to the Case Study in this chapter, and answer the questions below:

1. Should family members be allowed to witness field resuscitations? Why or why not?

2. What are your feelings regarding speaking with the family after resuscitation?

REFERENCES:

1. Wayne MA, Racht EM, et al. Prehospital management of cardiac arrest: how useful are vasopressor and antiarrhythmic drugs? *Prehosp Emerg Care.* 2002;6(1):72–80.

2. Montgomery WH. Prehospital cardiac arrest: the chain of survival concept. *Ann Acad Med Singapore.* 1992;21(1):69–72.

3. Wit AL. Cellular electrophysiologic mechanisms of cardiac arrhythmias. *Cardiol Clin.* 1990;8(3):393–409.

4. Kleber AG, Rudy Y. Basic mechanisms of cardiac impulse propagation and associated arrhythmias. *Physiol Rev.* 2004;84(2):431–488.

5. Rombola G, Colussi G, et al. Cardiac arrhythmias and electrolyte changes during haemodialysis. *Nephrol, Dial, Transplant.* 1992;7(4):318–322.

6. Bisogno JL, Langley A, et al. Effect of calcium to reverse the electrocardiographic effects of hyperkalemia in the isolated rat heart: a prospective, dose-response study. *Crit Care Med.* 1994;22(4):697–704.

7. Campieri C, Fatone F, et al. Terminal arrhythmia due to hyperkalemia corrected by intravenous calcium infusion. *Nephron.* 1987;47(4):312.

8. Letsas KP, Efremidis M, et al. Clinical characteristics of patients with drug-induced QT interval prolongation and torsade de pointes: identification of risk factors. *Clin Res Cardiol.* 2009;98(4):208–212.

9. Calkins T, Chan TC, et al. Review of prehospital sodium bicarbonate use for cyclic antidepressant overdose. *Emerg Med J.* 2003;20(5):483–486.

10. Lovecchio F, Berlin R, et al. Hypertonic sodium bicarbonate in an acute flecainide overdose. *Am J Emerg Med.* 1998;16(5):534–537.

11. Banai S, Schuger C. Magnesium sulfate is the treatment for torsades de pointes if the right dose is given. *Am J Cardiol.* 1990;65(3):266.

12. O'Connor N, Greene S, et al. Glucagon use in beta blocker overdose. *Emerg Med J.* 2005;22(5):391.

13. Doyon S, Roberts JR. The use of glucagon in a case of calcium channel blocker overdose. *Ann Emerg Med.* 1993;22(7):1229–1233.

14. *Advanced Cardiovascular Life Support Provider Manual (American Heart Association, ACLS Provider Manual).* Dallas: American Heart Association; 2007.

15. Dolinak D, Lew E, Matshes E. *Forensic Pathology: Principles and Practice.* Toronto: Academic Press; 2005.

16. Booth CM, Boone RH, et al. Is this patient dead, vegetative, or severely neurologically impaired? Assessing outcome for comatose survivors of cardiac arrest. *JAMA.* 2004;291(7):870–879.

17. Harvey L, Woollard M. Outcome of patients identified as dead (beyond resuscitation) at the point of the emergency call. *Emerg Med J.* 2004;21(3):367–369.

18. Jorgenson DB, Skarr T, et al. AED use in businesses, public facilities and homes by minimally trained first responders. *Resuscitation.* 2003;59(2):225–233.

19. Peberdy MA, Ottingham LV, et al. Adverse events associated with lay emergency response programs: the public access defibrillation trial experience. *Resuscitation.* 2006;70(1):59–65.

20. Kerber RE, Becker LB, et al. Automatic external defibrillators for public access defibrillation: recommendations for specifying and reporting arrhythmia analysis algorithm performance, incorporating new waveforms, and enhancing safety. A statement for health professionals from the American Heart Association Task Force on Automatic External Defibrillation, Subcommittee on AED Safety and Efficacy. *Circulation.* 1997;95(6):1677–1682.

21. Parish DC, Dinesh Chandra KM, et al. Success changes the problem: why ventricular fibrillation is declining, why pulseless electrical activity is emerging, and what to do about it. *Resuscitation.* 2003;58(1):31–35.

22. Desbiens NA. Simplifying the diagnosis and management of pulseless electrical activity in adults: a qualitative review. *Crit Care Med.* 2008;36(2):391–396.

23. Nagel EL, Fine EG, et al. Complications of CPR. *Crit Care Med.* 1981;9(5):424.

24. Beebe R, Funk D. *Fundamentals of Basic Emergency Care.* Albany: Delmar Cengage Learning; 2004.

25. Gobindram A, Clarke S. Cricoid pressure: should we lay off the pressure? *Anaesthesia.* 2008;63(11):1258–1259.

26. Ewart L. The efficacy of cricoid pressure in preventing gastro-esophageal reflux in rapid sequence induction of anaesthesia. *J Perioper Pract.* 2007;17(9):432–436.

27. Tintinalli, J. *Emergency Medicine: A Comprehensive Study Guide,* sixth edition. New York: McGraw-Hill Professional; 2003.

28. Haman L, Parizek P, et al. Precordial thump efficacy in termination of induced ventricular arrhythmias. *Resuscitation.* 2009;80(1):14–16.

29. Amir O, Schliamser JE, et al. Ineffectiveness of precordial thump for cardioversion of malignant ventricular tachyarrhythmias. *Pacing Clin Electrophysiol.* 2007;30(2): 153–156.

30. Davis SA. Cough-CPR and a new theory of blood flow. *Crit Care Nurse.* 1983;3(2):42–46.

31. Manoharan G, Evans N, et al. Comparing the efficacy and safety of a novel monophasic waveform delivered by the passive implantable atrial defibrillator with biphasic waveforms in cardioversion of atrial fibrillation. *Circulation.* 2004;109(13):1686–1692.

32. Bridy MA, Burklow TR. Understanding the newer automated external defibrillator devices: electrophysiology, biphasic waveforms, and technology. *J Emerg Nurs.* 2002;28(2):132–137.

33. Association A. *American Heart Association ACLS Resource Text; Professional for Instructors and Experienced Providers.* Dallas: American Heart Association; 2008.

34. LaRocco BG, Wang HE. Intraosseous infusion. *Prehos Emerg Care.* 2003;7(2):280–285.

35. DeBoer S, Seaver M, et al. Intraosseous infusion: not just for kids anymore. *Emerg Med Serv.* 2005;34(3):54, 56–63; quiz 119.

36. Sillberg VA, Perry JJ, et al. Is the combination of vasopressin and epinephrine superior to repeated doses of epinephrine alone in the treatment of cardiac arrest-A systematic review? *Resuscitation.* 2008;79(3):380–386.

37. Gueugniaud PY, David JS, et al. Vasopressin and epinephrine vs. epinephrine alone in cardiopulmonary resuscitation. *N Engl J Med.* 2008;359(1):21–30.

38. Upadhye S, Fernandes CM. Vasopressin versus epinephrine for out-of-hospital cardiopulmonary resuscitation. *CJEM.* 2005;7(1):48–50.

39. Ertmer C, Rehberg S, et al. Current place of vasopressin analogues in the treatment of septic shock. *Curr Infect Dis Rep.* 2008;10(5):362–367.

40. Maki DG. Low-dose vasopressin did not reduce mortality more than norepinephrine in septic shock. *ACP J Club.* 2008;149(3):14.

41. Ruggiero MS. Effects of vasopressin in septic shock. *AACN Adv Crit Care.* 2008;19(3):281–287.

42. Rea RS, Kane-Gill SL, et al. Comparing intravenous amiodarone or lidocaine, or both, outcomes for inpatients with pulseless ventricular arrhythmias. *Crit Care Med.* 2006;34(6):1617–1623.

43. Leeuwenburgh BP, Versteegh MI, et al. Should amiodarone or lidocaine be given to patients who arrest after cardiac surgery and fail to cardiovert from ventricular fibrillation? *Interact Cardiovasc Thorac Surg.* 2008;7(6):1148–1151.

44. Somberg JC, Bailin SJ, et al. Intravenous lidocaine versus intravenous amiodarone (in a new aqueous formulation) for incessant ventricular tachycardia. *Am J Cardiol.* 2002;90(8):853–859.

45. Dorian P, Cass D, et al. Amiodarone as compared with lidocaine for shock-resistant ventricular fibrillation. *N Engl J Med.* 2002;346(12):884–890.

46. Vukmir RB, Katz L. Sodium bicarbonate improves outcome in prolonged prehospital cardiac arrest. *Am J Emer Med.* 2006;24(2):156–161.

47. Vukmir RB, Bircher N, et al. Sodium bicarbonate in cardiac arrest: a reappraisal. *Am J Emerg Med.* 1996;14(2):192–206.

48. Moon SW, Lee SW, et al. Arterial minus end-tidal CO_2 as a prognostic factor of hospital survival in patients resuscitated from cardiac arrest. *Resuscitation.* 2007;72(2):219–225.

49. Arawwawala D, Brett SJ. Clinical review: beyond immediate survival from resuscitation-long-term outcome considerations after cardiac arrest. *Crit Care.* 2007;11(6):235.

50. Steiner LA, Balestreri M, et al. Predicting the response of intracranial pressure to moderate hyperventilation. *Acta Neurochir (Wien).* 2005;147(5):477–483; discussion 483.

51. Oertel M, Kelly DF, et al. Efficacy of hyperventilation, blood pressure elevation, and metabolic suppression therapy in controlling intracranial pressure after head injury. *J Neurosurg.* 2002;97(5):1045–1053.

52. Ramaraj R. Mild therapeutic hypothermia in patients after out-of-hospital cardiac arrest due to acute ST-segment elevation myocardial infarction. *Crit Care Med.* 2008;36(12):3280.

53. Foex BA, Butler J. Best evidence topic report. Therapeutic hypothermia after out of hospital cardiac arrest. *Emerg Med J.* 2004;21(5):590–591.

54. O'Brien E, Hendricks D, et al. Field termination of resuscitation: analysis of a newly implemented protocol. *Prehosp Emerg Care.* 2008;12(1):57–61.

CHAPTER 8

DISORDERS OF OXYGENATION

KEY CONCEPTS:

Upon completion of this chapter, it is expected that the reader will understand these following concepts:

- That respiratory failure results from the lungs' inability to diffuse oxygen into the blood
- The environmental, pulmonary, and cardiovascular causes for respiratory failure
- How treatment is aimed at improving diffusion while addressing the cause of respiratory failure

ANATOMY CONCEPTS:

Prior to reading this chapter the Paramedic student should be familiar with the following anatomy and physiology concepts:

- Respiratory gasses
- Gas exchange
- Alveolar capillary functions

The radio crackles to life: "Unit 24, respond to Wellspring Nursing Home for an 86-year-old male with shortness of breath." As the Paramedics arrive at the facility, the nursing supervisor briefs the crew as they make their way to Mr. Wilcox's room.

CRITICAL THINKING QUESTIONS

1. What are some of the possible causes of shortness of breath for an elderly male?
2. How is the fact that the patient is in a nursing home related to his trouble breathing?

OVERVIEW

Many people view suffocation with feelings of panic and fear. Oxygen is crucial to life; therefore, having it taken away is naturally a cause for concern. These concerns reflect the result of hypoxia, the inability of the respiratory system to get life-giving oxygen to the cells. By definition, this is called respiratory failure.

Chief Concern

Type I respiratory failure is the inability of the lungs to diffuse adequate oxygen into the blood. Type I respiratory failure, sometimes termed hypoxemic respiratory failure, is distinguished by a partial oxygen pressure (PaO_2) of less than 60 mmHg in the blood (**hypoxemia**).[1] Type I respiratory failure is sometimes termed hypoxemic respiratory failure. The etiology of Type I respiratory failure usually occurs because of structural damage to the patient's pulmonary tree (obstruction of a sufficient portion of the alveoli which in turn reduces arterial oxygenation) and/or blockage of the pulmonary circulation, which prevents diffusion of oxygen into the blood (Table 8-1).

Generally, elevated carbon dioxide levels are *not* appreciated in Type I respiratory failure, since even a small percentage of the functioning portion of the residual lungs is all that is necessary to excrete carbon dioxide. However, prolonged hypoxemia leads to respiratory fatigue. As a result, the patient's struggling respiratory efforts subsequently result in elevated carbon dioxide levels (hypercarbia) in the terminal stages of respiratory failure.

Respiratory Gasses

Type I respiratory failure is primarily a failure of gas exchange, specifically oxygen. Therefore, to understand Type I respiratory failure, it is important for the Paramedic to understand pulmonary gas exchange.

Ambient air is primarily made up of nitrogen (78%) and oxygen (20.98%). According to **Dalton's law**, the sum of partial pressures of each gas equals the total pressure of the gas mixture. Thus, if the total pressure of air at sea level, called the barometric pressure, is 760 mmHg, then the partial pressure of oxygen (at sea level) must be 160 mmHg (760 mmHg × 21% = 160 mmHg).

In the lungs, the partial pressure of oxygen contained in the venous blood is less than 160 mmHg. In fact, the partial

Table 8-1 Origins of Hypoxemic Respiratory Failure

- Emphysema
- Pulmonary edema
- Pulmonary embolism
- Acute asthma
- Pneumothorax

pressure of oxygen in venous pulmonary blood is approximately 70 to 100 mmHg, depending on the body's oxygen demand. The net difference between the two pressures (160 mmHg − 100 mmHg = 60 mmHg) creates a **pressure gradient**. This pressure gradient will result in a movement of gas from one area of high pressure to another area of lower pressure, via diffusion.

Note the inclusion of the condition "at sea level." If the patient is on the summit of a mountain at a height greater than 5,500 m, then barometric pressure would be one-half of that pressure at sea level, or 80 mmHg. A patient at that height might experience severe hypoxia and mountain sickness.

Other factors, such as temperature and acidity of the blood, also impact oxygen transfer. The impact of these additional factors, as well as the relationship between the partial pressure of oxygen and the saturation of hemoglobin by oxygen, is illustrated by an oxyhemoglobin curve (Figure 8-1).

Oxyhemoglobin Curve

Oxygen dissociates, or is released, from hemoglobin (Hb) whenever the oxygen concentration is low and a gradient exists, such as in the peripheral capillary beds where oxygen demand is the greatest. The availability of oxygen from hemoglobin is partly owed to the attraction that hemoglobin—specifically the binding of oxygen to the iron in the hemoglobin—had for oxygen when the hemoglobin was in the lungs.

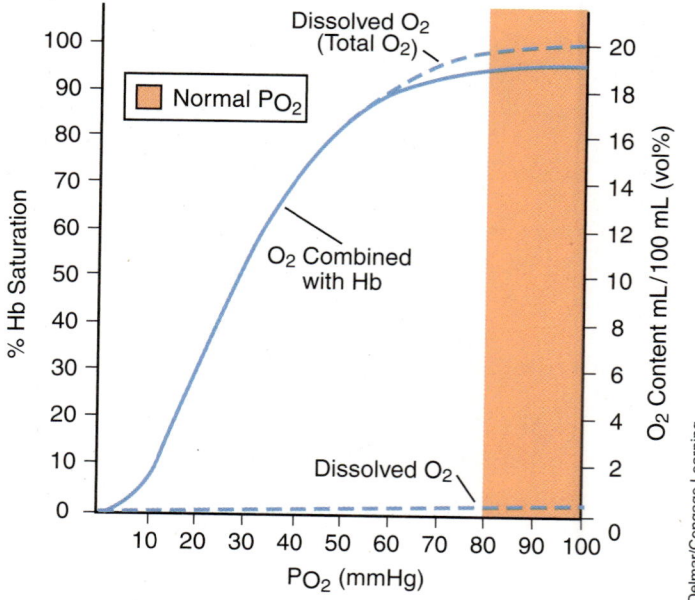

Figure 8-1 Oxyhemoglobin curve.

This **affinity** of oxygen for hemoglobin, the tendency to chemically react with and bind to hemoglobin in an endothermic redox reaction, can be affected by temperature and acid, as well as partial pressure of oxygen in the alveoli.[2] An increased temperature (e.g., as occurs during a fever) will decrease the affinity of oxygen for hemoglobin, shown by a shift of the hemoglobin curve to the right. Hypothermia will increase affinity and cause the curve to shift to the left.

In practical terms, the hemoglobin of the patient with a fever, read as a rightward shift of the oxyhemoglobin curve, will have a decreased affinity for oxygen, thus making it harder for the oxygen to bind to the hemoglobin. However, this condition makes it easier for the hemoglobin to release oxygen at the cellular level. In short, the tissues become much more effective at extracting oxygen from the blood, thus creating a larger difference in the alveolar oxygen gradient. This increased gradient helps to overcome the decreased affinity that oxygen has for the hemoglobin in the alveoli, ensuring the body gets the needed oxygen.

This tradeoff—increased oxygen gradient to overcome decreased affinity—has its limitations. Without supplemental oxygen, the patient will soon become hypoxic. Similarly, if the patient has acidosis (low pH) the oxyhemoglobin curve will shift to the right as well; this is known as the **Bohr effect**. Increased carbon dioxide, as seen in Type II respiratory failure, will also cause a rightward shift in the oxyhemoglobin curve.

Therefore, acidosis and hyperthermia cause oxygen dumping at the tissue level. Yet, these conditions also make it more difficult for hemoglobin to pick up oxygen at the alveolar level. To overcome the oxyhemoglobin shift to the right, the Paramedic must increase the partial pressure of oxygen through administration of higher-concentration oxygen (FiO_2). Failure to administer high-flow, high-concentration oxygen can result in tissue hypoxia and Type I respiratory failure.

PaO_2

A small percentage of oxygen is dissolved directly into the plasma, represented as **PaO_2**, and is a reflection of the partial pressure of oxygen in the blood. The PaO_2 is obtained by drawing an arterial blood sample and performing an arterial blood gas.

The importance of dissolved oxygen in the plasma, represented by the value PaO_2, should not be understated. In cases where there is a shortage of hemoglobin (e.g., due to hemorrhage) or where hemoglobin is bound by poisons (such as cyanide), increasing the percentage of oxygen delivered, via a nonrebreather mask, increases the amount of oxygen dissolved in blood plasma.

For example, an increase of the partial pressure of oxygen found in room air (160 mmHg) to the partial pressure of high-flow, high-concentration oxygen (706 mmHg) from a nonrebreather mask can have a dramatic impact on the volume of dissolved oxygen in the patient's blood. While this mechanism is not as effective as hemoglobin in transporting oxygen, it can be useful as a temporizing measure until more effective treatments can be instituted.

Total Oxygen Content

The total oxygen content of the blood, represented by the symbol CaO_2, is a combination of the amount of oxygen carried in hemoglobin, which can be measured by pulse oximetry, and the amount of oxygen dissolved in blood, measured in arterial blood gasses.[3]

Differential Diagnosis

The best approach to understanding the etiology of Type I respiratory failure is to take an outside to inside approach: It starts with oxygen in the atmosphere, then moves in through passage of oxygen into the lungs (ventilation), and then continues through diffusion of oxygen at the alveolar–capillary interface (respiration).

Whenever the fraction of inspired oxygen is low, decreased FiO_2, then hypoxia, may ensue. Common causes of low inspired oxygen include oxygen-poor environments (displacing gasses) and high altitudes. Classic examples of oxygen-poor environments include confined spaces such as manholes, holds of ships, and grain silos. Any environment that has less than 17% oxygen in the atmosphere should be considered an oxygen-poor environment. Individuals in these environments risk unconsciousness secondary to hypoxia and may have only minutes to escape the area (time of useful consciousness).

The density of a gas determines whether it is lighter than or heavier than air. In cases in which the gas is heavier than air (e.g., propane), the gas will displace oxygen, thus creating an oxygen-poor environment. The list of lighter than air gasses (aerosols) is short (Table 8-2). It can therefore be assumed that most other gasses are heavier than air and will displace oxygen. This is especially so in a confined space and can rapidly lead to hypoxia in the patient and a resultant loss of consciousness.

Table 8-2 Partial List of Lighter than Air Gasses

Acronym: 4H MEDIC ANNA	
H	Hydrogen
HC	Hydrogen cyanide
He	Helium
HF	Hydrogen fluoride
M	Methane
E	Ethylene
D	Diborane
I	Illuminating gasses (natural gas)
CO	Carbon monoxide
A	Acetylene
N	Neon
N	Nitrogen
A	Ammonia

High altitudes also reduce the oxygen available for diffusion in the lungs, as previously explained. Although there is not a true loss of oxygen, the percentage remains 21% (the change in barometric pressure), and thus the partial pressures result in a relative loss of available oxygen.

The second cause of alveolar hypoventilation can be barriers in the pulmonary tree, such as a foreign body airway obstruction. These causes actually create a Type II respiratory failure.

Other causes of alveolar hypoventilation are extrapulmonary. A classic example of an extrapulmonary cause of alveolar hypoventilation is an opiate overdose. An opiate overdose stimulates the μ receptors in the medulla and therefore suppresses respiration, which can lead to hypoxia.

Hypoxia from Type I respiratory failure should not be confused with other extrapulmonary causes of hypoxia such as hypermetabolic states or hypoperfusion, to name but two. In those cases, the lungs are functional; other circumstances have intervened to produce the hypoxia.

The third, and perhaps the most common, cause of Type I respiratory failure is impairment of the alveolar–capillary interface. The injury may be on the alveolar side of the interface or on the capillary side.

A common cause of impairment on the alveolar side of the interface is the development of pneumonia. Pneumonia acts as a physical barrier to gas exchange and physically displaces alveolar gas.[4,5] Functionally, pneumonia acts to increase **dead space**, that area in the lungs where gas does not exchange. This effectively removes whole portions of the lung from pulmonary function.

STREET SMART

A clot is made up of a cast of the blood clotting constituents. For example, when a pool of blood sets outside of the body a formed mass called a clot is created. A clot does not adhere to blood vessel walls and has a red currant jelly look. A thrombus, on the other hand, is a product of platelet adhesion to the inside of the blood vessel; in other words, it is a function of the coagulation cascade. A thrombus is often created due to injury or inflammation of the blood vessel in order to protect the blood vessel. Because the thrombus adheres to the blood vessel wall, portions of the thrombus can be torn off, becoming emboli, and float downstream. However, in common lay terms people often use clot and thrombus interchangeably.

Alternatively, the impairment can be on the capillary side of the interface. The pulmonary artery supplies the pulmonary capillaries with blood. An occlusion of the pulmonary artery by a blood thrombus or other obstacle is called a **pulmonary embolism (PE)**.

Pulmonary Embolism

Whenever an obstruction occurs in the pulmonary vasculature there is going to be a loss of respiration. Even though the lungs can tolerate a relatively large loss of function and still exhale enough carbon dioxide to maintain homeostasis, the lungs are unable to accommodate an even minor loss of functional lung without a dramatic impact on oxygenation.

There are a number of etiologies for pulmonary embolism, which can be remembered by the mnemonic FACCT (Table 8-3).

The F in FACCT stands for **F**at embolism from a fracture. When trauma occurs to a long bone, especially the femur, fat from within the bone (a substance resembling mercury or quick silver) can occasionally be seen among the bone fragments. This fat can also travel up the venous circulation and into the lungs, creating a pulmonary embolism in the process.[6–9]

The A in FACCT stands for an **A**ir embolism. An air embolism can occur when a neck wound is open to the environment. When the patient takes a breath in, creating a negative inspiratory pressure, air is drawn into the neck wound.

An air embolism can also occur during a diving emergency. In this situation, known as decompression sickness (DCS), air bubbles come out of solution during ascent from a deep dive.

In addition, an air embolism can occur when air is inadvertently injected into the bloodstream during intravenous access. The resulting venous air embolism is an iatrogenic complication of venous access. While a predominant cause of venous air embolism is central venous catheterization, other sources include high pressure mechanical ventilation and venous access during hemodialysis.

Childbirth, the C in FACCT, presents another source of embolism: amniotic fluid. During childbirth, amniotic fluid may inadvertently mix with maternal blood. Amniotic fluid is thought to be insoluble in blood and therefore creates an embolism that floats via the venous circulation into the pulmonary vasculature.[10–12] An amniotic fluid embolism (AFE) is a rare event.[13] Therefore, the Paramedic should consider other potential causes of hypoxia, profound hypotension, and dyspnea (such as internal hemorrhage) first.

Table 8-3 FACCT and Pulmonary Embolism

F	Fat embolism
A	Air embolism
C	Childbirth
C	Cancer
T	Thrombus

In the past, women taking oral contraceptives were at risk for PE, especially if the woman smoked cigarettes as well. Modern formulations of oral birth control, using lower doses of estrogen, have mitigated this hazard to some degree; however, it is still a risk.

Obesity is another risk factor for PE. Obesity is a national epidemic with a multitude of complications which accompany the condition; this is discussed in detail in Chapter 31 on bariatric medicine. Obese patients are also prone to PE secondary to peripheral insufficiency and venous stasis in the dependent limbs. Prolonged immobility in oversized chairs can cause a greater tendency to develop PE.

Cancer, the other C in FACCT, is also a risk factor for PE. On occasion, small clumps of cancer cells will break off from a tumor and float into the pulmonary vasculature, thereby creating a pulmonary embolism. Both lung and pancreatic cancer have been implicated in these pulmonary embolisms. However, current thinking suggests the problem may lie with hypercoagulability. **Hypercoagulability** is a state of increased tendency for **T**hrombus formation, the T in FACCT. Hypercoagulability in cancer patients may be owed to cancer therapies, such as radiation and chemotherapy, which on occasion activate the complement system as well as the coagulation cascade.

Thrombus

The most common source of pulmonary embolism is venous thromboembolism. Venous thromboembolism (VTE) occurs in approximately 15% of all PE. Factors thought to contribute to the formation of VTE, known collectively as **Virchow's triad**, are venous stasis (stagnant blood), a state of hypercoagulability, and inflammation or injury of the endothelial wall inside a vein.

The key to VTE may be hypercoagulability. Hypercoagulation states may be owed to deficiencies of vitamin C, either in diet or digestion; deficiency of antithrombin elements; blood disorders (dyscrasias) which include polycythemia, thrombocytopenia, and so on; and the use of estrogen.

Predisposing conditions for Virchow's triad include prolonged immobilization, obesity, and pregnancy. Medical bedrest is such a frequent source of PE that clinicians order special treatments, such as antiembolic stockings, alternating compression leg wraps, and heparin injections, to prevent PE from developing in patients.

Other conditions of prolonged immobilization, such as intercontinental air flights, increase the risk for PE. In fact, any situation in which a person sits with a bent knee for a prolonged period of time can cause a **deep vein thrombus (DVT)**. DVT can form in any of the deep veins of the legs, femoral or popliteal, or even the pelvic veins. DVTs are prone to form when blood flow from the lower extremities is hindered (e.g., by a bent leg).

There are no site-specific signs of a DVT. Generally the lower extremity, particularly the calf, becomes reddened, swollen, and painful to touch. Dilation of surface veins may also be appreciated as venous return attempts to bypass the obstruction using collateral circulation.

While the hospital clinician may actually measure the circumference of the calf at its midpoint and compare the measurement to the other calf, the Paramedic need only examine the patient's leg by grasping both calves approximately 10 cm below the tibial tuberosity and make a gross estimation of the equality in size of the two calves. If one calf feels physically larger, and the affected limb is painful and/or reddened, then the Paramedic should suspect the presence of a DVT.

Homans' sign, pain in the back of the knee with dorsiflexion of the foot on the affected side, has long been considered a cardinal sign of DVT. Although recent studies showing a false positive in 50% of patients without DVT make its reliability questionable, testing for Homans' sign remains standard in most DVT examinations (Figure 8-2).[14-16]

Various signs and symptoms are associated with a DVT, classified by the Scarvelis and Wells criteria (Table 8-4). The presence of two or more of these signs or symptoms should lead the Paramedic to a strong index of suspicion that a DVT may exist.

DVT occurs in about 1 hospitalized patient per 100 annually. Furthermore, approximately 1% to 5% of those patients

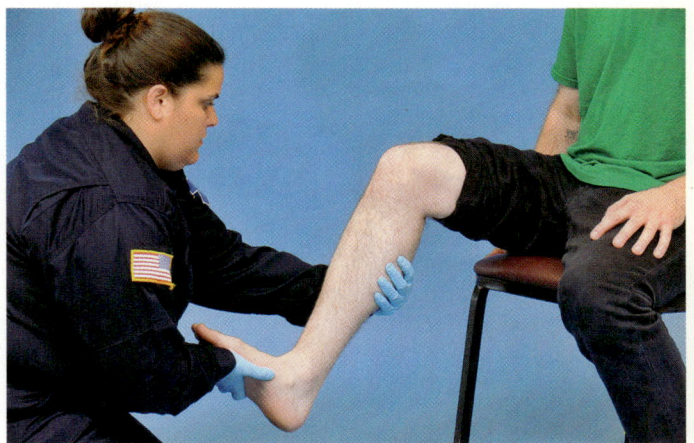

Figure 8-2 Testing for Homans' sign.

Table 8-4 Modified Scarvelis and Wells DVT Criteria

- Cancer under care
- Calf swelling (>3 cm)
- Cast over fracture
- Contraceptive use (birth control pill)
- Distended surface veins
- DVT in past medical history
- Pitting edema to affected limb
- Point tenderness in affected area
- Paralysis of limb
- Prolonged immobilization

will develop PE. While this percentage may not appear impressive, consider that 60% of PEs occur because of an embolus from a DVT. Therefore, a patient with a symptom complex indicative of PE should be examined for signs of a DVT.

Approximately 600,000 cases of PE occur annually in the United States, mostly in healthcare settings. Of those PE cases, approximately 1 in 10 (60,000) will lead to patient death.

Pulmonary Embolism Symptom Complex

The traditional triad of symptoms that indicate PE in a patient includes unexplained dyspnea, pleuritic type chest pain, and hemoptysis (Figure 8-3). Together these three signs are strongly suggestive of PE,[17] although individually they are less supportive of the suspicion of the disorder.

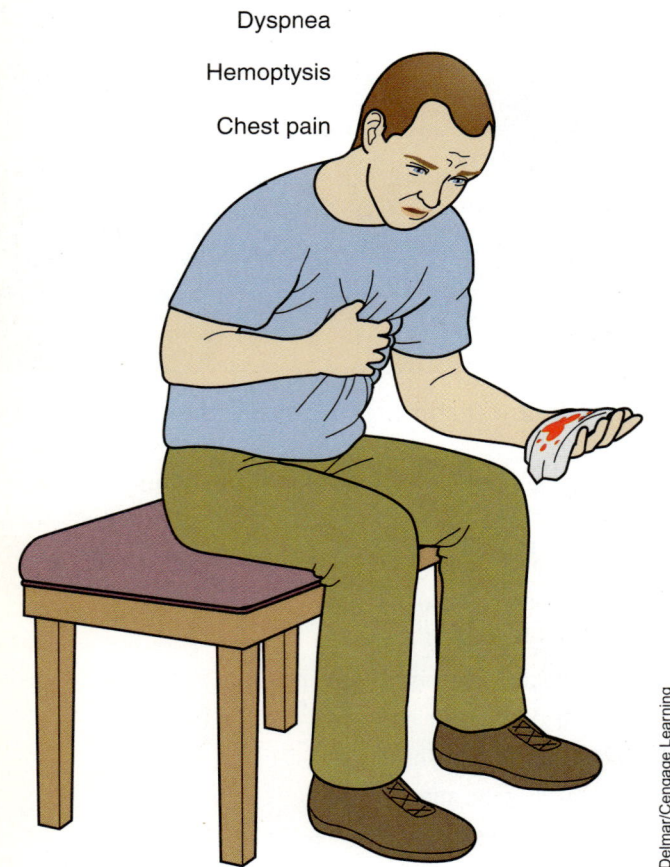

Dyspnea

Hemoptysis

Chest pain

Delmar/Cengage Learning

Figure 8-3 Triad of pulmonary embolism: dyspnea, chest pain, and hemoptysis.

The first sign, unexplained dyspnea and associated tachypnea, is evident in approximately three-quarters of patients with PE. However, shortness of breath is a constitutional sign (a sign suggestive of a number of other disorders and diseases) and therefore is not specific to PE.

Similarly, pleuritic type chest pain (pain that increases with deep inspiration without evidence of trauma) is common in patients with PE, occurring in approximately two-thirds of cases. However, pleuritic type chest pain is not specific to PE alone.

The last sign in the triad, hemoptysis (coughing up blood), is suggestive of PE but it is also suggestive of bronchitis, lung cancer, tuberculosis, and other more obscure etiologies. Furthermore, hemoptysis is only seen in approximately 13% of patients with PE. The more common sign, seen in over one-third of patients with PE, is a nonproductive cough.

12-Lead Electrocardiogram and Pulmonary Embolism

Paramedics follow the maxim that all pain from the nose to the navel is cardiac until proven otherwise. Therefore, the diagnosis of acute coronary syndrome must be considered even when there is a strong index of suspicion that the patient may be experiencing a pulmonary embolism. A prudent Paramedic should perform a 12-lead ECG in this case.

If the patient is experiencing a PE, the 12-lead ECG may show signs of right heart strain, or even acute cor pulmonale, with a large S wave in Lead I, Q wave in Lead III, and an inverted T wave in Lead III. This pattern, S1Q3T3, is seen in roughly 20% of PE cases.[18,19]

Regardless of the eventual diagnosis—PE or ACS—the patient may be a candidate for fibrinolytic therapy. The Paramedic should consider completing a fibrinolytic checklist in preparation for the hospital treatment.

V-Q̇ Mismatch

The key to successful oxygenation is the diffusion of oxygen across the alveolar–capillary membrane. If diffusion is disturbed then hypoxia will ensue. The two key components for diffusion are alveolar ventilation and pulmonary capillary perfusion. Therefore, hypoxia will occur when either alveolar ventilation or pulmonary capillary perfusion is disturbed.

There is typically a one-to-one relationship between the alveoli and the pulmonary capillaries. For illustrative purposes, the quotient one (1) is used to represent that alveolar ventilation is matched with a capillary in a 1:1 fashion. This is referred to as the ventilation to perfusion or **V-Q̇ match**.

If there is a mismatch, either due to less ventilation or loss of perfusion, then the patient is said to have a V-Q̇ mismatch (Figure 8-4). Any interference with either alveolar ventilation or capillary perfusion will result in blood passing by the lungs without becoming oxygenated, a process called **shunting**.

In a normal person, less than 10% of the blood volume passes through the lung fields without being oxygenated. **Atelectasis** is the failure of the alveoli to expand naturally

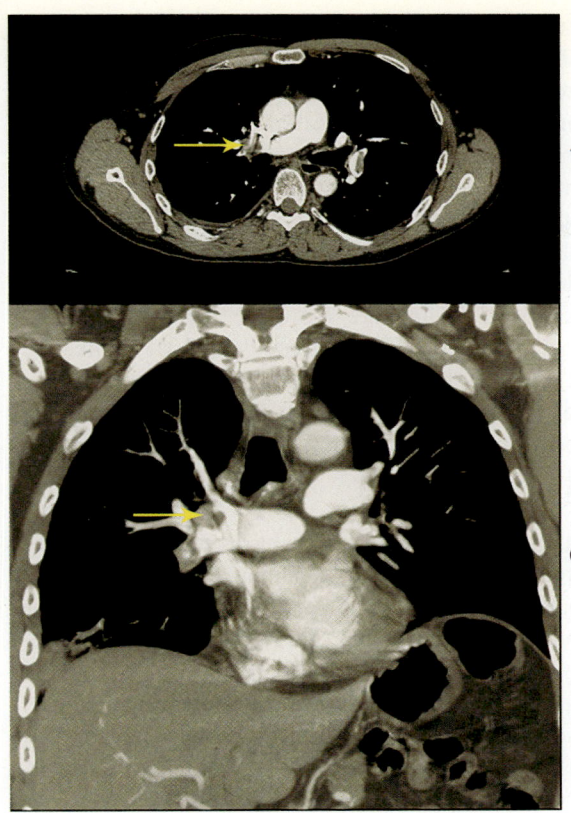

Figure 8-4 V-Q̇ mismatch in this patient is caused by the large pulmonary embolism seen on this CT scan of the chest (arrow).

Transverse

Coronal

Delmar/Cengage Learning

during inhalation. The base of the lungs is one of the most common locations of atelectasis. Basilar atelectasis is usually due to the abdomen compressing the base of the lungs. When the patient is asked to take a deep breath, or simply sigh, the rales (crackles) heard at the base of the lungs clear, indicating that the alveoli have been reinflated.

When the patient shunts more than 30% of his blood volume past the lung (representing a loss of one-third of the lung's capacity), then high-flow, high-concentration oxygen may not be able to reverse the hypoxia.

Treatment of Pulmonary Embolism

Symptoms of a pulmonary embolism can range from mild shortness of breath to cardiac arrest. A patient's survival from a PE is dependent on the Paramedic having a high index of suspicion that a PE may exist based on clinical presentation and aggressive treatment while en route to the hospital.

A cardinal sign of PE is persistent hypoxia (Type I respiratory failure) despite the administration of high-flow, high-concentration oxygen. Paramedics tend to rely on pulse oximetry (discussed in detail shortly) for estimations of oxygenation. These levels will remain relatively unchanged despite the administration of high-flow, high-concentration oxygen. However, high-flow, high-concentration oxygen should continue to be administered in any case despite the limited improvement of oxygen saturations. Additional oxygen is

being provided to the patient's body in the form of oxygen dissolved in plasma. This small addition to the blood's oxygen-carrying capacity may make a significant difference.

Survival for patients with a PE may be improved with administration of fibrinolytics in the hospital. The Paramedic should establish intravenous access and consider drawing blood samples. Hospital lab studies will include coagulation studies as well as studies for organ function, renal function, and liver enzymes.

The presentation of a patient with syncope, profound hypotension, and refractory hypoxia is ominous and suggests the presence of a saddle embolism. A **saddle embolism** is a large embolus that straddles the bifurcation of the pulmonary artery. As a result, there is a sudden loss of venous return, loss of preload, and a dramatic drop in cardiac output. The end result of a saddle embolism is often profound hypotension followed by cardiac arrest. Pulmonary embolism is the second most common cause of unexpected sudden death, behind sudden cardiac death.

Pneumonia

Noted physician William Osler called pneumonia the "old man's friend," referring to the disease as a common exit from mortal life for the elderly. Throughout history, pneumonia has been responsible for illness and death; in fact, in the 1900s pneumonia was one of the top three causes of death in the United States. Since that time, and with the advent of antibiotics and improvements in medical care, the death rates from pneumonia have dropped. It is now the eighth leading cause of death overall in the United States.

Pneumonia occurs whenever a microorganism (microbe) causes an infection (a discussion of these microorganisms follows shortly). Certain conditions that involve the loss of respiratory defenses can predispose a person to pneumonia. For example, pneumonia is more likely if the patient has aspirated. Aspiration, secondary to loss of airway control, can be caused by a number of factors including alcohol poisoning, stroke, or head injury. Aspiration pneumonia is more common in the elderly, the infirmed, and the inebriate.

Pneumonia can also be the result of exposure to chemicals (industrial, agricultural, or household). Chemicals found within the smoke of a cigarette, for example, can paralyze the cilia and bring the mucociliary escalator to a standstill. Cigarette smoke also tends to block the patient's cough reflex, further adding to the collection of mucus within the airways and creating the perfect breeding ground for microbes.

Geriatric patients are especially prone to **community acquired pneumonia (CAP)** because their mucociliary escalators are less effective and their immune systems are weakened. These patients, living in adult care facilities and the like, are exposed to bacteria that are highly virulent and resistant to certain antibiotics. As many as 2 to 5 million cases of CAP occur in the United States annually, and 30% of these patients will require hospitalization. The prevalence of CAP and its associated complications has helped make pneumonia the fourth or fifth (depending on race) leading cause of death among the elderly.

Etiology

The common thread in all pneumonia is the presence of an infectious microbe. Microbes are categorized as fungal, bacterial, or viral. Any microbes within these classifications are capable of producing pneumonia under the right conditions, from protozoa to viruses; however, some microbes are more likely than others to produce pneumonia.

For example, the yeast-like fungal infection pneumocystis jirovecii, formerly known as pneumocystis carinii, is more likely to seed in the patient who has been immunocompromised by the human immunodeficiency virus (HIV). Pneumocystis carinii pneumonia (PCP), identified early in the AIDS/HIV epidemic as an opportunistic infection among AIDS patients, can also occur in patients following organ transplant and in those who are being treated with immunosuppressive medications.

Viruses are also capable of causing pneumonia. Symptoms such as a dry cough, headache, and fever (flu-like symptoms) in a child may signal the start of respiratory syncytial virus (RSV) pneumonia. In fact, the majority of pneumonia cases in children, including influenza and adenovirus as well as RSV, are caused by viruses.

Severe Acute Respiratory Syndrome (SARS)

During the winter of 2002, in the Guangdong province of the People's Republic of China, a corona virus crossed over from an infection of either civets (a cat-like creature) or bats to infect humans. This corona virus was the source of severe acute respiratory syndrome (SARS). Like other zoonotic diseases before it—such as anthrax, Lyme disease, and plague—SARS struck a human population which had no protection, or natural immunity, to it.

Since SARS is transmitted from person to person, and with the advent of people travelling by jet, SARS quickly moved out of the Guangdong province to such locations as Toronto, Canada, where it caused over 8,096 cases and resulting in 774 deaths.[20-22] Its impact on the EMS community in Toronto served as an example of the dangers inherent in EMS. Over 850 Paramedics experienced approximately 1,115 exposures to patients with SARS, resulting in 436 Paramedics being held in home quarantine. During home quarantine, these Paramedics had to wear N95 masks to limit the spread of the disease and have their temperature taken twice a day. Despite these precautions, 62 Paramedics developed SARS-like illness and four required hospitalization. Fortunately, there were no fatalities among the Paramedics. Nonetheless, this case illustrates the need for vigilance around patients with respiratory symptoms.

Walking Pneumonia

A persistent severe cough, sometimes leading to coughing fits, that produces scant amounts of white sputum is consistent with the diagnosis of walking pneumonia. As the name implies, **walking pneumonia** is an incessant pneumonia that is not so debilitating as to require bedrest, although it is incapacitating, has a protracted recovery, and is often resistant to antibiotic therapy.

Walking pneumonia, also referred to as **primary atypical pneumonia (PAP)**, is often due to an infection of mycoplasma pneumoniae and affects primarily young adults. Mycoplasma pneumoniae is similar to a bacterium but lacks the bacterium's cell wall. It belongs to the class of microbes called mollicutes, the smallest independent microorganisms. Many antibiotics, such as penicillin, interfere with cell wall synthesis of bacteria and are therefore ineffective against mycoplasma pneumonia. It is estimated that 20% of the cases of walking pneumonia may be due to mycoplasma pneumonia and that outbreaks tend to occur in the fall. Fortunately, walking pneumonia has a very low mortality rate.

Bacterial Pneumonia

Bacteria, microorganisms that are abundant in the environment, are responsible for a large percentage of pneumonias (Table 8-5). For example, pneumococcal pneumonia is responsible for the largest percentage of bacterial pneumonias.[23-26] Over 35% of community acquired pneumonias are due to this gram-positive bacterium, formerly known as diplococcus pneumoniae because of its characteristic pairing of the sphere-like bacteria in cultures.

Pneumococcal pneumonia is responsible for over 175,000 patient hospitalizations in the United States annually and as many as 40,000 deaths. Pneumococcus can also lead to infections of the blood (bacteremias), as well as meningitis, with deadly results.

Currently there is a vaccine for pneumococcus, pneumonoccal polysaccharide vaccine (PPV23), which is effective against 23 of the 80 known serotypes of pneumococcus. Vaccination with PPV23 decreases the likelihood of pneumonia and meningitis, but it is not a perfect cure. Research continues in an effort to try to improve the vaccine.

Table 8-5 Other Pneumonia-Causing Bacteria

- Legionella pneumophila
  - Causative agent for Legionnaire's disease
  - More likely to strike patients over 50 years of age
- Haemophilus influenzae
  - Major causative agent of CAP
  - Decreased incidence with advent of Haemophilus influenzae conjugate vaccine (Hib)
- Human parainfluenza viruses (HPIV)
  - Also known as common cold
  - Causative agent in croup
  - Second to RSV for pneumonia in children
- Klebsiella, seen in alcoholics
- Chlamydia pneumonia
  - Proposed name: chalamydophila pneumoniae to prevent confusion with the STD chlamydia

Streptococcus pneumoniae, another gram-positive diplococcus, is a common agent causing pneumonia. Streptococcus, a frequent cause of ear infections (otitis media), acute sinusitis, endocarditis, and even pericarditis, often causes pneumonia after the patient has been weakened by a viral infection. In fact, streptococcus pneumoniae is part of the normal nasal flora in 5% to 10% of adults, and operates as a potential pathogen waiting for a weakness in the patient in order to flourish.

Drug-Resistant Streptococcus Pneumoniae

The virulence of streptococcus pneumoniae is owed to a number of factors. Among these is a polysaccharide capsule that is resistant to phagocytosis by white blood cells, including alveolar macrophages.

This resistance can be overcome by the antibiotic penicillin (PCN), discovered in 1928 by Sir Alexander Fleming. During World War II, penicillin was used widely to prevent infections in wounded soldiers as well as to combat gonorrhea (which was rampant at the time). Penicillin, and the next several generations of penicillins including penicillin G, penicillin V, and the semisynthetic ampicillin, dicloxacillin, and amoxicillin, were all effective against the beta-lactamase-producing streptococcus pneumoniae; without ß lactamase, bacterial cell walls are weakened.

Unfortunately, indiscriminate prescription of penicillins and noncompliant patients have led to the emergence of methicillin-resistant staphylococcus aureus (MRSA) and drug-resistant streptococcus pneumoniae (DRSP). Seven specific serotypes of streptococcus pneumoniae have become drug resistant.

Fortunately, the use of PPV23 has decreased the overall number of cases of streptococcus pneumoniae and correspondingly lowered the number of cases of DRSP. Paramedics, as part of their personal wellness plan, should consider being vaccinated with PPV23, not only for their personal wellness but also to prevent the spread of disease to patients under their care.

Penicillin Allergy

Many patients report an allergy to penicillin. In fact, an allergic reaction may occur in up to 10% of patients.[27,28] Fortunately, true anaphylaxis occurs in less than 0.01% of these patients. Unfortunately, with the large number of antibiotics similar to penicillin, cross-sensitivity is a possibility. Whenever a patient is on any antibiotic, a penicillin allergy should be highlighted in the patient's record.

CASE STUDY (CONTINUED)

The nurse explains that Mr. Wilcox is status post stroke and just returned from the hospital after being treated for a hip fracture. "This morning he didn't seem right. His blood pressure was down, he has a fever, and more importantly his oxygen saturation was 88%. We spoke to his doctor, who ordered 2 liters oxygen by nasal prongs. The doctor then requested that the patient be transported to the hospital for a chest X-ray."

CRITICAL THINKING QUESTIONS

1. What are the important elements of the patient's history that a Paramedic should obtain?
2. What is the symptom pattern for suspected nosocomial pneumonia?

History

The history of Type I respiratory failure primarily focuses on the Paramedic trying to ascertain the symptom complex (i.e., cough, chills, smoking history, activity at onset, etc.). Once the symptom complex is in hand, the Paramedic can compare it to a symptom pattern of common causes of respiratory failure and ascertain a diagnosis.

Pneumonia

The classic symptom complex associated with pneumonia is fever, cough, and shortness of breath, although there are other associated symptoms worth investigating. Patients suspected of having pneumonia will often complain of shortness of breath (dyspnea) even when placed on high-flow, high-concentration oxygen as a result of their persistent hypoxia.

The presence of a fever tends to compound the problem of hypoxia in patients by shifting the oxyhemoglobin curve to the right, making it harder for oxygen to on-load at the alveolar level. Paramedics who have the capability should record the patient's temperature as part of the vital signs and then appreciate the impact that fever has on the oxygen saturation.

Fever, an increase in the body's temperature due to a change in the thermoregulatory set point located in the hypothalamus, may be the result of pyrogens released by the bacterial infection. **Pyrogens** are, by definition, fever-producing substances released within the body. In this case, pyrogens are released from bacteria in the lungs during phagocytosis by white blood cells (macrophages). The specific pyrogen is a lipopolysaccharide (LPS) found on the cell wall of the bacteria which is released during the bacteria's destruction (lysis).

At this point, the remnants of the bacteria are considered endotoxins. **Endotoxins** not only act as pyrogens but also activate the inflammatory response system. Endotoxins also cause the release of nitric oxide (NO), a potent vasodilator which in sufficient quantities can lead to massive vasodilation and septic shock.

Shaking chills are often associated with fever. These chills (the medical term is "rigors") occur because the thermoregulatory set point of the hypothalamus has been reset higher by pyrogens. As a result, the body, which is cooler, actively increases body temperature by shivering (shaking chills) until the new body temperature is met.

Chest pain is often associated with pneumonia as well. Unlike the chest pain of acute coronary syndrome, the chest pain of pneumonia is pleuritic in nature. Pleuritic chest pain is sharp and originates from the pleura of the lungs.[29] Pleuritic chest pain can be differentiated from other chest pains because it worsens with a deep breath and is often aggravated by a cough.

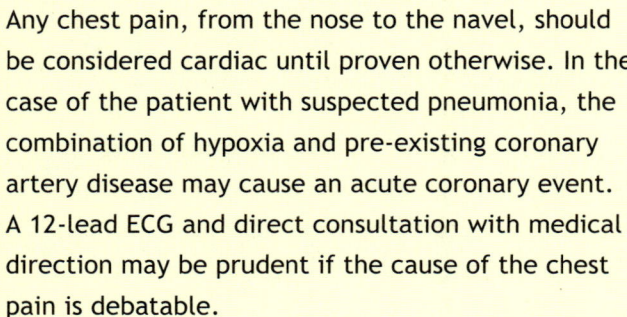

STREET SMART

Any chest pain, from the nose to the navel, should be considered cardiac until proven otherwise. In the case of the patient with suspected pneumonia, the combination of hypoxia and pre-existing coronary artery disease may cause an acute coronary event. A 12-lead ECG and direct consultation with medical direction may be prudent if the cause of the chest pain is debatable.

Productive Cough

A productive cough is the patient's effort at clearing the airway of secretions. The sudden, forceful expulsion of air clears the lower airways, as opposed to the sneeze which clears the upper airways. Coughing can be a single event but often is described as a series, or paroxysms, of coughs that leave the patient exhausted. These "fits" of coughing are usually involuntary. An acute onset of coughing is more suggestive of pneumonia.

Some patients will produce a rusty or greenish mucus in the sputum, indicating a bacterial infection. **Purulent sputum** (infectious secretions from the lungs) is actually drainage of the pneumonia. As pneumonia develops cellular debris, bacteria, and the like coalesce to form a pocket of pus called a **consolidation**. By its nature, a consolidation does not permit the exchange of gasses and leads to hypoxia. The patient's efforts to eliminate the consolidation, through a productive cough, are one defense mechanism which the body has against the bacterial invasion.

Some patients never have a productive cough yet still have pneumonia. A nonproductive cough can also be suggestive of many other disorders, including new onset pulmonary edema, asthma, and even a pulmonary embolism. Therefore, it should be noted in the medical record. A patient with a viral pneumonia, as well as patients with walking pneumonia, may be more prone to having a nonproductive cough.

Some patients also experience night sweats. While many people sweat at night, particularly women in menopause, **night sweats** (sweat that drenches the bedding and night clothes) is suggestive of an infectious process.

Other patients complain of unexplained weight loss. Such weight loss, in the case of pneumonia, is secondary to the increased metabolic demands placed upon the body by the infection.

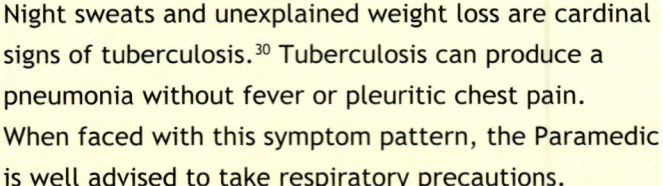

STREET SMART

Night sweats and unexplained weight loss are cardinal signs of tuberculosis.[30] Tuberculosis can produce a pneumonia without fever or pleuritic chest pain.

When faced with this symptom pattern, the Paramedic is well advised to take respiratory precautions.

Past Medical History

Aspiration is a common starting point for pneumonias. The past medical history should focus on the patient's risk of aspiration. Common events in which aspiration is a risk include past or present strokes, acute alcohol intoxication, and esophageal disorders including gastric esophageal reflux disease. Obese patients, as well as patients with sleep apnea, are prone to more occurrences of aspiration.

Once the infection has been seeded, it tends to proliferate in patients with weakened lungs or weakened immune systems. Patients with emphysema or chronic bronchitis are prone to pneumonias, as are patients with asthma. The combination of increased secretions, bronchospasms, and swelling of the airway tend to sequester secretions in the lungs, resulting in pneumonia.

Once the pneumonia has become established, it can flourish in patients with a weakened immune system. Patients with cancers, especially lymphoma and leukemia, as well as patients with diabetes are at particular risk for a severe pneumonia.

As a final point, those patients who are unable to "raise the sputum" are at greater risk for pneumonia. Patients with debilitating neuromuscular diseases that either diminish the muscles or affect the nerves—such as poliomyelitis, myasthenia gravis, and muscular dystrophy—are more prone to pneumonias.

In some cases, the patient is unable to raise the sputum because he is unwilling to breathe deeply for fear of inducing a coughing fit. Patients with recent abdominal, chest, or back surgeries often refuse to breathe deeply, even with the use of incentive spirometers, because of concerns about pain.

Use of opiates to relieve pain can help decrease patient anxiety and encourage deep breathing while also depressing respirations. The key to effective analgesic use is establishing a balance of pain management without respiratory depression. Overuse of opiates (such as fentanyl patches) can result in chronic hypoventilation and resultant pneumonia secondary to respiratory depression and atelectasis.

AMPLE

A careful medication history can help direct the Paramedic toward the correct diagnosis. The Paramedic can use the mnemonic AMPLE (Allergies, Medications, Past medical problems, Last oral intake, Events preceding the incident) as a guide when completing the patient's history. This information can be crucial in putting together a correct diagnosis.

For example, patients recently treated with macrolide antibiotics (such as azithromycin) or broad spectrum antibiotics (such as the class of fluoroquinolones) may have a community acquired pneumonia (CAP) that is resistant to these medications. Similarly, patients recently discharged from the hospital may have contracted a nosocomial infection, particularly if the patient was ventilator dependent while in the hospital.

CASE STUDY (CONTINUED)

From the doorway, the Paramedic notes that the patient appears pale and diaphoretic while lying in bed. His eyes are open yet not focusing on the Paramedic and he answers the nurse's questions with monosyllablic answers.

After introductions and a quick primary assessment, the Paramedic notes that the patient is drooling, which the nurse explains is a residual effect from his stroke. The nurse states that his lungs are "junky" at the apices and that he is tachypneic, tachycardic, and borderline hypotensive. The Paramedic's initial pulse oximetry readings are 88% on 4L nasal cannula.

CRITICAL THINKING QUESTIONS

1. What are the elements of the physical examination of a patient with suspected pneumonia?
2. Why is a chest X-ray a critical element for this patient?

Examination

The general impression a Paramedic may have from the pneumonia patient's doorway is of a patient who is ill. The combination of pallor (unnatural lack of color in the skin) and diaphoresis from the fever gives the patient the "sick look." Careful examination of the patient may reveal cyanosis as well.

After performing a primary assessment and addressing immediate life threats such as hypoxia, the Paramedic should obtain a thorough medical history. Based on this history, the Paramedic may begin to suspect the source of the patient's chief concern.

An assessment of breath sounds, particularly at the bases of the lungs as fluids flow downward, may reveal diminished breath sounds in areas of complete consolidation. If the infection has settled into the pleural space, then the collection of pus would be referred to as an **empyema**, a space occupying lesion which prevents the exchange of gasses and causes hypoxia. While a Paramedic cannot make that differentiation in the field, the result is the same.

Rales (crackles) at the bases can also be suggestive of pneumonia. These focal rales can be confused with the rales heard in pulmonary edema. However, pulmonary edema should be accompanied by the symptom complex associated with backward heart failure. This distinction is important as inappropriate treatment of pneumonia with furosemide, based on the presence of rales alone, has led to an increased mortality in those patients. The Paramedic should take the entire clinical picture into account before treating any patient. In other words, treatment should not be based upon a single assessment finding.

In cases of walking pneumonia and viral pneumonia, no rales may be appreciated at the bases. Therefore, the presence (or absence) of rales at the bases neither confirms nor denies a diagnosis of pneumonia.

In most instances, the patient with pneumonia will be hypermetabolic owing to the infection. Hypertension, tachycardia, and tachypnea, as well as a fever over 38°C (99°F), are common vital signs seen in patients with pneumonia (Table 8-6).

STREET SMART

The importance of personal protective equipment (PPE), particularly masks, cannot be overstated. Infectious respiratory diseases are passed primarily by droplet/aerosol. Therefore, the Paramedic should wear a mask and eye protection whenever assessing and treating a patient with respiratory complaints.

Pulse Oximeter

Hypoxia is the key finding in pneumonia that is cause for concern for a Paramedic. Paramedics seldom obtain arterial blood gasses from patients and thus largely depend on

Table 8-6 Clinical Indicators of Pneumonia

- Temperature > 38°C
- Tachycardia
- Rales (Crackles)
- Diminished breath sounds
- Productive cough
- Shaking chills

the pulse oximetry for a crude estimation of oxygen content in the blood, appreciating that the majority of the oxygen is bound to hemoglobin.

The pulse oximeter has a non-invasive probe with two light-emitting diodes (LED) that pass red (600 to 750 nm) and infrared (850 to 1,000 nm) light through a capillary bed to a photodiode across from the LED. Frequently, the probe is placed either on the patient's earlobes or fingertips for convenience.

Oxygenated blood, being a brighter red than deoxygenated blood, preferentially absorbs more infrared light while allowing red light to pass unimpeded. The pulse oximeter then compares the difference in the amount of light which passes through the capillary bed to the photodiode (the R/IR ratio) with established values on healthy patients. Using a microprocessor, it calculates a percentage of oxygen saturation of the hemoglobin.

Some pulse oximeters, using the signal variation with each pulse, average the pulsatile signal over 5 to 10 seconds to create a digital readout of a pulse rate. Recent pulse oximeters use digital signal processing (DSP) to filter extraneous signal artifact—including patient motion, low perfusion states, and electromagnetic interference—to produce a reliable reading. Use of special reflectance probes permits the application of the pulse oximeter probe on any tissue surface; for example, the forehead of the hypothermic patient may be used, and the patient packaged to maintain warmth of distal extremity.

Studies have shown a mean difference of less than 2% in oxygen saturation readings from a pulse oximeter when compared to simultaneously drawn arterial blood gasses when saturations are above 90%.[31] The accuracy of pulse oximetry saturation readings below 80% is dubious, with a variation of 5% on average, and clinical observation should guide empiric therapy.[32]

Another limitation of pulse oximetry is the presence of carboxyhemoglobin (COHb)—from carbon monoxide poisoning—and/or methemoglobin (MetHb)—the transformation of hemoglobin to ferric iron by poisons such as nitrates—in the blood. In those cases, the pulse oximeter will give a false positive (artificially elevated oxygen saturation readings). Similarly, patients in a sickle cell crisis (an acute vaso-occlusive emergency) may have errant pulse oximeter readings, as great as 8% in some cases.

Intravenous dyes (such as methylene blue, which is used in medical imaging and special therapy) can create falsely low SpO_2 readings for a short period of time (average 20 to 30 minutes). While the presence of acrylic nails does not interfere with pulse oximetry readings, the presence of blue, green, or black nail polish may interfere with the pulse oximeter.

The presence of a normal (>90%) SpO_2 reading does not automatically equate to absence of hypoxia. If the patient is anemic (lacking red blood cells)—for example, due to hemorrhage—the remaining hemoglobin can be saturated but remain less than the oxygen demands of the body, thus creating hypoxia in the cells.

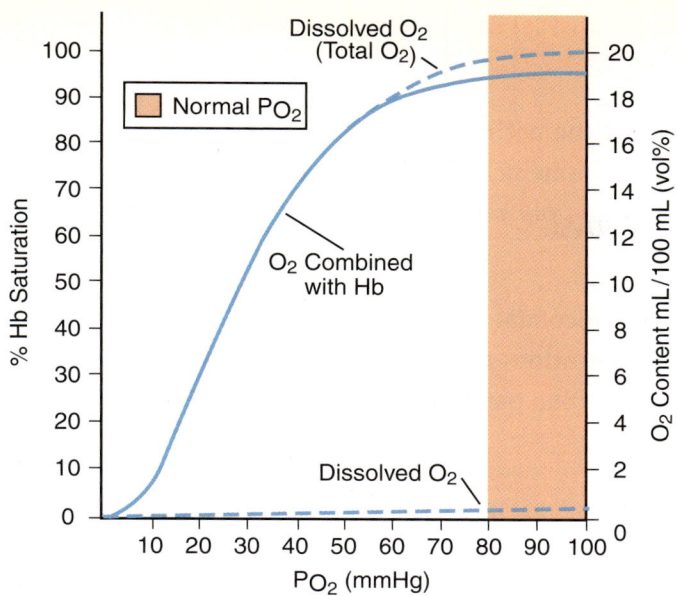

Figure 8-5 Oxyhemoglobin curve.

Perhaps the most important aspect regarding SpO_2 readings and hypoxia is understanding that the oxyhemoglobin curve is not a rounded curve but rather a sigmoid shape, similar to a ski slope (Figure 8-5). When SpO_2 drops below 90% then PaO_2 can be below 60 mmHg, with normal temperature and acidity. This is the definition of hypoxia. Continued small incremental drops in oxygen saturation can therefore produce dramatic decreases in oxygenation.[33]

Cyanosis

Cyanosis, another sign that Paramedics rely on as an indicator of hypoxia, is a bluish discoloration of skin. It can be observed peripherally, in the fingernails or toes, and centrally in the inside of the lips, the tongue, and the conjunctiva of the eyelids.

Peripheral cyanosis can be due to hypoxia, or it can be the result of poor circulation to the hands or feet. Raynaud's phenomena, an acute arterial spasm, can cause peripheral cyanosis.

Central cyanosis, on the other hand, is more likely due to hypoxia. Deoxygenated blood near the surface of the skin, particularly mucous membranes, can create a bluish hue to the skin.

Unfortunately, cyanosis is not a dependable sign of hypoxia. For cyanosis to exist, there has to be sufficient deoxygenated hemoglobin present. If the patient is profoundly anemic or has inadequate quantities of hemoglobin, perhaps secondary to hemorrhage, then cyanosis may not be observed.

Complicating the assessment of cyanosis is the combination of skin pigment and available lighting. These factors make observer reliability poor and the assessment of cyanosis somewhat suspect in some cases.

CASE STUDY (CONTINUED)

The nurse leaves to copy the chart while the crew prepares to transfer the patient to the stretcher. The Paramedic notices the dressing which covers the patient's recent hip surgery and the urine collection bag hanging from the rail.

The Paramedic shares with his partner that he suspects the patient has pneumonia, possibly acquired during his last hospitalization, and indicates that they should really get the patient to the hospital.

CRITICAL THINKING QUESTIONS

1. What is the significance of the wound dressing and the urine collection bag from the indwelling urinary catheter to this patient's condition?
2. What diagnosis did the Paramedic announce to his partner?

Assessment

In the face of the preceding clinical presentation, the Paramedic might suspect pneumonia as the cause of the patient's persistent low SaO_2 despite administration of high-flow, high-concentration oxygen. Regardless of the presenting symptom complex, a Paramedic faced with unresolved hypoxia following the administration of high-flow, high-concentration oxygen has to diagnosis the patient as having Type I respiratory failure.

It is critical that the Paramedic understand that little else, besides supportive care, can be done for this patient in the field and rapid transport is indicated.

The Paramedic is concerned about the persistent hypoxia while the patient is receiving oxygen by nasal cannula. Before transferring the patient to the stretcher, the Paramedic replaces the nasal cannula with a partial nonrebreather mask and adjusts the liter flow to 15 liters per minute.

CRITICAL THINKING QUESTIONS

1. What is the standard of care of patients with suspected nosocomial pneumonia?
2. What are some of the patient-specific concerns and considerations that the Paramedic should consider when applying this plan of care that is intended to treat a broad patient population presenting with nosocomial pneumonia?

Treatment

Normal oxygen delivery to tissues is approximately 1,000 mL per minute. At rest, the body's tissues use approximately 250 mL per minute. Therefore, the metabolic oxygen use at rest is normally one-quarter of the **VO$_2$ max**, the maximum oxygen consumption.

When the patient is hypoxic then she has reached the VO$_2$ max and any increase in cardiac demand will cause further deterioration. The importance of this relationship, between cardiac output and oxygen demand, is shown in the Fick equation. In the **Fick equation** the amount of oxygen delivered to the tissues (VO$_2$) equals the cardiac output (QT) times the arterial oxygen content minus venous oxygen content (VO$_2$ = CO × (CaO$_2$ − CvO$_2$).

The Fick equation shows that, even though oxygen content in both arterial and venous blood is being held constant, the increase in cardiac output increases the metabolic oxygen demand. Since Paramedics cannot measure either cardiac output or arterial oxygen content in the field, a rough approximation can be made using SaO$_2$ and systolic blood pressure. When the patient is asked to stand or walk, the cardiac output will increase, whereas the systolic blood pressure and the oxygen saturation will correspondingly decrease.

It is also important to keep the patient in a seated upright position. In the normal person, the ventilation (V) is approximately 4 L per minute and the normal perfusion (Q̇) is about 5 L of blood per minute. The resulting V-Q̇ ratio is approximately 4:5.

In the normal person in the seated position, the ventilation to perfusion match (V-Q̇ ratio) is greater than 1:1 at the apices, meaning that there is an almost perfect match of blood to air. The V-Q̇ ratio at the bases is less than 1:1.

When a patient is laid down, the V-Q̇ ratio falls to less than 1 throughout the lungs. Whenever the V-Q̇ ratio falls to less than 0.8 L/min, then ventilation decreases and oxygenation suffers.

En route to the hospital, the patient experiences worsening shortness of breath. The Paramedic reassesses the patient, which uncovers diffuse bilateral rales throughout the lower lung fields. They were previously isolated to the one lung. A drop in oxygen saturation (SaO$_2$) to less than 60 mmHg and a dramatic drop in blood pressure has occurred in the patient, which has resulted in a lapse of consciousness. While immediately taking action, the Paramedic suspects the patient has developed acute respiratory distress syndrome.

CRITICAL THINKING QUESTIONS

1. What are some of the predictable complications associated with pneumonia?
2. What are some of the predictable complications associated with the treatments for pneumonia?

Evaluation

Acute respiratory distress syndrome (ARDS) is an acute lung failure often associated with pneumonia. The key essential difference between Type I respiratory failure and ARDS is the increased permeability of the alveoli and the resultant acute pulmonary edema. ARDS should not be confused with congestive heart failure (CHF), although both can cause acute pulmonary edema (APE).

ARDS can also be the result of aspiration of stomach contents. The acidity in the aspirate triggers the same inflammatory mechanisms seen with pneumonia. The increased permeability is owed to a systemic release of chemical mediators, such as histamine, prostaglandins, and leukotrienes, as well as the activation of the complement system. Typically ARDS occurs in less than 72 hours from the initial lung injury (in this case, the pneumonia).

The resulting massive vasodilatation caused by these chemical mediators causes a severe drop in cardiac output. The loss of cardiac output, as illustrated in the Fick equation, dramatically worsens the cellular hypoxia.

The key to survival for these patients is aeration. In some cases, the use of **continuous positive airway pressure (CPAP)** in the spontaneously breathing patient may be sufficient to reverse hypoxia.

If there is a risk of aspiration, or the patient is unable to control the airway, then elective intubation should be performed. Endotracheal intubation with positive pressure ventilation returns collapsed alveoli to a functional state, and helps reverse hypoxia.

However, high ventilation pressures can result in barotrauma (destruction of alveoli) and thus worsen aeration of the lung. Ventilation with lower volumes (approximately 5 to 6 mL/kg) and lower pressure (less than 32 cm H_2O) is recommended if the Paramedic suspects ARDS. Studies have shown that low tidal volume ventilation improves survival compared with patients ventilated with conventional tidal volumes.[34–36]

The addition of positive end expiratory pressure (PEEP) may also be beneficial. However, its use does have drawbacks. The Paramedic should consider before using PEEP is the consequence of increased pressures within the thoracic from the PEEP. PEEP increases intrathoracic pressure and compresses the great vessels, including the less rigid vena cava. It also decreases venous return, resulting in decreased preload and decreased cardiac output.[37,38]

The goal of all respiratory therapy for these patients is to maintain adequate oxygenation, with SaO_2 greater than 85% and preferably at greater than 90%.

Fluids should be administered judiciously and only as necessary. If the patient remains hypotensive, then vasopressors such as dopamine should be considered after correcting any hypovolemia.

CASE STUDY CONCLUSION

Despite assistance with ventilation from a bag-valve-mask assembly, the patient remains unconscious and the Paramedic prepares to intubate the patient.

Leaning toward the front of the ambulance, the Paramedic shouts, "You better light it up!" The Paramedic intubates the patient while the din of the ambulance siren is heard.

CRITICAL THINKING QUESTIONS

1. What is the most appropriate transport decision that will get the patient to definitive care?
2. What are the advantages of transporting a patient with suspected acute respiratory distress syndrome to a hospital with critical care capabilities?

Disposition

Mortality rates for patients with ARDS average 40% and advance with age to 70%, especially if the patient does not receive the intense support provided in a critical care unit.

Rapid transport of the patient to a facility capable of treating this complex disease is critical.

CONCLUSION

Many disorders impair oxygenation and produce hypoxemia. The Paramedic must aggressively intervene in patients with impending respiratory failure and attempt to improve their oxygenation.

KEY POINTS:

- Type I respiratory failure is distinguished by a partial oxygen pressure (PaO_2) of less than 60 mmHg in the blood.

- Type I respiratory failure is primarily a failure of oxygen exchange.

- Causes of Type I respiratory failure include a low oxygen environment and impairments at the alveolar–capillary membrane.

- Gas exchange is dependent upon the differences in partial pressure of the gas in the lungs and the blood. Additional factors such as atmospheric pressure and concentration of oxygen in the air mixture affect exchange.

- The relationship between the partial pressure of oxygen and the saturation of hemoglobin by oxygen is illustrated by the oxyhemoglobin dissociation curve.

- Low oxygen environments occur secondary to the presence of other gasses or due to an increase in altitude.

- Impairments at the alveolar–capillary membrane can occur on the lung side or the blood side of the membrane.

- Impairments on the lung side cause shunting, where no gas exchange takes place but blood flow is normal.

- Impairments on the blood side cause dead space where ventilation is normal but blood flow through the capillary bed is interrupted.

- Pulmonary emboli may result from the release of fat following a fracture, air entering the vasculature, amniotic fluid following a birth, or a blood clot usually secondary to a change in venous return from the lower extremities.

- Unexplained dyspnea, pleuritic chest pain, and hemoptysis are common indicators for pulmonary embolus.

- Pneumonia is an infection in the lungs caused by a fungus, bacterium, protozoan, or virus.

- The usual symptoms associated with pneumonia are fever, cough, and shortness of breath.

- Even though oxygen content in both arterial and venous blood remains the same, any increase in cardiac output will increase metabolic oxygen demand.

- Acute respiratory distress syndrome is an acute lung failure often associated with pneumonia and characterized by the development of noncardiac pulmonary edema.

- Treatment of patients with acute respiratory distress is centered on improving oxygenation through the use of positive pressure as CPAP in the spontaneously breathing patient or intubation, ventilation, and PEEP.

REVIEW QUESTIONS:

1. What is the general cause of Type I respiratory failure?
2. What measurement of a gas mixture explains gas exchange?
3. What relationships are visualized by the oxyhemoglobin curve?
4. What is shunting as it relates to gas exchange?
5. What body components can become emboli?
6. What triad of complaints are indicators for a pulmonary embolus?
7. What does the Fick equation explain regarding metabolic oxygen demand?

CASE STUDY QUESTIONS:

Please refer to the Case Study in this chapter, and answer the questions below:

1. What conditions are likely to cause Mr. Wilcox's signs and symptoms?
2. Why is the Paramedic concerned with the drooling?
3. Under what conditions might the pulse oximetry reading be in error?
4. What concerns are suggested by the hip dressing? By the urine collection bag?
5. What actions should the Paramedic take when the patient decompensates?

REFERENCES:

1. Bordow R. *Manual of Clinical Problems in Pulmonary Medicine (Spiral Manual Series)*. Philadelphia: Lippincott Williams & Wilkins; 2005.
2. Bunn F. *Disorders of Hemoglobin: Genetics, Pathophysiology and Clinical Management*. New York: Cambridge University Press; 2001.
3. Marino P, Sutin K. *The ICU Book, third edition (ICU Book, 3E (Marino/ Lippincott))*. Philadelphia: Lippincott Williams & Wilkins; 2006.
4. Wolf GK, Arnold JH. Assessing the benefits of noninvasive ventilation: the tissue is the issue. *Crit Care Med.* 2008;36(1):349–350.
5. Haverkamp HC, Dempsey JA, et al. Treatment of airway inflammation improves exercise pulmonary gas exchange and performance in asthmatic subjects. *J Allergy Clin Immunol.* 2007;120(1):39–47.
6. Kao SJ, Yeh DY, et al. Clinical and pathological features of fat embolism with acute respiratory distress syndrome. *Clin Sci (Lond).* 2007;113(6):279–285.
7. de Feiter PW, van Hooft MA, et al. Fat embolism syndrome: yes or no? *J Trauma.* 2007;63(2):429–431.
8. Taviloglu K, Yanar H. Fat embolism syndrome. *Surg Today.* 2007;37(1):5–8.
9. Habashi NM, Andrews PL, et al. Therapeutic aspects of fat embolism syndrome. *Injury.* 2006;37 Suppl 4:S68–S73.
10. Moreno H. Management of critical haemodynamic complications of amniotic fluid embolism. *Int J Obstet Anesth.* 2008; 89(6):1079–1092.
11. Stafford I, Sheffield J. Amniotic fluid embolism. *Obstet Gynecol Clin North Am.* 2007;34(3):545–553, xii.
12. Sakuma M, Sugimura K, et al. Unusual pulmonary embolism: septic pulmonary embolism and amniotic fluid embolism. *Circ J.* 2007;71(5):772–775.
13. Moore, L. Amniotic fluid embolism. Available at: **http://www.emedicine.com/Med/topic122.htm**. Accessed January 30, 2008.
14. Cranley JJ, Canos AJ, et al. The diagnosis of deep venous thrombosis. Fallibility of clinical symptoms and signs. *Arch Surg.* 1976;111(1):34–36.
15. Sandler DA. Homans' sign and medical education. *Lancet.* 1985;2(8464):1130–1131.
16. Sternbach G. John Homans: the dorsiflexion sign. *J Emerg Med.* 1989;7(3):287–290.
17. Kruisman AE, et al. Comparison of the revised Geneva score with the Wells rule for assessing clinical probability of pulmonary embolism. *J Thromb Haemost.* 2008;6(1):40–44.
18. Punukollu G, Gowda RM, et al. Role of electrocardiography in identifying right ventricular dysfunction in acute pulmonary embolism. *Am J Cardiol.* 2005;96(3):450–452.
19. Ullman E, Brady WJ, et al. Electrocardiographic manifestations of pulmonary embolism. *Am J Emerg Med.* 2001;19(6):514–519.
20. Hawryluck L, Lapinsky SE, et al. Clinical review: SARS—lessons in disaster management. *Crit Care.* 2005;9(4):384–389.
21. Lapinsky SE, Granton JT. Critical care lessons from severe acute respiratory syndrome. *Curr Opin Crit Care.* 2004; 10(1):53–58.
22. Singer PA, Benatar SR, et al. Ethics and SARS: lessons from Toronto. *BMJ.* 2003;327(7427):1342–1344.

23. Robenshtok E, Shefet D, et al. Empiric antibiotic coverage of atypical pathogens for community acquired pneumonia in hospitalized adults. *Cochrane Database Syst Rev.* 2008;1:CD004418.

24. Mandell LA. Antimicrobial resistance and treatment of community-acquired pneumonia. *Clin Chest Med.* 2005;26(1):57–64.

25. Carratala J, Martin-Herrero JE, et al. Clinical experience in the management of community-acquired pneumonia: lessons from the use of fluoroquinolones. *Clin Microbiol Infect.* 2006;12 Suppl 3:2–11.

26. Ioachimescu OC, Ioachimescu AG, et al. Severity scoring in community-acquired pneumonia caused by Streptococcus pneumoniae: a 5-year experience. *Int J Antimicrob Agents.* 2004;24(5):485–490.

27. Solensky R, Earl HS, et al. Clinical approach to penicillin-allergic patients: a survey. *Ann Allergy, Asthma, Immunol.* 2000;84(3):329–333.

28. Anne S, Reisman RE. Risk of administering cephalosporin antibiotics to patients with histories of penicillin allergy. *Ann Allergy, Asthma, Immunol.* 1995;74(2):167–170.

29. Kass SM, Williams PM, et al. Pleurisy. *Am Fam Physician.* 2007;75(9):1357–1364.

30. Toth A, Fackelmann J, et al. Tuberculosis prevention and treatment. *Can Nurse.* 2004;100(9):27–30.

31. Barker SJ, Tremper KK. Pulse oximetry: applications and limitations. *Int Anesthesiol Clin.* 1987;25(3):155–175.

32. Carter BG, Carlin JB, et al. Accuracy of two pulse oximeters at low arterial hemoglobin-oxygen saturation. *Crit Care Med.* 1998;26(6):1128–1133.

33. Walls R. *Manual of Emergency Airway Management.* Philadelphia: Lippincott Williams & Wilkins; 2008.

34. Bream-Rouwenhorst HR, Beltz EA, et al. Recent developments in the management of acute respiratory distress syndrome in adults. *Am J Health-Syst Pharm.* 2008;65(1):29–36.

35. Girard TD, Bernard GR. Mechanical ventilation in ARDS: a state-of-the-art review. *Chest.* 2007;131(3):921–929.

36. Santacruz JF, Diaz Guzman Zavala E, et al. Update in ARDS management: recent randomized controlled trials that changed our practice. *Cleve Clin J Med.* 2006;73(3):217–219, 223–225, 229 passim.

37. Jellinek H, Krafft P, et al. Right atrial pressure predicts hemodynamic response to apneic positive airway pressure. *Crit Care Med.* 2000;28(3):672–678.

38. Jardin F. PEEP, tricuspid regurgitation, and cardiac output. *Intensive Care Med.* 1997;23(8):806–807.

CHAPTER 9

DISORDERS OF VENTILATION

KEY CONCEPTS:

Upon completion of this chapter, it is expected that the reader will understand these following concepts:

- The two types of respiratory failure
- How Type II respiratory failure exhibits carbon dioxide retention, whereas Type I does not
- That chronic obstructive pulmonary disease is the most common cause of Type II respiratory failure
- How to direct Type II respiratory failure assessment and treatment toward finding and improving airflow, effort of breathing, and surface area for diffusion

ANATOMY CONCEPTS:

Prior to reading this chapter the Paramedic student should be familiar with the following anatomy and physiology concepts:

- Pulmonary anatomy
- Neuronal control of respirations
- Physiology of ventilation

While standing by at the fairgrounds, two Paramedics are about to enjoy some fried dough when the radio crackles, "EMS arrival to Aid Station. 16-year-old female with shortness of breath. ETA in five minutes." While making their way back to the Aid Station, the two Paramedics talk about the possible causes of shortness of breath in a 16-year-old girl.

CRITICAL THINKING QUESTIONS

1. What are some of the possible respiratory related causes of shortness of breath?
2. How is the patient's shortness of breath possibly related to being at the fair?

OVERVIEW

The patient's decline from respiratory distress—and the agitation of hypoxia—to respiratory failure is highlighted by the lethargy that results from carbon dioxide retention. There are a number of reasons—some acute, some chronic—why a patient would start to retain carbon dioxide. However, the end game in every case, unless the Paramedic intervenes, is respiratory arrest.

Chief Concern

Type II respiratory failure is distinguished from Type I by the added feature of carbon dioxide retention, which tends to result from ventilation problems. The Paramedic should consider the concepts of respiratory physiology in order to understand the potential pathophysiology that could create Type II respiratory failure.

The initiation of a patient's breath occurs at the medulla oblongata and pons. Therefore, any depression of these centers of respiration (e.g., as a result of an opiate overdose) would slow ventilation, resulting in an increase in carbon dioxide.

The nervous signal travels down from the reticular formation in the medulla and along the spinal cord, exiting the spinal cord at the spinal nerves at the 3rd to 4th and 5th cervical vertebrae. Combined, these spinal nerves become the phrenic nerve; this nerve innervates the diaphragm, the primary muscle of respiration. Any interruption of these spinal nerves (the phrenic nerve), such as by traumatic spinal injury, would break off the signal traveling to the diaphragm and thus paralyze the patient's breathing. A traditional mnemonic to remember this fact goes "3–4–5 keeps a guy alive."

The phrenic nerve (originating from the cervical spinal nerves) and the intercostal nerves (originating from the thoracic spinal nerves) innervate other muscles that control respiration as well. Any neuromuscular disease, such as stroke, myasthenia gravis, Guillain–Barré, muscular dystrophy, polio, amyotrophic lateral sclerosis, or toxins like tetanus, may lead to difficulty with breathing, hypoventilation, and carbon dioxide retention.

Even chest wall deformities, such as pectus excavatum (funnel chest), pectus carinatum (pigeon breast), and scoliosis and kyphosis (both abnormal curvatures of the spine), can cause alteration in the mechanics of breathing. This alteration in breathing leads to hypoventilation and carbon dioxide retention.

However, the most common causes of Type II respiratory failure are the chronic obstructive pulmonary diseases. **Chronic obstructive pulmonary diseases (COPD)** all involve some disease process that creates an obstacle to free airflow in the airway.[1,2] The three primary obstructive pulmonary diseases are asthma, chronic bronchitis, and emphysema. Although each disease has a slightly different presentation, all three tend to cause retention of carbon dioxide as well as hypoxia (Type II respiratory failure).

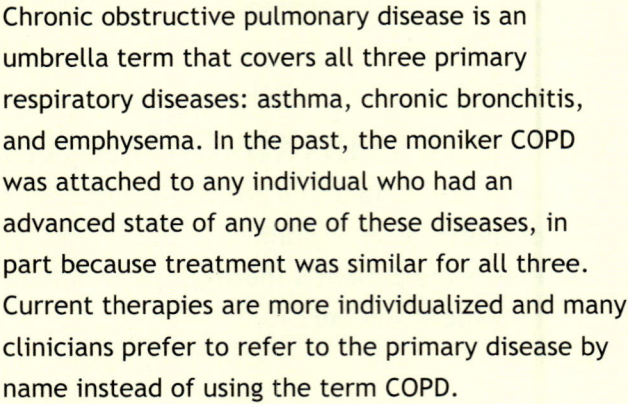

Pathophysiology of Type II Respiratory Failure

In all pathologies that lead to Type II respiratory failure, the common thread is the retention of carbon dioxide in the blood, or **hypercarbia**. A combination of reduced effort of breathing, increased resistance to airflow, and/or a decrease in the lung surface area available for diffusion leads to retention of the carbon dioxide generated by metabolism and results in hypercarbia.

Chronic Obstructive Pulmonary Diseases

The pathophysiology of the three primary respiratory diseases—asthma, chronic bronchitis, and emphysema—have three common pathological mechanisms, known as the three "S's": secretions, spasm and swelling (Figure 9-1).[3] The essential difference between these three diseases is the degree to which one of the three mechanisms predominates. These three mechanisms are the reason for an increase in airway resistance and a decrease in expired air, leading to carbon dioxide retention or hypercarbia.

Most respiratory disease is caused by stimulation of the respiratory tract by tobacco smoke, airborne pollutants, and/or microbes that cause infection. Once the respiratory tract is stimulated, the body's inflammatory system responds. This causes mast cells to release histamine, white blood cells to

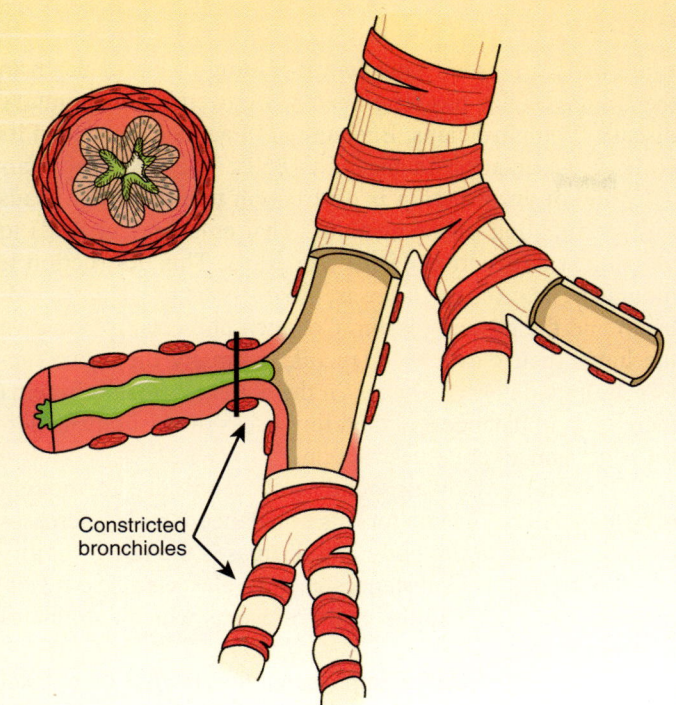

Figure 9-1 Secretions, spasm, and swelling.

Constricted bronchioles

migrate to the pulmonary tree, and chemical mediators such as leukotrienes and prostaglandins to be released. These actions produce the secretions, spasm, and swelling associated with respiratory disease.[4]

Secretions are the product of goblet cells that produce mucus, a viscous fluid containing mucins in a solution of electrolytes. These mucins protect the respiratory tree from damage by trapping particulate materials and microorganisms. These secretions are increased during the inflammatory response and may become thickened during hyperventilation, secondary to increased evaporation, and form into mucous plugs. These mucous plugs in turn block airways, trap air, and overdistend alveoli.

When stimulated by an exogenous source, such as an antigen or irritant, mast cells release histamine and basophils release leukotriene. These two chemical mediators dilate the venous pulmonary vasculature and increase blood vessel permeability, leading to edema and swelling.

The sudden constriction, or spasm, of the bronchioles (**bronchospasm**) is a key clinical finding in obstructive respiratory disease and leads to bronchoconstriction. This bronchoconstriction gives rise to wheezes appreciated by the Paramedic during the cardiopulmonary examination.

Bronchial Wheezing

Wheezing is the cardinal sign of acute respiratory distress that tends to grab the Paramedic's attention. The automatic assumption is usually that the wheezing is due to asthma. However, this is not always the case. The saying "not all that wheezes is asthma" is attributed to Dr. Chevalier Jackson

Table 9-1 ASTHMATIC

A	Asthma
S	Stasis (pulmonary embolism)
T	Toxins (inhaled gasses)
H	Heart (acute pulmonary edema)
M	Mechanical (partial foreign body obstruction)
A	Allergy
T	Trauma (pneumothorax)
I	Infection
C	Chronic respiratory disease

(1865–1958) and speaks to the multifactorial etiology of wheezing.[5] To remember all the potential causes of wheezing, the mnemonic ASTHMATIC (Table 9-1) can be used.

Of course, the most common source of wheezing is asthma, the **A** in ASTHMATIC; not surprisingly, asthmatics tend to wheeze. Asthma is a complex chronic disease which will be discussed in detail shortly.

Following a pulmonary embolism, blood flow in the area stops and stasis occurs. **S**tasis causes coagulation as well as localized inflammation, including swelling and bronchospasm. Therefore, auscultation directly over the area of stasis may reveal wheezing and/or rales (crackles).

Inhalation of gaseous poisons, or **T**oxins, even in small amounts, can cause direct damage to the epithelial lining of the bronchioles. Corrosive chemicals (such as chlorine) and irritating chemical vapors (such as phosgene or poisonous gasses of the type used in warfare) can create strong bronchospasms and wheezing. Bronchospasm in these cases results from a "reactive airway" and is typified by wheezing and severe shortness of breath.

Prolonged exposure to these same toxic chemicals, even in subclinical doses, will over time scar the bronchioles, a condition called bronchiolitis obliterans. The scars within the bronchioles then become a fixed airway obstruction and narrow the airway, resulting in wheezing during inhalation.

Swelling and accumulation of fluids in the lungs (pulmonary edema) can result from either cardiogenic (acute pulmonary edema) (i.e., **H**eart-related, secondary to acute pulmonary edema) or noncardiogenic (direct injury to the lung) causes. Sources of noncardiogenic pulmonary edema include sepsis, aspiration, and high altitude. Regardless of the cause of the pulmonary edema, as the patient's airway swells and thus narrows, wheezing may occur.

Another source of wheezing can be **M**echanical obstruction, such as an inhaled peanut, which narrows the airway. In these cases, the wheezing is typically focused. However, in small children it may be difficult to localize the source as the chest itself is small and sounds resonant throughout.

Any number of **A**llergens may cause anaphylatoxins (part of the complement system) to trigger the degranulation of mast cells. Degranulation in turn releases histamine, which increases capillary permeability, as well as basophils, which release leukotrienes that stimulate bronchoconstriction.

Trauma to the respiratory tree, pulmonary contusions, laryngeal trauma, barotrauma, burns, and so on, can cause physical injury as well as an inflammatory response leading to bronchoconstriction and wheezing.

Infections, such as croup or whooping cough, can also activate the inflammatory response, leading to bronchoconstriction and wheezing. Infectious disease should be distinguished by the sequela associated with the infection such as fever or a productive cough.

Finally, other Chronic respiratory diseases, most notably emphysema, have wheezes associated with their disease process. They too have a distinctive symptom complex.

Clearly there are many diseases, conditions, and disorders other than asthma which include wheezing as a symptom. A more complete patient history and physical is important to help differentiate them.

Bronchitis

Bronchitis is, by definition, an inflammation of the bronchi and is generally due to a viral infection. Secondary bacterial infections often accompany this viral infection. Occasional acute bronchitis is a fact of life for most people and only becomes problematic when it becomes chronic. **Chronic bronchitis** is inflammation of the bronchi, leading to a productive cough, for three months during two consecutive years.[6]

As a result of chronic inflammation, structural changes occur in the bronchial airways, such as loss of cilia, bronchial wall thickening, and an increase in the number of mucus-producing goblet cells. The collective result of these changes is airway narrowing, air trapping, and hyperinflation of the alveoli.

Emphysema

Emphysema, presently the fourth-leading cause of death in the United States, has long been recognized as a respiratory disease. Two physicians, Badham and Laennec, described its clinical presentation in the mid-1860s. The essential characteristic of **emphysema** is obstruction to airflow that leads to hyperinflation of the alveolus. That enlargement leads to permanent destruction of alveolar walls. This destruction is thought to be owed to elastases, proteins that break down collagen and the protein elastin. Collagen and elastin help give the lungs their elasticity or recoil. Normally these two factors are in balance. However, in the patient with emphysema there is an imbalance and therefore a loss of elasticity, hyperinflation, and alveolar destruction.

Oxygen-free radicals found in tobacco smoke are thought to be largely responsible for this imbalance. Smoke increases oxidative stress in the body and decreases the body's ability to detoxify reactive substances such as elastases. The resulting imbalance leads to the chain of events which culminates in emphysema.

A particular form of emphysema that involves the distal airways, including the alveolar sacs, can lead to the formation of blebs. **Blebs**, also called bullae, are bubble-like blisters on the pleural lining. These blebs, when under increased intrathoracic pressure (such as might occur during positive pressure ventilation) can rupture, leading to a spontaneous pneumothorax.

Cor Pulmonale

For some patients, the culmination of years of gradual respiratory failure is right-sided heart failure. The heart's right ventricle fails as a result of three insults that are directly related to the lungs.

As a result of chronic hypercarbia and/or hypoxia, the pulmonary vasculature constricts, leading to increased blood pressure within the pulmonary vascular bed, called **pulmonary hypertension**.[7] Pulmonary hypertension, in turn, increases the work of the right ventricle as it tries to send blood through to the left ventricle. The right ventricle, a low pressure pump, is not intended to pump against high resistance; therefore, the heart fails.

Further complicating matters are changes within, and a reduction of, the number of pulmonary vessels that carry the blood. This in turn leads to greater resistance to forward blood flow and subsequently increased right-sided heart failure.

Finally, as a result of the chronic hypoxia, the bone marrow produces greater and greater numbers of red blood cells to carry whatever oxygen is available. This condition, called **polycythemia**, increases the thickness (viscosity) of the blood, making it harder to pump and further taxing the right ventricle.

As the right ventricle fails, so does the left. As a result, the patient's cardiac output starts to plummet due to loss of preload in the left ventricle. This results in a backup of blood moving into the systemic circulation (backward failure) and loss of cardiac output (forward failure) terminating in **cor pulmonale**.[8–10]

Some patients with cor pulmonale may also manifest hemoptysis (the spitting up of blood). This occurs when blood spills into the airways because of pulmonary vessels that have ruptured under the pressure. Hemoptysis, although potentially a sign of cor pulmonale, is also seen in patients with tuberculosis. Therefore, respiratory precautions should be taken until the possibility of tuberculosis is eliminated.

Occasionally patients with cor pulmonale will complain of hoarseness. This hoarseness is secondary to compression of the left recurrent laryngeal nerve by the distended pulmonary artery that lies in close proximity.

The symptom complex associated with cor pulmonale is nonspecific and includes such constitutional signs as shortness of breath or dyspnea, unexplained weakness or malaise, and hypoxia as evidenced by cyanosis. Treatment of the disorder should focus on symptomatic relief and supportive care.

Cor Pulmonale, Diuretics, and Sympathomimetics

Acute pulmonary edema (APE), which on occasion occurs with cor pulmonale, is often treated with diuretics, such as loop diuretics (e.g., furosemide) or thiazide diuretics

STREET SMART

Acute cor pulmonale can occur because of a pulmonary embolism, which can cause instant increase in pulmonary resistance. As a result, the patient's blood pressure plunges precipitously. It is not important for the Paramedic to decide if an acute pulmonary embolism or chronic pulmonary hypertension was the cause of the cor pulmonale. The immediate pressing problem is the hypotension and associated repercussions.

STREET SMART

Although 90% of all cases of emphysema are believed to be due to tobacco smoke, it does not follow that all patients with emphysema are, or were, tobacco smokers. Occupational exposures to toxic chemicals, as well as life-long asthma, can lead to emphysema (Table 9-2). Paramedics must be sure to treat the patient without casting judgments on how the condition developed.

Table 9-2 Suspected Causes of Emphysema

- Cigarette smoking
  - Suspected in 80% to 90% of cases
- Alpha 1 antitrypsin deficiency (AAt)
  - Genetic
- Occupational dusts and chemicals
  - Pneumoconiosis
    - Coal miner's disease
    - Also known as black lung
  - Extrinsic allergic alveolitis
    - Also known as farmer's lung
  - Granulomatosis
    - Talc-induced lung disease
  - Asbestosis
    - Also known as white lung
  - Industrial chemicals
    - Popcorn packer's lung
- Fossil fuel air pollution

(e.g., hydrochlorothiazide (HCTZ)). These diuretics tend to cause a loss of potassium when creating diuresis (these are potassium-wasting diuretics).

Sympathomimetics, described shortly, used in the treatment of bronchospasm also tend to decrease intracellular potassium. The concomitant use of these two drugs could lead to profound hypokalemia, with a potential for cardiac dysrhythmia.

Tobacco Smoke

Tobacco smoke from cigarettes and cigars contains some 4,000 identified chemicals of which dozens are either toxic chemicals or known carcinogens. Tobacco smoke increases the risk of developing chronic bronchitis and/or emphysema by tenfold and triples the risk of dying from heart disease. While the lion's share of cancers attributed to smoking consists of cancer of the lungs, other cancers, such as throat cancer, have also been connected with cigarette smoke. Overall, 30% of all cancer deaths are attributed to tobacco smoke and 87% of lung cancer deaths are thought to be due to tobacco smoke.

The pathophysiology of tobacco smoke has been well researched. The tars and gasses both paralyze and destroy cilia, leading to a failure of the mucous elevator. Without the mucous elevator, the airway becomes clogged with phlegm that the patient attempts to expectorate (known as the proverbial smoker's hack). Compounding the problem is an increase in the number of goblet cells that produce the mucus. Ultimately, tobacco smoke exposure—either passive (secondhand) or active—increases inflammation, which leads to increased bronchial airway swelling.

Asthma

Asthma has been recognized as a medical condition for a long time. Greeks recognized the respiratory disorder associated with shortness of breath, mentioned in Homer's *Iliad*, and called it asthma (Greek for panting). Hippocrates, the father of medicine, spoke of spasms in breathing, a probable reference to asthma. In addition, possibly the oldest medical book in existence, the *Nei Ching*, written in about 1000 B.C. by Huang-Ti, describes what sounds like asthma being treated with Ma Huang plant, a source of the sympathomimetic ephedrine.

The American Thoracic Society defines **asthma** as an "increased responsiveness of the tracheobronchial tree," suggesting the spasmodic nature of asthma. The American Association for Respiratory Care describes asthma as a "common disease" affecting the bronchial tree and causing bronchospasm. The statement goes on to state ". . . the airways can become swollen or filled with mucus . . . ," in reference to the three pathological processes of lung disease.

Asthma has all three of the S's of obstructive respiratory disease, manifested by airway hyperirritability, reversible bronchospasm, and inflammation. Although the episodic nature of bronchospasm suggests it is an acute process (asthma attack) which subsides with time, the accepted wisdom is that asthma is a chronic disease whose history is punctuated with acute exacerbations.

The severity of asthma varies along a spectrum. In order to help provide structure, the National Heart, Lung, and Blood Institute created four classifications of asthma.[11] Healthcare providers use these classifications to treat patients along a therapeutic algorithm (Table 9-3).

The first classification is mild intermittent asthma. Patients who are symptomatic (i.e., they have a persistent cough, wheeze, chest tightness, or difficulty breathing less than twice a week) and have less than two nocturnal episodes a month are considered to have mild intermittent asthma. Key to the classification of mild intermittent asthma is that the patient remains asymptomatic between exacerbations.

The patient with mild persistent asthma, the next classification, has more frequent episodes. The patient is symptomatic three to six days a week and also has nighttime attacks approximately once a week. The patient with mild persistent asthma may note that activities have to be moderated or even curtailed because of the asthma. This is a key clinical finding that differentiates mild intermittent asthma from mild persistent asthma.

The patient with moderate persistent asthma is symptomatic on a daily basis. These patients may restrict activities, or avoid certain activities altogether, in order to circumvent an asthma attack. Furthermore, patients with moderate persistent asthma will have approximately one nighttime episode a week over the course of a month—some weeks will be symptom free, whereas during others patients will have night after night episodes. This crescendo–decrescendo pattern illustrates the chronic nature of asthma: sometimes better, sometimes worse, but never gone.

Table 9-3 Classifications of Asthma*

- Mild intermittent asthma
  - Brief exacerbations
  - Infrequent and less than twice a week
  - Asymptomatic between exacerbations
  - Nocturnal symptoms once a month or less
- Mild persistent asthma
  - Symptomatic three to six times a week
  - Exacerbations may impair activity
  - Nocturnal symptoms several times a month
- Moderate persistent asthma
  - Daily occurrences of symptoms
  - Daily use of rescue inhaler
  - Exacerbations may impair activity
  - Increasing frequency of nocturnal attacks weekly
- Severe persistent asthma
  - Continuous symptoms of cough, wheeze, chest tightness
  - Frequent, almost daily, nighttime symptoms
  - Key: limited physical activity secondary to asthma

Note: *Evidence of one attribute is sufficient for inclusion in that category.

Source: Based on a partial list from the National Heart, Lung, and Blood Institute guidelines.

The patient with severe persistent asthma has almost continuous symptoms including frequent nocturnal attacks. The lifestyle of these patients is profoundly affected and some might regard the asthma as out of control.

A key feature of persistent asthma—whether mild, moderate, or severe—is decreased lung compliance and the development of a fixed airflow obstruction. Over time these patients will develop emphysema as a result of air trapping and alveolar damage.

Treatment modalities for patients with asthma are often based upon classification.

Epidemiology

Although an adult can develop new onset asthma, classically asthma starts in childhood. It is the most common childhood disease, affecting over 4.8 million children in the United States alone.

An estimated 5% to 10% of the adult population in the United States has asthma, and that percentage is increasing. Asthma-related emergencies account for more than two million emergency department visits annually.

The number of new cases of asthma has increased by 40% in the last 10 years, leading to concerns about the etiology of asthma. Even though medical care has improved and new medications have been introduced, hospitalizations and deaths from asthma continue to rise, with a higher prevalence displayed among African Americans. A number of factors, including indoor pollution, have been attributed to this increase in asthma cases.

Although the majority of asthma attacks are managed successfully with rescue inhalers, many require emergency treatment. Between 2% and 20% of intensive care unit admissions are for asthma-related emergencies. However, even with emergency treatment and intensive care, between 1.1% and 7% of asthmatics (mostly children and African Americans, with African American youths between 15 and 24 years of age at greatest risk) will experience a fatal asthma attack.[12] This amounts to approximately 7,000 patients a year.

Risk factors for asthma include a family history, approximately 7% for each first degree family member, and atopy. **Atopy** is a genetic, IgE antibody-induced hypersensitivity to allergens found in approximately 50% of the population.[13,14] Although asthma is not always associated with atopy and atopy is not always associated with asthma, the relationship of atopy and asthma is strong, thus warranting its inclusion as a risk factor.

Adult onset asthma, unlike pediatric asthma, is not an IgE-mediated disease. Non-allergic asthma (intrinsic asthma) is related to coexisting sinusitis, drug allergies, and nasal polyps. Its exact mechanism is not well established but probably relates to an inflammatory pathway.

Asthma triggers can be broken down into two general divisions: extrinsic or intrinsic. Traditional allergens, such as pollen, mold, and animal dander, are examples of extrinsic triggers which induce an IgE-mediated reaction.

Recently, insects have been recognized as extrinsic triggers. Dust mites, feeding on bacteria in warm, moist environments and spread by forced air heating and air conditioning, have been identified as asthma triggers, as have cockroach droppings.

Examples of intrinsic triggers include irritants such as vapors from cleaning fluids and tobacco smoke. This list also includes occupational exposures to animal products, plastic resin, and certain metals. These pollutants, some of which can be carried in the air, are concentrated in hot humid days. Vigilant Paramedics are aware of the increased likelihood of asthma attacks during smog alerts.

Stress can also induce an asthma attack. Stressors such as an upper respiratory infection, exercise, and even emotional stress can trigger an asthma attack.

Aspirin has also been documented as inducing asthma (aspirin-induced asthma, sometimes abbreviated AIA). Paramedics should be cautious when administering aspirin to patients, even those with the symptom complex of acute coronary syndrome.

In some cases of patients with suspected acute coronary syndrome, use of a beta blocker may be indicated. The beta/adrenergic receptors in the bronchioles are responsible for bronchodilation. Administration of a beta blocker to block the beta/adrenergic receptors may inhibit bronchodilation and may lead to bronchospasm, an unintended effect.

Acute Exacerbation of Asthma

A key to airway inflammation in asthma is hyperresponsiveness of the airway. **Hyperresponsiveness** is the tendency of the bronchioles to narrow (bronchoconstrict) with the smallest of stimulus. The degree of hyperresponsiveness directly correlates to the severity of the asthma attack.

When making the diagnosis of asthma, hyperresponsiveness is measured by a challenge of inhaled histamine or methacholine, or even cold air, followed by measurements of peak expiratory flow.

An acute exacerbation of asthma can be biphasic. In the early phase, rapid onset asthma begins within as little as 15 minutes and as long as three hours. An initial trigger stimulates mast cells, macrophages, and/or T lymphocytes to release histamine, leading to increased capillary permeability, as well as other chemical mediators. These chemical mediators—eosinophilic chemotactic factor, leukotriene B, and neutrophil chemotactic factor—attract white blood cells, eosinophils, neutrophils, and basophils to the bronchioles. These cells, in turn, release more histamine (bradykinin and leukotrienes). Bradykinins and leukotrienes cause bronchoconstriction and are similar to histamine, although they are longer acting.

Up to 40% of patients with asthma have a late asthmatic reaction. In the later phase (slow onset asthma), bronchoconstriction and subsequent wheezing occurs in three to eight hours. These delayed asthma attacks are thought to be due to specific leukotrienes (LT4, LTD4, and LTE4) which are also called the slow reacting substances of anaphylaxis.

The combination of spasm, swelling, and secretions, seen in an asthma attack, result in airflow obstructions, increasing residual air volume left in the lungs. This residual air is essentially trapped. Since respiration (diffusion of gasses) has occurred, the air functionally acts like increased dead space.

Trapped air, if unable to be ventilated, cannot diffuse gasses and establishes a ventilation to perfusion mismatch (V to Q). Without respiration hypoxemia rapidly ensues, with PO_2 of less than 60 mmHg, as well as hypercarbia. Carbon dioxide in the blood increases the blood's acidity and shifts the oxyhemoglobin curve, which in turn stimulates increased ventilation. The patient, in an effort to increase ventilation, breathes hard. This increases the work of breathing, which creates more metabolic acids, worsening the acidosis.

Long-Term Effects

After years of repeated air-trapping episodes, physical changes start to occur in the bronchial airway. Smooth muscle in the bronchi starts to hypertrophy. Submucosal edema, as well as deposits of collagen under the basement membrane, combine to remodel the airway. As a result, increased air trapping hyperexpands the alveoli, which start to break down, leading to emphysema. The hyperinflated lungs in the thoracic cavity eventually cause the patient to become barrel-chested.

Asthma or Emphysema?

Asthma and emphysema have many features in common. Both can cause shortness of breath, wheezing, and coughing. Both can occur as a result of exposure to triggers such as cold air, infections, and exercise. Although an asthma attack is generally limited to a few hours, provided the patient obtains treatment, the shortness of breath associated with emphysema can last for weeks or even months.

Age might be considered as a difference between these diseases. Emphysema is generally a disease of the old and cigarette smokers, whereas asthma can affect patients of all ages, old and young alike.

The difference between asthma and emphysema is permanency. Asthma, while considered a chronic disease, does not cause permanent lung damage when it is suitably controlled with medications. Emphysema causes permanent damage to the alveoli.[15] Therefore, the patient with emphysema will need life-long supportive care.

Respiratory Acidosis

As hypoventilation occurs, the partial pressure of carbon dioxide ($PaCO_2$) builds, a by-product of metabolism, forming carbonic acid. As a result, hypercarbia occurs. Hypoventilation

Table 9-4 Causes of Acute Respiratory Acidosis

- Neuromuscular disease
  - Guillain–Barré syndrome
  - Muscular dystrophy
  - Amyotrophic lateral sclerosis (Lou Gehrig's disease)
  - Myasthenia gravis
- Airway obstructive disease
  - Asthma
  - Chronic bronchitis
  - Emphysema
  - Obesity hypoventilation syndrome (Pickwickian)

is believed to be caused by neuromuscular diseases or airway obstructions (Table 9-4).

Respiratory acidosis causes a shift in the oxyhemoglobin curve to the right. Therefore, the hemoglobin's affinity to oxygen is weakened. Acidosis at the cellular level means that oxygen will be more readily available for the tissues. Acidosis at the alveolar level means that oxygen will have difficulty attaching to the hemoglobin, resulting in hypoxemia. The shift of the oxyhemoglobin curve to the right lends more support to the importance of oxygen therapy for the patient in respiratory distress.

Hypoxic Drive

Normally, when the chemoreceptors in the aortic arch and carotid bodies sense rising carbon dioxide levels they send signals to the brain to breathe faster, to "blow off" the carbonic acid. However, persistent elevated carbon dioxide levels, as seen in patients with respiratory disease, tend to blunt the sensitivity of these chemoreceptors to the elevated carbon dioxide in blood ($PaCO_2$). In fact, these chemoreceptors sense an increase in the carbonic acid that causes patients with chronic lung disease to compensate. This compensation for increased carbonic acid occurs by retaining sodium bicarbonate to buffer the acid (compensated respiratory acidosis). The net result is that both the carbon dioxide and the circulating bicarbonate levels are elevated and the chemoreceptors sense a normal acid level (i.e., a pH within 7.35 and 7.45). As a result of this process, the patient's body comes to rely on hypoxia to stimulate breathing instead of elevated carbon dioxide levels.

In the past, Paramedics were concerned about administering high-flow, high-concentration oxygen to chronic lung disease patients for fear that the patient would stop breathing. Instead, they used special Venturi masks. However, the dangers of hypoxia outweigh the concern about respiratory failure/arrest. Any patient suspected of being hypoxic should not be deprived of oxygen.

Marissa is already at the aid station. From the door, the Paramedics can see she is in obvious distress. Her airway is open but she is laboring to breathe. She answers questions with only two words per breath and indicates that her rescue inhaler hasn't helped at all. While the first aid team places Marissa on oxygen, the Paramedics begin getting a history. Her difficulty began suddenly about 30 minutes ago while she was watching the demolition derby.

CRITICAL THINKING QUESTIONS

1. What are the important elements of the history that a Paramedic should obtain?
2. What is the symptom pattern for Type II respiratory failure?

History

A SAMPLE history (**S**igns and symptoms, **A**llergies, **M**edications, **P**ast history, **L**ast oral intake, and **E**vents leading up the emergency), which includes use of the mnemonic HAPISOCS (**H**istory of pulmonary disease, **A**ctivity at onset, **P**ain upon inspiration, **I**nfections, **S**moker, **O**rthopnea, **C**ough, **S**putum), can help the Paramedic establish the cause of the patient's shortness of breath. Armed with this knowledge of airway disease, the Paramedic can narrow the possible diagnosis.

The chief concern for the patient will be shortness of breath in most cases. Many patients with asthma are not aware of the degree of severity of their attack. In one study, over one-quarter of the patients underestimated the severity of their asthma. The patient's inability to accurately perceive the illness, as illustrated in several studies, should be taken into account when the Paramedic takes the patient's history.

To begin the history, the Paramedic should ask the patient if he has a history of pulmonary disease. Patients will often relate a childhood onset of asthma, although patients can have their first asthma attack in adulthood. Since asthma is a chronic disease with acute exacerbations, the frequency and timing of the patient's previous asthma attacks is important. If the asthma attacks are increasing in frequency or not resolving as easily as the previous attack, representing a crescendo pattern, the patient's asthma may be out of control.

Next, the Paramedic will determine the activity at the onset of symptoms. An asthma attack can be precipitated by such innocuous activities as climbing a flight of stairs (exercise), retrieving the newspaper outdoors (exposure to cold), and being exposed to other agents in the environment (pollen from plants and dander from animals).

Patients with asthma rarely complain of pain on inspiration, but rather complain of tightness in the chest. Since pain on inspiration would be more suggestive of pleurisy or pneumonia, its presence suggests an infectious etiology, perhaps viral in nature. This infection could be the trigger for the patient's reactive airway.

A careful patient history may uncover irritants in the environment, such as tobacco smoke (including secondhand smoke) and strong odors (suggestive of chemical irritants). A number of historical factors may lead the Paramedic to have a high index of suspicion of asthma (Table 9-5).

Table 9-5 History Leading to High Index of Suspicion of Asthma

- Symptomatic approach
  - Recurrent wheezing
  - Persistent cough
  - Awoke with cough
  - Recurrent shortness of breath
  - Recurrent chest tightness
- Generators
  - Exercise
  - Recent viral infection
  - Contact with animals
  - House dust mites
    - Exposure to unfamiliar mattresses, pillows, upholstered furniture
  - Mold
    - Damp basements and flooding
  - Smoke
    - Either tobacco or wood
  - Pollen
  - Change in weather
    - Smog alerts
  - Airborne chemicals
    - Agricultural household cleaners

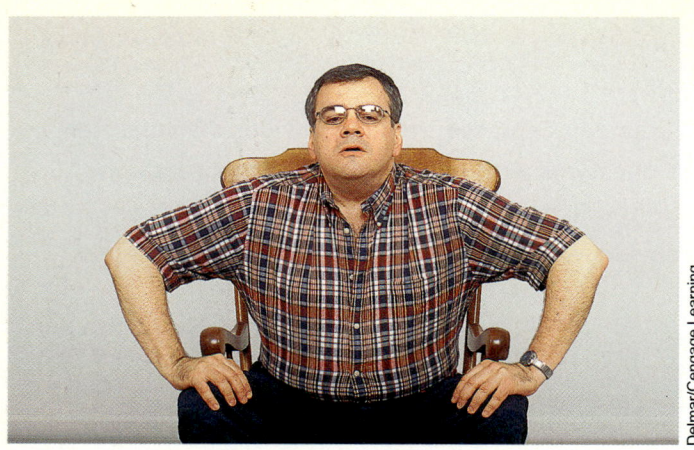

Figure 9-2 Tripoding associated with shortness of breath.

Putting a patient in a seated position improves her aeration. Many patients with asthma cannot tolerate a flat or even semireclined position during an attack. The classic **tripod position** is often witnessed during episodes of extreme shortness of breath (Figure 9-2). The presence of orthopnea suggests that the patient is maximizing ventilation by utilizing the patient's functional reserve capacity.

Since a cough is often associated with hyperresponsive airways, the presence of a persistent cough is suspicious. Some patients will have a cough that awakens them from sleep. This is the result of the body's natural circadian rhythm. The body's histamine levels are highest from 2 a.m. to 6 a.m., leading to a hyperresponsive airway. Nocturnal cough and/or wheezing are key diagnostic findings for asthma, although the Paramedic should consider acute pulmonary edema and/or gastroesophageal reflex disease (GERD) as potential etiologies.

Sputum production can be instrumental in ascertaining the etiology of a cough or wheeze. Sputum that is clear, white, or grey, called mucoid sputum, is the combination of mucus (produced by goblet cells) and cellular debris of macrophages and eosinophils. White–grey sputum is seen in patients with asthma or any acute upper respiratory infection (URI) or primary atypical pneumonia (walking pneumonia). Hyperventilation during an asthma attack dries the sputum and can give the sputum a stringy consistency.

Purulent sputum (i.e., infected sputum) may be yellow, green, or brown, depending on the bacterial infection. If the sputum is rusty colored then a pneumococcal pneumonia is likely.[16]

Serous sputum is pink-colored and seen in patients with acute pulmonary edema. The pink color is secondary to red blood cells forced out of the capillaries, into the alveolar space, and then into the sputum.

Smoking is a major contributing factor to respiratory diseases. Therefore, the Paramedic should obtain the patient's smoking history by asking how many packs of cigarettes the patient smokes a day and for how many years. For example, a patient smoking one-half a pack of cigarettes a day for the past

20 years would have a 10 pack-years history (1/2 × 20 = 10). Similarly, a patient smoking two packs a day for 10 years would have a 20 pack-years history. The risk of lung cancer and emphysema increases with each decade of smoking. A smoking history of greater than 10 pack-years is considered significant.

AMPLE

Allergies that can trigger asthma can be grossly categorized as due to environment, food, or drugs. Environmental allergies include pollen, dust, and other airborne pollutants. Like the patient with a heat emergency, the patient with asthma induced by an environmental allergen should be removed from the environment first.

The dander, urine, feces, and even saliva of any mammal, including cats, dogs, and rodents, as well as some birds, can be an allergen to a patient with asthma. The presence of these animals should be noted.

Another common household creature is the cockroach. Sensitivity to cockroaches and cockroach droppings has been found in inner city children with a history of asthma. The Paramedic should note the presence of cockroaches or unsanitary conditions that would attract cockroaches as well.

Approximately 2% of asthmatics are allergic to the chemical sodium bisulfite, which is used in commercial wines to preserve flavor. When added to food stuffs, especially canned foods, the sodium bisulfite releases sulfur dioxide which kills microbes.

Some patients claim an allergy to epinephrine, an endogenous chemical found in the body. In actuality, these patients are allergic to the sodium bisulfite preservative found in the aqueous epinephrine. Preservative-free epinephrine, though more expensive, is available for these patients.

When obtaining a medication history, the Paramedic should be mindful of any new prescriptions that might have triggered the asthma attack. Medications such as beta blockers and block bronchodilators can induce an asthma attack, as described earlier.

Aspirin and certain nonsteroidal anti-inflammatory drugs (NSAIDs) with crossover sensitivity to aspirin can induce asthma (aspirin-induced asthma, also called aspirin sensitive asthma). Aspirin-induced asthma typically occurs within one to three hours of ingestion of aspirin or other similar NSAID; many people with aspirin sensitivity have a cross-sensitivity to ibuprofen. These asthma attacks can be preceded by facial flushing and rhinorrhea.

AIA is thought to be the result of inhibition of cyclooxygenase 1 (COX-1), a chemical mediator that controls inflammation. The average age of patients with AIA (30 years) is associated with the development of nasal polyps. AIA is thought to occur in between 3% and 22% of adult onset asthmatics and 10% of pediatric asthma patients, and may be more common in patients with moderate to severe asthma. It should be noted that many over-the-counter (OTC) products contain acetylsalic acid. Many patients do not consider OTC products as medicine and therefore the Paramedic should ask specifically about any over-the-counter medicines used.

Corticosteroids—anti-inflammatory medications which are available in oral, solid, liquid, or inhaled forms—are typically prescribed to patients with persistent asthma. Steroids improve airway function, via reduced bronchial edema, by reducing inflammation.[17–19] The problems involved in using steroids, which tend to occur after months or years of use, include easier bruising, mood changes, and weight gain. However, these disadvantages are largely eliminated in inhaled corticosteroids which act directly on the mucosa without being absorbed systemically.

Some patients prematurely terminate their use of corticosteroids because of unwanted side effects. Examples of some of the more common side effects include increased appetite and associated weight gain, fluid retention with accompanying bloating and weight gain, and mood swings. Corticosteroids must be gently tapered over a period of time to prevent more severe side effects including acute unremitting exacerbation of asthma called status asthmaticus, which is discussed shortly.

Anti-inflammatory drugs that affect mast cells, such as cromolyn sodium, are also prescribed to patients with asthma. Effectively, these drugs stabilize mast cell membranes, preventing degranulization and/or inhibiting the release of chemical mediators from mast cells.

Xanthine compounds have been used to treat respiratory diseases for decades. Found in tea and coffee, as well as chocolate in the form of theobromine, xanthine compounds are thought to dilate the bronchi as well as decrease peripheral vascular resistance. The medicinal effects of coffee have led many to believe that coffee's popularity among patients with respiratory disease is owed to this effect.

Methylxanthines, in the form of theophyllines, are medications prescribed for long-term control of symptoms. Typically, a loading dose of the methylxanthine aminophylline would be 5 mg/kg infused intravenously over 30 minutes followed by a maintenance infusion of 0.5 mg/kg/hr. Although useful for some specific patient populations, methylxanthines are generally considered to be a second line drug because they are only about one-third as effective as the beta 2 agonists.

Furthermore, the difficulty in maintaining therapeutic serum concentrations—in part due to a number of factors that affect absorption and metabolism, as well as a narrow therapeutic window and the danger of toxicity—have caused methylxanthines to fall out of favor with many physicians. Signs of toxicity to methylxanthines are nausea, tremors, headache, and dysrhythmia.

Probably the most familiar medication that patients with asthma use are the inhaled beta 2 agonists in a metered dose inhaler; the action and use of this class of drugs will be discussed shortly. The metered dose inhalers each contain about 200 puffs (inhalations) per canister of medication. Even if the patient is prescribed use of the inhaler every morning, noon, and night, there should be sufficient medication for a

month. The Paramedic should be concerned if the patient is using more than one metered dose inhaler a month as this may indicate an overreliance on the medication and/or the need to change the patient's medication regime to include anti-inflammatory drugs. Use of two canisters a month has associated risks for hypokalemia and hyperglycemia, as well as other additional risks.

A new class of respiratory medications, the leukotriene modifiers, shows promise, especially as an alternative to inhaled corticosteroids in the patient with mild persistent asthma. These medications work as leukotriene receptor antagonists to prevent the long-acting inflammatory mediator from being effective.

Peak Flow Meter

Many patients are given a peak flow meter (Figure 9-3), a device that measures their airway's peak expiratory flow rate (the fast blast). The patient compares this value, obtained daily, with an ideal value, the personal best for that patient.

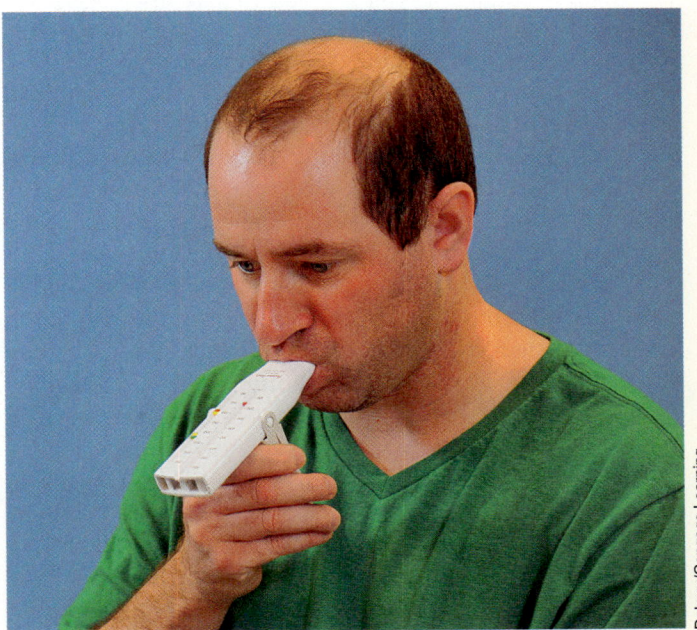

Figure 9-3 Peak flow meter.

Delmar/Cengage Learning

If the patient's peak expiratory flow rate is within 80% of her normal rate, then the patient is said to be in the green zone. Patients in the green zone have good control of their asthma and can resume normal activities of daily living without restriction, provided they take their medications as prescribed.

If the patient's peak expiratory flow rate is in the yellow zone, between 50% and 80% of her personal best, then caution is advised. The patient is encouraged to use the rescue inhaler, an inhaled beta/agonist, and to repeat use of the peak flow meter in 20 to 30 minutes. If there is no improvement in the peak expiratory flow rate, then the patient should seek medical attention.

A patient in the red zone, less than 50% of personal best, indicates a medical emergency. The patient is advised to contact either a personal physician or proceed to an emergency department. While waiting for further assistance, the patient is advised to use the rescue inhaler.

CASE STUDY (CONTINUED)

As the Paramedic continues his examination he notes that Marissa is becoming increasingly winded and complains that she would like to lie down, a request that causes some concern. People who are short of breath typically do not want to lie down.

CRITICAL THINKING QUESTIONS

1. What are the elements of the physical examination of a patient with suspected Type II respiratory failure?

2. Why is an end-tidal carbon dioxide reading a critical element in this examination?

Examination

The Paramedic's view from the doorway can be all telling for the patient with Type II respiratory failure. Type II respiratory failure is, by definition, an increase of carbon dioxide retention (hypercarbia).

The patient who is compensating will be awake and alert, although in varying degrees of distress (partially owed to the accompanying hypoxia). However, the patient who is decompensating (hypercarbiac) will appear drowsy. This somnolence is owed to carbon dioxide-induced narcosis. **Narcosis**, from the Greek *narke* meaning numbing, occurs whenever a drug, in this case carbon dioxide, anesthetizes the brain, particularly the reticular activating system of the brainstem, and induces a state of impaired consciousness ranging from stupor to coma.

Therefore, the patient who appears to be sleeping, or is difficult to arouse, may have hypercarbia and may be in imminent danger of respiratory arrest. Other clues of carbon dioxide narcosis include **head bobbing**, a rhythmic nodding of the head as the patient fights off sleep, and half-opened eyelids, where the patient appears to be half asleep.

The patient's position can also be telling. Patients in respiratory distress rarely lie supine. They prefer to be seated to allow the lungs to be suspended. This allows the abdominal pannus to descend, maximizing diaphragmatic excursion, in order to aerate the lungs more completely. To maximize this efficiency, many patients will sit in a tripod position, with the chest leaning forward and the upper body supported on the arms placed on the knees. Often patients with severe respiratory distress will be found seated in a straight back chair, such as the kind found at a kitchen table, and/or seated at the kitchen table with their elbows on the table supporting them.

The patient's speech is the next clue to the degree of respiratory distress. Patients able to complete full sentences in response to the Paramedic's open-ended questions are generally not in as much distress as the patient with choppy bursts of words (**word clusters**) or the patient who can only utter simple one-word responses (**monosyllabic answers**).

The remainder of the examination is generally performed in a head-to-toe fashion. **Nasal flaring**, the exaggeration of the nostrils (alae nasi), occurs early in respiratory distress as the body tries to enlarge the opening to allow more air passage.

While observing the oral cavity, the Paramedic might note either **open mouthed breathing** or **pursed lip breathing**. Both are forms of exaggerated ventilation. Patients generally do not utilize open mouth breathing unless they are in pain, have fear, or have air hunger, as they generally prefer to breathe through the nose instead.

Pursed lip breathing is a rescue technique taught to patients with lung disease. Pursed lip breathing creates an obstruction to exhalation, resulting in back pressure in the airways. In a sense, pursed lip breathing is similar to positive end expiratory pressure (PEEP), which is used to hyperinflate the lungs during resuscitation and thereby maximize the alveolar surface area for respiration. Properly performed pursed lip breathing can create between 5 to 10 cm H_2O PEEP.

Pursed lip breathing utilizes partially closed lips, such as when one is whistling, to slow exhalation and, more importantly, increase the time of exhalation to approximately two to three times longer than normal. Patients who are properly performing pursed lip breathing have the lips pursed in the center rather than puckered as if to whistle.

Generally inhalation is barely noticeable in patients, with minimal chest rise and no noise as air rushes into the chest cavity. However, the mechanics of respiration are altered in the patient with respiratory distress. This patient appears hunched over and pulls at every breath, using the sternocleidomastoid muscles (strap muscles) that run parallel to each other along the anterior neck to lift the sternum and the rib cage. The trapezius muscle, a large muscle that spans the neck and shoulder, pulls the shoulders upward to assist ventilation by expanding the chest cavity.

The three pairs of muscles called the scalenes originate at the posterior neck and wrap around to the first ribs. Contraction of the scalenes causes the first and second ribs to be elevated, thus increasing the chest cavity volume as well.

Together the sternocleidomastoid, scalene, and trapezius muscles are considered accessory muscles; in other words, they are only recruited to assist with ventilation in times of distress. These paired muscle groups tend to lift the upper chest cavity. When the accessory muscles are recruited by respiratory distress, their contraction is grossly visible in the neck and upper chest area.

The other accessory muscles of respiration are the intercostal muscles. The internal and external intercostal muscles are located between each rib and cause the ribs to bow, like leaf springs. The external intercostal muscles raise the ribs, increasing the chest cavity space. This augments the negative pressure created by the contraction of the diaphragm; therefore, the external intercostals help with inhalation. The internal intercostals bring the ribs together by collapsing the chest cavity and pushing air out. Therefore, the internal intercostal muscles are part of forced exhalation.

Forceful contraction of the intercostal muscles causes the ribs to appear more prominently and shallow depressions to become created between ribs. These depressions are named for their location on the chest wall: suprasternal retractions, supraclavicular retractions, and intercostal retractions.

Continuing the assessment triad of look, listen, and feel, the Paramedic should auscultate adventitious breath sounds. These additional breath sounds are superimposed over the natural ebb and flow of air in the chest.

Starting at the neck, auscultation of tracheal breath sounds may reveal **stridor**, a high-pitched sound that occurs when the upper airway is narrowed. The Paramedic should auscultate the trachea whenever a suspicion of upper airway stricture is present (i.e., audible stridor, burn patients, etc.).

Next, the Paramedic should auscultate the bronchial and bronchovesicular breath sounds appreciated over the lung fields, from apices to base and bilaterally. The most worrisome breath sound is silence. For the patient with asthma, silent lungs are an ominous sign of complete ventilatory collapse and imminent respiratory arrest.

Decreased breath sounds can have several meanings, depending on their position. Decreased breath sounds at the bases can imply consolidation, as with pneumonia, whereas decreased breath sounds at the apices can be suggestive of pneumothorax. Patients with advanced asthma can develop spontaneous pneumothoracies secondary to hyperinflation, or from assisted positive pressure ventilation to an already distended lung.

Although rales (crackles), either the higher pitched but soft fine rales, or the lower pitched louder sounds of coarse rales, are most often associated with heart failure, these sounds are the result of consolidation of secretions in the narrowing airway and can be present in the patient with asthma or emphysema.

Wheezing has always been strongly suggestive of asthma. Although many different conditions can cause wheezing, as noted earlier, the Paramedic should not ignore the presence of wheezing in the patient diagnosed with asthma. Some early warning signs of asthma can be observed in a head-to-toe assessment (Table 9-6).

Next, the Paramedic should palpate the patient's chest wall for symmetrical chest rise. Asymmetrical chest rise may be an indication of a spontaneous pneumothorax and bears further investigation. In some cases, chest rise is barely noticeable, implying that the chest cavity is already hyperinflated and there is no more room for expansion.

In advanced cases of asthma, and in cases of emphysema, the Paramedic may note that the patient has an increased anterior–posterior (AP) diameter. The normal chest depth should be about one-half of the chest width. Although this dimension changes slightly with age, the AP diameter should not be one to one. An increased AP diameter leaves the patient's chest appearing round or "barrel-chested."

Persistent Nonproductive Cough

A symptom Paramedics often overlook in patients is the presence of a persistent nonproductive cough that often occurs at night. This cough may be indicative of asthma. Patients who do not present with wheezing initially but rather with a

Table 9-6 Early Warning Signs of Asthma: from Head to Toe

- Headache
- Moodiness or irritability
- Nighttime waking
- Runny, stuffy nose
- Chin or throat itches
- Unexplained fatigue

dry hacking cough are diagnosed with cough-variant asthma. Cough-variant asthma is generally responsive to standard asthma therapies, such as inhaled beta/agonists.

Vital Signs

Patients with dyspnea, regardless of the etiology, will be hyperdynamic. Tachycardia, along with tachypnea, are to be expected as the patient attempts to resolve the buildup of carbon dioxide and reverse hypoxia by circulating blood through the lungs faster. Epinephrine, the sympathetic neurotransmitter that stimulates the sympathetic nervous system, is responsible for the hyperdynamic state. Epinephrine also stimulates vasoconstriction, noted in the elevated blood pressures which are observed as well.

Diagnostic Examination

The simplest diagnostic test that can be performed on a patient experiencing an asthma attack is pulse oximetry.[20] Assuming good perfusion, the pulse oximeter can help identify underlying hypoxia.

Pulse oximetry is very helpful in identifying hypoxia. In one study, up to 85% of patients who were hypoxic by pulse oximetry did not feel short of breath, and in some cases the hypoxia was not recognized by physical examination. Based on this data, the benefits of pulse oximetry are clear.

Therefore, pulse oximetry should be utilized whenever the patient's presentation may lead to a finding of hypoxia. Persistent hypoxia in the face of high-flow, high-concentration oxygen, as shown by the pulse oximeter, is a reliable indicator of poor outcomes and is correlative with hospital admission.

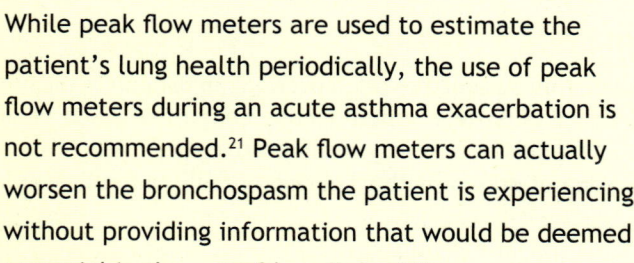

STREET SMART

While peak flow meters are used to estimate the patient's lung health periodically, the use of peak flow meters during an acute asthma exacerbation is not recommended.[21] Peak flow meters can actually worsen the bronchospasm the patient is experiencing without providing information that would be deemed essential in the out-of-hospital setting.

Respiratory Sinus Arrhythmia

The changes of intrathoracic pressure—compressing and releasing the great vessels and in particular the vena cava—result in a slight variation in cardiac rhythm and output. The resultant variability in heart rhythm, called the **respiratory sinus arrthythmia**, is recognized on the ECG as a variation between the cardiac complex, specifically the R-to-R intervals.

As a result, the heartbeat is closer together during inspiration and further apart during exhalation. This relationship emphasizes the interconnectedness of the cardiopulmonary systems (i.e., matching ventilation with perfusion). During periods of hypercarbia, the ventilation-to-perfusion match is lost and the result is less effective heartbeats and respirations.

12-Lead Electrocardiogram

Another tool of the Paramedic, the 12-lead electrocardiogram, can also provide diagnostic information. Increased intrathoracic pressures during an acute asthma attack can decrease venous return to the left ventricle. The resultant back pressure into the lung fields creates pulmonary hypertension and backward failure into the right ventricle. The right ventricle, a low pressure pump, begins to strain under the additional load. This strain, manifested on the 12-lead ECG as **P pulmonale**, is a right atrial abnormality. It appears on the 12-lead ECG as tall peaked P waves in leads II, III, and aV, with a > 2.5 mm, and a prominent positive P wave in precordial Lead V1. Right axis deviation, secondary to right ventricular hypertrophy, is also seen in patients with pulmonary diseases. A right axis deviation is seen when the QRS in Lead I is negative and the QRS in Lead III and Lead aVF are positive.

Capnography

Capnography is another valuable diagnostic tool for assessing the severity of asthma and other pulmonary diseases.[22] **Capnography** measures the amount of carbon dioxide in expired air.

During the beginning of exhalation, air from dead space in the trachea, that area where no gas exchange occurs, passes over the sensor, resulting in a zero reading. This portion of the graph is referred to as phase one. As deeper alveolar air passes over the sensor, the carbon dioxide reading typically rises until it reaches its peak and plateaus out in phases two and three. Subsequent inhalation of carbon dioxide-free air causes the reading to plummet in what is phase zero.

The carbon dioxide reading at the end of exhalation, the end-tidal carbon dioxide ($EtCO_2$), is usually greatest and ranges between 35 and 37 mmHg. The difference between the carbon dioxide in the blood (the $PaCO_2$) and the end-tidal carbon dioxide (the $EtCO_2$) is usually within 5 mmHg. Thus, the $EtCO_2$ can be used as an indirect measurement of $PaCO_2$.[23]

Capnography, providing a waveform, is preferable to a capnometer, which provides a digital readout as it displays a normal "square" waveform for the patient with normal lung function. For the patient with air trapping secondary to bronchospasm, phase two and phase three are prolonged, resulting in a shark fin-like waveform (Figure 9-4).

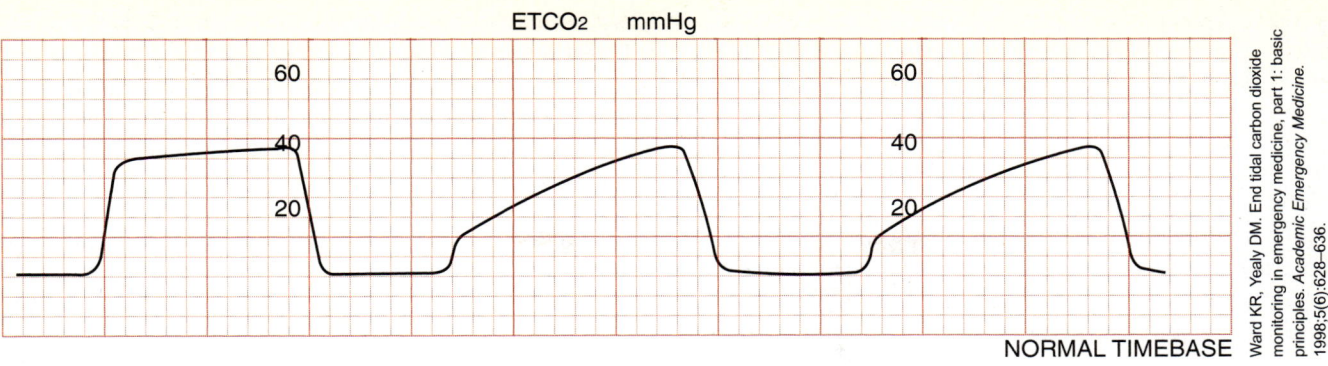

ETCO2   mmHg

NORMAL TIMEBASE

Ward KR, Yealy DM. End tidal carbon dioxide monitoring in emergency medicine, part 1: basic principles. *Academic Emergency Medicine.* 1998;5(6):628–636.

Figure 9-4   Shark fin waveform of asthma on a patient's capnograph.

CASE STUDY (CONTINUED)

While the Paramedics prepare to treat Marissa, her friends relate that she has a history of asthma and that she had tried to use her rescue inhaler earlier, apparently without success. One of the friends hands the rescue inhaler over to the Paramedic. The expiration date of the metered dose inhaler expired six months ago.

CRITICAL THINKING QUESTIONS

1. What is the significance of the elevated end-tidal carbon dioxide level?
2. What does the use of a rescue inhaler suggest?

Assessment

Based on the symptom complex presented (elevated carbon dioxide levels and concomitant hypoxia), the Paramedic's diagnosis would be Type II respiratory failure likely secondary to reactive airway disease.

The critical clinical decision the Paramedic has to make is the patient's degree of respiratory distress. Respiratory distress can be divided into respiratory distress, respiratory failure, and respiratory arrest. The division between distress and failure is premised on the patient's level of consciousness. Regardless of whether the faltering level of consciousness is secondary to carbon dioxide narcosis or hypoxia, the Paramedic must institute dramatic life-saving measures to forestall the inevitable respiratory arrest that will result if action is not taken.

CASE STUDY (CONTINUED)

As the Paramedic proceeds with treatment, he requests that the dispatcher expedite an ambulance to the scene and advise the ambulance to prepare for an imminent respiratory arrest. With the aid of an EMT on scene, medical control is contacted as the two Paramedics start care.

CRITICAL THINKING QUESTIONS

1. What is the standard of care of patients with suspected Type II respiratory failure?
2. What are some of the patient-specific concerns and considerations that the Paramedic should consider when applying this plan of care that is intended to treat a broad patient population presenting with acute respiratory failure?

Treatment

Treatment for the patient with an exacerbation of asthma focuses on the dynamic hyperinflation of the lungs, not on the difficulty with respiration. Resolving the bronchospasm, a first priority, will improve ease of respiration, ventilation, and reverse hypercarbia.

The treatment options for the patient with asthma are as simple as remembering the ABCs (airway, breathing, circulation), drugs, and emergency transportation. While the ABCs are easy to remember, the order of treatment must be individualized to the patient's needs and evolving condition.

For the crashing asthmatic who is rapidly deteriorating and either is facing or is in respiratory arrest, control of the airway is critical. Although the problem is with the lower airway rather than the upper airway, the patient who cannot control the upper airway must be endotracheally intubated.

The Paramedic's decision whether or not to intubate can be based on a simple ABC decision tree. If the patient is at risk for **A**spiration (A), worsening **B**ronchospasm (B), and/or **C**ardiac compromise (C), then intubation should be considered. The clinical indicators for emergency intubation include evidence of respiratory fatigue (somnolence), persistent tachypnea, silent lungs, and bradycardia.

Complications associated with intubation of the patient with an acute exacerbation of asthma include pneumothorax, aspiration, and worsening bronchospasm.

Simple pneumothorax is possible secondary to high airway pressures created by positive pressure ventilation (discussed shortly) and is more likely in the patient with COPD and blebs.

All prehospital patients can be assumed to have full stomachs. Positive pressure ventilation, especially without cricoid pressure, established in preparation for intubation can lead to gastric distention, regurgitation, and aspiration.

Finally, the introduction of an endotracheal tube into the trachea (a mechanical stimulus) can lead to further bronchospasm and a worsening condition. Prior to intubation, premedicating the patient with 1.5 mg/kg of lidocaine may help decrease airway reactivity and prevent bronchoconstriction.[24,25]

If the patient is to be intubated, then the Paramedic should use the largest diameter endotracheal tube that the patient will tolerate in order to improve laminar airflow and minimize any resistance created by the endotracheal tube to ventilation. Intubation of the patient with asthma has ominous implications. Approximately 16.5% of patients who have asthma and are intubated breathe their last breath while on a ventilator.

Next, the Paramedic should focus on the quality of breathing. Caution should be exercised if assisted ventilations are utilized. Manual ventilation with a positive pressure device, such as a bag–mask assembly, can lead to breath stacking. With breath stacking, each positive pressure ventilation increases the intrathoracic pressure, leading to cardiac compromise and a risk for a spontaneous pneumothorax.

When ventilating the patient with an asthma attack, the Paramedic can expect increased airway pressures and decreased airway compliance. Instead of increasing the force of ventilation to overcome airway pressure, the Paramedic should use smaller than usual volumes, in the 6 to 8 cc/kg range, and slower breaths that allow for prolonged exhalation, somewhere between 6 to 10 breaths per minute. If the bag–mask assembly is equipped with a "pop–off" valve, the valve should be disabled.

While Paramedics have a tendency to overventilate the patient in extermis, the current concept in ventilation of the patient with asthma is **permissive hypercarbia**.[26–28] Patients can tolerate elevated carbon dioxide levels better than was previously assumed, provided that any hypoxia is corrected. The effect of hypercarbia is sedation and carbon dioxide narcosis. The sedated patient is more likely to tolerate intubation and manual ventilation.

The goal of permissive hypercarbia is to maintain the $PaCO_2$ between 45 and 55 mmHg while maintaining low airway pressures (approximately 30 to 35 cm H_2O). With an increased inspiration to exhalation ratio of 1:4 or 1:6, the patient has a greater chance of recovering from the asthma attack.

The use of continuous positive airway pressure (CPAP) for patients with asthma is somewhat controversial. The theory is that the airways are mechanically stented up, with about 5 to 8 cm H_2O pressure, thus overcoming the bronchoconstriction. In essence, CPAP is thought to work like pursed lip breathing. Randomized clinical trials in the field may provide better evidence of the utility of this approach in the future.[29,30]

With the multiple attendant risks associated with intubation and manual/mechanical ventilation of the patient with asthma, the decision to intubate should be considered carefully (Table 9-7). If at all possible, the Paramedic should avoid this course of action.

Oxygen therapy is a cornerstone of respiratory disease treatment. The implications of acidosis, secondary to carbon dioxide retention, and its impact on the oxyhemoglobin curve impart a higher importance to the provision of oxygen therapy. Normally a pulse oximetry reading of 92% or more is acceptable. However, if the patient is pregnant, a child, or has other comorbidities such as coronary artery disease or diabetes, then a reading of 96% or greater should be the goal.

Paramedics frequently forego intravenous access in a patient with mild respiratory distress, depending instead on inhaled medications to provide symptomatic relief. However, if there is any concern for cardiovascular compromise, or

Table 9-7 Indications for Intubation of the Patient with Asthma

- Diminished level of consciousness (somnolence)
- Severe hypoxia in the face of 100% oxygen
- Severe respiratory failure manifested by $PaCO_2 > 55$ mmHg
- Cardiac or respiratory arrest

the use of steroids is anticipated, then intravenous access is necessary. Paramedics should exercise caution when infusing intravenous solutions to avoid the complication of acute pulmonary edema.

Short-Acting Beta 2 Agonist

When treating a patient with asthma, it is important to understand that the patient's difficulty lies with bronchoconstriction. Neither positive pressure ventilation nor intubation will help to resolve bronchoconstriction.

Bronchoconstriction is the result of contraction of the muscular bands that wrap around the bronchioles in a crisscross pattern. The purpose of these muscles is to narrow airways and prevent contaminates from entering the alveoli. In some circumstances (such as patients with respiratory diseases), these bronchi are hyperresponsive to even benign stimuli, causing abnormal airway narrowing, air trapping, and hyperinflation of the alveoli.

These smooth muscles in the bronchi are controlled by dual innervations from the sympathetic and the parasympathetic nervous system. Sympathetic stimulation, by means of epinephrine, would cause muscular relaxation in the bronchi. Specifically, epinephrine stimulates the enzyme adenyl cyclase. This enzyme catalyzes the conversion of ATP—the energy source for the cellular ion exchange—into cyclic AMP. As a result of decreased ATP, there is a calcium influx into the cell and relaxation of bronchial muscle.

Epinephrine was found to be an effective bronchodilator in the past. For this reason, epinephrine was one of the first treatments of respiratory distress. Some physicians still advocate for the use of epinephrine in select cases of respiratory distress, especially those unresponsive to newer medications. However, epinephrine is generally not considered a first line medication because of its potential for excessive cardiac stimulation.

Currently, the first line treatment for bronchoconstriction is a class of drugs called sympathomimetics. **Sympathomimetics** are drugs that imitate the effect of the natural bronchodilator epinephrine (the neurotransmitter of the sympathetic nervous system), but do not have the same undesirable side effects (Table 9-8). The sympathomimetics work so effectively that they are referred to as rescue drugs.

Current sympathomimetics are more beta selective, meaning that these drugs preferentially attach to beta 2 receptors in the lungs rather than beta 1 receptors in the heart. This leads to less cardiac stimulation in general, and reduces the

Table 9-8   Side Effects of Sympathomimetic Medications

- Tachycardia
- Hypertension
- Muscle cramps
- Hypokalemia

risk of coronary artery vasoconstriction in particular. Because these drugs preferentially chose beta 2 receptors, these beta 2 adrenergic receptor agonists are called **beta agonists**.

These beta agonists can be given via many routes. Although the preferred route for drug administration is inhaled, as will be discussed in more detail shortly, some of these drugs can also be administered orally or intravenously.

The side effects of beta-selective sympathomimetics (beta 2 agonists) primarily involve the effects of epinephrine. For example, during the fight or flight response (adrenaline rush) glucose is liberated from glycogen as needed. Therefore, when select-elective beta agonists are administered, the patient may experience hyperglycemia. Other side effects include hypokalemia (as potassium is forced into the cells), increased lactic acid production (secondary to skeletal muscle tremors), and even a headache.

One of the most common initial side effects of beta 2 agonist use is an increase in wheezing. As the particles of medicine bombard the walls of the hyperresponsive airway, the initial response is to constrict. This bronchoconstriction should only last moments before the medication takes effect. The onset of medication effect is generally within 15 minutes.

A new formulation of albuterol named levalbuterol, which uses the R isomer of albuterol, has been used to treat patients with asthma. Touted as having fewer side effects than standard albuterol, such as tremors and tachydysrhythmia, it has been prescribed to patients with a history of tachydysrhythmias and in some pediatric cases.

STREET SMART

Paramedics prefer drugs that can be used for multiple functions, thus limiting the number of drugs to be carried. Some examples of multi-use drugs are beta-selective sympathomimetics. For example, some of these drugs, depending on the formulation, can be used to reverse hyperkalemia (which may occur with crush injury) and to slow labor (tocolysis) in obstetric cases.

Drug Interactions with Sympathomimetics

Many psychiatric medications, such as tricyclic antidepressants and monoamine oxidase inhibitors (MAOIs), work with agonist—or block antagonist—neurotransmitters in the brain, such as norepinephrine, with concurrent systemic side effects.

The mode of action of the antidepressant medication MAOI, for example, works to block an enzyme that breaks down norepinephrine, thus increasing norepinephrine levels in the brain. The additional epinephrine in the body tends to lead to vasoconstriction and hypertension in this patient population, necessitating close medical monitoring. Coadministration of sympathomimetic medications and MAOI could potentially lead to dangerous increases in circulating catecholamines (epinephrine), leading to profound hypertension, hypertensive crisis, and stroke. Because these psychiatric medications tend to augment the effects of these sympathomimetic medications, their use is generally reserved for emergencies and then only with close medical monitoring.

Anticholinergics

The parasympathetic nervous system's effects are in opposition to the effects of the sympathetic nervous system. The parasympathetic nervous system creates bronchoconstriction for the patient with respiratory disease. The primary neurotransmitter for the parasympathetic nervous system is acetylcholine. Drugs that interfere with the parasympathetic neurotransmitter are called **anticholinergics**.

Anticholinergics, such as atropine, prevent an increase in the intracellular cyclic GMP, a second intracellular messenger like cyclic AMP, and thus act as an antagonist to the effects of epinephrine, although via a slightly different mechanism. This distinction allows the Paramedic to understand how the patient can be tachycardic, secondary to hypoxia-induced epinephrine secretion, and still be bronchoconstricted from parasympathetic stimulation, which is an apparent contradiction.

Atropine sulfate is the quintessential anticholinergic medication that blocks muscarinic receptors, specifically the M_3 receptors located in the lungs. This action prevents bronchoconstriction and mucous secretion, leading to dry mouth.

It should be noted that atropine, and atropine-like derivatives, do not cause bronchodilation. Therefore, atropine helps to sustain the action of bronchodilators, such as the sympathomimetics mentioned earlier.

As with epinephrine, there are newer formulations of atropine-like drugs that produce better airflow. Some of these have a half-life of two hours. The newest parasympathetic blockers have up to 20 times more affinity to muscarinic receptors. Like the sympathomimetics, atropine and many of its derivatives can be given via inhalation or intravenously.

Anticholinergics, such as Ipratropium, can cause modest improvement in ventilation when given in combination with a sympathomimetic. While its onset of action is upward of 20 minutes, the patient's improvement may only be sustained if repeated doses are used.

The newer formulations of anticholinergics, when inhaled, do not cross into the blood. This is a significant advantage as it limits the drug's systemic anticholinergic effects. However, when compared side by side, the two drugs have like effects on lung volume and airway resistance. In addition, atropine has been shown to be more effective in larger airways.

Although the use of an anticholinergic and sympathomimetics together is useful for patients with chronic obstructive pulmonary disease, there is some controversy about their concomitant use in patients with an exacerbation of asthma. However, the use of sympathomimetics (rescue inhalers) for patients with asthma remains a mainstay of medical therapeutics.

Conversely, some patients are sensitive to sympathomimetics, such as albuterol, and cannot tolerate the side effects. For those patients, an anticholinergic, such as Ipratropium bromide, is prescribed along with anti-inflammatory medications or methylxanthines.

It should be noted that patients on these anticholinergic medications have decreased vagal tone and thus decreased vagally mediated airway reflexes. These vagally mediated airway reflexes help to bronchoconstrict and protect the airway from irritants, including gastric reflex. As a result, these patients may be more prone to aspirations and aspiration pneumonitis.

Nebulized Medications and Peanut Allergies

Some nebulized inhaled medications contain lecithin. Lecithin, a chemical isolated from egg yolks, soy beans, or peanuts, is used as a food additive and in the pharmaceutical production of certain inhalers. Therefore, caution should be observed when administering any inhaler to a patient with an allergy to any of the potential sources of lecithin for fear of triggering an allergic reaction.

Many "rescue" inhalers are lecithin-free. However, the Paramedic should review the list of inert ingredients as well as the active ingredients in any preparation before administration as well as obtain a medical history which includes the patient's allergies.

STREET SMART

Occasionally patients with a history of asthma may be inadvertently prescribed a beta blocker medication and, as a result, may experience bronchoconstriction. Anticholinergics, such as Ipratropium bromide, are the drug of choice for these patients.

Anti-Inflammatory Medicines

Synthetic systemic steroids administered in the field supplement the naturally occurring hormone cortisol in the patient's body. Cortisol, supplied from the adrenal cortex, is a potent immunosuppressant that can be used to treat allergies and asthma. Steroids can help reduce inflammation, thereby improving airway function and preventing future reoccurrence of asthma attacks. For these reasons, Paramedics often offer patients steroids for their asthma while in the field.

Although the administration of anti-inflammatory medications in the field does not offer the patient immediate relief from the symptoms, respiratory diseases are inflammatory in nature. Early administration of anti-inflammatory medication serves to reduce the degree of inflammation over time. A Cochrane meta-analysis (a statistical analysis of several studies) of anti-inflammatory steroid administration showed that early steroid use decreases the severity of illness and reduced hospital admissions.[31,32]

Although steroids have many positive effects, especially for the patient with respiratory disease, they do have drawbacks. For example, administration of steroids can lead to immunosuppression, leaving the patient vulnerable to infections, a problem for patients with concurrent respiratory infections. Steroids can also decrease glycogen formation, promote glycogenolysis, and lead to hyperglycemia. Patients with hyperglycemia are more prone to infections.

Most Paramedics administer steroids intravenously. Although medical opinions vary, corticosteroids should be considered whenever the patient has moderate to severe persistent asthma, is experiencing recurrent asthma without complete resolution following self-administration of repeated doses of a rescue inhaler, or the patient is at risk for status asthmaticus (discussed shortly).

Paramedics tend to not administer medications orally because of the risk of vomiting as well as the patient's inability, or unwillingness, to swallow a pill while short of breath. However, some studies have suggested that oral administration of steroids is as effective as intravenous administration, with peak plasma levels within 15 minutes. Oral administration should be considered, in part because it offers deferred venous access, which is advantageous in some pediatric cases.

Alternatively, some Paramedics may opt to administer steroids to patients with moderate to severe symptoms via a metered dose inhaler. High dose inhaled corticosteroids (ICS) can be as effective as intravenous systemic corticosteroids and may be quicker to administer than systemic corticosteroids. Furthermore, inhaled corticosteroids deposit the medications directly on the site of inflammation and may avoid some of the systemic complications that are associated with intravenous systemic steroids. Again, this method offers the opportunity to defer venous access in some pediatric cases.

Regardless of the route chosen, research has suggested that early administration of steroids, within one hour of onset of symptoms, can reduce the severity and/or length of an asthma attack in children.

Aerosol Medication Delivery Methods

The endgame of respiratory care during an acute asthma attack is to relieve bronchoconstriction. To do that, medication must get to the pulmonary tree through either inspired air or the bloodstream.

The easiest method of drug delivery to the lungs, via inspired air, is to take the medication and aerosolize it. The process of aerosolizing a drug is called nebulization, from the Latin *nebula*, meaning mist. Early physicians and pharmacists prescribed volatile aromatic solutions which would off-gas vapors, which would then be inhaled by asthma patients. The forerunner of the modern nebulizer, the atomizer, was used to treat asthma in the 1930s.

There are currently two delivery platforms for the administration of inhaled asthma medications in the prehospital setting: the metered dose inhaler and the small volume nebulizer. Although Paramedics tend to prefer using the small volume nebulizer, the metered dose inhaler—when properly used in cases of mild to moderate asthma—can be equally as effective. In fact, a Cochrane style meta-analysis of studies comparing the small volume nebulizer against the metered dose inhaler showed little difference between the two devices in terms of the amount of medication the patient received. The single factor that motivated providers to use one device rather than the other was hand-to-inhalation coordination. This analysis lends support to the practice of EMT-assisted medication administration and its potential efficacy in the field. Between 4 to 10 puffs of albuterol via a metered dose inhaler with a spacer is equivalent to 2.5 mg of albuterol via small volume nebulizer (SVN).[33]

Metered Dose Inhaler

The **metered dose inhaler (MDI)**, first launched in 1956, is a device that holds medication suspended in an aerosol inside a pressurized canister (Figure 9-5). When the MDI is actuated by compression of the plastic trigger—or actuator—on the inhaler, a specific amount of medication, measured by means of a metering valve, is released into the air. This mist is then inhaled into the lungs for direct absorption into the bronchioles.

Before providing the MDI, often referred to as the "inhaler" by patients, it should be shaken three to four times to evenly disperse the suspension (the medication) within the propellant. The patient should then exhale. The Paramedic removes the cap from the MDI and, with the inhaler upright, places the mouthpiece about two finger breadths away from

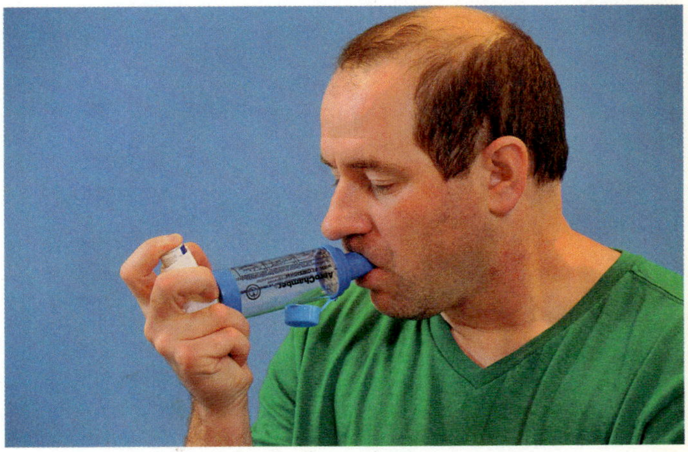

Delmar/Cengage Learning

Figure 9-5 Anatomy of inhaler with aerochamber.

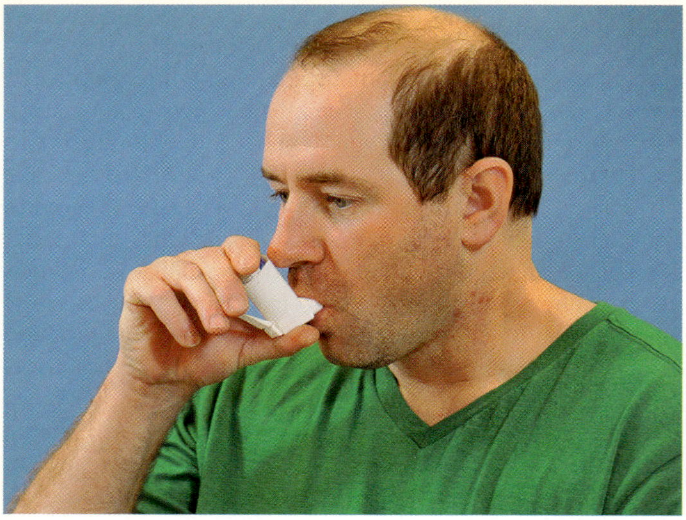

Figure 9-6 Use of MDI inhaler.

the patient's open mouth. This distance is important, as the optimal inspired particulate size is less than 5 microns (Figure 9-6). Use of the MDI in this manner allows the larger particles to drop or "rain out" in the air instead of in the mouth, leaving only the smaller medication particles to be inhaled.

To obtain maximum efficiency of the MDI, the Paramedic must time the actuation of the MDI to begin as the patient takes a slow breath, over a three to five second count. Once the medication is inhaled, then the patient should attempt to hold her breath for a count of 10 (10 seconds) before exhaling. Breath-holding allows the medication to reach to the alveolar level. The patient should wait a minimum of 30 seconds between each use. Remember to store the MDI canister at room temperature.

Dry powder inhalers operate differently. The patient is instructed to place the mouthpiece in between the teeth and inhale quickly. At present, dry powder inhalers are not commonly used by Paramedics.

STREET SMART

In the past, most MDIs used ozone-depleting chlorofluorocarbons (CFC) as the propellant. These CFC-containing propellants were banned in 1978 with the notable exception of medical devices such as the MDI. The exception provided pharmaceutical companies with the opportunity to research and develop alternative medication delivery platforms. Currently non-CFC-containing MDIs are being developed. Some use dry powder instead of an aerosol whereas others are using hydrofluoroalkanes (HFA) as the propellant.

Spacers

Because some patients, particularly the very young and the very old, have difficulty with timing ventilation with the MDI, a device called a **spacer** was developed. A spacer is simply a reservoir that allows the mist from the MDI to be suspended until the patient is ready to inhale. When properly used, a spacer can increase the MDI's efficiency by as much as 20%.[34]

Spacers often "whistle" when the patient inhales too quickly, thus encouraging the patient to take a slow deep breath. Some pediatric spacers come with a small face mask so a child using it does not have to place the mouthpiece between the teeth.

Small Volume Nebulizer

Many Paramedics prefer to use the small volume nebulizer for respiratory medication administration. As the name suggests, the **small volume nebulizer (SVN)** takes a small volume of solution and creates a medical aerosol via nebulization. Although ultrasonic nebulizers do exist, Paramedics primarily use the jet small volume nebulizer.

In some circumstances, the SVN has advantages over the MDI in the field. Use of the MDI requires that patients be able to hold the device in front of them, coordinate hand to breath when actuating the MDI, as well as hold a breath for 10 seconds. The SVN, on the other hand, delivers the medication as long as the patient is breathing and resting comfortably or can be mechanically ventilated. Although it takes upward of 10 to 20 minutes to deliver a single treatment, the SVN allows continuous patient monitoring throughout the duration of the treatment. Finally, the SVN allows the Paramedic to administer multiple medications with the same medication delivery platform. Often a beta 2 agonist is mixed with an anticholinergic medication.

The SVN is designed to deliver a fine mist, with mass median aerodynamic diameter less than 5 microns and preferably between 1 and 3 microns, into the lungs. To accomplish that, most SVNs must be run at a precise liter flow of 7 to 8 lpm. Compressed gas flow rates may not deliver the prescribed medication dose (**Skill 9-1**).

The jet small volume nebulizer operates by using the Bernoulli's principle through a Venturi device. When a compressed gas flows through a tube it creates pressure on the sides of the tube. When the compressed gas reaches a smaller diameter tube called a jet, the velocity increases and the pressure decreases, thus creating a vacuum (Bernoulli's principle).

In an SVN, compressed air is forced through a narrowed opening, or jet, and creates a negative pressure. This negative pressure in turn aspirates fluid from the medication bowl at a precise rate and pushes it into the inner tube where it is ejected against a baffle inside the nebulizer, smashing the droplets into a fine mist. The resulting mist is then carried out to the patient.

Before starting an SVN, the Paramedic may consider wearing an N95 mask. Aerosols from the SVN are carried deep into the lungs and then exhaled into the ambient air shared with the Paramedic. Lung infections, such as tuberculosis, held in the lungs could thus be carried on the exhaled air.

Assembly of the small volume nebulizer starts with instilling medication(s) into the medicine bowel (an optimal volume is 3 cc). The average SVN will dispense approximately 3 cc of medication within seven (7) minutes at 7 lpm.[35]

For a step-by-step demonstration of Use of the Small Volume Nebulizer, please refer to Skill 9-1 on page 258.

While SVNs are effective, research has shown that current SVNs deliver less than 10% of medication within the respirable range to the bronchioles. However, some claim that upward of 40% of the medication can be delivered with certain devices. A small volume nebulizer can even be placed in line, between the mask and bag assembly, in order to deliver the medication with assisted ventilation (Figure 9-7).

Some physicians think that continuous bronchodilator therapy is more effective than intermittent therapy. Repeated bronchodilator treatments may be in order for patients with severe bronchoconstriction as evidenced by a visible increase in the work of breathing; for example, accessory muscle use, productive cough, or lack of improvement with standard therapy.

The Paramedic should exercise caution if the patient's heart rate increases 20% above the baseline for the first treatment or the patient is suspected to be hypokalemic. Extreme caution should be observed if the patient is suspected of having cardiac involvement with the asthma (cor pulmonale) or if the wheezing is thought to be cardiac in origin.

Mucokinetic Drugs

In cases of severe intractable asthma and end-stage COPD, mucous plug formation can be practically problematic. The combination of increased mucous production (secondary to an increased number of goblet cells), increased mucous

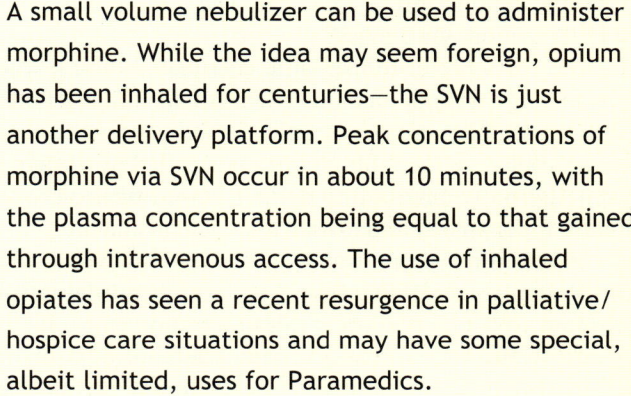

viscosity (secondary to dehydration owed to rapid respirations), ineffective cough (secondary to exhaustion), and abnormal ciliary function results in tenacious secretions that obstruct smaller, bronchoconstricted airways.

Phlegm (sputum) is made up of water and mucus, a proteinaceous chemical compound that is nearly clear. Any color present in the phlegm is owed to bacteria and/or leukocytes. **Mucokinetic** drugs are medications that thin and liquefy viscous phlegm for removal by suctioning or expectoration.

To open plugged airways, and to improve ventilation, Paramedics provide pulmonary toilet to their patients. **Pulmonary toilet** is the combination of deep breathing, coughing, medications to reduce secretions, and respiratory treatments with bronchodilators that result in a productive cough, thus clearing the airway and improving ventilation. Good pulmonary toilet prevents atelectasis and promotes deep alveolar aeration.

Diluents

Humidification of secretions through the use of aerosolized solution can help to liquefy those secretions, making it easier to either expectorate (cough up) or suction the airway-blocking phlegm.

Patients commonly use water to help liquefy viscous respiratory secretions. However, Paramedics tend to use

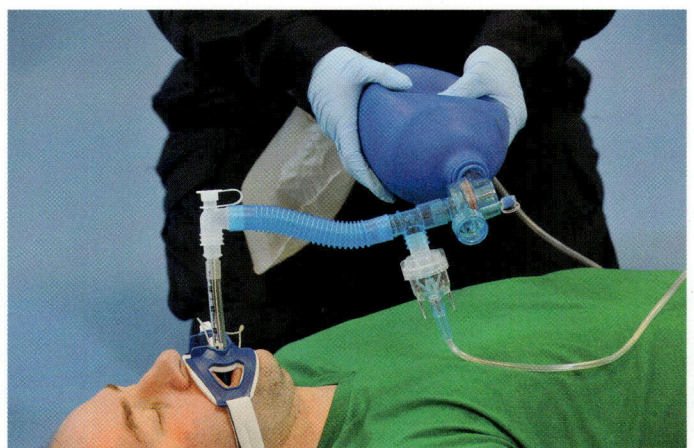

Delmar/Cengage Learning

Figure 9-7 A small volume nebulizer can be placed in line between the BVM and endotracheal tube in an intubated patient.

saline solutions. Normal saline (0.9% sodium chloride in sterile water) is well tolerated as it is physiologic, creating the same osmotic pressures in the patient as plasma. In that way, saline neither adds nor withdraws fluids from the systemic circulation.

Hypotonic one-half normal saline (0.45% sodium chloride in sterile water) is thought to have better penetration in the distal bronchioles and alveoli and is therefore the solution of choice for patients with asthma. The two methods commonly used to add humidity to the patient's airway are the large volume nebulizer and bland aerosol administration via the small volume nebulizer.

The **large volume nebulizer**, also called the "humidifier," is a sterile glass or plastic container filled with sterile solution that attaches to an oxygen regulator or directly to an oxygen source outlet. It has a Venturi device which aerosolizes the solution in the container. The mist is then delivered to the patient via a mask.

Paramedics prefer to use large corrugated tubing when using the large volume nebulizer. The small lumen of standard oxygen tubing creates turbulence and causes the vapor to form droplets in the tubing (a process called rain out).

An alternative method to deliver humidification to the patient's upper airway and to help break up the mucous plugs is to deliver either sterile water or sterile saline via a small volume nebulizer, called a **bland aerosol administration**. The intent of a bland aerosol administration is to deliver moisture to the upper airways. Bland aerosol administration can be helpful for patients with subglottic edema (e.g., following smoke inhalation) or post-extubation edema. The aerosol generated by the SVN should have a mass median aerodynamic diameter (MMAD) of greater than 5 microns. In an emergency, a jet small volume nebulizer can be used, although large volume nebulizers are more effective.

Mucolytics

Mucolytics, also called expectorants, are drugs that can help to dissolve mucus, promote coughing, and allow for better pulmonary toilet by the Paramedic. Mucolytics break down mucin, a glucose-covered protein which gives mucus its thickness, into more soluble strands.

An example of a mucolytic medication is the drug N-acetylcysteine. Acetylcysteine is generally reserved for patients with severe atelectasis secondary to mucous plugging, as seen in the patient with COPD. The usual dosage is 3 to 5 mL of 20% solution. When administered via nebulizer, its effect can peak within one minute and last for over 10 minutes.

CASE STUDY (CONTINUED)

The Paramedics begin a nebulizer treatment of a beta 2 agonist medication plus a parasympatholytic medication. They also initiate venous access in case of need. Marissa tries to use the nebulizer as directed but she becomes increasingly somnolent with minimal chest rise. Upon reassessment, the Paramedic notes that her lung sounds are now silent.

CRITICAL THINKING QUESTIONS

1. What are some of the predictable complications associated with acute respiratory distress secondary to reactive airway diseases?

2. What are some of the predictable complications associated with the treatments for acute respiratory distress?

Evaluation

In the past, asthma was thought to be a single event of bronchospasm (i.e., asthma attack). It is now known that asthma is a chronic disease with acute exacerbations. For this reason, patients with asthma must be consistently monitored to prevent another flareup.

Status Asthmaticus

When the patient's condition steadily worsens despite treatment with beta 2 agonists, the patient is at risk for **status asthmaticus**. Appreciating the chronic nature of asthma, status asthmaticus is typically the culmination of days, or even weeks, of unremitting asthma. Unresolved, status asthmaticus leads to profound hypercarbia with respiratory failure and then respiratory arrest secondary to acidosis. Patients who are at high risk for status asthmaticus display certain distinguishing characteristics (Table 9-9).

The patient with status asthmaticus has severe intractable bronchospasm, often associated with hypercarbia. These patients are unresponsive to standard adrenergic drug therapy and still have persistent dyspnea. The patient with status asthmaticus is more likely to have trouble between the hours of midnight and 6 a.m. Some have attributed this variation to the increase in histamine in the body that occurs as a normal part of circadian rhythm.

A street definition of status asthmaticus might be wheezing for 30 to 60 minutes after a rescue inhaler was used (regardless of whether administered by either the Paramedic or the patient). This lack of airway responsiveness to treatment has been attributed to a combination of mucous plugging, excessive airway edema, and/or inflammation. Therefore, treatments are focused on resolving those issues.

Sudden Onset Asthma

Sudden onset asthma (SOA), a frightening form of fulminate asthma, is a rare form of asthma in which the patient rapidly deteriorates into respiratory arrest despite aggressive medical treatment.[36] Although theories vary as to the etiology of sudden onset asthma, some suggest it is actually an anaphylactic reaction. It is histologically distinct from asthma, with neutrophils exceeding eosinophils.

The rapid deterioration in sudden onset asthma, also called "sudden asphyxia asthmatics," occurs in less than three hours from the onset of symptoms, with intubation being the inevitable result. Approximately 10% of patients with asthma fall into this category, with males predominant among the population. These rapid near-fatal asthma attacks are often preceded by exposure to specific allergens, such as aspirin or beta blockers, or a stressful event. While adolescents (10 to 14 years) constitute the largest group of fatal asthma cases, the single best indicator for sudden onset asthma is a previous episode of sudden onset asthma, lending credence to the importance of a good history.

Physical Examination

The patient's mental status should be the Paramedic's first indication of status asthmaticus. As the patient begins to develop significant hypercarbia, the patient will become somnolent from carbon dioxide-induced narcosis. In this case, it may be necessary for the Paramedic to secure the patient's airway at this point with an endotracheal tube.

Assessing the chest next, when a patient is in status asthmaticus the lungs may be so hyperinflated that it is difficult for the Paramedic to appreciate air movement with a stethoscope. The presence of a silent chest in a patient with asthma is an ominous finding, with a higher frequency of silent chest occurring in patients who will experience SOA.

If air movement is heard, it is not unusual for the Paramedic to detect asymmetry. This asymmetry may due to the effects of mucous plugging and the resultant atelectasis. The Paramedic should suspect the presence of a foreign body obstruction, most likely right side, if unilateral breath sounds are appreciated.

If diminished breath sounds are heard at the apices, then the Paramedic should be concerned that the patient has developed a pneumothorax. If unresolved, a simple pneumothorax can evolve into a life-threatening tension pneumothorax. Therefore, if the Paramedic suspects a pneumothorax, he should palpate the patient's upper chest and neck for the presence of crepitus, a sign of subcutaneous emphysema secondary to an air leak in the pleura.

When the intrathoracic pressures increase, secondary to air trapping and hyperinflation, the venous return to the heart decreases. Without adequate preload, the heart's cardiac output is diminished. This drop in systolic pressure is most notable during inspiration (systolic pressure drops 10 to 15 mmHg with each breath). This phenomenon is called **pulsus paradoxus**. Although Paramedics may not make note of the change in blood pressure, the waxing and waning of the pulse is noticeable. The term "paradoxus" refers to the presence of a heartbeat, verified by heart sounds, without the presence of a corresponding pulse. This represents a paradox.

When pulsus paradoxus is present, careful assessment may also reveal the presence of Kussmaul's sign. **Kussmaul's sign** is an increase in jugular venous distention (JVD) noted with each inspiration as well. Together, pulsus paradoxus and Kussmaul's sign is suggestive of high intrathoracic pressures.

Table 9-9 Patients at High Risk for Status Asthmaticus

- Prior near-fatal attack
- Pneumothorax associated with asthma
- Two or more hospitalizations for asthma in one year
- Current use of steroids
- Sudden cessation of steroid use
- History of intubation with asthma

Treatment

Securing the patient's airway may be the Paramedic's first order of business for the crashing asthmatic (see the indications listed earlier). When the patient is still semiconscious and able to resist the intubation, the Paramedic should consider medication-facilitated intubation.

If the Paramedic so chooses, lidocaine 1.5 mg/kg should be administered to blunt the bronchospastic response to the intubation. It must be remembered that the time of onset of action for lidocaine can be as much as 5 minutes from intravenous administration.

Arguably, ketamine is the drug of choice for medication-facilitated intubation.[37–39] While providing unconsciousness and analgesia, as well as being an amnesic, it also provides bronchodilation while leaving the airway reflexes relatively intact. Furthermore, ketamine can be given to the patient even if the patient is hemodynamically unstable, as ketamine stimulates the cardiovascular system, raising blood pressures and heart rates.

Unfortunately, ketamine is also known for causing emergence reactions, including hallucination, extracorporeal experiences, and a gamut of feelings ranging from euphoria to fear. However, only 10% to 30% of adults experience emergence reactions following the use of ketamine. These reactions can be controlled with benzodiazepines. With long-term sedation occurring immediately after intubation, emergence reaction is not a concern for the Paramedic.

Small Volume Nebulizer and Intubation

Administration of respiratory medications via an endotracheal tube requires Paramedics to place the largest endotracheal tube tolerable. Larger endotracheal tubes decrease resistance and increase laminar airflow into the lungs.

Critical care units routinely administer respiratory medications to intubated patients on mechanical ventilators. The Paramedic can also apply these lessons from "the unit" in the field. When placing a nebulizer "in-line" (in the ventilation pathway), it is best if the nebulizer can be placed at approximately 30 cm from the endotracheal tube. This additional tubing is, in effect, a spacer that allows the medication mist to accumulate between ventilations.

Mechanical difficulties with using an in-line SVN, such as keeping the medication bowl perpendicular to the supine patient, sometimes makes it impractical for field use. However, studies have shown that the use of an MDI in mechanically ventilated patients can produce the same results as an SVN. The Paramedic needs to only interrupt ventilation for a few seconds to attach an MDI with a 30 cm (12 inch) length of corrugated respiratory tubing, deliver a dose of medication, and then resume ventilation.

Parenteral Adrenergics

Inhaled beta 2 agonists may be ineffective if severe bronchoconstriction prevents the drug from entering the alveoli. In those cases of severe asthma, an alternative route (the parenteral route) should be considered. The parenteral route allows the sympathomimetics to reach the bronchial muscles via the capillary route, instead of through the airways, to cause smooth muscle relaxation and subsequent bronchodilation.

Epinephrine, the principal sympathomimetic, has been used as a treatment for life-threatening asthma for nearly a century. Administered subcutaneously at a dose of 0.3 to 0.5 mg, epinephrine effects begin within 5 to 10 minutes, reaching peak plasma levels within 20 to 30 minutes. Because epinephrine peaks in approximately 20 minutes, a repeat dose should be administered at 20-minute intervals.

Parenteral epinephrine can also be administered intramuscularly, a route preferred by some Paramedics for its ease of administration.

Some medical authorities advise caution whenever administering epinephrine to patients over age 40 or those with known coronary artery disease (CAD). It is feared that a combination of increased cardiac oxygen demand (MvO_2) created by the resultant tachycardia and coronary artery vasoconstriction could induce myocardial ischemia.[40] However, other medical authorities argue, with the support of several studies, that the danger of myocardial ischemia is outweighed by the threat of respiratory failure.

Another beta/adrenergic agonist bronchodilator that can be given subcutaneously is terbutaline sulfate, at a dose of 0.25 mg commonly injected into the deltoid. Although hypothetically terbutaline could be effective in optimizing beta-receptor stimulation without concurrent cardiac effects, clinical studies have shown that subcutaneously injected terbutaline does not have a preferential beta/adrenergic effect. Therefore, epinephrine is often the preferred adrenergic agent.

Intravenous Adrenergics

Intravenous epinephrine is generally reserved for use in life-threatening emergencies. Such an emergency is evidenced by altered mental status, pending respiratory arrest, and/or an ominous bradycardia that forebodes a cardiopulmonary arrest, and/or after inhaled beta/agonists have failed.

Caution is advised whenever epinephrine is administered intravenously for fear of potential cardiac complications. However, at least one study showed that the risks for this limited subpopulation of patients with asthma were offset by the benefits.

In those instances, the epinephrine may be administered intravenously by either bolus or infusion (infusion being the preferred method). A typical epinephrine infusion starts with a loading dose of between 50 mcg and 1,000 mcg (1 mg). An epinephrine dilution of 1:10,000 typically used for an intravenous bolus has 100 mcg/mL.

The loading bolus is followed by an infusion of 1 to 4 mcg per min, titrated to effect with careful attention paid for tachycardia, hypertension, and dysrhythmia.

Intravenous Anticholinergics

Atropine, the quintessential anticholinergic, can be given intravenously to patients in status asthmaticus who cannot receive these anticholinergics via aerosol inhalation. If given intravenously, atropine can be effective in preventing further bronchoconstriction, but it is not effective for the cough produced by asthma.

Because atropine can cross the blood barrier when nebulized, with resultant sedation, the use of nebulized atropine cannot be advocated. Ipratropium bromide should be used instead.

Magnesium

When faced with a "crashing asthmatic" patient, some physicians and Paramedics "throw the kitchen sink" at the patient. Typically in medicine, and in paramedicine, one treatment is administered and then the patient's response to that treatment is measured. If the patient responds, then the treatment is continued. If the patient does not respond, the treatment may be discontinued and/or another treatment instituted.

In the case of the rapidly decompensating patient with asthma, multiple treatments are initiated more or less simultaneously. These include oxygen, sympathomimetics administered either subcutaneously or intramuscularly, an anticholinergic corticosteroid, and magnesium. Magnesium can be given either intravenously or through nebulization. This alternative route of administration can be helpful if the patient is in cardiovascular collapse, or is vasculopathetic, and venous access cannot be obtained.

Intravenous magnesium directly affects the bronchial smooth muscle and does not depend on nervous system receptors. After administration of 1 to 2 grams of magnesium sulfate, the Paramedic should expect to see an improvement in pulmonary function almost immediately.[41]

Magnesium needs to be infused slowly, over 10 to 20 minutes, to avoid the attendant vasodilation that could lead to profound hypotension. Careful hemodynamic monitoring of the patient during the intravenous administration is important. If the patient should become hypotensive, this may be due to either the progressive acidosis or the drug effect. The magnesium should be slowed or stopped and the patient observed for changes.

Heliox

Heliox is a breathing gas composed of helium and oxygen. It is used because helium molecules, which are smaller than nitrogen molecules, are theoretically able to slide past narrowed bronchioles with oxygen (so-called slippery oxygen). Because of the smaller molecular size there is less turbulence in the airway, allowing for a more laminar airflow. Although a review of several studies did not recommend the routine use of heliox, it is potentially beneficial for patients with profound bronchoconstriction and should be considered for patients with impending respiratory failure.

CASE STUDY CONCLUSION

Both Paramedics work furiously to try to stabilize Marissa while en route to the hospital. Fortunately, since the EMT at the first aid station had called ahead and gave the emergency department an early warning, the "crash" room is ready and waiting for their arrival.

CRITICAL THINKING QUESTIONS

1. What is the most appropriate transport decision that will get the patient to definitive care?
2. What are the advantages of alerting the hospital before transporting a patient with suspected respiratory failure?

Disposition

Patients with status asthmaticus, who are unresponsive to standard therapies, may need inhaled anesthetics (such as halothane or isoflurane) which can only be administered in the operating room or intensive care unit.

Once the bronchospasm is controlled, many of these patients are extubated in as little as 12 hours. Unfortunately, a number of these patients never have their bronchospasm resolved. As a result, these patients die of complications of asthma.

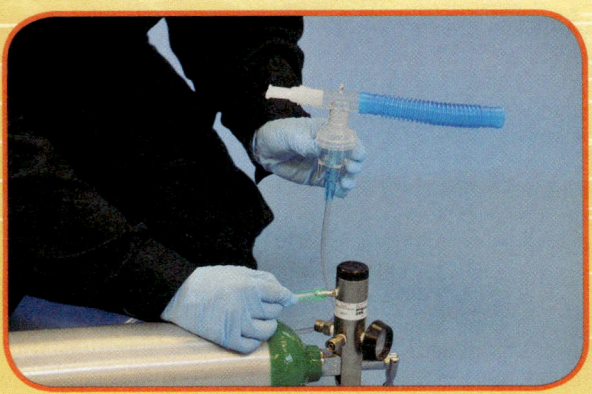

1 Assemble the nebulizer components and attach them to an oxygen source.

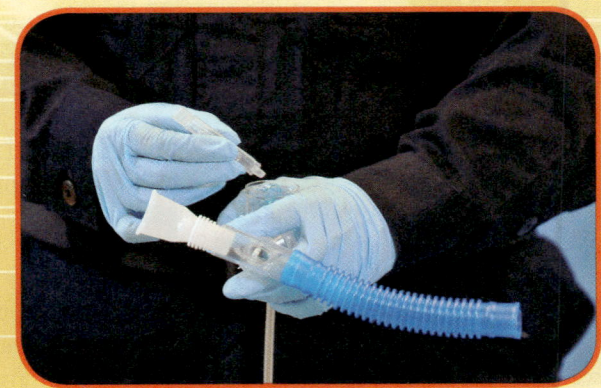

2 Instill the appropriate medication into the chamber.

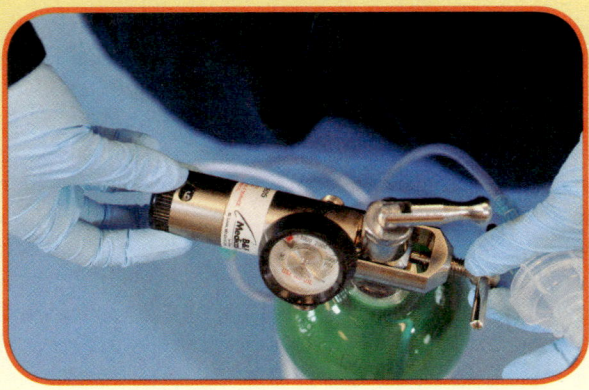

3 Set the oxygen flow rate to 6–8 liters per minute.

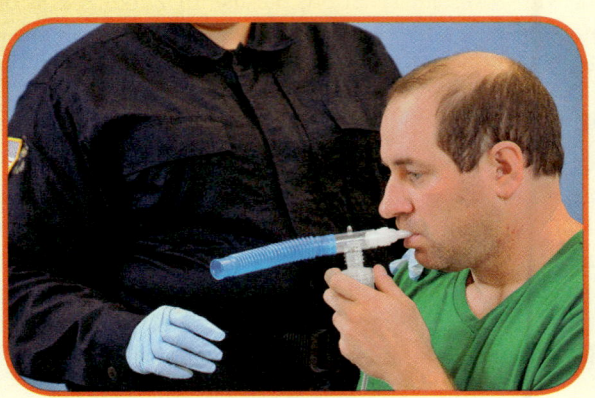

4 Instruct the patient to place the mouthpiece in the mouth with a good seal.

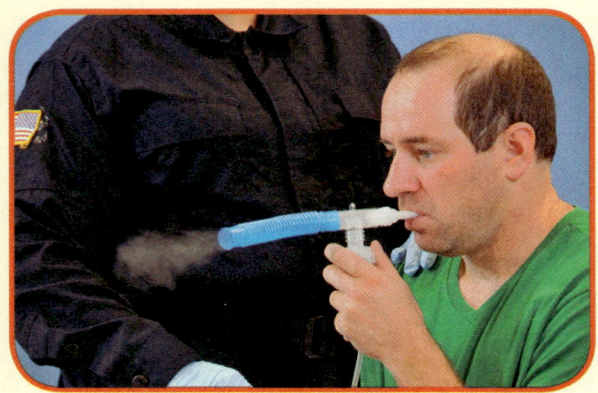

5 Instruct the patient to inhale as deeply as possible and fully exhale.

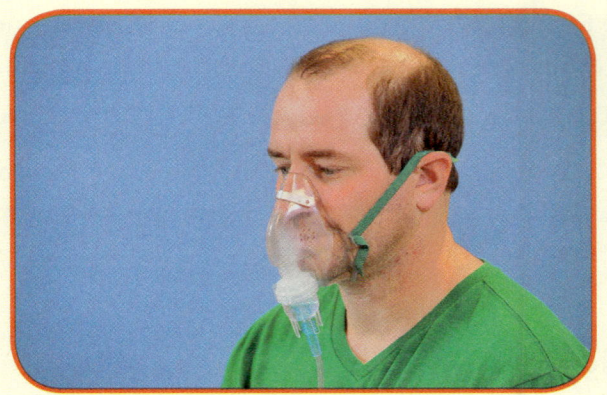

6 Some patients will perform better using a face mask rather than a mouthpiece for delivery of aerosolized medication, though its effectiveness is questionable.

Delmar/Cengage Learning

CONCLUSION

This chapter reviewed disorders of ventilation. It is important for the Paramedic to remember that ventilation and oxygenation, while intertwined, are two separate physiologic processes that both need to be addressed when caring for the patient that has a chief concern related to difficulty breathing.

KEY POINTS:

- Impairment of airflow leads to CO_2 retention, the differentiation between Type I and Type II respiratory failure.

- Although neuromuscular and muscular-skeletal defects can lead to impaired airflow and diffusion, the most common cause is one of the chronic obstructive pulmonary diseases.

- The primary difference between the various chronic obstructive pulmonary diseases is the predominance of either excessive secretions, spasms, or swelling of the airway.

- Chronic bronchitis is characterized by irreversible airway changes and chronic productive cough.

- Emphysema is characterized by distended, inelastic alveoli which reduce space for diffusion, leading to potential weakened areas that may lead to pneumothoraxes and increase air trapping.

- Emphysema is associated with right-sided heart failure due to pressure changes in the pulmonary artery and an excessive production of red blood cells, which make up the body's attempt to counter hypoxemia.

- Asthma is a chronic disease with exacerbations characterized by airway hyperirritability, reversible bronchospasm, and inflammation.

- Wheezing is a common sign of airway swelling but is not specific to asthma.

- Difficulty in exhaling leads to air trapping which, over time, alters the shape of the chest, causing a condition called barrel chest.

- Respiratory acidosis occurs secondary to rising carbon dioxide levels. Patients exposed long term to a high carbon dioxide level acclimate to it and thus respond to a low oxygen level as the stimulus to breathe, called hypoxic drive.

- In taking a history, the Paramedic should utilize mnemonics to help the patient recall information about the present incident, past medical history, and specifically the history of pulmonary disease and exposures.

- In performing the exam, the Paramedic should complete an initial exam followed by a full cardiopulmonary systems exam. This exam should include peak flow result, full vital signs, monitor lead, and 12-lead plus capnography.

- Oxygen is the cornerstone of treatment for COPD.

- Other medications are directed to counter spasm, mobilize or reduce secretions, and/or reduce or prevent inflammation.

- Emergency medication can be delivered in aerosol form or intramuscularly, subcutaneously, and intravenously.

- Positive pressure ventilation may be required to ensure adequate gas flow but places the patient at risk for pneumothorax and aspiration.

- Patients unable to control their airway, experiencing a worsening of their bronchospasm, or at risk for cardiac complications are candidates for endotracheal intubation.

REVIEW QUESTIONS:

1. What general mechanism causes carbon dioxide retention?
2. What three mechanisms characterize chronic obstructive respiratory diseases?
3. How is emphysema related to heart failure?
4. What three conditions characterize an asthma exacerbation?
5. What is the stimulus to breathe in a patient with long-term hypercarbia?
6. How does the capnography waveform of a patient with air trapping differ from that of a patient without air trapping?
7. What are the risks of positive pressure to the patient with emphysema?

CASE STUDY QUESTIONS:

Please refer to the Case Study in this chapter, and answer the questions below:

1. What indicators in the history and exam tend toward the development of status asthmaticus in Marissa?
2. What interventions exist for the field treatment of status asthmaticus?

REFERENCES:

1. Stephens MB, Yew KS. Diagnosis of chronic obstructive pulmonary disease. *Am Fam Physician.* 2008;78(1):87–92.
2. Celli BR. Update on the management of COPD. *Chest.* 2008;133(6):1451–1462.
3. Briggs DD, Jr. Chronic obstructive pulmonary disease overview: prevalence, pathogenesis, and treatment. *J Manag Care Pharm.* 2004;10(4 Suppl):S3–S10.
4. Holgate ST. Pathogenesis of asthma. *Clin Exp Allergy.* 2008;38(6):872–897.
5. Jackson C. *The Life of Chevalier Jackson: An Autobiography.* New York: Kessinger Publishing, Llc; 2008.
6. Chung KF, Pavord ID. Prevalence, pathogenesis, and causes of chronic cough. *Lancet.* 2008;371(9621):1364–1374.
7. Elwing J, Panos RJ. Pulmonary hypertension associated with COPD. *Int J Chron Obstruct Pulmon Dis.* 2008;3(1):55–70.
8. Shujaat A, Minkin R, et al. Pulmonary hypertension and chronic cor pulmonale in COPD. *Int J Chron Obstruct Pulmon Dis.* 2007;2(3):273–282.
9. Greyson CR. Pathophysiology of right ventricular failure. *Crit Care Med.* 2008;36(1 Suppl):S57–S65.
10. Kale P, Fang JC. Devices in acute heart failure. *Crit Care Med.* 2008;36(1 Suppl):S121–S128.
11. Borish L, Culp JA, Asthma: a syndrome composed of heterogeneous diseases. *Ann Allergy, Asthma, Immunology.* 2008;101(1):1–8; quiz 8–11, 50.
12. Wenzel S. Severe/fatal asthma. *Chest.* 2003;123(3 Suppl): 405S–410S.
13. Wenzel S. Mechanisms of severe asthma. *Clin Exp Allergy.* 2003;33(12):1622–1628.
14. Wenzel, S. Pathology of difficult asthma. *Paediatr Respir Rev.* 2003;4(4):306–311.
15. Quon BS, Gan WQ, et al. Contemporary management of acute exacerbations of COPD: a systematic review and metaanalysis. *Chest.* 2008;133(3):756–766.
16. Harwell JI, Brown RB. The drug-resistant pneumococcus: clinical relevance, therapy, and prevention. *Chest.* 2000;117(2): 530–541.
17. Larj MJ, Bleecker ER. Therapeutic responses in asthma and COPD. Corticosteroids. *Chest.* 2004;126(2 Suppl):138S–149S; discussion 159S–161S.
18. Suissa S, Ernst P. Inhaled corticosteroids: impact on asthma morbidity and mortality. *J Allergy Clin Immunol.* 2001;107(6):937–944.
19. Scarfone RJ, Friedlaender E. Corticosteroids in acute asthma: past, present, and future. *Pediatr Emerg Care.* 2003;19(5):355–361.
20. Sole D, Komatsu MK, et al. Pulse oximetry in the evaluation of the severity of acute asthma and/or wheezing in children. *J Asthma.* 1999;36(4):327–333.
21. Kallstrom TJ. Evidence-based asthma management. *Respir Care.* 2004;49(7):783–792.

22. Kupnik D, Skok P. Capnometry in the prehospital setting: are we using its potential? *Emerg Med J.* 2007;24(9):614–617.

23. Bhende MS, LaCovey DC. End-tidal carbon dioxide monitoring in the prehospital setting. *Prehosp Emerg Care.* 2001;5(2):208–213.

24. Butler J, Jackson R. Best evidence topic report. Lignocaine as a pretreatment to rapid sequence intubation in patients with status asthmaticus. *Emerg Med J.* 2005;22(10):732.

25. Zelicof-Paul A, Smith-Lockridge A, et al. Controversies in rapid sequence intubation in children. *Curr Opin Pediatr.* 2005;17(3):355–362.

26. Hemmila MR, Napolitano LM. Severe respiratory failure: advanced treatment options. *Crit Care Med.* 2006;34 (9 Suppl):S278–S290.

27. Kavanagh BP, Laffey JG. Hypercapnia: permissive and therapeutic. *Minerva Anestesiol.* 2006;72(6):567–576.

28. Oddo M, Feihl F, et al. Management of mechanical ventilation in acute severe asthma: practical aspects. *Intensive Care Med.* 2006;32(4):501–510.

29. Sullivan R. Prehospital use of CPAP: positive pressure = positive patient outcomes. *Emerg Med Ser.* 2005;34(8):120, 122–124, 126.

30. Kallio T, Kuisma M, et al. The use of prehospital continuous positive airway pressure treatment in presumed acute severe pulmonary edema. *Prehosp Emerg Care.* 2003;7(2):209–213.

31. Vuillermin P, South M, et al. Parent-initiated oral corticosteroid therapy for intermittent wheezing illnesses in children. *Cochrane Database Syst Rev.* 2006;3:CD005311.

32. Edmonds ML, Camargo CA, Jr., et al. Early use of inhaled corticosteroids in the emergency department treatment of acute asthma. *Cochrane Database of Syst Rev.* 2003;3:CD002308.

33. Stein SW. Estimating the number of droplets and drug particles emitted from MDIs. *AAPS PharmSciTech.* 2008;9(1):112–115.

34. Buxton LJ, Baldwin JH, et al. The efficacy of metered-dose inhalers with a spacer device in the pediatric setting. *J Am Acad Nurse Pract.* 2002;14(9):390–397.

35. Rau JL. Design principles of liquid nebulization devices currently in use. *Respir Care.* 2002;47(11):1257–1275; discussion 1275–1278.

36. Restrepo RD, Peters J. Near-fatal asthma: recognition and management. *Curr Opin Pulm Med.* 2008;14(1):13–23.

37. Denmark TK, Crane HA, et al. Ketamine to avoid mechanical ventilation in severe pediatric asthma. *J Emerg Med.* 2006;30(2):163–166.

38. Allen JY, Macias CG. The efficacy of ketamine in pediatric emergency department patients who present with acute severe asthma. *Ann Emerg Med.* 2005;46(1):43–50.

39. Lau TT, Zed PJ. Does ketamine have a role in managing severe exacerbation of asthma in adults? *Pharmacotherapy.* 2001;21(9):1100–1106.

40. Cydulka R, Davison R, et al. The use of epinephrine in the treatment of older adult asthmatics. *Ann Emerg Med.* 1988;17(4):322–326.

41. Rowe BH, Camargo CA, Jr. The role of magnesium sulfate in the acute and chronic management of asthma. *Curr Opin Pulm Med.* 2008;14(1):70–76.

CHAPTER 10

DISORDERS OF BRAIN FUNCTION

KEY CONCEPTS:

Upon completion of this chapter, it is expected that the reader will understand these following concepts:

- That any change in consciousness may be labeled a seizure, so it is important to differentiate seizures from other life-threatening processes
- The importance of the patient's history and the Paramedics' need to search for medic alert tags and protect themselves
- How prehospital care is directed toward ending the patient's seizure, supporting body processes, and protecting the patient from harm

ANATOMY CONCEPTS:

Prior to reading this chapter the Paramedic student should be familiar with the following anatomy and physiology concepts:

- Neuroanatomy of the reticular activating system
- Neurotransmitters of the brain
- Neuroreflexes

Since the start of the holiday season, two Paramedic teams have been assigned to the mall. As the team is patrolling, they hear someone shouting, "Help! She's passed out! Help!" Both Paramedics grab their gear and move toward the commotion. They observe a twenty-something female convulsing on the floor.

CRITICAL THINKING QUESTIONS

1. What are some of the possible causes of convulsions in a young woman?

2. What immediate actions should the Paramedics take to safeguard this patient?

OVERVIEW

Any impairment of a patient's level of consciousness can be an indication of a serious underlying physical condition. The etiologies for an altered mental status are numerous. In some cases, the cause is a chronic condition without resolution. It is the Paramedic's responsibility to analyze the clinical picture—differentiating chronic issues from critical ones—to determine life threats and to treat emergent conditions accordingly.

Review of Neurophysiology of Consciousness

To work out the potential etiology of an altered mental status, it is helpful for the Paramedic to study the neurophysiology of consciousness. Consciousness consists of two components—wakefulness and self-awareness, with its attendant condition of perception.

Wakefulness is a function of the brain's **reticular activating system (RAS)**. The RAS is perfectly located in the brainstem between the medulla oblongata and the midbrain. The RAS accepts signals from the **afferent nerves** (stimulation from the senses), sending them upward to the cerebral cortex for interpretation. Descending fibers of the RAS control respirations and cardiac functions, and are able to increase both respirations and cardiac functions in preparation for danger (i.e., the fight or flight reflex), if necessary.

Wakefulness and sleep are part of the body's **circadian rhythm**, cyclic phenomena necessary for the body's rejuvenation. The reticular activating system connects the body, via sensory input, to the outside world.

Wakefulness does not constitute consciousness. Consciousness is a state of knowing, an awareness of the outside world that is a product of cognition. As a sentient being (able to sense the world), the body must take that information and make it meaningful in order to be conscious.

At the first level, the brain distinguishes itself from the world (self-awareness). Secondly, the brain attempts to establish a spatial relationship (location). Finally, the brain attempts to establish a temporal relationship (place in time). These three levels of consciousness—person, place, and time—are foundational to consciousness.

Consciousness assumes that the person is arousable. Arousal, the condition of being able to stimulate the cerebral cortex via the RAS and receiving a response, falls along a continuum starting with alertness and ending in coma.

The classic descriptions of decreased levels of cortical interaction are lethargy, stupor, and coma. With lethargy, the patient is able to be aroused with verbal stimulus. The stuporous patient is arousable with pain and opens her eyes. The comatose patient does not arouse (open the eyes) to even painful stimuli. These patients are said to be in a vegetative state. Initially, Paramedics tend to use the classic descriptions when caring for a patient with an altered mental status. They

use the Glasgow coma scale later to establish a baseline for other healthcare providers. Thus, the key difference between stupor and coma is eye opening.

Chief Concern

A seizure results in an altered mental status. Since seizures are widely misunderstood by the public, any syncope may be labeled as a seizure.[1,2] The difficulty for the Paramedic is in trying to ascertain if there truly was a seizure or if another, potentially life-threatening disease process is occurring.

A **seizure**, by definition, is an involuntary contraction of voluntary muscles (sometimes called a fit or convulsion) caused by some insult to the central nervous system and the brain. A common malady, it is thought that one in ten people (10%) will experience a seizure in their lifetime.[3] These pathology producing insults can be grossly categorized as either intracranial or extracranial.

There are many extracranial etiologies for convulsions. The Paramedic is responsible for distinguishing intracranial etiologies from extracranial ones. One mnemonic to help the Paramedic remember the major etiologies of a convulsion is "HIT + 1." In the mnemonic, there are five H's, one I, and five T's, plus epilepsy (Table 10-1).

The first extracranial cause of convulsions to be considered is **H**ypoxia. Hypoxia can have many origins, as described in the previous chapters, and the Paramedic has many treatment

Table 10-1 HIT + 1

- Hypoxia
- Hypoglycemia
- Heat exhaustion
- High fever
- Heart-related
- Iatrogenic
- Trauma
- Tumor
- Toxemia of pregnancy
- Toxicology
- Tremens
- Epilepsy

options to treat hypoxia. Resolution of hypoxia is one of the Paramedic's chief priorities.

Following hypoxia as an extracranial cause of convulsions is **H**ypoglycemia. Commonly, hypoglycemia engenders thoughts of diabetes and the various treatments available for diabetes that can cause hypoglycemia. However, there are many other causes of hypoglycemia, including liver disease, alcoholism, pancreatic tumors called insulinomas, endocrine disorders such as hypopituitarism, drugs such as chloramphenicol, obesity surgery, postgastrectomy syndrome, and certain genetic disorders. Routine supportive care dictates that a Paramedic ascertain the blood sugar level of any patient with an altered mental status (a simple point of care procedure) and act accordingly. The Paramedic must treat the three high priority conditions in the field (Figure 10-1).

The next two conditions in the list, **H**eat exhaustion and **H**igh fever (both topics covered extensively in chapters on infectious disease and outdoor emergencies), have a commonality—hypoxia. An increase in body temperature alters the oxyhemoglobin curve, thus altering oxygen affinity for hemoglobin, which can lead to hypoxia with subsequent seizure activity.[4,5]

Infections also carry the potential for meningitis, either viral or bacterial. Any patient with a seizure and a fever should be considered a potential meningitis case; therefore, the Paramedic should take appropriate infectious disease precautions, such as wearing mask, goggles, and even a gown.

Hypoperfusion is the common link in **H**eart-related causes of convulsions. Whether it is a run of ventricular tachycardia, new onset atrial fibrillation, or a heart block, all dysrhythmia alters hemodynamics and can result in pancerebral hypoperfusion and subsequent seizure activity.

Iatrogenic causes are those causes of altered mental status induced by the Paramedic. For example, if the patient was hypoxic and dependent on oxygen, then a disconnected oxygen mask could create oxygen deprivation leading to hypoxia and subsequent seizure. Iatrogenic etiologies of convulsive disorders lend credence to careful monitoring of all medical procedures, in keeping with *primum non nocere* or "first, do not harm."

Trauma, as a source of seizures, has two potential etiologies. The first etiology is extracranial and involves hypoxia as well as hypoperfusion secondary to hemorrhage or other traumatic pathology. The other etiology is due to direct injury to the brain (traumatic brain injury). These pathologies are described in detail in subsequent chapters.

Although almost one-half of patients with brain **T**umors, both cancerous and benign, seek medical attention for a headache, for another third a seizure is the first presenting sign. Seizures can occur in 50% of cases of brain tumors of the cerebral cortex. For this reason, brain cancer must be ruled out for any adult with new onset seizures.

A convulsing pregnant patient is a clinical challenge for most Paramedics. Although some women who are pregnant may also have a history of seizures, the specter of **T**oxemia

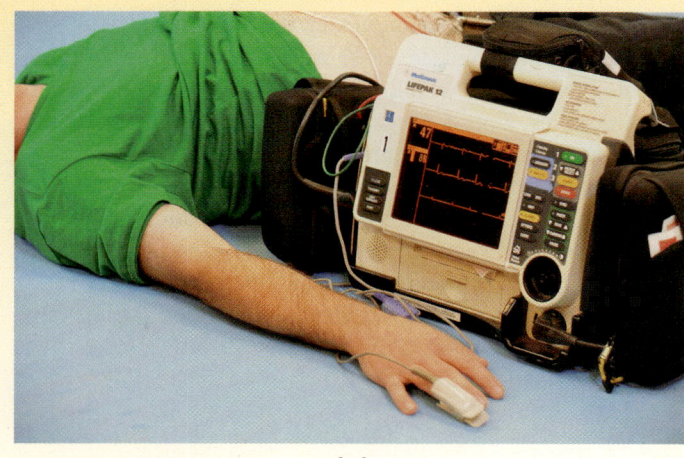

(a)

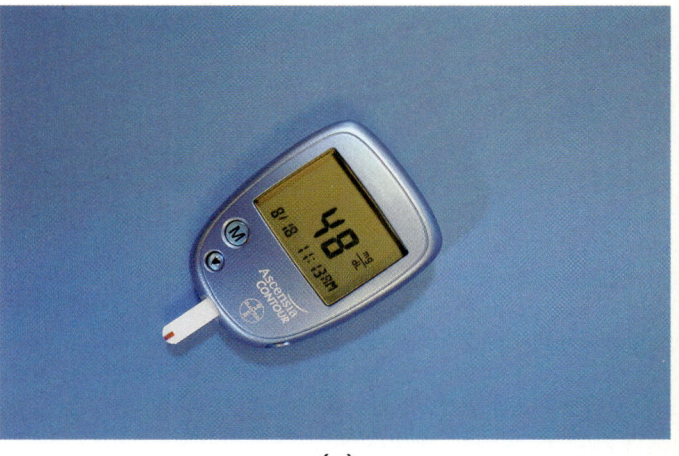

(b)

(c)

Delmar/Cengage Learning

Figure 10-1 Rule out the top three H's in initial assessment. (a) Hypoxia. (b) Hypoperfusion. (c) Hypoglycemia.

of pregnancy must be considered.[6] Toxemia of pregnancy (eclampsia) shares a common pathway with trauma and tumors, increased intracranial pressure, and/or cerebral hypertension. Preeclampsia and eclampsia are discussed in the chapters on pregnancy.

Toxic substances can poison the brain, interfere with cerebral function, and cause seizures. Some more common toxicological agents which can cause seizures are the sympathomimetics. These drugs, such as cocaine and methamphetamine, stimulate the sympathetic nervous system.

Tremens or **Delirium tremens**, also known as the rum fits, is often mistaken for a true convulsive disorder, although it is not one. Delirium tremens occurs during alcohol withdrawal. Alcoholic patients can also seize as a direct result of brain trauma, subdural hematomas sustained during falls. The differential diagnosis of these two variant conditions is difficult to make in the field.

STREET SMART

Although the terms "convulsion" and "seizure" are commonly used interchangeably by the public, seizure connotes an epileptic seizure whereas convulsion would be any new and unexplained event. Although the public often uses the term "seizure" to describe any episode of unconsciousness, spasms, and even strokes, the Paramedic should not take that to mean that the patient has the diagnosis of epilepsy.

Psychogenic Non-Epileptic Seizures

Some psychiatric patients with depression, post-traumatic stress disorder (PTSD), or personality disorders will somatize their distress as psychogenic non-epileptic seizures, formerly known as **pseudoseizures**.

Several findings, or lack thereof, are suggestive of a psychogenic non-epileptic seizure. For example, the lack of signs of incidental self-injury, lack of incontinence, and the ability to provoke spontaneously are suggestive of psychogenic non-epileptic seizure. Some patients will manifest avoidance behaviors, such as sitting before falling to the ground in order to avoid injury. For others, the trigger for the seizure is an emotional or situational event. Other behaviors suggestive of psychogenic non-epileptic seizures include crying during the seizure, side-to-side head movements, thrusting pelvic movements, dystonic posturing, and closed eyes during the seizure.[7–10]

Epileptic patients tend to bite their tongue on the side. However, the patient with suspected psychogenic non-epileptic seizures will bite his tongue on the tip, not the sides.

Psychogenic non-epileptic seizures, often termed pseudoseizures, are a form of coping mechanism. The seizure is the patient's way of responding to intolerable stress or emotion. This patient population often has a history of physical and/or sexual abuse or other extreme psychosocial stressor (for example, PTSD).

It should be emphasized that these seizures are not intentional, meaning the patient does not make a conscious decision to seize. Although maladaptive, it is counterproductive for the Paramedic to confront the psychiatric patient regarding psychogenic seizures.

After the Paramedic rules out life-threats, these patients need reassurance and supportive care. The long-term prognosis for these patients is poor. One study showed that after 10 years of psychiatric care, 71% of this patient population continued to have seizures.

Epilepsy

References to epilepsy have been found dating back to Mesopotamia that mentioned the "falling disease" and accurately described aura and convulsions. Later, the Greeks referred to the condition as the "sacred" disease. Among the early Greeks, epilepsy was seen as a disease bestowed on mortals by the gods until Hippocrates suggested that it was a disorder with a natural cause.

However, the public considered patients with epilepsy to be overtaken by spirits—some were even declared witches. Confusion was so widespread about the cause of epilepsy that some states forbid marriage and even authorized sterilization of patients with epilepsy until the mid-1800s when three prominent English neurologists correctly attributed seizures to abnormal nervous discharge.

The origin of the term "epilepsy" speaks to its past, from the Greek word meaning to "seize or attack," implying that the soul was under attack. Yet it is actually a brief excessive discharge of neurons. An epileptic seizure, or epileptic attack, is defined as a "transient occurrence of signs and/or symptoms due to abnormal, excessive or asynchronous neural activity of the brain" by the International League Against Epilepsy. Epilepsy is not a single disease but a reoccurring symptom of a number of underlying disorders characterized by a history of two or more unprovoked seizures.

Epilepsy affects approximately 2.7 million Americans, or 8.2 per 1,000 of the general population.[11,12] Nearly 150,000 people are given the diagnosis of epilepsy every year. Epilepsy has no regard for sex, age, race, or national origin—it occurs in all populations.

Classification of Seizures

Seizures can be grossly divided into two classifications: generalized and focal seizures. Focal seizures can be further broken down into simple partial seizures and complex partial seizures. During a simple partial seizure, the patient remains conscious. During a complex partial seizure, the patient does not remain conscious.

Focal seizures include focal sensory or focal motor seizures. Automatisms, unconscious repetitious actions, are an example of focal motor seizure. **Narcolepsy**, excessive daytime sleepiness, is another example of a focal motor seizure. Paramedics are generally not called to the scene of a patient experiencing a focal seizure.

Simple partial seizures and complex partial seizures can progress to generalized tonic–clonic seizures, a process called secondary generalization. From a practical point of view, the difference between these is academic for a Paramedic.

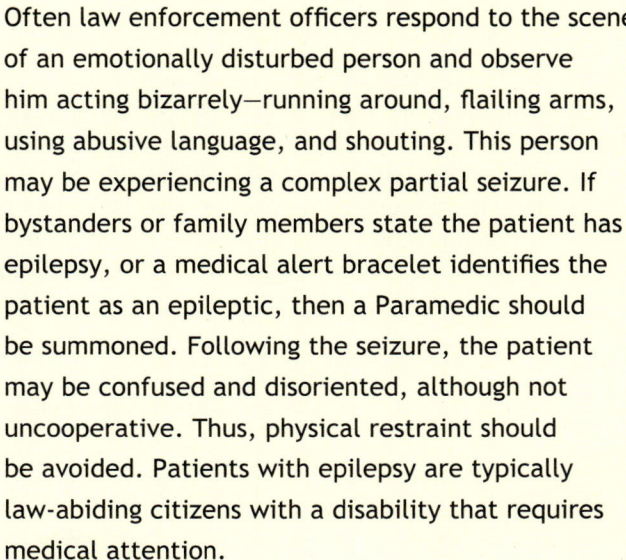

STREET SMART

Often law enforcement officers respond to the scene of an emotionally disturbed person and observe him acting bizarrely—running around, flailing arms, using abusive language, and shouting. This person may be experiencing a complex partial seizure. If bystanders or family members state the patient has epilepsy, or a medical alert bracelet identifies the patient as an epileptic, then a Paramedic should be summoned. Following the seizure, the patient may be confused and disoriented, although not uncooperative. Thus, physical restraint should be avoided. Patients with epilepsy are typically law-abiding citizens with a disability that requires medical attention.

Generalized Seizure

Generalized seizures begin with a loss of consciousness and proceed to affect the entire cerebral cortex (i.e., both hemispheres). Generalized seizures are further classified as atonic, absence, and tonic–clonic.

An **atonic seizure**, formerly referred to as a drop attack, involves sudden loss of muscle tone and a collapse of the patient to the ground. Atonic seizures occur without any warning and can result in severe head and/or facial trauma. Anti-epileptic drugs are at times ineffective, requiring the patient to wear a helmet for safety.

Absence seizures, also called petit mal seizures, cause a lapse of consciousness, manifest by a staring gaze, without loss of motor tone and often last only a few seconds. In a true generalized seizure, the absence seizure affects the cerebral hemispheres (consciousness) but does not affect the cerebellum where motor tone is maintained. The only outward manifestation of the seizure may be rapidly blinking eyes before the patient resumes whatever she was doing exactly where she left off.

Absence seizures can occur so frequently that they interrupt activities of daily living and necessitate medication. Absence seizures are commonly triggered by bright or flashing lights (the flicker effect which induces these photoepileptic seizures) or other strong sensory input such as sudden loud noises.

Like the focal seizure, the patient with an absence seizure can manifest automatisms. **Automatisms** are repetitive unconscious movements such as lip smacking, eyelid fluttering, and finger tapping. In one study, 44% of patients with absence seizures had secondary automatisms.

Tonic–Clonic Seizure

Within the brain, and its billions of nerve cells, there are two chemical factors that are in balance. The first chemical factor is the excitatory neurotransmitters, which decrease the neurons' membrane potential by allowing more sodium into the cell. In opposition to this factor are the inhibitory neurotransmitters, such as gamma aminobutyric acid (GABA), which increase the membranes' potential by allowing potassium to enter the neuron.

When these two factors are imbalanced, then abnormal neuronal discharge occurs, leading to widespread misfirings and "electric storm" (a tonic–clonic seizure). **Tonic–clonic seizures**, formerly known as grand mal seizures, have four distinct phases: aura, tonic, clonic, and postictal.

For some patients, the first indication that a seizure is impending is a sensation called the **aura**. The aura can be a perception of light or smell. Some patients describe the sensation as if going down a tunnel or falling into a hole. Others describe hearing voices or smelling strange odors. The patient may tell the Paramedic that she is lightheaded or dizzy, or has nausea, which is another prelude to a convulsion. Patients with epilepsy also describe this as a feeling of déjà vu.[13] An aura can last for seconds or for several minutes. In some cases, the patient, feeling an aura and understanding its implications, is able to sit or lie down before falling. In fact, an aura is a simple partial seizure that secondarily generalizes to the entire body. A description of the aura can help the neurologists narrow the probable source of the seizure in the brain. In other cases, the aura is self-limiting and the patient returns to normal. However, not all patients experience an aura. Many patients state they never have any warning before a seizure.

The patient next proceeds to the tonic–clonic phase, or a convulsion. In the **tonic phase**, all of the body's muscles contract and the body appears to get stiff. At this point, the patient has lost consciousness and is unresponsive to verbal stimuli.

If the patient inhales just prior to the tonic phase, air will be forced out of the lungs. This air, crossing the partially closed glottis, will produce a shrill sound, euphemistically called the "epileptic cry." Hearing this sound led some people in the past to think that a spirit had entered the body.

Air, while continuing to rush out of the body, blows spittle out of the mouth, creating an appearance of foam.

Some people witnessing this foaming at the mouth assumed that the patient had rabies, since rabid mammals foam at the mouth.

During the tonic phase there is no breathing. The muscles of respiration are contracted and frozen, and the patient may become transiently hypoxic as evidenced by cyanosis. With this forceful contraction of muscles comes the loss of postural tone, and the patient typically falls to the ground.

The next phase, referred to as the **clonic phase** (from the Greek *klonos*, meaning turmoil), is a series of random contractions of muscles. The clonic phase typically lasts one to two minutes and rapidly wanes as the patient becomes exhausted. During the clonic phase, the patient may resume ineffective gasping respirations. The patient's "color" may return as the cyanosis seen in the tonic phase resolves.

During this phase, the patient may become incontinent of urine, provided the bladder has urine. The Paramedic may witness the patient's eyes roll back into the head, eyelid fluttering, drooling, chewing motions, lip smacking, hand waving, and a general twitching of the extremities. However, not every patient experiences the tonic phase nor does every patient experience the clonic phase. Nonetheless, most demonstrate both the tonic and the clonic phases.

Following the tonic–clonic phase, the patient enters the **postictal period** (ictal from the Latin *ictus*, meaning to strike). While awaiting the postictal period, the patient should be placed in the lateral recumbent position, also known as the recovery or coma position. This allows the patient's airway to drain any blood or sputum (Figure 10-2). The brain, now

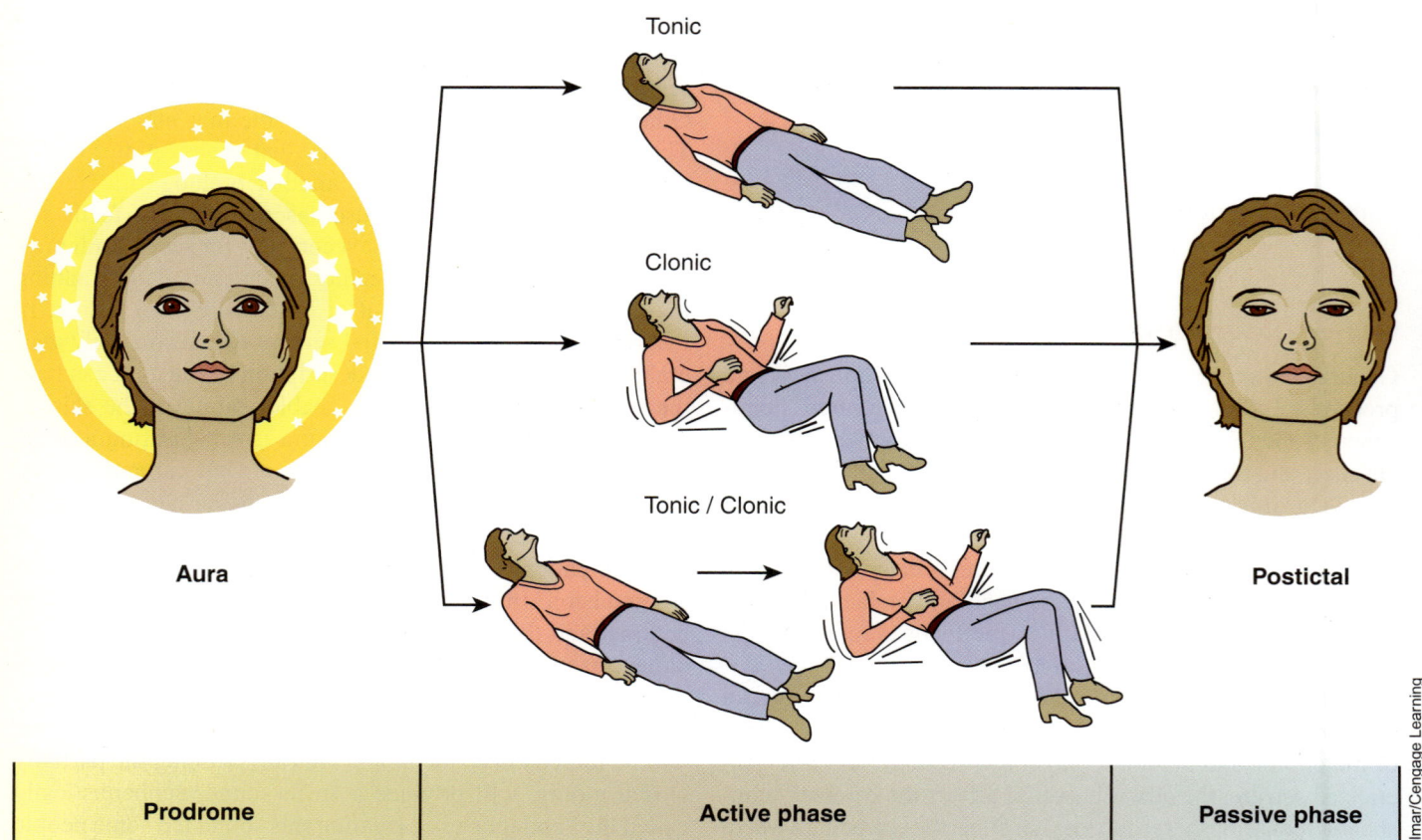

| Prodrome | Active phase | Passive phase |

Figure 10-2 Progression of seizure.

in a period of recovery, slowly regains its functions including wakefulness and then consciousness. Typically, the patient will go through the stages of consciousness starting with stupor, lethargy, and then alertness.

A seizure is a physically challenging episode after which many patients complain of feeling tired and just wanting to go to sleep. The postictal period typically lasts from between 15 to 30 minutes but can last up to several hours in some cases.

Pediatric Seizures

Although seizure disorders span the patient's lifetime, some seizure disorders are associated with childhood, the period from childbirth to adolescence. Hypoxia can be a cause of seizures in a newborn and routine resuscitation measures should be instituted whenever a seizure occurs. In some instances, the newborn's respirations are depressed because the mother was addicted to opiates, which crossed the placental barrier once ingested. However, the use of naloxone should be avoided.[14,15] Imprudent use of naloxone in the addicted mother's newborn can precipitate seizures.

Hypoglycemia, a possible cause of seizures in the newborn, can usually be ruled out through simple point of care testing. Repeated episodes of hypoglycemia, some associated with seizures, may suggest that the child has an inborn error of metabolism and requires further follow-up.

An infantile spasm, known as West syndrome, is a form of epilepsy seen in infancy, typically within three to six months. It is characterized by arching of the infant's torso when waking. Infantile spasms are self-limiting, usually resolve by age 5, and are commonly associated with cerebral palsy. Children with West syndrome often develop other forms of epilepsy later in life.

Febrile seizures are probably the most common seizure disorder associated with childhood. Febrile seizures occur early in the patient's fever history, typically when the fever is greater than 102°F.[16] It closely resembles a generalized seizure. A febrile seizure generally lasts only for a couple of minutes as a rule, after which the child will regain consciousness.

The care for a seizing child is basic. The Paramedic should place the child down on the floor or bed, either on his side or stomach, and allow the seizure to run its course. All objects should be removed from the child's mouth and the child should not be restrained.

Meningitis is a cause for Paramedic concern in a patient who has not had a prior seizure but has one now. Children, particularly toddlers, are prone to middle ear infections (otitis media) and can subsequently develop meningitis if the infection extends into the brain. These children may seize as a result of either the fever or the meningitis. Critical clues of meningitis include nuchal rigidity, photophobia, and projectile vomiting.

Parents are frequently concerned as to whether their child will develop epilepsy. However, less than 2% to 5% of children with a febrile seizure will develop epilepsy. Furthermore, those without certain risk factors, such as cerebral palsy or another seizure within 24 hours, have less than a 1% chance of developing epilepsy later.

Another common concern is brain damage. Several large studies have shown that children with febrile seizures do not have any intellectual impairment, now or in the future, as a result of the febrile seizure.

As previously mentioned, febrile seizures typically occur in children between the ages of 6 months to 5 years. Approximately 1 in 25 children will have a febrile seizure, and a toddler who has a febrile seizure has a 30% chance of having another one at some point.[17]

Children tend to outgrow febrile seizures. However, a child can develop epilepsy, triggered by the fever. Differentiating a febrile seizure from an epileptic seizure is difficult in the field. For this reason, pediatric seizure patients should be seen by a physician for further medical evaluation.

Absent seizures, a form of partial seizure, are often identified in school-age children. These seizures involve a loss of consciousness, witnessed as staring off, without loss of motor tone (i.e., the patient remains seated and upright). Dismissed by some as simply inattention, enlightened teachers will recognize the disorder and properly send the student for medical attention. The typical age of onset is 3 to 10 years. Approximately 40% of these affected children will spontaneously resolve the issue during their teenage years.

Juvenile myoclonic epilepsy, also known as jerk epilepsy, is seen in 7% of all epilepsy patients and is thought to be inherited. Juvenile myoclonic epilepsy is highlighted by myoclonic spasms of the limbs that usually occur after waking. Spasms of the legs can cause the patient to fall, without any loss of consciousness. However, upward of 80% of patients with juvenile myoclonic epilepsy will go on to have a generalized seizure.[18]

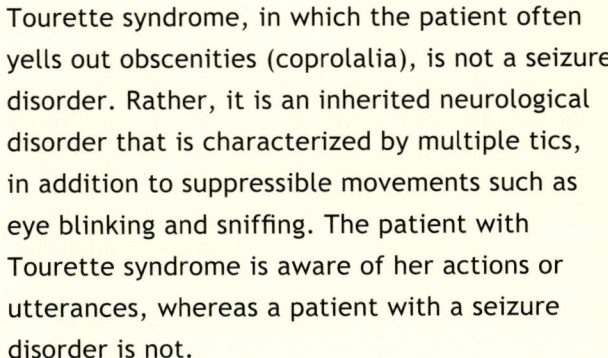

STREET SMART

Tourette syndrome, in which the patient often yells out obscenities (coprolalia), is not a seizure disorder. Rather, it is an inherited neurological disorder that is characterized by multiple tics, in addition to suppressible movements such as eye blinking and sniffing. The patient with Tourette syndrome is aware of her actions or utterances, whereas a patient with a seizure disorder is not.

Upon arriving at a small cluster of patrons, the Paramedics see a young woman lying supine on the floor. While taking cervical spine stabilization, the team learns that the woman looked fearful and then laid down on the floor. She then appeared to tense up and let out a shrill cry. No one in the crowd knows the woman, so the Paramedics continue with the primary assessment.

The Paramedics find that the woman is rigid, has a patent airway, and is breathing shallowly. She has strong regular peripheral pulses and no signs of overt bleeding. Blood sugar is 124 mg/dL and pulse oximetry is 94%. The patient is becoming more responsive and is able to answer questions about herself.

CRITICAL THINKING QUESTIONS

1. What are the important elements of the history that a Paramedic should obtain?
2. What is the symptom pattern for a seizure?

History

The first priority when caring for a patient who has experienced a seizure is ensuring the ABCs. Following the primary assessment, the Paramedic should be confident that the patient has an airway, is not hypoxic, is not hypotensive, and is not hypoglycemic. Further history taking and physical examination should exclude all of the pathologies represented by the mnemonic HIT+1.

Once the Paramedic is confident that the patient experienced an epileptic seizure, then the focus of the medical history is to try and determine the seizure's trigger (those events that initiate a seizure).

Subtherapeutic anti-epileptic drug levels are the most common trigger for a seizure. The patient's anticonvulsant levels may be depressed for a number of reasons including changes in liver or renal function (affecting the anticonvulsant pharmacodynamics), changes in gastrointestinal function (affecting the anticonvulsant pharmacokinetics), or simply a change in medication to a generic formulation.

Missed doses of medication, intentional or otherwise, and other issues of noncompliance, such as dementia, can also lead to subtherapeutic anticonvulsant levels in the patient. Other triggers include sleeplessness, fatigue, and alcohol and drug use, as well as emotional stressors such as worry and strong emotions such as anger. Hormonal changes associated with the menstrual cycle and pregnancy can affect the patient's seizure threshold as well.

Seizures can also be triggered by external stimuli that affect the senses, such as hot water, light touch, and flashing lights (i.e., photosensitivity). Photosensitivity is predicted in about 25% of patients with epilepsy.

Next, the Paramedic should attempt to obtain the patient's seizure history. The patient should be asked if this seizure is the same as previous seizures. If it is different, the patient should explain what makes it different. A change in the

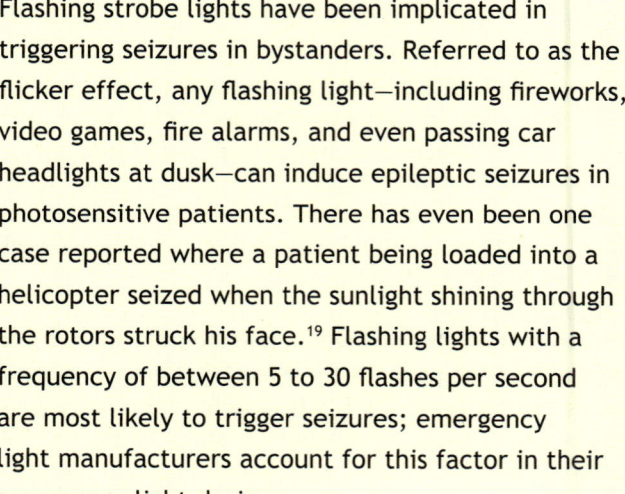

STREET SMART

Flashing strobe lights have been implicated in triggering seizures in bystanders. Referred to as the flicker effect, any flashing light—including fireworks, video games, fire alarms, and even passing car headlights at dusk—can induce epileptic seizures in photosensitive patients. There has even been one case reported where a patient being loaded into a helicopter seized when the sunlight shining through the rotors struck his face.[19] Flashing lights with a frequency of between 5 to 30 flashes per second are most likely to trigger seizures; emergency light manufacturers account for this factor in their emergency light designs.

seizure experience suggests either a change in the pathology or perhaps a new pathology has developed.

The patient should be queried about the frequency of the seizures as well as their typical duration. Increasing numbers or duration of seizures suggests a crescendo pattern. Recurrent, serial, or crescendo seizures may indicate insufficient plasma levels of anti-epileptic medications. It has been suggested that up to one-third of seizures cannot be controlled with current medications.

The majority of new onset convulsions are not epileptic, but rather the result of some occurrence that lowered the patient's seizure threshold (Table 10-2).

Table 10-2 Etiology of New-Onset Convulsion

- Unknown 24%
- Alcohol 20%
- Stroke 13%
- Tumor 10%
- Drug 10%
- Remainder Epilepsy

Table 10-3 Medications Thought to Induce Seizures

- Theophylline/aminophylline
- Meperidine HCl
- Isoniazid
- Clonazapine
- Phenothiazines
- Beta–Lactam antibiotics
- Tricyclic antidepressants (TCA)
- Antidysrhythmics
  - Lidocaine HCl
- Selective serotonin reuptake inhibitors (SSRI)
- Beta blockers
- Prescription drugs for malaria

Medication

Many drugs that disturb the brain's metabolic balance can temporarily lower a patient's seizure threshold (Table 10-3). The patient will experience a self-limiting seizure condition which will resolve when the medication is withdrawn.

Most patients with epilepsy are on one of five major categories of anti-epileptic drugs: barbiturates, hydantoins, benzodiazepines, succinimides, or carboxylic acids.

The therapeutic goal of all anticonvulsive medications is to stop seizures without causing debilitating side effects, such as lethargy. It should be noted that anti-epileptic drugs do not "cure" epilepsy, but rather control the number of seizures. Control of seizures, via raising the seizure threshold, can be achieved by either blocking electrolytes, such as sodium, from entering the cell, and thus lowering the membrane potential, or by enhancing the inhibitory effect of the neurotransmitter GABA.

The key to seizure control with any anticonvulsant is to maintain therapeutic drug levels. When the drug level drops, thus lowering the seizure threshold, then the patient may experience what is referred to as a **breakthrough seizure**.

The great majority of breakthrough seizures are due to noncompliance with the medications. In some cases, the absence of pathology (seizures) equates to no need for medicine. These patients may be aware of the numerous studies that indicate that as many as three-quarters of patients with epilepsy may be in long-term remission. In addition, up to one-third of patients simply stop the medication(s) because of the medication's noxious side effects, especially lethargy.

Some patients stop their medications because they do not want to be labeled as "epileptic." The diagnosis of epilepsy can adversely affect activities of daily living (ADL) (e.g., driving restrictions or limited occupational opportunities). Finally, financial and/or health insurance concerns can play into the patient's decision to stop taking medication.

Barbiturates

The first anticonvulsant was phenobarbital, marketed in 1912 as an anticonvulsive medication under the name Luminal®. It had the advantage of a long half-life which promoted long-term seizure control. Barbiturates are thought to enhance the inhibitory neurotransmitter GABA.

In low doses, barbiturates (a central nervous system depressant) are effective as anxiolytics and anticonvulsants. However, at higher doses barbiturates act as hypnotics, leading to profound sedation and even coma. Barbiturates, as a class, can be divided into three further groups: long acting, short acting, and ultra-short acting.

Patients on barbiturates often develop a tolerance to the drug and require escalating doses to obtain the therapeutic effect. At high doses, barbiturates can induce respiratory depression and apnea, making continued use dangerous for the patient.

The next generation of anticonvulsant which enhanced the inhibitory neurotransmitter GABA was carbamazepine. Originally released in 1953, carbamazepine was re-released in 1997 as a once daily anticonvulsant.

Another drug similar to carbamazepine is oxcarbazepine. The active metabolite of both of these drugs, after first pass metabolism in the liver, is phenobarbital.

Hydantoins

The next class of drugs, released around 1939, was the hydantoins. The hydantoins, such as phenytoin, are low cost and effective anticonvulsants that cause less sedation than barbiturates.

The drug fosphenytoin, the pro-drug of phenytoin, is converted by the liver to phenytoin. Fosphenytoin can be

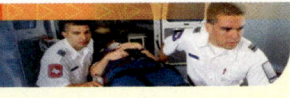

STREET SMART

Anti-epileptic drugs, such as phenytoin, can cause swollen gums and yellowed teeth. Proper dental care can help the patient to reduce or eliminate this side effect.

given intravenously, thus eliminating the pain and burning associated with intravenous administration of phenytoin.

The mechanism of action for hydantoins, such as phenytoin, is sodium channel blockade. This quality also makes this drug a potent antidysrhythmic.

Benzodiazepines

Benzodiazepines—including clonazepam, diazepam, and lorazepam—suppress seizure activity—particularly in the cortex, thalamus, and limbic areas—by enhancing the GABA neurotransmitters.

Introduced in the 1960s, benzodiazepines were thought to be the replacement for barbiturates. There are upward of 20 benzodiazepine derivatives in the market. One of the key advantages of benzodiazepines is their relative safety. The therapeutic index (lethal dose versus therapeutic dose) of benzodiazepines is large. Unless taken in combination with other sedatives, such as alcohol, overdose from benzodiazepines is rare.[20,21]

All benzodiazepines are lipophilic, meaning they cross the blood-brain barrier readily, and therefore are an effective anticonvulsant in an emergency. Like barbiturates, benzodiazepines can be divided into three groups: long acting, intermediate acting, and short acting.

Different formulations of benzodiazepines offer special advantages. For example, diazepam can be given rectally in the seizing patient, whereas midazolam can be absorbed through the buccal mucosa. All benzodiazepines can be given intravenously and most can be given intramuscularly as well.

Unfortunately, many of the benzodiazepines suffer from the same problem as barbiturates, namely tolerance and respiratory depression. Tolerance is thought to be due to a phenomenon called **neural adaptation**. This occurs whenever a neuron is constantly stimulated. As a result, the neuron becomes less responsive to the drug over time. Neural adaptation is not the same phenomenon as habituation, in which an increase in the number of receptors requires larger doses to obtain the same therapeutic effect. A new drug that theoretically does not cause tolerance to develop, called clobazam, is under study by the FDA in the United States.

Succinimides

In 1958, ethosuximide was introduced as a new anticonvulsant. Although all succinimides slow nerve conduction, its exact mechanism of action is unknown. It is thought to involve voltage ion gates, particularly T-type calcium channels.

Carboxylic Acids

The mechanism of action of valproic acid (VPA), released in 1963, is different than its predecessors. Valproic acid works by interfering with GABA transaminase, the enzyme that breaks down the inhibitory neurotransmitter GABA. In effect, it elevates the levels of GABA.

The discovery of valproic acid as an anticonvulsant was a serendipitous finding. At the time, valproic acid was being used as a carrier for other chemicals that were thought to be possible anticonvulsant agents. True to scientific principle, it was administered as a stand-alone drug to ensure that there was no interference with the other chemical preparation's mechanism of action.

Together succinimides, or carboxamides, and valproic acid provide anti-epileptic coverage superior to either drug alone. They are often prescribed together for that reason. Later formulations of VPA dissolve in the stomach faster and cause less stomach upset. These improvements have led to better patient compliance.

VPA and its related drugs are known teratogenic agents (e.g., congenital malformations). They are generally not prescribed to women of childbearing age without a careful assessment of risk versus benefit. Some of the teratogenic effects, such as neural tube disorders, may be relieved by the coadministration of folic acid.

New Anticonvulsants

Newer anticonvulsants have attempted to replicate GABA (such as felbamate and gabapentin), enhance GABA synthesis, or prevent its breakdown (vigabatrin) in an effort to elevate GABA levels. Other anticonvulsant formulations have complex actions. For example, topiramate is an enhancer of GABA levels while also working as a sodium channel blocker.

Originally used as antibiotics, the sulfonamides (sulfa drugs) have seen a new use as anticonvulsants. Following extensive experience with the drugs in Japan, sulfonamides are now being used in the United States.

STREET SMART

Antibiotics have been known to interact with anticonvulsants, lowering the patient's seizure threshold. There have been reports of an interaction between erythromycin and anticonvulsants, causing complications such as breakthrough seizures. As many of these drugs end up being metabolized in the liver, competition, particular for the cytochrome pathway, may result in erratic anticonvulsant levels.[22]

Neurostimulators

In the future, seizures may be controlled by way of **electroneurostimulators**. Electroneurostimulators use a system of probes placed on the brain's surface that are attached to a generator/computer assembly. The device takes continuous, real time, electroencephalograms (EEG) and detects spikes. When a spike is detected, an electrical stimulus is applied to the brain, via the electrodes, to neutralize the irritable focus.

In 1997 the federal Food and Drug Administration allowed the use of a vagus nerve stimulator for patients who are pharmacoresistant. The implanted **vagus nerve stimulator** periodically sends electrical stimulus to the brain, via the vagus nerve, to discharge and neutralize irritable sites in the brain that could induce a seizure (Figure 10-3). After one year, 45% of patients in one study reported fewer seizures after the vagus nerve stimulator was implanted.[23,24]

Past Medical History and Comorbid Factors

Seizures are the result of a massive pancerebral discharge of neurons which results from stimulation of a trigger. Normally, a combination of excitatory and inhibitory neurotransmitters control cerebral function. If there is a deficit of inhibitory neurotransmitters, or an abundance of excitatory neurotransmitters, in one area, then that area could stimulate a cascade of neuronal stimulation. For example, an irritable neuron that prematurely discharges and starts an electrical storm of chaotic firings across the brain could be likened to the ectopic focus in the heart, often induced by myocardial ischemia, which starts ventricular fibrillation.

The balance of inhibitory and excitatory neurotransmitters prevents seizures (that electrical storm) from occurring. Any influence which upsets that balance will likely lower the patient's threshold, causing a seizure.

Any disease that alters cerebral blood flow, causing cerebral hypoperfusion, can lower the patient's seizure threshold. Such a disease is therefore a comorbid factor for epilepsy. Cardiac dysrhythmias (e.g., congestive heart failure and cardiac arrest) can reduce blood flow to either the cerebral cortex or the hippocampus, resulting in seizure activity.

Similarly, cerebrovascular disease (stroke) can be epileptogenic. Strokes, whether hemorrhagic or ischemic, have been implicated in 22% to 69% of seizures in the elderly.

Seizures have many causes. Chief among them is inadequate drug levels of the anti-epileptic drug. Many of these anticonvulsants are affected by the liver. Liver disease can alter both the pharmacokinetics and pharmacodynamics, resulting in subtherapeutic drug levels.

Intuitively, traumatic brain injury that alters cerebral circulation could lead to epilepsy. The direct effects of trauma on the brain (e.g., a collection of blood within the skull) and the secondary effects of inflammation on the brain can lower the patient's seizure threshold, making it likely the patient will experience a seizure. Prophylactic anticonvulsive medications for traumatic brain injury are not generally indicated. However, once a seizure does occur then intravenous benzodiazepines are the drug of choice.[25,26]

The brain uses the largest percentage of blood oxygen. Therefore, any pulmonary disease that can produce hypoxia, up to and including respiratory arrest, can lead to epilepsy. Sleep apnea, with upper airway obstruction, is one syndrome that has been specifically linked to epilepsy. A combination of airway obstruction (leading to apnea and hypoxia) and sleep deprivation leads to a lowered seizure threshold.

Finally, infections of the brain (e.g., encephalitis and/or meningitis) from a number of infectious diseases—including syphilis, Lyme disease, tuberculosis, malaria, and so on—can lower the patient's seizure threshold (Table 10-4).

Last Meal

The patient's diet may also be part of the treatment plan. The ketogenic diet, first advocated in the 1900s, is a diet high in fat and low in carbohydrates, leading to ketosis.[27] This "starvation diet" was made famous by Dr. Atkins. However, fasting (starvation) has been effective in controlling seizures since the Middle Ages. The ketogenic diet offers the pediatric patient a drug-free existence with satisfactory seizure control; this is a key treatment with children who have poor medication compliance.

Events Preceding the Seizure

The history of the events preceding the patient's present illness (seizure) should focus on establishing or disproving the presence of, or possibility of, infection or toxic exposure.

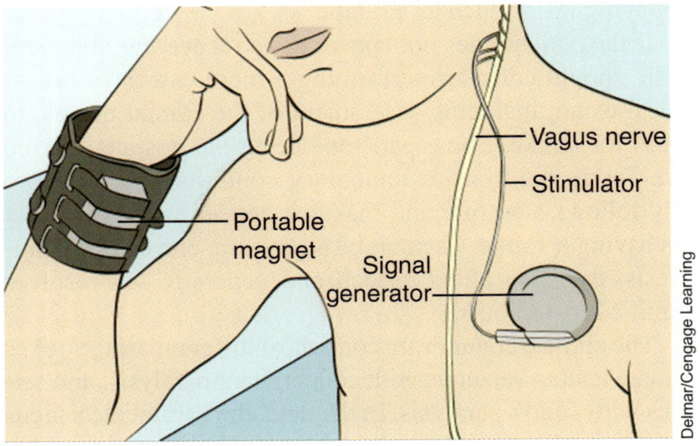

Figure 10-3 Vagal nerve stimulator.

Table 10-4 Comorbidities Associated with Epilepsy

- Brain tumors
- Cardiac disease
- Cerebrovascular disease
- Liver disease
- Traumatic brain injury
- Inflammatory disorders
- Pulmonary disease
- Infections

Any inhaled substance—be it cocaine, methamphetamines, carbon monoxide, or cyanide—can induce seizures through hypoxia. Removal of the patient from the environment and the provision of oxygen can go a long way toward preventing further seizures.

Reported symptoms such as fever or chills should lead the Paramedic to suspect an infection. The complaint of a stiff neck, or sensitivity to light (photophobia), should alert the Paramedic to the possibility of meningitis. In that case, all appropriate precautions should be taken.

Witnesses

Reliable eyewitnesses on scene who witnessed the seizure can provide vital insights into the possible source of the seizure. The Paramedic's questioning should focus on what the patient was doing at the onset of the seizure and whether there was any provocation; for example, is the patient withdrawing from alcohol (delirium tremens), was the patient using illicit drugs (intoxication), has the patient been sleep deprived?

Next, the Paramedic should ask the bystander if he witnessed any unusual behavior in the patient prior to the start of the tonic–clonic phase, such as arrested speech or repetitive movements such as eye blinking or lip smacking. The Paramedic should ask if a part of the patient's body appeared to tremble before the entire body trembled. This progressive spread of the convulsions from one point across the body is called the **Jacksonian march**. The presence of a Jacksonian march suggests the spread of the electrical storm from one point of the cerebral cortex across the entire brain, a partial complex seizure with secondary generalization.

Finally, the Paramedic should ask the witness to describe the patient's seizure, including the presence or absence of cyanosis, vomiting, tongue biting, or incontinence.

CASE STUDY (CONTINUED)

The young woman's convulsion had drawn a crowd of onlookers. After completing their primary assessment and vital signs, the Paramedics elect to move the patient to the safety and privacy of the security office where they can perform their examination. Mall security officers help clear a path for the patient, who is placed in a wheelchair and rolled to the office.

CRITICAL THINKING QUESTIONS

1. What are the elements of the physical examination of a patient with suspected seizure disorder?
2. Why is a cranial nerve examination a critical element in the neurological examination?

Examination

The first focus of the Paramedic's physical examination during the primary assessment is to assess and treat a patient's underlying hypoxia, hypoglycemia, or hypoperfusion. These three elements are essential to brain function. The secondary physical examination then proceeds in a head-to-toe fashion, eliminating opiate ingestion, head injury, stroke, and meningitis.

First, it is important to establish the patient's level of consciousness. Initially the patient will be comatose, but after a time the patient's mental status should improve. The Paramedic should repeatedly ask and then state the time and location of the patient. This action helps to reorient the patient as well as establish a trend. The Glasgow Coma Scale (GCS) can be helpful in objectively documenting this trend.

Next, the patient's scalp should be examined for any evidence of trauma, suggesting a possible head injury, including contusions or lacerations. The ears and nose should also be examined for evidence of ottorrhea or rhinorrhea.

Focusing on the eyes, the Paramedic should examine the pupils. Constricted pupils suggest the use of opiates, or could be evidence of a pontine hemorrhage, a brainstem stroke that may cause the patient to deteriorate quickly.

Conversely, dilated pupils may be suggestive of hypoxia or increased intracranial pressure. Normally, a patient's gaze reflexively moves in the opposite direction of the way the head is turned. When the patient's gaze is fixed when the head is turned, called **doll's eyes** (Figure 10-4), then the Paramedic should suspect a brainstem injury. A fixed lateral gaze is suggestive of either intracranial hemorrhage or another space occupying lesion such as a tumor.

If the patient does not appear to be recovering, the Paramedic should consider performing a more extensive neurological exam, including assessment of the cranial nerves, to assess for stroke. Some patients during the postictal period have Todd's paralysis, a temporary condition that immediately follows a seizure and makes it appear as if the patient was having a stroke. The paralysis, or more correctly a hemiparesis, can also affect speech and generally self-resolves within 24 to 48 hours.

The clinical conundrum consists of differentiating strokes that can lead to seizures, with concomitant paralysis, and seizures with Todd's paralysis. In the field, the Paramedic's focus should be a disorder of cerebral circulation ruling out stroke, hoping for the best but treating for the worst.

Normal (reflex present)

Head rotated
to the right

Abnormal (reflex absent)

Head rotated   Eyes follow
to the right

Delmar/Cengage Learning

Figure 10-4 Doll's eyes.

Table 10-5 Partial List of Meningeal Signs and Symptoms

- Symptoms
  - Nausea
  - Chills
  - Headache
  - Photophobia
  - Nuchal rigidity
- Signs
  - Projectile vomiting
  - Fever
  - Seizure
  - Kernig's sign
  - Brudzinski's sign

The patient's extremities should be examined for signs of injury. Particular attention should be given to the shoulders. Shoulders occasionally become injured, even dislocated, during the fall immediately preceding the tonic–clonic phase. The forearms should also be examined for needle bruises, called track marks, indicative of illicit drug use. The shins should also be examined for distribute bruises in various stages of healing, which could indicate frequent falls secondary to seizures.

Meningeal Signs

Seizures can be a secondary symptom of a more severe, potentially life-threatening illness: the infection known as meningitis. Meningitis manifests with many clinical symptoms, collectively referred to as **meningeal signs** (Table 10-5). Headache and neck stiffness (**nuchal rigidity**) are the most common complaints associated with meningitis.[28]

If meningitis is suspected (e.g., fever and seizures), the patient should be assisted with lifting her head off of the pillow, assuming no spinal injury is suspected. Meningeal irritation will cause the patient's legs to lift involuntarily, a condition called **Brudzinski's sign**.

Next, the Paramedic should have the patient, while lying supine, flex her hips and then passively extend her knees. Pain with extension, called **Kernig's sign**, is another indication of meningeal irritation.

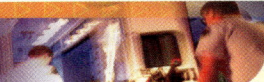

PROFESSIONAL PARAMEDIC

Patients are not their disease. In describing someone with epilepsy, the Paramedic should say, "The patient has a history of epilepsy" rather than saying that "The patient is an epileptic."

CASE STUDY (CONTINUED)

The woman's medic alert bracelet identifies her as a patient with epilepsy. Mall security, after finding her identification in her wallet, discovered her name was Sarah and tried to contact relatives. The patient is becoming increasingly coherent as time progresses, and is asking "What happened?"

CRITICAL THINKING QUESTIONS
1. What is the significance of the history of epilepsy?
2. What other possibilities should the Paramedics consider for the cause of the convulsion?

Assessment

Before diagnosing that a patient has a disorder of brain function, the Paramedic needs to determine that a seizure, and not simply syncope, occurred.

While limbs may twitch and extremities may shake during a syncope, the patient generally regains consciousness and composure quickly. However, the patient who is postictal may take several minutes, and up to 30 minutes, to become fully conscious, awake, and alert. In addition, the patient with syncope is not usually incontinent nor is there any residual paralysis (Todd's paralysis). The differential diagnosis of syncope versus seizure is difficult to ascertain in the field. The key difference is that a faint (syncope) is rapid in onset, without an aura, and the recovery is spontaneous and quick.

Syncope, the loss of oxygenated blood to the brain, should be addressed as a medical emergency. If a determination cannot be made, then the Paramedic should assume that the event was a syncopal episode and treat the patient accordingly.

Treatment

Generalized seizures are usually self-limiting. If the patient is seizing, then the Paramedic's first order of business is to protect the patient by removing hard objects from the immediate vicinity, such as objects that could serve as strike surfaces. The Paramedic should also loosen any ties around the neck that might be constrictive.

Physical restraint of the seizing patient is not necessary or indicated. A soft object such as a pillow or rolled-up coat could be placed under the patient's head to prevent head injury. Under no circumstances should any objects, such as spoons, be forced into the patient's mouth.

The majority of patients in the postictal period are lethargic, since their brains are recovering from the electrical storm that just occurred. For these patients, the Paramedic only needs to provide a supportive, protective environment in which to recover.

While providing a supportive and protective environment during the postictal period, the Paramedic's care should focus on the primary assessment. If possible, and as the seizure subsides, the patient should be rolled into a lateral recumbent position (the recovery position) to allow passive drainage of secretions and to prevent aspiration. The Paramedic should suction as needed with a Yankauer suction tip to clear secretions collecting in the buccal pocket.

Use of the oropharyngeal airway is generally discouraged as it can stimulate retching and vomiting, potentially leading to aspiration. Use of the nasopharyngeal airway could be considered, especially if the patient's recovery seems slow or there is a concern about a repeated seizure (Figure 10-5).

The application of oxygen in the immediate postictal period may reverse hypoxia associated with the seizure or other unknown etiologies, such as carbon monoxide poisoning.

The postictal patient may be witnessed to frequently yawn in an effort to re-establish normal respiratory function. The use of the bag–mask assembly is generally not indicated

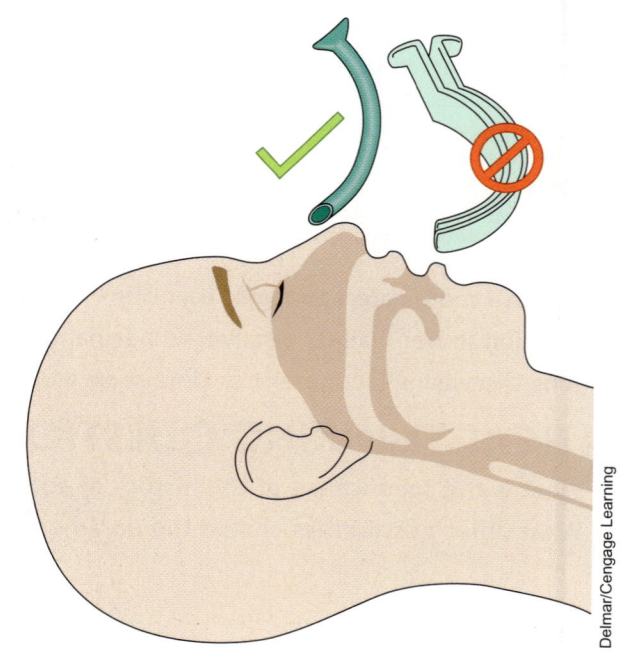

Figure 10-5 Use of the nasopharyngeal airway is recommended over the oropharyngeal airway in the postictal patient.

unless there is concern about respiratory failure (e.g., as manifested by bradypnea).

Most patients who are postictal following a seizure are hyperdynamic, with elevated blood pressures and heart rate, secondary to a surge of adrenaline that occurs during the seizure. These indicators of physiological function should normalize as the patient recovers.

The presence of a bradycardia, hypertension, and irregular respirations (Cushing's triad) should raise suspicion of increased intracranial pressure.[29] Increased intracranial pressure could be secondary to head injury, intracranial hemorrhage, or another space-occupying lesion such as a tumor.

The presence of hypertension and tachycardia can also be a manifestation of hypoglycemia. As a point of care, the Paramedic should perform blood glucose analysis and immediately treat hypoglycemia.

If the postictal patient is unable to maintain an airway independently, eliminating the possibility of oral glucose administration, then the Paramedic will need to use intravenous access for administration of dextrose solution.

The patient who falls from a standing position to the ground generally does not require spinal immobilization unless indicated by trauma above the clavicle or point tenderness to the posterior midline of the neck.[30,31] Paramedics can elect to take manual cervical spine control while waiting for the patient to recover, thus averting the need for spinal immobilization. If the patient does not recover, and/or remains unable to cooperate with the examination, it may be prudent to provide spinal immobilization.

Certain patient populations, such as patients with Down syndrome and the elderly, are prone to spinal injuries. All precautions should be taken to ensure the spinal cord's integrity in these populations. The greatest percentage of seizures are breakthrough seizures secondary to noncompliance with medications. The axiom in medicine is that "seizures beget seizures." The risk of a reoccurrence is greater if the patient seized during sleep or has a history of frequent seizures.

CULTURAL/REGIONAL DIFFERENCES

Some regions elect to administer a long-acting benzodiazepine intravenously whereas others utilize a shorter-acting drug given intramuscularly. Some areas utilize Diastat™, a benzodiazepine administered per rectum. If using Diastat™, the Paramedic should remember to protect the patient's modesty.

CASE STUDY (CONTINUED)

Suddenly the patient becomes unresponsive and slips down in the wheelchair. Moving her to the floor, the Paramedics reassess her. Her assessment shows that her vital signs are 168/88, pulse 118 and regular, and respirations are 20 and irregular but with good chest movement. The Paramedics are turning her to her left side when she begins lip smacking and then displays tonic rigidity.

CRITICAL THINKING QUESTIONS

1. What are some of the predictable complications associated with status epilepticus?
2. What are some of the predictable complications associated with prolonged seizure activity?

Evaluation

Constant re-evaluation is important in patients who present with a disorder of brain function.

Status Epilepticus

During a seizure, the ensuing electrical storm rapidly depletes the brain's stores of oxygen and glucose, the essential substrates for cerebral function. When a seizure reoccurs in the already exhausted brain, which is starved of oxygen and glucose, it can lead to irreparable damage. The injured brain suffers additional damage from cerebral anoxia, which can lead to permanent brain injury and even death.

Brain injury from continuous or repetitive seizures, a condition called status epilepticus, can occur within five minutes. By definition, **status epilepticus** is one continuous seizure, as evidenced by electroencephalogram (EEG). The more pragmatic definition is a seizure that lasts for greater than 30 minutes.[32]

In many instances, the patient cannot physically sustain a continuous tonic–clonic seizure, owed in part to muscle fatigue. In those instances, the Paramedic may witness a pattern of repeated seizures of declining intensity.

As the patient fatigues, the shaking declines to a tremor and then eventually stops. However, the absence of muscle activity does not represent the end of the seizure. Instead, the end of a seizure is marked by increasing consciousness during the postictal period. The patient who remains unconscious or in a prolonged postictal state, a state called **prolonged twilight**, is still seizing. Close examination of the patient in prolonged twilight may reveal automatisms.

The pathophysiology of status epilepticus is the result of ineffective ventilation, acidosis, and hyperthermia. Ineffective ventilation causes hypercarbia (carbon dioxide retention) as well as hypoxia. The hypercarbia (coupled with the metabolic acidosis created by the muscle activity) and the heat produced by the muscle activity (resulting in hyperthermia) all impact the oxyhemoglobin curve and further worsen hypoxia. As the acidosis worsens, acid-mediated vasodilatation occurs and the patient experiences hypoperfusion, evident by hypotension. In combination, hypoxia, hypoglycemia, and hypotension generate conditions that are noxious for cerebral survival. In this case, aggressive resuscitation is critical.

Every year some 20% of patients with status epilepticus do not survive, with some dying despite aggressive resuscitation efforts. Very old patients, as well as the very young (neonates), are especially vulnerable to a fatal status epilepticus.

The Paramedic's primary objective in status epilepticus is to stop the seizure activity. The most effective agents to do so are benzodiazepines. Diazepam is the drug of choice.[34] First introduced to the public in 1961, the intravenous administration of diazepam can terminate the majority of cases of status epilepticus.

Midazolam is an alternative medication for status epilepticus. However, diazepam is preferred because midazolam takes three times longer to reach peak therapeutic effect, or two to three minutes, when compared with diazepam.

Patients prone to status epilepticus may have been prescribed Diastat®, a gel form of diazepam that is packaged with a rectal introducer (Figure 10-6). With a three-year shelf life, Diastat® is generally reserved for epileptic emergencies. Diastat® is packaged with two doses, as a twin pack, for a second administration if the first is not effective.

In cases of refractory status epilepticus, either an infusion of midazolam or phenytoin is indicated. The loading dose of phenytoin is 20 mg per kg infused slowly at 50 mg per minute to prevent hypotension. Cardiac monitoring is essential during the administration of phenytoin because it acts like a sodium channel blocker (class I antidysrhythmic).[35]

Sudden Unexpected Death in Epilepsy

Occasionally a Paramedic dispatched to the scene of a seizure is confronted with a cardiac arrested patient. The sudden, nontraumatic death of a patient with epilepsy has no known etiology. Some possible causes include autonomic nervous stimulation (i.e., catecholamine surges), effects leading to dysrhythmia, and respiratory changes including pulmonary edema and/or central apnea.

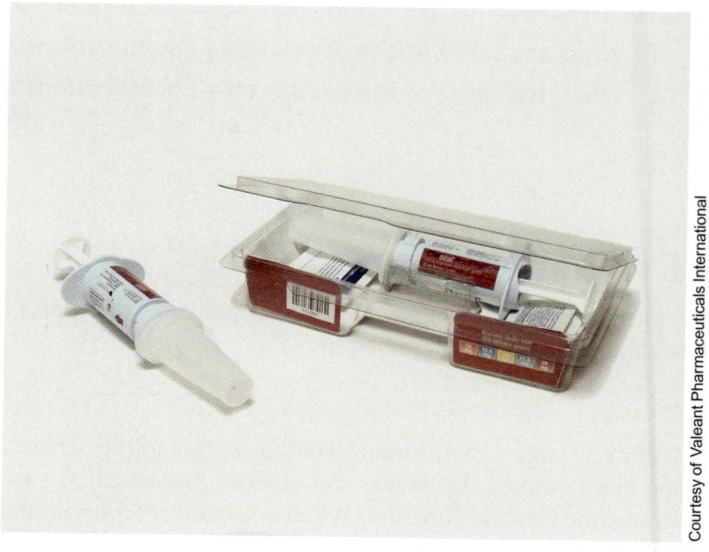

Figure 10-6 Diastat®.

Courtesy of Valeant Pharmaceuticals International

While the mall security officer calls for ambulance support, the Paramedics proceed to treat the patient's seizure activity with diazepam. Although the medication is effective in stopping the patient's motor activity, she remains unresponsive.

Sarah responds well to a second dose of IV benzodiazepine and is transported to the community hospital while still postictal. During a later transport to the same hospital, the Paramedics learn that Sarah is being treated with antibiotics for a strep throat. Her seizure is diagnosed as a breakthrough seizure and the neurologist is working with her primary physician to order a different antibiotic and monitor levels of her anti-seizure medications.

CRITICAL THINKING QUESTIONS

1. What is the most appropriate transport decision that will get the patient to definitive care?
2. Why does this patient need definitive care immediately?

Disposition

The decision to treat and transport the patient with status epilepticus is a foregone conclusion. However, other patients who have experienced a seizure may or may not be willing to agree to further medical evaluation.

Patients who have any injuries (such as a head injury), who are having difficulty staying awake, who seem to have visual difficulties, or who are vomiting—all signs of a head injury—should be encouraged to seek medical attention.

Seizures during pregnancy represent a special case. Although it is possible to be a patient with a history of epilepsy who has seized, a unique condition called toxemia of pregnancy can also cause seizures (toxemia of pregnancy is discussed in Chapter 36). All pregnant patients who have seized should be encouraged to seek further medical attention.

Patients at higher risk for cranial pathologies, including those with cancer, those on anticoagulants, or those with meningeal signs, should be encouraged to seek further medical attention.

Patients with a history of epilepsy often refuse further care and transportation. These patients spontaneously regain consciousness within five minutes and have no signs of serious injury from the fall. Paramedics, frequently after consultation with medical control, may permit these patients to refuse care after ensuring informed consent.

If the patient has an increase in the duration or frequency of her seizure, crescendo pattern, or an abnormal postictal period, then the patient should be encouraged to seek further medical attention.

If the patient does refuse care and/or transportation, the Paramedic should ensure that any hypoxia has been resolved and that hypoglycemia does not exist.

CONCLUSION

Our consciousness, our awakened sense of self, defines our being and any alteration in consciousness has grave implications for the patient. Although most seizures are self-limited and benign, the Paramedic must keep an open mind to other possibilities. The Paramedic should treat the patient for the worst case scenario, with the hope that the seizure is merely an inconvenience to the patient and that, with proper treatment, the patient can have a seizure-free existence.

KEY POINTS:

- Wakefulness does not constitute consciousness.

- Three levels—person, place, and time—are foundational to consciousness.

- A seizure is an involuntary contraction of voluntary muscles caused by some insult to the central nervous system and the brain.

- Delirium tremens, which are not true seizures, occur during alcohol withdrawal.

- Psychiatric patients with specific histories may experience psychogenic non-epileptic seizures, formerly known as pseudoseizures.

- Epilepsy is not a single disease but a reoccurring symptom of a number of underlying disorders characterized by two or more unprovoked seizures.

- Seizures can be grossly divided into two classifications: generalized and focal seizures.

- Control of seizures can be achieved by either blocking electrolytes or by enhancing the inhibitory effect of the neurotransmitter GABA.

- The Paramedic's care should focus on the primary assessment while providing a supportive and protective environment.

- The greatest percentage of seizures are breakthrough seizures secondary to noncompliance with anticonvulsant medications.

- Status epilepticus is best defined as a seizure that lasts for greater than 30 minutes.

REVIEW QUESTIONS:

1. In what order should the Paramedic assess the three levels foundational to consciousness?
2. What are the causes of seizures?
3. What disorders can masquerade as epileptic seizures?
4. What classifications exist for seizures?
5. What are the mechanisms of action for anticonvulsant medications?
6. For patients with an epileptic history, what is the most likely cause of seizures?
7. What is status epilepticus?

CASE STUDY QUESTIONS:

Please refer to the Case Study in this chapter, and answer the questions below:

1. What are some clues to differentiating seizures from other changes in consciousness?
2. What is an explanation of Sarah's elevated vital signs during her postictal stage?
3. What physiological risks is Sarah subject to as her seizure continues?

REFERENCES:

1. Adams SM, Knowles PD. Evaluation of a first seizure. *Am Fam Physician.* 2007;75(9):1342–1347.

2. Morley JE. Falls—where do we stand? *Mod Med.* 2007;104(1):63–67.

3. Cavazos JE. Seizures and epilepsy. Available at: **http://www .emedicine.com/neuro/TOPIC415.htm**. Accessed July 12, 2008.

4. Giardina B, Messana I, et al. The multiple functions of hemoglobin. *Crit Rev Biochem Mol Biol.* 1995;30(3):165–196.

5. Somero GN. Temperature as a selective factor in protein evolution: the adaptational strategy of "compromise". *J Exp Zool.* 1975;194(1):175–188.

6. Leeman L, Fontaine P. Hypertensive disorders of pregnancy. *Am Fam Physician.* 2008;78(1):93–100.

7. Adams SM, Knowles PD. Evaluation of a first seizure. *Am Fam Physician.* 2007;75(9):1342–1347.

8. LaFrance WC, Jr. Psychogenic nonepileptic seizures. *Curr Opin Neurol.* 2008;21(2):195–201.

9. Reuber M. Psychogenic nonepileptic seizures: answers and questions. *Epilepsy Behav.* 2008;12(4):622–635.

10. Binder LM, Salinsky MC. Psychogenic nonepileptic seizures. *Neuropsychol Rev.* 2007;17(4):405–412.

11. Kobau R, Zahran H, et al. Epilepsy surveillance among adults—19 states, behavioral risk factor surveillance system, 2005. *MMWR Surveill Summ.* 2008;57(6):1–20.

12. Hauser WA, Beghi E. First seizure definitions and worldwide incidence and mortality. *Epilepsia.* 2008;49 Suppl 1:8–12.

13. Wild E. Deja vu in neurology. *J Neurol.* 2005;252(1):1–7.

14. McGuire W, Fowlie PW. Naloxone for narcotic-exposed newborn infants. *Cochrane Database Syst Rev.* 2002;4:CD003483.

15. Guinsburg R, Wyckoff MH. Naloxone during neonatal resuscitation: acknowledging the unknown. *Clin Perinatol.* 2006;33(1):121–132, viii.

16. Chadwick DJ, 2nd. Febrile seizures: an overview. *Minn Med.* 2003;86(3):41–43.

17. Berg AT. Febrile seizures and epilepsy: the contributions of epidemiology. *Paediatr Perinat Epidemioly.* 1992;6(2):145–152.

18. Willmore LJ. Treatment of benign epilepsy syndromes throughout life. *Epilepsia.* 2001;42 Suppl 8:6–9.

19. Cushman JT, Floccare DJ. Flicker illness: an underrecognized but preventable complication of helicopter transport. *Prehosp Emerg Care.* 2007;11(1):85–88.

20. Gaudreault P, Guay J, et al. Benzodiazepine poisoning. Clinical and pharmacological considerations and treatment. *Drug Saf.* 1991;6(4):247–265.

21. Isbister GK, O'Regan L, et al. Alprazolam is relatively more toxic than other benzodiazepines in overdose. *Br J Clin Pharmacol.* 2004;58(1):88–95.

22. Patsalos PN, Froscher W, et al. The importance of drug interactions in epilepsy therapy. *Epilepsia.* 2002;43(4):365–385.

23. Ramani R. Vagus nerve stimulation therapy for seizures. *J Neurosurg Anesthesiol.* 2008;20(1):29–35.

24. Ardesch JJ, Buschman HP, et al. Vagus nerve stimulation for medically refractory epilepsy: a long-term follow-up study. *Seizure.* 2007;16(7):579–585.

25. Singhi S, Singhi P, et al. Status epilepticus: emergency management. *Indian J Pediatr.* 2003;70 Suppl 1:S17–S22.

26. Meierkord H, Boon P, et al. EFNS guideline on the management of status epilepticus. *Eur J Neurol.* 2006;13(5):445–450.

27. Hartman AL, Gasior M, et al. The neuropharmacology of the ketogenic diet. *Pediatr Neurol.* 2007;36(5):281–292.

28. Herf C, Nichols J, et al. Meningococcal disease: recognition, treatment, and prevention. *Nurse Pract.* 1998;23(8):30, 33–36, 39–40 passim.

29. Fodstad H, Kelly PJ, et al. History of the cushing reflex. *Neurosurgery.* 2006;59(5):1132–1137; discussion 1137.

30. Peery CA, Brice J, et al. Prehospital spinal immobilization and the backboard quality assessment study. *Prehos Emerg Care.* 2007;11(3):293–297.

31. Brouhard R. To immobilize or not immobilize: that is the question. *Emerg Med Serv.* 2006;35(5):81–82, 84–86.

32. Costello DJ, Cole AJ. Treatment of acute seizures and status epilepticus. *J Intensive Care Med.* 2007;22(6):319–347.

33. Feen ES, Bershad EM, et al. Status epilepticus. *South Med J.* 2008;101(4):400–406.

34. Garcia Penas JJ, Molins A, et al. Status epilepticus: evidence and controversy. *Neurologist.* 2007;13(6 Suppl 1):S62–S73.

35. Craig S. Phenytoin poisoning. *Neurocrit Care.* 2005;3(2):161–170.

CHAPTER 11

DISORDERS OF CEREBRAL CIRCULATION

KEY CONCEPTS:

Upon completion of this chapter, it is expected that the reader will understand these following concepts:

- How headache, weakness, and other mental and physical abnormalities can be related to a stroke but may also be caused by conditions that are treatable and reversible in the field
- That strokes may occur in patients at any age from newly born to the elderly
- How symptoms of stroke are related to the location of injury and any related inflammation or edema
- That most treatments for disorders of cerebral circulation are time dependent

ANATOMY CONCEPTS:

Prior to reading this chapter the Paramedic student should be familiar with the following anatomy and physiology concepts:

- Cerebral circulation
- Neuroanatomy

The Paramedic unit is called to the downtown campus of the state university for a 61-year-old female who has developed a sudden headache and weakness. Upon their arrival, the two Paramedics find Dr. Spencer, a well-known biology professor, seated on the front steps to the biology building.

Dr. Spencer is leaning forward with her eyes covered by her left hand. Her teaching assistant states that they were walking and discussing the day's lab setup when Dr. Spencer complained of a sudden headache and stumbled. Although she didn't fall, the assistant had to help her to the steps.

CRITICAL THINKING QUESTIONS

1. What are some of the possible causes of sudden headache?

2. How could the sudden headache be related to the patient's weakness?

OVERVIEW

A loss of consciousness is of concern for a patient under any circumstances. The implications of syncope range from minor bruising as a result of a fall when fainting, to permanent life-long disability as a result of a stroke. In every case, the Paramedic's diligence in determining the underlying cause of the syncope and providing appropriate supportive care can lessen the disorder's effects.

Chief Concern

Estimates suggest that every year over one-half million people in the United States will have a stroke, sometimes called a brain attack. Stroke is a devastating disease and is the third leading cause of death in the United States. In fact, approximately one-third of stroke victims die within one year of the event.[1]

Stroke is also the leading cause of disability in the United States with over four million stroke survivors presently receiving supportive care. In addition, the number of strokes is expected to double in the next 20 years, owed to an increased number of patients with diabetes and an increased aged population.

In terms of lost years of productivity, medical care, and other direct and indirect costs, strokes are estimated to cost the country between $43 billion and $51 billion annually. In addition, approximately one-third of all stroke patients will require assistance with their self-care and assisted living after a stroke.

Differential Diagnosis

The initial presentation of a patient with syncope is strongly suggestive of stroke. Stroke, a neurovascular disease that can lead to permanent disability, is discussed in detail shortly. However, a number of nonvascular conditions can also create stroke-like symptoms. Many of these conditions are life-threatening and must be ruled out before the Paramedic entertains making a diagnosis of stroke. In one study, the initial diagnosis of stroke, made in-hospital for patients admitted to the stroke unit, was incorrect in 13% of cases.

One cause of syncope the Paramedic always needs to consider is hypoglycemia. Hypoglycemia—whether diabetic in origin or alcohol induced, for example—can generate a gross clinical presentation of stroke.[2,3] The associated confusion, as well as aphasia and/or hemiplegia, are seen in both stroke and hypoglycemia patients.

Conversely, hyperglycemia, with its attendant hyperosmolarity, can present with focal neurological deficits such as aphasia, hemiparesis, and homonymous hemianopia; these patient conditions are defined shortly.[4]

Generally, the symptoms seen in space-occupying lesions, such as tumors and abscesses, tend to be more gradual. However, a sudden change, such as the development of a subdural hemorrhage, can also create stroke-like symptoms.

Todd's paralysis, secondary to unwitnessed seizures, is another common condition that manifests with similar signs of a stroke. Post-ictal patients can also manifest confusion and transient focal neurological signs such as automatisms. These signs are often mistaken for cerebellar stroke signs. Confusing the issue, many of these seizure patients have previously had a stroke, thus muddying the assessment picture. In addition, a number of toxic exposures, such as carbon monoxide poisoning, can have stroke-like presentations (Table 11-1).

Stroke

A **stroke** results when there is an interruption of blood flow to the brain, resulting in loss of function. This loss of function results in permanent disability and can profoundly affect the patient's life.

Table 11-1 Differential Diagnosis of Stroke

- Physiologic
  - Hypoxia
  - Hypoglycemia
  - Hyperglycemia
  - Hypotension
  - Hypertensive emergency
- Space-occupying CNS lesions
  - Tumor
  - Subdural bleeds
- Infectious
  - Herpes simplex
  - Encephalitis
  - Meningococcal meningitis
  - Poisoning
- Uremia
- Toxicology
- Headaches
  - Migraine mimicking stroke
- Psychiatric disorders
  - Conversion disorder
    - Functional hemiparesis

Cerebral Physiology

The brain is the most metabolically active tissue in the body. Although it makes up only 2% of the total body weight, the brain consumes between 15% and 20% of the body's cardiac output, 30% of the blood glucose, and as much as 50% of the oxygen while at rest. However, even with this tremendous appetite, the brain does not store any glucose or oxygen. Therefore, it needs a continuous supply, even if that means depriving other areas of the body.

The normal cerebral blood flow (CBF) is 50 to 60 mL for every 100 grams of tissue every minute. This oxygen- and glucose-laden blood arrives at the brain via two interconnected systems. The main supply of blood comes from the internal carotid arteries; it moves through the carotid canal in the skull and connects with the circle of Willis. The circle of Willis is a series of blood vessels that connect to one another to form a ring. Not every person has a complete ring. This interconnectedness serves to provide collateral circulation to the brain in the event one blood vessel becomes narrowed or blocked.

The other major blood vessel that enters the circle of Willis is the basilar artery. The basilar artery arises from the vertebral arteries, which are branches of the subclavian artery. The vertebral arteries—two arteries that run parallel to one another within the vertebral column—provide blood to the brainstem. They join together, at about the level of the medulla oblongata, to form the basilar artery.

Pathophysiology of Stroke

By definition, a stroke is an interruption in cerebral blood flow that results in a disability. That interruption can occur because of either a blockage of a blood vessel or a rupture of a blood vessel. In either case, distal blood flow is interrupted and cerebral ischemia ensues.

Over 75% to 80% of strokes are due to an occlusion, leading to distal **ischemic strokes**.[5] The remaining 20% to 25% of strokes are due to rupture of blood vessels (an aneurysm) and are classified as **hemorrhagic strokes** (Figure 11-1).

Ischemic strokes can be further divided into two classifications that have one feature in common—a blood clot.

The origin of the blood clot indicates the usefulness of these divisions.

If the blood clot developed somewhere in the body, other than the cerebral circulation, then the stroke is classified as an **embolic stroke**. Approximately 20% of strokes fall into this category. Most embolic strokes are of a cardiac or arterial origin.[6] Clots formed in the venous circulation would be filtered out in the pulmonary tree (pulmonary embolisms) and would never reach the cerebral circulation. The only exception is in patients who have a patent foramen ovale. A patent foramen ovale is a defect in the atrial septal wall which allows blood to flow from the right atrium directly to the left atrium without going through the lungs. In this situation, a systemic embolism could cause a stroke. Auscultation should reveal a loud holosystolic murmur, similar to the murmur of a mitral regurgitation, if a patent foramen ovale is present.

Cardiac Embolism

Under normal conditions, blood does not clot inside the heart. However, if there is sluggish blood flow, then blood clots can form. These clots would enter into the arterial circulation and potentially could enter into the cerebral circulation.

Atrial fibrillation is one condition in which blood clots form in the heart (Figure 11-2). When the heart goes into atrial fibrillation, the atrium does not contract effectively but

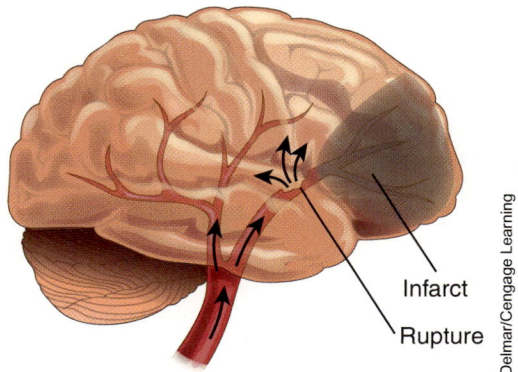

Figure 11-1 Hemorrhagic stroke.

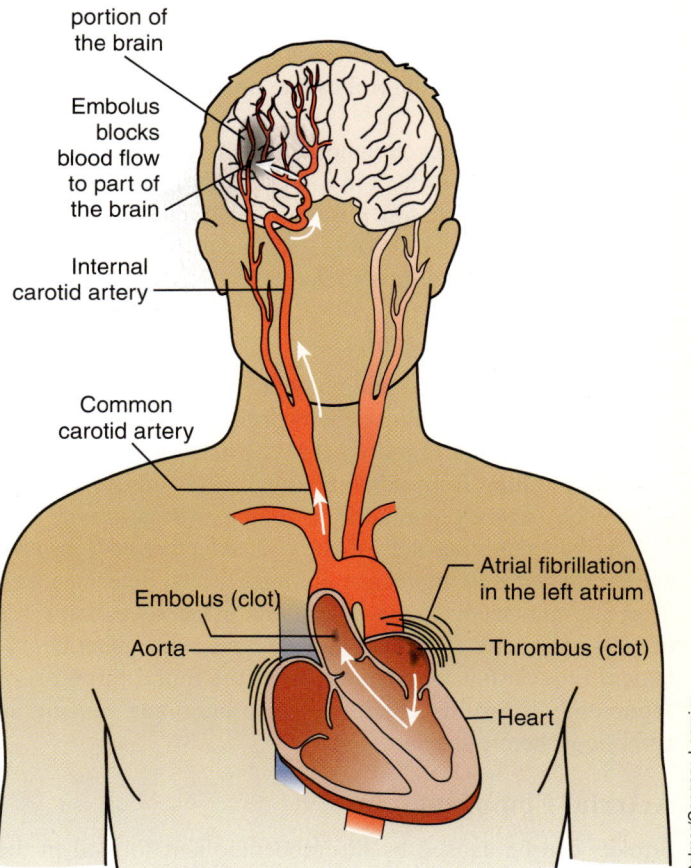

Figure 11-2 Atrial fibrillation and stroke.

instead quivers. Blood found inside the quivering atriums tends to clot and attach to the walls of the atriums (also called the mural), and those form **mural thrombi**.[7] The likelihood of mural thrombi increases when there is associated mitral valve disease, such as mitral stenosis.

If the heart returns to normal, through either electrical or chemical cardioversion, and the atrium contract normally, mural thrombi on the walls of the atrium become dislodged and float upstream to the brain.

In cases of advanced mitral valve prolapse, thromboembolism can occur with downstream complications such as stroke. The characteristic machinery murmur of the mitral regurgitation can best be heard over the point of maximal intensity (PMI) at the apex of the heart.

Another condition in which altered blood flow is the common variable is prosthetic valves. Prosthetic valves, particularly earlier mechanical models, would disturb blood flow, creating eddies where a thrombus could form. Patients with prosthetic valves are often placed on anticoagulants to prevent this complication. However, if the patient's anticoagulant levels drop below the therapeutic range (e.g., due to noncompliance), then thrombi could form and be released upstream to the brain.

Acute Myocardial Infarction

Following a myocardial infarction, a weakness in the ventricular wall, called an **aneurysm**, can occur, The aneurysm, an outpouching in the wall, is a low flow area where a thrombus can form. If the thrombus extends into the ventricular flow, a portion of the mural thrombus can break off and become a cerebral embolism.

Mural thrombus occurs more often in anterior wall acute myocardial infarctions than in inferior wall acute myocardial infarctions. For this reason, it is reasonable for a Paramedic to use a 12-lead electrocardiogram to rule out an acute coronary event for any patient with a stroke.

Endocarditis and Stroke

Endocarditis is an inflammation of the heart's innermost lining. Typically endocarditis results from an infection within the heart, such as from strep throat (rheumatic fever). The resultant swelling from inflammation creates intraventricular turbulence and the potential for thrombus formation.

While examining the patient with infective endocarditis, the Paramedic may appreciate elevated fevers, petechiae, and heart murmurs secondary to vegetations on the valves. Upwards of 20% of patients with endocarditis have subsequent neurological sequela (such as emboli from the mural thrombi) or septic emboli floating upstream to the brain and causing an embolic ischemic stroke.

Arterial Embolism

Strokes can be caused by thromboembolism formed in the arteries that service the brain. Starting at the source, the first artery arising from the heart is the aorta.

Any **aortic outflow obstruction** (e.g., the narrowing of the artery due to hypertrophic cardiomyopathy) can lead to the development of thromboembolism. **Hypertrophic cardiomyopathy** is thought to be a congenital defect in the genes that leads to hypertrophy of the myocardium and compression of the ventricular chamber. This remodeling of the ventricle can lead to valvular disorders, as well as thromboembolism and strokes. The first symptom of hypertrophic cardiomyopathy for some patients is sudden cardiac death during athletic events.[8–10]

The main supply for cerebral circulation is the carotid artery. Carotid artery disease has long been implicated in stroke. Atherosclerosis, the same disease process that causes acute coronary occlusions, can also occur in the carotid arteries. When atherosclerotic plaques develop in the carotid arteries, narrowing the lumen of the carotids, they restrict cerebral blood flow to the brain. Fortunately, collateral blood flow from the other carotid artery and/or the vertebral arteries through the circle of Willis may compensate for this loss. Unfortunately, the narrowing of the carotid arteries can go unnoticed until the plaque ruptures, sending an embolus downstream to lodge in the terminal arterioles. This thrombus now occludes the blood flow, leading to distal cerebral ischemia or stroke. Upwards of 25% of ischemic strokes are thought to be caused by carotid emboli. Therefore, a carotid artery examination should be part of every stroke evaluation.

When a patient has suspected carotid artery disease (a critical lesion that narrows the carotid artery by 50% to 70%), then a carotid endarterectomy may be indicated. A **carotid endarterectomy** clears the interior (endo) wall of the carotid of any plaque. Alternatively, stents (mechanical scaffolding) can be placed inside the lumen of the artery to maintain patency.

Vertebral Embolism

Generally, the cerebral cortex is involved in a stroke. When the vertebral arteries are involved, then the result is a brainstem stroke. The two vertebral arteries, combining into the basilar artery at the base of the skull, supply blood to the brainstem. When these arteries are occluded, the result is an infarction of the brainstem.

One of the more common symptoms of brainstem stroke is vertigo. **Vertigo** is a feeling of things spinning around which is often dismissed as a disorder of the inner ear.

A primary feature of a brainstem stroke will be peripheral cranial nerve involvement on one side of the body (the side with the stroke) and weakness on the opposite or contralateral side of the body. An example of the symptom pattern associated with a brainstem stroke would be a drooping eyelid (ptosis), with pinpoint (miosis) pupils and contralateral weakness.

When the stroke is a hemorrhage in the pons, frequently due to an aneurysm of smaller arterioles, the effect can be devastating. A pontine hemorrhage (i.e., bleeding into the pons) affects the reticular activating system, leading to coma.

It essentially cuts off the brain from the spinal cord, leading to quadriplegia. The characteristic sign of a pontine hemorrhagic stroke is pinpoint pupils with unresponsiveness and generalized flaccidity. Pontine hemorrhage also mimics opioid overdose but does not respond to naloxone.

When an embolic occlusion affects the basilar artery, the result is brainstem ischemia with resultant quadriplegia and respiratory failure. If left untreated, the respiratory arrest can lead to death.

Patients surviving this catastrophic event have an active and intact brain that is housed inside a body completely paralyzed from head to toe, a condition called **locked-in syndrome**. The opposite of a persistent vegetative state, the patient with locked-in syndrome is capable of sensing and understanding what is going on around him but is incapable of movement.

STREET SMART

A symptom pattern of vertigo, ringing in the ears called tinnitus, and changes in hearing are seen in Ménière's disease, secondary to changes in inner ear pressure. Vertigo may also be a sign of an impending stroke.

Ischemic Strokes
Thrombotic Strokes

In older patients, the majority of ischemic strokes (over 60%) are caused by a thrombus which arises from atherosclerotic lesions within blood vessels inside the brain (Figure 11-3). In younger patients, these thrombotic strokes are more often due to vasoconstriction (secondary to drugs like cocaine) or coagulopathies (such as sickle-cell disease or polycythemia). Regardless of the mechanism, the effect is the

same—occlusion of a blood supply to the brain, leading to distal cerebral ischemia. A correlation exists between stroke location, by blood vessel, and stroke symptoms (Table 11-2).

Lacunar Strokes

Micro-occlusions of small blood vessels can result in microscopic areas of ischemia at the terminus of arterioles. Symptoms of these smaller strokes are often attributed to senility and old age and manifest as a gradual and general decline in mental function.

The tissue in these micro-strokes will eventually progress to necrosis and form a cavity. Then, fluid filling the resulting cavity will form a lake, or **lacunar infarct**. These lacunar infarcts are often only appreciated during the patient's autopsy.

Watershed Strokes

The body, like the brain, depends on a constant supply of oxygen-rich, glucose-laden blood to function. Whenever either of those substances are absent (as occurs with hypoxia and hypoglycemia) or blood flow is reduced (such as with hypoperfusion), then ischemia will occur.

However, unlike the rest of the body, the brain is acutely sensitive to any hypoxia, hypoglycemia, or hypoperfusion. In conditions of prolonged deprivation, and in as little as six minutes, pancerebral ischemia will begin.

Even when these conditions are reversed, permanent injuries, via stroke, can occur. These strokes, called **watershed strokes**, are the direct result of hypoxia, hypoglycemia, or hypoperfusion.

Neurophysiological Changes of an Ischemic Stroke

Following an ischemic stroke, chemical changes occur within the brain tissue as it progresses from ischemia to injury to infarction. Neurochemicals released from the stroke cause further damage. Regardless of the etiology—embolic or thrombotic—the pathophysiology remains the same. An area

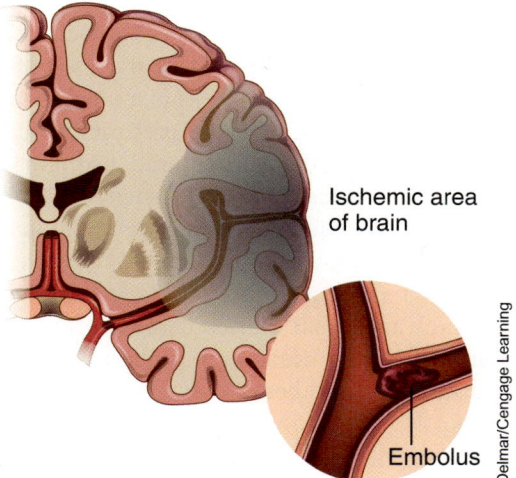

Ischemic area of brain

Embolus

Delmar/Cengage Learning

Figure 11-3 Thrombotic stroke.

Table 11-2 Large Vessel Correlation to Stroke Symptoms

• Anterior cerebral artery
○ Contralateral lower extremity and face
• Middle cerebral artery
○ Aphasia
○ Contralateral hemiparesis
• Vertebral/basilar
○ Ipsilateral
○ Ataxia
○ Diplopia
○ Vertigo

of the brain is deprived of a blood supply and ischemic changes occur.

Initially, the area immediately distal to the occlusion becomes injured, then ischemic, and then infarction occurs or the ischemia cascades. As bordering tissue starts to become affected, increasing areas of hypoperfusion lead to a series of ring-like zones of damage. This process is called **ischemic penumbra**, and long-term tissue viability is a function of reperfusion of these border areas (Figure 11-4).[11]

The ultimate effect of a stroke, or damage, is a function of time as ischemic penumbra develops and the stroke progresses, or evolves. It may take days before the full evolution of a stroke declares itself and the residual damage is known. When no further neurological deterioration is noted, the stroke is said to be completed.

The clinical goal of therapy is to minimize the neuronal damage. Although the tissue at the core of the stroke (infarction) is often lost, connected tissues may be salvaged with aggressive intervention. However, these interventions must occur within a narrow three hour window to attain any appreciable recovery of the ischemic tissue. Therefore, it is critical to ascertain, as close as possible, the onset of the symptoms and the progression of the stroke.

During the three-hour window, the ischemic cascade continues. Initially, during hypoperfusion, local vasodilatation occurs and unoccluded arterioles in surrounding tissue start to provide collateral circulation. Unfortunately, if cerebral blood flow to the affected tissues falls below 50%, then neuronal tissue activity stops and electrical silence ensues. Without cerebral blood flow, the neurons begin to convert from aerobic respiration to anaerobic respiration within minutes, leading to an increase in intracellular levels of calcium (Ca^{++}) and sodium (Na^+).

Simultaneously, and as a result of loss of ATP (which in turn leads to failure of the sodium–potassium pump), excitatory neurotransmitters (such as glutamate) are released and an imbalance between excitatory and inhibitory neurotransmitters occurs. The key to this release is the influx of calcium into the neuron. This imbalance of neurotransmitters is the source of the seizures.

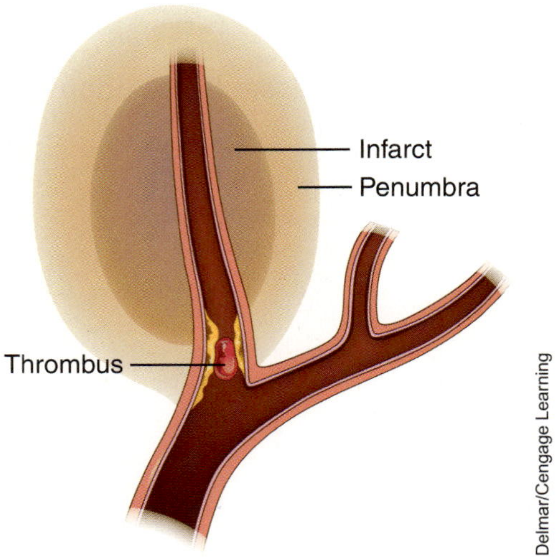

As anaerobic metabolism continues and intracellular acids accumulate, with a resultant metabolic acidosis and inflammation, cellular death begins. Although the inflammatory response occurs within one hour, cellular death does not start for several hours. It peaks in about 12 hours and, unabated, can continue for 48 hours.

Prognosis and Mortality

The prognosis for an ischemic stroke depends on a number of factors including premorbid factors, the vessel involved, and the severity of the stroke, as well as post-stroke complications, such as aspiration. The treatment of stroke patients, in order to improve the prognosis, is discussed in more detail later in the chapter.

The overall mortality for an ischemic stroke in the 30 days following the event is about 19% with a one year survival of 77%. Populations at particular risk are African Americans, possibly owed to pre-existing hypertension, and the elderly. Although strokes tend to affect the elderly (approximately 75% of strokes), strokes can affect persons of all ages, even children.

Hemorrhagic Strokes

Hemorrhagic strokes can occur because of a ruptured cerebral aneurysm or as the consequence of an arteriovenous malformation. They result in either an intracerebral hemorrhage or a subarachnoid hemorrhage.

Although small blood vessels can weaken and rupture due to microvascular disease, such as occurs with diabetes mellitus, the majority of ruptured cerebral aneurysms are found in large vessels, such as the internal carotids. These aneurysms, small out-pouches called berry aneurysms, typically involve the anterior portion of the circle of Willis (approximately 85%). They are heralded by headaches, nausea, impaired vision, and even loss of consciousness.

Some 50% of patients who suffer a ruptured cerebral aneurysm had warning symptoms, such as a headache, 10 to 20 days before the stroke. These symptoms are the result of small leaks in the cerebral aneurysm, called sentinel bleeds, and indicate that the aneurysm is expanding and preparing to rupture.

Approximately 60% of ruptured cerebral aneurysms occur during physical exertion, such as defecation or coitus, and are the result of a sudden increase in blood pressure. Bleeding from a cerebral aneurysm can either enter into the brain (intracerebral) or the subarachnoid space. The cerebral aneurysm causes a mass effect, which will be discussed shortly. Bleeding into the subarachnoid space causes a subarachnoid hemorrhage, which will also be discussed shortly.

Patients at risk for a ruptured cerebral aneurysm include those on anticoagulants, those with coagulopathies, and those who use recreational drugs such as cocaine.

Figure 11-4   Ischemic penumbra of stroke.

Delmar/Cengage Learning

Arteriovenous Malformation

The other source of intracerebral hemorrhage is from a cerebral **arteriovenous (AV) malformation**. An AV malformation is a congenital anomaly that appears like a tangled bundle of blood vessels, called a nidus (Latin for nest). It is prone to bleeding at the union where the higher pressure arterioles meet with the low pressure venuoles.

> ### STREET SMART
>
> A genetic disorder called hereditary hemorrhagic telangiectasia has a tendency to cause recurrent nosebleeds (epistaxis) as well as strokes. Even a simple nosebleed can be an omen of future events.

The incidence of intracranial hemorrhage is about 18,000 cases per year in the United States. Of those, 80% of cases of intracranial hemorrhage are secondary to ruptured aneurysms.[12] Intracranial hemorrhage is analogous to sudden cardiac death. An estimated 25% of cardiac patients die without warning and 10% of patients with hemorrhagic stroke die without any warning signs. Even if the patient survives the initial insult, the prognosis remains poor. Nearly 60% of patients with intracranial hemorrhage die within 30 days, a significant number when compared to the 19% of patients with ischemic strokes who die within 30 days.

The high mortality is attributed, in part, to the incidence of re-bleeds. Re-bleeds are a major complication with a 50% to 80% mortality rate.

A high percentage of patients, almost 50%, experiencing an intracranial hemorrhage complain of a headache. A sudden new onset seizure, especially in a middle-aged hypertensive patient, is also highly suggestive of an intracranial hemorrhage.

Intraparenchymal Bleeding

Blood from an AV malformation leak or a ruptured cerebral aneurysm can follow either into the meningeal spaces, such as the subarachnoid or subdural spaces, or it can bleed into the brain tissues directly.

Patients with either a subarachnoid hemorrhage or a subdural hemorrhage, described in more detail shortly, tend to have a more dramatic presentation. These types of hemorrhage also have more catastrophic consequences.

Alternatively, bleeding directly into the brain tissue itself (**intraparenchymal bleeding**) tends to occur very slowly. Patients may notice a progressively worsening weakness or increasing problems with coordination. This occurs because intraparenchymal bleeding happens most frequently in the cerebellum and the pons.

Subarachnoid Hemorrhage

When either an arteriovenous malformation or an intracerebral aneurysm ruptures, they can bleed into the subarachnoid space, creating a **subarachnoid hemorrhage (SAH)**.

The classic sign of a subarachnoid hemorrhage is the **thunderclap headache**. This sudden, severe headache—often starting in the back of the head—is often described by patients as the worst headache they have ever experienced.[13–15] A subarachnoid hemorrhage can lead to compression of the brain and subsequent stroke symptoms (Figure 11-5).

The initial effect of the subarachnoid hemorrhage observed by the Paramedic can range from the alert patient, who may be vomiting, to the patient who is seizing, to the patient who is unconscious and unresponsive with absent brainstem reflexes (i.e., midposition pupils unresponsive to light, presence of doll's eyes, and a cough when the carina is stimulated by a suction catheter).

The symptom complex associated with a subarachnoid hemorrhage includes the thunderclap headache, nausea, and meningeal signs (such as nuchal rigidity, as a result of blood running between the meninges which cover the brain and the spinal cord). Photophobia, another meningeal sign, is also associated with subarachnoid hemorrhage.

The first symptom, the thunderclap headache, may be the only complaint the patient voices. Upwards of 10% of patients who complain of the "worst headache in their life" have a subarachnoid hemorrhage. The Hess and Hess

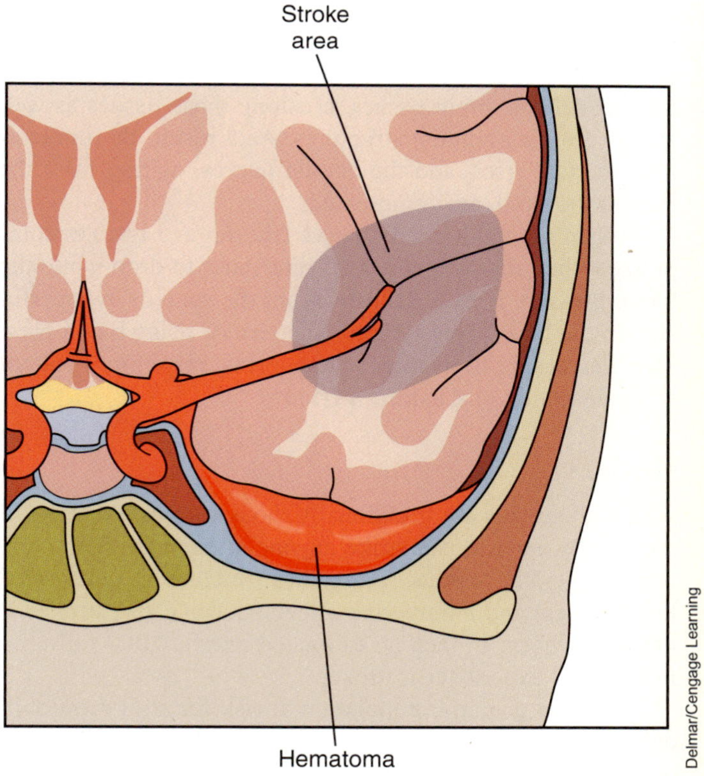

Figure 11-5 Subarachnoid hemorrhage and stroke.

Table 11-3 Hess and Hess Scale of SAH Severity

Grade	Symptom Pattern	Long-Term Survival
I	Asymptomatic	70%
	Minimal headache	
	Slight nuchal rigidity	
II	Moderate headache	60%
	Nuchal rigidity	
	Negative neurological deficit	
III	Stuporous	50%
IV	Stuporous	20%
	Hemiparesis	
	Decerebrate posturing	
V	Coma	10%
	Decerebrate posturing	

scale (Table 11-3) has been used to rate the severity of the subarachnoid hemorrhage and its relationship to long-term survival.

Neurophysiological Changes of a Hemorrhagic Stroke

When either an AV malformation or an aneurysm bleeds, a blood clot (hematoma) can form in the subarachnoid space, the epidural space, or the subdural space. These hematomas act as **space-occupying lesions**. They exert pressure onto adjunct delicate brain tissues, crushing those tissues as well as compressing adjunct structures. As a result, the intracranial pressure rises, and the cranial nerves, exiting from the base of the skull, are compressed.

When the tenth cranial nerve (the vagus nerve) is compressed, then the patient's heart rate starts to drop while the blood pressure rises reflexively from the state of hypoperfusion in the brain. This symptom pattern of rising blood pressure, decreasing heart rate, and abnormal respiratory pattern is the definition of **Cushing's triad**.

Pediatric Strokes

Although strokes are traditionally thought of as a disease of the elderly, strokes can strike anyone at any age. For example, congenital cardiac anomalies (including malformed heart valves) and intrauterine infections can cause strokes in the newly born. In fact, an estimated one in 4,000 full-term infants will experience a stroke.

Another pediatric population at risk for stroke are children with sickle-cell disease. When red blood cells sickle during sickle-cell crisis, the abnormal shape prevents easy passage through capillary beds, including cerebral capillary beds, thus leading to stroke.[16,17]

Children and young adults have a higher incidence of trauma-related injuries than older individuals. During the resuscitation phase, blood products may be administered. The combination of intravenous fluids and blood products can create hypercoagulability, clot formation, and subsequent strokes.

Finally, children can have a congenital arteriovenous malformation which ruptures (e.g., during the stress of childbirth), causing a stroke.

STREET SMART

Children with cerebral palsy will present with partial paralysis, a sign of brain damage that could have occurred in utero, during childbirth, or as the result of brain injury during trauma. Perinatal arterial ischemic stroke is the most common cause of cerebral palsy.

Mimics of Strokes

Several conditions may have a similar presentation as a stroke but will have a different etiology. For example, when the seventh cranial nerve (the facial nerve) becomes inflamed, secondary to Lyme disease or herpes simplex, a nerve palsy will develop. This condition is called **Bell's palsy** and results in a facial droop (Figure 11-6).

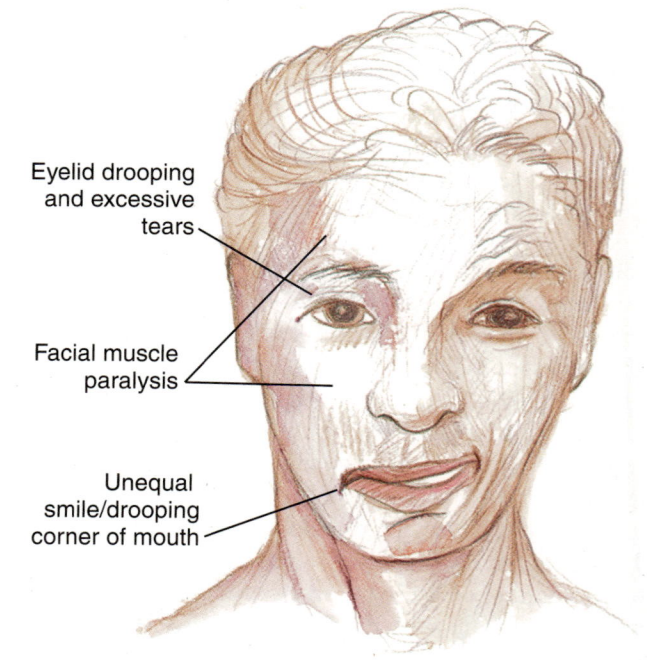

Eyelid drooping and excessive tears

Facial muscle paralysis

Unequal smile/drooping corner of mouth

Delmar/Cengage Learning

Figure 11-6 Bell's palsy.

As mentioned previously in Chapter 10 on disorders of brain function, approximately 13% of patients with generalized seizures will have unilateral weakness during the post-ictal period. This condition, called Todd's paralysis, typically lasts just a few minutes but can last for several days.

Thoracic outlet syndrome, a rare congenital anomaly, leaves the patient, typically a middle-aged female, with feelings of weakness and paresis in one hand. **Thoracic outlet syndrome** is a group of disorders which affects both nerves, hence causing the neurological deficits as well as effects upon the blood vessels. The symptoms are caused by intermittent compression of the brachial nerve plexus and/or the subclavian and vertebral artery. Because the occlusion is positional, elevating the affected limb above the shoulder will produce pallor in the hand.

CASE STUDY (CONTINUED)

Professor Spencer has an extensive medical history that includes hypertension and hypercholesterolemia. Although she has never experienced chest pain, she does tell the Paramedics that she had a "fluttering" in her chest about one week ago but it went away without further developments.

CRITICAL THINKING QUESTIONS

1. What are the important elements of the history that a Paramedic should obtain?
2. What is the symptom pattern for suspected stroke?

History

The beginning of an ischemic stroke is often heralded by a sudden onset of a neurologic deficit that may wax and wane over the course of the early phase. Although some patients,

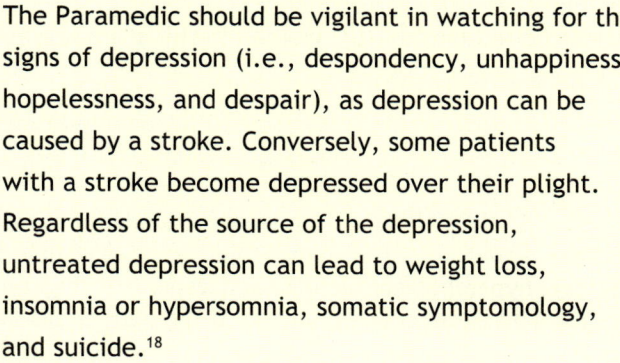
approximately 5%, dramatically present with a seizure as their initial sign, another 30% of patients present with headache as a chief concern. However, the principal symptoms of a stroke include numbness or weakness of part of the body, especially on one side; slurred speech; or a partial loss of vision. Any neurological symptom should be noted by the Paramedic and thoroughly investigated.

Other symptoms suggestive of a stroke include unusual clumsiness, such as repeatedly dropping a drinking glass or the inability to button a shirt. Falls in the elderly are particularly worrisome, as a stroke can impair one's gait, leading the patient to stumble and fall.

The OPQRST mnemonic can be helpful in establishing the symptom pattern surrounding the suspected stroke. After establishing the patient's chief concern, the Paramedic should establish the quality of those symptoms.

The patient's activity at the time of onset of symptoms may have initiated, or provoked, the stroke. For example, strenuous physical activity or emotional stress may have caused a rupture of an AV malformation or cerebral aneurysm. In some cases, particularly in the case of an embolic stroke, the onset occurs during sleep and it is impossible to establish an exact time of onset of the patient's symptoms.

It is also important to ascertain the quality of the symptoms. If the symptoms were sudden and abrupt, or stuttering, this may be suggestive of a migrating embolism. In some cases, the patient may have noticed a gradual weakness that progressed over minutes or even hours, suggesting the evolution of the stroke.

Some patients will self-prescribe medications, such as analgesics, in an attempt to relieve a headache secondary to a hemorrhagic stroke. However, there is little a patient can do for himself in the case of an ischemic stroke. Instead of stressing what the patient did to seek relief, and aggravating the patient's sense of helplessness, the Paramedic should focus on the nature of the patient's symptoms. The patient should be asked if the symptom was persistent or if it appeared to be self-resolving without medical intervention.

Following questions about the nature of the symptom, the Paramedic should focus on the severity of the impairment the stroke has created. For example, many patients call for EMS because their symptoms prevented them from accomplishing their activities of daily living (ADL).

Finally, the Paramedic should establish the exact time of onset of symptoms as exactly as possible. Many strokes occur while the patient sleeps in the early hours of the morning, when blood pressure is lowest. It has been suggested that the sudden increase in blood pressure when one awakens causes the embolism to break free and create an ischemic stroke. Instead of establishing when the symptoms started, the Paramedic should focus on determining when the patient was last observed to be normal (symptom-free). This information may be available from a reliable observer.

Past Medical History

A past stroke is often an indicator of future strokes. A careful history of past strokes—including residual symptoms such as aphasia, ataxia, dysarthria, confusion, and diplopia—should be elicited from the patient (Table 11-4). Next, the Paramedic should gather further history of neurological events such as migraine headaches, dementia, and other neurological conditions such as Bell's palsy, for example.

Since atherosclerosis is the common link between stroke and acute coronary syndrome, it is appropriate to get a cardiac history as well. A history of acute coronary syndrome—and coronary artery procedures such as coronary artery bypass graft (CABG) and angioplasty, with or without stent placement—is suggestive of systemic atherosclerosis.

The Paramedic should ask if the patient has a history of hypertension (HTN), and if so how it is being treated. Acute hypertension has been implicated in ruptured cerebral aneurysm. If the patient has a history of hypertension, then a careful medication history should be obtained, including compliance with prescribed medications.

Table 11-4 Effects of Stroke

- Right-sided stroke
  - Paralysis on contralateral side (left)
  - Paresthesia in contralateral side (left)
  - Loss of left lateral gaze
  - Excessive talking
  - Slurred monotone speech
  - Difficulty swallowing
  - Difficulty recognizing familiar faces
  - Short attention span
- Left-sided strokes
  - Paralysis on contralateral side (right)
  - Paresthesia in contralateral side (right)
  - Loss of right lateral gaze
  - Difficulty speaking
  - Inability to read or write
  - Difficulty with purposeful movements
- Brainstem strokes
  - Double vision
  - Loss of sensation to face
  - Unilateral dilated pupil
  - Difficulty swallowing
  - Loss of fine motor control
- Cerebellar strokes
  - Ataxia (drunken staggers)
  - Slurred speech
  - Tremors
  - Abnormal eye movements (nystagmus)

STREET SMART

Women who have had a spontaneous abortion may temporarily have hypercoagulability (see the HELLP syndrome in Chapter 36). Women in this state are at risk for a stroke.

The SAMPLE history should be rounded out with questions about allergies, comorbid diseases (such as diabetes), hypercholesterolemia, and especially cigarette smoking. The Paramedic should ask if the patient has had a history of heart valve disease or atrial fibrillation in the past as well.

Initial examination of Dr. Spencer shows that she is swallowing her saliva, respiration is adequate at 14 breaths per minute, and her radial pulse rate is 68 beats per minute. However, Dr. Spencer's blood pressure was elevated at 210/100. Dr. Spencer has an asymmetrical smile, weakness on the left side, and is unable to repeat a simple sentence.

CRITICAL THINKING QUESTIONS

1. What are the elements of the physical examination of a patient with suspected stroke?
2. Why is a blood glucose measurement a critical element in this examination?

Examination

The Paramedic's physical examination of the patient with a suspected disorder of cerebral circulation should focus on three major areas following the primary assessment: (1) identifying potential mimics of stroke, (2) assessing the severity of the patient's neurologic deficits following the stroke (especially those that might be life-threatening), and (3) identifying any comorbid illness that might complicate the patient's condition.

Primary Assessment

The Paramedic should pay particular attention to the airway. Loss of airway control, either partial or complete, can lead to aspiration and pneumonia, which are both potentially preventable complications of stroke. The saying goes, "If he is drooling on the outside, then he is drooling on the inside." Definitive airway control is absolutely essential.

Following assessment and treatment of the airway, the Paramedic should assess respirations. The presence of bradypnea or tachypnea is concerning. Rapid shallow breathing, like when a dog pants, could be evidence of central neurogenic hyperventilation, which is seen with increased intracranial pressure.

Next, the Paramedic assesses the patient's respiratory pattern. Irregular respirations (Cheyne–Stokes) are another respiratory pattern suggestive of increased intracranial pressure.

Finally, the Paramedic should assess for the presence of hypoxia. Pulse oximetry readings should be greater than 90% and maintained above that level at all times.[19] If the Paramedic is confident that the patient's airway is patent and the patient has adequate oxygenation and ventilation, the next order of business would be obtaining vital signs.

Although vital signs can be nonspecific for the ischemic stroke, it is important for the Paramedic to establish baseline values to trend the patient's condition. Hypertension can be particularly problematic for the stroke patient; therefore, the blood pressure should be re-assessed every five to ten minutes as conditions permit.

Many Paramedics include point of care testing of blood glucose as part of the vital signs. Hypoglycemia can create a clinical picture similar to stroke. As one of the essential substrates of cerebral metabolism, along with oxygen, hypoglycemia should be treated immediately.

STREET SMART

Although rare, an embolism from a dissecting thoracic aneurysm may cause a stroke. Signs of a dissecting thoracic aneurysm include unequal pulses in the upper extremities and/or unequal blood pressures in a patient with severe sharp or tearing chest pain that radiates to the back.

Vectored Physical Examination

Using a head-to-toe fashion, the Paramedic should next perform a thorough trauma examination of the patient's head and neck. This is followed by a cardiovascular examination and then a neurological examination.

The first two examinations—focused trauma and cardiovascular—are intended to rule out stroke. For example, a subdural hematoma secondary to a fall can mimic a stroke. The neurological examination is performed to support the presumptive diagnosis of stroke.

A focused trauma examination of the patient's head, looking for deformities, contusions, abrasions, and so on, as well as rhinorrhea and ottorrhea, can help the Paramedic eliminate trauma. While the Paramedic continues to palpate the patient's neck, she should also assess for point tenderness (suggesting spine injury) and nuchal rigidity. Nuchal rigidity is a meningeal sign. Other meningeal signs include pain upon movement of the neck (Kernig's sign) as well as photophobia (fear of light secondary to the experience of pain when the eyes are exposed to bright light). The presence of meningeal signs should alert the Paramedic to the possibility of meningitis and prompt her to take appropriate protective measures.

Next, the Paramedic should assess the patient for the presence of a bilateral carotid pulse and carotid bruit. The carotids are a common source of emboli and the absence of a pulse and/or the presence of a bruit suggests an atherosclerotic process may be present in the carotids. Gentle, non-occlusive pressure should be applied when palpating or auscultating the carotids.

If time permits, and if the Paramedic is suspicious of a brainstem involvement (i.e., diplopia or ataxia), then the patient's posterior neck proximal to the vertebrae should be auscultated for a vertebral bruit. Astute patients, prior to experiencing a brainstem insult, may complain of a humming in their ears. This humming is due to the vibration of the vertebral artery against the spine that is subsequently transmitted, via bone, to the ears.

Proceeding to the chest, the Paramedic should perform a thorough cardiovascular examination. The heart should be auscultated for irregularities in rhythm as well as murmurs that may be suggestive of a patent foramen ovale, or incompetent aortic or mitral valves.

Recording an ECG is also important. The presence of new onset atrial fibrillation is highly suspicious in the face of a symptom pattern suggestive of stroke. Unless the patient is grossly symptomatic, rhythm conversion—via either chemical or electrical cardioversion—is not advised.

Following completion of the vital signs examination, the Paramedic should proceed to a stroke assessment. There are a number of excellent stroke examinations, or stroke scales, in use. Some, such as the Cincinnati Stroke Scale or the Miami Emergency Neurologic Deficit Exam, are quick and are excellent screening tools for rapid decision making. Others, such as the National Institute of Health Stroke Scale, are more complete.

Cincinnati Stroke Scale

The **Cincinnati Stroke Scale (CSS)** is an excellent screening tool for stroke in the field. Based upon the findings, the Paramedic can make a rapid transportation decision in the field.[20,21]

The CSS uses only three criteria to make a determination: facial symmetry, extremity weakness, and speech. To assess speech, the patient is asked to repeat a simple statement such as "The sky is blue in Cincinnati," or "You can't teach an old dog new tricks." If the patient can repeat the phrase clearly, an assumption is made that the patient can hear, comprehend, and articulate; each is a complex neurological process.

The patient is then asked to smile. Any asymmetry of the face, such as a crooked smile, is suggestive of a stroke. However, here the Paramedic is cautioned. Some people have previously suffered injury to the facial nerve (e.g., trauma or Bell's palsy). Immediately after asking the patient to smile, the Paramedic should ask family members if the smile is normal. If no one is available to ask, then the patient can be given a mirror and asked if his smile is normal.

Finally, the patient should be asked to place his arms extended forward with the palms straight up, in supination, and to close his eyes. If there is motor weakness, then one hand will start to drift and rotate inwards. This movement is termed pronator drift (Figure 11-7).

Los Angeles Stroke Scale

Another prehospital stroke scale used in the field is the **Los Angeles Stroke Scale (LASS)**.[22,23] This scale has the advantage of including time of onset of symptoms as well as point of care blood glucose testing, two essential pieces of the stroke patient's assessment (Table 11-5).

Miami Emergency Neurologic Deficit (MEND) Exam

The University of Miami has also created an abbreviated advanced examination for patients with a suspected stroke called the **Miami Emergency Neurologic Deficit (MEND) Exam**.

The MEND Exam includes a quick assessment of the patient's mental status, cranial nerves, and extremities as well as prompts for treatment and an abridged fibrinolytic checklist (Table 11-6).

National Institutes of Health Stroke Scale (NIHSS)

The 15-item **National Institutes of Health Stroke Scale (NIHSS)** focuses on six areas during the assessment of the patient suspected of having a stroke: level of consciousness, visual fields, facial palsy, speech, motor function, and thought processes.[24–26]

The NIHSS is more comprehensive than other "screening" stroke scales, and serves as a valuable foundation for continued stroke assessment.

Although many Paramedics do not perform the NIHSS, a neurological examination that is inclusive of some of its elements can help the physician establish the baseline and may have predictive value for the patient.

Table 11-5 Los Angeles Prehospital Stroke Scale

Los Angeles Prehospital Stroke Scale
1) Age over 45 years
2) No prior history of seizure disorder
3) New onset of neurologic symptoms in last 24 hours
4) Patient was ambulatory prior to event
5) Blood glucose between 60 and 400
6) Facial smile
7) Grip
8) Arm weakness

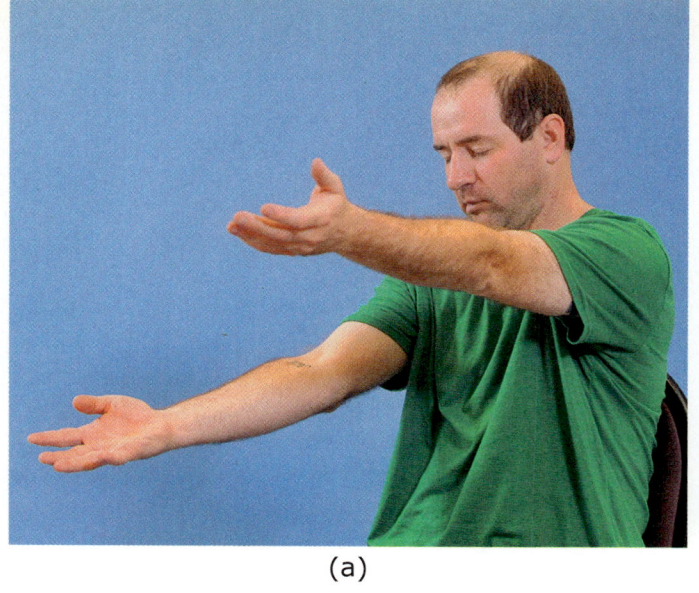

(a)

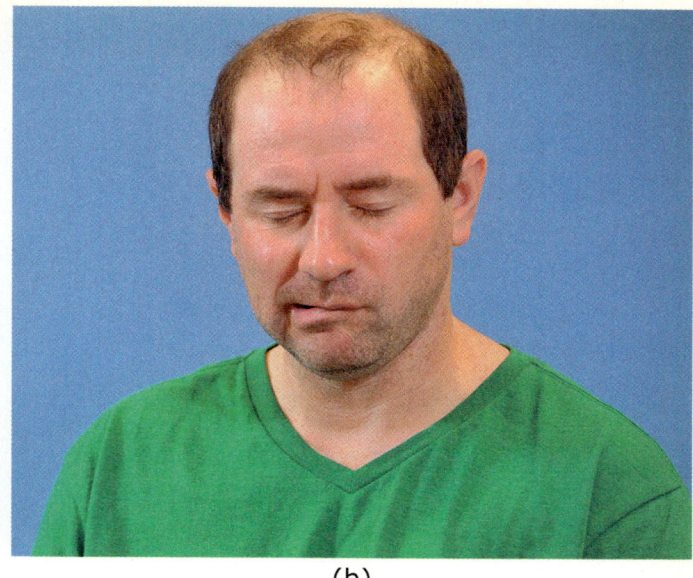

(b)

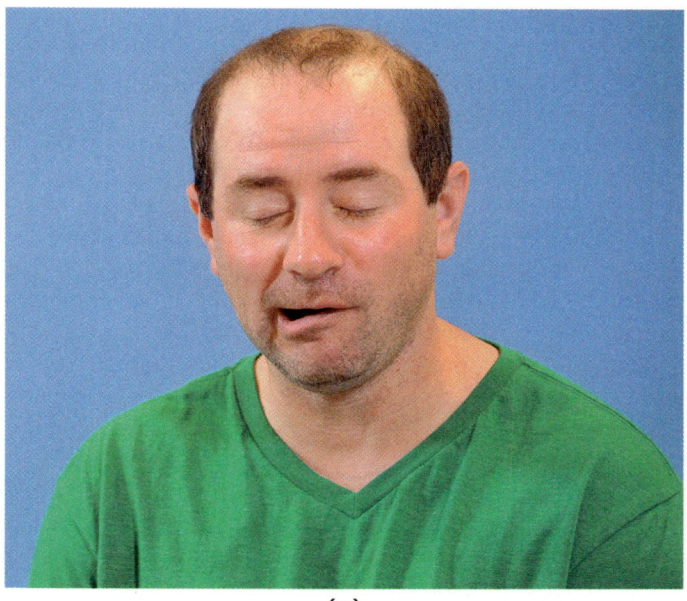

(c)

	Normal	**Abnormal**
Arm drift	Both arms move equally or not at all.	One arm drifts compared to the other.
Facial droop	Both sides of the face move equally.	One side of the face does not move at all.
Speech	Patient uses correct words without slurring.	Patient uses inappropriate words, slurs, or is mute.

(d)

Delmar/Cengage Learning

Figure 11-7 (a) Arm drift. (b) Facial droop. (c) Speech. (d) Cincinnati Stroke Scale.

Level of Consciousness

The patient's level of consciousness is first assessed in all patients suspected of having a stroke. Consciousness in the NIHSS is graded similarly to the AVPU (**A**lert, **V**oice, **P**ain, **U**nresponsive) scale used by EMS. The alert patient, one that is oriented and interactive with the environment, is given a zero score in the NIHSS, whereas the stuporous patient who can be aroused with verbal stimuli is awarded a one. The patient requiring repeated stimulation or painful stimulation to respond is given a score of two and the unresponsive patient, or patient who postures with reflex movements, is awarded a three.

Visual Fields and Cardinal Gazes

Next, the Paramedic assesses the patient's visual fields for defects by asking the patient to follow the Paramedic's finger with her eyes through the six cardinal gazes. Asking the patient to follow a finger as it traces the star of life in the front of the patient will put the patient through the necessary horizontal, vertical, and diagonal ocular movements.

Finally, the Paramedic should ask the patient to follow the finger to the bridge of the patient's nose to test convergence. The Paramedic should report any loss of vision in any field (loss of gaze).

Table 11-6 MEND Stroke Scale

- Mental status
  - Level of consciousness (AVPU)
  - Speech (clarity)
  - Questions (orientation)
  - Commands (eye opening)
- Cranial nerves
  - Facial droop
  - Visual fields
  - Horizontal gaze
- Limbs
  - Leg drift (leg lift)
  - Sensation (extremities)
  - Coordination (finger to nose or heel to shin)

Loss of the same half of a visual field in both eyes (e.g., both right sides of the two visual fields) is called **homonymous hemianopia** and is a typical sign of an occipital lobe stroke. Patients with homonymous hemianopia often have a gaze preference, and they tend to look toward the side with the stroke. Patients with homonymous hemianopia may be startled as the Paramedic approaches because they have lost the ability to distinguish objects, or people, approaching them from the affected side.

Another passive test for homonymous hemianopia is to have the patient read a short passage. Patients with homonymous hemianopia often lose their place when reading, because of loss of a visual field, and complete only one-half of the sentence.

Patients with homonymous hemianopia may exhibit a phenomenon called visual neglect. With visual neglect, the patient's brain does not compensate for homonymous hemianopia. A classic example of visual neglect is the man who only shaves one-half of his face or the patient who can only describe objects on one-half of the room.

Some patients who have had a stroke will complain of double vision or **diplopia**. This condition is owed to a microvascular stroke of the nucleus that controls the ocular muscles. If the double vision is worse when the patient looks up (vertical diplopia), then the fourth cranial nerve is involved (trochlear nerve palsy). In contrast, if the double vision is worsened when looking to the left, then the sixth cranial nerve (abducens nerve palsy) is involved.

Some patients experience a phenomenon called **agnosia** (meaning without knowledge). Visual agnosia is the inability to recognize familiar faces or items. Agnosia is not blindness; the patient is able to see and describe objects, but just cannot recognize them.

Prosopagnosia, a form of agnosia, is the inability to recognize familiar faces. This form of agnosia is not dementia since the patient remembers familiar people, such as family members. However, he cannot identify them visually.

Facial Palsy

Facial droop, a typical finding in stroke, is so characteristic of the disorder that it is included in most stroke scales. Yet, over 75% of isolated facial droop in patients is attributed to Bell's palsy, an inflammation of the facial nerve.[27] To differentiate Bell's palsy from the paralysis attributed to stroke, the Paramedic should ask the patient to raise her eyebrow. The patient with Bell's palsy cannot raise her eyebrow, whereas the patient experiencing a stroke can.

Another sign of stroke is the patient's ability to completely close the eyelids. The patient with Bell's palsy will not be able to close her eyes. Finally, the patient with Bell's palsy may have excessive tearing from the affected side as well.

It should be noted that upwards of 20% of patients with Bell's palsy have a permanent facial droop. The patient or the patient's family should be asked if the current facial droop is new or pre-existing.

Speech and Aphasia

Aphasia is the inability to comprehend or to utter speech, not the inability to utter sounds. It is another stereotypical sign of stroke. There are several types of aphasia. **Expressive aphasia**, also called Broca's aphasia, is the patient's inability to communicate. While the patient may form words, the speech is grammatically incorrect and somewhat telegraphic, meaning the speech comes in short stucco bursts of words. Anyone who has had a word on the "tip of the tongue" but cannot remember it is experiencing, in a small way, what the patient with expressive aphasia is feeling. The speech of a patient who has expressive aphasia can be characterized as flat, without normal inflections and emphasis.

Expressive aphasia is the result of injury to an area of the left frontal lobe, called Broca's area, and is often associated with hemiplegia and hemiparesis. These symptoms are often right-sided, as speech is in the left hemisphere in 90% of the population.

Patients with expressive aphasia may be prone to sudden outbursts of crying, screaming, and yelling as they try to express themselves and become increasingly frustrated with their inability to do so. The Paramedic can best handle the patient's low frustration level with tolerance and an understanding of the patient's plight.

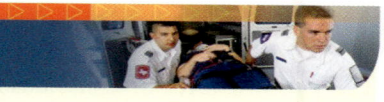

STREET SMART

The patient with expressive aphasia may maintain rote speech (i.e., yes or no, counting, swearing, etc.). Therefore, the Paramedic should endeavor to ask open-ended questions. Closed questions will only elicit an automatic response and will not be helpful when assessing the patient's speech.

Alternatively, **receptive aphasia** (also called Wernicke's aphasia) is the patient's inability to comprehend the spoken word. Receptive aphasia is also called fluent aphasia, meaning that the patient's speech is clear and understandable—just incomprehensible.

The condition can be described by the patient as being a "stranger in a strange land," where nothing makes sense and the speech of others sounds like gibberish. The patient with fluent aphasia rambles on with meaningless words and may create neologisms, a word coined with a new meaning.

The speech of a patient with receptive aphasia is semantically inappropriate (i.e., without meaning to the context of the conversation), but the articulation is clear. Jabberwocky, a non-sensical poem written by Lewis Carroll, is an example of how a patient with Wernicke's aphasia might speak. These patients are often unaware of the impairment (a condition called anosognosia) and will ramble on with wordy and even pressured speech. Unlike expressive aphasia, patients with receptive aphasia seldom have associated hemiplegia or hemiparesis.

Global aphasia occurs when the patient's stroke, involving more global aspects of the cerebral cortex, impairs the patient's ability to both comprehend and to respond to conversation.

Motor and Cerebellar Function

A sudden loss of motor function, particularly acute weakness on one side of the body, is an archetypal symptom associated with a stroke. However, any sudden unexplained weakness can be associated with stroke. The Paramedic should ask the patient to grasp two fingers of each of the Paramedic's hands with his own hands and to squeeze. Alternatively, the patient can be asked to shrug his shoulders against resistance. An unequal hand grasp or shoulder shrug is indicative of weakness.

The stroke symptom pattern may include **monoparesis** (a weakness in just one limb) or **quadriparesis** (a weakness in all four extremities), as well as **hemiparesis** (weakness in one side of the body). Any abrupt and unexplained weakness may signify a stroke in development.

Before proceeding to assess cerebellar functions, the Paramedic should ascertain handedness—that is, whether the patient is right handed or left handed. Patients, sometimes unknowingly, compensate for a weakness on one side, particularly if that weakness is on the nondominant side. Knowing the patient's handedness can help the Paramedic grossly discern compensation and more accurately determine disability.

Cerebellar strokes primarily affect motor function, especially fine motor functions. Alcohol also affects cerebellar motor function. For this reason, the misdiagnosis of intoxication may be inappropriately applied to the stroke patient.

Patients who have experienced a cerebellar stroke may exhibit slurred speech, a loss of balance, and a staggering gait similar to drunken staggers when walking (this condition is called **ataxia**). The patient may also have **nystagmus**, a flickering extraocular eye movement (EOM) observed when

Figure 11-8 Romberg test.

assessing the cardinal gazes. Some patients may even experience hiccups.

Assessment of cerebellar function can be as simple as asking patients to run their heels up the shin of the opposite leg to the knee while lying on the stretcher. However, the classic cerebellar test is called the **Romberg test**. Although there are variations of the Romberg test (e.g., heel-to-toe walking), they all test the patient's ability to stand in a steady upright position with the eyes closed (Figure 11-8). To have the patient perform the Romberg test, the Paramedic should ask the patient to stand with her feet together and eyes closed. It is important that the patient close her eyes tightly to prevent sensory feedback that will help her compensate. A positive Romberg test occurs when the patient starts to sway, demonstrating truncal instability. This may be indicative of a cerebellar stroke.

Often the Paramedic will grasp the patient by the shoulders and give her a slight push on the shoulder to see if she will compensate. The Paramedic must be prepared to catch the patient if she should start to fall.

Higher Cortical Functions

Occlusions of the cerebral arteries can lead to stroke in the cerebral cortex. Damage to the cerebral cortex may be evidenced by deterioration of higher cortical functions.

The first evidence of cortical injury may be noted during the rapid stroke survey. Specifically, this is the patient's inability to carry out simple or learned purposeful movement, which is called **apraxia**. An example of apraxia would be the patient's inability to shake the Paramedic's hand, even if the Paramedic takes the patient's hand in her own hand. Other examples of apraxia would be the patient's inability to write down his own name and difficulty with following simple commands such as following a penlight. The presence of apraxia suggests that the patient may have difficulty with performing the simplest activities of daily living.

The effects of some strokes can be subtle but debilitating. Although these strokes do not impair the activities of daily living (ADL), such as feeding, toileting, and so on, they do affect the patient's quality of life.

The patient with a stroke may be unable to do the math to balance a checkbook (dyscalculia) or read simple instructions (dyslexia). Dysgraphia, the inability to write, is associated with loss of fine motor control. Another subtle sign is the patient's inability to tie her own shoes.

Although many of these patients learn how to compensate for their impairment (e.g., wearing slippers rather than shows), these "mini-strokes" fortell future strokes. Therefore, the patient should receive a complete medical evaluation.

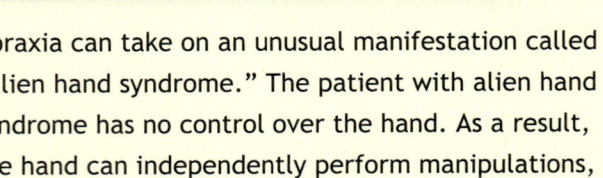

STREET SMART

Apraxia can take on an unusual manifestation called "alien hand syndrome." The patient with alien hand syndrome has no control over the hand. As a result, the hand can independently perform manipulations, such as unbuttoning a shirt, without conscious control.[28] Often the patient is unaware of the hand's activity unless it is brought to his attention.

Sensory Loss

Another typical finding in stroke is loss of feeling, or **paresthesia**, in the extremities. Paresthesia can be either an abnormal feeling, like "pins and needles," or a lack of feeling, like the extremity is "asleep." Although many patients have experienced a paresthesia, typically as a result of resting a limb on a nerve, the paresthesia associated with stroke is prolonged.

However, there are many other causes of chronic paresthesia including nerve conduction disorders, Lyme disease, multiple sclerosis, and even hyperventilation syndromes. Therefore, while the presence of paresthesia should be medically evaluated, the presence of paresthesia alone should not be equated with stroke.

Stroke in Evolution

Some patients experience a sudden loss of function not directly adjunct to the ischemic area, but rather in an area that is connected by neuronal pathways. This loss of function is called **diaschisis** (Table 11-7). Diaschisis, also called neural shock, is thought to be due to edema and inflammation from the ischemic tissue and may resolve spontaneously as the edema and inflammation subside. During this period of inflammation and recovery, the Paramedic sees the patient's symptoms wax and wane as the stroke evolves

and eventually terminates. Often it takes 48 to 72 hours for a stroke to fully evolve and the final neurological effects to manifest. For this reason, the Paramedic often cannot know the eventual outcome, or residual effect, of the patient's stroke in the field.

Table 11-7 Neuroanatomic Approach to Stroke

The following chart of symptoms is suggestive of the location of the arterial occlusion in the four major stroke syndromes. This chart is intended to be illustrative of the symptom patterns of these strokes.

- Anterior cerebral artery (ACA)
  - Primarily affects the frontal lobe
  - Loss of judgment
    - Disinhibition
      - Left hemisphere
  - Contralateral weakness in legs
    - Ataxia
  - Urinary incontinence
    - Left hemisphere
- Middle cerebral artery (MCA)
  - Primarily affects the temporal lobe
  - Contralateral hemiparesis
    - Weakness in upper extremity
    - Facial droop
  - Ipsilateral hemianopsia
  - Agnosia
  - Aphasia
    - Receptive
    - Expressive
  - Neglect
- Posterior cerebral artery
  - Primarily affects occipital lobe
  - Vision
    - Visual agnosia
  - Impaired memory
- Vertebrobasilar artery
  - Cranial nerve functions
    - Vertigo
    - Diplopia
    - Dysphagia
  - Cerebellar functions
    - Ataxia
  - Brainstem functions
    - Syncope

During the course of the patient history, the patient's assistant relates that the professor had the flu, and suggests that maybe these symptoms are related to the virus she had. The Paramedic reassures her that, while that was a possibility, it would be more prudent to transport the professor to the emergency department for a medical evaluation.

CRITICAL THINKING QUESTIONS

1. What other conditions can mimic a stroke?
2. Why did the Paramedic suggest that the patient be transported?

Assessment

Based on the presenting symptom pattern, the Paramedic may postulate that the patient is having an ischemic stroke. However, without further testing the Paramedic must limit the prehospital diagnosis to a disorder of cerebral circulation.

Professor Spencer is becoming more and more unresponsive as time goes on and the Paramedic is becoming more concerned about her inability to maintain her airway, as well as the alterations in her breathing pattern.

CRITICAL THINKING QUESTIONS

1. What are some of the predictable complications associated with acute stroke?
2. What are some of the predictable complications associated with the treatments for acute stroke?

Treatment

Any obtunded patient (a patient with a Glasgow coma scale less than eight) should be electively intubated, if possible, to protect the patient's airway and prevent possible aspiration.[29,30] In some cases, the use of medication-facilitated intubation may be necessary if the patient's protective airway reflexes are still intact.

Regardless of the method of intubation—elective or medication-facilitated—lidocaine 1.0 mg to 1.5 mg/kg administered intravenously should be considered prior to the intubation. Lidocaine used prior to intubation is thought to blunt the rise in intracranial pressure that occurs during instrumentation of the throat, although there is some controversy about this practice.[31–34]

After ensuring that the patient has an adequate airway, the Paramedic should assess for the adequacy of ventilation and respiration. The use of high-flow, high-concentration oxygen has been a subject of debate in medical circles, generated by concerns about the creation of oxygen-free radicals and lipid perioxidation during cellular hypoperfusion, both of which are associated with poor outcomes.

Contrary opinion, supported by research, suggests that hyperoxia via high-flow, high-concentration oxygen improved—if even transiently—the neurological outcomes of stroke patients. It is safe to say that hypoxia—before, during, and after the intubation, and at any time during patient care—should be avoided and a steady oxygen state of greater than 92% to 95% SaO_2 should be maintained.

It is difficult to distinguish hemorrhagic strokes from ischemic strokes in the field. If a hemorrhagic stroke is suspected and the patient is grossly symptomatic (i.e., Cushing's triad), then the patient should be treated as if there is a traumatic brain injury.

Controlled hyperventilation will help to control hemorrhage in the patient via reduced carbon dioxide levels and subsequent vasoconstriction. Unfortunately, the resulting vasoconstriction is not localized and hyperventilation can lead to pancerebral hypoperfusion, leading to worsening ischemia. Therefore, hyperventilation should be carefully considered and utilized only if necessary.

Blood oxygen levels are affected by both acid levels, controlled by ventilation, and temperature. This relationship is demonstrated in the oxyhemoglobin curve. After controlling for ventilation, the Paramedic should also make efforts to control hyperthermia, in order to ensure optimal oxygenation.

Even a modest rise in the patient's core temperature can have an adverse effect (such as oxygen-free radical production and blood-brain barrier breakdown). Therefore, patient care should include efforts to maintain the patient's core temperature in a normothermic range (98.0°F to 98.6°F). Typically, simple techniques, such as removing the patient from the warm environment, are sufficient and active cooling is not necessary.

The brain does not tolerate hypoxia or hypoglycemia well. Glucose, as a substrate, is so essential that the brain does not need insulin to uptake the glucose for metabolism. Without adequate glucose, the brain malfunctions, leading to stroke-like symptoms and/or seizures. Seizures in the stroke patient are particularly problematic, as they lead to increased intracranial pressure and/or worsening ischemia. For these reasons, glycemic control is crucial. The patient's blood glucose should be minimally at 80 to 100 mg/dL with a goal of maintaining the patient's euglycemic state (i.e., normal glucose levels). Administration of either oral glucose, provided the patient can control the airway, or 25 grams of glucose intravenously is the current standard of care.

Hyperglycemia is also problematic, as studies have shown increased morbidity and mortality for stroke patients with hyperglycemia. Therefore, glucose-containing intravenous solutions, such as dextrose 5% in sterile water, should be avoided.

Currently, the prehospital administration of insulin is rare, owed in part to the difficulty of storing insulin in the field. Minimally, the Paramedic should report hyperglycemia.

As mentioned earlier, seizures are problematic for the patient with a suspected stroke. In one study of 1,640 cases of patients with stroke, the initial presenting symptom was a seizure in 5.4% of cases. Other estimates run as high as 10%, and it has been suggested that stroke is the most common cause of new onset seizures in the elderly.

Currently, prophylactic seizure control, using a benzodiazepine, is not indicated. However, if the patient with a suspected stroke does seize, then use of benzodiazepines to promptly resolve the seizures is in order.

Hypertension, defined as systolic pressure greater than 170 mmHg and/or diastolic pressure greater than 100 mmHg, is not uncommon for the patient with stroke. It has been suggested that upwards of 80% of patients are hypertensive. This initial hypertension is thought to be neuroprotective, part of the autoregulation of cerebral blood flow, and often spontaneously resolves within days.

Hypertension becomes problematic, and deserving of treatment, when the elevated blood pressure results in a hypertensive emergency. Unresolved hypertension can result in end-organ damage (e.g., heart failure) and/or dissecting aortic aneurysm.

Patients with systolic pressures over 200 mmHg or diastolic pressures greater than 120 mmHg may be treated with a beta blocker, such as labetalol, or nitrates.

Finally, the patient should be positioned on the stretcher with the head in a neutral position, permitting venous outflow. Some controversy exists regarding whether the patient should be transported with the head elevated, to decrease intracranial pressures, or supine, to optimize cerebral blood flow.

Paramedicine and the Future

Paramedics may be involved in early administration of neuroprotective agents in the future. For example, intravenous administration of calcium channel blockers early in the course of a stroke may help to attenuate the calcium influx and improve membrane stability. Similarly, the use of glutamate receptor antagonists to block excitotoxicity events—a state where the excitatory neurotransmitter overstimulates the neurons, leading to premature cell death or apoptosis—may be authorized. The window of opportunity for the administration of these drugs is narrow (only one or two hours). It is possible that Paramedics administering these treatments offers great promise for reducing patients' neurological damage.

Another drug therapy being considered early in the treatment for stroke during the hyperacute phase is magnesium administration. Magnesium both inhibits the release of glutamate and blocks the N-methyl d-aspartate (NMDA) receptors that attract glutamate for attachment. Magnesium has the added bonus of being a potent vasodilator, thus increasing collateral blood flow to the area surrounding the lesion and decreasing the amount of penumbra.

As emphasized earlier, tight glycemic control is critical. In the future, Paramedics may administer an infusion of glucose, insulin, and potassium (GIK) to patients with acute strokes to help maintain euglycemia (i.e., normal blood glucose levels in the blood). This treatment has shown promise in acute myocardial infarctions.

CASE STUDY (CONTINUED)

Suddenly, Dr. Spencer regains movement and some strength in her right side. Her speech becomes clear and her questions indicate the high level of curiosity for which she is well known as a professor.

The Paramedic speaks with her about her past medical complaints and she says that she had had a mini-stroke three months ago. At that time, she was started on aspirin therapy and an antihypertensive medication.

CRITICAL THINKING QUESTIONS

1. What are some of the predictable complications associated with acute stroke?
2. What are some of the predictable complications associated with the treatments for acute stroke?

Evaluation

The sudden resolution of stroke symptoms is suggestive of a transient ischemic attack. The **transient ischemic attack (TIA)**, known to the lay public as a "mini-stroke," is a temporary cessation of blood flow in the brain that leads to a temporary focal neurological deficit. This disturbance in blood flow may be due to a traveling embolism, a thrombus that has disintegrated, or a vasospasm.

Generally, a TIA only lasts a few minutes (typically 10 minutes), but can last up to several hours.[35,36] The occurrence of a TIA should prompt the Paramedic to reassess the patient with particular attention given to the possibility of seizure. The seizure patient may initially present as confused and stroke-like, with Todd's paralysis, then spontaneously resolve. Thus, the evidence would suggest that the patient may have had a TIA.

Although the diagnosis of a TIA as opposed to a stroke may initially bring relief to the patient and the patient's family (in some instances, the patient may even refuse further medical treatment), the patient still needs medical evaluation. Approximately one-third of patients presenting with a TIA will have a stroke within 90 days.[37,38]

Factors that suggest the patient with a TIA will go on to develop a stroke include age greater than 60 years and initial presentation with hemiparesis or aphasia, especially if the symptoms lasted over one hour and/or there is a history of hypertension or diabetes.

CASE STUDY CONCLUSION

During the course of the transport, the Paramedic contacts medical control. After their conversation she advocates that the patient may prefer to go to the nearby stroke center. The patient and the Paramedic confer and mutually agree to divert her to the stroke center.

CRITICAL THINKING QUESTIONS

1. What is the most appropriate transport decision that will get the patient to definitive care?
2. What are the advantages of transporting a patient with suspected stroke to these hospitals, even if that means bypassing other hospitals in the process?

Disposition

In 1992, a stroke trial by the National Institute of Neurological Disorders (NINDS) demonstrated that the use of tissue plasminogen activator (t-PA) was an effective treatment option for patients experiencing an ischemic stroke if the patient received the treatment within three hours of onset of symptoms. Since that landmark study, hospitals have been organizing into stroke centers, complete with special teams that respond to "stroke alerts." Currently, the American Stroke Association, a subsidiary of the American Heart Association, supports rapid transport of patients who may benefit from fibrinolytics to stroke centers.

Rapid Transport

This concept—stroke or "brain attack" as an emergency—is a major paradigm shift for both medicine and paramedicine. Brain damage, once assumed inevitable for the patient with a stroke, can be prevented in as much as 50% of cases under certain conditions.

New research has also produced the MERCI system, a clot retrieval system with a 48% success rate for recanalization. Using the same or similar technologies used in the cardiac catheterization lab, specially trained neurosurgeons are capable of performing cerebral endovascular embolectomy to remove clots and/or carotid endocardectomy to reopen occlusions.

Futures in Stroke Care

Research in stroke care has been expanding and new therapies are currently in trials. These new techniques include the use of induced hypothermia, hyperbaric chambers, and stem cells.

Dr. Krieger of the Cleveland Clinic is presently studying the use of induced hypothermia in the care of stroke patients.[39,40] The concept is simple: The damage from a stroke is owed to ischemic changes, which can be slowed if the patient becomes hypothermic. Using alcohol rubs and paralytics to prevent shivering, Dr. Krieger's team is reporting upwards of 50% of patients recovering neurologically intact.

Another promising therapeutic treatment could be hyperbaric oxygen. Although initial studies of hyperbaric oxygen with high-flow, high-concentration oxygen were disappointing, new studies with room air only or room air and hemoglobin-based oxygen carriers are promising.

Finally, researchers from the University of South Florida under the leadership of Dr. Saberg have been using stem cells. These stem cells, recovered from umbilical cords, are infused intravenously into patients with stroke. The reports have been that upwards of 80% of patients with residual effects from a stroke fully recovered if they received the stem cells within 24 hours of the onset of symptoms.

These developments underscore the importance of thorough evaluation and rapid transport of patients with suspected stroke to a stroke center for immediate medical treatment.

CONCLUSION

The signs and symptoms of a stroke can vary based upon the specific territory of the brain affected by the stroke. Patients who have a TIA that resolves are at a much higher risk for subsequent massive stroke. The Paramedic needs to constantly re-evaluate the improving stroke patient to allow early detection of a sudden worsening of the patient's stroke.

KEY POINTS:

- Sudden weakness or syncope can result from vascular or nonvascular conditions.

- Stroke, or brain attack, results from an interruption of blood flow to the brain.

- The brain does not store oxygen or glucose and must have a continuous supply.

- Interruption can occur from bleeding or from blockage of arteries.

- Bleeding may occur into the meningeal spaces (subarachnoid hemorrhage, subdural hematoma, epidural hematoma) or directly into the brain parenchyma.

- Any part of the brain can be affected by a stroke. Different signs and symptoms reflect the area of the brain which is damaged.

- As with cardiac tissue, a portion of brain tissue dies during a stroke, but surrounding tissue becomes injured (ischemic penumbra).

- The time frame from initial tissue death until surrounding tissue is no longer suffering injury (ischemic cascade) is called evolution.

- Several different stroke scales exist as screening tools.

- Vectored physical assessment includes level of consciousness, motor exam, and sensory exam.

- Transient ischemic attacks are a temporary cessation of blood flow to the brain, resulting in stroke-like symptoms which resolve suddenly.

- The American Stroke Association suggests that patients with TIA or stroke be transported to facilities capable of timely administration of treatments.

REVIEW QUESTIONS:

1. What vascular disorders can result in sudden weakness and/or syncope?
2. What nonvascular disorders can result in sudden weakness and/or syncope?
3. What signs/symptoms would you find in a patient with interrupted blood flow to the following areas:
   - Right side of cerebrum
   - Left side of cerebrum
   - Cerebellum
   - Brainstem
4. How do neuroprotective drugs work?
5. What are the differences between the Cincinnati Stroke Scale, the Los Angeles Stroke Scale, the Miami Emergency Neurologic Deficit Exam, and the National Institutes of Health Stroke Scale?

6. Describe the difference in patient presentation for a patient with receptive aphasia versus one with expressive aphasia.

7. What is the maximum time frame from symptom start to the safe administration of t-PA?

 CASE STUDY QUESTIONS:

Please refer to the Case Study in this chapter, and answer the questions below:

1. What signs and symptoms will help determine a list of differential diagnoses?

2. What factors in Dr. Spencer's history signal a likely stroke within the next 90 days?

 REFERENCES:

1. Becker, JU, MD. Stroke, ischemic. Available at: **http://www.emedicine.com/EMERG/topic558.htm**. Accessed March 7, 2009.

2. Ng CL. Diagnostic challenge—is this really a stroke? *Aust Fam Physician.* 2006;35(10):805–808.

3. Ginsburg BY, Hoffman RS, et al. Comment on "Is prehospital blood glucose measurement necessary in suspected cerebrovascular accident patients?" *Am J Emerg Med.* 2006;24(6):757–758; author reply 758–759.

4. Kagansky N, Levy S, et al. The role of hyperglycemia in acute stroke. *Arch Neurol.* 2001;58(8):1209–1212.

5. Quinn TJ, Dawson J, et al. Past, present and future of alteplase for acute ischemic stroke. *Expert Rev Neurother.* 2008;8(2):181–192.

6. Di Tullio MR, Homma S. Mechanisms of cardioembolic stroke. *Curr Cardiol Reps.* 2002;4(2):141–148.

7. Ferro JM. Atrial fibrillation and cardioembolic stroke. *Minerva Cardioangio.* 2004;52(2):111–124.

8. Miller MA, Gomes JA, et al. Risk stratification of sudden cardiac death in hypertrophic cardiomyopathy. *Nat Clin Pract Cardiovasc Med.* 2007;4(12):667–676.

9. Pigozzi F, Rizzo M. Sudden death in competitive athletes. *Clin Sports Med.* 2008;27(1):153–181, ix.

10. Germann CA, Perron AD. Sudden cardiac death in athletes: a guide for emergency physicians. *Am J Emerg Med.* 2005;23(4):504–509.

11. Lo EH. A new penumbra: transitioning from injury into repair after stroke. *Nat Med.* 2008;14(5):497–500.

12. Nassisi D, MD. Stroke, hemorrhagic. Available at: **http://www.emedicine.com/EMERG/topic557.htm**. Accessed March 7, 2009.

13. Savitz SI, Edlow J. Thunderclap headache with normal CT and lumbar puncture: further investigations are unnecessary: for. *Stroke.* 2008;39(4):1392–1393.

14. Moussouttas M, Mayer SA. Thunderclap headache with normal CT and lumbar puncture: further investigations are unnecessary: against. *Stroke.* 2008;39(4):1394–1395.

15. Schwedt TJ. Clinical spectrum of thunderclap headache. *Expert Rev Neurother.* 2007;7(9):1135–1144.

16. Carpenter J, Tsuchida T, et al. Treatment of arterial ischemic stroke in children. *Expert Rev Neurother.* 2007;7(4):383–392.

17. Bernard TJ, Goldenberg NA, et al. Treatment of childhood arterial ischemic stroke. *Ann Neurol.* 2008;63(6):679–696.

18. Carota A, Bogousslavsky J. Poststroke depression. *Adv Neurol.* 2003;92:435–445.

19. Carlson KA, Jahr JS. A historical overview and update on pulse oximetry. *Anesthesiol Rev.* 1993;20(5):173–181.

20. Available at: **http://www.strokecenter.org/trials/scales/cincinnati.html**. Accessed March 7, 2009.

21. Lindsell CJ, Alwell K, et al. Validity of a retrospective National Institutes of Health Stroke Scale scoring methodology in patients with severe stroke. *J Stroke Cerebrovasc Dis.* 2005;14(6):281–283.

22. Llanes JN, Kidwell CS, et al. The Los Angeles Motor Scale (LAMS): a new measure to characterize stroke severity in the field. *Prehosp Emerg Care.* 2004;8(1):46–50.

23. Ramanujam P, Guluma KZ, et al. Accuracy of stroke recognition by emergency medical dispatchers and Paramedics—San Diego experience. *Prehosp Emerg Care.* 2008;12(3):307–313.

24. Spilker J, Kongable G, et al. Using the NIH Stroke Scale to assess stroke patients. The NINDS rt-PA Stroke Study Group. *J Neurosci Nurs.* 1997;29(6):384–392.

25. Kasner SE. Clinical interpretation and use of stroke scales. *Lancet Neurol.* 2006;5(7):603–612.

26. Available at: **http://www.ninds.nih.gov/doctors/NIH_Stroke_Scale_Booklet.pdf**. Accessed March 7, 2009.

27. Tiemstra JD, Khatkhate N. Bell's palsy: diagnosis and management. *Am Fam Physician.* 2007;76(7):997–1002.

28. Muangpaisan W, Srisajjakul S, et al. The alien hand syndrome: report of a case and review of the literature. *J Med Assoc Thai.* 2005;88(10):1447–1452.

29. The Brain Trauma Foundation, The American Association of Neurological Surgeons, The Joint Section on Neurotrauma and Critical Care. Glasgow coma scale score. *J Neurotrauma.* 2000;17(6-7):563–571.

30. Davis DP, Vadeboncoeur TF, et al. The association between field Glasgow coma scale score and outcome in patients undergoing Paramedic rapid sequence intubation. *J Emerg Med.* 2005;29(4):391–397.

31. Robinson N, Clancy M. In patients with head injury undergoing rapid sequence intubation, does pretreatment with intravenous lignocaine/lidocaine lead to an improved neurological outcome? A review of the literature. *Emerg Med J.* 2001;18(6):453–457.

32. Brucia JJ, Owen DC, et al. The effects of lidocaine on intracranial hypertension. *J Neurosci Nurs.* 1992;24(4):205–214.

33. Yano M, Nishiyama H, et al. Effect of lidocaine on ICP response to endotracheal suctioning. *Anesthesiology.* 1986;64(5):651–653.

34. Weingart S. Additional thoughts on the controversy of lidocaine administration before rapid sequence intubation in patients with traumatic brain injuries. *Ann Emerg Med.* 2007;50(3):353.

35. Hadjiev DI, Mineva PP. A reappraisal of the definition and pathophysiology of the transient ischemic attack. *Med Sci Monit.* 2007;13(3):RA50–RA53.

36. Caplan LR. Transient ischemic attack: definition and natural history. *Curr Atheroscler Rep.* 2006;8(4):276–280.

37. Wu CM, McLaughlin K, et al. Early risk of stroke after transient ischemic attack: a systematic review and meta-analysis. *Arch Intern Med.* 2007;167(22):2417–2422.

38. Giles MF, Rothwell PM. Prediction and prevention of stroke after transient ischemic attack in the short and long term. *Expert Rev Neurother.* 2006;6(3):381–395.

39. Hammer MD, Krieger DW. Acute ischemic stroke: is there a role for hypothermia? *Cleve Clin J Med.* 2002;69(10):770, 773–774, 776–777 passim.

40. Gupta R, Jovin TG, et al. Therapeutic hypothermia for stroke: do new outfits change an old friend? *Expert Rev Neurother.* 2005;5(2):235–246.

CHAPTER 12

DISORDERS OF THE PERIPHERAL NERVOUS SYSTEM

KEY CONCEPTS:

Upon completion of this chapter, it is expected that the reader will understand these following concepts:

- That peripheral nervous system disorders do not usually present as emergencies
- How progression of acute disorders or exacerbation of chronic ones may lead to airway and breathing difficulties
- Why attention to comfort is an essential component of care for patients with peripheral nervous system disorders

ANATOMY CONCEPTS:

Prior to reading this chapter the Paramedic student should be familiar with the following anatomy and physiology concepts:

- Peripheral nervous system anatomy
- Parasympathetic innervations
- Neuromuscular junction

Medic 12 is responding to an emergency transfer of an intubated patient in respiratory failure from the Auburn Memorial emergency department to BC Medical Center. During the trip, the Paramedics discuss various reasons for transferring a patient with respiratory failure a half hour away to the tertiary care center. Upon arrival at the ED, the two Paramedics grab their stretcher, oxygen, monitor, and transport ventilator and enter the ED.

They are greeted by the charge nurse who directs them to the patient in bed 5. "This is Mrs. Smith. She is a 35-year-old female who came in with respiratory distress and weakness. Dr. Hardy thinks she has a neurological disorder and wants to transfer her up to BC Medical Center for a higher level of treatment. He intubated her for respiratory failure."

The Paramedics introduce themselves to Mr. and Mrs. Smith. After a brief explanation to Mrs. Smith regarding their need to ask her husband some questions, they begin to interview Mr. Smith.

CRITICAL THINKING QUESTIONS

1. What are some of the possible causes of unexplained weakness?
2. How is trouble breathing related to the weakness?

OVERVIEW

Paramedics should have a fundamental understanding of peripheral nervous system disorders. Although many are chronic disorders in which the Paramedic may simply be called upon to treat complications of the condition, in other cases the Paramedic may be faced with a patient who has not yet been diagnosed with a specific condition. In either case, a fundamental understanding of these conditions will help Paramedics in their assessment and management of the patient.

Chief Concern

The division between the central nervous system and peripheral nervous system is distinct from an anatomical standpoint; however, from a functional standpoint the lines are blurry. For the purpose of discussion in this textbook, peripheral nervous system disorders are those disorders that manifest peripherally and may involve sensory deficits, motor deficits, or movement disorders. Although the brain may be primarily responsible for the disorder, the limbs may actually display the symptoms peripherally. Before discussing the specific disorders, a review of the patient's anatomy is in order.

Peripheral Nervous System Anatomy

The nervous system is made up of literally millions of nerves that function to control the body's operations, receive sensory input about internal functions and external stimuli, and maintain the body's balance. The central nervous system, discussed in Chapter 10, consists of the brain and spinal cord. The peripheral nervous system consists of the nerves that originate in the brain (cranial nerves) or spinal cord (spinal nerves) and reach out to the body. In order to discuss disorders of the peripheral nervous system, we must first review the anatomy and functional divisions of the peripheral nervous system.

Nerve Anatomy

Each nerve cell is made up of three parts: the dendrite, the body, and the axon (Figure 12-1). The dendrite receives information from other nerves and transmits it to the cell body in the form of a series of electrical impulses that travel down the dendrite toward the cell body. Each nerve cell may have multiple dendrites, each receiving information from different sources. The cell body receives and processes all of these signals and develops an appropriate output action. The third part of the nerve cell, the axon, takes the output action developed by the cell body and transmits that signal down the axon. Axons and dendrites can be long; in fact, the axons that originate from the lower spinal cord and operate the muscles in the sole of the foot can be several feet long. While there can be multiple dendrites per nerve cell, there is only one axon. Signals are conducted along the dendrite and axon in the form of a series of electrical pulses that are generated by the movement of electrolytes in and out of the cell.

Nerve fibers are covered in a connective tissue formed by layers of Schwann cells. This layer serves to electrically insulate the nerve fiber by creating a sheath around it (Figure 12-1). These types of nerves, called myelinated nerves, are typically fast-conducting nerves because of the layered insulation. Alternatively, groups of nerves can be surrounded as a group by Schwann cells without the formation of an individual myelin sheath. These slower-conducting nerves are called unmyelinated nerves. For example, cutaneous sensory nerves are typically unmyelinated nerves. The gross nerves that can be seen by the naked eye are actually composed of thousands of specific nerve fibers or neurons bundled together.

The junction between two nerve cells is called a synapse (Figure 12-2). The nerve that contributes an axon to the synapse is called the presynaptic nerve and the nerve that contributes a dendrite to the synapse is called the postsynaptic nerve. As the electrical impulse travels to the end of an axon, it causes the release of a chemical neurotransmitter stored in vesicles from the end of the axon. This mechanism utilizes calcium within the cell to release the neurotransmitter in the vesicles into the synapse. If the patient has low serum calcium (hypocalcemia), this may produce a feeling of weakness or affect nerve transmission. The neurotransmitter then travels the short distance across the synapse to receptors on the dendrite of the next nerve. The neurotransmitter binds to appropriate receptor sites specific for that neurotransmitter. Upon binding with the receptor site, electrolyte ions either rush in or out of the cell, developing an action potential and generating an impulse that will travel down the dendrite. Enzymes in the synapse act on the neurotransmitter to disengage it from the receptor site after enough time has passed to generate the action potential in the postsynaptic nerve. The neurotransmitter is taken up and recycled by the presynaptic nerve, readying the nerve to transmit another impulse.

Many different types of neurotransmitters are used depending on the function of the nerve. For example, the brain uses dopamine, norepinephrine, and serotonin for various functions affecting movement and level of consciousness. Acetylcholine is used in motor nerves at the neuromuscular junction, or the interface between the motor nerve axon and the muscle. Some neurotransmitters are used to inhibit the effects of other neurotransmitters by either binding to the receptor and not causing a nerve discharge or binding to different receptors on the dendrite that slow or cancel out the effects of a different neurotransmitter. For example,

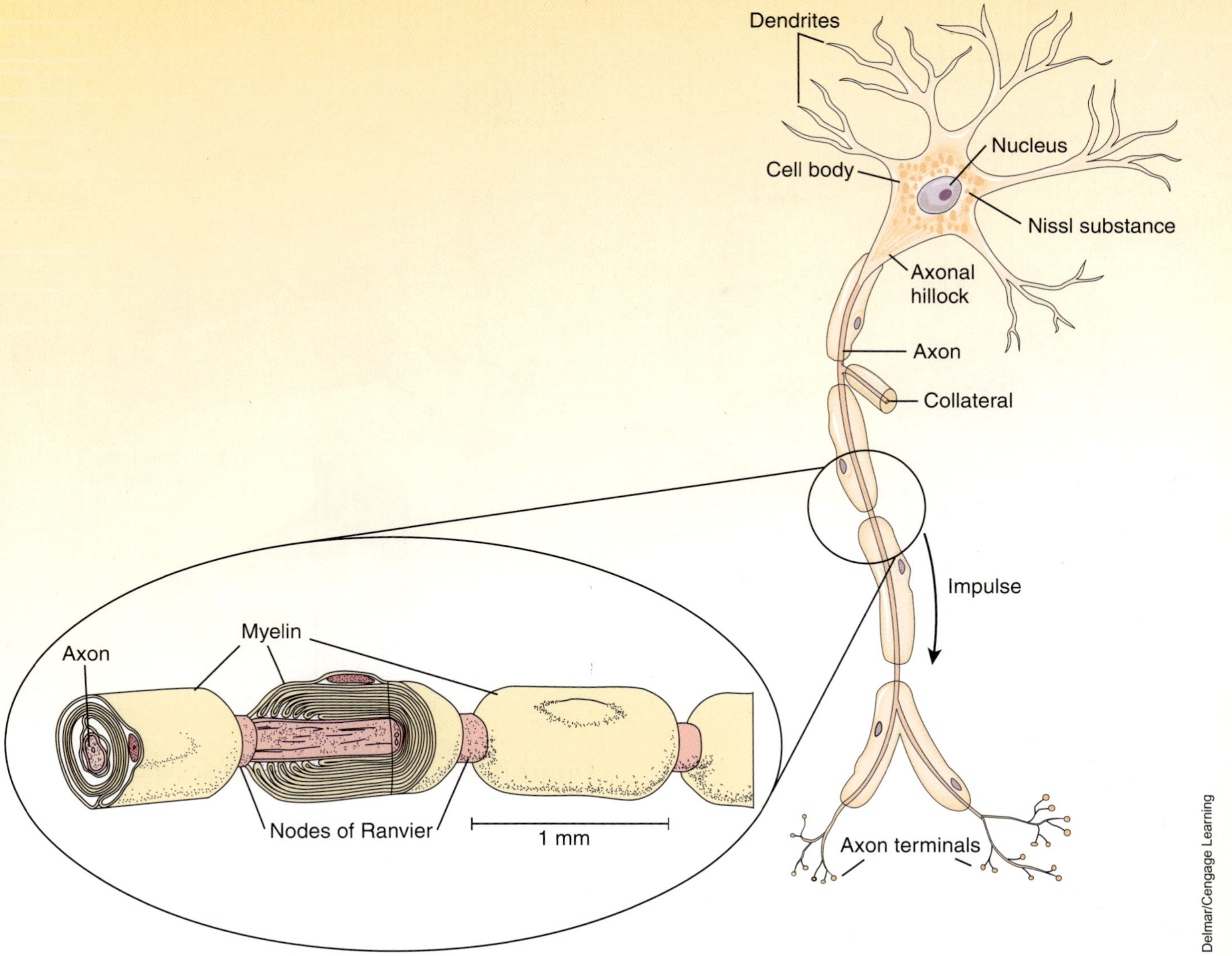

Figure 12-1 Anatomy of a nerve cell.

endorphins are neurotransmitters that inhibit nerve action. Endorphins act to decrease pain stimulus from sensory neurons. Several of the medications administered by Paramedics, such as diazepam (Valium®), act on the synapse to either inhibit or enhance the action of neurotransmitters.

As previously mentioned, the neuromuscular junction is the interface between the motor nerve and the muscle (Figure 12-3). As it reaches the muscle, the axon of the motor nerve branches into multiple unmyelinated fibers that form the motor end plate. When the motor impulse travels down the motor axon and reaches the motor end plate, acetylcholine is released from vesicles in the motor end plate and travel across to the receptors on the muscle. When the receptors become active, calcium is released within the muscle to cause muscle fiber contraction. Thus, the patient who has hypocalcemia may complain of weakness due to the lack of calcium needed to produce adequate muscle contraction. The motor end plate is a clinically significant area as this is where all neuromuscular blockade agents used in medication-facilitated intubation

act to produce paralysis.[1] Of interest, a single motor neuron can cause an action in up to 25,000 muscle fibers!

Functional Divisions

Although the nervous system is divided anatomically into the central and peripheral nervous system, in reality the peripheral nervous system is a seamless continuation of the central nervous system. From a functional perspective, the nervous system can be divided into two main functional divisions: the somatic nervous system and the autonomic nervous system. The somatic nervous system is distributed among the skin and musculoskeletal system and is responsible for voluntary body actions (e.g., movement). The autonomic nervous system is distributed among the organs and blood vessels and is responsible for the body's automatic functions (e.g., cardiac activity and digestion). Certain areas of the body feature crossover of the two functional systems; for example, autonomic nerves that control the diameter of arterioles in the forearm skin may be close to the somatic nerves that detect pressure on the skin over that arteriole.

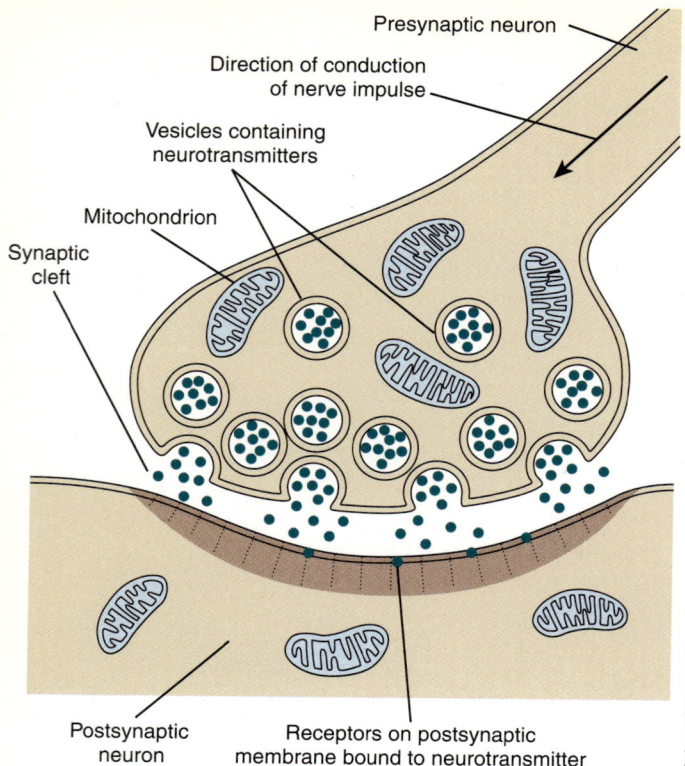

Figure 12-2 Neurotransmitters are chemicals used to transmit impulses between nerves.

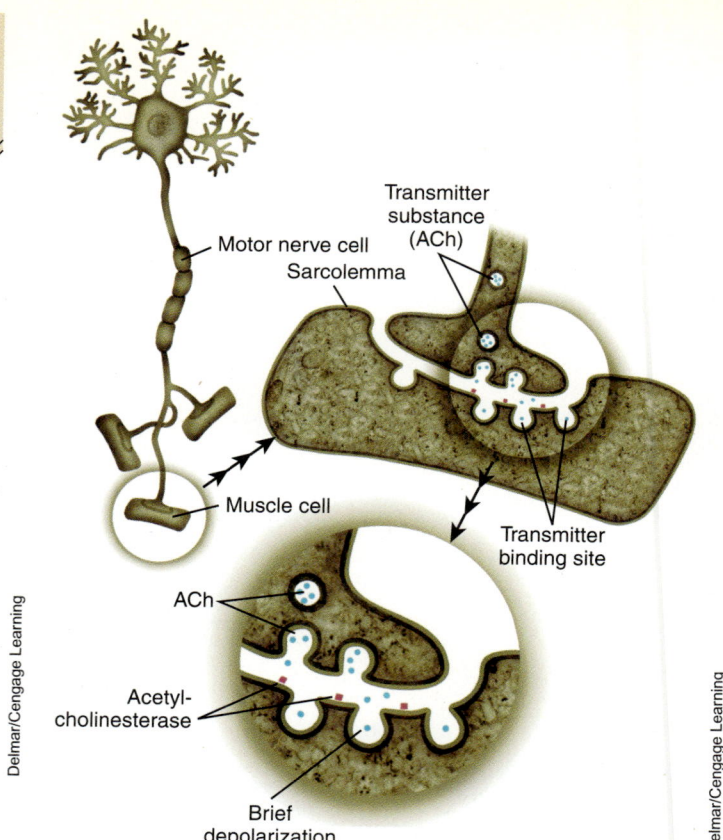

Figure 12-3 The neuromuscular junction.

The somatic nervous system contains three types of neurons: motor neurons, sensory neurons, and interneurons. The motor neurons carry impulses from the brain to muscle cells producing muscle contraction (i.e., movement). Sensory neurons carry impulses from the sensory organs in the skin back to the spinal cord and then up to the brain. Interneurons are neurons that serve as a relay between sensory and motor neurons and are generally located in the spinal cord. These interneurons are responsible for the reflex arc that allows the body to react to a dangerous stimulus that is likely to damage tissue. For example, suppose a person accidently puts her hand down on a hot electric coil on a stove that she did not realize was on. The sensory nerves sense that this stimulus can cause significant tissue damage and race a signal up to the spinal cord. If this sensory input had to travel up to and be processed by the brain as an indicator of a destructive stimulus, by the time the brain reacted, it would be too late and the person's hand would be severely burned. However, at the same time the impulse is transmitted to the brain, the interneuron rapidly causes a set of motor neurons to fire, producing the movement that allows her to quickly remove her hand from the stove. This often occurs before the sensation of pain is registered in the brain. This reflex arc limits the damage caused by destructive stimuli (Figure 12-4).

The somatic nervous system is organized into pairs of nerve roots that leave the spinal cord at discrete levels and pass through the spaces between the vertebrae laterally. There are 8 cervical nerve roots, 12 thoracic nerve roots,

5 lumbar nerve roots, and 5 sacral nerve roots. The sensory distribution of these nerve roots starts at the back and wraps around to the front, forming approximately horizontal slices of the body. For the limbs, the spinal nerves intertwine into a nerve plexus where individual nerve fibers from one spinal nerve root join with nerve fibers from other spinal nerve roots to form peripheral nerves that provide motor and sensory function for specific areas of the extremity. The brachial plexus, located in the axilla, is formed from the cervical spinal nerves C4 to C8 and produces the radial, ulnar, medial, and musculocutaneous nerves that provide sensory and motor coverage for the upper extremity (Figure 12-5).

The autonomic nervous system is functionally subdivided into the sympathetic and parasympathetic nervous systems (Figure 12-6). The sympathetic nervous system is responsible for the fight or flight response, which prepares the body to face a dangerous situation. The parasympathetic nervous system is responsible for the "rest or digest" response; it acts to improve the movement of material through the digestive tract and counteracts sympathetic system response. These two divisions of the autonomic nervous system are constantly acting to maintain a balance of the body's automatic functions. Although most people focus on the actions of these two systems, there is also a sensory component to both the sympathetic and parasympathetic divisions of the autonomic nervous system. The sensory nerves obtain sensory input from the organs and blood

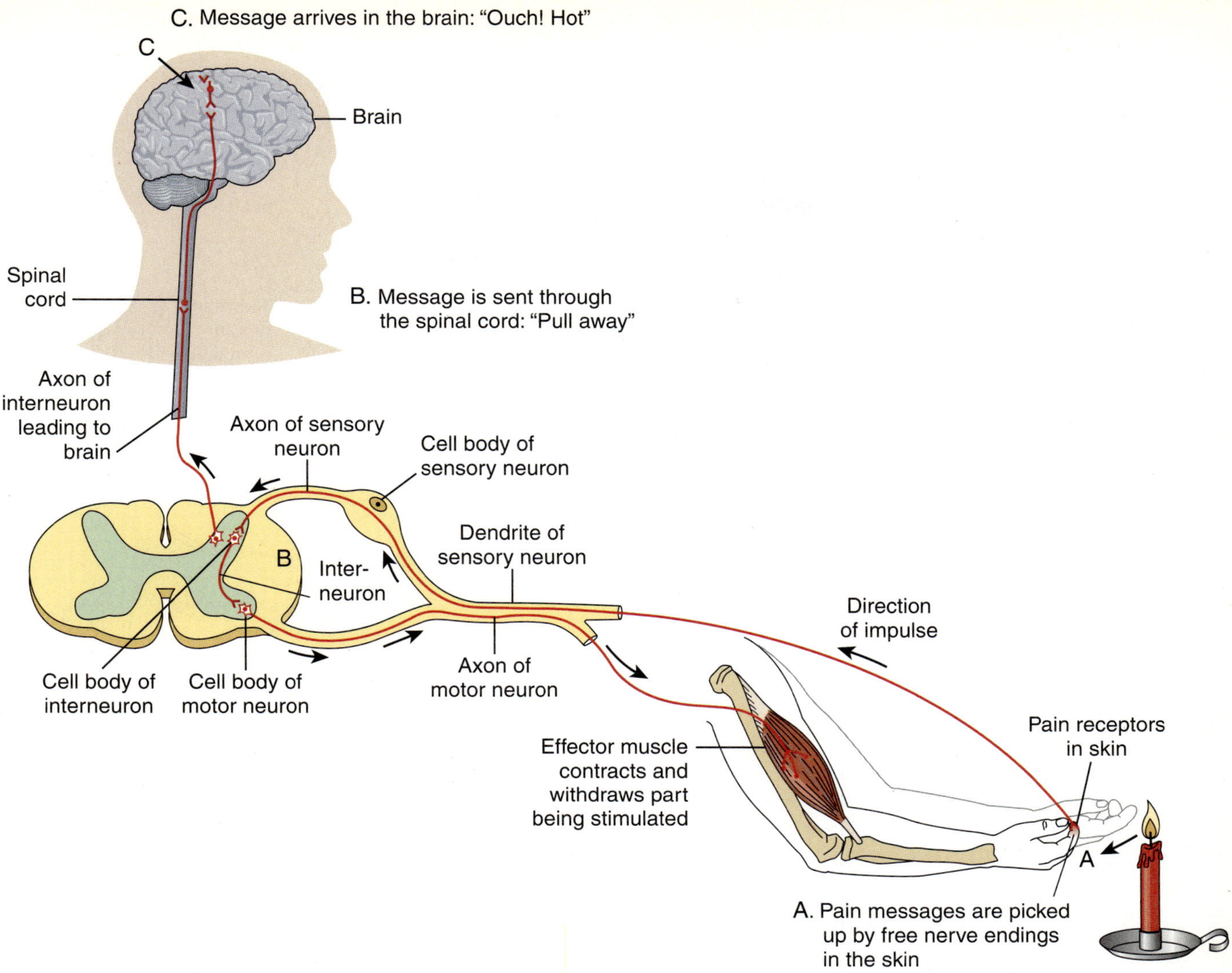

Figure 12-4 The reflex arc provides an expedited response when a dangerous condition is sensed by the sensory nerve.

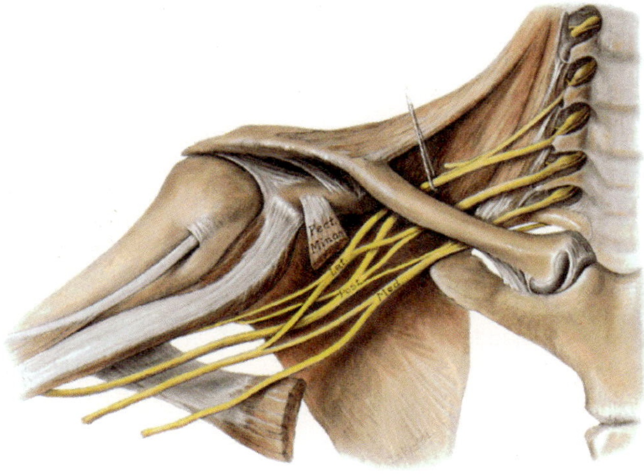

Figure 12-5 The brachial plexus is formed from nerve fibers that come from spinal nerves C4 to C8 and develop into the peripheral nerves of the upper extremity.

vessels. Referred pain occurs because of some crossover in sensory impulses between the autonomic and somatic nervous systems at the spinal cord level. For example, a sensation of pain from an abdominal organ (e.g., the gallbladder) may come in for relay up to the brain and cross over with sensory nerves that normally transmit information from an area innervated by the somatic sensory nerves (e.g., the right shoulder). The brain interprets the signals as pain either in the right shoulder only, in the right upper quadrant only, or as both, depending upon the crossover of specific nerve fibers in the system.

Nerve Maps

The peripheral nervous system can be mapped in two ways that are both related to the course of the nerves after they leave the spinal cord. The first is a dermatome mapping (Figure 12-7) that maps the body surface in relation to the spinal nerve that receives sensory information from that area. The second mapping describes the territories of the peripheral nerves that form

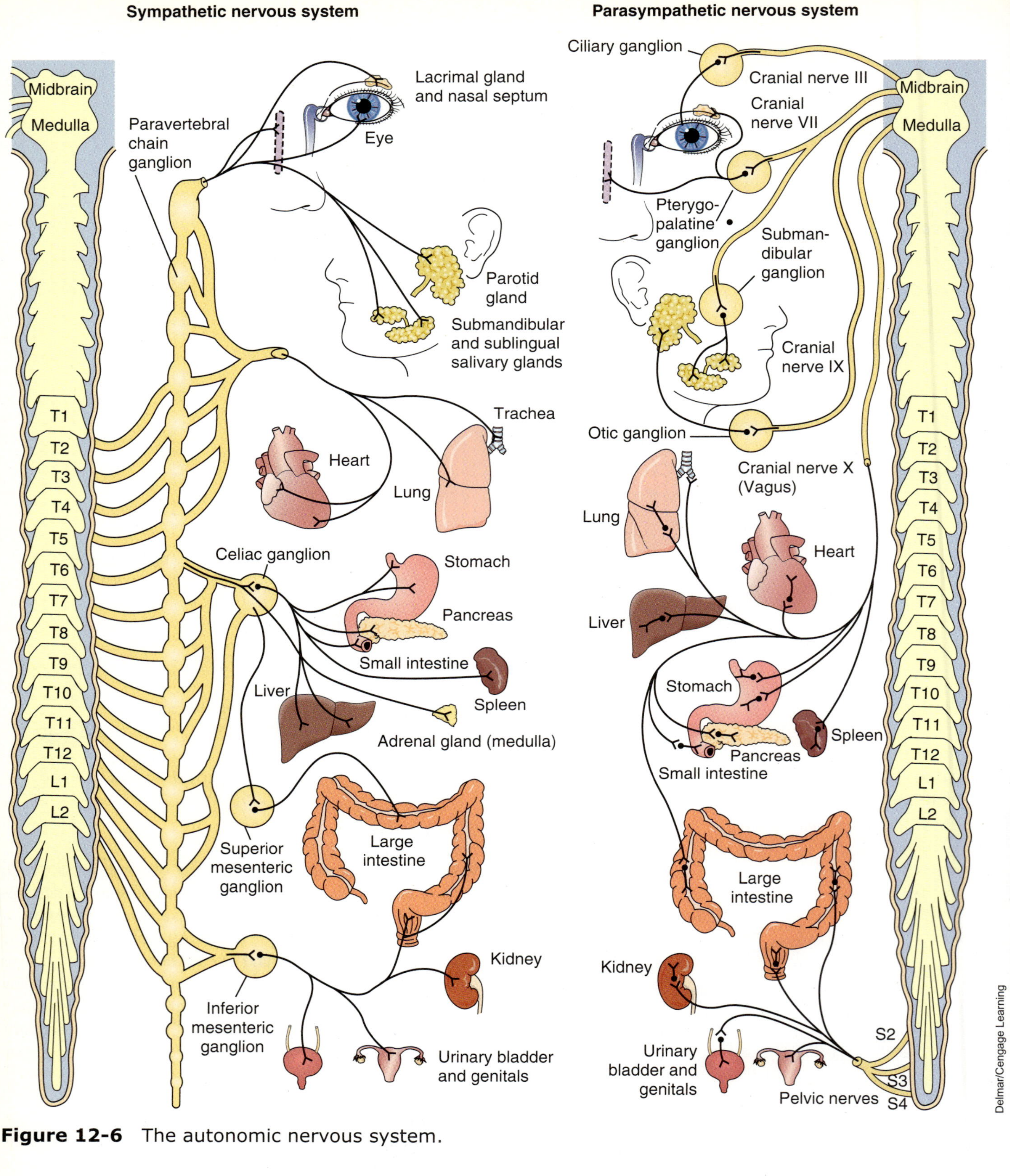

Figure 12-6 The autonomic nervous system.

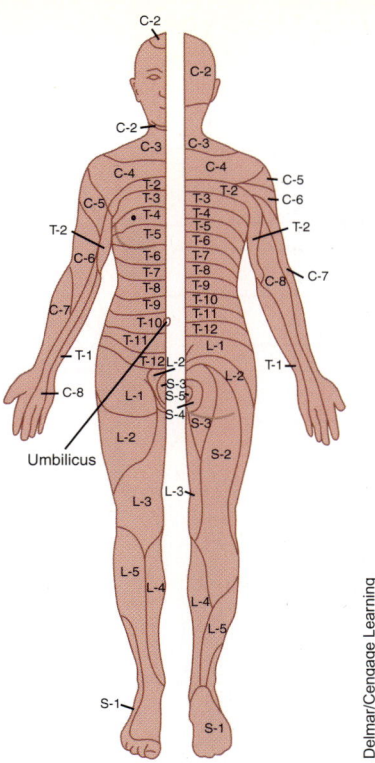

Figure 12-7 The surface dermatomes.

in the nerve plexuses supplying the extremities (Figure 12-8). Both diagrams assist the Paramedic with the sensory examination in determining areas of deficit in the event of a spinal injury or peripheral nerve injury.

Pathophysiology of Peripheral Nervous System Disorders

Peripheral neuropathies are generalized disorders of the peripheral nerves. In these disorders, the nerve is damaged in such a way that signal transmission is either delayed or lost. Although many of these are bilateral disorders that affect the more distant nerves first, the neuropathy can be local if caused by a localized exposure to a substance. There are many causes of peripheral neuropathies—infections, medications, toxic substances, HIV, and side effects of chemotherapy and radiation treatment. However, peripheral neuropathies most commonly develop secondary to poorly controlled diabetes, renal disease, alcoholism, or liver disease.[2] In general, peripheral neuropathies produce stocking and glove distribution paresthesia (tingling feeling of pins and needles). In other words, they do not follow dermatome or peripheral nerve maps but instead cover a territory similar to placing a glove on a hand or a stocking on a foot. Peripheral neuropathies typically start out distal (peripherally) and progress inward in a proximal fashion. Peripheral neuropathies can also produce pain that may be difficult to treat with traditional NSAIDs, acetaminophen, or opioid medications.

Many peripheral nerves travel either through bony canals or through muscular structures that may narrow with injury,

localized edema from overuse, or skeletal muscle hypertrophy. Compression of the nerve at those points slows nerve conduction and produces paresthesia distally in the distribution of the nerve (Figure 12-8). The condition can progress to the point where motor function is affected, and atrophy of muscles supplied by the peripheral nerve occurs. The most common locations for nerve entrapment are the medial nerve in the wrist's carpal tunnel (Figure 12-9), the ulnar nerve at the elbow, and the deep peroneal nerve at the fibula head. In severe cases, surgical intervention (e.g., a carpal tunnel release for carpal tunnel syndrome) is required to decompress the nerve. However, most patients can improve with modifications of their work environment.

Complex regional pain syndrome (CRPS), also known as **reflex sympathetic dystrophy (RSD),** is a condition that produces severe and intense burning pain in an extremity.[3] The exact pathophysiology of this condition is still unknown, although it is thought to be somehow maintained by the sensory portion of the autonomic nervous system. The patient typically reports that the pain began gradually after an injury, surgery, or casting of a limb. Other conditions that produce peripheral nerve injury are also associated with the development of CRPS. The patient may report the presence of pain from a non-painful stimulus (e.g., light touch on the affected limb) or pain that is out of proportion to the stimulus. These findings are called **allodynia** and **hyperalgesia,** respectively. Because of the autonomic system involvement, the pain may also have limb edema, changes in skin color, or changes in skin temperature related to changes in blood flow to the extremity. Although many patients with this condition suffer from anxiety and depression, the evidence does not suggest that patients who suffer from this condition have underlying mental illness.[4]

The neuropathies previously discussed generally affect one limb or affect limbs asymmetrically. The most common peripheral neuropathy that affects the limbs symmetrically is **Guillain-Barré syndrome.**[4] Guillain-Barré syndrome is an autoimmune condition in which the body's immune system is triggered to attack the myelin sheath in peripheral motor nerve fibers, causing significantly slowed nerve conduction. Its cause is believed to be a preceding viral illness, although some bacteria have also been associated with the condition. In the late 1970s, an outbreak of Guillain-Barré syndrome in patients after an influenza vaccination led to increased surveillance, with continued evidence to suggest a possible link between the vaccine and Guillain-Barré syndrome.[4] Guillain-Barré syndrome is a progressive condition that produces symmetrical ascending muscle weakness and then paralysis that will generally begin at the patient's legs and progress to the arms and trunk (i.e., an ascending paralysis). In some patients, the cranial nerves are also affected. In extreme cases, patients with intercostal muscles and diaphragm involvement can develop hypercapnia and respiratory failure from poor ventilation. The deep tendon reflexes are lost early on and the patient may become so weak that he cannot sit without falling over. On some occasions, sensory neurons are involved in the disease and the patient will develop symmetric paresthesia. The most common complication of

Radial, dors. antebrach. cut. (C5-6)
Lateral antebrachial cutan. (C5-6)
Medial brachial cut. (C8-T1)
Palmar
Radial, superficial (C6-8)
Palmar
Palmar, digital
Median (C5-8)
Palmar, digital
Lat. fem. cut. (L2-S2)
Com. peroneal lat. sural cut. (L4-S1)
Sup. (L4-S1) peroneal
Sural, lateral dorsal cut. (S1-2)
Deep peroneal (L4-5)
Supra-clavicular (C3-4)
Axillary sup. lat. cut. (C5-6)
Intercosto-brachial (T2)
Medial brachial cut. (T1-2)
Last thoracic nerve (T12)
Superior cluneal (post. div. of L1-3)
Middle cluneal (post. div. of S1-3)
Lumboinguinal, of genitofemoral (L1-2)
Lat. cut. branch of iliohypogastric (L1)
Ilioinguinal (L1)
Ant. fem. cutaneous (L2-3)
Saphenous, med. crural cut. (L3-4)
Post brach. cut.
Inf. lat. cut.
Post. antebrach. cut.
Medial brachial cut. (C8-T1)
Lateral antebrachial cutan. (C5-6)
Dorsal
Radial, superficial (C6-8)
Dorsal digital
Proper palmar digital
Median (C5-8)
Proper palmar digital
Lat. fem. cut. (L2-3)
Post. fem. cut. (S1-3)
Com. peroneal, lat. sural cut. (L4-S2)
Sup. peroneal (L5-S1)
Sural (S1-2)
Lateral dorsal cut.
Lateral calcaneal
Tibial, medial calcaneal (S1-2)
Medial plantar
Lateral planta
Saphenous
Sural
Tibial
Delmar/Cengage Learning

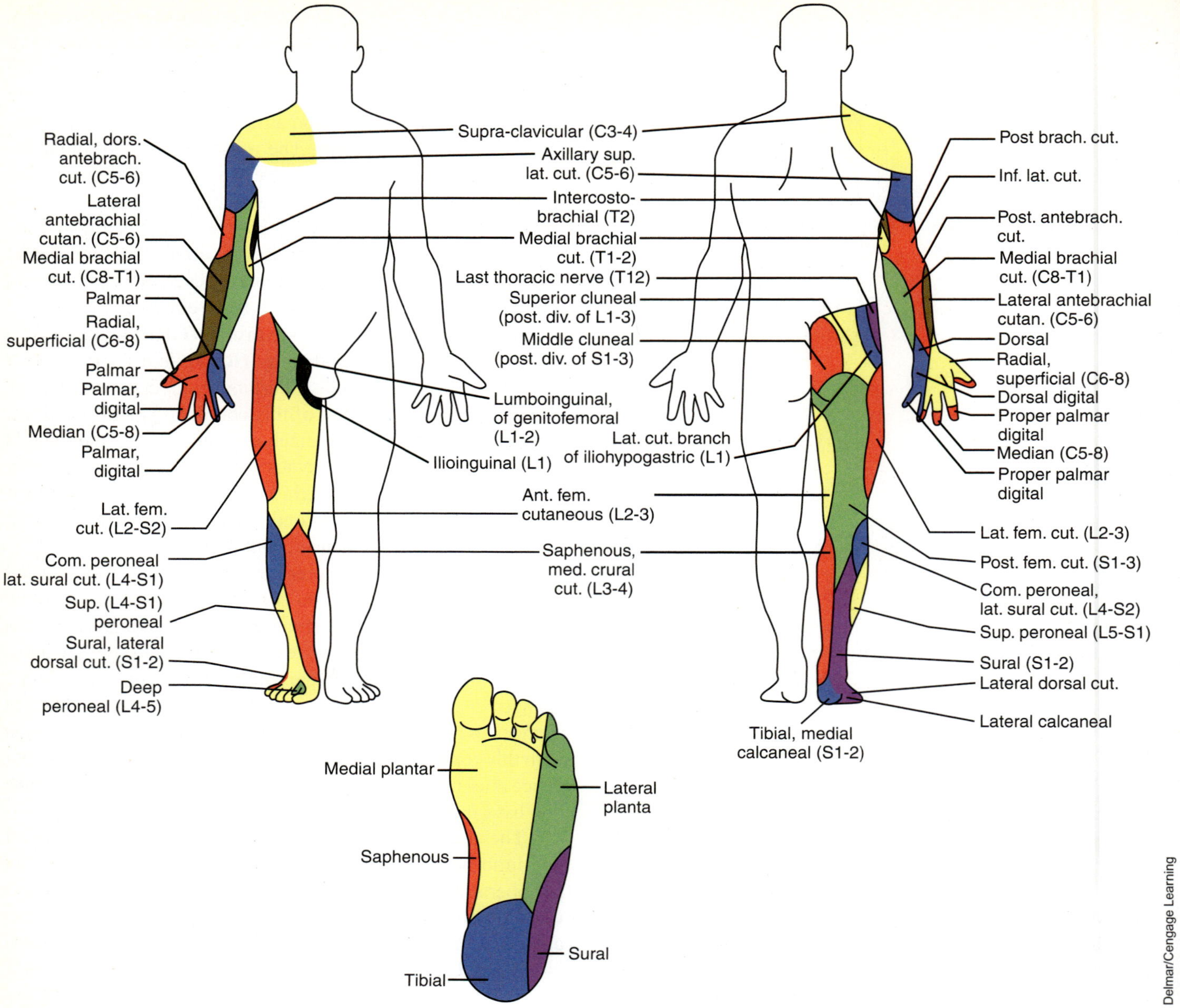

Figure 12-8 Peripheral nerve maps.

STREET SMART

The Paramedic may think the patient with new onset Guillain-Barré syndrome is having a stroke (i.e., unable to sit up) or is suffering a spinal cord injury (i.e., unable to move legs). In either case, the Paramedic should assume the condition is the worst case scenario and treat accordingly.

Transverse carpal ligament (flexor retinaculum)
Carpal canal
Median nerve
Delmar/Cengage Learning

Figure 12-9 Inflammation of the tendons that pass through the carpal tunnel causes compression of the medial nerve in the tunnel, producing the characteristic paresthesias and pain.

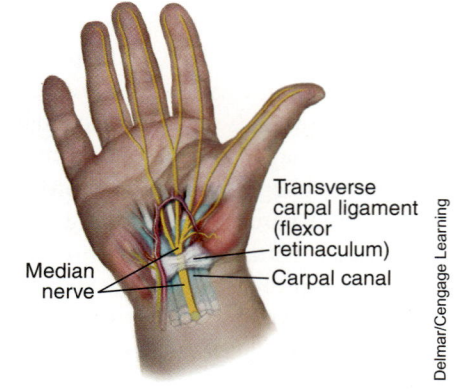

History

As previously discussed, peripheral neurological conditions can present with a variety of complaints. By performing a thorough history, the Paramedic may be able to narrow down the paramedical differential diagnosis.

History of Present Illness

Often it is helpful for the Paramedic to narrow down the patient's most significant or troublesome concern and start from there. When there are multiple areas of concern, it is also helpful to question the patient in a way that develops a timeline as to when different concerns began, ended, and whether they were present constantly or intermittently. Following the OPQRST AS/PN mnemonic, the Paramedic should ask the patient to describe when the symptoms first occurred; what actions provoke or worsen the symptoms; what the symptoms feel like, specifically where they are located; what steps relieve the symptoms; and any other associated symptoms the patient may have. The Paramedic should attempt to correlate the patient's sensory symptoms with the dermatome (Figure 12-7) and peripheral nerve maps (Figure 12-8). Do motor symptoms worsen with activity or time, or are they constant? Was there a preceding event in the last few weeks, including illness, vaccination, or trauma? For focal complaints that appear related to a peripheral nerve distribution, what does the patient do for employment or activities at home that may exacerbate the symptoms? Pertinent negatives may include the absence of sensory symptoms if the chief concern is of motor weakness, or absence of motor symptoms if the chief concern is primarily sensory.

Past Medical/Surgical, Family, and Social History

The Paramedic should explore the patient's past medical history, focusing on the neurological system and related systems. The patient should be questioned about past strokes, chronic neurological diseases, and head or spinal trauma. The patient should also be asked about a past medical history of hypertension, diabetes, and renal diseases, as these may cause peripheral neuropathies, strokes, or vascular issues that may have led to the present neurological concern. The Paramedic should determine if any of these conditions run in the patient's immediate family. Finally, the Paramedic should elicit a social history including the patient's tobacco, alcohol, and drug use as well as occupational and exposure history.

CASE STUDY (CONTINUED)

The Paramedic excuses herself and starts to review the emergency department chart while her partner begins to switch over the monitoring equipment for transport. In the chart, the emergency physician documented that Mrs. Smith had bilaterally weak upper and lower extremities, with no motor in the lower extremities and minimal power in her hands but no motor at her shoulders.

The chart indicated her respiratory rate was slow and she had very shallow breathing with an initial room air pulse oximetry of 85%. Mrs. Smith was incoherent. The emergency physician intubated Mrs. Smith shortly after arrival for respiratory failure. An arterial blood gas performed after she was intubated revealed a pCO_2 of 120 mmHg. The Paramedic was almost to the end of the chart when Dr. Salerno greeted her at the desk.

CRITICAL THINKING QUESTIONS

1. What are the elements of the physical examination of a patient with suspected neuromuscular disease?
2. Why is the end-tidal carbon dioxide reading a critical element in this examination?

Examination

Once the primary assessment is completed and the patient's life-threatening conditions have been addressed, the Paramedic can perform a focused physical examination. Given the variability of the chief concern related to the peripheral nervous system, an appropriate examination may range from a limited examination of an affected extremity to a complete neurological system examination. Other related systems that should be examined include the cardiovascular and musculoskeletal systems, depending on the patient's chief concern.

From a neurological standpoint, the patient should be examined for sensation in all extremities as well as the trunk if extremity sensory deficits are found. The area of sensory deficit may point toward either a peripheral nerve problem, a spinal nerve problem if in a dermatome distribution, or a situation not related to a specific nerve distribution. Muscle strength and equality is examined both distally and proximally, comparing both left and right upper and lower extremities to each other. Deep tendon reflexes may be more brisk than usual if there is an issue with central control of the muscles or may be decreased if there is muscle weakness. A brief cranial nerve exam may indicate a more central problem involving the cranial nerves as well as issues with airway protection and gag reflex.

From a circulatory standpoint, the Paramedic should assess the peripheral pulses for strength and equality, and the heart for new murmurs and regularity of rhythm. The Paramedic should also palpate the abdomen for a pulsatile mass that may indicate an abdominal aneurysm.

CASE STUDY (CONTINUED)

The Paramedic and Dr. Salerno briefly discuss Mrs. Smith's history and presentation to the emergency department. Dr. Salerno states she suspects that Mrs. Smith developed Guillain-Barré syndrome and is transferring her to BC Medical Center for evaluation and treatment with either immunoglobulin or plasmaphoresis, neither of which can be done at this hospital. Both of these treatments attempt to counteract the autoimmune nature of the disease, halting neuron destruction.

CRITICAL THINKING QUESTIONS

1. What is the significance of the diagnosis of Guillain-Barré syndrome?
2. What significance is the diagnosis of any neuromuscular disease?

Assessment

Although many neurologic conditions have a subtle onset, some present with very classic patterns of symptoms that suggest a particular condition. For example, a patient who presents with progressive paralysis that starts in the legs and moves upwards toward the arms and torso is often suggestive of Guillain-Barré. A patient who has multiple sclerosis may have intermittent or patchy complaints or sudden blindness in one eye. A patient who develops muscle fatigue rapidly after repetitive movement is consistent with myasthenia gravis. The key to narrowing the paramedical differential diagnosis is detailing the history as much as reasonably possible.

CASE STUDY (CONTINUED)

The Paramedic and EMT transfer Mrs. Smith to their stretcher after attaching their monitoring equipment and setting up their transport ventilator. After making sure Mrs. Smith is adequately sedated for the trip, they load Mrs. Smith into the ambulance and start for the BC Medical Center emergency department.

CRITICAL THINKING QUESTIONS

1. What is the importance of monitoring this patient?
2. Why is it necessary to adequately sedate the patient?

Treatment

Since many of the peripheral neurological disorders discussed are chronic in nature, the Paramedic may only be needed to offer comfortable transport. However, with patients who develop an exacerbation or complication of their chronic disease, the Paramedic may need to intervene. For example, a patient's respiratory effort may be inadequate and will need to be supported with positive pressure ventilation by either a bag–valve mask or intubation. Patients with other chronic neurologic disorders may develop respiratory failure from pneumonia or sepsis from a urinary or skin infection. Patients suffering from movement disorders may fall and require splinting of extremities or spinal motion restriction with a cervical collar and long spine board if indicated by the history and examination.

During transport, the Paramedic constantly monitors Mrs. Smith's end-tidal carbon dioxide, pulse oximetry, blood pressure, and heart rate. Mrs. Smith's vital signs remain steady during the 30-minute transport to BC Medical Center. During the course of the transport the patient starts to cough, causing the pressure alarms to alert the Paramedic.

CRITICAL THINKING QUESTIONS

1. What are some of the predictable complications associated with Guillain-Barré syndrome?
2. What are some of the predictable complications associated with the transport of intubated patients?

Evaluation

The amount of monitoring performed during transport is highly dependent on the patient's chief concern and condition. A critically ill individual will require intensive monitoring of her vital signs and respiratory status during the transport and require intervention by the Paramedic if a change occurs. A patient with an isolated peripheral neuropathy without cardiopulmonary involvement, however, may only require repeat vital signs and neurologic checks during transport. If analgesia was provided for painful conditions, the Paramedic should evaluate the effect of the analgesia and re-dose the patient if appropriate.

CASE STUDY CONCLUSION

Mrs. Smith is transported to the BC Medical Center emergency department where she is evaluated by the emergency department staff and admitted to the medical intensive care unit. The neurologist confirms that she has developed Guillain-Barré syndrome and begins immunoglobulin treatment. Mrs. Smith slowly improves and is discharged two weeks later to a ventilator-dependent unit at a local rehabilitation hospital. The strength of her respiratory muscles improved by the time of discharge, and she was expected to recover enough function to not require the ventilator.

CRITICAL THINKING QUESTIONS

1. What is the most appropriate transport decision that will get the patient to definitive care?
2. What are the advantages of transporting a patient with suspected neuromuscular disease to these hospitals, even if that means bypassing other hospitals in the process?

Disposition

The discussion in this chapter has focused on many chronic conditions that the Paramedic may encounter. Those that are stable and chronic can be managed by any emergency department. However, critically ill patients should be brought to the closest appropriate emergency department for evaluation and stabilization. Although the first diagnosis of many of these illnesses is challenging, the Paramedic should focus on the identifying life- or limb-threatening conditions, controlling pain, and providing comfortable transport to an appropriate facility.

CONCLUSION

Some neuromuscular diseases impair the patient's ability to adequately breathe and may require intervention by the Paramedic to prevent hypoxemia and hypercarbia. The Paramedic may be the first healthcare provider a patient with a new onset neuromuscular disorder encounters who has the ability to positively impact the patient's medical care.

▶ KEY POINTS:

- Peripheral neuropathies result from ineffective nerve signal transmission.

- Complex regional pain syndrome or reflex sympathetic dystrophy may follow an injury, surgery, or cast removal and results in severe pain in the extremity.

- Guillan-Barré syndrome is an autoimmune condition that causes an ascending weakness and paralysis.

- Multiple sclerosis is an inflammatory disorder that produces a scattered symptom picture due to irregular demyelination.

- Poliomyelitis is a viral disease which destroys motor neurons.

- Post-polio syndrome is a condition that develops in patients who have recovered from polio.

- Amyotrophic lateral sclerosis is an irreversible disease that destroys the motor neurons, causing movement, balance, and cranial nerve dysfunction.

- Myasthenia gravis is an autoimmune disorder that affects the function of the acetylcholine receptors at the neuromuscular junction.

- Parkinson's disease results from a decrease in dopamine in specific regions of the brain responsible for movement.

- Huntington's disease is a genetic disorder resulting in loss of motor neurons.

- Since these disorders are chronic, the Paramedic should begin the history with the patient's most significant or bothersome concern.

- The Paramedic should assess both motor and sensory systems.

- Peripheral nervous system disorders place the patient at risk for falls, respiratory failure, and pulmonary, urinary, and skin infections.

▶ REVIEW QUESTIONS:

1. In complex regional pain syndrome, what signs and symptoms result from autonomic nervous system involvement?

2. What is the pattern of paralysis in Guillan-Barré syndrome?

3. What are the emergent problems for patients with exacerbation of their multiple sclerosis?

4. What is the symptom progression in amyotrophic lateral sclerosis?

5. Which drugs should be used cautiously by a patient with myasthenia gravis?

6. What are the movement disorders in Parkinson's disease?

7. What emergent considerations exist for a patient with Huntington's disease?

CASE STUDY QUESTIONS:

Please refer to the Case Study in this chapter, and answer the questions below:

1. Is Guillan-Barré syndrome contagious? Why or why not?

2. Why should the Paramedics explain to Mrs. Smith their need for interviewing Mr. Smith?

3. What considerations should the Paramedics have for positioning Mrs. Smith?

REFERENCES:

1. Nathan N, Odin I. Induction of anaesthesia: a guide to drug choice. *Drugs.* 2007;67(5):701–723.

2. Ziegler D. Painful diabetic neuropathy: treatment and future aspects. *Diabetes/Metab Res Rev.* 2008;24 Suppl 1:S52–S57.

3. Albazaz R, Wong YT, et al. Complex regional pain syndrome: a review. *Ann Vasc Surg.* 2008;22(2):297–306.

4. Miller A. Guillain-Barré syndrome. Available from: **http://www .emedicine.com/emerg/topic222.htm**. Accessed May 19, 2008.

5. Vender RL, Mauger D, et al. Respiratory systems abnormalities and clinical milestones for patients with amyotrophic lateral sclerosis with emphasis upon survival. *Amyotroph Lateral Scler.* 2007;8(1):36–41.

6. Grob D, Brunner N, et al. Lifetime course of myasthenia gravis. *Muscle Nerve.* 2008;37(2):121–129.

7. Lacomis D. Myasthenic crisis. *Neurocrit Care.* 2005;3(3): 189–194.

8. Juel VC. Myasthenia gravis: management of myasthenic crisis and perioperative care. *Semin Neurol.* 2004;24(1):75–81.

9. Rusyniak DE, Nanagas KA. Organophosphate poisoning. *Semin Neurol.* 2004;24(2):197–204.

10. Brodsky MA, Smith JA. Exacerbation of myasthenia gravis after tourniquet release. *J Clin Anesth.* 2007;19(7):543–545.

11. Jankovic J. Parkinson's disease: clinical features and diagnosis. *J Neurol, Neurosurg Psychiatry.* 2008;79(4):368–376.

CHAPTER 13

DISORDERS OF GLUCOSE METABOLISM

KEY CONCEPTS:

Upon completion of this chapter, it is expected that the reader will understand these following concepts:

- How multiple hormones keep blood glucose levels within a specific range
- That low blood glucose levels (hypoglycemia) can be a medical emergency, leading rapidly to convulsions and death
- How high blood glucose levels (hyperglycemia) lead to alterations in fluid and electrolyte levels, causing confusion, shock, cardiac arrhythmias, and death
- That diabetes mellitus is the usual cause of glucose metabolism abnormalities; although medications, physical conditions such as pregnancy, and environmental factors such as alcoholism can also alter glucose levels.

ANATOMY CONCEPTS:

Prior to reading this chapter the Paramedic student should be familiar with the following anatomy and physiology concepts:

- Endocrine system
- Hormonal control of glucose metabolism
- Electrolyte balance

CASE STUDY:

Andros Ambulance Company is dispatched in emergency mode to Tower Apartments for a 49-year-old diabetic male found confused. En route to the scene, the Paramedics review the potential causes of diabetic emergencies and the algorithms for their treatment. One Paramedic cautions the other not to get tunnel vision; persons with diabetes can suffer other complications and injuries as well.

CRITICAL THINKING QUESTIONS

1. What are some of the possible diabetic-related emergencies?
2. What are other conditions that could mimic a diabetic-related emergency?

OVERVIEW

Paramedics encounter patients with disorders of glucose metabolism on a regular basis. Patients with these disorders, including hyperglycemia (high blood glucose) and hypoglycemia (low blood glucose), can have a variety of clinical signs and symptoms and frequently require prompt diagnosis and treatment in the field. The Paramedic plays a crucial role in assuring proper management of glucose disorders during an emergency, and may at times serve as the only contact a patient has with the healthcare field. This chapter will discuss the basic science behind glucose use and metabolism, the common causes of both hyperglycemia and hypoglycemia, and the appropriate treatment for each of these conditions.

Chief Concern

Since glucose is an essential substrate for brain function, it is imperative that the body maintain a steady supply of glucose. However, too much of anything can be as detrimental to the patient's health as too little, and the results of excess glucose can be pathological. Whether the patient has hyperglycemia or hypoglycemia, the Paramedic must support the body's own systems while transporting the patient to definitive treatment.

Overview of Glucose Metabolism

Carbohydrates are the main fuel source for the human body. Approximately half of all daily caloric intake is in the form of carbohydrates, both simple and complex.[1] Simple carbohydrates (also known as simple sugars), such as sucrose, lactose, glucose, and maltose, are found in foods such as fruits, table sugar, and milk. Complex carbohydrates, including starches and cellulose, are long chains of simple sugars connected by chemical bonds. They are derived from vegetables, nuts, and whole grains. These complex carbohydrates are broken down during the process of digestion and the component simple sugars are either used immediately as energy sources or stored for later periods of fasting. By far the most abundant and most important of the simple sugars is glucose.

Glucose ($C_6H_{12}O_6$) is the main substrate (source) for energy production in the human body and is utilized by every organ system. Although some organs are also capable of using proteins and fat as supplemental energy sources when the body's glucose levels are low, the brain and red blood cells rely exclusively on glucose to survive.[2] Therefore, changes in circulating blood glucose levels can have a significant impact on neurologic and cognitive functioning.

Since the brain and red blood cells exclusively utilize glucose as an energy source, and since most other organ systems preferentially use glucose over other nutritional substrates, there must be a constant supply provided to these organs in order for them to survive and function properly. One's diet is the body's source of glucose, but it is certainly not practical or feasible for a person to eat 24 hours per day simply to provide

a constant source of glucose. Therefore, the body has a well-developed system for glucose management, through storage and "on time" utilization, involving the small intestine, liver, brain, and pancreas. The coordination of these organs and the hormones they produce allow human beings to eat at discrete times during the day or night and still maintain a consistent glucose supply around the clock.

In the process of digestion, complex carbohydrates such as starches and cellulose are broken down into their simple sugars (glucose, fructose, and galactose), a process called **catabolism**.[3] These simple sugars are absorbed from the lining of the small intestine into the bloodstream and eventually transported throughout the body.

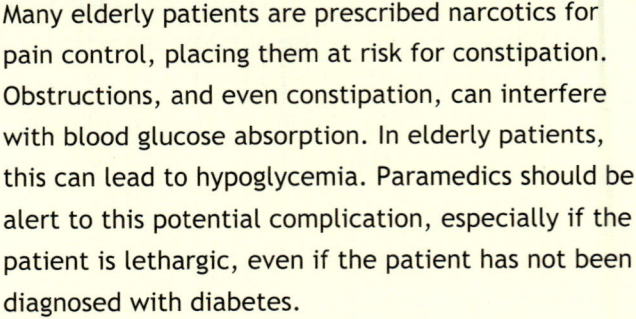

STREET SMART

Many elderly patients are prescribed narcotics for pain control, placing them at risk for constipation. Obstructions, and even constipation, can interfere with blood glucose absorption. In elderly patients, this can lead to hypoglycemia. Paramedics should be alert to this potential complication, especially if the patient is lethargic, even if the patient has not been diagnosed with diabetes.

As individual cells come into contact with blood, and the blood glucose therein, they use the hormone **insulin** to help transport the glucose from the bloodstream into the cell, where it is then used as an energy source (Figure 13-1). To be precise, insulin does not physically transport glucose into the cell. Instead, insulin opens pores in the cell wall, which then allows glucose (a relatively large molecule) to pass into the cell.[2]

Excess glucose that is not immediately used by the body is converted into **glycogen** (a chemical compound composed of long chains of glucose molecules connected together) and stored in the liver (25%) and skeletal muscles (75%).[3]

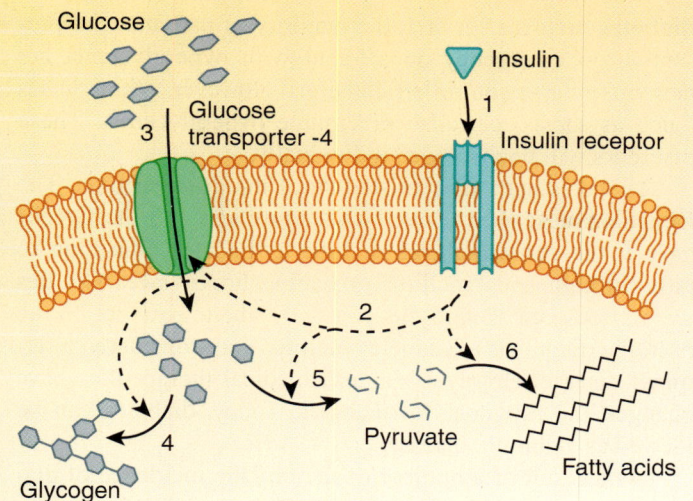

Figure 13-1 Glucose metabolism.

In order for an individual to maintain a stable blood glucose level, within a relatively narrow range, without eating constantly, the body must be able to store, release, and use glucose as needed. This is accomplished through the use of a pair of hormones: insulin and glucagon.

Insulin is produced in the beta cells within the islets of Langerhans found in the pancreas. These specialized cells produce and secrete insulin in response to increased blood sugar levels. When an individual ingests glucose in the form of dietary intake (i.e., enterally) or when glucose is delivered via an injection route, or intravenously (i.e., parenterally), the blood sugar rises and the pancreas responds by secreting insulin into the bloodstream to lower the blood sugar. As it circulates, insulin binds to insulin receptors on the surface of body cells, permitting those cells to then absorb glucose from the blood. This is somewhat analogous to using a key to open a door. The end result is that the blood sugar drops as the sugar enters the cells.

Insulin is also used to help store glucose in the form of glycogen by directing the formation of glycogen, a linking of multiple glucose molecules. These glycogen molecules are stored in the liver and skeletal muscle until the body has use for them. The relationship between glucose and insulin is direct: as glucose increases in the bloodstream from ingestion or injection, insulin is secreted. As glucose levels fall, insulin secretion is inhibited so as not to precipitate hypoglycemia.

Insulin also stimulates **lipogenesis**, the creation of triglycerides from fatty acids and glycerol, which are in turn bound to high density lipoproteins. This triglyceride and lipoprotein unit is stored in adipose tissue cells for use during periods of starvation. The liberation of glucose and its by-products from adipose tissue is discussed shortly. Finally, insulin is also crucial in the protein synthesis process. Insulin prevents the body from breaking down muscles (i.e., catabolism) for use as a source of energy.

Certain medications inhibit the release of insulin, including hydrochlorothiazide (diuretic), beta blockers, calcium channel blockers (both antihypertensives), and phenytoin (anticonvulsant). Other medications increase the production of insulin, and thus lower the blood sugar, including salicylates (found in any aspirin-containing medication) and glucagon.

When blood glucose levels decrease below a certain minimum level, such as while fasting overnight during sleep or in times of starvation, the body is able to mobilize glucose from the glycogen stores, and synthesize (produce) glucose from other nutrient sources, such as fats and proteins. Both the mobilization and synthesis of glucose is directed by the hormone glucagon.

Glucagon is produced in alpha cells of the islets of Langerhans in the pancreas. It is secreted in response to low blood glucose levels (hypoglycemia) or when the body's demands for glucose are increased, such as during strenuous exercise. In the liver and skeletal muscle, glucagon breaks down glycogen into its component glucose molecules in a process known as **glycogenolysis**. Glucose released from the glycogen in the liver by glucagon can be circulated throughout the body and used by all types of body cells. Those skeletal muscles, however, can only use glycogen stored in the skeletal muscle. This is particularly important during strenuous exercise as the muscle cells can release and then use their own stores of glucose.

At times when glucose stores are low and carbohydrate intake is limited, the body is able to synthesize glucose from amino acids (components of proteins) and even fat. These proteins and fats can either be from dietary sources or from the body's own stores, such as muscle and body fat tissue. The process of breaking down fat into free fatty acids and glucose, called **gluconeogenesis**, can provide energy to the body in times of prolonged starvation.

Glucagon also stimulates the **ketogenic pathway**. Glucagon can help convert free fatty acids into ketoacids and other ketonic bodies, which in turn are metabolized in the liver into energy.

The other counterregulatory hormone is epinephrine. Epinephrine has multiple effects on metabolism including suppression of insulin and stimulation of glucagon. Epinephrine also stimulates the mobilization of fatty acids (lipolysis of stored triglyceride), which can result in ketone production.

Range of Blood Glucose

Blood glucose levels can fluctuate dramatically. However, the typical range of blood glucose in the body is between a low of 70 to 80 mg/dL and a high of 120 and 140 mg/dL. Although experts differ on the lower limit of normal blood glucose, whether it is 70 or 80 mg/dL, it is not the number alone that should be used to determine if a patient has hypoglycemia, but rather the entire clinical picture.

On the opposite end of the glucose spectrum is hyperglycemia. Generally, a blood sugar over 120 to 140 mg/dL is considered elevated, though patients can transiently have a blood sugar over 180 mg/dL.

Impaired Glucose Metabolism

The process of glucose production, storage, and utilization is very complex and requires an intricate balance of hormones and coordination between several organ systems in order to maintain a constant energy supply to the body cells. Impairment in any of these organs or their hormones can result in significant disease, thereby causing considerable health consequences. For instance, failure of the pancreas to produce insulin results in inappropriately high blood glucose levels, as seen in diabetes mellitus type 1.[4] This and other disorders of glucose metabolism will be discussed in the following sections.

Diabetes Mellitus

The normal random blood glucose level is 70 to 113 mg/dL, although the upper limit can extend to 180 mg/dL within two hours of starting a meal.[5] Hyperglycemia is the term used to describe abnormally elevated levels of circulating blood glucose.

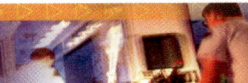

PROFESSIONAL PARAMEDIC

Paramedics draw what are called "random" blood glucose levels. During the course of a day, the patient's blood glucose should not vary widely (i.e., the blood glucose should be maintained within a range), and therefore testing for hypoglycemia can occur at any time. A random blood glucose test is not the same as a fasting glucose test, which is a test performed to detect diabetes.

Patients with hyperglycemia may have a variety of clinical presentations depending on the degree of hyperglycemia and the patient's other comorbidities (i.e., other diseases that often accompany diabetes). Most patients experience no symptoms at all, and may be surprised to know their blood glucose level is elevated. Others may have minimal symptoms, such as increased thirst or urination, due to the diuretic effect of glucose in the blood. In both of these instances, the glucose elevation is likely to be mild to moderate (<200 mg/dL). More significant elevations in glucose above 200 mg/dL tend to be associated with dramatic and serious patient presentations. For example, altered mental status, ranging from simple confusion to coma, may be the result of profound hyperglycemia. Although the elevated glucose level is ultimately responsible for these mental status changes, it is the effects of hyperglycemia, such as profound dehydration and electrolyte disturbances, that stimulate changes in the patient's mental abilities.

Although there are multiple causes of hyperglycemia, the most common cause encountered in the United States is diabetes mellitus. In fact, the majority of patients who present to an emergency department with hyperglycemia are new onset or uncontrolled diabetics. However, other causes (such as sepsis) can also precipitate hyperglycemia. These disorders will be discussed individually.

Diabetes may have existed since the dawn of time. The Egyptians described it over 4000 years ago and the Greeks gave it the name diabetes mellitus ("diabetes" meaning to pass through and "mellitus" meaning honey sweet).[6] Flies were often seen around the urine of diabetic patients. In the past, the diagnosis of diabetes mellitus was considered a terminal disease. However, modern medical therapeutics have changed the prognosis of diabetes. Today, diabetes can be viewed as a chronic disease.

As a result of a number of factors, the incidence of diabetes is growing. The Centers for Disease Control and Prevention (CDC) indicate that the number of Americans with diabetes increased from 5.6 million to 15.8 million between 1980 and 2005, with approximately 40% of these people age 65 or older.[7] (The worldwide demographics are somewhat different, with the majority of diabetics between 45 to 64 years old).[8] This astonishing increase in the number of diabetics across the country has had a profound effect on the healthcare system, including emergency medicine and emergency medical services. For example, the average annual medical cost for a nondiabetic is approximately $2,700, whereas the average annual medical cost for a diabetic can be $10,000. Many of these medical costs can be attributed to the complications of diabetes including end-stage renal disease, cardiovascular disease, and nontraumatic lower extremity amputations secondary to vascular insufficiency. Diabetes is the leading cause of blindness and the fourth leading cause of death overall in the United States.[7]

The increase in the incidence of diabetes has been largely attributed to the increase in patient obesity. Patients with obesity tend to develop diabetes as a complication of their obesity. This problem is so prevalent that a new term—diabesity—has been created to describe diabetes secondary to obesity.

Diabetes should not be thought of as a single disease but rather a group of chronic metabolic disorders whose key characteristic is hyperglycemia. However, there are numerous different names for the same or similar conditions (Table 13-1). To standardize the nomenclature, the American Diabetes Association (ADA) simplified the classification of diabetes in 1997. The general classifications of diabetes are type 1, type 2, gestational, and other specific types. The majority of patients with diabetes mellitus either have impaired production of

Table 13-1 Nomenclature of Diabetes

Old Names	Juvenile diabetes (JD)	Adult onset diabetes (AODM)
	Insulin dependent (IDDM)	Non-insulin dependent (NIDDM)
New Term	Type 1	Type 2

insulin and are classified type 1, or have cellular resistance to circulating insulin and are classified as type 2.

Type 1 Diabetes Mellitus

Type 1 diabetes, also referred to as insulin-dependent diabetes mellitus, affects approximately 10% of patients with diabetes and results from a lack of insulin produced in the pancreas.[9] In most cases, this disorder is due to a lack of insulin-producing islet cells. It is thought that patients may have a genetic predisposition to developing type 1 diabetes. Under normal circumstances, an increase in blood glucose would result in increased insulin production and secretion, thereby directing glucose uptake, utilization, and storage. The type 1 diabetic, however, is unable to respond to such a glucose load, and the net result is hyperglycemia. The majority of patients with type 1 diabetes are diagnosed when they are children, with peak onset at age 13, and require life-long management of their glucose levels and their symptoms. Although the clear majority of patients develop type 1 diabetes as children, it can occur later in life (i.e., in patients as old as 70 years of age or older).

Type 1 diabetes may be the result of an autoimmune disease in which the patient's own immune system attacks the islets of Langerhans. It has been suggested that this autoimmune response may be the result of an infection with Coxsackie virus. Another theory suggests that type 1 diabetes may be the result of a genetic malfunction in a gene called Lmp2. Another theory suggests type 1 diabetes is the result of malfunctioning cyotoxic "killer" T cells. Research into the exact etiology is ongoing.

Since their bodies cannot produce an adequate supply of insulin to meet the body's metabolic demands, patients with type 1 diabetes require supplemental insulin. Most patients with type 1 diabetes require daily insulin injections based on their blood glucose level as it fluctuates during the day and following meals. Many also take insulin daily, which helps maintain a steady baseline blood glucose concentration.

Types of Insulin

Normally a patient's pancreas will produce, as a basal rate, one unit of insulin an hour and the liver will eliminate that insulin within 10 to 15 minutes. Patients with type 1 diabetes do not make insulin; therefore, these patients will need supplemental insulin for the rest of their lives. The difficulty lies in trying to artificially maintain a correct level of insulin.

Since its discovery in 1923, pharmaceutical companies have developed over 20 different types of insulin, each with its own quality that makes it superior to other insulin for a specific use. What differentiates these insulins is usually the onset of action, the peak time, and the duration of action. For example, rapid-acting insulin works within 15 minutes to lower blood sugar and its hypoglycemic effect peaks in one hour. Rapid-acting insulin may be used when a patient's blood glucose fluctuates quickly; this patient is sometimes referred to as a "brittle diabetic." Short-acting insulin (i.e., regular insulin) is typically used approximately one half hour before a meal so that it peaks when digestion peaks the blood sugar in two to three hours. Short-acting insulin lasts about six to eight hours, or the time between daytime meals.

Intermediate-acting insulin, such as NPH and Lente, are mixed with materials that slow absorption. This insulin will peak in about 10 hours and will last 10 to 16 hours, or about the time between dinner and breakfast. Some patients prefer to use intermediate-acting insulin, particularly Lente, because it can control the blood sugar all day. These patients may supplement their intermediate-acting insulin if they unexpectedly eat a large meal.

The last classification of insulin is long-acting insulin. Ultralente, an example of long-acting insulin, works within six to eight hours and lasts for 20 hours or more. Like intermediate-acting insulin, long-acting insulin is usually taken either at bedtime or in the morning (Table 13-2).

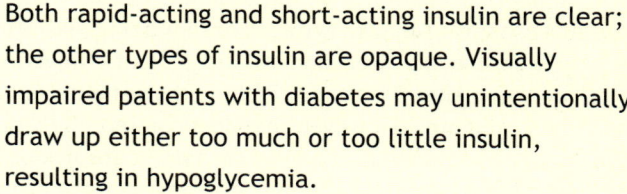

STREET SMART

Both rapid-acting and short-acting insulin are clear; the other types of insulin are opaque. Visually impaired patients with diabetes may unintentionally draw up either too much or too little insulin, resulting in hypoglycemia.

In order to achieve satisfactory blood glucose control, the patient with diabetes will often match different insulins to eating patterns, glucose monitoring, and activities of the day. For example, rapid-acting insulin may be given immediately following a meal to prevent a spike in blood glucose levels, whereas very long-acting insulin may be taken at bedtime to avoid nocturnal hypoglycemia.

STREET SMART

Insulin must be either refrigerated or used within 30 days if it is at room temperature. Furthermore, insulin denatures rapidly in high temperatures. For these reasons, insulin is not a medication that would be practical for use in routine Paramedic practice.

Insulin Administration

The most common administration method for insulin is injection, using an insulin syringe. An insulin syringe can come in 13 unit (U13), 50 unit (U50), or 100 unit (U100) barrels with a microfine needle between 27 and 31 g that may be 1/8 to 1/2 inch in length.

Table 13-2 Properties of the Different Types of Insulin

Insulin	Brand	Onset	Peak	Duration
Rapid Acting				
Lispro	Humalog®	Within 15 minutes	45 minutes to 1½ hours	3½ to 4½ hours
Aspart	Novolog®	Within 15 minutes	1 to 3 hours	3½ to 4½ hours
Short Acting				
Regular	Humulin R	Within 1 hour	2 to 3 hours	3 to 6 hours
Zinc	Semilente	1 to 3 hours	5 to 10 hours	10 to 16 hours
Intermediate				
NPH or zinc	Lente	2 to 4 hours	4 to 12 hours	12 to 18 hours
Long Acting				
Extended zinc	Ultralente	6 to 10 hours	8 to 20 hours	20 to 24 hours
Very Long Acting				
Glargine	Lantus	1 to 4 hours	6 to 8 hours	24 hours
Detemir	Levemir	1 to 4 hours	6 to 8 hours	24 hours

A number of insulin injection aids are on the market. These aids use spring-loaded syringes or stabilizing platforms that help improve the precision of the patient's injection. Typical injection sites for insulin include the patient's upper arms, thighs, and hips. However, the most common injection site may be the abdomen as it allows the fastest absorption.

A novel approach to insulin injection has been the invention of the insulin pen. It has the appearance of a regular pen, but the barrel of the pen has a prefilled cartridge with 150 to 130 units of insulin. Using a dial, the patient dials in the desired amount of insulin and then depresses a plunger to inject the insulin.

A complication of repeated insulin injections at one spot is the development of scar tissue at that site which impedes absorption. In an effort to eliminate the needle, and subsequent complications, the insulin jet injector was created. The insulin jet injector uses a microfine blast of compressed air to send a spray of insulin subcutaneously.

Perhaps the development with the greatest potential is inhaled insulin.[10,11] Inhaled insulin is a fine dry powder that is absorbed through the oral or nasal mucosa or absorbed into the lungs (Figure 13-2). Exubera® is an example of an FDA approved inhaled insulin. Although Exubera has been discontinued by the manufacturer, its production provided an example of an alternative delivery platform for insulin. Other platforms are currently in development.

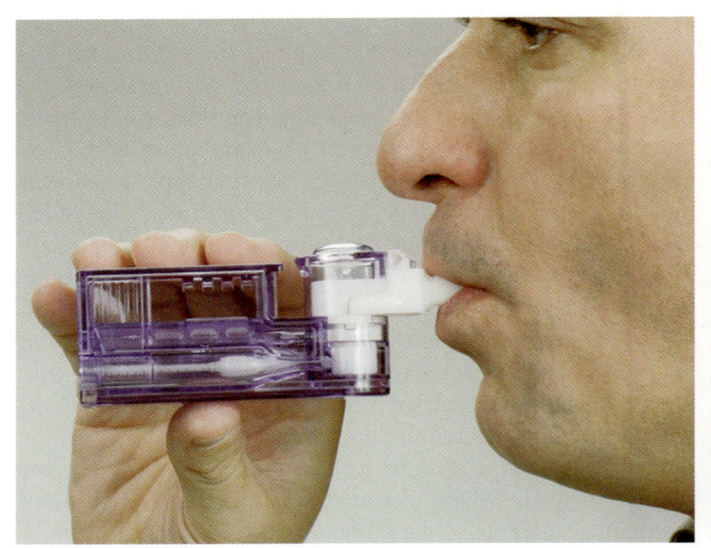

Figure 13-2 Inhaled insulin.

Insulin Pumps

One of the revolutionary devices that have simplified life for many diabetic patients is the insulin pump. This external device holds a volume of insulin that is injected via Teflon catheter into the patient's subcutaneous tissue. Approximately the size of an electronic pager, the insulin pump can deliver varying amounts of insulin according to the patient's meal pattern and activity levels (Figure 13-3). Future units may

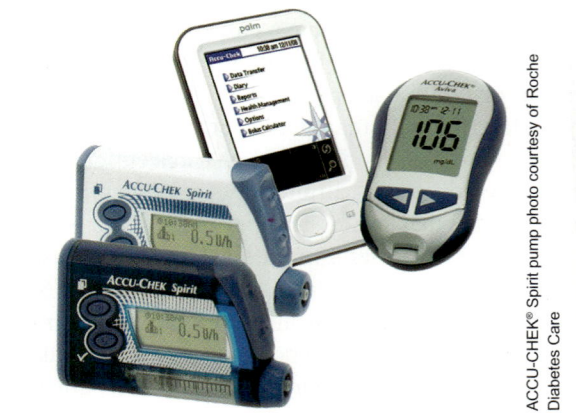

Figure 13-3 Insulin pump.

also be capable of determining the blood glucose and will be, in essence, an artificial pancreas.

These insulin pumps are attached to the waistband of a pair of pants, a bra, or a garter belt, and are so common that the Paramedic should investigate the presence of an insulin pump on any unconscious patient with diabetes. The insulin pump will continue to deliver insulin even if the patient is hypoglycemic.

To disconnect the insulin pump, the Paramedic should first remove the tubing from the unit. A luer lock typically connects it and a simple twist is all that is needed for its release.

The next generation of insulin pumps may be surgically implanted and will deliver a basal dose of insulin. The pumps will administer additional insulin via a patient controlled telemetry unit.

Type 2 Diabetes Mellitus

In contrast to type 1 diabetes in which the body has a lack of insulin, patients with type 2 diabetes do not have this concern (although that can occur later in the disease's development). Rather, type 2 diabetes is notable for the presence of **insulin resistance**. These patients, who account for approximately 80% to 90% of all diabetics, produce insulin normally in response to elevated glucose. However, the body cells are unable to use insulin due to resistance at the cells' insulin receptors. In other words, patients with type 2 diabetes produce sufficient amounts of insulin but are unable to use it. As a result, the glucose in the blood is not absorbed into the cells and remains in the bloodstream, causing hyperglycemia. Interestingly, many patients with type 2 diabetes actually have elevated insulin levels due to their persistent hyperglycemia and the pancreas' response to hyperglycemia.

The onset of type 2 diabetes typically occurs in adulthood, since cells may develop insulin resistance as they age, and the resistance increases with age. Type 2 diabetes is strongly correlated with obesity since adipose (fat) cells naturally have lower numbers of insulin receptors.[12,13] Unlike type 1 diabetes, type 2 diabetes has a strong genetic predisposition, and most patients cite a family history of the disease.

The treatment of type 2 diabetes may begin with diet modification and exercise, but may require the use of medications

collectively known as oral hypoglycemic agents. These medications, including the biguanides (i.e., metformin), sulfonylureas (i.e., glipizide and glyburide), and thiazolidinediones (i.e., rosiglitazone and piaglitazone) work to decrease glucose absorption from the GI tract, decrease gluconeogenesis in the liver, stimulate insulin secretion, and decrease insulin resistance in body cells.

Insulin Resistance

Type 2 diabetes arises from one of three sources or a combination therein. In some patients, the pancreas response to a rising blood sugar level is delayed. For others, the pancreas produces too little insulin for the demand. For yet others, the body's cells do not respond to the insulin produced. This last condition, called insulin resistance, is the hallmark of type 2 diabetes.

To respond to the insulin resistance, the pancreas attempts to compensate and overproduces insulin, a condition called hyperinsulinemia. This increased insulin in the bloodstream promotes fat storage and has several other pathologic effects.

Insulin, as a chemical, acts to increase atherosclerosis. Insulin can also prevent the breakdown of clots and leads to microthrombi. Elevated insulin levels also cause an increase in plasma calcium levels, which in turn increase vascular tone. This results in hypertension. The cumulative effect of the hyperinsulinemia is an increased risk of acute coronary syndrome and stroke.

Treatment

The first generation of oral hypoglycemic agents used to treat type 2 diabetes were the sulfonylureas, such as orinase and diabinese. The sulfonylureas encourage insulin release from the pancreas as well as increase the uptake of glucose in insulin resistant cells. This class of oral hypoglycemic medications has many interactions with other medications (alcohol, MAO inhibitors, salicylates, etc.) and they were problematic for patients with renal disease, a common complication of diabetes.

The next two generations of oral hypoglycemic medications were improvements on the sulfonylureas.[14,15] These medications (glucotrol, diabeta, and micronase, for example) encouraged insulin release from the pancreas but could also, in rare cases, cause profound hypoglycemia.

The next group of oral hypoglycemic medications—the biguanides, alpha–glucosidase inhibitors, and thiazolidinediones—approached glucose control from a different perspective. Instead of encouraging the pancreas to release more insulin, these medications decreased the cell's resistance to insulin, thereby making insulin more effective.

Several other oral hypoglycemic agents are either on the market or currently being researched, including meglitinides and DPP-4 inhibitors. With the increase in type 2 diabetes, a more effective and perhaps more varied approach to glucose control will be needed.

The net result of all oral hypoglycemic medications is a decrease in circulating blood glucose and improved glucose uptake into the cells. Patients with type 2 diabetes may eventually decrease their own insulin production late in the course of the disease. This results in insulin deficiency similar to that seen with type 1 diabetes. When this occurs, these patients require supplemental insulin in addition to their oral hypoglycemic agents.

STREET SMART

Insulin taken by mouth (PO) would seem to be the most effective means of controlling blood sugar. However, insulin is a complex polypeptide that is broken down by the stomach's acid and rendered impotent if administered orally.

Gestational Diabetes

Gestational diabetes is defined as an elevation in a woman's blood glucose levels that begins during pregnancy. The American Diabetes Association estimates that approximately 4% of pregnant women are diagnosed with gestational diabetes.[16] Although the causes of gestational diabetes are not completely understood, there are many similarities between gestational diabetes and type 2 diabetes, including insulin resistance and increased weight.

In the case of the pregnant woman, hormones secreted by the placenta are responsible for insulin resistance. Therefore, most women resolve their hyperglycemia after they give birth.

Undiagnosed or poorly controlled diabetes during pregnancy causes major birth defects in 5% to 10% of pregnancies. In addition, it may be responsible for 15% to 20% of miscarriages. Several other complications of pregnancy are also associated with diabetes during pregnancy, including a large baby or fetal macrosomia. As a result of fetal macrosomia, the infant's head may be too large to be delivered through the mother's pelvic opening, thus requiring delivery by Cesarean section.

Infants born of diabetic mothers are also prone to infantile hypoglycemia on delivery, particularly if the mother was hyperglycemic before childbirth. The infant's blood sugar should be checked, usually by heelstick, if the infant remains lethargic following delivery.

There is a small subset of women, about 2%, who will remain diabetic following pregnancy. In addition, as many as 50% of women with gestational diabetes will subsequently develop type 2 diabetes within 10 years. However, with careful control of blood sugar through diet, exercise, and occasionally insulin therapy, this disorder can be avoided. In contrast to treatment for type 2 diabetes, oral hypoglycemic agents are never used in cases of gestational diabetes, and in fact are contraindicated in pregnancy.

Prediabetes

Some patients may be diagnosed with prediabetes. Prediabetes is a condition of chronic hyperglycemia that does not reach the level of diabetes but has many of the same complications associated with it. Prediabetes is usually diagnosed by an impaired fasting glucose or impaired glucose tolerance test. The incidence of prediabetes is increasing along with the increased prevalence of obesity. It is estimated that 40% of adults from age 40 and beyond may be prediabetic. Prediabetics risk developing type 2 diabetes within 10 years.

Complications of Diabetes

Abnormal metabolism secondary to diabetes can have a number of negative systemic impacts including disease in the cardiovascular, neurological, and renal systems. These diabetes-related complications exceed $100 billion of healthcare dollars annually in the United States alone.[6]

Besides lowering blood sugar, insulin also affects nitric oxide. Nitric oxide, the active ingredient in nitroglycerin, is a local vasodilator that also inhibits smooth muscle proliferation within the tunica media. Inhibition of insulin, such as occurs during insulin resistance, results in vasoconstriction and accelerated vascular disease. Approximately three-quarters of patients with diabetes also have hypertension or are under treatment for hypertension.

Under these conditions, the patient experiences accelerated vessel disease, which can progress to coronary artery disease. Patients with diabetes are at greater risk for acute coronary syndrome, hypertension, and heart failure. For this reason, the American Diabetes Association recommends that patients with diabetes and identified cardiac risk factors take aspirin daily.[17,18]

Another common complication of diabetes is nervous system disease. Some 70% of patients with diabetes have some nervous system complication, ranging from peripheral neuropathy to blindness. Peripheral neuropathy can be as mild as impairment of sensation in the hands and feet and range to severe pain in the extremities. Approximately one-third of diabetic patients over age 40 have peripheral neuropathy. These sensations—which have been described as burning, tingling, or numbness—often take a stocking or glove distribution and end abruptly. The loss of sensation prevents that patient from experiencing pain when the foot is injured. Coupled with poor peripheral circulation secondary to accelerated vessel disease, these injuries can result in serious ulcers and infections. Over one-half of nontraumatic amputations (82,000 annually) are due to diabetes-related foot ulcers.

Diabetic neuropathy affects all of the nerves in the body, including the nerves that innervate the heart. With decreased pain sensation, patients with diabetes may experience a "silent MI." The first indication of threatened acute myocardial infarction in this population may be unexplained fatigue and weakness or dysrhythmia.

Another associated neuropathy is blindness. Diabetes is the leading cause of blindness in adults in the United States.[19,20] Blindness can be preceded by periods of vision loss secondary to capillary hemorrhage in the vitreous of the eye.

Finally, patients with diabetes are at a greater risk for kidney disease. Diabetes is also the leading cause of kidney failure; approximately one-half of new cases of kidney failure each year are the result of diabetes.

Factors such as poor glycemic control, hypertension, and dietary changes (especially diets high in protein) cause a series of changes in the kidneys that impair glomerular filtration. This can lead to nephron damage and subsequent kidney failure.

Hyperglycemia

Both type 1 and type 2 diabetes involve hyperglycemia. This common condition leads to common complications. As the blood sugar rises, it acts as an osmotic diuretic, pulling fluids from the tissues and into the bloodstream. The kidneys, in turn, expel the excess fluid as urine. Shortly thereafter, the now-dehydrated cells send out signals indicating the patient should start to increase his intake of water, a condition called **polydipsia**.

As blood sugar levels continue to rise, the glucose reaches the renal threshold, about 170 to 200 mg/dL, and the glucose is spilled into the urine. This glucose in the urine (glycosuria) pulls water with it along with several essential elements needed for body metabolism—sodium, potassium, magnesium, and phosphate. This large amount of urine production forces the patient to void often, a condition called **polyuria**.

While the blood sugar is climbing, the body's cells continue to go without needed glucose and the cells send out signals requesting it. In an effort to respond to the starvation, the patient is constantly hungry and tries to eat more, a condition called **polyphagia**.

Without glucose for energy, the patient suffers lethargy, weakness, and ease of fatigue. These symptoms, plus the "3 Poly's" (polyuria, polyphagia, and polydipsia), may lead the Paramedic to suspect the patient has diabetes. However, the patient is often unaware of the condition, sometimes for as long as six years. Usually it takes a dramatic event, such as pain, to cause the patient to seek medical attention. For example, fluid shifts within the body often cause problems in fluid-sensitive organs such as the intestines. The initial presentation of a patient with new onset diabetes mellitus may be for abdominal pain.

Typically, hyperglycemia is not a concern for the Paramedic and is not treated aggressively in the prehospital setting. However, there are two extreme conditions—diabetic ketoacidosis (DKA) and hyperglycemic hyperosmolar nonketotic syndrome (HHNS)—which may require the Paramedic's intervention.

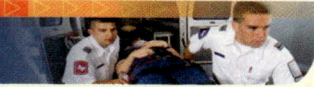

Diabetic Ketoacidosis

A life-threatening complication of uncontrolled hyperglycemia is **diabetic ketoacidosis (DKA)**. This condition, characterized by profound hyperglycemia, severe dehydration acidosis, and mental status changes, can be the presentation of new onset diabetes or can occur in a known diabetic who is poorly compliant with the treatment regimen or who has some other physical stressor that causes the blood glucose to rise.

The diagnosis is made based on the presence of high blood glucose levels, ketone bodies in the blood, and urine acetone and acidosis. Diabetic ketoacidosis occurs almost exclusively in type 1 diabetic patients, but may occasionally be seen in type 2 diabetics as well. Annually, DKA is responsible for the hospitalization of over 100,000 patients, and has a mortality rate approaching 5%.[21]

Although there are several potential causes of DKA, including infections (such as pneumonia or urinary tract infections), myocardial infarction, drug or alcohol use, and trauma, the most common cause is medication noncompliance.

Pathophysiology

In a quest to provide glucose to the glucose-starved cells, the body resorts to alternate energy pathways. One source of energy is the conversion of muscle into its primary constituents—amino acids. This process is called proteolysis. These amino acids are, in turn, converted into glucose in the liver. However, without insulin this energy production only worsens the hyperglycemia. Concurrently the body starts to break down adipose tissue, via lipolysis, releasing fatty acids that can be oxidized for energy.

Although these processes—proteolysis, lipolysis, cellular dehydration, and so on—are complicated enough, it must be understood that these processes occur concurrently, and not consecutively. The result is a rapid increase in blood serum glucose to toxic levels in a matter of days.

The crucial problem in diabetic ketoacidosis is due to the ketones produced by these alternative energy pathways. Normally, the body produces a small amount of ketones which the liver metabolizes. During DKA, the liver is overwhelmed by the demands to produce energy and to neutralize the ketones.

The result is ketosis, or the buildup of ketone bodies in the bloodstream. Ketones, as an acid, lead to a condition called metabolic acidosis. As it is important for the metabolism to operate in a narrow pH range, the body attempts to compensate (Figure 13-4).

Hyperosmolar Nonketotic Syndrome

Hyperosmolar nonketotic syndrome (HONKS), also known as **hyperglycemic hyperosmolar nonketotic syndrome (HHNS)**, is sometimes confused with DKA but is actually much different. Patients with HONKS may have extremely high blood glucose levels (>600) and profound dehydration (up to 9 L), but do not typically become acidotic, and may not produce ketones.[22]

HONKS is thought to be the result of pancreatic failure coupled with renal insufficiency. The impaired insulin production, from the pancreatic failure, leads to profound

hyperglycemia, with values as high as 800 to 1,000 mg/dL of blood glucose. This pancreatic failure may be caused by epinephrine-induced depression of insulin function.

Elevated epinephrine may be the result of infections (such as pneumonia or urinary tract infection), stroke, acute myocardial infarction, and even gastrointestinal bleeding. Even certain medications, such as hydrochlorothiazide, furosemide, phenytoin, and beta blockers, can help lead to HONKS.

Normally the body would spill the glucose. However, the compounding complication of renal insufficiency decreases glycouria and results in extreme elevations of blood glucose.

Similar as to what occurs with DKA, extreme hyperglycemia leads to osmotic diuresis with body fluid losses as high as 8 to 12 liters. These staggering fluid losses lead to profound electrolyte imbalances, most notably hypokalemia.

Unlike DKA, the patient with HONKS does not experience ketosis. Minimal secretion of insulin during the episode provides sufficient insulin to stave off lipolysis and prevent the use of the ketogenic pathway for energy production.

Most of the time, those afflicted are elderly patients requiring care from others, either in nursing facilities or in the homes of family or friends (although there are reports of pediatric HONKS as well). The hyperglycemia and dehydration develop over the course of several days to weeks, unlike DKA, which usually presents within three days. Unfortunately, because HONKS develops so gradually, it may go undetected for a long time. HONKS may lead to coma in about 10% of cases and often has a high mortality rate (20% to 60%).[23]

As a result, the patients with HONKS are more severely dehydrated and present almost exclusively with some degree of mental status change or lack of responsiveness. Because of this, there may be greater need for careful airway monitoring during transport to the emergency department. The remainder of the treatment, however, is the same as for DKA: measure blood glucose and initiate IV normal saline (Table 13-3).

Hypoglycemia

Although patients with diabetes must be concerned with controlling blood glucose levels to prevent hyperglycemia, they must also be cautious to avoid overtreating and precipitating hypoglycemia, a complication becoming more frequent with the addition of more diabetic treatment agents. Hypoglycemia is defined as a serum blood glucose level less than 50 mg/dL

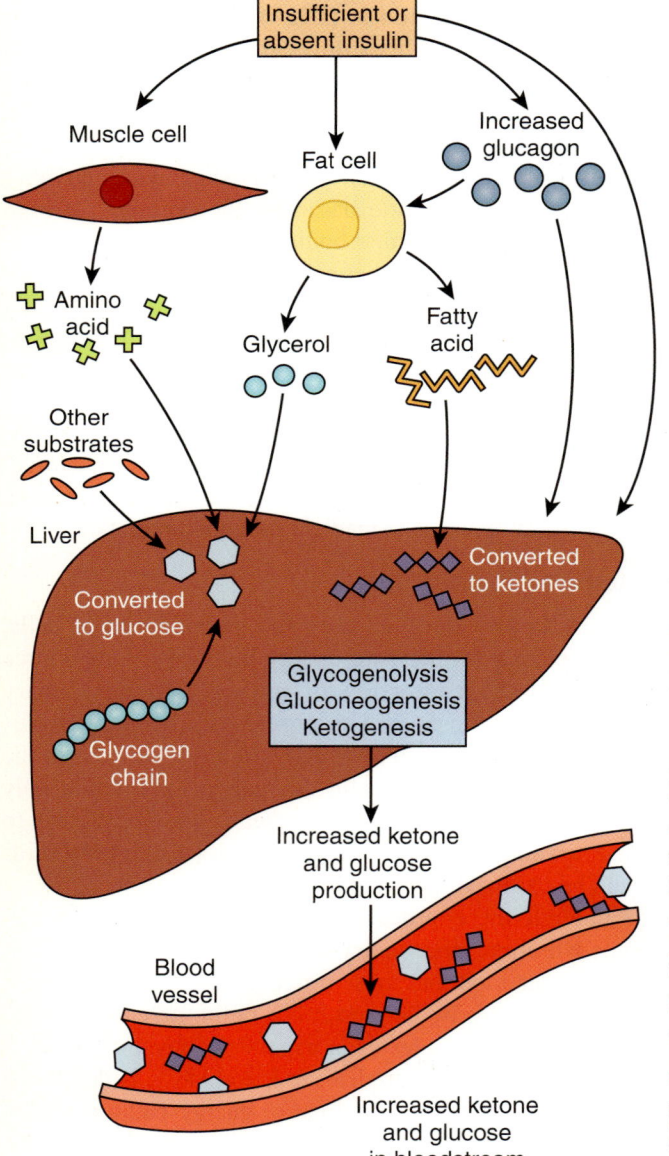

Figure 13-4 Diabetic ketoacidosis.

Table 13-3 DKA versus HONKS

Feature	DKA	HONKS
Median age at onset	40s	60s
Neurological deficits	Uncommon	Common
Nausea and vomiting	Common	Uncommon
Cramps	Common	Uncommon
Shortness of breath	Common	Uncommon
Thirst and dehydration	Common	Common

associated with signs and symptoms such as tachycardia, sweating, tremulousness, and/or altered mental status.

Although this condition is seen most frequently as a complication of diabetes treatment, sepsis, renal failure, and pancreatic tumors can all cause hypoglycemia (Table 13-4).

As described earlier in this chapter, glucose is the sole energy source for the brain and red blood cells. Therefore, while other cells are able to use alternate fuel sources (fats, protein) in times of glucose deficiency, the brain is unable to do so. As a result, the cells of the brain cease to function properly and patients exhibit alterations in mental status (from confusion to coma), neurologic deficits, and/or psychiatric manifestations.

The neurologic deficits associated with hypoglycemia may be so profound as to mimic an acute stroke. The most recent American Heart Association and American Stroke Association guidelines for early management of stroke include early blood glucose testing to exclude hypoglycemia as a potential confounder.[24] In addition to the mental status changes and neurologic deficits, prolonged hypoglycemia may result in severe cardiovascular collapse, such as cardiac arrhythmias or even cardiac arrest. Therefore, fingerstick blood glucose testing should be obtained in any patient presenting with altered mental status, neurologic deficit, new or unexplained psychiatric disorder, or cardiovascular collapse.

In addition to the neuropsychiatric effects of hypoglycemia, there are several potential systemic (body wide) effects, which should be investigated as clues to detect hypoglycemia. When the body is devoid of glucose, the sympathetic nervous system is stimulated, releasing epinephrine (the "rescue hormone"). This results in increased heart rate, sweating, tremor, nausea, and weakness. These physical findings can help aid the Paramedic's diagnosis of hypoglycemia when placed in the correct context based on a patient's history and hypoglycemia.

Although these symptoms are very useful as a diagnostic aid, they are not present all the time, and may even be blocked by other medications such as beta blockers, which prevent tachycardia. The best approach, when in doubt, is for the Paramedic to measure a fingerstick glucose level and treat with a high index of suspicion that hypoglycemia exists if

Table 13-4 Potential Causes of Hypoglycemia

- Diabetes related
  - Accidental insulin overdose*
  - Intentional overdose of insulin or oral antihypoglycemic
  - Antihyperglycemic agents such as sulfonylureas
  - Starvation**
- Sepsis
  - Pulmonary infection
  - Urosepsis
  - Skin infections
- Pregnancy***
- Medications
  - Salicylate overdose, such as aspirin
  - Beta blocker overdose
- Alcohol intoxication
- Chronic renal failure

Notes:

*Blindness is a complication of diabetes.

**Obesity is associated with type 2 diabetes; dieting is one means of controlling diabetes.

*** This is more likely to happen in early pregnancy.

the blood glucose reading is low. The change in glucose as a result of intravenous dextrose administration is minimal. In a risk–benefit analysis, it is better to administer the dextrose than risk cerebral injury.

The majority of patients with low glucose seen and treated by EMS personnel will be hypoglycemic because of their medications. A common situation involves an insulin-dependent diabetic who takes the usual insulin dose without an appropriate sized meal or snack. This frequently occurs at bedtime when diabetics typically take their long-acting insulin, but can occur with short-acting insulin bolus at meal times as well. Without at least a small carbohydrate load to offset the bolus of insulin, the blood glucose can plummet rapidly and trigger the response described earlier. Because of this, it is extremely important for a Paramedic to review a patient's insulin use when evaluating for a hypoglycemic emergency. Most of these patients respond favorably to a glucose load, which will be discussed in further detail later in this chapter.

The addition and expansion of oral hypoglycemic agents as treatment for type 2 diabetes has generated several new classes of non-insulin therapy. Unlike insulin, these medications do not require a carbohydrate load at the time of, or shortly after, administration. However, many of these drugs, particularly the sulfonylureas, are capable of causing hypoglycemia, but with much less predictability than insulin itself. The class of medications known as sulfonylureas (i.e., glipizide, glyburide) function by increasing insulin production in the pancreas. Insulin can then be secreted in response to carbohydrate ingestion. The end result is similar to insulin injections in that the amount of circulating insulin is increased, which will cause increased absorption of glucose from the bloodstream. The remainders of the oral hypoglycemic medications act by reducing insulin resistance in the body cells. Although they can cause hypoglycemia, it is much less often a problem compared to use of the sulfonylureas.

It must be remembered that while most of the medication-induced hypoglycemic episodes are unfortunate side effects within the regular course of diabetes treatment, these medications can be—and sometimes are—used as drugs of abuse, self-harm, and suicide. Therefore, it is important to determine the number of pills ingested, the time they were taken, and the purpose.

STREET SMART

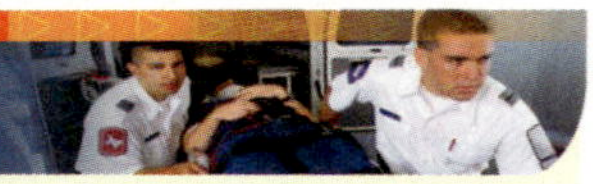

In the past, psychiatrists would purposely induce hypoglycemia (i.e., insulin shock or insulin coma) in an attempt to treat schizophrenia. This practice was abandoned with the advent of neuroleptic drugs.

In addition to medication-induced hypoglycemia, several illnesses and diseases can increase circulating insulin levels, thus causing low glucose levels. Excess insulin is metabolized and eliminated via the kidney. Patients with kidney disease are at risk of having abnormally high insulin levels since their kidneys cannot break down and eliminate the circulating insulin. This then further decreases the patient's blood glucose levels, and can result in significant hypoglycemia. This can be particularly dangerous if these patients are taking insulin injections, and their insulin dosage may need to be adjusted to compensate for their kidney failure.

Liver failure can also contribute to hypoglycemic episodes. In healthy people, the liver is stimulated to undergo gluconeogenesis and glycogenolysis when the cells of the brain

sense low blood glucose. However, if a patient has a damaged liver—either from chronic causes such as hepatitis or cirrhosis, or acute ones as seen in toxic ingestions—he or she may not be able to release glucose from the liver to increase the blood level. In addition, the person may not be able to respond to glucagon administered as treatment for hypoglycemia. Alcoholics are especially at risk since their livers are usually damaged. In addition, they tend to be malnourished as most of their calories are from alcohol and not from other sources. Therefore, EMS and emergency department staff should keep an open mind when treating alcoholics who are behaving in a bizarre manner and consider hypoglycemia as a potential cause.

Although very rare, certain types of pancreatic tumors may precipitate episodes of hypoglycemia. Insulinomas are tumors that chronically produce and secrete insulin into the bloodstream.[25] These tumors can be very difficult to diagnose, but should be considered in patients who have chronically low blood glucose levels, especially if they are not taking any medications which would lower glucose. Insulinomas are a special class of pancreatic tumors, and should not be confused with the more common form of pancreatic cancer, which does not increase the risk of hypoglycemia.

Special Case of Alcoholic Ketoacidosis

Alcoholic ketoacidosis (AKA) is an anomaly of glucose disorders. The patient presents with the signs and symptoms of DKA yet is hypoglycemic. AKA is a distinct syndrome seen in patients with a history of chronic alcoholism.

Although the pathophysiology is not completely understood, in essence AKA is a competition within the liver between the metabolism of ethanol alcohol and the production of glucose via gluconeogenesis (Figure 13-5). As a result, partial products of metabolism, including ketonic acids, are produced, without the hoped for glucose. Patients with AKA will be dehydrated, malnourished, and hypoglycemic. Therefore, the patient must be treated for hypoglycemia as well as dehydration.

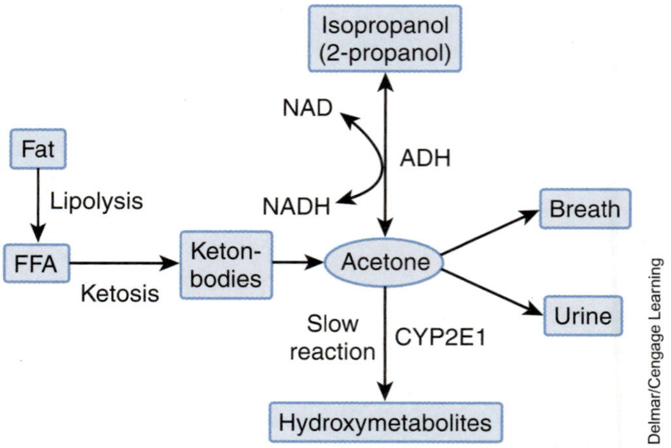

Figure 13-5 Ketoacidosis from the fat metabolism.

The Paramedics are met on scene by three EMTS from a BLS engine company codispatched with them. The providers are brought to Apt. 2D by the building superintendent. When they knock on the door, they are answered with a grunt. As they enter they take note of the apartment, which has expensive furniture and knick knacks but looks as if it hasn't been cared for in several days. Mr. Joslin is lying supine on a bed. There is an emesis basin nearby with bile-colored liquid in it.

One EMT searches the apartment to find Mr. Joslin's medications and, if possible, information on his past history. Another EMT begins interviewing the building superintendent. The Paramedics begin their assessment.

CRITICAL THINKING QUESTIONS

1. What are the important elements of the history that a Paramedic should obtain?
2. What is the symptom pattern for suspected diabetic emergency?

History

The suspicion of a diabetic emergency is based on the patient presentation, particularly if he has an altered mental status. Treatment should be focused on the immediate relief of the complications of disorders of glucose metabolism. However, of equal importance is obtaining a history which helps to identify the cause of the disorder so that it may be prevented in the future.

Hypoglycemia

An important element in the history of a patient with hypoglycemia is the time of the last meal. A fasting hypoglycemia usually occurs just before mealtime. In contrast, postprandial hypoglycemia typically occurs two to four hours after a meal. However, postprandial hypoglycemia is cause for concern. This hypoglycemia may be due to insulin overdose, which could be accidental or the result of a pancreatic cancer or insulinoma. The more likely cause of hypoglycemia is either a missed meal or a meal that is high in proteins and fats but low in simple carbohydrates.

STREET SMART

Bariatric surgery for obesity can lead to a form of reactive hypoglycemia. This alimentary induced hypoglycemia typically occurs within one to three hours after a meal.

The hypoglycemic effects of ethanol alcohol should not be underestimated. Any patient who appears intoxicated should be suspected of having hypoglycemia and tested for blood glucose.

Diabetic Ketoacidosis

The classic triad of symptoms of type 1 diabetes are the three "poly's"—polyuria, polydipsia, and polyphagia. In fact, some cases of juvenile onset diabetes are first suspected after episodes of nocturia and enuresis (bedwetting).

As the blood glucose climbs to dangerous levels, the patient will experience generalized weakness, lethargy, and nausea with vomiting. In addition, some patients initially present with abdominal pain.

The most common underlying reason for the development of DKA is an infection, with urinary tract infections (UTI) being the largest source of infection. Therefore, the patient's history should include questions about fever and chills.

Noncompliance with insulin regimens is the next leading cause of DKA. Undiagnosed diabetes is a relatively minor source of DKA (i.e., approximately 15% of cases), as other symptoms tend to encourage the patient to seek medical attention.

The initial presentation of HONKS includes altered mental status, with drowsiness, delirium, and even coma.[26] Some patients with HONKS may demonstrate stroke-like symptoms, such as hemiparesis or visual disturbances, and may even convulse. Like DKA, the patient with HONKS will have polyuria and polydipsia. However, unlike DKA, patients with HONKS usually do not have abdominal pain.

According to the superintendent, Mr. Joslin is a chemistry teacher and lives alone. His sister had called asking that someone please check on her brother as he had a history of diabetes and she hadn't been able to reach him by phone. The superintendent found Mr. Joslin like this and called 9-1-1. The EMT states that he found insulin in the refrigerator along with pill bottles labeled atenolol and micronase.

Mr. Joslin is verbally responsive and has an open airway with a fruity odor to his breath. He is breathing deeply and rapidly and feels warm to the touch. The last blood sugar reading noted on his glucometer was dated yesterday afternoon and was 289. He appears to have vomited but there is no evidence of food in the vomitus.

CRITICAL THINKING QUESTIONS

1. What are the elements of the physical examination of a patient with suspected acute coronary syndrome?
2. Why is a blood glucose reading a critical element in this examination?

Examination

Hypoglycemia, diabetic ketoacidosis, and hyperosmolar hyperglycemic nonketotic syndrome can all present with altered mental status. Therefore, it is imperative that the Paramedic immediately ascertain the patient's blood glucose while simultaneously attending to the airway.

Measuring Blood Glucose

The amount of glucose circulating through the bloodstream can be measured either in a laboratory using a whole blood specimen, or on a smaller device known as a glucometer. A **glucometer** (Figure 13-6) is a handheld device that requires less than a drop of blood to measure the patient's glucose level. The blood is usually obtained from the patient's finger using a thin lancet to pierce the skin after it has been cleaned with an alcohol swab. Typically, the first drop of blood is wiped away and the next drop is used for measurement. Results are reported within one to two minutes, although new glucometers can give results in as quickly as 10 to 15 seconds. Most diabetics own their own glucometer, as it is important for them to monitor their daily blood glucose levels. In some states, basic level EMTs are permitted to use or assist with the use of glucometers. In other states, however, only advanced level EMTs or Paramedics are allowed to practice this skill. Regardless of who obtains the fingerstick glucose level, this information can be very important in the diagnosis and management of a glucose disorder.

A number of factors affect the accuracy and performance of a glucometer.[27] Altitude, humidity, and ambient temperature can have effects on the test strips. A patient's hematocrit can also have an impact on the glucometer reading. Patients with higher hematocrit readings (e.g., patients with emphysema who are polycythemic) will generally register lower blood glucose. Conversely, those patients with low hematocrits (i.e., patients with anemia) may have higher than average blood glucose readings. For these reasons, it is important that the Paramedic obtain a complete history and take that history into account when treating the patient with a suspected glucose disorder.

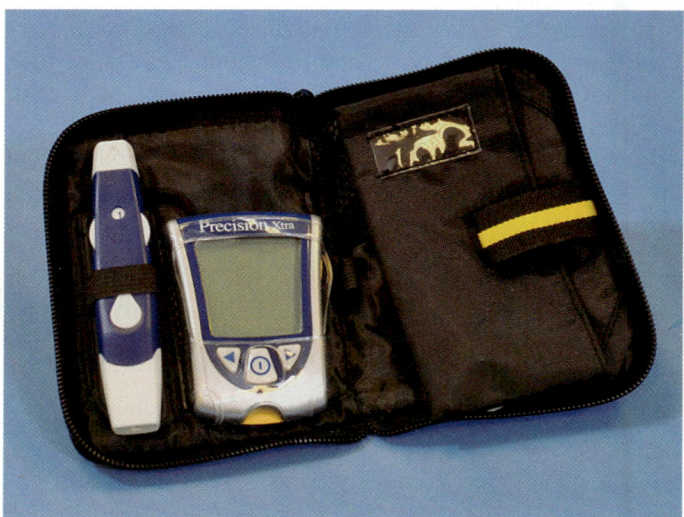

Figure 13-6 Glucometer.

Delmar/Cengage Learning

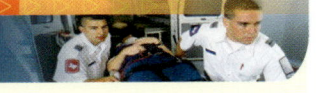
As much as a 15% variation can exist between glucose readings obtained from whole blood (by fingerstick) versus glucose readings obtained from plasma (obtained during intravenous access). Furthermore, blood glucose readings from a fingerstick may be inaccurate if the patient's peripheral capillary bed is shut down by catecholamine release during hypoglycemia. For these reasons, it is important that the Paramedic consider not only the glucometer reading but the entire clinical picture.

Hypoglycemia

The symptom pattern associated with hypoglycemia is the result of the release of a catecholamine such as epinephrine. These symptoms, which are the result of sympathetic stimulation, are called **neuroglycopenic** symptoms. However, the diagnosis of hypoglycemia can be the result of other diseases besides diabetes. For example, Addison disease, adrenal crisis, alcoholism, and hypopituitarism can also cause hypoglycemia.

The hypoglycemic diabetic patient, with neuroglycopenic symptoms, will often present with restlessness and agitation, as well as tremors and shakiness. The patient may even become combative. The patient's skin will be pale, cool, and diaphoretic. Hemodynamically, the patient will be hyperdynamic, with tachycardia and hypertension. This state may give rise to anginal chest pain and/or dysrhythmias.

Hypoglycemic Unawareness

Patients with chronic diabetes (i.e., ongoing for greater than 10 years) may not present with the classic symptom pattern of catecholamine release. For a variety of reasons, including neuropathy and beta blocker therapy, the normal response is blunted and the patient may not have recognizable signs of hypoglycemia. In some cases, the patient may become unconscious from hypoglycemia, never realizing that he was hypoglycemic. Additional signs of hypoglycemia in those patients may include yawning, perioral numbness, and heaviness in the legs. Even if the patient states that he is feeling fine, it is prudent to verify blood glucose if there is any suspicion of hypoglycemia.

Diabetic Ketoacidosis

The symptom pattern associated with diabetic ketoacidosis is the result of dehydration and acidosis. The dehydration, the consequence of osmotic diuresis, results in soft or sunken eyes that lack luster, dry mucous membranes in the mouth, a furrowed tongue, and generally poor skin turgor. The decrease in body water, particularly circulating blood volume, can cause tachycardia and postural hypotension. In addition, loss of electrolytes—particularly potassium and magnesium—during diuresis impacts muscle tone and leads to weakness.

Compensation for acidosis, created during ketosis, leads to the characteristic hyperpnea and tachypnea of breathing called Kussmaul's respiration. In fact, EMS may have been called because the patient complained of shortness of breath. Acetone, a by-product of acetoacetic acid (a ketonic acid), may also be detected, though not all people can smell acetone due to genetic predisposition.[28]

Beyond the Kussmaul's respiration, acetone breath, and signs of dehydration, the Paramedic may note the patient's altered mental status. An altered mental status is a key sign of decompensated diabetic ketoacidosis.

Hyperosmolar Nonketotic Syndrome

The presentation of HONKS in a patient is one of profound dehydration without ketosis. Because the patient's pancreas is still secreting minimal amounts of insulin, the patient avoids ketosis. Kussmaul's respiration and acetone breath only occur when ketosis occurs.

The key finding that should raise the Paramedic's suspicion of HONKS is altered mental status and extreme hyperglycemia. As a result of the hyperglycemia, the patient's mental status may range from mild confusion to delirium to coma. The patient may also be observed to experience partial or generalized seizures. Myoclonus, a twitching of muscles secondary to hypokalemia, may also be witnessed.

Patients with HONKS often present with concurrent tachycardia secondary to extreme dehydration and may be orthostatic (i.e., experiencing syncope when they stand).

However, orthostatic vital signs may not be evident in this patient population if regulatory mechanisms remain intact.

A head, eyes, ears, nose, and throat (HEENT) examination may reveal sunken eyes, dry mucous membranes, and a furrowed tongue. These are all signs of dehydration. A complete neurological examination may also reveal loss of visual fields, such as peripheral vision or a nystagmus.

CASE STUDY (CONTINUED)

The patient's blood glucose reading comes back "too high to read." The Paramedic takes a moment and reflects upon the symptom complex the team has assembled and his knowledge of hyperglycemic emergencies. He suspects that the patient is in diabetic ketoacidosis.

CRITICAL THINKING QUESTIONS

1. What is the significance of the elevated blood glucose?
2. What diagnosis did the Paramedic announce to the superintendent to relay to the family?

Assessment

The Paramedic's diagnosis of a disorder of glucose metabolism, either hypoglycemia or hyperglycemia, is based upon an accurate history and physical. For example, the diagnosis of hypoglycemia is based upon Whipple's triad (neuroglycopenic symptoms, report of low blood glucose, and symptomatic relief with administration of glucose).

Differentiation between HONKS and DKA in the prehospital setting is not as important as the understanding that the patient is experiencing a disorder of glucose metabolism in the form of hyperglycemia. Patients with untreated DKA have mortality rates as high as 20% whereas patients with untreated HONKS can have mortality rates as high as 70%.

CASE STUDY (CONTINUED)

Based on the initial findings, one EMT is instructed to use a BVM to assist ventilations with supplemental oxygen. One Paramedic sets up for IV access and a check of the blood glucose level. The other Paramedic sets up the cardiac monitor for ongoing monitoring and a 12-lead ECG. The Paramedic elects to start physiologic stabilization while on scene, knowing that working in the back of the ambulance on narrow and poorly maintained city streets can be difficult at best.

CRITICAL THINKING QUESTIONS

1. What is the standard of care of patients with suspected hyperglycemia?
2. What are some of the patient-specific concerns and considerations that the Paramedic should consider when applying this plan of care that is intended to treat a broad patient population presenting with diabetic emergency?

Treatment

Although hyperglycemia cannot be resolved in the field, the Paramedic must be prepared to treat the complications associated with hyperglycemia as well as offer care that supports the patient's efforts to compensate for the effects of hyperglycemia.

Hyperosmolar Nonketotic Syndrome

Fortunately, the treatment for HONKS and DKA is essentially the same in the prehospital setting. After assuring an adequate airway, the Paramedic should establish intravenous access and start a bolus of normal saline. It is common to replace one-half the estimated body fluid loss (usually between 8 and 12 liters) in the first 12 hours of patient care. However, unless transport time is prolonged, the Paramedic will likely administer 1 to 2 liters of normal saline during her patient contact. Saline bolus should be limited when or if the blood glucose drops below 250 mg/dL. If possible, the Paramedic should draw a pre-infusion blood sample for later analysis.

If the patient should experience a convulsion, standard anticonvulsant medications (such as diazepam or midazolam) are effective in limiting the seizure activity. If the patient is in a coma, then airway management is of paramount importance. Unlike DKA, there is no empirical evidence to support the routine use of sodium bicarbonate.

Diabetic Ketoacidosis

As vomiting is often associated with diabetic ketoacidosis, the Paramedic must be prepared to suction the patient's airway as needed and, perhaps more importantly, prevent vomiting by the administration of antiemetics. If a decreased level of consciousness imperils the patient's airway, the Paramedic must be prepared to secure the airway. This may include the use of endotracheal intubation.

The Paramedic should also be prepared to support the patient's ventilation. Kussmaul's respiration can lead to respiratory distress and exhaustion, with a resultant increase in acidosis and subsequent peripheral vasodilation. This profound vasodilation, in turn, leads to hypotension and hypoperfusion.

As electrolyte imbalances are a concomitant complication of diabetic ketoacidosis, the Paramedic should place the patient on the ECG monitor and obtain intravenous access. The patient in diabetic ketoacidosis may have as much as a 5 or 6 liter fluid deficit; therefore, intravenous administration of 1 to 2 liters of normal saline is appropriate, provided there are no contraindications such as pulmonary edema.[29–31] Subsequent fluid boluses may be given in 200 cc doses. The administration of a fluid bolus has the twofold advantage of diluting hyperglycemia as well as diluting acidosis. After administration of 1.5 liters of normal saline, the blood glucose may drop by as much as 20%.

Hyperglycemia is particularly problematic for the patient with borderline heart function, which often occurs in patients with diabetes. The glucose-laden blood is difficult for the heart to pump. The administration of a normal saline bolus can dilute the blood, making it easier for the heart to pump and helping the heart to recover from its failure.

Finally, the administration of a fluid bolus can help to increase distal perfusion and therefore decrease the formation of lactate acidosis, which is created during anaerobic respiration. Therefore, a fluid bolus can help to decrease the formation of acid and the patient's acid load.

Hypoglycemia

Once hypoglycemia has been identified, treatment should begin immediately with some form of glucose. If a patient is awake, alert, and able to swallow without aspirating, the patient should take some form of oral glucose, such as a tablespoon of sugar or honey, hard candy, fruit juice, carbonated beverage (not diet), or even jelly beans. The Paramedic may elect to use three or more glucose tablets or a tube of glucose (each approximately 15 grams).

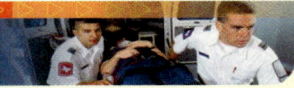

Most diabetics, especially those taking insulin, are aware of when their blood sugar is dropping and will take in sugar-laden foodstuffs on their own without needing to call for EMS assistance. The one drawback to oral administration of glucose is that it immediately stimulates the pancreas to release insulin, which may negatively counterbalance the effects of the glucose load. However, most experts recommend at least attempting oral replacement if it is safe to do so.

Patients with altered mental status or for whom administration of oral glucose would be unsafe should receive dextrose intravenously as a bolus. A common formulation is D_{50} (dextrose 50%) in single-dose packages. One amp of D_{50} supplies 25 grams of dextrose, which may be enough to return the patient's blood glucose levels to normal. If the patient's blood glucose is borderline, some Paramedics administer half the dose (i.e., administer 12.5 grams of the 25 grams of 50% dextrose). If a patient is profoundly hypoglycemic and does not respond completely to one amp, or if the blood glucose measured 10 minutes after D_{50} administration is still low, a second bolus may be given.

Intravenous Access

Due to changes in the venous blood vessel, secondary to diabetes, intravenous access may be difficult for the Paramedic to obtain. Further complicating the situation, administration of a bolus of viscous solution requires a large bore access.

High-concentration glucose, D_{50}, is not only viscous, but it also creates a high osmotic pressure. If D_{50} infiltrates the intravenous site, the high osmotic pressure will draw fluid from surrounding cells, resulting in necrosis. Understanding this phenomenon, venous access patency is critical. Venous access at either the antecubital space or the back of the hand (areas with tendons or nerves) should be avoided. At every instance when D_{50} is being administered, the patency of the venous access must be confirmed, usually by flashback, and the site closely observed for infiltration during administration.

Glucagon

If a patient does not have IV access or if attempts at IV access will significantly delay therapy, glucagon may be administered intramuscularly or subcutaneously. Although it does not directly raise blood glucose levels like dextrose, glucagon stimulates glycogenolysis in the liver, resulting in the breakdown of glycogen into glucose molecules that are then released from the liver. Therefore, glucagon only works if the patient has sufficient glycogen stores in the liver. Fasting, malnourished, alcoholic, or anorexic patients may not have adequate glycogen stores.

The typical dose of glucagon is 1 mg/mL for an adult or one-half of that dose for children (i.e., 0.5 mg for children less than 55 kg). Pregnant women or nursing mothers can also use glucagon as it is an FDA category B medication.

Glucagon, as a naturally occurring or endogenous hormone, and its diluents must be mixed in the field prior to administration. It may take 10 to 20 minutes before blood glucose is elevated to minimal acceptable levels. Therefore, it is imperative that the Paramedic's attempts at either venous or intraosseous access continue.

A study published in the *Annals of Emergency Medicine* in 1991 established glucagon as a safe and effective therapy for hypoglycemia in the prehospital setting.[32] In this study, patients given glucagon had an average increase in serum glucose from 33 mg/dL to 133 mg/dL, and an average improvement in Glasgow coma scale (GCS) from 9 to 13 after approximately nine minutes. Since that time, glucagon

has been a standard of care for prehospital treatment of hypoglycemia when intravenous access cannot be obtained. In fact, some experts recommend using glucagon, in conscious patients, instead of oral glucose or even intravenous dextrose since it can be administered quickly without needing to start an IV and produces favorable results.[33, 34]

Some patients complain of nausea and vomiting, particularly with higher doses or glucagon-administrated rapid intravenous bolus. Because of its positive inotropic and chronotropic effect on the heart, the patient may also experience tachycardia and hypertension. Overall, glucagon administration is relatively safe. Glucagon has a large therapeutic window, with an LD_{50} of 100 to 200 mg/kg. Administration of glucagon is a relative contraindication for patients with a pheochromocytoma, an epinephrine-secreting tumor, because it could cause a secondary hypoglycemia.

Once a patient has been given replacement glucose, regardless of route, the Paramedic should repeat a fingerstick glucose level 10 minutes following treatment to be certain the blood glucose is increasing appropriately (Figure 13-7). Many physicians and diabetes experts recommend at least 13 minutes of observation and another fingerstick to watch for rebound hypoglycemia.

Thiamine Administration

Thiamine administration in hypoglycemia has been debated in the medical and prehospital literature. Patients who are thiamine deficient due to malnourishment are at risk of developing Wernicke's encephalopathy when given a large glucose load (Wernicke's encephalopathy is discussed in Chapter 15 on disorders of addiction). However, not all hypoglycemic patients are malnourished or thiamine deficient; in fact, this population is most likely a very small minority of patients. Patients who are alcohol dependent and obtain many of their calories from alcohol are among this group. Therefore, thiamine should not be administered routinely to patients presenting with hypoglycemia unless it can be established that their low blood sugar is due to prolonged starvation or malnourishment.[35]

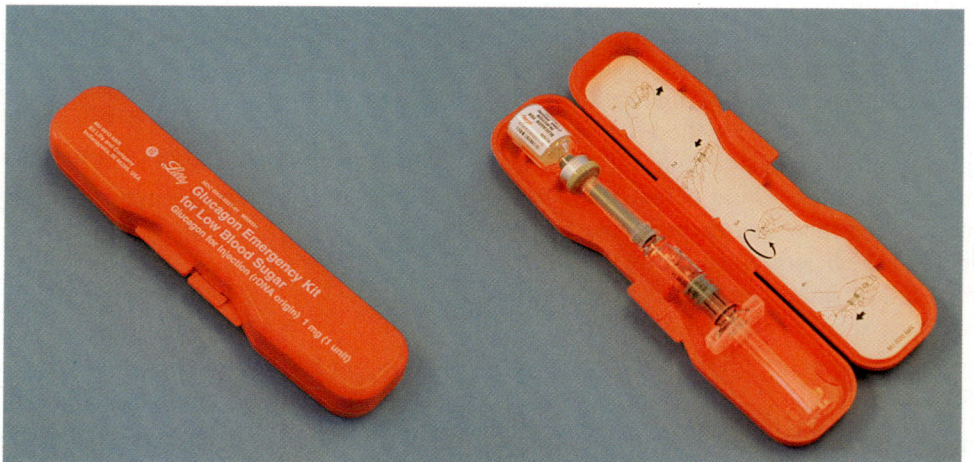

Figure 13-7 Glucagon kit.

The cardiac monitor shows a wide complex rhythm with a normal PR interval and peaked T waves. While the Paramedic is obtaining the 12-lead ECG, Mr. Joslin becomes responsive only to pain. The monitor shows ventricular tachycardia with pulses still present. One Paramedic says to the other, "This will be an interesting case for the monthly review. Hand me some sodium bicarbonate."

CRITICAL THINKING QUESTIONS

1. What is the significance of the rhythm change that occurred during transport? Why did the rhythm change occur?

2. What other issues should the Paramedic anticipate during transport?

Evaluation

Hyperkalemia is a common complication of DKA and the leading cause of death among patients with the condition. During DKA, the acidosis causes the potassium to move out of the cells and into the bloodstream, causing hyperkalemia. Hyperkalemia, acidosis and hypoxia secondary to a shift in the oxyhemoglobin curve contrive to irritate the heart, which results in ventricular tachycardia.

Hyperkalemia should be suspected when peaked T waves, with or without a depressed ST segment, are noted on the ECG. In extreme cases, the QRS may widen until it takes a sine wave-like appearance. Untreated extreme hyperkalemia can lead to ventricular dysrhythmia and even asystole. The use of competitive electrolytes such as sodium bicarbonate and calcium chloride may be in order in these cases.

After administration of sodium bicarbonate, Mr. Joslin's QRS complex narrows and the T waves start to flatten. During the 10-minute transport to the emergency department, Mr. Joslin receives a bolus of intravenous fluid and becomes increasingly more responsive. His initial blood sugar of today, 497, drops to 389; his breathing slows to 20 breaths per minute, and he is switched to a nonrebreather mask. He is transferred to an ED stretcher with report given.

Later that day, the crew calls to inquire about Mr. Joslin. The physician reports that he has a urinary tract infection, which likely led to his episode of DKA. The potassium was initially 6.9 upon admission to the ED and he is currently receiving an IV of insulin and potassium which will be switched to normal saline when his blood sugar reaches 200 mg/dL.

CRITICAL THINKING QUESTIONS

1. What is the most appropriate transport decision that will get the patient to definitive care?

2. What are the advantages of treating a patient with complications secondary to diabetic ketoacidosis while transporting the patient to the hospital?

Disposition

A controversial decision in the treatment of hypoglycemia is whether or not to transport the patient to an emergency department for evaluation. As stated earlier, many patients with diabetes can sense when their blood sugar is low and will eat something to bring it back to normal, without involving EMS or requiring hospital evaluation. However, for those patients who request EMS assistance, the choice remains for the Paramedic whether or not to transport to the ED. Most patients, if given the choice, would prefer to refuse further medical attention rather than go to a hospital. However, there are no well-established guidelines that address this issue, despite a great deal of research in this area.[36]

The key issue is the patient's ability to rationally refuse transport (i.e., whether the patient has capacity, a critical element of consent). The patient must be able to understand the consequences of the decision. Some Paramedics use an "ABC" approach to decide if the patient has capacity. At first, the Paramedic assesses the patient's **A**ffect. Next, the Paramedic should assess the patient's **B**ehavior. An agitated patient may still be hypoglycemic. Lastly, the Paramedic should assess the patient's **C**ognition (i.e., does the patient demonstrate evidence that he has good mentation)?

One caveat, however, is that any nondiabetic who presents with hypoglycemia should be transported for ED evaluation because the cause of the low glucose level may not be readily apparent. Additionally, any diabetic patient who routinely takes oral hypoglycemic agents should be transported for evaluation since the possibility of rebound hypoglycemia after treatment is much higher and less predictable than for patients taking insulin alone.

The question remains, however, whether or not it is safe for the Paramedic to release, without further medical evaluation, an insulin-dependent diabetic patient who has resolved hypoglycemia. This question was studied and answered in a 2003 study published in the *American Journal of Emergency Medicine*.[37] In this study, patients were followed-up 24 hours after their episodes of hypoglycemia for which they were not transported to an emergency department. Each of the patients studied returned to a normal glucose level and mental status. Of these patients, 91% had no complications after their on-scene treatment, and only 3% (totaling one patient) had a serious complication which required subsequent hospitalization. The authors concluded that it is safe for Paramedics to treat uncomplicated hypoglycemia in insulin-dependent diabetic patients and then discharge them without transport to an emergency department. However, the patient must not be left alone after treatment. The patient must have an adult present

Table 13-5 Pediatric Dosages (0.5 to 1 g/kg) for the Different Dextrose Solutions

Dextrose Solution	Volume for 0.5 g/kg to 1 g/kg
D_5	8 to 16 mL/kg
D_{10}	4 to 8 mL/kg
D_{25}	2 to 4 mL/kg
D_{50}	1 to 2 mL/kg

or immediately available for the next 12 hours to watch for signs of rebound hypoglycemia. The patient must also be eating a meal containing both carbohydrates and proteins to provide longer lasting glucose than the D_{50} administered by the Paramedic. Finally, the patient should be otherwise healthy and without complaint along with a reasonable explanation (e.g., missed meal, increased activity) for the episode of hypoglycemia.

Pediatric Considerations

Hypoglycemia in children is slightly different than in adults. Like adults, children who take insulin are susceptible to episodes of hypoglycemia if they do not ingest an appropriate-sized meal or snack at the time of their insulin injections. However, hypoglycemia can also occur in nondiabetic children, particularly those who are vomiting or have decreased their oral intake due to illness. Since the most common manifestations of hypoglycemia in children are altered mental status and seizure, it is recommended that fingerstick glucose be measured in any pediatric patient presenting with these symptoms. For those children who are hypoglycemic and symptomatic, treatment should be initiated with D_{10}, D_{25}, D_{50}, or glucagon by EMS (Table 13-5). For the hypoglycemic child requiring dextrose, the doses are 4 mL/kg of dextrose 10% solution or 2 mL/kg of dextrose 25% solution intravenous bolus.[38] Unlike adults, all children who are hypoglycemic should be evaluated in an emergency department regardless of resolution of symptoms or hypoglycemia.

CONCLUSION

The recognition and treatment of both hyper- and hypoglycemia begins in the field. Routine measurement of fingerstick glucose levels and the appropriate response can have a significant impact on the outcome of these patients. Although the definitive treatment will usually take place in the hospital setting, Paramedics may be able to treat some episodes of hypoglycemia in the field without requiring transportation of the patient to an ED. It is important for the Paramedic to review all state and local protocols to determine the scope of practice in those jurisdictions.

KEY POINTS:

- Carbohydrates fuel the body under normal conditions.

- Insulin opens pores in the cell, allowing glucose to enter and lowering blood sugar.

- Insulin is produced in the beta cells of the islets of Langerhans within the pancreas.

- Insulin also promotes fat storage for times of starvation.

- Common medications may increase or decrease the release of insulin for the pancreas.

- Glucagon, a counterbalance to insulin, is produced in the alpha cells of the islets of Langerhans.

- Glucagon increases blood sugar levels through glycogenolysis and gluconeogenesis.

- Blood sugar levels generally range from 70 to 140 mg/dL (depending upon lab). A blood sugar level greater than 140 mg/dL is considered hyperglycemia; lower than 70 mg/dL is considered hypoglycemia.

- Signs and symptoms of hyperglycemia may range from asymptomatic to altered mental status, dehydration, and electrolyte abnormalities.

- Diabetes mellitus is the most common cause of hyperglycemia in the United States.

- Diabetes is not a singular disease but a collection of metabolic derangements.

- Type 1 diabetes results from lack of insulin production in the pancreas.

- Persons with type 1 diabetes must take insulin on a daily basis.

- Insulin comes in many varieties depending upon onset, peak of action, and duration of action.

- Insulin syringes are marked in units.

- Insulin pumps can administer bolus doses of insulin and basal doses of insulin.

- Type 2 diabetes results from insulin resistance.

- The pancreas can increase its production of insulin, resulting in hyperinsulinemia. In diabetes, cells do not respond to the insulin increase in blood sugar.

- Treatment is aimed at increasing cellular response to the insulin.

- Pregnant women may experience gestational diabetes resulting from hormonal alterations causing insulin resistance.

- Complications of diabetes range from vascular damage to neuropathy and blindness.

- Diabetic ketoacidosis (DKA) results from the body using fats for fuel, leading to elevated blood sugar and ketone production. DKA occurs most often in type 1 diabetes and presents with polydipsia, polyuria, and polyphagia.

- Hyperosmolar, nonketotic syndrome (HONKS) results from pancreatic and renal insufficiency.

- Both DKA and HONKS cause profound dehydration and electrolyte disorders.

- HONKS develops more gradually than DKA.

- Hypoglycemia develops rapidly, leading to altered mental status, convulsions, and death unless the patient is rapidly administered sugar.

- Patients with a history of alcoholism may present with signs of ketosis, dehydration, and hypoglycemia (an unusual combination called alcoholic ketoacidosis).

- Hyperkalemia is a complication of DKA.

- Transport of the treated hypoglycemic patient depends upon the type of diabetes, the patient's ability to understand the refusal of further care processes, and the availability of an adult to monitor the patient posttreatment.

REVIEW QUESTIONS:

1. How does insulin function in the utilization of carbohydrates and storage of fats?
2. Describe the relationship between insulin and glucagon.
3. What are the signs and symptoms of hyperglycemia? Hypoglycemia?
4. How does type 1 diabetes differ from type 2 diabetes? What is gestational diabetes?
5. Explain the function of oral hypoglycemic agents.
6. How are DKA and HONKS similar to each other? How do they differ?
7. Explain the development of hyperkalemia during DKA.
8. List conditions that should be present for a patient with a treated hypoglycemic reaction to refuse further medical care.

CASE STUDY QUESTIONS:

Please refer to the Case Study in this chapter, and answer the questions below:

1. In addition to blood sugar alterations, what other likely complications can cause confusion in this patient?
2. What does the scene tell you?
3. How does the beta blocker atenolol affect insulin? How does micronase affect insulin?
4. What is the relevance of emesis without evidence of food in it?
5. Describe the relationship between Mr. Joslin's ECG results and serum potassium levels.
6. How does an illness such as a urinary tract infection lead to DKA?

REFERENCES:

1. Groff JL, Gropper SS. *Advanced Nutrition and Human Metabolism,* third edition. Belmont: Wadsworth/Thomson Learning; 2000.
2. Horton R, Moran L, Perry M, Rawn D, Scrimgeour, G. *Principles of Biochemistry,* fourth edition. Alexandria, VA: Prentice Hall; 2005.
3. Berne RM, Levy MN. *Physiology*, fourth edition. St. Louis: Mosby, Inc.; 1998.
4. Hingorjo MR, Syed S, et al. (2007). Current trends in type 1 diabetes mellitus—stem cells and beyond. *J Pak Med Assoc.* 2007;57(12):603–606.
5. American Diabetes Association. Available at: **http://www .diabetes.org**. Accessed March 7, 2008.
6. **http://en.wikipedia.org/wiki/Diabetes_mellitus**. Accessed March 7, 2008.

7. Centers for Disease Control and Prevention. Available at: **http://www.cdc.gov**. Accessed March 7, 2008.

8. World Health Organization. Available at: **http://www.who.int**. Accessed March 7, 2008.

9. Cotran RS, Kumar V, Collins T. *Robbins' Pathological Basis of Disease,* sixth edition. Philadelphia: W.B. Saunders Company; 1999.

10. Arnolds S, Heise T. Inhaled insulin. *Best Pract Res Clin Endocrinol Metab.* 2007;21(4):555–571.

11. Setter SM, Levien TL, et al. Inhaled dry powder insulin for the treatment of diabetes mellitus. *Clin Ther.* 2007;29(5):795–813.

12. Ioannidis I. The road from obesity to type 2 diabetes. *Angiology.* 2008;59(2 Suppl):39S–43S.

13. Guilherme A, Virbasius JV, et al. Adipocyte dysfunctions linking obesity to insulin resistance and type 2 diabetes. *Nat Rev: Mol Cell Biol.* 2008;9(5):367–377.

14. Bell DS, Yumuk V. Frequency of severe hypoglycemia in patients with non-insulin-dependent diabetes mellitus treated with sulfonylureas or insulin. *Endocr Pract.* 1997;3(5):281–283.

15. van Staa T, Abenhaim L, et al. Rates of hypoglycemia in users of sulfonylureas. *J Clin Epidemiol.* 1997;50(6):735–741.

16. Adams HP, et al. Guidelines for the early management of adults with ischemic stroke. *Stroke.* 2007;38:1655–1711.

17. Leitao CB, Krahe AL, et al. Aspirin therapy is still underutilized among patients with type 2 diabetes. *Arq Bras Endocrinol Metabol.* 2006;50(6):1014–1019.

18. Faragon JJ, Waite NM, et al. Improving aspirin prophylaxis in a primary care diabetic population. *Pharmacotherapy.* 2003;23(1):73–79.

19. Rosenberg EA, Sperazza LC. The visually impaired patient. *Am Fam Physician.* 2008;77(10):1431–1436.

20. Tumosa N. Eye disease and the older diabetic. *Clin Geriatr Med.* 2008;24(3):515–527, vii.

21. Wolfson AB. *Harwood-Nuss' Clinical Practice of Emergency Medicine*, fourth edition. Philadelphia: Lippincott Williams & Wilkins; 2005.

22. Levine SN, Sanson TH. Treatment of hyperglycaemic hyperosmolar non-ketotic syndrome. *Drugs.* 1989;38(3):462–472.

23. Magee MF, Bhatt BA. Management of decompensated diabetes. Diabetic ketoacidosis and hyperglycemic hyperosmolar syndrome. *Crit Care Clin.* 2001;17(1):75–106.

24. Adams HP, et al. Guidelines for the early management of adults with ischemic stroke. *Stroke.* 2007;38:1655–1711.

25. Halfdanarson TR, Rubin J, et al. Pancreatic endocrine neoplasms: epidemiology and prognosis of pancreatic endocrine tumors. *Endocr-Relat Cancer.* 2008;15(2):409–427.

26. Small M, Alzaid A, et al. Diabetic hyperosmolar non-ketotic decompensation. *Q J Med.* 1988;66(251):251–257.

27. Eastham JH, Mason D, et al. Prevalence of interfering substances with point-of-care glucose testing in a community hospital. *Am J Health-Syst Pharm.* 2009;66(2):167–170.

28. Laffel L. Ketone bodies: a review of physiology, pathophysiology and application of monitoring to diabetes. *Diabetes Metab Res Rev.* 1999;15(6):412–426.

29. Cardella F. Insulin therapy during diabetic ketoacidosis in children. *Acta Biomed.* 2005;76 Suppl 3:49–54.

30. Bevacqua JE. Diabetic ketoacidosis in the pediatric ICU. *Crit Care Nurs Clin North Am.* 2005;17(4):341–347, x.

31. Harris GD, Fiordalisi I. Physiologic management of diabetic ketoacidemia. A 5-year prospective pediatric experience in 231 episodes. *Arch Pediatr Adolesc Med.* 1994;148(10):1046–1052.

32. Vukmir RB, et al. Glucagon: prehospital therapy for hypoglycemia. *Annals of Emergency Medicine.* 1991;20:375–379.

33. Vermeulen MJ, et al. Subcutaneous glucagon may be better than oral glucose for prehospital treatment of symptomatic hypoglycemia. *Diabetes Care.* 2003;26(8):2472–2473.

34. Carstens S, Sprehn M. Prehospital treatment of severe hypoglycaemia: a comparison of intramuscular glucagon and intravenous glucose. *Prehosp Dis Med.* 1998;13(2-4):44–50.

35. Bledsoe BE. No more coma cocktails. Using science to dispel myths & improve patient care. *JEMS.* 2002;27(11):54–60.

36. Steinmetz J, et al. Hypoglycaemia in patients with diabetes: do they prefer prehospital treatment or admission to hospital? *Eur J Emerg Med.* 2006;13:319–320.

37. Lerner EB, et al. Can Paramedics safely treat and discharge hypoglycemic patients in the field? *Am J Emerg Med.* 2003;21(2):115–120.

38. Kwon KT. Metabolic and endocrine disorders. In: Wolfson AB, et al, ed. *Harwood-Nuss' Clinical Practice of Emergency Medicine,* fifth edition. Lippincott, Williams & Wilkins, Philadelphia, PA. 2010.

CHAPTER 14

DISORDERS OF HOMEOSTASIS

KEY CONCEPTS:

Upon completion of this chapter, it is expected that the reader will understand these following concepts:

- How the body regulates its internal environment to maintain balance (homeostasis)
- That the endocrine system secretes hormones that interact with all body systems
- That hormones can directly cause an action or can stimulate another organ to release a chemical that will cause an action
- How the body's inability to maintain homeostasis may be the cause of—or the result of—critical illness or injury

ANATOMY CONCEPTS:

Prior to reading this chapter the Paramedic student should be familiar with the following anatomy and physiology concepts:

- Endocrine system
- Feedback mechanisms

"Medic 702, please respond to 5275 Malderboro Hill Road, upper left apartment, for a 45-year-old female with altered mental status."

"Altered mental status calls are so challenging," says the senior Paramedic. "There are so many conditions that can cause that. Remember that CME lecture last month on endocrine emergencies? Many of those conditions cause altered mental status and are so tough to figure out!" Both partners quietly reflect on that CME session while responding to the scene.

CRITICAL THINKING QUESTIONS

1. What are some of the possible causes of altered mental status?
2. Are there some basic disorders that can cause altered mental status?

OVERVIEW

Homeostasis is the body's ability to maintain a state of internal balance. This occurs through many complex mechanisms that maintain adequate blood sugar, temperature, vital signs, hormone levels, and metabolism. A healthy body can automatically handle significant stress while maintaining homeostasis. However, at times the body's balance can be disrupted. Pituitary, adrenal, thyroid, and electrolyte disorders all affect homeostasis. These imbalances can cause serious damage to the body, especially in critically ill patients. Therefore, the Paramedic must understand the mechanisms of homeostasis in order to successfully manage these complex patients.

Chief Concern

Homeostasis is maintained in the human body through several complex mechanisms that regulate metabolism, temperature, blood chemistry, and glucose levels. The major types of disorders affecting homeostasis are pituitary disorders, adrenal disorders, thyroid disorders, and fluid and electrolyte disorders. The pituitary, adrenal, and thyroid glands (Figure 14-1) are part of the endocrine system and secrete various hormones that help regulate the body's systems.

Pituitary Disorders

The pituitary gland, located at the base of the brain, is referred to as the master gland because it secretes hormones that control other glands (e.g., the thyroid). The hormones produced by the pituitary regulate growth, reproduction, and development. Key hormones secreted by the pituitary include **thyroid stimulating hormone (TSH)**, which controls the thyroid gland; **adrenocorticotropic hormone (ACTH)**, which controls the adrenal gland; and **antidiuretic hormone (ADH)**, also known as vasopressin, which signals the kidneys to absorb water. Although congenital deficiency in pituitary hormones can cause growth and development issues, development of **hypopituitarism** as an adult is often caused by decreased blood flow to the pituitary, tumor compression of the pituitary, subarachnoid hemorrhage, traumatic brain injury, inflammation of the pituitary gland, or (in women) necrosis of the pituitary after childbirth. Many of the signs and symptoms that develop are similar to problems associated with the target glands controlled by the pituitary. These signs and symptoms may develop acutely, and the patient may decompensate acutely if the event occurs suddenly (e.g., as with a subarachnoid hemorrhage). More often, however, the symptoms develop gradually over a period of time as the hormones are depleted and not replaced. This can lead to vague complaints from the patient. Many patients with a history of traumatic brain injury will develop some degree of hypopituitarism over 3 to 12 months after the injury.[1]

Symptoms are related to the specific hormone deficiency. For example, deficiency of the thyroid stimulation hormone will cause signs and symptoms similar to hypothyroidism

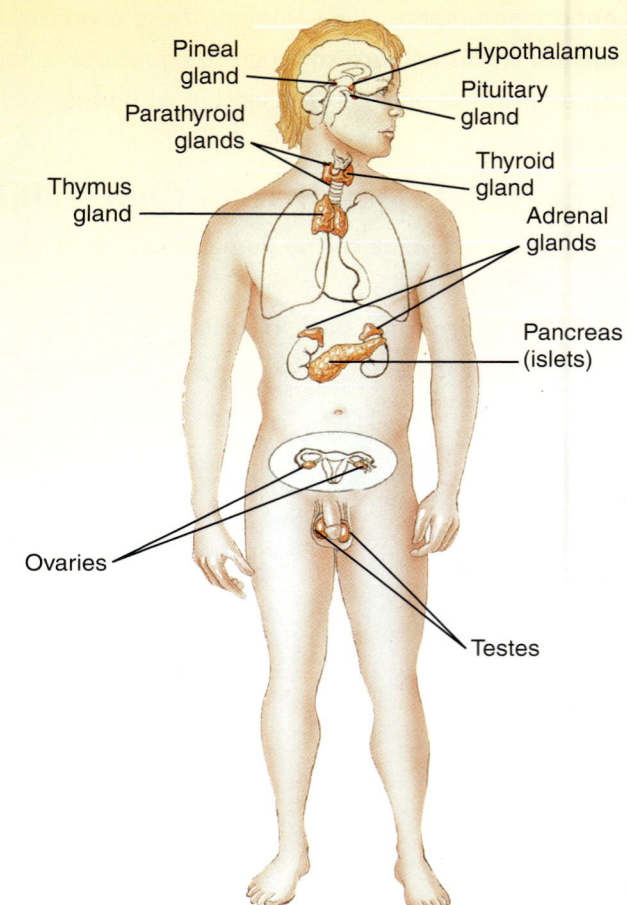

Endocrine system: Pituitary, thyroid, parathyroid, thymus, adrenal and pineal glands, as well as portions of hypothalamus, pancreas, liver, kidneys, skin, digestive tract, ovaries, testes, and placenta. Also included are hormonal secretions from each gland.

Delmar/Cengage Learning

Figure 14-1 The pituitary, adrenal, and thyroid glands are part of the endocrine system.

and deficiencies of adrenocorticotropic hormone will cause signs and symptoms similar to **hypoadrenalism**, or decreased adrenal gland function. Deficiencies in antidiuretic hormone, or vasopressin, will cause a condition known as **diabetes insipidus**. Much of the fluid filtered by the kidneys is normally reabsorbed into the bloodstream. The amount of fluid absorbed is controlled by antidiuretic hormone. If antidiuretic hormone is deficient, the patient will produce excessive urine that is very dilute. This condition can be severe enough that the patient becomes hypotensive when her fluid intake is far exceeded by her urinary output. Patients often have polyuria and polydipsia, very similar to patients who develop elevated blood glucose levels. However, in patients with diabetes insipidus the blood glucose is normal or only mildly elevated—not to the extent to produce polyuria and polydipsia.

Adrenal Disorders

The adrenal glands sit on top of the kidneys (Figure 14-1) and serve to regulate several body systems. The adrenal gland is divided into two distinct areas: the medulla and the cortex (Figure 14-2). The centrally located medulla manufactures and secretes epinephrine and norepinephrine into the bloodstream in response to activation by the sympathetic nervous system. This enhances sympathetic nervous system stimulation. The outer cortex layer of the adrenal gland secretes three different types of **steroids** which control glucose production, protein, and fat metabolism; as well as maintain salt balance, vascular tone, cardiac contractility, and reproductive cycles. The androgens are responsible for the reproductive cycles in both males and females. **Glucocorticoids** are responsible

for the actions that assist the body in responding to stresses (Table 14-1), whether physical, emotional, external (e.g., trauma), or internal (e.g., infection). If the glucocorticoids are low, the patient may develop cardiovascular collapse and shock in response to any stress placed on the body.[2,3] Finally, aldosterone is the primary **mineralocorticoid** produced by the adrenal gland and is responsible for increasing sodium and water reabsorption in the kidneys while causing the release of potassium in the urine. The absorption of sodium and water from the urine helps to maintain an adequate intravascular fluid volume and therefore maintain blood pressure.

Adrenal disorders can occur due to either an excess of adrenal hormones or a decrease of adrenal hormones. **Cushing's syndrome** occurs when there is an excess of adrenal hormones, causing hypertension, elevated blood glucose, insulin resistance, and hypokalemia (low potassium). Patients with Cushing's syndrome develop weight gain with fat deposits in their trunk (referred to as truncal obesity) as well as in the upper back (sometimes referred to as a buffalo hump), a rounded face referred to as a moon face (Figure 14-3), and hyperpigmentation. Cushing's syndrome can be caused by an increase in steroid production by the adrenal glands but can also be seen in patients who are on chronic steroid medications. Cushing's syndrome develops gradually over time, and

Table 14-1 Glucocorticoid Actions

- Stimulate glucose production and decrease cell use
- Inhibit the effects of insulin
- Increase red blood cell and platelet levels
- Perform anti-inflammatory effects on the body
- Maintain vascular tone
- Maintain cardiac contractility

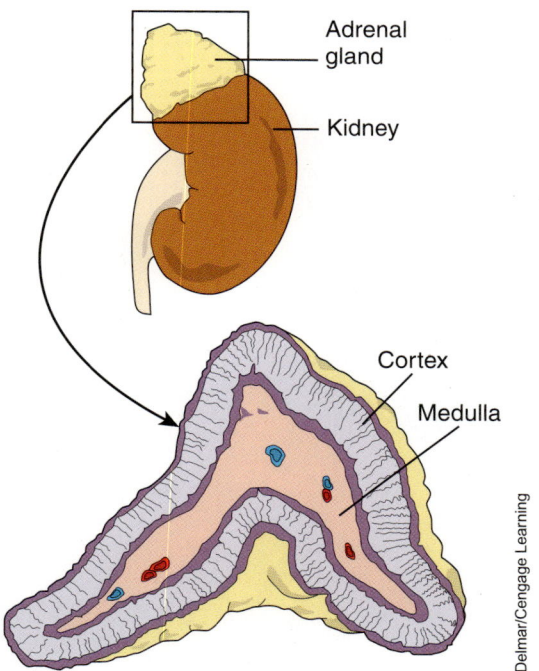

Figure 14-2 The adrenal glands are located atop both kidneys and are divided into the central medulla and the surrounding cortex.

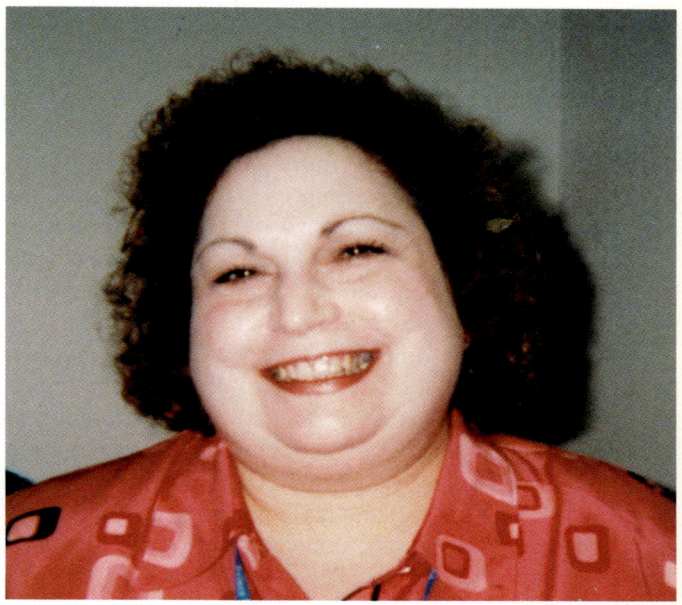

Figure 14-3 A patient with Cushing's syndrome.

by itself does not produce emergent issues for the Paramedic. However, patients may present to EMS with complaints related to exacerbations of their hypertension or hyperglycemia.

In contrast, a patient who develops adrenal insufficiency can present to EMS as severely ill and in shock. Addison's disease is a condition in which the adrenal gland chronically does not produce enough steroids. In an acute setting, adrenal insufficiency occurs most often in patients who were on chronic steroids (e.g., prednisone) and who stopped the steroids suddenly. Once a patient has been on high dose steroids for longer than two weeks, the adrenal glands produce a smaller amount of natural glucocorticoids, and eventually halt production. With a sudden decrease in externally supplied glucocorticoids, the patient will develop adrenal crisis and become severely hypotensive.[4]

This condition will not respond to intravenous fluids and vasopressor support. Other causes of an adrenal crisis include hemorrhage in the adrenal gland or a clot that disrupts the blood supply to the adrenal glands. Head trauma which damages the pituitary gland and affects ACTH production may also cause adrenal crisis. In addition, adrenal crisis may occur in a patient with chronic adrenal insufficiency who faces an acute stress (e.g., trauma, surgery, or illness) that exceeds the adrenal glands' ability to compensate for the stress.

Unfortunately, many of these patients will either not know that they have adrenal insufficiency or will not be able to communicate that to the Paramedic. Patients who have adrenal insufficiency often complain of fatigue, anorexia, and unexplained weight loss and have a baseline low blood pressure, orthostatic blood pressure changes, thin hair, and chronic electrolyte imbalance. Again, patients with adrenal insufficiency may develop an adrenal crisis if their body is stressed beyond its capability to handle the stress.

Thyroid Disorders

The thyroid gland, located in the neck just anterior to the larynx (Figure 14-1), is a small gland controlled by the pituitary gland that is responsible for controlling the body's rate of energy production and function. The thyroid may either produce an overabundance of hormone, increasing metabolism, or produce less hormone, decreasing metabolism. Metabolism may also be increased by other substances that mimic thyroid hormones such as those often found in weight loss preparations or thyroid replacement medications. In contrast with the adrenal gland, the Paramedic may experience emergent conditions in patients with both hyperthyroidism and hypothyroidism.

A **goiter** is an enlargement of the thyroid gland that may be caused by inflammation, cancer, or overproduction of hormone. Goiters are classified as nontoxic if they do not produce symptoms or changes in serum thyroid hormone levels. If the goiter is associated with symptoms or overproduction of thyroid hormone, it is called a toxic goiter. Some goiters can grow very large and become uncomfortable if the airway or larynx is compressed; however, they are not usually painful.

Hyperthyroidism can occur for several reasons, including problems with the pituitary gland; inflammation of the thyroid gland that may be caused by radiation, infection, trauma, or autoimmune disease; or drug use. Hyperthyroidism induced by autoimmune disease is called **Graves' disease**.

Sympathetic nervous system activity is increased in hyperthyroidism, producing an increased heart rate and blood pressure. The first indication of hyperthyroidism in a patient may be palpitations or a supraventricular tachycardia.[5,6] Patients with hyperthyroidism often complain of heat intolerance (such that they prefer cooler environments), palpitations, unexplained weight loss, sweating, tremors, nervousness, weakness, and fatigue. Some patients will develop an enlarged and visible thyroid gland or exophthalmos (Figure 14-4). **Exophthalmos** associated with Graves' disease is the bilateral protrusion of the eyes and retraction of the eyelids due to deposits of connective tissue behind the eyes.

A rare and potentially life-threatening form of hyperthyroidism is thyroid storm. **Thyroid storm** occurs due to an elevation in thyroid hormones and is often precipitated by a specific event, such as surgery or an infection. The sympathetic response is extreme, producing significant hypertension and tachycardia. In this state of significantly increased metabolism, the patient becomes hyperthermic, agitated, tremulous, and psychotic. Patients with thyroid storm eventually become hypotensive and comatose before death. However, it is estimated that only 1% of patients with hyperthyroidism will develop thyroid storm.

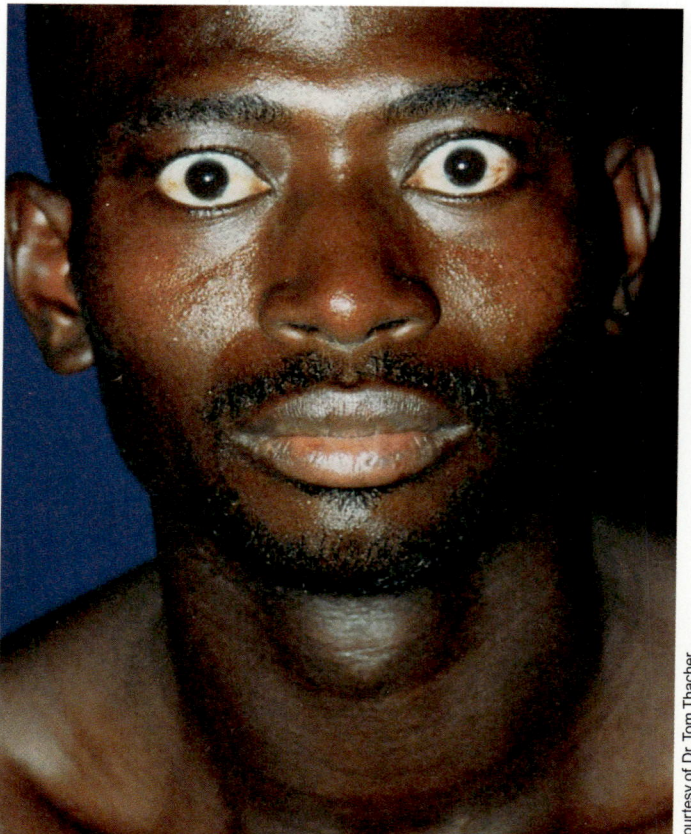

Figure 14-4 A patient with hyperthyroidism.

On the opposite end of the spectrum is **hypothyroidism**, in which there is a decreased amount of circulating thyroid hormone. Hypothyroidism typically develops gradually over time and may be difficult to detect due to its insidious nature. The decreased circulating hormones decrease the patient's metabolism and produce many effects which are opposite of hyperthyroidism. Hypothyroidism can occur for many reasons including burnout of the thyroid after autoimmune disease or inflammation that has markedly increased hormone production. This condition ultimately destroys the thyroid cells.

Hypothyroidism can also occur as a side effect of certain medications, due to removal of the thyroid for either cancer or for hyperthyroidism, and for unknown reasons. Iodine deficiency may also cause functional hypothyroidism as iodine is a key element involved in production of thyroid hormones. Finally, patients on thyroid hormone replacement who are not compliant with taking their medication may also develop hypothyroidism when they stop taking their medication.

Patients who develop hypothyroidism often complain of general fatigue, unintended weight gain, intolerance of the cold, depression, and constipation. Their skin becomes dry, rough, and waxy, and the patients may develop a peripheral neuropathy. Many times patients who are diagnosed with depression can point to hypothyroidism as an organic cause.

In **myxedema coma**, a severe and rare form of hypothyroidism, the patient develops altered and often depressed mental status, hypothermia, hypoglycemia, and bradycardia.[7,8] The patient will develop nonpitting periorbital and peripheral edema that occur from changes in the soft tissues. The patient may also present with decreased deep tendon reflexes. Myxedema coma often occurs in elderly patients. However, it can also occur in younger patients on thyroid replacement hormones who suddenly stop taking their medication for a long period of time.

Electrolyte Disorders

Almost two-thirds of the body consists of water. Several different salts are dissolved within that water, both in the intracellular fluid and the extracellular fluid. These salts, called electrolytes, act in many ways to turn electrical impulses into mechanical action, generate the electrical impulses that drive the heart, shift fluids between the different body compartments, and allow materials to be transported across cell membranes.

Proper function of the body is dependent upon maintaining the proper concentration of the different electrolytes in the extracellular and intracellular fluid. Regulation of electrolyte balance depends heavily on the hormones produced by the different endocrine glands, the function of the kidneys, and water intake by the patient. The concentration of any substance dissolved in water is affected by the amount of that substance as well as the total amount of fluid (Figure 14-5a–d) and is determined by dividing the amount of the electrolyte by the fluid volume. It is estimated that, with normal renal function, the average adult needs to drink 2 to 3 liters of water daily in order to replace fluid losses from urine, sweating, respiration, and feces.

The four electrolytes most applicable to Paramedic practice are sodium, potassium, magnesium, and calcium. The patient may exhibit conditions related to a serum (blood) electrolyte concentration that is either lower than normal (hypo-) or higher than normal (hyper-). Although each of these electrolytes is presented individually, more often than

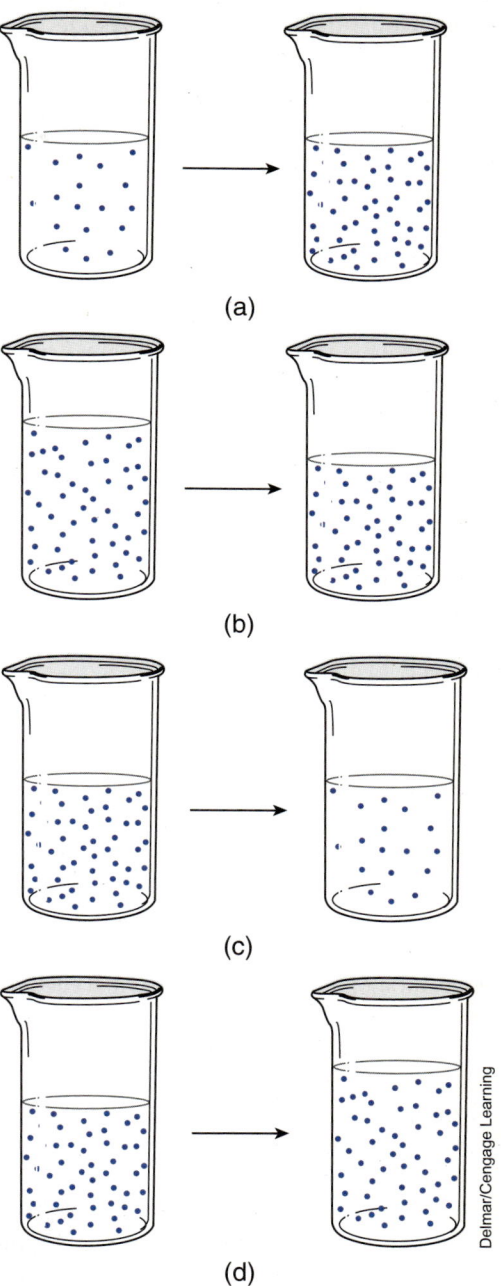

(a)

(b)

(c)

(d)

Delmar/Cengage Learning

Figure 14-5 The concentration of an electrolyte depends on the amount of the electrolyte and the amount of fluid. The concentration increases (a) if the amount of electrolyte increases and water stays the same or (b) if the amount of the electrolyte stays the same but the amount of water decreases. The concentration decreases if (c) the amount of electrolyte decreases and the water stays the same or (d) the amount of electrolyte stays the same but the amount of water increases.

not more than one electrolyte is affected by the pathophysiology of the patient's acute condition.

Sodium

Sodium (Na^+) is an electrolyte that normally has a higher concentration in the extracellular fluid than in the intracellular fluid. In extracellular fluid, the normal concentration of sodium is between 135 and 150 mEq/L, whereas the normal concentration of sodium in intracellular fluid is less than 10 mEq/L. Sodium is used by the body to remove or retain water through the action of aldosterone in the kidney. If the body retains sodium, the concentration of sodium increases slightly, drawing additional water from the urine produced by the kidneys. If the body increases the amount of sodium excreted into the urine, the patient will release additional water in the urine.

Hyponatremia is a less-than-normal blood concentration of sodium. This can be caused by either increasing the amount of water, as happens when a patient ingests significantly greater than the 2 to 3 liters of water required to maintain fluid and electrolyte balance (i.e., water intoxication) or when sodium is lost faster than water, as in profuse and prolonged sweating often seen in heat emergencies.

The symptoms associated with hyponatremia are related to the rate of decrease in concentration as opposed to the actual value. A patient who experiences a sudden decrease in sodium concentration will experience symptoms at a higher concentration than a patient who undergoes a gradual decline in sodium concentration.

Hyponatremia causes altered mental status; confusion; lethargy or fatigue; anorexia, or loss of appetite; and muscle cramping.[9] In later stages, the patient may become comatose or develop seizures. The coma and seizures occur due to the difference between the sodium concentrations in the brain cells compared with the sodium concentration in the blood. As the blood concentration of sodium decreases, the concentration of sodium in the brain tissue remains relatively constant. This difference in sodium concentration produces a gradient that encourages water to move from the blood into the cerebral cells. This causes the brain cells to swell which, in turn, causes the agitation, coma, seizure, and death associated with hyponatremia.[10]

Hypernatremia is a higher-than-normal serum concentration of sodium. Hypernatremia can be caused by either water loss or an increase in total sodium content. In the vast majority of cases, hypernatremia is due to volume loss and dehydration, especially in bedridden nursing home patients with altered thirst mechanisms and an inability to ingest fluids on their own. As discussed earlier in this chapter, diabetes insipidus can produce profound hypernatremia due to water loss through the kidneys.

As with hyponatremia, the development and severity of symptoms is related to the rate of rise in sodium concentration as opposed to the actual value. The patient may present with a generalized increase in muscle tone, fever, altered mental status, coma, and seizures.

In severe hypernatremia, in which the serum sodium concentration is higher than the sodium concentration in brain cells, water may shift from the brain cells into the blood.

This causes shrinking of the cells and can lead to either a cerebral hemorrhage or thrombus if the shrinkage is significant enough to overstretch the bridging veins between the dura and the brain. Patients with hypernatremia generally can undergo volume replacement with IV fluids. However, if the concentration of sodium drops too quickly, the nerve fibers in the brainstem can demyelinate, or lose their layer of insulation, and disrupt nerve impulse conduction.[11,12,13]

Potassium

Potassium (K^+) is a second important electrolyte that works with sodium to change the electrical potential of nerve cells and is important in the cardiac conduction system. The normal extracellular concentration of potassium is 3.5 to 5.0 mEq/L and the normal intracellular concentration of potassium is 100 to 150 mEq/L. Potassium is excreted into the urine through the kidneys.

Patients with a low potassium level are said to have **hypokalemia**. Patients who develop hypokalemia often do so from potassium losses due to diuretics. Potassium can also be lost through the gut in patients with significant diarrhea. Potassium is also transiently shifted from the serum into the cells during albuterol nebulizer treatments and insulin administration, thus decreasing serum potassium. Since potassium is essential for proper nerve conduction, hypokalemia may affect the heart as well as the nervous system.

Patients who have hypokalemia often complain of general malaise, weakness, fatigue, paresthesias, and cramps. In addition, these patients may develop tachycardias, orthostatic hypotension, and decreased reflexes. A number of electrocardiographic changes are associated with hypokalemia (Table 14-2 and Figure 14-6). Hypokalemia may also cause, or enhance the effects of, digitalis as well as worsen the signs of digitalis toxicity.

Table 14-2 ECG Effects of Hypokalemia

- T wave flattening
- U wave development
- ST depression

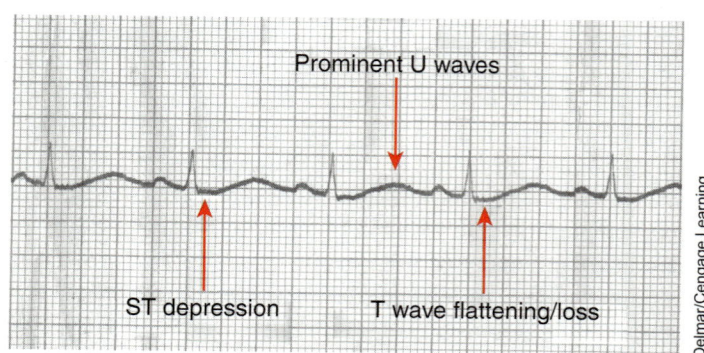

Figure 14-6 An ECG of a patient with severe hypokalemia. Note the features listed in Table 14-2.

Hyperkalemia is a higher-than-normal level of potassium in the blood. Hyperkalemia often develops in the setting of renal insufficiency or renal failure when the kidney is not able to secrete the usual amount of potassium into the urine. Hyperkalemia may also develop in some patients who are in diabetic ketoacidosis because the elevated blood glucose level and relatively low insulin level cause potassium to shift from the cells into the bloodstream. Patients will tolerate chronic potassium elevations better than acute elevations in the serum potassium concentration.

Hyperkalemia can produce symptoms of weakness, paresthesias, depressed or absent deep tendon reflexes, ascending paralysis, nausea, vomiting, and diarrhea. Hyperkalemia can also cause life-threatening ECG changes (Table 14-3 and Figure 14-7) which predispose the patient to ventricular fibrillation, torsades de pointes, complete heart block, and asystole.[14,15]

Table 14-3 ECG Changes Observed in Hyperkalemia

Serum Potassium Concentration	ECG Changes
>5.5 mEq/L	• With acute hyperkalemia, one may see any of these changes • Changes may be absent or delayed in chronic hyperkalemia
6.5 to 7.5 mEq/L	• Tall, peaked T waves • Shortened QT interval • Prolonged PR interval
7.5 to 8.0 mEq/L	• Widened QRS • Flattening of the P wave
10 to 12 mEq/L	• QRS-T complex degrades into a sine wave pattern

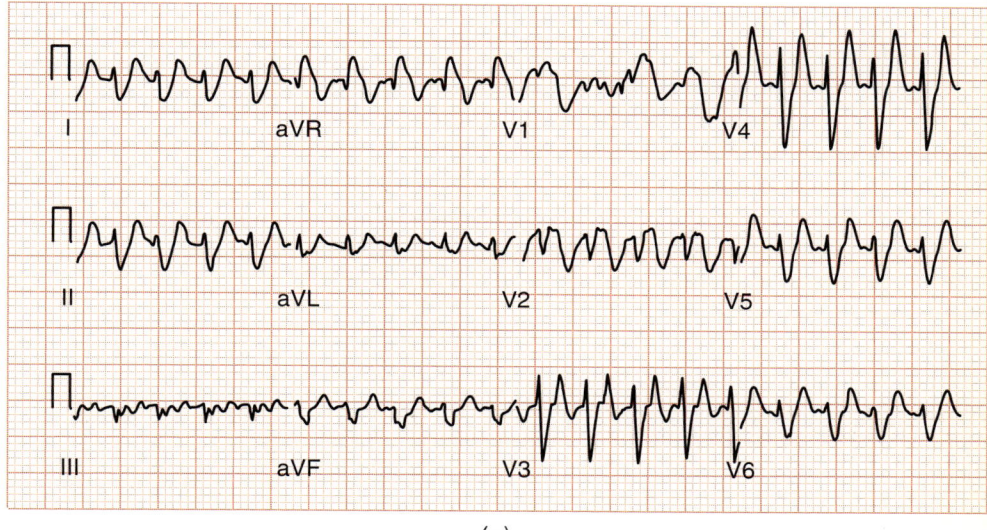

(a)

(b)

Figure 14-7 The electrocardiogram of a patient with severe hyperkalemia as a result of diabetic ketoacidosis (a) before treatment exhibiting the widened QRS and near sine wave pattern and (b) after treatment showing normalization of the ECG.

Delmar/Cengage Learning

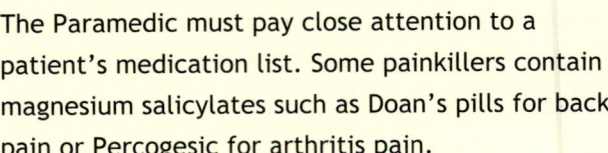
The Paramedic must pay close attention to a patient's medication list. Some painkillers contain magnesium salicylates such as Doan's pills for back pain or Percogesic for arthritis pain.

and in pregnant women to treat preeclampsia and seizures (see Chapter 37). Excessive intake can also occur in the setting of a bowel obstruction or chronic constipation when additional magnesium is absorbed into the bloodstream from the gut (Table 14-4). Although inadequate magnesium elimination most often occurs in the setting of acute renal failure, it can also occur if the patient has chronic constipation. As with the other electrolytes, the development of symptoms depends more on how quickly the serum magnesium concentration rises than the actual concentration.

Calcium

Calcium is essential for muscle contraction, cardiac contraction, and intracellular functions. The bones and teeth are made up of calcium and are also used to store calcium. The normal extracellular concentration of calcium is 8.7 to 10.4 mg/dL. Serum levels of calcium are actually regulated by three different hormones which balance the normal breakdown and regeneration of bone and the concentration of calcium in the blood. Excess calcium is cleared by the kidneys into the urine.

Hypocalcemia is an abnormally low level of calcium in the blood. Hypocalcemia may develop acutely in

---

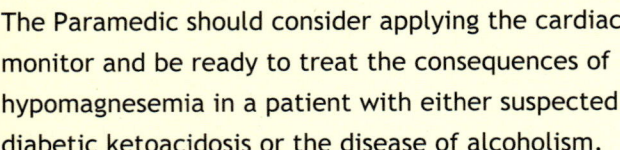
Unless the patient's potassium is known to be low or normal, the Paramedic should consider treating any patient with renal failure who is in cardiac arrest for hyperkalemia. Typically sodium bicarbonate, a competitive electrolyte, is administered to counteract the effects of the hyperkalemia.

Magnesium

Magnesium (Mg^{++}) is another important electrolyte that plays a significant role in both central and peripheral nervous tissue; production of energy, proteins, and DNA in the cell; and in the binding of hormones to their cell receptors. The normal extracellular concentration of magnesium is 1.5 to 2 mEq/L and an intracellular concentration is approximately 40 mEq/L. Magnesium is absorbed in the small intestine and excreted in both the stool and the urine.

Hypomagnesemia is a state of low magnesium levels in the blood. Hypomagnesemia can be caused by excessive loss of magnesium in diarrhea or excessive loss of magnesium in the urine. Hypomagnesemia can occur in chronic alcoholics both due to malnutrition and alcohol-related diuresis. Hypomagnesemia can also occur in DKA or in poorly controlled diabetic patients with chronic hyperglycemia from diuresis due to elevated serum glucose.

Symptoms associated with hypomagnesemia include generalized weakness, muscle cramps, vertigo, and depression. The patient may experience tachycardias, torsades de points, nystagmus, ataxia, decreased deep tendon reflexes, irritability, altered mental status, disorientation, combativeness, and seizures. Hypomagnesemia is often closely associated with hypokalemia, which explains the overlap in symptoms and signs.[16]

The Paramedic should consider applying the cardiac monitor and be ready to treat the consequences of hypomagnesemia in a patient with either suspected diabetic ketoacidosis or the disease of alcoholism.

Conversely, **hypermagnesemia** is an elevated magnesium level in the blood. Hypermagnesemia can be caused by either excessive intake of magnesium or an inability to excrete magnesium. Excessive intake can be from ingesting magnesium replacement tablets or can occur during intravenous magnesium infusions. Paramedics use intravenous magnesium infusions to treat certain dysrhythmias (see Chapter 5)

Table 14-4 Effects of Hypermagnesemia and the Approximate Serum Magnesium Level

Serum Magnesium Concentration	Effects
3.5 to 5 mEq/L	• Nausea, vomiting, skin flushing, weakness, lightheadedness • If acute elevation: decreased level of consciousness, respiratory depression, cardiac arrest
5 to 6 mEq/L	• Decreased or absent deep tendon reflexes • Vasodilation and shock
8 to 10 mEq/L	• Arrhythmias (especially atrial fibrillation and intraventricular conduction delay) • Flaccid paralysis of skeletal muscle
Over 10 mEq	• Asystole, complete heart block • Respiratory failure • Stupor, coma • Death

trauma, sepsis, acute pancreatitis, hyperventilation, and renal failure. Certain medications can also decrease the serum calcium concentration. Symptoms associated with hypocalcemia include paresthesia around the mouth and fingertips, muscle weakness, and fatigue. Hypocalcemia can cause depressed myocardial contractility, hyperactive deep tendon reflexes, and seizures. Hypocalcemia can also cause carpal spasms, in which the forearm muscles contract and put the patient's wrists into a spastic position. Hypocalcemia can also prolong the QT interval on the electrocardiogram.[17,18]

Hypercalcemia, an elevated level of calcium in the blood, can be caused by increased absorption of calcium from the intestinal tract, often due to an increase in the regulatory hormones and inadequate clearance of excess calcium from the kidneys, as seen in renal failure. Hypercalcemia is also seen in some malignancies, either related to the cancer itself or associated with the breakdown of bone due to metastatic bone cancer. As with the other electrolytes, development of symptoms is associated with the rate of change as opposed to the actual serum concentration. The patient who has hypercalcemia will often complain of nausea and vomiting, abdominal or flank pain related to a new kidney stone, constipation, weakness, headaches, lethargy, and depression. The patient may develop altered mental status, hypertension, bradycardia, and increased deep tendon reflexes. Stupor and coma can occur with higher serum calcium levels.

STREET SMART

Some patients with anginal pain will self-medicate with antacids, many of which contain calcium. Even though these antacids do not resolve the underlying cardiac pain, the patient continues to take them in the hope they will, while denying the cardiac origin of the pain.

CASE STUDY (CONTINUED)

Medic 702 arrives on scene, and the Paramedics grab their gear and head up to the left upper apartment. Mr. George answers the door with a somewhat relieved look on his face. The Paramedic notices a toddler hooked to Mr. George's leg and they hear the crying of a small baby.

"I am glad you are here, I'm not sure what is happening with my wife," Mr. George says. "She has been acting strange the last few days and I have had my hands full with a toddler and a newborn," he says, pointing at the car seat carrier on the floor with their second child.

Mr. George leads the medics to the bedroom where they find Mrs. George mumbling unintelligible sounds. "She has been up the last two nights and would not settle down. She seemed to get more confused, but this morning she was just like this. I have not been able to get her to say anything straight. She has been shaking and feels very warm."

"Did you check her temperature?" one Paramdic asks as she opens up her bag.

"No, we don't have a thermometer," Mr. George replied.

The Paramedic attempts to get Mrs. George's attention, but is unable to obtain a further history. The Paramedic then turns to Mr. George to obtain a history. Mrs. George had delivered their second child four months ago during an uncomplicated delivery. She has no prior medical conditions, and does not drink alcohol nor use tobacco or other recreational drugs. She has been losing weight since the pregnancy faster than she had with her first child. She has not complained of a fever, cough, or other infectious symptoms. She has not been tolerating the summer warmth as well as she usually does and has been sweating a lot.

CRITICAL THINKING QUESTIONS

1. What are the important elements of the history that a Paramedic should obtain?
2. Does the symptom complex match with any symptom pattern?

History

In patients who present with altered mental status or level of consciousness, a thorough history can be key to determining the source of their symptoms. Family, friends, and other witnesses provide important pieces of the history when the patient is unable to provide a reliable history.

When compiling the history of a patient's present illness, it is important for the Paramedic to attempt to determine the specific symptoms the patient is experiencing. With many of these conditions, there is an overlap of both the symptoms the patient experiences and signs that develop. Fatigue is also a common symptom associated with many of the conditions discussed previously. Although using open-ended questions is the best way to start the interview, the Paramedic may have to ask the patient specific yes or no questions to help obtain a better history. The timing and duration of the symptoms are also important in narrowing the paramedical differential diagnosis as some conditions take longer to develop whereas others are more acute.

The past medical history may be helpful as well, especially in cases in which a patient knows he or she has hypo- or hyperthyroidism or adrenal insufficiency. Recurrent history of similar symptoms may also point toward a source. A patient with undiagnosed hyperthyroidism may have had several episodes of supraventricular tachycardia that are becoming more frequent. That piece of history may lead the Paramedic to keep hyperthyroidism in her paramedical differential. The SAMPLE mnemonic is also helpful in prompting the Paramedic to obtain key elements of the history, including the patient's allergies, medications, last meal, and events leading up to the request for assistance.

A history of substance abuse—including alcohol, illegal substances, and abuse of prescription medications—is important to elicit in any patient with altered mental status. The altered mental status may be due to recent ingestion of those substances or may be due to withdrawal from those substances. Asking about past psychiatric history is also important. Altered mental status may be related to a patient's prior psychiatric history, especially if the events leading up to the call for assistance were similar to prior episodes. It is often helpful for the Paramedic to ask how the present episode is different than prior episodes.

CASE STUDY (CONTINUED)

The Paramedic performs a rapid physical examination on Mrs. George. She appears mildly agitated, and is making unintelligible sounds. Her airway appears patent; she is breathing fast and is markedly tachycardia with a bounding radial pulse. Mrs. George's skin feels warm and dry and her mucous membranes are also dry. When the Paramedic looks at Mrs. George's face, she thinks Mrs. George's eyes are a little more prominent than they should be and her eyelids do not appear to cover her entire eyes. Mrs. George has a small bulge in the center of her anterior neck.

The EMT records Mrs. George's vitals as a blood pressure of 180/100, heart rate of 140 beats per minute, a respiratory rate of 22 per minute, a room air pulse oximetry of 99%, and a tympanic temperature of 104°F (39°C). A blood glucose performed when the Paramedic starts the intravenous line is 102 mg/dL. A 12-lead electrocardiogram reveals a sinus tachycardia at 140 bpm with normal intervals.

CRITICAL THINKING QUESTIONS

1. What are the elements of the physical examination of a patient with suspected thyroid disorder?
2. Why are a blood glucose and a 12-lead ECG critical elements in this examination?

Examination

The Paramedic's physical examination of a patient with altered mental status first focuses on ensuring a patent airway, providing adequate oxygenation and ventilation, and maintaining adequate circulatory status. Once the primary assessment is performed and any life-threatening issues are resolved, the Paramedic can move on to the secondary examination. The patient's general appearance may provide some clues as to any issues that might be present in the endocrine system. The Paramedic should observe the patient for moon face, truncal obesity, or "buffalo hump," as these suggest Cushing's syndrome. A general increase in pigmentation along with thin hair suggests adrenal insufficiency. Exophthalmos and a visible thyroid suggest hyperthyroidism. Nonpitting periorbital and tibial edema along with waxy skin suggests hypothyroidism.

The neurologic examination may reveal a change from baseline mental status, disorientation, and confusion. Muscle strength should be symmetric, although it may be weaker than normal. Reflexes may be increased or decreased from normal, but are also symmetric. Sensation is usually intact. The cranial nerves are also often functioning normally, although a

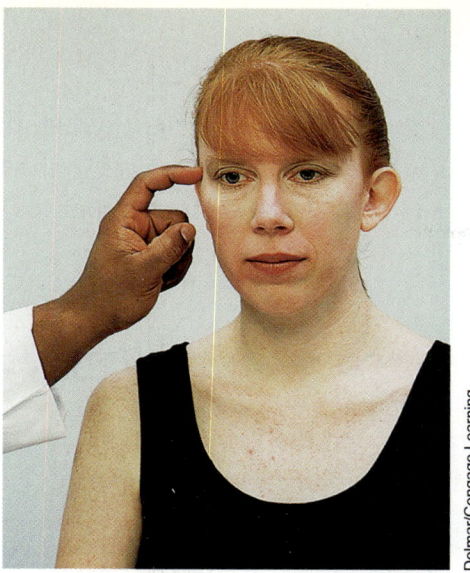

Figure 14-8 Chvostek's sign is elicited by tapping the facial nerve where it exits the skull just anterior to the ear.

hypotension that is unresponsive to treatment suggests either adrenal crisis or myxedema coma. The pulmonary exam is generally normal except in rare cases where the patient's tachycardia causes heart failure. The abdominal examination is often unremarkable. From a psychiatric standpoint, the Paramedic should assess the patient's affect, speech pattern, thought processes, and insight. Many of the conditions discussed in this chapter will mimic psychiatric disorders and may be difficult for the Paramedic to discern from a psychiatric condition.

The Paramedic should obtain a rapid blood glucose level on every patient with any change from the normal mental status. Hypoglycemia should be treated. The electrocardiogram may show changes which suggest hyperkalemia, hypokalemia, or hypocalcemia. For Paramedics who carry a rapid blood chemistry machine, the analysis may confirm the presence of an electrolyte disorder.

patient who has hypocalcemia will twitch the facial muscles when the facial nerve is tapped (Figure 14-8). This is called **Chvostek's sign**.

The Paramedic's cardiovascular examination may show tachycardia or bradycardia. New hypertension may be associated with hyperthyroidism or hyperaldosteronism, while

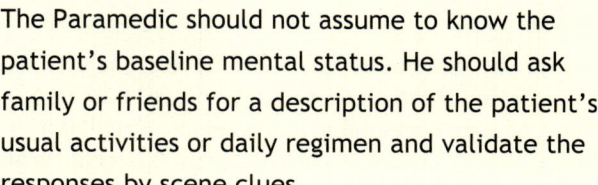

STREET SMART

The Paramedic should not assume to know the patient's baseline mental status. He should ask family or friends for a description of the patient's usual activities or daily regimen and validate the responses by scene clues.

CASE STUDY (CONTINUED)

Mr. George denies that his wife has had any recent illness and denies knowledge of substance abuse. However, Mr. George states his wife has been losing weight rapidly after her delivery and was not tolerating the summer heat, whereas usually she has no problem. She is now delirious and not able to communicate. She is hyperthermic, tachycardic, and hypertensive, suggesting a state of increased metabolism.

The Paramedics discover one major finding during the physical examination that suggests a cause for Mrs. George's altered mental status: an enlargement of her thyroid gland that the Paramedic is able to observe without palpation, as well as the exophthalmos. It appears that Mrs. George may have developed hyperthyroidism after her recent pregnancy, which has worsened to the point that she has developed thyroid storm.[19]

CRITICAL THINKING QUESTIONS

1. What is the significance of the patient's hyperdynamic hemodynamics?
2. What explanation would the Paramedic announce to the patient's husband for the symptoms?

Assessment

The list of conditions that can cause altered mental status is long; however, the combination of a relatively sudden decline in mental status, weight loss, and a hyperdynamic state, coupled with an enlarged thyroid and exophthalmos, suggests thyroid storm.[19]

Although maintaining a high index of suspicion that Mrs. George's problem is related to her thyroid, the Paramedic understands that there are other possibilities and elects to provide supportive care in the form of high-flow, high-concentration oxygen and intravenous fluids. In addition, she seeks medical advice for further treatment.

CRITICAL THINKING QUESTIONS

1. What is the standard of care for patients with an endocrine disorder, such as suspected thyroid storm?
2. What are some of the patient-specific concerns and considerations that the Paramedic should consider when applying this plan of care that is intended to treat a broad patient population presenting with thyroid storm?

Treatment

In many of the conditions discussed in this chapter, Paramedic care is supportive and focuses on maintaining a patent airway, adequate breathing, and adequate circulation. The Paramedic should ensure a patent airway by using airway adjuncts or intubation, if necessary. In addition, the Paramedic should apply supplemental oxygen if the patient is hypotensive, hypoxic, or in respiratory distress. Hypotensive patients should receive fluid resuscitation with normal saline up to a volume of 2 liters. If the patient remains hypotensive, the Paramedic should consider adding a vasopressor medication (e.g., dopamine or norepinephrine). For patients who remain hypotensive despite adequate intravenous fluids and vasopressor medications, the Paramedic should consider intravenous steroids (e.g., methylprednisolone 125 mg or hydrocortisone 100 mg).

Tachycardia from hyperthyroidism may respond better to intravenous beta blockers (e.g., metoprolol) rather than calcium channel blockers. This is due to the fact that the beta blockers inhibit the peripheral conversion of the thyroid hormone into the actual compound that produces the signs and symptoms of hyperthyroidism. As with all patients who present with altered mental status, the Paramedic should administer intravenous glucose to treat hypoglycemia and consider administering naloxone in the setting of suspected patient overdose.

Despite the administration of intravenous fluids and high-flow, high-concentration oxygen, Mrs. George starts to develop chest pain and some shortness of breath. The 12-lead ECG fails to reveal any specific pattern of ischemia that would be suggestive of acute coronary syndrome, although Mrs. George does fit the profile for a patient with cardiac disease.

Electing to withhold the nitroglycerin, the Paramedic instead contacts medical control. The attending emergency physician, overhearing the conversation between the Paramedic and the emergency medicine resident, suggests administering a beta blocker.

CRITICAL THINKING QUESTIONS

1. What are some of the predictable complications associated with thyroid storm?
2. What are some of the predictable complications associated with the treatments for thyroid storm?

Evaluation

During transport, the Paramedic continuously monitors the patient's airway patency, adequacy of ventilation, and effectiveness of the circulatory system. The airway is especially important in patients who have altered mental status as the patient may not be able to protect the airway in the event of vomiting or increased oral secretions.

CASE STUDY CONCLUSION

Medic 702 pulls into the emergency department at Memorial Hospital. The Paramedics bring Mrs. George into the ED. After going through the triage process, they transfer Mrs. George to room 21 and provide a report to the RN assigned to Mrs. George. After filling out and leaving their prehospital care report, they briefly talk to the emergency physician about thyroid storm before leaving the emergency department.

CRITICAL THINKING QUESTIONS

1. What is the most appropriate transport decision that will get the patient to definitive care?
2. What are some other possible complications that could occur as a result of the thyroid storm?

Disposition

Although patients who present with some of the conditions discussed in this chapter may ultimately require care at a tertiary care hospital, most of these conditions can be handled in a local community hospital. Electrolyte disorders can be effectively managed with either electrolyte replacement or through medications or dialysis to decrease elevated serum concentrations. Therapy for the other endocrine conditions can be initiated at the community hospital and followed after discharge. Most patients the Paramedic encounters with altered mental status should be transported to the closest appropriate hospital emergency department.

CONCLUSION

The body hosts an amazingly complex collection of interrelated systems that maintain homeostasis. As discussed in this chapter, these mechanisms can easily become disrupted in critically ill patients. Disorders of these homeostatic mechanisms can also have profound effects on the patient and produce seemingly unrelated signs and symptoms. The Paramedic may be the first healthcare provider to encounter the patient who has a disorder of her homeostatic mechanisms.

KEY POINTS:

- The body uses complex mechanisms to regulate itself.

- The pituitary gland secretes hormones that control other glands.

- Adrenal glands secrete epinephrine and norepinephrine from the medulla and steroids from the cortex.

- The thyroid gland secretes hormones that control energy use and metabolism.

- Too much or too little thyroid hormone in a patient can cause life-threatening conditions.

- Hyponatremia can occur secondary to excessive water intake or increased sodium loss. Hyponatremia can lead to seizures.

- Hypernatremia can occur due to excessive sodium movement into the vascular system but most often occurs due to volume loss and dehydration. Hypernatremia can also cause seizures.

- Hypokalemia occurs when potassium is lost through diuretic use or diarrhea. Albuterol lowers potassium levels. Low potassium can cause general malaise and cramps.

- Hypokalemia alters ECG tracings and can enhance digitalis toxicity.

- Hyperkalemia occurs with renal insufficiency or diabetic ketoacidosis. High potassium levels can cause cramps, nausea, and sensory nerve changes.

- Hyperkalemia can cause life-threatening ECG changes.

- Hypomagnesemia is associated with hypokalemia and can lead to torsades de pointes.

- Hypermagnesemia occurs secondary to alterations in bowel function and can cause life-threatening dysrhythmias.

- Hypocalcemia is associated with trauma, sepsis, acute pancreatitis, and hyperventilation. It depresses myocardial contractility.

- Hypercalcemia is seen with excessive intake or endocrine dysfunction.

- Endocrine dysfunction often leads to a change in mental status. It is important for the Paramedic to know the patient's baseline.

REVIEW QUESTIONS:

1. What mechanisms does the body use to maintain homeostasis?

2. What types of hormones are secreted by the pituitary gland?

3. What signs and symptoms are seen in each of the following:
   - Excessive thyroid hormone
   - Deficient amount of thyroid hormone

- Excessive adrenal steroids
- Deficient amount of adrenal steroids
4. What conditions can cause torsades de pointes?
5. What patients are at risk for developing the following disorders?
   - Hyponatremia
   - Hypernatremia
- Hypokalemia
- Hyperkalemia
- Hypocalcemia
- Hypercalcemia
- Hypomagnesemia
- Hypermagnesemia

CASE STUDY QUESTIONS:

Please refer to the Case Study in this chapter, and answer the questions below:

1. What signs and symptoms suggest Mrs. George's final diagnosis?

2. What specific event may have triggered the condition in Mrs. George?

3. What is the mechanism of action for the beta blocker administered to Mrs. George?

REFERENCES:

1. Dusick JR, Wang C, et al. Chapter 1: pathophysiology of hypopituitarism in the setting of brain injury. *Pituitary* May 15, 2008 (epub ahead of print).
2. Marik PE, Pastores SM, et al. Recommendations for the diagnosis and management of corticosteroid insufficiency in critically ill adult patients: consensus statements from an international task force by the American College of Critical Care Medicine. *Crit Care Med.* 2008;36(6):1937–1949.
3. Runer ER, Brennan JR, et al. Adrenal insufficiency in a patient with severe hypotension caused by bilateral adrenal hemorrhage. *Endocr Pract.* 2002;8(4):307–310.
4. Chin R. Adrenal crisis. *Crit Care Clin.* 1991;7(1):23–42.
5. Vlase H, Lungu G, et al. Cardiac disturbances in thyrotoxicosis: diagnosis, incidence, clinical features and management. *Endocrinologie.* 1991;29(3–4):155–160.
6. Woeber KA. Thyrotoxicosis and the heart. *N Engl J Med.* 1992;327(2):94–98.
7. Kwaku MP, Burman KD. Myxedema coma. *J Intensive Care Med.* 2007;22(4):224–231.
8. Jordan RM. Myxedema coma. Pathophysiology, therapy, and factors affecting prognosis. *Med Clin North Am.* 1995;79(1):185–194.
9. Gross P. Treatment of hyponatremia. *Intern Med.* 2008;47(10):885–891.
10. Lin M, Liu SJ, et al. Disorders of water imbalance. *Emerg Med Cli North Am.* 2005;23(3):749–770, ix.
11. Huq S, Wong M, et al. Osmotic demyelination syndromes: central and extrapontine myelinolysis. *J Clin Neurosci.* 2007;14(7):684–688.
12. Kumar S, Fowler M, et al. Central pontine myelinolysis, an update. *Neurol Res.* 2006;28(3):360–366.
13. Kraft MD, Btaiche IF, et al. Treatment of electrolyte disorders in adult patients in the intensive care unit. *Am J Health-Syst Pharm.* 2005;62(16):1663–1682.
14. Dittrich KL, Walls RM. Hyperkalemia: ECG manifestations and clinical considerations. *J Emerg Med.* 1986;4(6):449–455.
15. Freeman K, Feldman JA, et al. Effects of presentation and electrocardiogram on time to treatment of hyperkalemia. *Acad Emerg Med.* 2008;15(3):239–249.
16. Tong GM, Rude RK. Magnesium deficiency in critical illness. *J Intensive Care Med.* 2005;20(1):3–17.
17. Diercks DB, Shumaik GM, et al. Electrocardiographic manifestations: electrolyte abnormalities. *J Emerg Med.* 2004;27(2):153–160.
18. Janeira LF. Torsades de pointes and long QT syndromes. *Am Fam Physician.* 1995;52(5):1447–1453.
19. Casey BM, Leveno KJ. Thyroid disease in pregnancy. *Obstet Gynecol.* 2006;108(5):1283–1292.

CHAPTER 15

ADDICTION DISORDER— ALCOHOLISM

KEY CONCEPTS:

Upon completion of this chapter, it is expected that the reader will understand these following concepts:

- The understanding that alcoholism is a multifactorial, chronic disease
- The ways the disease of alcoholism affects all of the body's vital organs including the brain, heart, lungs, and digestive organs, as well as altering endocrine, hematologic, and neurologic functions
- The ways deprivation of ethanol alcohol may lead the alcoholic to seek more toxic substances
- The recognition that alcohol withdrawal and acute alcohol poisoning are medical emergencies

ANATOMY CONCEPTS:

Prior to reading this chapter the Paramedic student should be familiar with the following anatomy and physiology concepts:

- Neurotransmitters
- Alcohol metabolism

The Paramedics are called by the police to a house on LeCuyler and Main Streets for a middle-aged male patient exhibiting bizarre behavior. The corner of LeCuyler and Main is located in the residential district of town, known for small, well-kept, one-family houses. Upon arrival, the crew finds a male with slurred speech and a yellow cast to his skin and eyes. He is yelling and swinging at the air wildly in apparent anger at something unseen.

CRITICAL THINKING QUESTIONS

1. What are some of the possible causes of the patient's bizarre behavior?
2. How is slurred speech related to the bizarre behavior?

OVERVIEW

Delirium is a temporary or transient state of acute confusion, often brought on by a number of medical and/or psychiatric conditions. Delirium abates when the medical condition is corrected.[1]

Chief Concern

The patient with delirium often has an inability to focus on the task at hand and is easily distracted, shifting his attention from one stimulus to another. Delirium is also associated with memory impairment and acute disorientation. However, delirium should not be confused with dementia.[2–4] **Dementia** is a progressive and permanent deterioration of a patient's mental function, whereas delirium is an acute short-term, and potentially reversible, impairment of cognitive function that has a wide range of potential causes (Table 15-1).

The patient with delirium can present with a range of abnormal behaviors and emotions ranging from agitation to somnolence to overt psychotic behaviors. All of these behaviors are linked to fear and confusion.

Table 15-1 Differential Diagnosis for Delirium

I	Infection
W	Withdrawal
A	Acute metabolic causes (hypoglycemia)
T	Trauma
C	Central nervous system (seizures)
H	Hypoxia
D	Deficiencies (vitamin)
E	Endocrine (hyperglycemia)
A	Acute vascular disorders (migraine)
T	Toxins and drugs
H	Heavy metal poisoning

STREET SMART

Paramedics should exhibit caution when approaching the patient who appears tranquil but who was reported to be agitated moments before. If emotionally labile, the delirious patient will manifest the spectrum of emotions, fitfully shifting from tearfulness to euphoria and back again.

Alcoholism

The use of alcohol dates back in recorded history almost 8,000 years. In fact, an Egyptian papyrus dating from 5,000 B.C. describes a brewery. As a staple food, alcoholic beverages in the form of beer, wine, and distilled spirits have been a part of life since ancient times. As a side effect, alcoholism has accompanied it. **Alcoholism** is a chronic disease that is thought to have genetic, psychosocial, and environmental influences. The disease, if left untreated, is progressive and can be fatal.

The term "alcoholism" is relatively new (coined within the last 100 years), although the problem has been recognized for centuries. Early theories suggested alcoholism was a sign of a patient's moral weakness or a psychiatric disease. In the 1950s, the American Medical Association recognized alcoholism as a disease and applied a medical model of assessment and treatment to the problem.

The *Diagnostic and Statistical Manual of Mental Disorders*, fourth edition (DSM-IV), of the American Psychological Association defines alcoholism (paraphrased) as "maladaptive" use of alcohol with "clinically significant impairment." This definition includes development of tolerance and withdrawal, which are both discussed in this chapter. The key to the definition of alcoholism is persistent use of alcohol with full knowledge of the physical, social, and psychological harm that will occur.

Alcoholism, as a disease, is characterized by several key features. The patient with alcoholism must have an inability to control her consumption of alcohol. In addition, the alcoholic patient is constantly driven to find alcohol and preoccupied with drinking. Next, the patient with alcoholism must have experienced adverse consequences as a result of drinking. These consequences can be to one's health, which occurs almost invariably, or to one's lifestyle. The patient with alcoholism will typically have impaired interpersonal relationships, difficulty with work, and a number of legal and financial impairments that all are owed to drinking. Finally, alcoholism as a syndrome manifests as distortions in the patient's reasoning, with the patient rationalizing the drinking and seeking solace in spirits rather than people.

Scope of the Problem

Of the 160 million Americans of drinking age, an estimated 7 million or so are considered alcoholics (i.e., they drink one-half pint of hard liquor or the equivalent in other alcoholic beverages daily).[5]

To keep the problem of alcohol consumption in perspective, consider some of its residual effects. Estimates indicate one in three rapes, two in five assaults, and three in five cases of child abuse involve alcohol. An estimated 25,000 Americans will die each year in alcohol-related

Table 15-2 CAGE Alcohol Assessment Tool

- Have you ever tried to **C**ut down on your drinking?
- Are you easily **A**nnoyed when people criticize your drinking?
- Do you ever feel **G**uilty about your drinking?
- Do you need an "**E**ye opener" in the morning?

crashes; in other words, one out of two motor vehicle fatalities is alcohol related.

Alcoholism is not exclusive to any one race, creed, ethnic origin, or profession. Anyone can suffer from its effects. Dr. John Ewing, of the University of North Carolina, developed the CAGE questionnaire (**C**ut down drinking, **A**nnoyed by comments, **G**uity about drinking, **E**ye opener needed) to help identify those patients at greatest risk for alcoholism. A "yes" to any of four simple questions (Table 15-2) is suggestive of alcoholism and warrants further investigation.

Some common misconceptions about alcoholism are that alcoholics are unemployed, only drink inexpensive wines, and have a distinctive appearance. However, individuals with alcoholism exist in all walks of life and social and economic classes. Some alcoholics have developed elaborate schemes to conceal their alcoholism, denying there is a problem, and still manage to remain functional in society.

Pharmacokinetics of Ethanol

Ethyl alcohol, or ethanol, is a sedative–hypnotic drug that can be likened to benzodiazepines; each is capable of being replaced by the other to prevent withdrawal. Like benzodiazepines, ethanol can also cause physical dependence.[6,7]

Medically, ethanol has been used in the past variously to treat vomiting secondary to seasickness (using iced champagne) and as an antiseptic to prevent "putrefaction." Ethanol, for medicinal purposes, is known under the term "*spiritus frumenti*." It could be obtained from grain (such as whiskey) with strength of approximately 50%. Gin, containing the oil of juniper, was an effective diuretic used to treat a disease called dropsy, currently known as heart failure.

Nonmedical alcoholic beverages were often laced with various aromatics, such as oil of turpentine and even lead acetate, to give them flavor. Alcohol is also found in many preparations, from perfumes and colognes to antiseptic mouthwashes and over-the-counter medications.

Alcohol is a molecule that consists of two carbon atoms and various formulations that include a hydroxyl group (represented by OH). The abbreviation for ethyl alcohol is the abbreviation of ethyl and OH, or EtOH.

Alcohol diffuses easily through membranes, including the mucous membranes along the entire digestive tract, with approximately one-third adsorbed in the stomach. Once absorbed, the alcohol quickly distributes to all compartments of the body, including the brain through the blood–brain barrier. It is evenly distributed and reaches its peak within 30 to 60 minutes.

Alcohol is metabolized in the liver by alcohol dehydrogenase into acetaldehyde which, in turn, is transformed by aldehyde dehydrogenase. About 95% is excreted into the urine, with the remaining 5% excreted in the lungs, as well as through sweat and saliva.

Pharmacodynamics

Ethanol acts in various ways in the central nervous system: as an antagonist to acetylcholine within the brain (thereby affecting cognition) and as an agonist for the inhibitory neurotransmitter GABA. This last effect, GABA agonist, is responsible for depression of the brainstem and the resulting respiratory depression.[8]

It should be noted that EtOH binds to a different site on the GABA receptor than do either barbiturates or benzodiazepines. Thus, whenever either of these drugs are used in combination with EtOH, the cumulative effect on the brainstem is compounded and respiratory depression is more profound.

Alcohol's effect on the GABA receptors indirectly causes an increase in the release of dopamine, which affects the pleasure center of the brain (the limbic system). This effect is thought to cause the patient's psychological addiction to alcohol.

Finally, alcohol acts as an antagonist to the excitatory neurotransmitter glutamate, through its NMDA receptor. This leads to impaired learning.

The effects of alcohol are often dose related. For example, alcohol can stimulate respirations at low doses and suppress respirations at high doses. As a drug, alcohol is a peripheral vasodilator, leading to the sense of warmth when ingested. However, in reality it increases heat loss and the risk of hypothermia for susceptible individuals.

Tolerance and Dependence

Through its effects on the limbic system, alcohol lowers inhibitions. In some cases, these lowered inhibitions lead to violence, including assaults and rape. The effects progress to a loss of coordination, leading to falls, and eventually to sedation, unconsciousness, and respiratory suppression, owed to its effects on the brainstem.

Despite these potentially adverse outcomes, some people continue to drink, imbibe (often to excess), and eventually start to develop a dependence on the drug. The mechanism for dependence is the same mechanism of dependence to benzodiazepines and other CNS depressants.

A normal liver is able to detoxify approximately 13 to 25 milligrams per deciliter of alcohol per hour. The liver of the alcoholic patient, via upgrades to its enzyme systems, eventually becomes capable of detoxifying 30 to 50 milligrams per deciliter of alcohol per hour.[9] At this point, the patient has developed a physical tolerance to alcohol. Neuronal adaptation occurs as well, requiring the patient to drink in ever-increasing amounts of alcohol in order to obtain those same effects as experienced previously.

Chronic heavy drinking leads to an irreversible drug-induced brain syndrome typified by a clouded sensorium, disorientation, and diminished intellectual capacity. The characteristic sign of this syndrome is blackouts, states of amnesia that occur following the binge. Many of these patients resort to confabulation (the creation of falsehoods) to compensate for their loss of memory or amnesia. For example, they may fill in the defects of memory with embellished tales. This filling-in of the memory gaps with fictitious stories is called confabulation.

Drug Interaction with Alcohol

The treatment plan for detoxification of patients with alcoholism can include the use of the drug disulfiram (Antabuse). Antabuse, when taken along with even a small amount of alcohol, causes severe abdominal pain, nausea, and vomiting. This discourages the patient from further drinking by utilizing the classic operant conditioning technique of using a negative stimulus to modify behavior.

Inadvertently, healthcare providers may prescribe drugs to patients that have a similar disulfiram-like reaction. Drugs that will cause a disulfiram-like reaction (i.e., abdominal pain, nausea, and vomiting) include metronidazole (Flagyl) used to treat trichomonas infections, chlorpropamide (Diabinese) as an oral hypoglycemic agent, and antibiotics in the sulfonamide and cephalosporin class.

Unfortunately, many intoxicated patients also have abdominal pain, secondary to pancreatitis, nausea, and vomiting. A careful drug history will help the Paramedic differentiate the symptoms associated with intoxication from a potential disulfiram-like drug reaction (Table 15-3).

Fetal Alcohol Syndrome

A particularly troubling development due to maternal drinking is **fetal alcohol syndrome**.[10] Alcohol can lead to birth defects in 30% to 50% of infants born to mothers who drink alcohol during pregnancy. This condition occurs to the children of women who drink during pregnancy, especially during the fourth to sixth weeks of pregnancy. Children with fetal alcohol syndrome can be recognized by their wide-set eyes, flat bridge of nose, and small cheek bones. These children suffer from hyperactivity, mental retardation, and often have difficulty with social integration.

Health Implications of Chronic Alcoholism

The long-term effects of excessive alcohol ingestion on health are devastating. Diseases of the central nervous system, as well as the cardiac, endocrine, hepatic, and digestive systems (particularly pancreatic) are common.

Pancreatitis

Acute attacks of **pancreatitis**, an inflammation of the pancreas typified by a sudden severe pain in the epigastric area that radiates to the back, commonly occur anywhere from one to two hours to several days after a bout of drinking. The inflamed pancreas excretes trypsin to meet the challenge of breaking down the ingested alcohol. Trypsin, a powerful digestive enzyme, causes tissue damage and bleeding in the intestinal tract.

In the case of chronic pancreatitis, the inflamed pancreas can no longer produce enzymes. The fats and proteins subsequently pass through the gastrointestinal system unchanged. Without fats and proteins, the patient enters into a state of malnutrition. The characteristic thin "stick" arms and legs of the patient with chronic alcoholism is owed to muscle wasting and reallocation of scarce protein and fat reserves to the core of the body. In advanced cases of chronic pancreatitis, the tail of the pancreas—where the insulin is produced—is affected. The resultant loss of the islets of Langerhans makes the patient functionally a diabetic.

The most menacing result of chronic alcoholism is liver disease. Excessive alcohol ingestion can eventually damage the liver in three ways: fat accumulation in the liver (fatty liver or steatohepatitis), inflammation of the liver (alcoholic hepatitis), and scarring of the liver, leading to cirrhosis. Cirrhosis of the liver, attributed as the cause of death in 75% of alcoholics, impairs the liver's ability to function by obstructing blood flow through the liver.[11,12]

Jaundice and Liver Disease

Under normal conditions, the Kupffer cells, part of the reticuloendothelial system within the liver, would recycle aged thrombocytes (red blood cells). Kupffer cells normally break down the RBC, via phagocytosis, releasing the bound hemoglobin. In turn, this hemoglobin is broken down into iron and bilirubin. Bilirubin is then usually excreted in the bile.

The breakdown of erythrocytes (red blood cells) in the liver produces about 250 to 350 mg of bilirubin (an insoluble waste) every day. Bilirubin usually travels in the blood, bound to albumin. To be excreted, this bilirubin must be made soluble. Using an enzyme (glucuronyl transferase), the liver takes up the bilirubin and makes it soluble. The now-soluble bilirubin drains into the hepatic duct, which then joins the

Table 15-3 Drug Interactions with Alcohol

- Prolonged action
  - Antihistamines
  - Barbiturates
  - Benzodiazepines
  - Opiates
  - Phenothiazines
- Shortened half-life
  - Propranolol
  - Isoniazid
  - Phenobarbital
  - Phenytoin
  - Warfarin

cystic duct in the gallbladder. Traveling via the common bile duct, it then drains into the duodenum of the small intestine via the ampulla of Vater. After joining other waste products in the bowels, the bilirubin is metabolized by intestinal bacteria, which turns the stool brown.

In the diseased liver, the bilirubin excretion is diminished by three factors. First, the Kupffer cells of the liver may fail to break down the red blood cells and release the bilirubin. Next, the diseased liver's impaired protein synthesis decreases the amount of albumin that can attach to the bilirubin, allowing bilirubin to accumulate in the bloodstream. Finally, the bilirubin that is made soluble and stored in the gallbladder may be sequestered because the enlarged liver may impinge on the common bile duct that drains the gallbladder.

These three factors, when combined, can increase the levels of circulating bilirubin in the blood, a condition called **hyperbilirubinemia**. Jaundice is evident whenever elevated levels of bilirubin, or hyperbilirubinemia, are present in the blood.

Jaundice, defined as the yellowish color in the sclera, or whites of the eyes, and/or a yellowish tinge to the skin (also called **icterus**), is evident with hyperbilirubinemia. Icterus is easily detectable in the sclera, under normal light conditions, even at low levels such as 2 to 2.5 mg/dL. **Pruritus**, an itchiness that is present secondary to the buildup of bile salts under the skin (which is often worse on the hands and feet), is also often associated with jaundice. Finally, the stools, lacking the conjugated bilirubin, become clay-colored.

STREET SMART

Bilirubin aids in the digestion and absorption of fats. Without bilirubin, fat is not absorbed and is passed with the stool. Alcoholic patients often have foul smelling diarrhea caused by fats called steatorrhea.

Alcoholic Liver Diseases

People who abuse alcohol are at risk for developing **alcoholic liver diseases**. Depending on the longevity of the alcoholism, each patient may have one or more of these associated diseases.

Early in the history of alcoholism, the patient may experience fatty changes in the liver, alcoholic hepatitis, and/or cirrhosis of the liver. At this stage, the effects of alcoholism are likely to be reversible. As the alcoholism progresses, chronic changes, such as fibrosis, can lead to permanent liver damage and eventually liver failure.

Fatty Liver Disease

Whenever excessive alcohol is present in the body, it signals the liver's cells to inhibit the breakdown of fatty acids while also increasing the synthesis of fatty acids, resulting in increased fatty acids. The resultant accumulation of fatty acids is converted to fat within the hepatic cells.

These globules of fat become stored in vacuoles within the liver cells, a process called **steatosis**, which distends the hepatic cells. This distention impairs circulation and distribution of blood within the liver. Eventually this causes the liver cells to swell (hepatocyte ballooning) and to rupture. Subsequently, fibrotic tissue replaces the necrotic liver cells, leading to permanent changes within the liver.

Alcoholic Hepatitis

Chronic alcohol intoxication can eventually lead to **alcoholic hepatitis**, a complex inflammatory–immunological response that is the result of oxidation of alcohol.

There are three metabolic pathways to oxidize alcohol and all produce acetaldehyde. Acetaldehyde, a reactive metabolite from the breakdown of alcohol, damages the hepatic cell membranes, altering the hepatic cells' function and structure. Specifically, alcoholic hepatitis alters cell function by causing the hepatic cells to enter into an abnormal hypermetabolic state, producing heat instead of ATP.

Furthermore, the metabolism of alcohol leads to the generation of oxygen-free radicals. These oxygen-free radicals—superoxides and hydroperoxides—lead to further inflammation and cell death. Consistent with its inflammatory origin, alcoholic hepatitis causes fever, swelling of the liver called **hepatomegaly**, and impairment of liver function.

In extreme causes, alcoholic hepatitis can lead to coagulopathy disorders and portal hypertension; both these disorders are discussed shortly.

Liver Cirrhosis

Liver cirrhosis is a chronic degenerative disease of the liver first described by Rene Laennec, the inventor of the modern stethoscope. In fact, a micronodular disease of the liver is called "Laennec's cirrhosis."

Chronic alcohol abuse interferes with the liver's metabolism of fats, proteins, and carbohydrates. The resultant damage to the hepatocytes leads to inflammation, scarring, and fibrosis of the liver.[13,14] These changes result in impaired hepatic flow and eventually liver failure. However, alcoholism is not the only cause of liver cirrhosis. Certain diseases (e.g., hepatitis C), as well as drugs and toxins, can cause liver cirrhosis as well.

Regardless of its etiology, the impact of cirrhosis on the liver's functions are vast and include coagulopathies, encephalopathy, and portal hypertension, to name only a few.

Androgens

The liver modifies and/or inactivates certain hormones. In the cirrhotic liver, the levels of estrogen (following conversion of androgens to estrogen) are higher and levels of circulating testosterone are lower. The result leads to hypogonadism and feminization, as evidenced by the development of breasts in men (a condition called gynecomastia).

Hyperinsulinemia

The alcoholic patient is prone to hypoglycemia because of decreased oral intake of foodstuffs (hypophagia), altered fat metabolism, and the creation of inhibitory metabolic by-products in the oxidation of alcohol. These factors combine to promote hypoglycemia, inhibit glycogen production (i.e., glycogenesis), and limit gluconeogenesis, the production of glucose from substrates like glycerol and amino acids. The compound effect of these three factors results in hypoglycemia.

Conditions Associated with Liver Disease

Impaired Protein Synthesis

One of the body's first casualties of liver failure is impaired protein synthesis. The liver is responsible for producing a number of protein-related items: albumin (a major blood protein), many globulins that are involved in immunity and coagulation (including prothrombin and plasminogen), and the blood-clotting factors. Without the capacity to produce these essential proteins, the patient will suffer hypoproteinemia (causing coagulopathies) and hypoalbuminemia (causing ascites).

Ascites

Without oncotic pressure created by blood proteins (i.e., colloidal osmotic pressure, or COP), fluid in the blood shifts into the peripheral tissue, a phenomenon known as third spacing. Therefore, alcoholic patients with hypoalbuminemia frequently have peripheral swelling and another development called ascites. Ascites, the presence of fluid in the peritoneal cavity, occurs because liver cirrhosis creates blood backup into the portal artery (portal hypertension) and subsequently sequesters blood in the abdomen.[15] This sequestered blood, without benefit of either hydrostatic pressure or colloidal osmotic pressure, leaks plasma-like fluid into the peritoneal cavity. Initially, the patient's abdomen will appear to be slightly distended, with impairment of diaphragmatic excursion. The patient may complain of shortness of breath as well as abdominal heaviness in this stage.

The Paramedic can assess ascites in the patient by noting flank bulging on inspection when the patient is turned and shifting dullness to percussion as well. Eventually the fluid buildup is so noticeable in the patient's abdomen that the Paramedic appreciates a fluid wave when the patient rolls onto his side. It is possible for the patient to accumulate up to 25 liters of transudate, the low protein plasma-like fluid in the abdominal cavity. This degree of fluid shift, from the intravascular to the interstitial space, stimulates the kidneys (through the renin-angiotensin-aldosterone mechanism) to retain fluids. It also stimulates the sympathetic nervous system.

In extreme cases (e.g., when the ascites cause severe shortness of breath), a surgical procedure called paracentesis may be performed to drain the fluid from the abdomen. Alternatively, an artificial portacaval shunt will be placed to lessen portal hypertension by diverting blood past the liver to the inferior vena cava.

Coagulopathy

Several coexisting circumstances, ineffectual Kupffer cells, and impaired protein synthesis create coagulopathy disorders in the patient with liver failure. The Kupffer cells, mentioned earlier in the discussion on jaundice, are also responsible for clearing any activated coagulation factors that remain in the blood. Circulating coagulation factors that are not removed are still capable of stimulating the coagulation cascade.

The liver in failure also fails to synthesize proteins, including new coagulation factors. In fact, all of the coagulation factors except von Willebrand's factor are created in the liver. Compounding the problems of hemostasis created by the liver is the indirect effect that the enlarged liver has on the spleen. Typically, the spleen sequesters approximately 30% of the available circulating platelets. Portal hypertension, which occurs in liver disease, can cause as much as 90% of the available platelets to be sequestered in the spleen, with the portal vein draining both the mesenteric and splenic veins. The resulting relative thrombocytopenia (drop in blood cells) leaves the rest of the body at risk for abnormal bleeding.

These factors all combine to create activation of the coagulation cascade in some parts of the body while at the same time failing to adequately provide fibrinolysis in other parts of the body. This results in an imbalance of hemostasis. This pathological phenomenon is called disseminated intravascular coagulation (DIC).[16,17] Patients with DIC are at great risk of intracerebral hemorrhages (such as chronic subdural hematomas) and gastrointestinal bleeding.

Portal Hypertension and Esophageal Varices

Normally the portal system is a low pressure system that allows the mesenteric and splenic veins to drain through the liver. With the cirrhotic changes associated with liver disease, blood flow is impeded and blood backs up into the portal vein, a condition called portal hypertension. The blood then backs up into the mesenteric veins (including the esophageal veins) and the splenic vein. In some patients, this backup of blood recanalizes the umbilical veins. These umbilical veins, which resemble writhing snakes, are visible under the surface of the patient's skin. Fittingly, this condition is called caput medusa (Latin for head of Medusa, the goddess with serpents for hair).

The presence of caput medusa should raise the Paramedic's suspicion of a potentially more life-threatening condition: esophageal varices. **Esophageal varices**, distended veins in the esophagus, are the result of portal hypertension. Some veins that line the esophagus drain into the left gastric vein which, in turn, drains into the portal vein. When the portal vein is distended (portal hypertension), then blood backs up into these delicate veins in the throat, distending them to over twice their normal diameter.

If a sudden increase in intra-abdominal pressure was to occur, such as during retching and vomiting, these distended veins (varices) could rupture. The resultant bleeding can be life-threatening, especially if the bleeding is associated with a coagulopathy. Bleeding esophageal varices is a medical emergency which may require either banding (to ligate the offending blood vessel) or sclerotherapy. **Sclerotherapy** is a process of injecting the vein with a caustic substance that causes blood clot formation or thrombosis. When the clot forms, the bleeding stops. The medical treatment for threatened rupture of esophageal varices in the field can include the use of beta blockers and/or nitrates to artificially lower the patient's blood pressure to prevent rupture and potentially life-threatening exsanguination.[15–20]

Renal Failure

Many patients with end-stage hepatic failure (approximately 50%) have concomitant renal failure. This renal failure may be due to the combination of renin and sympathetic nervous system-induced vasoconstriction, or from direct renal insult from toxins that would normally be detoxified in the liver.

Regardless of the etiology, acute tubular necrosis can occur in the kidneys, leading to acute renal failure (ARF). This condition is called **hepatorenal syndrome**.

Patients with hepatorenal syndrome produce scant amounts of concentrated, and often malodorous, urine and retain nitrogen waste products. The accumulation of these nitrogenous wastes is a condition called **azotemia**. Occasionally, these wastes are excreted through the sweat glands and form crystals on the skin after the sweat evaporates, called **uremic frost**. The manifestations of azotemia (uremia) include confusion, orthostatic hypotension, and total body edema called **anasarca**.

Although hepatorenal syndrome is rare (occurring in only about 10% of hospitalized liver failure patients), the mortality from the syndrome is high (approaches 90%). Kidney dialysis or kidney transplant are the patient's best hopes for survival.[21]

Hyponatremia

The complication of hyponatremia often compounds the problem of renal failure and/or liver failure. **Hyponatremia**, a state of low sodium, is the result of changes in the blood's osmolarity. Osmolarity of the blood is partly a function of the amount of blood proteins (particularly albumin) in the blood, which creates COP. These blood proteins are primarily created in the liver. When albumin levels drop (for example, the COP is affected), the osmolarity drops. When the osmolarity drops, then fluids shift from the intravascular space to the interstitial space. The intravascular volume becomes depleted with a resultant loss of effective blood volume.

With diminished blood volume the renin–angiotensin–aldosterone mechanism of the kidneys responds and fluids are retained. The patient thus experiences water overload. The result of this fluid retention is dilution of the blood, including the sodium, and hypo-osmolar hyponatremia. The problem of hyponatremia, secondary to water overload, is compounded by the use of diuretics prescribed for the treatment of ascites and/or anasarca.

When the patient's sodium falls to less than 135 mmol/L of blood, secondary to water intoxication, osmotic shifts start to occur in the brain. The resulting cerebral edema increases intracranial pressure (ICP), leading to complaints of headache, projectile vomiting, and seizures.

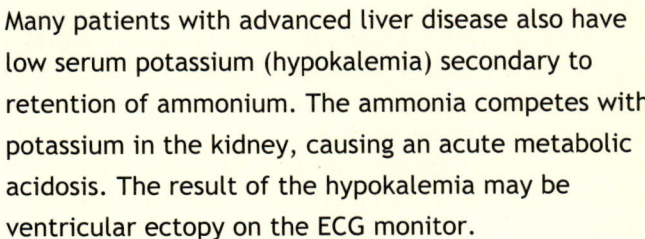

Strict fluid restrictions are typically observed during intravenous therapy of the patient with ascites and/or anasarca unless ensuing hypotension presents a risk to cerebral perfusion.

Cerebral Syndromes

The average person has sufficient stores of the water-soluble vitamin thiamine (B-1) for approximately one month. This supply is constantly being replenished as long as the patient maintains a proper diet. However, the alcoholic patient often fails to eat well, preferring to substitute high caloric alcoholic beverages for food. In the process she fails to ingest needed nutrients, particularly thiamine. The resultant thiamine deficiency, also called beriberi, has impacts on both the cardiovascular system (wet beriberi) and the nervous system (dry beriberi). During wet beriberi, the thiamine deficiency causes vasodilation, activation of the renin-angiotensin-aldosterone mechanism, and fluid retention. This fluid overload stresses the heart and leads to heart failure.

Thiamine deficiency has a dramatic effect upon both the central and peripheral nervous systems. The deficiency initially leads to altered glucose metabolism and neurogeneration, as well as resultant cerebral atrophy in the long term.

Wernicke-Korsakoff Syndrome

The loss of specific brain functions which can be attributed to thiamine deficiency is described in **Wernicke–Korsakoff syndrome** (WKS).[22–24] Carl Wernicke first described a syndrome that included loss of gaze, ataxia, and mental confusion in 1581. If left untreated, Wernicke's encephalopathy would gradually develop into Korsakoff's psychosis. Later in the nineteenth century, it became apparent that the two syndromes had a common thread—thiamine deficiency.

Initially, thiamine deficiency tends to impact both the central and peripheral nervous systems. The alcoholic patient tends to experience peripheral polyneuropathies, which include paresthesia, numbness, and weakness.

Central nervous system involvement includes focal deficits with impacts to the ocular motor centers. This results in impairment of eye movement, manifested by nystagmus, gaze palsy, and even ophthalmoplegia (paralysis of the eyes). Other central nervous system impairments include cerebellar signs, such as ataxia (drunken staggers without intoxication). The presence of ataxia can be assessed by administering the Romberg's test. Over time, the alcoholic patient will progress to central nervous system impairment as a result of degeneration of both the neuron's axons as well as the myelin sheath that protects each axon.

This permanent neurodegeneration, secondary to the thiamine deficiency, leads to Korsakoff's syndrome. **Korsakoff's syndrome**, also known as Korsakoff's psychosis, involves behaviors that can be attributed to a severe impairment of memory such as anterograde and retrograde amnesia. To make up for the loss of memory, these patients often resort to confabulation, the creation of sometimes intricate tales to fill in defects in their memory. These patients genuinely believe that what is being said is true, despite being presented evidence to the contrary. Typically in confabulation, short-term memory is most affected while long-term memory remains intact.

Simple examinations of the eyes (cardinal gazes) can help the Paramedic identify Wernicke's encephalopathy. Simple three item memory tests can help the Paramedic to distinguish Korsakoff's psychosis from Wernicke's encephalopathy. The key difference between these two syndromes is that Wernicke's encephalopathy is temporary and can be cured relatively quickly with the administration of thiamine. However, Korsakoff's psychosis is permanent. Thiamine should be administered whenever alcoholism is suspected in order to reverse the symptoms associated with Wernicke's encephalopathy.

Wernicke-Korsakoff Syndrome and Glucose Administration

Administration of glucose-containing solutions, either dextrose 5% in sterile water as an infusion or dextrose 25 grams intravenous bolus, to reverse hypoglycemia in patients with alcoholism was thought to leave the patient at risk for thiamine deficiency. It was also thought that the glucose could potentially exacerbate Wernicke-Korsakoff syndrome. For this reason, many Paramedics would coadminister from 100 mg to 500 mg thiamine either intravenously or intramuscularly whenever dextrose was administered, reasoning that the thiamine was benign and could potentially protect the patient from WKS. However, thiamine is not without its dangers. Several cases of anaphylaxis due to the preservatives in the intravenous thiamine solution have been reported.[25–27] Furthermore, intravenous administration of thiamine does not immediately repair the damage of prolonged thiamine deficiency, particularly to the nervous system. Therefore, when balancing the benefits of prehospital administration of thiamine (which is negligible) against the risk of anaphylaxis, many EMS systems have stopped the practice of thiamine administration.

Many alcoholic patients also suffer from hypomagnesemia. Without magnesium, thiamine is rendered ineffective, making it imperative to correct the magnesium levels first. Finally, WKS is relatively rare in the United States thanks, in part, to vitamin fortified foods.

If WKS is strongly suspected following physical examination of a patient with alcoholism, then 50 to 100 mg thiamine may be administered either intravenously or intramuscularly. Re-examination of the patient may show an improvement in ocular signs but may not necessarily show improvements in memory.

Acute Liver Failure

Liver failure can take from months to years to occur, with all of the complications discussed previously. A patient with a rapid deterioration of liver function is said to be in **acute liver failure**. Acute liver failure is a medical emergency, with an associated high mortality rate despite modern medical therapeutics.

Patients with acute liver failure, also known as fulminant hepatic failure, routinely have coagulopathy (discussed earlier) and/or hepatic encephalopathy. Hepatic encephalopathy often brings these patients to the attention of Paramedics.

Drug overdose, accidental or intentional, is the leading cause of acute liver failure, and the leading offender is acetaminophen. During metabolism of acetaminophen, the liver produces a more toxic metabolite that is usually neutralized by intrahepatic glutathione. If the patient ingests a large dose of acetaminophen, the active metabolite overwhelms the reserves of intrahepatic glutathione, leading to hepatic toxicity.

Alternatively, the patient may have ingested a therapeutic dose of acetaminophen in addition to alcohol, even in moderate amounts. In that case, both the alcohol and the acetaminophen are competing for the same intrahepatic glutathione and the result is a relative toxicity.

Although acetaminophen presents the single largest cause of acute liver failure, viral infections—including hepatitis A and B, herpes, and cytomegalovirus—can also cause acute liver failure. Another etiology of acute liver failure is idiosyncratic hypersensitivity reactions to drugs such as antibiotics, antivirals, antidepressants, antiepileptics, and Antabuse®, to name just a few. Also, several well-known toxins—from mushrooms, cyanobacteria, and organic solvents—can cause acute liver failure. Even heat stroke has been known to cause acute liver failure.

At present, while artificial liver support systems are being developed, the best chance of survival lies with orthotopic (donated) liver transplant. Patients receiving a liver transplant have between a 60% to 80% chance of one year survival.

Hepatic Encephalopathy

Hepatic encephalopathy occurs when either the liver fails to clear toxins from the blood or the patient develops a portal systemic shunt, secondary to portal hypertension, that causes blood to bypass the liver. Regardless of the etiology of the toxins, **hepatic encephalopathy** is a potentially reversible metabolic derangement which affects the brain, causing it to dysfunction.

Ammonia

The key metabolite that has been implicated in hepatic encephalopathy is ammonia.[28,29] Elevated ammonia levels in the blood (**hyperammonemia**) can lead to cerebral edema, increased intracranial pressure, and death.

Ammonia is a naturally occurring by-product of protein catabolism by bacteria in the intestine. Normally, the amino acids and ammonia absorbed from the intestines would then proceed to the liver via the mesenteric veins. The liver then detoxifies the ammonia, via the urea cycle (discovered by Krebs), with N-acetylglutamate. The resulting urea is primarily excreted in the urine, with a small amount excreted in the sweat.

With the development of liver cirrhosis and subsequent portal hypertension, the flow of blood is impeded and alternative pathways opened. These new pathways, called portacaval anastomosis, allow blood to bypass the liver (portacaval shunt) and enter into the systemic circulation without undergoing first-pass detoxification of ammonia and other toxins. Subsequently, ammonia levels build to toxic levels.

Ammonia can build, even if the patient is on a low protein diet, because of blood present inside the gastrointestinal tract. This blood, secondary to GI bleeding, contains proteins. These blood proteins are broken down into ammonia and, using the portacaval shunts, bypass the liver to enter the systemic circulation. Ammonia readily crosses the blood–brain barrier, where it causes cellular edema (particularly of astrocytes), global cerebral edema, and increasing intracranial pressure.

The patient's mental status changes associated with cerebral edema are progressive. The changes have, by medical consensus, been divided into four neuropsychiatric grades. The first stage represents minimal hepatic encephalopathy and is characterized by shortened attention span and similar mental deficits. Infections can also trigger hepatic encephalopathy. When the body responds to an infection (e.g., a spontaneous bacterial peritonitis secondary to bacterial infection of ascitic fluid), the immunologic response includes immunoglobins (proteins) which are broken down in the attack. Thus, ammonia levels rise and hepatic encephalopathy ensues. This is often the only overt sign of infection.

As the hyperammonemia levels climb, in the second stage, the patient starts to become apathetic with occasional displays of inappropriate behavior. Often the patient will have difficulty following simple commands. At the third stage, the patient becomes stuporous but remains responsive to verbal stimuli. At this point, the patient is markedly confused and disoriented. Finally, in stage four, the patient is comatose, and will experience marked increases in intracerebral pressure, leading to transtentorial herniation and death.

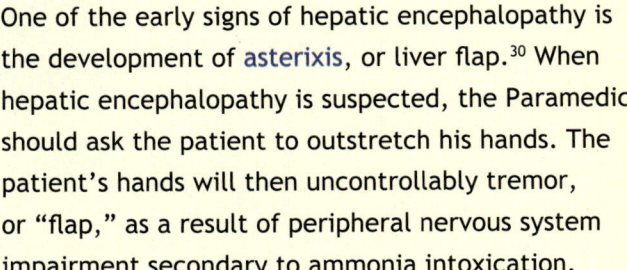

STREET SMART

One of the early signs of hepatic encephalopathy is the development of asterixis, or liver flap.[30] When hepatic encephalopathy is suspected, the Paramedic should ask the patient to outstretch his hands. The patient's hands will then uncontrollably tremor, or "flap," as a result of peripheral nervous system impairment secondary to ammonia intoxication.

Cerebral Edema

Cerebral edema (excess fluid on the brain), secondary to ammonia intoxication, leads to increased intracranial pressures. This in turn leads to transtentorial herniation through the foraman magnum. Alternatively, hypo-osmolarity, secondary to hyponatremia associated with hepatorenal syndrome, can lead to free fluids shifting from the blood into the brain and creating cerebral edema, transtentorial herniation, and death.

Compounding the concern for cerebral edema is the complication of cytotoxic mechanisms at work in the brain. Normally, the blood–brain barrier would impede toxins, which normally would be detoxified in the liver, from entering the brain. With liver disease the integrity of the blood–brain barrier is compromised, particularly with the accumulation of ammonia. These poisons enter the brain, alter brain metabolism, create toxic oxygen products (oxygen-free radicals), and weaken cell membranes. This results in the release of cell-destroying lysozymes and a host of other cytotoxic mechanisms.

When signs and symptoms of hepatic encephalopathy (i.e., acute liver failure) occur within 28 days, etiologies other than alcohol must be considered. Potential causes of acute liver failure include acetaminophen overdose, acute viremia from hepatitis, Reye's syndrome, and an idiosyncratic reaction to medication.[31]

Acute Alcohol Poisoning

Any substance, even water, taken in excess can be toxic, and alcohol is no exception (Table 15-4). **Acute alcohol poisoning** is ingestion of excessive quantities of alcohol within a short period of time, leading to a peak alcohol level greater than 0.40 grams per deciliter.

Individuals at risk for alcohol poisoning come in all ages. However, the majority are males (over 80%), and the rate is highest among unmarried persons. The Centers for Disease Control and Prevention estimates that approximately 300 to 400 deaths a year occur directly because of alcohol poisoning. In addition, alcohol contributes to another 1,000 deaths. Patients most at risk for alcohol poisoning are inexperienced drinkers between the ages of 35 and 54, not the chronic alcoholic who has developed a tolerance to alcohol.

In one study of acute alcohol poisoning, where the majority of victims were males with a mean age of 53 years, the BAC was found to be 0.36 mg/dL, with the highest being 0.68 mg/dL. Children may also be at risk of acute alcohol poisoning with ingestion of seemingly small amounts of alcohol and a BAC as low as 0.10 mg/dL.

High blood alcohol levels essentially anesthetize the brain, suppressing protective airway reflexes as well as causing autonomic dysfunction. This autonomic dysfunction can lead to hypotension, hypothermia, and hypoventilation, with a resultant cardiovascular collapse if untreated.

Treatment of Alcohol Overdose

In the not too distant past, noxious stimulants (such as ammonia inhalants) were used to arouse the patient. Hot beverages, such as black coffee, were used to keep the patient stimulated.

The airway is the Paramedic's first priority when treating a suspected alcohol overdose. The easiest technique for airway control, assuming no spinal injury is present, is to roll the patient into the recovery position (left lateral recumbent) and allow the airway to drain naturally with suctioning as needed. The majority of alcohol poisonings can be treated with these simple techniques.

If the patient is deeply obtunded (responding to painful stimuli) it may be necessary for the Paramedic to intubate the patient to protect the airway and prevent aspiration. It may also be necessary to use a short-acting sedative, such as etomidate, to facilitate the intubation if the patient has a weak gag reflex.

In the past, gastric lavage (in lay terms, "pumping the stomach") was performed if the ingestion occurred within the past four hours. It should be noted that Paramedics generally do not use lavage unless the ingestion occurred less than one hour ago or the patient is completely obtunded.[32]

Table 15-4 Blood Alcohol Concentration to Clinical Presentation

Blood Alcohol Concentration	Behavior	Symptoms	
0.01 to 0.12	Euphoria	Loss of inhibition	Loss of fine motor control Shortened attention span
0.10 to 0.25	Lethargy	Somnolence	Memory impairment Ataxia
0.25 to 0.40	Stupor	Difficult to arouse	Lack of muscle coordination Lapses of consciousness Incontinence Risk of aspiration
0.35 to 0.50	Coma	Unconsciousness	Depressed reflexes Hypothermia Respiratory depression Risk of CNS collapse

After the Paramedic places the nasogastric tube, the stomach contents should be evacuated. Following that, a gavage (irrigation) of the stomach may be ordered. Unless mixed ingestion is suspected, activated charcoal should not be administered. It does not absorb alcohol well and could result in an aspiration if the patient vomits.

In the past, Paramedics used large bore orogastric tubes, called Ewald tubes, to "pump the stomach." However, the efficacy of this practice has been questioned and the use of large bore orogastric tubes has fallen out of favor.

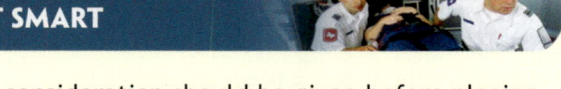

STREET SMART

Careful consideration should be given before placing a nasogastric tube if the patient is a chronic alcoholic with a potential for esophageal varices.

After ensuring airway patency, the Paramedic should consider the patient's respiratory status. If the patient is hypoventilating, the Paramedic may need to support the ventilation with a bag–valve mask, while being constantly vigilant for signs of vomiting.

The Paramedic should also consider establishing intravenous access to check blood glucose levels, administer fluids as needed, and use as an access point for medication administration in case of seizure.

Ingestion of large quantities of alcohol is thought to be one of the causes of idiopathic atrial fibrillation. This phenomenon, also called holiday heart syndrome, may be due to the increased levels of epinephrine which occur during the period of intoxication and leads to heart stress and tachycardias.

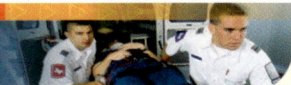

STREET SMART

Acute intoxication increases the secretion of insulin and can cause hypoglycemia even in the nondiabetic patient. The Paramedic should perform a point of care blood glucose analysis on acutely intoxicated patients.

Ethylene Glycol, Methanol, and Isopropyl Poisoning

The term "alcohol" represents a group of organically obtained chemical compounds that all have a hydroxyl group (-OH) attached. Alcohols in the alcohol family include ethylene glycol, methyl alcohol (methanol), glycerol, and isopropyl alcohol.[33]

Ethyl alcohol, with the abbreviation Et for ethyl and OH for the hydroxyl group, or EtOH, is the popular substance used in alcoholic beverages. EtOH is strongly attracted to water (hydrophilic) and therefore distributes easily to all compartments of the body, including the brain.

Isopropyl alcohol, another alcohol with strong solvent properties, is used as a cleaner and as a gasoline additive in dry gas. It binds with water in the gasoline and, because of alcohol's lower freezing temperature, prevents fuel line freeze-up. Although isopropyl alcohol can be used as a "rubbing" alcohol, the commercially available isopropyl alcohol is actually ethyl alcohol that has been denatured to render it unfit for consumption.

Methyl alcohol is a simple, sweet tasting alcohol that is extremely volatile, and thus prone to give off a distinctive odor. It is used in antifreeze, fuels, and as a biofuel. As a naturally occurring alcohol, also called wood alcohol or wood spirits, it can be produced by destructive distillation of wood. Ingestion of wood alcohol is probably most noted for its ability to cause blindness. During the detoxification process, the liver converts methyl alcohol into formic acid and formaldehyde, the substance used in embalming, which affects the optic nerve.

One form of denatured alcohol, via the use of methyl alcohol in the mixture with ethyl alcohol to denature it, is called methylated spirits. Manufacturers purposely denature ethyl alcohol to avoid paying liquor excise taxes to the federal government. Use of filters, such as bread, does not remove the impurities in the denatured alcohol. Poverty stricken alcoholics have been known to drink the gelled alcohol found in Sterno®, a canned heating fuel, by straining it through a sock or even a loaf of French bread to retrieve the alcohol. This filtration process does not work and, as a result, the patient ingests the methyl alcohol used to denature the ethyl alcohol.

Ethylene glycol is a particularly dangerous form of alcohol. The use of ethylene glycol as an antifreeze for radiators and as a deicer for aircraft lead to its wide distribution. Unfortunately, children and house pets may ingest the sweet ethylene glycol and become poisoned. Ethylene glycol is highly toxic in amounts of approximately 1 to 1.5 mL per kilogram of body weight. As little as 30 milliliters, or two tablespoons, can potentially cause death in a patient. Ingestion can rapidly lead to liver failure.[34] Toxicity occurs because the liver converts ethylene glycol, via oxidative reactions, into glycolic acid, and thereby induces a metabolic acidosis.

The symptoms of ethylene glycol poisoning are initially similar to alcohol intoxication (i.e., confusion, ataxia, hallucinations, and slurred speech). As the ethylene glycol is metabolized, the metabolic acidosis phase starts. In about 6 to 12 hours, the cardiopulmonary impacts become evident. The poisoned patient will initially experience hypertension and tachycardia, with associated muscle spasms linked with hypocalcemia (the end product oxalic acid binds available free calcium).

If left untreated, ethylene glycol becomes fatal within 24 to 36 hours. Oxalic acid forms with calcium to become calcium oxalate, causing kidney failure as well as general muscle weakness, heart failure, and death.

Gastric lavage or the use of syrup of ipecac is not indicated for the treatment of ethylene glycol ingestion. Ethylene glycol is rapidly absorbed in the stomach, making these

The presentation of an intoxicated person, without the typical odors associated with an alcoholic beverage, might lead a Paramedic to suspect ethylene glycol poisoning.

time-consuming treatments ineffective. Instead, the treatment of ethylene glycol poisoning focuses on the reversal of the metabolic acidosis and the prevention of the production of toxic metabolites in the liver. Sodium bicarbonate, approximately 50 to 100 mEq, can be used to reverse the metabolic acidosis, as well as increase the elimination of glycolic acid via the kidneys. However, this action may worsen hypocalcemia. If sodium bicarbonate is administered, then the

Paramedic must focus on maintaining ventilation, including hyperventilation, as needed.

Another potential prehospital treatment of ethylene glycol poisoning is the administration of ethyl alcohol. The ethyl alcohol competes with the ethylene glycol for the enzyme alcohol dehydrogenase, which inhibits the formation of toxic metabolites. Ethanol may be administered intravenously, orally, or via nasogastric tube if the patient is unwilling or unable to drink. The therapeutic goal is to reach and maintain a blood alcohol level of approximately 0.1 to 0.15 mg/dL.

Fomepizole inhibits the enzyme alcohol dehydrogenase and has received U.S. FDA approval as a treatment for ethylene glycol poisoning. Although expensive (up to $3,000 per patient), it has been shown to be safe and effective, and can potentially eliminate the need for hemodialysis.[35]

If the ethylene glycol poisoning has progressed to the point of renal complications and/or metabolic acidosis, then it may be necessary to use hemodialysis.

CASE STUDY (CONTINUED)

Using a calm approach and quiet voices, the two Paramedics are able to calm the man and place him in their ambulance. One Paramedic develops rapport with the patient and begins an assessment while the other confers with the police officer.

The officer reports that the patient's wife had given the man an ultimatum to stop his drinking or she was leaving. To her knowledge, the patient last had a drink two days ago. He had tried to stop drinking many times in the past but always resumed when life became stressful.

CRITICAL THINKING QUESTIONS

1. What are the important elements of the history that a Paramedic should obtain?
2. What is the symptom pattern for acute alcohol withdrawal?

History

Taking a history from a patient with alcoholism can be a challenge. Early changes of hepatic encephalopathy, and a tendency toward defensiveness regarding alcoholism, can leave the patient irritable and difficult to communicate with on an interpersonal level.

Taking a History

Before taking a medical history from the patient, the Paramedic should remove the patient from the alcohol and distance the patient from any family, or others, who may agitate him. The safety and sanctuary of the ambulance is often the best place for a Paramedic to take a history and perform a physical examination.

The history should be as short as possible, concentrating on important information. However, it may be necessary for the Paramedic to repeat certain questions, as the patient may have problems with short-term memory.

If the patient appears to get angry when asked a certain question, the Paramedic should not attempt to force an answer. For example, if the patient does not want to answer the question "When was your last drink?" the Paramedic should explain the need for the information and try to reword the question in a nonthreatening manner.

The Paramedic should also attempt to remain nonjudgmental but firm with the patient about the need for medical evaluation and treatment. If the patient asks questions, honesty is the best policy. The Paramedic should not agree or disagree with statements the patient may make regarding the use of alcohol.

Symptom Complex

After primary assessment has ruled out hypoxia and hypoglycemia as possible etiologies for the altered mental status, the Paramedic should proceed with a careful history to try and ascertain the symptom complex.

One of the most characteristic symptoms associated with hepatic disease is pruritis, an itchy feeling not relieved by scratching. In one study, 40% of patients with diagnosed liver disease complained of pruritus. Pruritus is often limited to the lower extremities but may progress to the body's trunk. However, pruritus may also be induced by drugs (e,g., the phenothiazines) or other causes of cholestasis.

Often an acute infection will cause the patient with alcoholic liver disease to decompensate. Of particular concern is bacterial peritonitis. The patient should be questioned regarding fevers, sweats, and chills, as well as abdominal pain, which could all be symptoms of an infection. However, a great number of associated symptoms (e.g., anorexia) are not specific to alcoholic liver disease and can also be seen in other diseases.

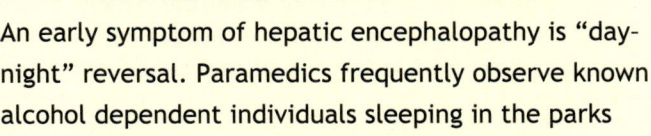

STREET SMART

An early symptom of hepatic encephalopathy is "day-night" reversal. Paramedics frequently observe known alcohol dependent individuals sleeping in the parks during the day and frequenting the bars at night.

Allergies and Pertinent Past Medical History

As per routine, the patient should be asked about diagnosis of various chronic diseases such as diabetes. Many alcoholic patients have a codiagnosis of seizures, which may have been the result of head injuries or prior attempts at alcohol withdrawal.

Another common coexistent disorder with alcoholism is pancreatitis. Even if undiagnosed, the presence of right upper quadrant abdominal pain following a bout of drinking is highly suggestive of pancreatitis.

Finally, the Paramedic should ask the patient if he has vomited bright red blood (hematemesis) as opposed to spitting up blood (hemoptysis). Hematemesis is suggestive of esophageal varices, another comorbidity of alcoholic liver disease.

Medications and Last Meal

The Paramedic should elicit a careful drug history, concentrating on the patient's new prescriptions, changed prescriptions, or noncompliance with prescribed medications. For example, the addition of a benzodiazepine, in an attempt to self-medicate during withdrawal, may actually potentiate even a small amount of alcohol. Alcohol can also shorten the acute liver failure-life of certain drugs. For example, alcohol taken with phenytoin may shorten the acute liver failure-life of phenytoin, with a potential for subsequent breakthrough seizures.

The dietary status of alcoholics is always cause for concern. The combination of anorexia with the patient's tendency to substitute high calorie alcoholic beverages for food that can provide proper nutrition can lead to malnutrition and vitamin deficiencies, particular if the diet has a lack of thiamine.

While asking the patient about his last meal, the Paramedic should also ask about the patient's last drink and the possibility of ingestion of non-ethyl alcohols such as antifreeze or "moonshine." If the patient is resistant to answer the question, an alternative question may be posed about drinking mouthwash or over-the-counter medications that contain alcohol.

Like the patient with emphysema who is asked about his "pack-years" of tobacco smoking, the alcoholic should be asked about his number of drinks a week and the number of years of drinking. If the patient is reticent to disclose that information, the Paramedic can pose an alternative question, such as the occurrence and number of blackouts the patient has experienced.

Events Preceding

Questions about events preceding the arrival of the Paramedics should focus on trauma (including falls, with subsequent head injury) or assaults (with head injury). Some alcoholics develop chronic subdural hematomas (i.e., reoccurring brain bleeds) as a result of liver disease and subsequent coagulopathy. Therefore, the patient should be asked about any falls or assaults that have occurred in the past 30 days.

Family and friends can offer insight into the patient's mental status. They may report that they have observed subtle changes in the patient's personality or thinking. These mental status changes may be indicative of early liver disease secondary to alcoholism.

CASE STUDY (CONTINUED)

The Paramedics' initial assessment shows the man to be aware of his surroundings with an open airway, adequate breathing, and no obvious bleeding. He is confused as to what day it is and is convinced that someone is chasing him. He is tachycardic, hypertensive, and diaphoretic.

CRITICAL THINKING QUESTIONS

1. What are the elements of the physical examination of a patient with suspected acute alcohol withdrawal?
2. Why is a neurological examination a critical element in this examination?

Examination

After completing the primary assessment of the patient and taking a history, the Paramedic should proceed with a head-to-toe assessment of the patient, starting with a set of vital signs. It is characteristic of a patient with alcoholic liver disease to be hyperdynamic, secondary to the stimulation of the renin-angiotensin-aldosterone mechanism as well as the release of epinephrine.

Alterations of this hyperdynamic pattern—hypertension, tachycardia, and tachypnea—may be indicative of other pathologies, such as increased intracranial pressure, and warrant further investigation.

Head-to-Toe Examination

The continued physical examination of the patient with alcoholic liver disease should proceed in a head-to-toe fashion, with careful attention paid to the signs of trauma. After examining the the patient's scalp for injury, as well as examining the ears and nose for drainage, the Paramedic should examine the eyes. The presence of jaundice in the sclera and/or the conjunctiva may be indicative of liver cirrhosis. The patient's eyesight should also be examined for visual acuity. Poor vision may be suggestive of the impending blindness which occurs when the optic nerve is poisoned by methyl alcohol.

After examining the eyes, the Paramedic should sit back and make a general assessment of the patient's face, the neck, and the upper chest for the presence of spider nevi. Spider nevi, also known as spider telangiectasias, are small bundles of blood vessels that appear as a red dot in the center with vessels radiating outward, like a spider's web. The growth of these bundles of new blood vessels, or angiogenesis, is secondary to high estrogen levels, and is seen in about one-third of patients with alcoholic liver disease.

During the examination, the Paramedic may note a musty sweet odor on the patient's breath. This fetid breath, called **fetor hepaticus**, is a mixture of ammonia, thiol, a sulfur compound, and volatile ketones on the breath.[36] Another consequence of elevated estrogen levels in males with alcoholic liver disease is **gynecomastia** or breast enlargement.

Abdominal Exam

Upon gross inspection, the abdomen of the patient with alcoholic liver disease will appear distended. This distention may be the result of hepatomegaly, splenomegaly, and/or ascites. Closer examination of the skin by the Paramedic may reveal snake-like veins on the surface, secondary to umbilical vein distention, or caput medusa.

Auscultation of the abdomen may reveal a venous hum in the epigastric region secondary to portal hypertension and portacaval shunting. The Paramedic may appreciate the border of the distended liver when palpating the left upper quadrant. This is often described as being like a pencil rolling under the fingers. Palpation of the right upper quadrant may elicit some point tenderness from the enlarged spleen (i.e., splenomegaly).

Finally, the Paramedic may appreciate the presence of ascites, the protein-containing fluid that leaks into the peritoneal cavity, in the abdomen. Mild ascites may be noted by fluid accumulation in the flanks when the patient is lying supine. Substantial accumulations of ascites can occur and appear as a fluid wave when the patient is turned or the abdomen is tapped.

Extremities

The patient with chronic alcoholic liver disease often has characteristically thin arms, sometimes described as stick-like, secondary to muscular atrophy. The Paramedic should ask the patient to hold out his hands in front of him with the arms outstretched and dorsiflex the wrist. The hands of the patient with alcoholic liver disease, particularly those patients with hepatic encephalopathy, will tend to tremor in a flapping motion. This phenomenon, called a **liver flap**, is not reserved to the wrists but can also be seen in the foot, hips, and even the tongue.

Examination of the palms of the patient's hands may reveal **palmar erythema** (i.e., liver palm), or redness of the palms. Palmar erythema is characterized by mottling of the palms which blanches under pressure. Patients sometimes complain of a throbbing in the hands. Like gynecomastia, palmar erythema is thought to be due to elevated estrogen levels.

CASE STUDY (CONTINUED)

The patient has calmed down and is asking for his wife. He is concerned that she will think he has relapsed (i.e., "is off the wagon") and is drinking again. The Paramedic reassures him that he will speak to the patient's wife but first they need to take care of him.

CRITICAL THINKING QUESTIONS

1. Why does the patient need immediate care?
2. What diagnosis did the Paramedic announce to the patient's wife?

Assessment

A patient symptom complex, such as the one presented in the Case Study, and the resultant physical examination findings would suggest an addiction disorder related to alcoholism and the associated pathology of alcohol cirrhosis.

CASE STUDY (CONTINUED)

Appreciative of the Paramedic's concern, the patient agrees to some rudimentary treatments, such as an intravenous access. While the patient states that he is calm, saying repeatedly "I am all right, I am all right," his darting eyes and concerned look telegraph to the Paramedic that he is still anxious and apparently fearful of something.

CRITICAL THINKING QUESTIONS

1. What is the standard of care of patients with suspected acute alcohol withdrawal?
2. What are some of the patient-specific concerns and considerations that the Paramedic should consider when applying this plan of care that is intended to treat a broad patient population presenting with acute alcohol withdrawal?

Treatment

Treatment of the alcoholic patient with an altered level of consciousness should focus on eliminating obvious etiologies such as hypoxia and hypoglycemia. After instituting protective measures—such as airway management and endotracheal intubation, as needed—the next concern is maintaining adequate cerebral perfusion. Cerebral perfusion is a function of the mean arterial pressure (MAP) minus the intracranial pressure (CPP = MAP − ICP). If the MAP is insufficient to maintain cerebral perfusion (i.e., less than 60 mmHg), then vasopressor support may be necessary to maintain an adequate systemic blood pressure.

Conversely, increased intracranial pressure, secondary to ammonia-induced cerebral edema, may reduce cerebral perfusion. Efforts to decrease intracranial pressures through the use of diuretics may be considered, but any ensuing hypotension will be more devastating to the patient.

Psychological First Aid

Fear is the key factor that leads to the agitation of the delirious patient. Through careful manipulation of the environment, the Paramedic can reduce the patient's anxiety and agitation.

To begin, the Paramedic must provide the patient with emotional support and continuous reorientation to reality. Through clear and concise communications, the Paramedic should reinforce the time, the date, and the situation, including repeated introductions of all the providers. If the patient is hearing or sight impaired, then the Paramedic should ensure that the patient's hearing aids, glasses, and any other assistive technologies are available.

Patients are often frightened of chaotic and confusing scenes. The Paramedic should make efforts to either defuse and deescalate the scene or move the patient to an unambiguous environment, like the back of the ambulance.

To aid the patient with identifying environmental clues which help reorient the patient, the Paramedic can ensure there is adequate lighting, decrease ambient noise by removing unnecessary personnel, and turn down the volume on the radio.

CASE STUDY (CONTINUED)

Although the patient has been tremulous throughout the transport, he suddenly starts to shake uncontrollably. The Paramedic immediately realizes that the patient is experiencing a convulsion most likely related to his alcohol withdrawal. After taking initial basic measures to protect the patient, the Paramedic prepares to sedate the patient to prevent further seizures.

CRITICAL THINKING QUESTIONS

1. What are some of the predictable complications associated with acute alcohol withdrawal?
2. What are some of the predictable complications associated with the treatments for convulsions related to acute alcohol withdrawal?

Evaluation

Acute alcohol withdrawal is a potentially life-threatening emergency, particularly if the patient has a history of prior attempts at alcohol withdrawal. It is estimated that every year over two million Americans will experience alcohol withdrawal, yet less than 20% will be medically monitored during their withdrawal. When those patients who choose to withdraw alone have unexpected and/or unmanageable withdrawal symptoms, they will call for EMS.

Pathophysiology of Alcohol Withdrawal

Alcohol enhances the inhibitory neurotransmitter GABA, leading to its sedative effects in large doses. Chronic alcohol abuse results in desensitization of the GABA receptors in the brain to alcohol, requiring ever increasing amounts of alcohol to get the same effect (i.e., a tolerance to alcohol is developed).

Alcohol also inhibits the excitatory neurotransmitter NMDA. Chronic alcohol abuse results in the upregulation of NMDA receptors as the brain tries to balance the sedative effects of alcohol. When the patient suddenly stops abusing alcohol, the excitatory NMDA receptors are no longer inhibited and the inhibitory GABA receptors are no longer stimulated, resulting in a collective effect of overstimulation of the brain.

Symptom Pattern

Alcohol withdrawal causes both psychological and physical symptoms in varying degrees according to the extent of the patient's alcohol addiction and the number of prior attempts at detoxification. The repeated detoxification efforts' impact on alcohol withdrawal is embodied in a phenomenon called "kindling." Kindling is the result of the impact of repeated prior detoxification on the brain. Each detoxicification tends to increase the patient's desire for alcohol, witnessed as increasingly obsessive thoughts about drinking. The kindling phenomena also suggests that with each attempt at alcohol withdrawal the patient will become increasingly more symptomatic, with a corresponding increase in the risk of convulsions as well as long-term neurological disability.

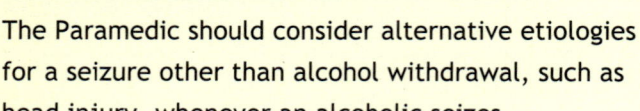

STREET SMART

The Paramedic should consider alternative etiologies for a seizure other than alcohol withdrawal, such as head injury, whenever an alcoholic seizes.

The severity of alcohol withdrawal can range from mild to debilitating to deadly. The patient with mild to moderate withdrawal may have feelings of anxiety, shakiness, and emotional lability ranging from excited to depressed. Patients with mild to moderate alcohol withdrawal may also experience visual and/or tactile hallucinations, but otherwise are coherent and interactive with their surroundings.

Collectively, the symptom pattern associated with alcohol withdrawal can be summarized as **autonomic hyperactivity**. The patient may experience profuse sweating (particularly of the hands and face), tachycardia, and hypertension, as well as hand tremors and nausea (with or without vomiting) as a result of autonomic overstimulation.[37–39]

Patients in withdrawal may also complain of a pulsating headache. Headaches are a particularly problematic symptom for the Paramedic, as the headache may be associated with alcohol withdrawal or an intracranial hemorrhage brought on by hypertension.

Delirium Tremens

Severe alcohol withdrawal results in confusion, delirium, and seizures. This triad of symptoms is referred to as the **delirium tremens (DT)**. Although a myriad of factors—such as heavy alcohol abuse, age, liver function, and previous withdrawal seizures—combine to make a withdrawal severe, the presence of confusion, delirium, and/or seizures signals a potentially life-threatening event. Even with current technologies and medications, the mortality from the DT is between 1% and 5%.

The DT is a disorder that includes psychotic behaviors, including hallucinations, and a disconnection with the patient's surroundings. Generalized tonic–clonic seizures may also occur; these seizures earned the DT the nickname the "rum fits."

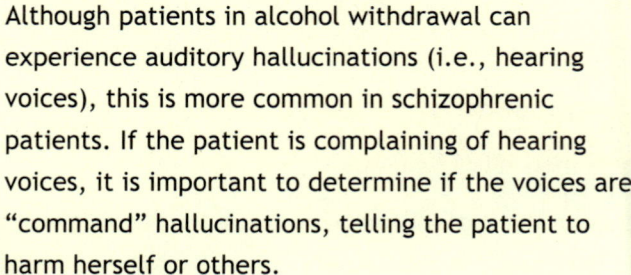

STREET SMART

Although patients in alcohol withdrawal can experience auditory hallucinations (i.e., hearing voices), this is more common in schizophrenic patients. If the patient is complaining of hearing voices, it is important to determine if the voices are "command" hallucinations, telling the patient to harm herself or others.

The first symptoms of withdrawal generally occur about 6 to 12 hours after the patient stops drinking. During this period, the patient becomes increasingly restless (autonomic hyperactivity) and starts to have the general physical symptomology of withdrawal.

During the next 6 to 12 hours, the patient may start to experience the psychological symptoms of withdrawal or

alcoholic hallucinosis (i.e., auditory, tactile, and visual hallucinations). Characteristic hallucinations ascribed to alcohol withdrawal are a feeling of insects under the skin, the sound of ringing bells, or walls that seem to move. These hallucinations are genuinely frightening to the patient.

Treatment

The focus of prehospital treatment of the patient with severe alcohol withdrawal focuses on decreasing the autonomic stimulation and correcting any fluid deficits. A combination of hyperthermia, profuse diaphoresis, and unremitting vomiting may leave the patient in withdrawal acutely hypovolumic. If that is the case, intravenous administration of isotonic fluid may be indicated.

The Paramedic must exercise caution when resuscitating the patient in withdrawal as the typical signs of hypoperfusion (tachycardia) may be the result of alcohol withdrawal.

The mainstay of pharmacological treatment of alcohol withdrawal has been benzodiazepines. Benzodiazepines have the twofold advantage of treating the symptoms of alcohol withdrawal syndrome as well as preventing seizures.

Typically, diazepam is used in the prehospital setting. This is in part because of its safety profile but also because of its relatively longer acute liver failure-life, preventing the rebound that is seen with shorter-acting sedatives.

Alternatively, the benzodiazepine lorazepam can be used. Lorazepam is the drug of choice for patients who have difficulty metabolizing drugs, such as those patients with liver failure or the elderly. Lorazepam has the added bonus of being able to be administered intramuscularly without concerns for erratic absorption seen with other benzodiazepines administered intramuscularly.

The traditional concerns of respiratory depression are less problematic for the patient in alcohol withdrawal. The Paramedic's focus of treatment should remain on normalizing the patient's vital signs. On occasion, the patient in delirium tremens is so agitated that additional pharmacological support is needed. In those cases, the drug of choice is haloperidol. It is important to administer the benzodiazepine to stop seizures associated with alcohol withdrawal first, since haloperidol is known to lower the seizure threshold. The patient may therefore be at risk of experiencing a seizure. In some EMS systems, haloperidol is withheld entirely if the patient has a history of seizures, in order to prevent drug-induced seizure activity.

Autonomic hyperactivity may also strain the heart. The use of beta blockers as an adjunctive therapy could be considered to decrease the myocardial oxygen demand. Caution should be taken to ensure that the patient does not have a mixed addiction of alcohol and cocaine. Administration of a beta blocker to a patient on cocaine can create an alpha receptor surge, leading to hypertensive crisis.

STREET SMART

When the symptoms of alcohol withdrawal become intolerable, the alcoholic patient may choose to self-medicate with alcohol. The Paramedic should emphasize that these symptoms can be controlled with benzodiazepines and the patient does not have to resume drinking.

CASE STUDY CONCLUSION

The Paramedic administers a benzodiazepine to control the seizure. The patient is brought to the emergency department where his alcohol withdrawal can be medically monitored. He is quickly admitted to a detoxification unit.

CRITICAL THINKING QUESTIONS

1. What is the most appropriate transport decision that will get the patient to definitive care?
2. What are the advantages of transporting a patient with suspected acute alcohol withdrawal to these hospitals, even if that means bypassing other hospitals in the process?

Disposition

The patient with alcoholic liver disease has a complex multisystem pathology. Although at times this is difficult, these patients must be directed to medical care to prevent further deterioration of their condition.

CONCLUSION

Addiction disorders are common across all socioeconomic boundaries, leaving no group unaffected. Withdrawal from some substances can cause significant physical problems, which may develop into life-threatening conditions. Although an addiction disorder may not be immediately apparent to the Paramedic, it should be considered in the paramedical differential for any patient with altered mental status or delirium.

KEY POINTS:

- Delirium is a transient state caused by medical or psychiatric conditions.

- Alcoholism is a chronic disease that can be fatal.

- A key feature of alcoholism is the patient's inability to control the consumption of alcohol, resulting in adverse consequences and distorted reasoning.

- Coexistent problems with alcoholism include seizures, pancreatitis, and hematemesis.

- Treatment of the patient with alcoholism and an altered level of consciousness begins with focusing on reversible causes, for example hypoglycemia.

- Careful manipulation of the environment can reduce the patient's fear and agitation.

- Ethanol acts in different ways throughout the different parts of the central nervous system.

- Alcohol consumption can induce birth defects in the developing fetus.

- Excessive alcohol consumption is implicated in several forms of liver disease, leading to abnormal bleeding and altered fluid balance.

- Acute alcohol poisoning impairs both cardiovascular and respiratory systems.

- Ethanol is the alcohol component of alcoholic beverages. Other forms of alcohol may be ingested with fatal results.

- Many alcoholic patients experience seizures.

- Emergency treatment of the alcoholic patient should focus on prevention or mitigation of hypoxia and/or hypoglycemia.

- Withdrawal from alcohol is a medical emergency leading to autonomic hyperactivity, delirium tremens, and seizures.

- Benzodiazepines are the emergency treatment of choice for alcohol withdrawal.

REVIEW QUESTIONS:

1. What three key features characterize alcoholism?
2. What is the mechanism of action of ethanol?
3. How does the ingestion of alcohol by a pregnant woman affect the fetus?
4. Name three liver diseases related to the ingestion of ethanol.
5. How does alcohol ingestion affect fluid balance?
6. Describe alcohol poisoning as it relates to respiratory and cardiovascular collapse.
7. What Paramedic observation may lead to investigation of the ingestion of ethylene glycol?
8. Name signs and symptoms of delirium tremens.
9. How are delirium tremens treated in the field?

Please refer to the Case Study in this chapter, and answer the questions below:

1. What assessments led the Paramedics to conclude that their patient was in withdrawal and not suffering from alcohol poisoning?

2. What signs and symptoms point toward alcoholism in this patient?

3. What comorbidities or injuries are likely to be present in a patient with alcoholism?

4. Would you consider beta blockers for tachycardia and hypertension? Why or why not?

REFERENCES:

1. Kirshner HS. Delirium: a focused review. *Curr Neurol Neurosci Rep.* 2007;7(6):479–482.

2. Milisen K, Braes T, et al. Cognitive assessment and differentiating the 3 Ds (dementia, depression, delirium). *Nurs Clin North Am.* 2006;41(1):1–22, v.

3. Arnold E. Sorting out the 3 D's: delirium, dementia, and depression. *Nursing.* 2004;34(6):36–42; quiz 43.

4. Antai-Otong D. Managing geriatric psychiatric emergencies: delirium and dementia. *Nurs Clin North Am.* 2003;38(1):123–135.

5. Zimberg S. *The Clinical Management of Alcoholism.* New York: Brunner Routledge; 1982.

6. Falk JL, Samson HH. Schedule-induced physical dependence on ethanol. *Pharmacol Rev.* 1975;27(4):449–464.

7. Littleton J, Little H. Current concepts of ethanol dependence. *Addiction.* 1994;89(11):1397–1412.

8. Morrow AL, VanDoren MJ, et al. The role of GABAergic neuroactive steroids in ethanol action, tolerance and dependence. *Brain Res: Brain Res Rev.* 2001;37(1–3):98–109.

9. Flomenbaum N, Goldfrank L, et al. *Goldfrank's Toxicologic Emergencies.* New York: McGraw-Hill Professional; 2006.

10. Floyd RL, O'Connor MJ, et al. Recognition and prevention of fetal alcohol syndrome. *Obstet Gynecol.* 2005;106(5 Pt 1):1059–1064.

11. Haberman PW, Weinbaum DF. Liver cirrhosis with and without mention of alcohol as cause of death. *Br J Addict.* 1990;85(2):217–222.

12. DiMaio VJ. Sudden, unexpected death due to massive, nontraumatic intra-abdominal hemorrhage in association with cirrhosis of the liver. *Am J Forensic Med Pathol.* 1987;8(3):266–268.

13. Tilg H, Day CP. Management strategies in alcoholic liver disease. *Nat Clin Pract: Gastroenterol Hepatol.* 2007;4(1):24–34.

14. Bergheim I, McClain CJ, et al. Treatment of alcoholic liver disease. *Dig Dis.* 2005;23(3–4):275–284.

15. Laleman W, Landeghem L, et al. Portal hypertension: from pathophysiology to clinical practice. *Liver Int.* 2005;25(6):1079–1090.

16. Peck-Radosavljevic M. Review article: coagulation disorders in chronic liver disease. *Aliment Pharmacol Ther.* 2007;26 Suppl 1:21–28.

17. Levi M. Disseminated intravascular coagulation. *Crit Care Med.* 2007;35(9):2191–2195.

18. Shah VH, Kamath P. Management of portal hypertension. *Postgrad Med.* 2006;119(3):14–18.

19. Burroughs AK, Panagou E. Pharmacological therapy for portal hypertension: rationale and results. *Semin Gastrointest Dis.* 1995;6(3):148–164.

20. Nader A, Grace ND. Pharmacological prevention of rebleeding. *Gastrointest Endosc Clin N Am.* 1999;9(2):301–310.

21. Cardenas A, Arroyo V. Hepatorenal syndrome. *Ann Hepatol.* 2003;2(1):23–29.

22. Sechi G, Serra A. Wernicke's encephalopathy: new clinical settings and recent advances in diagnosis and management. *Lancet Neurol.* 2007;6(5):442–455.

23. Donnino MW, Vega J, et al. Myths and misconceptions of Wernicke's encephalopathy: what every emergency physician should know. *Ann Emerg Med.* 2007;50(6):715–721.

24. Lindberg MC, Oyler RA. Wernicke's encephalopathy. *Am Fam Physician.* 1990;41(4):1205–1209.

25. Johri S, Shetty S, et al. Anaphylaxis from intravenous thiamine—long forgotten? *Am J Emerg Med.* 2000;15(5):642–643.

26. Stephen JM, Grant R, et al. Anaphylaxis from administration of intravenous thiamine. *Am J Emerg Med.* 1992;10(1):61–63.

27. Wrenn KD, Slovis CM. Is intravenous thiamine safe? *Am J Emerg Med.* 1992;10(2):165.

28. Abou-Assi S, Vlahcevic ZR. Hepatic encephalopathy. Metabolic consequence of cirrhosis often is reversible. *Postgrad Med.* 2001;109(2):52–54, 57–60, 63–65 passim.

29. Gerber T, Schomerus H. Hepatic encephalopathy in liver cirrhosis: pathogenesis, diagnosis and management. *Drugs*. 2000;60(6):1353–1370.

30. Smaga S. Tremor. *Am Fam Physician*. 2003;68(8):1545–1552.

31. Gill RQ, Sterling RK. Acute liver failure. *J Clin Gastroenterol*. 2001;33(3):191–198.

32. Gaar GG. Gastrointestinal decontamination for acute poisoning by ingestion. Prevention of absorption of toxic compounds. *J Fla Med Assoc*. 1994;81(11):747–749.

33. Litovitz T. The alcohols: ethanol, methanol, isopropanol, ethylene glycol. *Pediatr Clin North Am*. 1986;33(2):311–323.

34. Davis DP, Bramwell KJ, et al. Ethylene glycol poisoning: case report of a record-high level and a review. *J Emerg Med*. 1997;15(5):653–667.

35. Vasavada N, Williams C, et al. Ethylene glycol intoxication: case report and pharmacokinetic perspectives. *Pharmacotherapy*. 2003;23(12):1652–1658.

36. Shimamoto C, Hirata I, et al. Breath and blood ammonia in liver cirrhosis. *Hepatogastroenterology*. 2000;47(32):443–445.

37. Lussier-Cushing M, Repper-DeLisi J, et al. Is your medical/surgical patient withdrawing from alcohol? *Nursing*. 2007;37(10):50–55; quiz 55–56.

38. Puz CA, Stokes SJ. Alcohol withdrawal syndrome: assessment and treatment with the use of the Clinical Institute Withdrawal Assessment for Alcohol-revised. *Crit Care Nurs Clin North Am*. 2005;17(3):297–304.

39. Ebell MH. Benzodiazepines for alcohol withdrawal. *Am Fam Physician*. 2006;73(7):1191.

CHAPTER 16

TOXICOLOGICAL EMERGENCIES

KEY CONCEPTS:

Upon completion of this chapter, it is expected that the reader will understand these following concepts:

- The recognition that any chemical can have adverse effects on the body
- That different classes of chemicals cause classic pictures of signs and symptoms called toxidromes
- The realization that, due to a decrease in the function of their organs, the elderly suffer greater adverse effects from toxic exposures

ANATOMY CONCEPTS:

Prior to reading this chapter, the Paramedic student should be familiar with the following anatomy and physiology concepts:

- Neurotransmitters
- Central nervous system function

Medic 7 is dispatched to the industrial district of their service area for a possible chemical exposure. As they respond to the scene, the Paramedics discuss a recent professional development lecture on poisoning and chemical exposures. They talk about what they will need to do before they make contact with the patient.

As they arrive at the scene, they notice an engine company is already there. The officer in command directs them to the rear of the building, where there is a loading dock. He reports a 47-year-old male patient opened a drum of an unknown chemical and soon thereafter became short of breath and vomited. The chemical was identified by MSDS sheets and the patient has been decontaminated.

CRITICAL THINKING QUESTIONS

1. What are some of the possible causes of toxicology-related shortness of breath?
2. How is trouble breathing related to the vomiting?

OVERVIEW

Toxicology is the study of the harmful effects that different chemicals—both natural and man-made—have upon the body. Therefore, it encompasses a wide variety of potential toxins and an equally wide spectrum of clinical effects. A toxin is any substance that can cause harmful physical effects when a person is exposed to it. Toxins may (1) produce little to no clinical effect; (2) produce very serious effects, such as leukemia or liver carcinoma, but not until years after exposure; or (3) produce immediate and life-threatening effects. The effects from a patient's exposure to a toxin depend on the potency of the toxin, the route of exposure, and the dose. This chapter will discuss those toxins which can produce recognizable clinical symptoms that the Paramedic may be able to identify, and those requiring specific prehospital interventions.

There is no completely accurate data available on poisonings. The best available data comes from the American Association of Poison Control Centers (AAPCC) Toxic Exposure Surveillance System (TESS) database.[1] This database of all the calls handled by all the poison control centers across the country is published every year. Although an average of 1.4 million calls are covered in each report, there are still thousands (if not millions) that never get reported to the poison control centers and never make it into this database. Among the data that is received, the majority of calls (>50%) are for children, of whom the majority of exposures are minor and deaths rare. The majority of deaths in the annual TESS reports involve adults, from both intentional and unintentional exposures. The agents associated with the most deaths in the TESS report tend to be over-the-counter analgesics (such as acetaminophen) and antidepressant medications. Medication errors by healthcare professionals, as well as industrial exposures, account for a small but notable percentage of the deaths. The disparity between adults and children in terms of the severity of their exposures is likely related to the fact that adults are much more likely to take a massive overdose or be exposed to industrial toxins.

Chief Concern

Different toxins will produce different effects on different body systems, through many different mechanisms of action. The Paramedic should consider several general principles with all potential exposures.

Route of Exposure

The route of exposure may determine whether or not a specific toxin will have any significant effects. The routes of exposure for toxins are very similar to the routes of medication administration: ingested, inhaled, transdermal, and injected (Figure 16-1). In general, injected or inhaled toxins have the most immediate effect. Further, certain toxins are much more effective by one route than another; for example, heroin is a potent opiate that can cause respiratory arrest when injected or inhaled, but has virtually no absorption across the skin.[2] Other toxins, such as nerve agents or pesticides, are toxic through any route of exposure. Another reason why the route of exposure is important is that it can help the Paramedic determine whether or not the patient may need to be decontaminated. An agent such as a pesticide, with a great deal of dermal absorption, requires that the patient have the skin washed off prior to any other care in order to decrease further absorption of the toxin and also lessen the risk of exposure to others.

Time of Exposure

The time of exposure is important in determining both the need for decontamination and need for other treatment. It can also help to determine whether or not the patient will develop any serious effects from the exposure. In general,

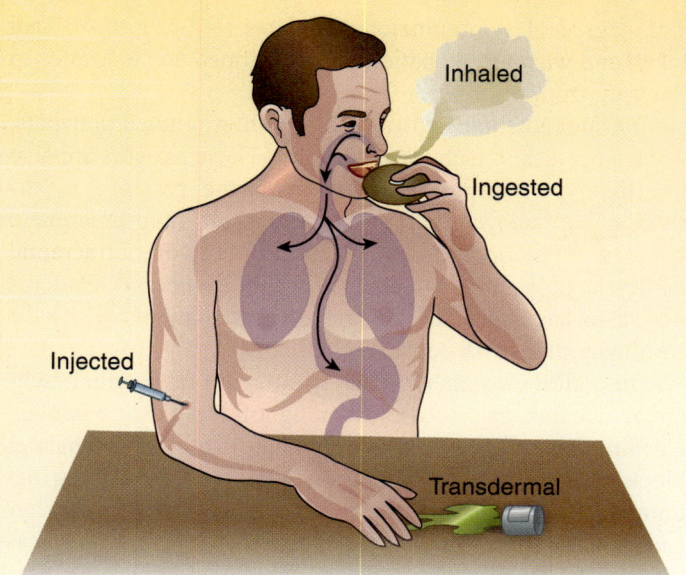

Figure 16-1 The four routes of toxin exposure.

this factor is most important for ingested toxins, but it does matter with exposure via other routes as well. A patient who recently ingested a massive amount of a potentially serious toxin, such as a tricyclic antidepressant medication, may need aggressive decontamination of the GI tract upon reaching the hospital. Likewise, a patient exposed to a nerve or pesticide agent will need **antidotes** (a substance to counteract a form of poisoning) within a very short time frame depending on the specific toxin in order to prevent death or weeks of paralysis. Time can also help determine whether or not a patient will develop any serious symptoms, as a person who is several hours out from a reported ingestion and has not developed any symptoms at all may be "safe" after a set period of time.

Toxidromes

Certain classes of toxins will produce a series of classic physical exam findings. These are known as **toxidromes**. Toxidromes may be apparent to the Paramedic during the patient's examination and may be helpful in guiding prehospital treatment. The four classic toxidromes are sympathomimetics, anticholinergics, cholinergic toxidromes, and opiates (Table 16-1).

Opiate and sympathomimetic toxidromes are some of the most commonly encountered drug intoxications that a Paramedic will encounter. Although the cholinergic toxidrome is rare, Paramedics need to be able to identify it, primarily because of its implications for either a pesticide exposure or a nerve agent exposure. As noted in Table 16-1, there is some overlap between the symptoms of sympathomimetic and anticholinergic toxidromes. The presence of moist or diaphoretic skin can help the Paramedic differentiate between the two toxidromes. It is important for the Paramedic to be able to identify opiate and cholinergic toxidromes as they will require specific antidotes to be administered in the field.

Table 16-1 Commonly Encountered Toxidromes

- Sympathomimetics (cocaine, amphetamines)
  - Agitation/altered mental status
  - Hypertension
  - Tachycardia
  - Dilated pupils
  - Moist skin
  - Hyperthermia
- Anticholinergics (tricyclic antidepressants, antihistamines, antipsychotics)
  - Agitation/altered mental status ("Mad as a hatter")
  - Tachycardia
  - +/− hypertension
  - Dilated pupils ("Blind as a bat")
  - Dry skin ("Dry as a bone")
  - Flushed ("Red as a beet")
  - Hyperthermic ("Hot as a pistol")
- Cholinergic toxidromes (organophosphate pesticides, nerve agents)
  - Diarrhea/diaphoresis
  - Urination
  - Miosis (small pupils)
  - Bronchorrhea, bradycardia, bronchospasm
  - Emesis
  - Lacrimation (crying)
  - Salivation (drooling)
- Opiates (heroin, morphine, methadone, fentanyl, oxycodone, hydrocodone, codeine)
  - Small (pinpoint) pupils (not present with newer opiates)
  - Decreased respirations
  - Decreased level of consciousness

Sympathomimetics

Sympathomimetics are drugs that stimulate the sympathetic nervous system, commonly referred to as the fight or flight syndrome. Stimulation of the sympathetic nervous system will cause the body to release the hormones epinephrine and norepinephrine. The result is an elevated pulse, blood pressure, and respiratory rate; a heightened sense of alertness; and increased blood flow to the muscles. All of this is designed to help the body protect itself in dangerous situations. Drugs that stimulate the sympathetic nervous system will cause similar effects, although in large enough doses they can cause harmful side effects as well.

There is some overlap between the toxidrome for sympathomimetic (Figure 16-2) and anticholinergic poisoning. In both cases, hypertension, tachycardia, and altered mental status can occur. Seizures can also occur in both cases. The

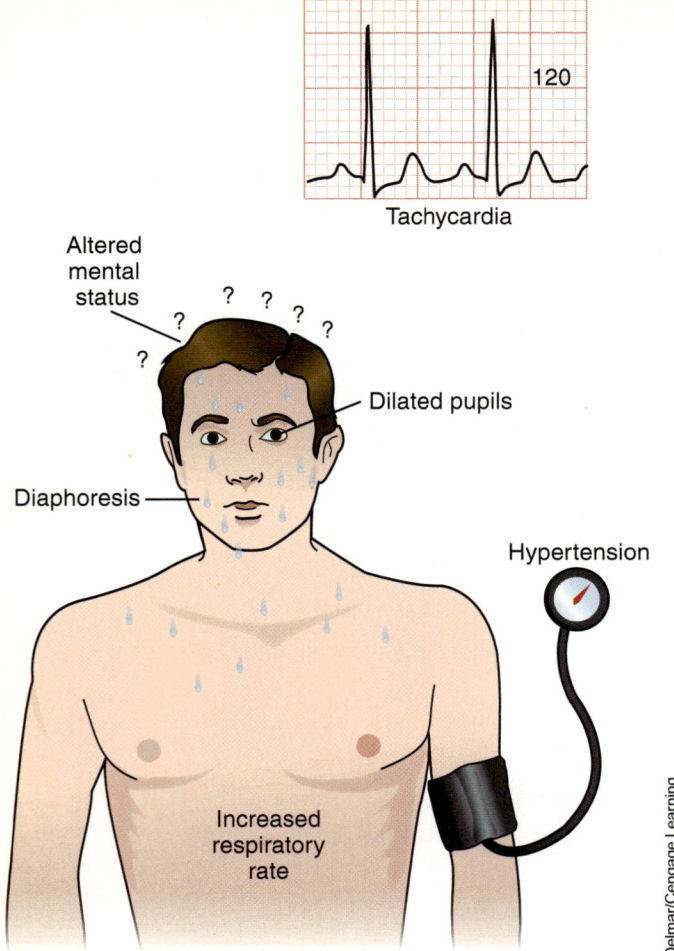

Figure 16-2 Sympathomimetic toxidrome.

The degree of symptomatology relates to the dose of drug taken and whether the patient has developed any tolerance to the drug from prior use.

Serious poisoning will manifest with an agitated, delirious, hypertensive, and tachycardic patient. These patients are also usually hyperthermic. The degree of the patient's hypertension and tachycardia can be severe and may precipitate other medical conditions (myocardial infarction, intracranial hemorrhage, pulmonary edema, aortic dissection). Patients may also have seizures. In severe cases, patients will have cardiovascular collapse and arrhythmias.[3]

In addition to arrhythmias from acute myocardial ischemia, cocaine can cause widening of the QRS complex. Cocaine is similar to lidocaine, which is a sodium channel blocking agent. In massive doses, cocaine can prolong the duration of the QRS complex, simulating ventricular tachycardia. In a patient with known or suspected cocaine intoxication, the Paramedic may consider giving sodium bicarbonate 1 to 2 mEq/kg, especially if she is not responding to the typical treatment for ventricular tachycardia. Sodium bicarbonate will overcome the sodium channel blockade and may narrow out the QRS complex.[4]

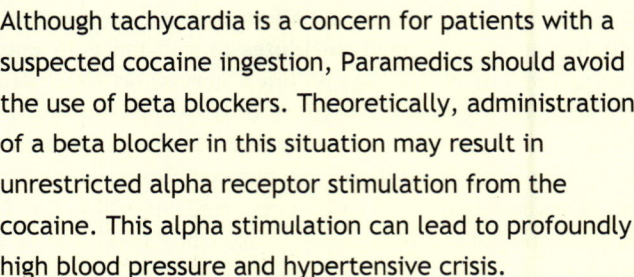

PROFESSIONAL PARAMEDIC

Although tachycardia is a concern for patients with a suspected cocaine ingestion, Paramedics should avoid the use of beta blockers. Theoretically, administration of a beta blocker in this situation may result in unrestricted alpha receptor stimulation from the cocaine. This alpha stimulation can lead to profoundly high blood pressure and hypertensive crisis.

biggest clue between them on physical exam is that an anticholinergic patient will have dry skin and mucous membranes whereas the sympathomimetic patient will not and often is diaphoretic.

Several drugs can cause sympathomimetic effects. Some of them, such as albuterol and epinephrine, are commonly used by Paramedics. However, the drugs Paramedics will most often encounter that cause a sympathomimetic toxidrome are cocaine and methamphetamine. Of all the sympathomimetic drugs, reports indicate cocaine is the most commonly abused drug.

Sympathomimetic toxidrome features have already been reviewed. When treating the patient who is experiencing a sympathomimetic toxidrome, the Paramedic has two primary concerns: treating the physiological results of the toxidrome and maintaining the safety of both the providers and the patient.

There is a broad spectrum along which patients with sympathomimetic poisoning will present, ranging from a mildly anxious, tachycardic patient to a patient who is delirious, seizing, or having an acute myocardial infarction.

A major concern when treating a patient with a sympathomimetic toxidrome is safety, for both providers and patients. These patients, as previously stated, can be very agitated and combative. They often require physical restraints for safety and transport. One of the effects of sympathomimetics, which is not easily appreciated except via lab tests, is that they frequently have a significant metabolic acidosis. Between increased physical activity, increased metabolism, and direct toxic effects to muscle cells by the drugs involved, severely intoxicated patients generate a great deal of lactic acid. This is a normal by-product of physical activity. When the level of exertion exceeds the body's ability to get oxygen-rich blood to the area, such as during intense exercise, the muscle cells switch to anaerobic metabolism, meaning they begin to use a form of metabolism that does not require oxygen. The by-product of this is lactic acid, which builds up as activity increases and is felt by the patient as muscle cramps, pain, and fatigue. The body's first immediate response is to increase the respiratory rate and depth to decrease carbon dioxide, helping to balance out the drop in pH caused by increased acid production. When a very agitated patient is restrained, either by straps or by being held down by several persons, there may be some compromise of the patient's respirations. Even a slight decrease in the patient's respiratory effort may cause the pH to drop suddenly and cardiac arrest to ensue. The survival for this type of cardiac arrest (restraint-associated cardiac arrest) is very poor. A patient with severe sympathomimetic intoxication may have a pH of 7.0. However, to help keep the pH from dropping any lower, the body increases respirations to decrease the carbon dioxide levels (sometimes down to 10 to 15 mmHg), which has the effect of keeping pH up. When the respirations are impaired during struggle and restraint, the pH can drop to 6.7 quickly, at which point cardiac arrest often occurs. ACLS drugs do not work well at low pH.[5,6] Although it was thought that the use of tasers to immobilize patients would decrease the need for Paramedics to use restraints and increase overall safety, there have been reports of deaths involving tasers as well.[7–11]

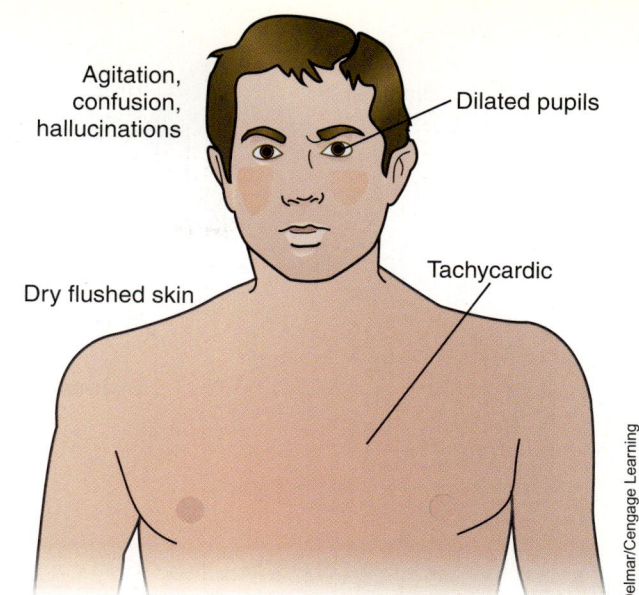

Figure 16-3 Anticholinergic toxidrome.

Anticholinergics

Organophosphate pesticides and nerve agents produce their symptoms by creating overactivity of the cholinergic, or parasympathetic, nervous system. Anticholinergic toxins counteract the activity of the parasympathetic nervous system. As such, the clinical presentation is nearly the opposite of that seen with nerve agents or pesticides.

Anticholinergic agents typically work in the neurons by blocking the binding of acetylcholine. Muscarinic and nicotinic branches of the parasympathetic nervous system, although termed "anticholinergic agents," are more accurately described as antimuscarinic.

Anticholinergic poisoning almost always occurs by ingestion of the toxin. Most commonly, it is due to a medication, although persons who ingest jimsonweed can also get anticholinergic symptoms. Medications that most commonly cause anticholinergic symptoms are tricyclic antidepressants (amitriptyline, nortriptyline), antihistamines (diphenhydramine), atropine, and a slew of other less common medications.

Patients with anticholinergic poisoning will often be agitated, confused, and sometimes will even hallucinate (Figure 16-3). They will generally be flushed and tachycardic, with dry skin and dilated pupils. Severe anticholinergic poisoning may cause seizures. In addition, many of the medications that cause anticholinergic symptoms, such as tricyclic antidepressants, also can cause cardiac arrhythmias and hypotension.

Cholinergic Toxidrome

With the current uncertain global situation, and concerns regarding terrorism at an all-time high, recognition and treatment of potential casualties from chemical weapons has received a great deal of attention. Although the overall likelihood of a chemical weapons attack using nerve agents is extremely low, the Paramedic nevertheless needs to

be able to recognize this specific toxidrome. In addition to nerve agents, a group of commonly used pesticides called **organophosphates** can produce a cholinergic toxidrome.[12] Treatment for both is the same, although there may be subtle differences in the clinical presentations.

The autonomic nervous system is composed of two subdivisions—the sympathetic (SNS) and parasympathetic (PNS) nervous system—that continually balance many body functions. The primary transmitter in the PNS is a molecule called acetylcholine. Acetylcholine (ACh) is released from the end of one neuron and migrates across the synapse to the end of the other neuron, triggering the firing (depolarization) of that neuron and sending out signals for muscle contraction. The specific part of the PNS involved in muscle contraction is called the nicotinic part of the PNS. The other parts of the PNS that involve ACh include smooth muscle (such as sweat glands, tear ducts, GI, and bronchial smooth muscle) and the vagus nerve of the heart. This is referred to as the muscarinic part of the PNS. Both parts of the PNS will be stimulated by additional ACh release. ACh doesn't last long normally; after it triggers a depolarization, it is broken down by an enzyme called **acetylcholinesterase**, or ACh-ase. Both nerve agents and organophosphates block ACh-ase. As a result, ACh is not broken down in the synapse. Therefore, it keeps telling the next neuron to depolarize. The initial result is overstimulation of the affected systems: in the nicotinic region, it causes muscle twitching called **fasciculation**; in the muscarinic side, it causes overstimulation of the glands and vagus nerve (causing bradycardia, bronchospasm, bronchorrhea, vomiting, diarrhea, sweating, and salivation). Eventually, the nerves can no longer continue depolarizing and stop sending any signals out. This causes paralysis of the muscles. If the patient has managed to survive this far, the patient will die of respiratory arrest if not promptly treated (Figure 16-4).

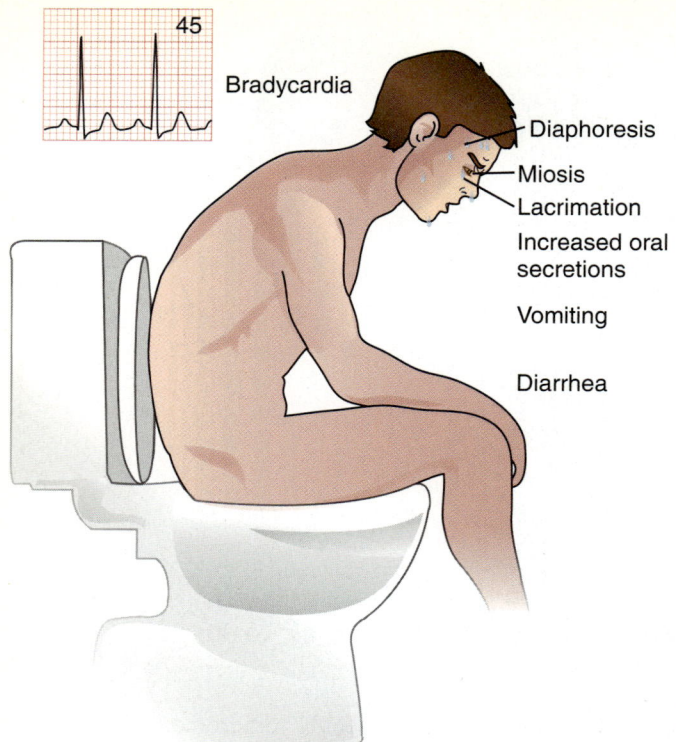

Figure 16-4 Cholinergic toxidrome.

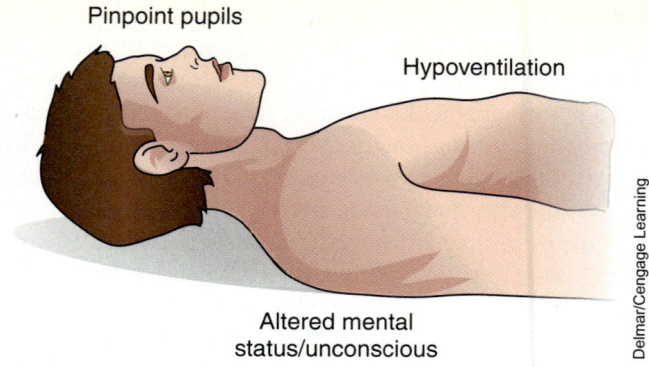

Figure 16-5 Opiate toxidrome.

Organophosphate pesticides (OP) generally produce the classic cholinergic toxidrome remembered using the DUMBELS mnemonic (**D**iarrhea/diaphoresis, **U**rination, **M**iosis, **B**ronchorrhea/bradycardia/bronchospasm, **E**mesis, **L**acrimation, **S**alivation). Depending on the degree of exposure, onset may be rapid or may be more subtle. Workers in agriculture are most likely to be exposed, and those in high-risk jobs are required to be monitored, although it is likely that some are not being monitored out of legal concerns. With OP, the exposure route is most often dermal (as these agents absorb well through skin) or inhalational. In addition to the typical toxidrome, respiratory muscle weakness develops, as well as seizures. If these occur, respiratory failure resulting in death may follow.

Opiate Toxidrome

Opiates are drugs that are derived from, or related to, morphine. They are used as painkillers and rank among the most commonly prescribed drugs in the United States today. The most common illicit form of opiate is heroin. Prescription opiates include methadone, fentanyl, oxycodone, codeine, and hydrocodone. Frequently, these opiates are combined with acetaminophen. Both heroin and the prescription drugs can cause physical dependence and psychological addiction. Because of the phenomenon of tolerance, patients need higher and higher doses of the drug over time to achieve the same effects. When someone who is addicted to opiates requires pain medication, then much larger doses of pain medication may be required to achieve symptom relief. Heroin is typically injected IV or snorted, like cocaine. The other opiates are generally in pill, liquid, or occasionally transdermal patch form.

The opiate toxidrome includes slow respiration, decreased level of consciousness, and constricted pupils (Figure 16-5). Although this is true for morphine, heroin, and codeine, some of the newer opiates (oxycodone, methadone) may not cause constricted pupils.[13] The newer opiates, which are generally in pill or patch form, have been associated with cardiac arrhythmias and seizures in overdose. Hypotension may be present, but it is not common unless there has been a massive overdose.

Sedatives and Hypnotics Toxidrome

Sedative-hypnotics are drugs used primarily for treatment of anxiety and sleep disorders, although they have also been used to treat muscle spasm, seizures, and alcohol withdrawal. The two main classes are (1) benzodiazepines, which include diazepam and midazolam; and (2) barbiturates, such as pentobarbital and phenobarbital. Benzodiazepines are much more commonly prescribed. Other agents, such as carisoprodol, are also classified as sedative-hypnotics.

All these drugs have certain effects in common: decreased level of consciousness, decreased respiratory rate, and (if severe enough) decreased blood pressure (Figure 16-6). The patient may present along a spectrum from appearing slightly lethargic with slurred speech to deep coma and able to be intubated without any additional medications being needed. The patient's pupils are typically normal sized to dilated. Patients can be hypothermic because they frequently are unconscious and in an exposed state for several hours. Even if inside a house, if the patient has been lying on a floor uncovered for several hours he may still be hypothermic. Although most of the benzodiazepines are safe, in terms of not causing respiratory arrest even in large doses, mixing two or more sedating drugs (including a benzodiazepine and alcohol) can cause respiratory depression. Death typically occurs due to respiratory failure and aspiration.

Carbon Monoxide Toxidrome

Carbon monoxide poisoning is the most common poison-related cause of death in the United States each year. Carbon monoxide (CO) is a colorless, odorless gas that is the

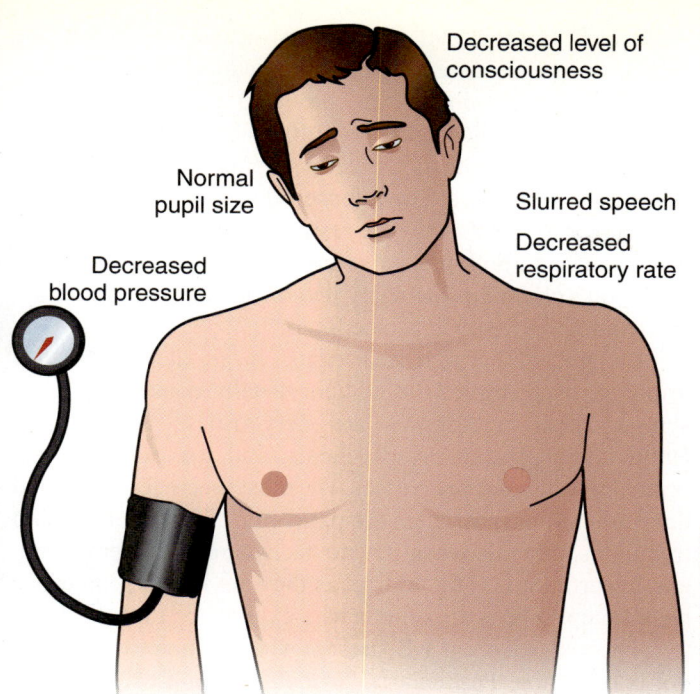

Figure 16-6 Effects of sedative and hypnotic medication overdose.

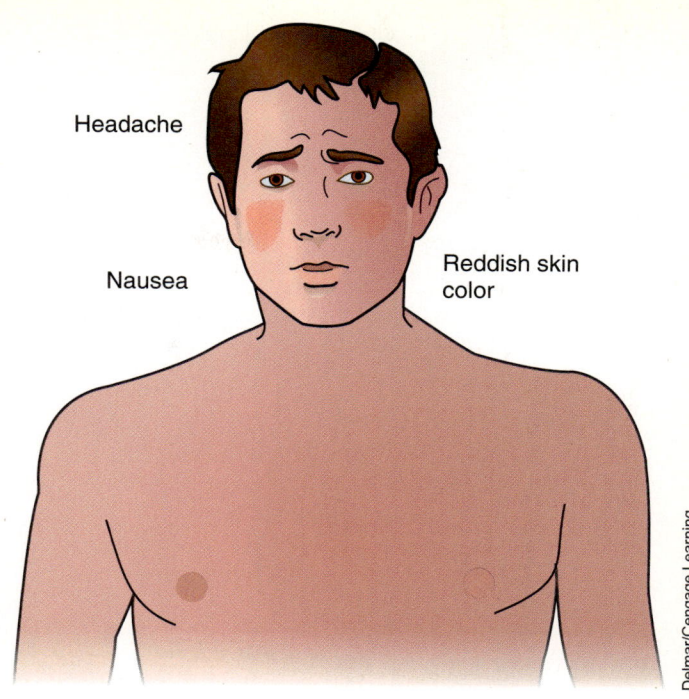

Figure 16-7 Signs and symptoms of carbon monoxide poisoning.

by-product of combustion. It can be generated by auto or other combustion engine exhaust; wood burning stoves; house fires; gas-powered generators; or paint stripper (methylene chloride). It occurs more commonly during the winter months. Although the use of CO monitors in houses have somewhat decreased the incidence of this poisoning, it still remains one of the most common toxicologic emergencies.

Symptoms of CO poisoning range from headache and nausea (leading patients to often be misdiagnosed as having the flu) to coma, seizures, myocardial infarction, and cardiac arrest. In some cases (such as the person sitting in a running car in a closed garage), CO poisoning may be obvious; in other cases, the patient may appear to be only mildly ill, or may present with altered mental status or stroke-like symptoms (Figure 16-7).

There is no reliable way for the Paramedic to diagnose carbon monoxide poisoning in the field.[14–16] If CO detection equipment is available, then measurement of CO in the ambient air may yield a clue as to whether there is at least the potential of CO exposure. Co-oximeters are a developing technology that may be used as a screening tool to identify patients at a scene with an elevated carboxyhemoglobin level. The presently available co-oximeters overestimate the carboxyhemoglobin level, making those devices an excellent tool to identify those patients at most risk for carbon monoxide poisoning.

Toxic Alcohols Toxidrome

Alcohol refers to a group of chemicals that have widespread uses as solvents, cleaning agents, disinfectants, mouthwash, medications, and deodorants. Ethyl alcohol, or ethanol

(abbreviated as EtOH), is the ingredient in alcoholic beverages such as beer, wine, and liquor. The amount of ethanol varies by drink; beer generally has the least amount of alcohol per unit volume, hard liquor like whiskey and vodka the most. Proof refers to the percentage of ethanol by volume—the higher the proof, the more ethanol in the product. Other common and important alcohols are methyl alcohol (methanol), found in windshield washer fluid; ethylene glycol, found in antifreeze; and isopropyl alcohol (isopropanol), used in rubbing alcohol. These last three (methanol, ethylene glycol, and isopropanol) are called "toxic" alcohols. That is, while ethanol in moderation has minimal toxic effects, the "toxic" alcohols all cause varying degrees of problems from severe intoxication to blindness, kidney failure, metabolic acidosis, and death (Figure 16-8).

Ethanol is the most commonly abused drug in the United States. Alcoholism is the state of physical and psychological dependence on ethanol. Users of ethanol, like other drugs, exhibit tolerance, meaning that the more a person drinks, over time, the less effect the ethanol has, requiring the person to consume higher and higher doses before showing signs of intoxication. Heavy regular drinkers will develop a physical dependence on ethanol and will show withdrawal symptoms when they decrease or cease their drinking.

Methanol can be toxic with ingestion of very small amounts. Although methanol is broken down in the liver by the same enzymes that break down ethyl alcohol, methanol is broken down into formaldehyde and formic acid. Both of these compounds are toxic and affect the brain, eyes, and gastrointestinal tract. Patients can permanently lose their eyesight after ingesting a small volume of methanol.

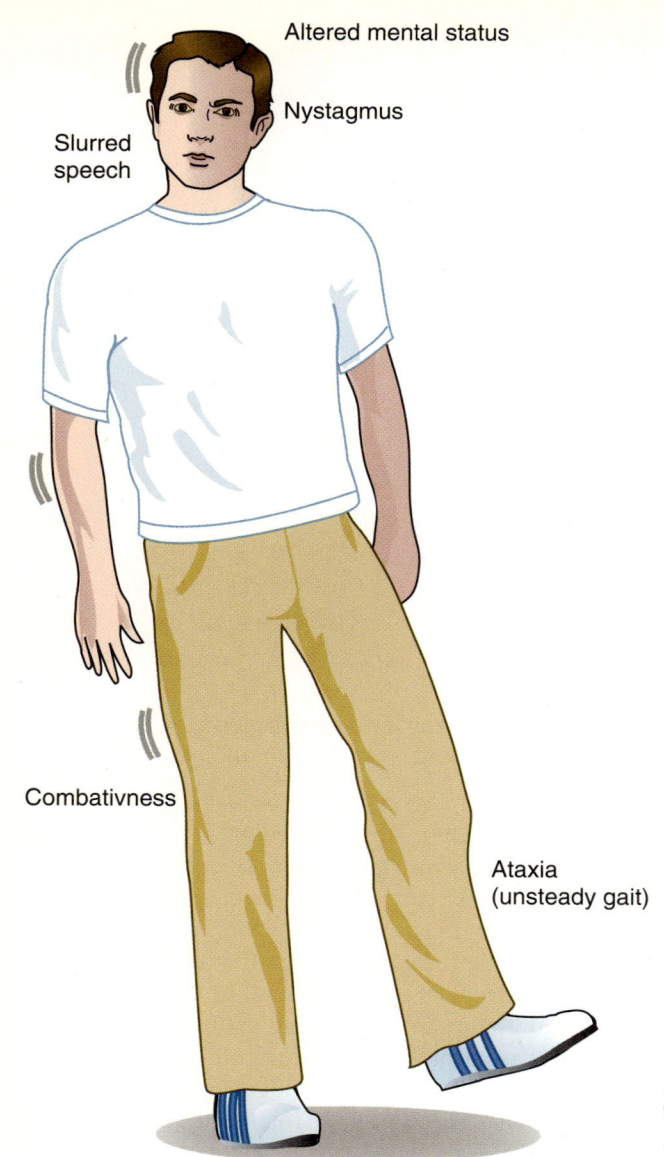

Altered mental status

Nystagmus

Slurred speech

Combativness

Ataxia (unsteady gait)

Delmar/Cengage Learning

Figure 16-8 Effects of the toxic alcohols.

Isopropyl alcohol, found in rubbing alcohol and other compounds, is approximately three times more potent than ethanol. It produces the same signs and symptoms; however, it is not usually ingested in toxic amounts. Chronic alcoholics sometimes substitute isopropyl alcohol for ethanol if they have difficulty obtaining ethanol.

Ethylene glycol is a primary ingredient in radiator cooling fluid and is an extremely toxic substance that can cause acute renal failure and acidosis. As with the other alcohols, ethylene glycol is metabolized by an enzyme in the liver into two toxic substances: glycoaldehyde and glycolic acid. The patient can become profoundly acidotic due to the glycolic acid. Oxalate crystals can form in the urine, kidneys, and blood, decreasing the kidneys' ability to filter the blood and sending the patient into acute renal failure.

Signs of intoxication with any of the alcohols look the same: slurred speech, ataxia, altered mental status,

nystagmus (erratic eye movements when looking to the sides), and (with severe enough intoxication) unresponsiveness or coma. Alcoholics are prone to trauma from falls, motor vehicle accidents, and assault. Alcoholics often are not compliant with medications or treatments for other medical conditions. Chronic alcohol abuse often results in liver disease and cirrhosis. One of the results of chronic liver disease is a decrease in both platelets (the blood's clotting cells) and the blood's clotting proteins, which means that minor trauma can result in more serious bleeding.

Ethanol withdrawal can occur if an alcoholic stops drinking, or decreases the amount usually consumed. Early symptoms of withdrawal are nervousness and tremor. Hallucinations, seizures, psychosis, and hyperthermia can occur as withdrawal progresses. The most severe form is called delirium tremens, in which the patient is indeed delirious and tremulous, but also has severe tachycardia, hypertension, and hyperthermia. The "DT's," as they are known, can cause death in up to 10% of patients who experience them.[17]

The toxic alcohols will present with signs similar to ethanol intoxication. Particularly for methanol and ethylene glycol, patients who present later after ingestion can have coma and severe metabolic acidosis, which will present with rapid respirations, hypotension, and occasionally dysrhythmias.

Special Considerations

As with most other medical conditions, the elderly are more susceptible to problems relating to poisoning and overdose. Underlying heart, lung, or kidney disease can complicate any poisoning or ingestion. Even at typical recommended doses, elderly patients can have toxic side effects from common medications; for example, they may have delirium or urinary retention from antihistamines, which have anticholinergic effects. In the colder months, they may be more susceptible to carbon monoxide poisoning as they may use alternate heating sources to save money. In addition, the rate of alcohol abuse among the elderly may be higher than in younger age groups. The elderly take more medications and are susceptible to drug interactions and side effects.

Children generally present differently than adults in terms of poisoning. The majority of reported poisonings are in children under age 12, the majority of those in children less than age 6. Many are exploratory ingestions and do not result in the massive quantities of pills ingested by adults. However, children are more likely to ingest nonpharmaceutical substances. Many pills or medications that are harmless in adults when taken in the prescribed dose can be serious or fatal in children. Older children may take deliberate, suicidal ingestions. Often, the precise agents ingested or amounts ingested cannot be determined.

Paramedics treating pregnant patients face the unique challenge of treating both the mother and unborn child. Any significant poisoning in the mother can have deleterious effects on the child. Some poisonings, such as carbon monoxide, can affect the fetus even more than the mother. Occasionally, a pregnant patient overdoses in an attempt to terminate the pregnancy.

Although the Paramedic understands that the exposure occurred and that the patient was decontaminated, she seeks out more information about the chemical involved and the route of exposure. She asks to see the MSDS and then elects to call poison control for more information.

CRITICAL THINKING QUESTIONS

1. What are the important elements of the history that a Paramedic should obtain?
2. What is the symptom pattern for the major toxidromes?

History

The Paramedic should be sure to obtain several important elements in the history of any potentially poisoned patient. The first question should ascertain what substance the patient was exposed to, if known. However, there are potential problems in this approach. The patient or bystander may not know what the patient was exposed to, or the patient may willfully conceal that information, particularly if the patient is suicidal or fears that there may be legal repercussions to disclosing the information. Sometimes, physical clues at the scene, such as paraphernalia of drug abuse, may help the Paramedic make a determination. In the event of any unknown exposure, the Paramedic must perform a quick search of the house to locate any pill bottles. If a patient is visiting another person's house, then identifying any medications that person is taking may also provide clues. A particularly useful clue, in the case of ingestion, is whether or not the medication is a sustained release (SR, ER, or XL on bottle).

The next element is the route of exposure, which is generally easily apparent (ingestion of pills, "track marks" suspicious for IV drug abuse, paint around the lips of someone abusing inhalants). The patient's time of exposure is crucial, both in determining the need for antidotes and for the patient's further management in the hospital. An example is patients with medication ingestions. Several medications, including cardiac medications such as verapamil, are manufactured in what is known as sustained release preparations, meaning they are designed to slowly dissolve in the stomach over many hours. As such, an overdose on a sustained-release product may not produce immediate symptoms. Other medications, such as acetaminophen, do not produce immediate symptoms; however, over a period of several hours they will produce liver damage unless treated with an antidote.[18] Time of exposure is very important; whenever possible, the Paramedic should attempt to determine this from the patient or bystanders.

Additional important information the Paramedic should acquire that is specific to poisonings is determination of the amount of toxin the patient was exposed to (i.e., "I swallowed a full bottle" vs. "I swallowed two"). Although this can be difficult for the Paramedic to determine, and a patient may willfully conceal this information, it is still worth trying. Bringing all pill bottles from the scene to the hospital with the patient may help the hospital determine the amount of a potential ingestion.

The timing of the ingestion is critical to determine, as certain antidotes are time sensitive. The treatment for certain medications (e.g., acetaminophen) depends upon a blood level that is time dependent, and the threshold for treatment changes over time. It is important to attempt to confirm the time of ingestion from another source besides the patient, as many patients who ingest with the intent of self-harm may not be forthcoming with the time of ingestion. Talk with bystanders, family, and any other potential source that can help narrow down a time frame for the patient's ingestion or confirm the patient's story.

The Paramedic should also try to determine why the exposure happened. A person who developed symptoms because he accidentally took a blood pressure pill instead of a cholesterol pill is different from an intentional suicidal ingestion. Specifically, in the instance of a suspected suicidal ingestion, the patient should not be allowed to refuse transport.[19,20]

Finally, the Paramedic should ascertain any decontamination or treatment that occurred prior to her arrival. Some patients still have ipecac or activated charcoal at home in the bathroom, even though the use of ipecac is being discouraged. If someone already called a poison control center, one of these substances may have been administered to the patient.[21] Any vomiting is important to note, as it may have partially decontaminated the patient in the setting of ingestion. In the case of a suspected contamination, such as an industrial chemical exposure, external decontamination (removing the patient's clothes and copiously washing them with water) is a critical step and takes priority over everything else—even airway issues. A patient who is contaminated with a chemical, meaning chemical residue is present on his person, can in turn expose others to the chemical and turn responders into patients. Precise decontamination needs depend on the chemical. All other relevant history (past medical history, meds, allergies) should be obtained as well. Details related to specific poisonings discussed in this chapter will be addressed.

The Paramedics find their patient wrapped in a disposable rescue blanket, naked because he had been thoroughly decontaminated. He is in obvious respiratory distress, has copious secretions and is unable to answer questions. His exam shows vital signs: BP 88/50, pulse 44, with respirations of 36. His skin is cool and diaphoretic, and his pupils measure 1 mm and are unreactive. An assessment of his lungs reveals both diffuse rales and wheezes, and he has twitching of the muscles in his face and extremities.

CRITICAL THINKING QUESTIONS

1. What are the elements of the physical examination of a patient with suspected acute poisoning?
2. Why is a cardiovascular examination a critical element in this examination?

Examination

The same general principles of physical examination apply to exposures as they do to other patients. The one difference, however, is the potential danger to the Paramedic as he carries out his patient assessment. For the safety of the medical crew, unless one is working as part of a HAZMAT team and is taking appropriate precautions, the patient must be decontaminated before the Paramedic makes contact with the patient.

Scene safety is of paramount importance in caring for the intoxicated patient, as some intoxicated patients are belligerent and combative. Glucose and oxygen saturation should be measured as soon as feasible.[22–24] If the patient is severely obtunded and concern exists for airway protection, then the Paramedic should consider intubation. Above all, the Paramedic should not ascribe to the patient with altered mental status the label of "just drunk," even if the patient smells like alcohol. The patient may have head trauma, be hypoglycemic, or have another cause for the altered mental status.

The Paramedic rapidly assesses the patient's airway, breathing, and circulation and immediately corrects any deficiencies. The remainder of the physical examination looks for evidence of both a toxidrome and for trauma that may have occurred during a fall or assault. The Paramedic should ensure that other problems are not missed by focusing an exam on detecting a specific toxin or toxidrome. There is nothing to say that an agitated, sympathomimetic-appearing patient does not have a stab wound to the flank and is hypoxic, or that the opiate overdose is not in fact hypoglycemic. The Paramedic should think of the toxidromes as an addition to the standard physical exam, and not a replacement. In all cases of altered mental status, the Paramedic should remember to check glucose and pulse oximetry, as these are also immediately treatable causes of altered mental status.

Based on the physical findings, the Paramedic suspects an organophosphate-like poisoning. The patient is manifesting the classic symptom pattern of the cholinergic toxidrome and the MSDS confirms the chemical is an organophosphate.

CRITICAL THINKING QUESTIONS

1. What is the symptom pattern for cholinergic toxidrome?
2. Based on the suspected toxidrome, why did the Paramedic avoid the use of succinylcholine?

Assessment

The materials safety data sheet can provide the Paramedic with important information about the substance, precautions, effects of exposure, and any specific treatment considerations.

In the absence of a clear toxidrome, the specific agent may be difficult for the Paramedic to determine based on history and physical alone.

The Paramedic decides to electively intubate the patient, avoiding the use of succinylcholine in the process and simultaneously administering an antidote of atropine IM.

CRITICAL THINKING QUESTIONS

1. What is the national standard of care of patients with suspected organophosphate poisoning?
2. What are some of the patient-specific concerns and considerations that the Paramedic should consider when applying this plan of care that is intended to treat a broad patient population presenting with acute cholinergic poisoning?

Treatment

After history taking and examination, there are some general principles the Paramedic should follow that are common to all poisonings. Scene safety, as with all other complaints, takes precedence. For poisonings, this is particularly important; both EMS and other medical personnel/responders may become casualties themselves if they enter a contaminated environment.[25] An inappropriately decontaminated patient may also contaminate the Paramedics and hospital staff. Although this issue is particularly important for chemical weapons agents (such as nerve agents, cyanide, and mustard), decontamination is important for any toxin that causes dermal or inhalational exposure. One need not be on a farm or in an industrial area to have a contaminated scene.

Methamphetamine labs can be found in any setting and are potential sources of chemical exposure. The specific manner of decontamination differs based on the agent, although if nothing else is available copious irrigation with water is recommended. Decontamination should precede all other care, including evaluation of ABCs in the appropriate patient.

Basic ABCs are unaltered in the poisoned patient, except in the previously noted instance of a patient who needs external decontamination. Supplemental oxygen should be administered as indicated. Since several of these poisonings can lead to cardiac arrhythmias, the Paramedic should place all suspected or known poisoned patients on a cardiac monitor and obtain a 12-lead ECG. The Paramedic should perform a fingerstick glucose as part of the initial assessment if the patient presents with altered mental status. The IV access should be obtained using an isotonic crystalloid solution, with an adequately sized catheter for both medication and fluid bolus administration.

In addition to all standard treatment for altered mental status, including checking blood glucose, the Paramedic's primary goal should be airway management and ventilatory support if there is suspicion of trauma. Severely intoxicated patients can often be intubated without the use of any other drugs. If opiates are suspected, naloxone 1 to 2 mg may be given prior to intubation and titrated until the patient's respirations are adequate.[26,27] The Paramedic should give the patient IV fluids if hypotension is present and a blanket to help maintain the patient's body heat. If the exact toxidrome is not known, the Paramedic should remember that help can be obtained, anywhere in the country, from a poison control center by dialing the national hotline: 1-800-222-1222.

The focus thus far on decontamination has been **external decontamination**. In the treatment of ingested poisons, however, **internal (gastric) decontamination** is frequently discussed. In the prehospital environment, this will take the form of either administration of an emetic agent, such as ipecac, or an agent to prevent absorption of an ingested toxin, such as with activated charcoal. Use of ipecac has largely been discouraged; the vomiting can persist for hours after it is administered and it does not offer any benefit over charcoal in most cases. However, charcoal is difficult to administer in the ambulance. In EMS services with short transport times, no gastric decontamination need be considered, although it may be of benefit for services with longer transport times. Antidotes for certain toxins are commonly carried in the Paramedic's drug box. Antidotes will be discussed under specific toxin management.

Sympathomimetics

Treatment of a patient with sympathomimetic poisoning involves making sure both the Paramedics and patient are safe, giving IV fluids, and, if the patient is hyperthermic, applying ice packs and other cooling measures. The Paramedic should use IV benzodiazepines (diazepam, lorazepam, midazolam) to prevent agitation and seizures. These drugs are also generally very effective in lowering the patient's blood pressure and pulse. If a patient appears to be having an acute myocardial infarction, then aspirin should be administered. Beta blockers, if they are included in the regional protocols, should be avoided. Cocaine has both alpha and beta agonist properties, and beta blockers will work on the beta effects (slowing heart rate), leaving the alpha effects of cocaine (vasoconstriction) unopposed. As a result, giving beta blockers to someone acutely intoxicated with cocaine can cause the patient's blood pressure to rise sharply and has been associated with sudden death.

Anticholinergic Agents

Treatment for anticholinergic symptoms involves protecting the patient and the EMS providers from harm. Agitation and seizures can both be treated with IV benzodiazepines, such as diazepam, lorazepam, or midazolam. If the patient is markedly hyperthermic (temp > 102°F or 40°C) then cooling measures, such as icepacks, may be used. For those toxins causing arrhythmias or hypotension, such as tricyclic antidepressants, there is further specific treatment: IV fluids for hypotension, and IV sodium bicarbonate 1 to 2 mEq/kg bolus for wide complex tachycardia caused by tricyclic antidepressants.

Organophosphate Pesticides/Nerve Agents

Management of potential nerve or OP agent exposure is time critical but also different from the majority of other poisonings. Given that dermal absorption is one of the primary routes of exposure for both, decontamination must be the first step taken. Scene safety will involve the Paramedic staging upwind from the potential site of exposure, wearing appropriate personal protective equipment (PPE), and decontaminating the patient(s) appropriately. In the event of a chemical weapons attack, the Paramedic may have to treat several patients at once. Despite this, all patients need to be decontaminated prior to further treatment or transport.

Treatment of nerve or OP agent poisoning involves administration of two medications, atropine and 2-PAM, in addition to supportive care. As these patients are often seizing, in respiratory distress, or in various stages of paralysis, they often require intubation. Bronchial secretions can be copious, appearing similar to those in acute pulmonary edema, so the patient may require frequent suctioning. The Paramedic should administer IV fluids as there is often significant fluid loss (remember, the patient may present with salivation, vomiting, diarrhea, and diaphoresis).

The medications most commonly used to treat these patients are atropine and pralidoxime, or 2-PAM. Atropine is an anticholinergic drug, meaning it antagonizes the effects of ACh. Unlike for bradycardia, there is no limit to the dose of atropine that can be administered; the endpoint is not pupil size or heart rate but rather the drying up of secretions. Some patients have required in excess of 100 mg of atropine to treat nerve agents.[28,29] Pralidoxime is important not because it will result in rapid improvement the way atropine will, but because it will prevent the nerve agent or OP from binding permanently to the ACH-ase. Depending on the agent, it will bind permanently to the ACH-ase anywhere from a few minutes to several hours after exposure. Then, even if the patient initially survives, she will have profound weakness and may even need to be on a ventilator for weeks. The pralidoxime helps unbind the nerve or OP agent from the ACH-ase molecule and therefore helps to shorten the length of time the patient will have symptoms. Typically, the quicker the medication is given, the better. To that end, the Mark I kits, which contain 2 mg of atropine and 2 g of pralidoxime, have been made available to several municipalities in the wake of the terrorists attacks of 9/11 (Figure 16-9). Previously, these kits were issued to members of the military. Diazepam is also a component of the kit, and is used in the event of seizures. The Paramedic may use diazepam in doses of 5 to 10 mg IM or IV to treat seizures in these patients.

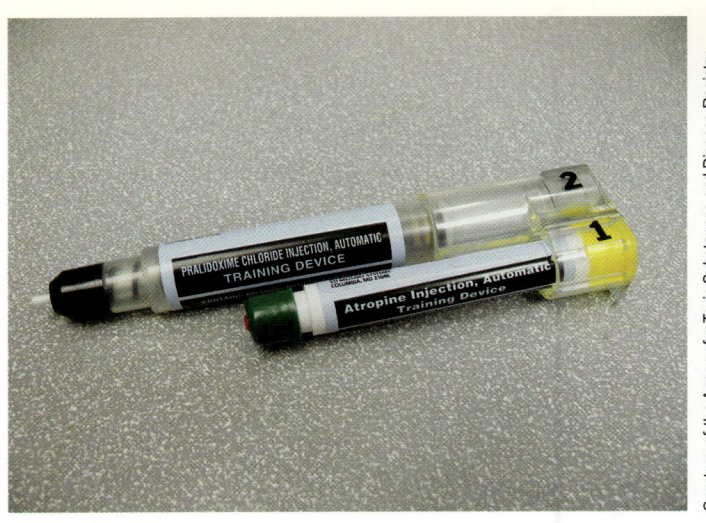

Figure 16-9 Mark I kit.

One drug the Paramedic should avoid is succinylcholine (SCh). Although some systems use SCh to facilitate intubation, SCh will cause paralysis by triggering constant firing of the neurons until they cannot fire any more, resulting in the muscles becoming refractory to any further signals. Without any incoming signals telling the muscles to contract, paralysis ensues. This is very similar to the way the nerve agents work. SCh is also broken down by ACH-ase; as a result, in a nerve or OP agent-poisoned patient, the SCh will last for hours to days, causing a prolonged paralysis.

Opiates

Treatment of suspected opiate poisoning involves all the typical initial steps in evaluating and managing the patient with altered mental status. Ventilatory assistance is often needed. The antidote for opiates is the opiate antagonist naloxone, which displaces opiates from the receptors in the CNS. Naloxone often has dramatic effects, with a comatose patient in respiratory arrest becoming alert within one to two minutes. However, this effect varies by both dose of naloxone and the type of opiate. Heroin typically responds quickly to small doses of naloxone, while methadone may require up to 10 mg of naloxone. If heroin use is suspected, the recommended starting dose is 0.4 mg of naloxone; if an oral opiate, such as methadone, is ingested, it may take up to 10 mg of naloxone. On rare occasions, patients may require a continuous IV infusion of naloxone. Naloxone should be titrated to an increase in respiratory rate sufficient to cease ventilatory assistance. If opiate overdose is suspected, then naloxone should be given before intubation.

Naloxone can be given IM, SC, IV, SL injection, or intranasal. Typical doses are 0.4 to 2 mg. For patients who are breathing spontaneously, but may need to have their level of consciousness gradually raised, naloxone 2 mg can be nebulized in much the same way as albuterol. Patients who are physically dependent on opiates may develop acute withdrawal symptoms, which manifest as muscle cramps, vomiting, goosebumps, and diarrhea. Frequently, these patients are also agitated upon awakening. Rapid reversal of the opiates may result in a combative patient, which may cause a safety issue for the Paramedics.

There have been isolated reports of patients having seizures, pulmonary edema, or cardiac arrest after receiving naloxone. These effects are most likely not from the naloxone itself; rather, patients may mix drugs. A patient who has taken a heroin/cocaine mixture can manifest with acute cocaine toxicity after the opiate has been reversed. Several opiates (heroin, methadone, and propoxyphene) can cause pulmonary edema that may not be evident in a patient in respiratory arrest until the patient wakes up and starts taking deeper breaths. The pulmonary edema may become clinically apparent. Pulmonary edema that develops in this setting is a noncardiogenic pulmonary edema, and treatment includes respiratory support with CPAP or intubation and mechanical ventilation. Nitrates, furosemide, and other pharmacologic treatments for cardiogenic pulmonary edema should not be used to treat pulmonary edema from naloxone use. None of these events happen with any great frequency. Overall, naloxone is a very safe drug when used appropriately.

Naloxone lasts for 30 to 40 minutes, whereas most opiates last for significantly longer. Therefore, if a patient is given naloxone, wakes up, and refuses transport, there is a risk that when the naloxone wears off the patient will become sedated or even suffer respiratory arrest again. All patients who receive naloxone for an opiate overdose should be transported so they can be observed for recurrent symptoms.

With the advent of newer opiates that come in an oral or patch form, the telltale "track marks" of an IV drug user may not be present. The patches, generally fentanyl, are flesh colored and may be hidden anywhere on the body. If fentanyl patches are the suspected cause of the patient's overdose, the Paramedic needs to perform a careful head-to-toe examination.

Sedative-Hypnotics

The antidote for benzodiazepine overdose is flumazenil. This drug briefly gained attention 10 to 15 years ago as a potential addition to the "coma cocktail."[30] However, cases of seizures after administration of flumazenil were reported, generally in patients who ingested another drug that can cause seizures, which happened after the benzodiazepines were reversed by flumazenil. If flumazenil is given and this does occur, the Paramedic should give larger doses of benzodiazepines to overcome the flumazenil. In general, however, flumazenil should be avoided unless the overdose is clearly known to be an isolated benzodiazepine overdose, which unfortunately is rarely known with certainty.

Carbon Monoxide

The Paramedic's treatment in the case of carbon monoxide first involves scene safety, as the EMS providers can become symptomatic as easily as the patients. Therefore, if there is suspected atmospheric CO then appropriately trained personnel with self-contained breathing apparatus (SCBA) should be the ones initially entering the scene. Once the patient has been extricated, the Paramedic can initiate the initial primary and

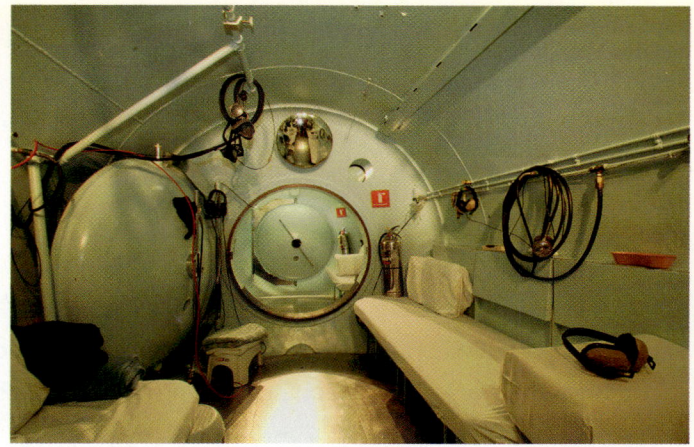

Delmar/Cengage Learning

Figure 16-10 A hyperbaric chamber.

secondary survey and appropriate interventions. For example, patients extricated from a fire may have burns, traumatic injuries, or hemodynamic instability from cyanide poisoning. The initial steps in resuscitation are unchanged. Prehospital treatment for CO poisoning involves high-flow, high-concentration oxygen via a tight fitting nonrebreather mask, bag-valve mask, or endotracheal tube. Any concerns regarding CO poisoning should be related to the receiving hospital.

One of the available treatments for carbon monoxide poisoning is "diving" the patient in a hyperbaric chamber (Figure 16-10). The patient is put in a **hyperbaric chamber** that increases pressure from 1 atmosphere (standard atmospheric pressure) to 2.8 atmospheres. The Paramedic administers 100% oxygen to the patient within the chamber. Under the increased pressure, a higher concentration of oxygen can be achieved in the tissues than at normal atmosphere. This has the effect of decreasing the percentage of blood bound to carbon monoxide (carboxyhemoglobin). Although there is some debate as to how much this ultimately benefits patients, if there is a center equipped for delivering hyperbaric oxygen in the transport area and the patient is stable for transport, then the Paramedic should strongly consider transporting the patient to the hyperbaric chamber-equipped hospital.[31,32]

Toxic Alcohols

If the patient who is intoxicated or in alcohol withdrawal requires intravenous dextrose to treat hypoglycemia, the Paramedic should administer thiamine 100 mg IM or IV immediately prior to or after dextrose is recommended. Some alcoholics are malnourished, and may be thiamine deficient. Thiamine is needed for metabolism of glucose, and a large bolus of glucose may cause significant enough depletion of thiamine to cause Wernicke's syndrome, which is acute onset of confusion, nystagmus, and ataxia.[33] If left untreated, then a condition called Korsakoff's psychosis, with permanent memory loss, can result. Although these conditions are rare, alcoholics are at higher risk for the condition. Therefore, thiamine is recommended.

When providing treatment for other toxic alcohol ingestion, the Paramedic should aggressively support the patient's airway, breathing, and circulation. The enzymes which metabolize all of the other alcohols have a greater affinity for ethanol than the other alcohols. For many years, the patient who suffered either an ethylene glycol or methanol ingestion was given ethanol, either orally or intravenously, so the enzyme would preferentially break down the ethanol and not convert the ethylene glycol or methanol into their toxic metabolites. While fomepizole is now administered as a treatment for methanol and ethylene glycol toxicity, it is possible the Paramedic may encounter a patient who is on an intravenous infusion of ethanol during a transport from a small community hospital to a tertiary care center if the community hospital does not have fomepizole available.

CASE STUDY (CONTINUED)

The patient remains bradycardic and has copious secretion from his endotracheal tube, thus requiring frequent suctioning. The Paramedic elects to coadminister the 2-PAM medication along with an additional dose of atropine.

CRITICAL THINKING QUESTIONS

1. What are some of the predictable complications associated with acute organophosphate poisoning?
2. What are some of the predictable complications associated with the treatments for acute organophosphate poisoning?

Evaluation

During transport, the Paramedic should monitor the patient's airway for patency, the vital signs for stability, and the ECG for interval changes that indicate worsening effects of the substance. The patient who is initially talking on scene may become obtunded and require airway management. The patient's vital signs may change in a way that requires Paramedic intervention to continue to resuscitate the patient. An ECG that shows a widening of the QRS complex or prolonging of the QT interval can signal a patient who may develop a life-threatening dysrhythmia. In cases where the Paramedic has administered a specific antidote, he should observe the patient for her response to the antidote and signs that additional dosing of the antidote is required.

CASE STUDY CONCLUSION

When Medic 7 arrives at the hospital, the patient is initially brought into the decontamination area to determine if further decontamination is required. The patient is then transferred to the emergency department staff.

After several days in the intensive care unit, the patient is weaned off the ventilator and is improved enough for discharge. Eventually the owners of the industrial plant are cited for improper storage of hazardous chemicals.

CRITICAL THINKING QUESTIONS

1. What is the most appropriate transport decision that will get the patient to definitive care?
2. What are the advantages of transporting a patient with suspected organophosphate contamination to a hospital with decontamination capabilities?

Disposition

Patient disposition depends largely on local or regional resources. Patients who have been exposed to industrial or other hazardous materials should be taken to an emergency department with the capability to continue to decontaminate the patient in the event of hasty scene decontamination. Patients involved in a mass casualty situation, as can occur with acts of terrorism, may need to be distributed to many different emergency departments or transported to a temporary hospital to decrease cross-contamination with other patients. Patients who have expressed the intent to harm themselves or others may require transport to an emergency department with psychiatric capabilities. It is important to note that if the patient is unstable or severely obtunded, he should be transported to the nearest emergency department, even if there is a concern the patient is suicidal. The patient's medical condition takes priority over the psychiatric condition in the case of an intentional ingestion or trauma. Once the patient is medically stabilized, then he can be transferred to a psychiatric emergency department.

"Rescue 7, respond low priority to 5327 Brook Road, cross streets Duey and Howe, for a 65-year-old male complaining of severe leg pain." Two Paramedics start the ambulance and drive to the scene. As they make the mile and a half trip from the ambulance station to Brook Road, the Paramedics discuss the types of conditions that may cause leg pain.

CRITICAL THINKING QUESTIONS

1. What are some of the possible causes of severe leg pain?
2. How is the patient's age related to these causes?

OVERVIEW

A fairly large list of potential causes of nontraumatic extremity pain exists (Table 22-1). Within this list are many chronic conditions that are either chronic painful conditions or conditions that can become worse in certain situations. The Paramedic's key action is to recognize patients who may have an emergent cause of nontraumatic extremity pain and identify those patients to the emergency department staff. The emergent conditions, which can present with nontraumatic extremity pain, include an acute arterial or venous occlusion, nontraumatic hip fracture, septic arthritis, osteomyelitis, and fasciitis. The Paramedic should always question the patient and bystanders about potential trauma, including mechanisms that appear to be minor.

Chief Concern

The Paramedic's greatest concern regarding vascular disorders are emergent conditions that present with a patient's complaint of nontraumatic extremity pain, specifically those conditions put the limb in jeopardy. Although most such complaints are not immediately limb-threatening, there are instances in which the patient's limb function can be permanently damaged without proper treatment.

Acute Vascular Occlusion

An **acute vascular occlusion** occurs in an extremity when a blood vessel is either occluded (blocked) or the inner diameter is acutely reduced to the point where blood flow past the obstruction is minimal. When the patient's arterial blood flow to an extremity cannot keep up with the body's demand for oxygen and nutrients, the cellular metabolism changes over to anaerobic metabolism, in which oxygen is not required to produce energy. Besides the inefficiency of this process, acids are produced that make it difficult for the body to continue

Table 22-1 Conditions That May Cause Nontraumatic Extremity Pain

- Arterial occlusion
- Venous occlusion
- Osteomyelitis
- Arthritis
  - Septic, gout, rheumatoid, osteoarthritis
- Slipped capital femoral epiphysis
- Rhabdomyolysis
- Bursitis
- Tendonitis
- Flexor tenosynovitis
- Paronychia
- Gangrene
- Fasciitis
- Pathologic fractures

to produce the energy needed for cell survival. After several hours of ischemia, tissue death starts to occur in the limb, leading to permanent disability and damage.[1]

An **acute arterial occlusion** is caused by an embolus lodging in the vessel and occluding (or partially occluding) the arterial supply to an extremity. Although the limb's arterial system has a significant amount of **collateral circulation**—a network of smaller vessels that can keep blood flowing to the extremity around an injury or occlusion—this may not be sufficient to avoid limb ischemia.

The embolus occurs in one of three mechanisms. Certain patients have developed peripheral vascular disease, or narrowing of the arteries to the extremities, gradually over time. This occurs in the same patients at risk for cardiovascular diseases: those who are obese, who smoke, or who have diabetes, hypertension, and/or high cholesterol. In these patients, the vessel is narrowed by cholesterol deposits along the side walls (Figure 22-1). At some point, a piece of the plaque breaks off and occludes the vessel downstream, decreasing blood flow to the rest of the limb.[2]

A second mechanism involves patients who have a history of atrial fibrillation. A patient who develops atrial fibrillation is at risk for developing clots in his atria because the blood in the atria is not propelled out of the atria efficiently and can pool and coagulate. The clots may be propelled out of the atria and into the central circulation at any time, most often if the atrial fibrillation resolves and normal blood flow resumes. Although these newly embolized blood clots most often head for the brain and can cause a stroke, at times they will be propelled into the central circulation toward the lower extremities until they lodge in the medium and small blood vessels supplying the legs. For this reason, many patients who develop atrial fibrillation are placed on long-term anticoagulation, such as either warfarin or clopidogrel, to help prevent this phenomenon.

A third mechanism that can cause an acute arterial occlusion is dissection of an abdominal aortic aneurysm that extends into the iliac or femoral artery on the affected side. The vessel may either be occluded by a flap of the inner wall of the vessel that falls over the lumen, or by plaque that is embolized from the area of rupture that lodges downstream. Pain from an acute arterial occlusion results from the limb

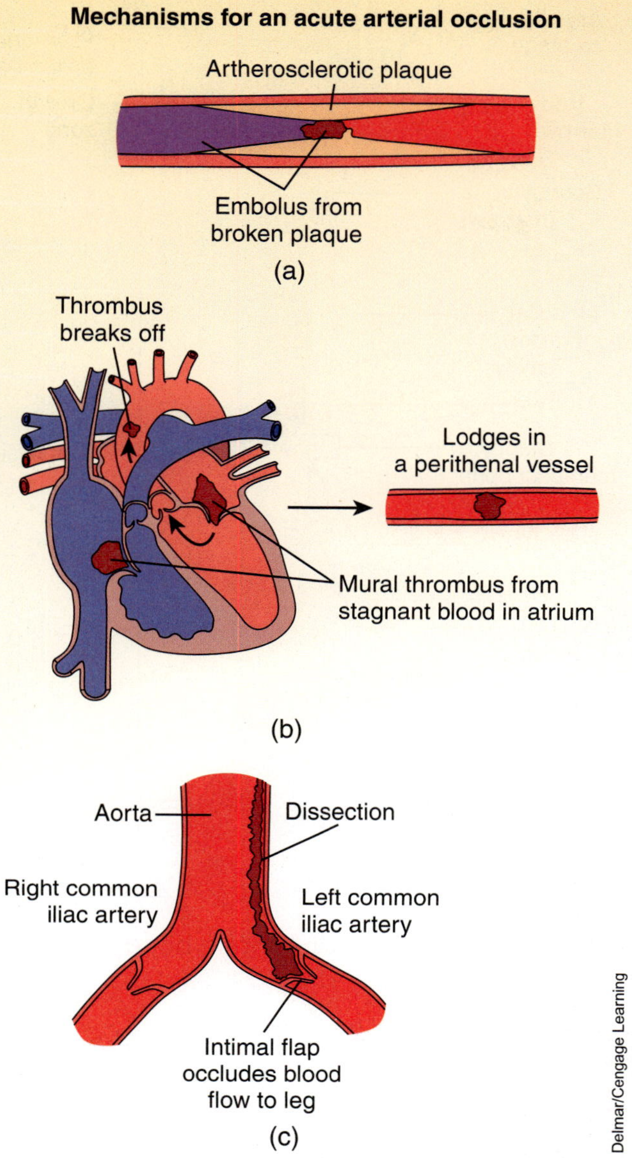

Mechanisms for an acute arterial occlusion

Artherosclerotic plaque

Embolus from broken plaque

(a)

Thrombus breaks off

Lodges in a perithenal vessel

Mural thrombus from stagnant blood in atrium

(b)

Aorta

Dissection

Right common iliac artery

Left common iliac artery

Intimal flap occludes blood flow to leg

(c)

Delmar/Cengage Learning

Figure 22-1 Mechanisms for an acute arterial occlusion. (a) Embolus occludes a narrowed peripheral vessel. (b) A patient with atrial fibrillation embolizes a clot from the heart, which lodges in a narrowed vessel. (c) In an abdominal aortic dissection, the intimal (innermost layer) flap occludes the iliac artery.

STREET SMART

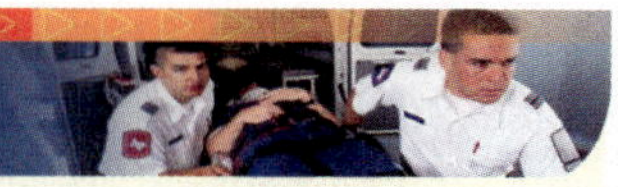

Paramedics often use the five P's in assessment of a possible acute arterial occlusion: **P**ain, **P**aresthesia, **P**aralysis, **P**allor, and **P**ulselessness.

ischemia and the buildup of lactic acids in the extremity distal to the occlusion, which together provide a generalized, severe ache.

On the venous side of the circulation, an embolus can occlude the outflow of blood from an extremity. Since venous circulation is a low pressure system, it is difficult for blood to flow from the lower extremities back to the heart without assistance. This assistance occurs by flexion and relaxation of the leg muscles as well as from the negative intrathoracic pressure that develops during the inspiratory phase of respiration. As a result of the low pressure system, blood tends to pool in the legs. For active people, this is not an issue as the normal muscular contraction in the legs does not allow the blood to pool in the deeper veins. However, for someone who has difficulty ambulating, had recent surgery, or had a recent orthopedic injury and has a casted or splinted lower extremity, the patient may not be able to keep the blood moving out of the extremity.[3,4]

If the blood pools, it is at risk for developing a clot or thrombus in that extremity. Generically, this is termed a **venothromboembolus (VTE)**. When this occurs in the deeper and larger extremity veins, this is called a **deep venous thrombosis (DVT)**. Risk factors for developing a lower extremity DVT include the factors mentioned previously, certain genetic issues with coagulation that make that individual more likely to produce clots and not dissolve them efficiently, pregnancy, oral contraceptives, and prolonged travel without breaking to walk or stretch.[5]

Although DVTs can occur in the upper extremities, this is not as likely to happen since the blood often does not pool in the upper extremities. In fact, even debilitated patients will often move their upper extremities. The biggest risk factor for an upper extremity DVT is a central venous catheter that is placed in either the internal jugular vein in the neck or in the subclavian vein under the clavicle. These catheters tend to develop clots around the outer lumen of the catheter (the portion within the vessel), which can occlude outflow of blood from the upper extremity.

The pain associated from a venous occlusion originates from the significant edema that can occur in that extremity, which stretches pain receptors in the tissues in the leg. The edema is from capillary leak of plasma that cannot return to the heart via the venous system due to the occlusion, and either uses the lymphatic system to return or becomes interstitial fluid remaining in the extremity. In extreme cases, this edema can also compress the arterial supply to the extremity and produce the same problems as an acute arterial occlusion.

As opposed to an acute arterial occlusion, where the risk of damage is from ischemia from lack of blood flow, the risk of DVT is embolization of a portion of the DVT that travels into the lung, becoming a pulmonary embolus (PE). The overwhelming majority of PEs originate from a lower extremity DVT.[6] An acute arterial occlusion will produce permanent damage to the lower extremity within a few hours. Although a DVT will produce pain and discomfort, it generally does not compromise the extremity in and of itself. If a PE develops, however, it can be a life-threatening event.

Fractures

Most fractures result from trauma to an extremity. In some cases, however, the force required to produce a fracture is minimal and may seem innocuous. These are called pathological fractures. In patients who do not have normal cognition (e.g., an elderly person with dementia or a younger person who is mentally handicapped), it may be difficult to elicit a history of trauma or to localize the source of extremity pain. The Paramedic should always look for a traumatic origin, no matter how minor the pain appears to the Paramedic.

As people age, the calcium content in their bones decreases, leading to bones that are more brittle than usual. Although this condition can be decreased with an appropriate diet while young, weight-bearing exercise (e.g., walking), and medications that help enhance the deposit of calcium in the bones, it is still a condition that affects many older individuals. In some cases, osteoporosis is severe enough that placing one's weight off center or too forcibly on a lower extremity can cause a fracture. The two common places for a pathologic fracture to develop in a patient who has osteoporosis are in the hip and the spine. These types of spine fractures rarely cause any neurologic symptoms or damage; however, they can be quite painful.

Pathologic fractures can also occur due to metastasis of cancer from a primary site to bone. Many types of cancer spread either through the blood or through the lymphatic system to locations distant from the primary site of the tumor. Tumors that metastasize to bone start small and then become destructive as the tumor grows inside the bone. Eventually, these tumors disrupt the bone's ability to bear weight, producing a fracture. In the extremities, this type of pathologic fracture occurs most commonly in the humerus, femur, or pelvis. Pain from a pathologic fracture of the pelvis can produce referred pain down into the lower extremity.

One injury affecting adolescents that produces leg pain is a **slipped capital femoral epiphysis (SCFE)**. The metaphysis is the shaft of the bone, the epiphysis is the end of the bone, and the growth plate is located between those parts of the bone (Figure 22-2). The growth plate is a softer portion of the bone that stays open until the late teenage years. For that reason, the growth plate is a common location for fractures in children. In SCFE, the proximal end of the femur becomes displaced from the femoral shaft at the growth plate (Figure 22-3). Although both young males and females can develop a SCFE, it is at least twice as common in boys as girls. Obesity is also a risk factor for SCFE, due to the extra stress placed on the femur.[7] SCFE can develop acutely, often while running, or it can develop gradually over a short period of time. The child may complain of pain anywhere in the upper part of the lower extremity down to the knee and is often only able to walk with a limp, if he is able to walk at all.

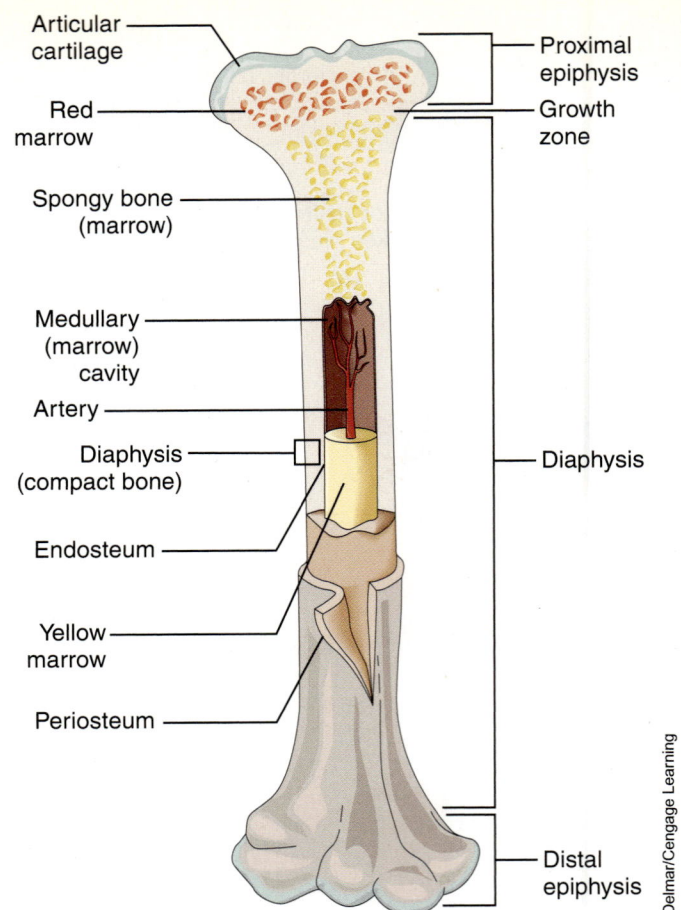

Figure 22-2 Sections of a long bone.

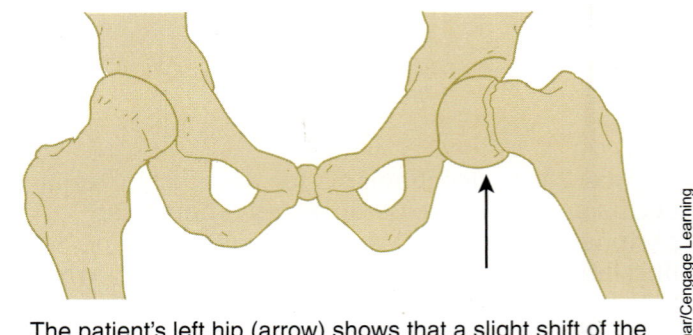

The patient's left hip (arrow) shows that a slight shift of the head of the femur has occured through the growth plate.

Figure 22-3 Slipped femoral capital epiphysis.

Soft Tissue Infections

Cellulitis is an infection of the superficial layers of the skin, producing an area of redness called **erythema** (Figure 22-4). This area can spread locally, producing an even larger area of erythema. Streaking, called **lymphangitis**, can also occur from the area of infection, indicating its lymphatic spread. Swelling of the extremity often results due to the reactive changes that occur as the body attempts to contain and fight the infection, and can easily be confused with a DVT. The source of the infection is often the spread of bacteria into a small break in the skin at the affected area. Patients with a history of diabetes, especially poorly controlled diabetes, are at higher risk for developing cellulitis from minor damage to the skin. Cellulitis can also occur as an abscess develops in the skin and the infection spreads outside the abscess capsule. Uncomplicated cellulitis does not produce fever or chills. Although generally not a life-threatening condition, cellulitis is a potential cause of sepsis in patients with compromised immune systems and patients at the extremes of age.

A deeper soft tissue infection that can be life-threatening is necrotizing fasciitis (i.e., flesh-eating bacteria) (Figure 22-5). Fasciitis occurs as a result of the spread of bacteria into the body's deeper tissue layers. Necrotizing fasciitis often occurs when bacteria travels into the deeper soft tissues of the body, below the skin, and into the facial planes that surround the muscles and body cavities.

Fasciitis can occur anywhere in the body, but most often appears in the lower extremities. The bacteria can reach this deep through either direct trauma (e.g., penetrating trauma to an extremity) or if a surface infection spreads deeper. In patients with risk factors, bacteria can spread through breaks in the skin without producing a surface infection. Several risk factors include immunosuppressive medications, long-term antibiotics, diabetes, renal failure or transplant, abdominal infections, HIV and AIDS, deep trauma, and intravenous or injection drug abuse.

Bullae, or blisters, can form in the skin, and the discharge from the area is often grayish and foul smelling rather than the greenish discharge normally associated with pus. Gangrene, or tissue death, can occur, causing the skin to turn purple or black. As the infection worsens, it can lead to sepsis and death. The facial planes are connected and provide a means for the rapid spread of the infection throughout the extremity and into the trunk. The signs and symptoms may be the same as in cellulitis; however, the patient with fasciitis usually complains of severe pain in the area of the deeper infection. These patients also tend to have high fevers and appear ill during the examination. Hypotension may develop as part of the sepsis from the infection.

Soft tissue infections can also affect the tendons. One specific tendon infection that can cause significant disability, a **flexor tenosynovitis**, is an infection of the tendons in the hand and forearm (Figure 22-6). This is most often caused by minor injury to the finger or hand. An untreated minor infection of a finger—whether from a laceration, cracked skin, or minor penetrating injury—can spread into the tendon sheath that surrounds the tendon and then up the tendon into the hand.

Injection from a high pressure gun (e.g., paint or grease gun) can inoculate the deeper tissues and tendons with bacteria that will rapidly grow and spread. Injection injuries often are taken to the operating room within 24 hours so a hand surgeon or orthopedist can surgically clean out the wound and prevent infection. Patients who have developed a flexor tenosynovitis also are taken to the operating room within a few hours for surgical washout of the infection.[8,9]

Another soft tissue infection is a cutaneous abscess, the formation of a collection of pus just under the skin (Figure 22-7). Often cutaneous abscesses develop from a plugged sweat duct or an ingrown hair follicle that traps

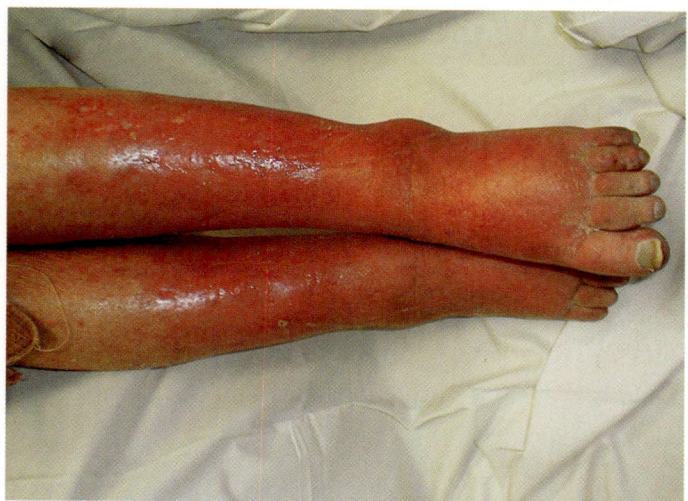

Figure 22-4 Cellulitis.

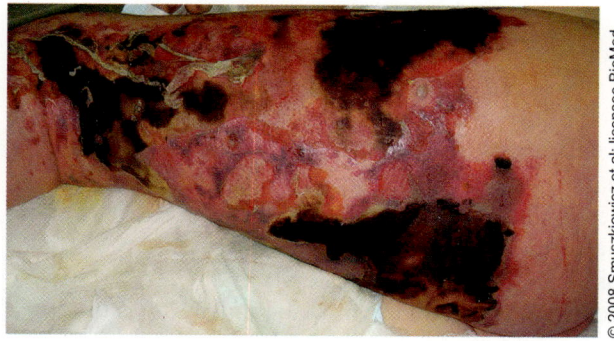

© 2008 Smuszkiewicz et al; licensee BioMed Central Ltd.:Late diagnosed necrotizing fasciitis as a cause of multiorgan dysfunction syndrome: A case report. Cases Journal 2008, 1:125. doi:10.1186/1757-1626-1-125

Figure 22-5 Necrosis can occur from necrotizing fasciitis.

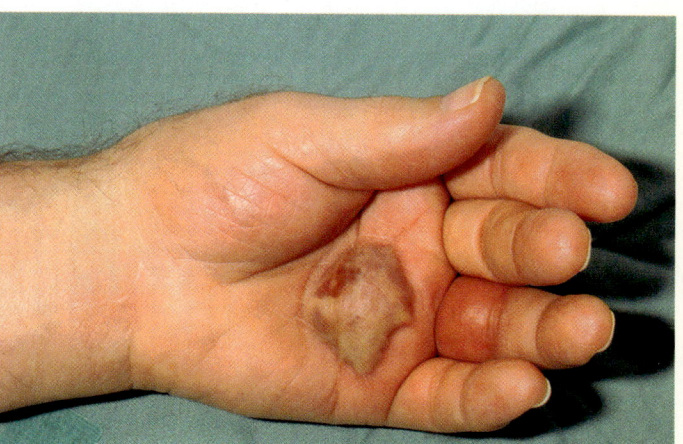

Figure 22-6 Flexor tenosynovitis occurs from spread of an infection into a digit's tendon sheath or from a high pressure injection injury.

surface bacteria in an environment that encourages growth of the bacteria. Erythema can develop around the abscess, which may represent a surrounding cellulitis, or may be secondary to the inflammatory process that the body uses to fight the infection. **Paronychia** (Figure 22-8) is a cutaneous abscess located around a nail bed, most often in the hand. Bacteria is transmitted to the cuticle from individuals who bite their fingernails or cuticles.[10] A paronychia may also develop through cracked skin or if the fingernails are cut too short. The physician or mid-level provider (physician's assistant or nurse practitioner) treats a cutaneous abscess by making an incision into the abscess and washing out the pus.

Bone and Joint Infections

Surface infections that spread into deeper tissues can spread as deep as the bone and cause **osteomyelitis**, or an infection of the bone. Osteomyelitis can also occur when deep skin ulcers, commonly occurring in patients with poorly controlled diabetes or vascular insufficiency, become infected. In addition. osteomyelitis can occur in patients after trauma to an extremity or fracture repair. Osteomyelitis can be difficult to treat and typically requires several weeks of antibiotic treatment. The Paramedic may encounter a patient undergoing her initial episode or, alternatively, a patient with known osteomyelitis who presents with worsening pain. Pain that is worsening may indicate either progression of the infection or inadequate analgesia.

Infection can spread to the tissues inside a joint space, causing a septic arthritis or septic joint. This can occur by direct spread, either from a cutaneous infection or an injury that penetrates the capsule surrounding a joint. More often, however, the infection spreads as bacteria travels through the blood and infiltrates the joint. The knee and hip are most often affected in this manner, although infection can occur in any joint. Infected joints are often warm, erythematous, and swollen. The patient may also complain of constitutional symptoms (e.g., fever, chills, sweats, or shaking). A patient who has developed a septic joint typically requires surgical intervention to open the joint and wash out the infection, followed by the use of long-term antibiotics.

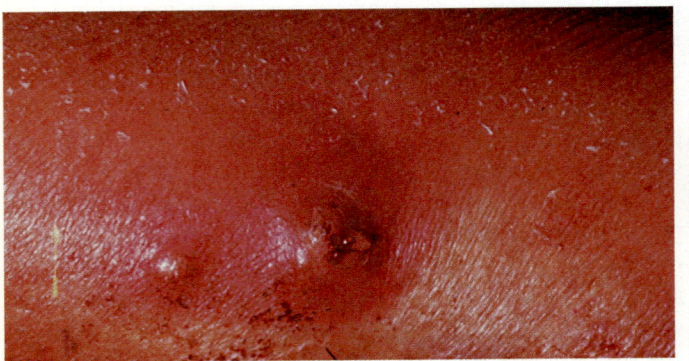

Figure 22-7 A cutaneous abscess with surrounding cellulitis.

CDC/Bruno Coignard, M.D.; Jeff Hageman, M.H.S.

CULTURAL/REGIONAL DIFFERENCES

Gonococcal arthritis is an infectious (septic) type of arthritis that occurs with those patients infected with gonorrhea. It affects women more often than men and is more common in younger people. The condition can present as a skin rash with multiple joint involvement or as an infection of a single joint. Its presentation can be confused for Lyme disease, and is prevalent in the northeast and the Great Lakes region.

Rhabdomyolysis

Rhabdomyolysis, the breakdown of muscle, is a condition that is most often associated with crush injury, electrical injury, or prolonged soft tissue compression (e.g., the elderly patient who is found after lying on the floor of his apartment for several days after a fall), although it can occur from a variety of causes.

Rhabdomyolysis can also occur in patients who have exercised to the point of muscle breakdown or as a side effect of some medications (including the statin class of medications used to treat high cholesterol) and illicit substances (e.g., cocaine).[11–13] In addition, rhabdomyolysis can be seen in patients who fight against physical restraint. On rare occasions, mild rhabdomyolysis may be seen in patients who have undergone repeated discharges with a taser. However, it is not

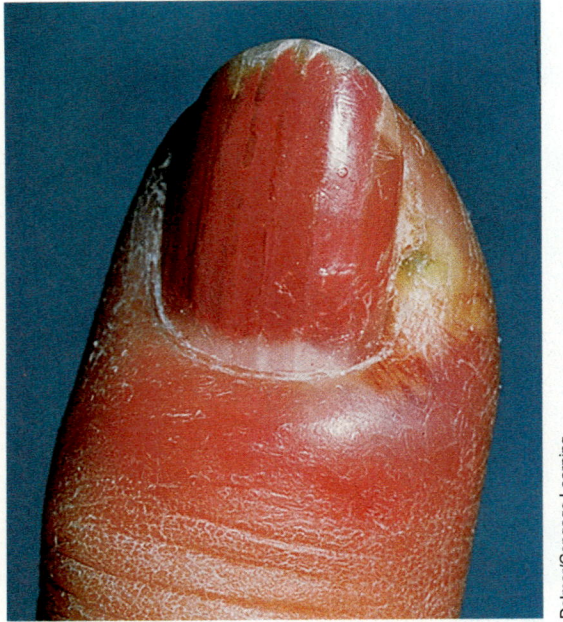

Figure 22-8 Paronychia is an infection adjacent to a nail cuticle.

Delmar/Cengage Learning

clear if rhabdomyolysis occurs from the muscle contraction that happens with repeated discharge or from restraint used after the patient was apprehended.[14,15]

Patients most often complain of severe muscle aching (proximal muscle groups around the hips and shoulders more than distal muscle groups) and cramping, as well as cola-colored urine. Rhabdomyolysis can cause renal failure, acidosis, and hyperkalemia.

Pathophysiology of Chronic Causes of Extremity Pain

The previous discussion covered the emergent causes of extremity pain. However, the Paramedic will also encounter patients who have conditions that produce extremity pain that is more chronic in nature and not life- or limb-threatening. The three causes of chronic extremity pain discussed here are arthritis, bursitis, and tendonitis.

Arthritis

Arthritis is a general term indicating inflammation of a joint, which can occur due to many different causes. As previously discussed, infection that spreads into the joint is one cause of arthritis. Although other types of arthritis can be painful and affect a patient's quality of life, they are generally not life- or limb-threatening. The three types of arthritis covered here are osteoarthritis, rheumatoid arthritis, and gout.

Osteoarthritis occurs when the cartilage that cushions the bones, making up the joint, wears out and becomes thin. As the cartilage thins, the bony surfaces impact each other, causing changes within the bone that initiate inflammatory changes within the joint. At this point, the patient will feel some discomfort and stiffness with use, especially at that joint's extremes of the range of motion. In some joints, spurring (an abnormal outgrowth of bone) can occur; if so, that may also enhance inflammation. Eventually, the cartilage may wear down to the point where the two bones that make up the joint are in contact with each other, causing severe pain.

Rheumatoid arthritis is an inflammatory disease where the body's immune system attacks both the tissue in the capsule surrounding the joints as well as the cartilage within the joint. This causes an inflammatory arthritis characterized by joint swelling, pain, and stiffness. Although rheumatoid arthritis can be caused by an infection that triggers the immune response, in many cases a clear cause is unknown. Rheumatoid arthritis can last for a few months to a lifetime. In extreme cases, the patient's joints become deformed (Figure 22-9) and the tendons weaken, predisposing the patient to dislocations from minor trauma.

Gout, a common form of inflammatory arthritis, is caused by the deposit of uric acid crystals in the joint fluid in the joint capsule. This can be a very painful and debilitating condition and, if left untreated, can cause joint destruction. The crystals in the joint produce an inflammatory response that is responsible for the pain and destruction. The joint becomes warm and swollen, and the skin over the joint may become erythematous, making it difficult to differentiate from a septic joint. The joints most often affected by gout include the great toe, the knee, the wrist, and the thumb.[16] Men are affected more than women, with men experiencing gout starting in their thirties and forties whereas women are affected more in their fifties.

Bursitis

Bursa are small sacs of fluid located around the major joints that provide support and cushioning for tendons that act on that joint (Figure 22-10). Bursa are often connected to the

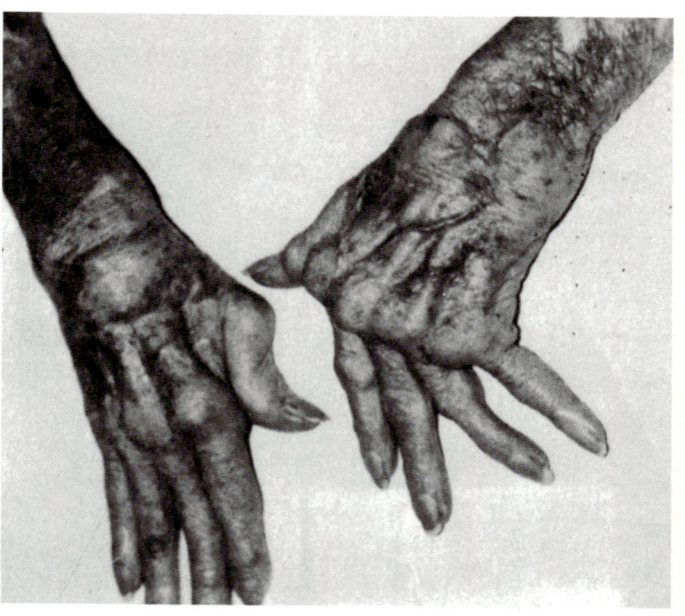

Figure 22-9 Ulnar deviation of the fingers from late stage rheumatoid arthritis.

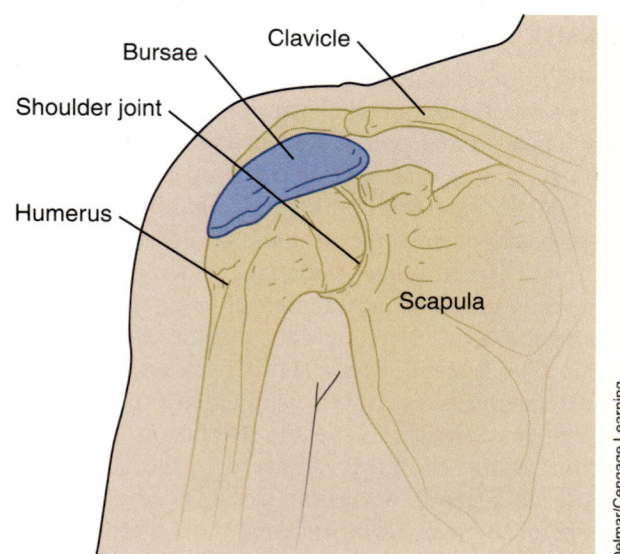

Figure 22-10 The fluid-filled bursa of the shoulder reduce friction and support the tendons in moving the joint.

joint capsule, and the fluid in the bursa is the same as the fluid in the joint. **Bursitis** is an inflammation of a bursa sac, often from repetitive motion and stress on that joint. Bursitis can cause mild swelling around a joint and pain with movement of the affected joint.

Tendonitis

Tendonitis is an inflammation of a tendon often caused by either a minor injury or repetitive motion of a joint. The tendon swells within its sheath, causing it to rub against the inner surface of the sheath, producing pain with movement of the affected joint. This often occurs in the upper extremity, but can also occur in the lower extremity. In some cases, the pain can be severe with small amounts of movement.

Fibromyalgia

Fibromyalgia is a painful syndrome that includes muscular pain, digestive disorders, chronic headaches, and even sleep disorders that may affect 3% to 6% of the population. The cardinal symptom of fibromyalgia is exhaustion that is coupled with muscle pain. Although fibromyalgia has only recently come to the public's attention, descriptions of fibromyalgia symptoms date back to the seventeenth century. Abnormally low serotonin levels have been implicated as a cause of fibromyalgia.

CASE STUDY (CONTINUED)

When the ambulance arrives, Mrs. McCarthy opens the door and motions the Paramedics to come in. Mr. McCarthy is sitting at the table in obvious pain, rubbing his right lower leg. The Paramedics introduce themselves. On interview, Mr. McCarthy states that his leg pain started suddenly about three hours ago and was worse than his usual pain. He took his oral analgesic and was hoping that it would work, but the pain is becoming worse, so he asked his wife to call for an ambulance. He has had pain in the past from "circulation problems" in his legs, but this is much worse. He has a history of diabetes, hypertension, and renal insufficiency. He has not had any fevers, chills, sweats, or skin ulcers. Mr. McCarthy also denies having chest pain, trouble breathing, or trauma.

CRITICAL THINKING QUESTIONS

1. What are the important elements of the history that a Paramedic should obtain?
2. What is the symptom pattern for deep venous thrombosis?

History

The circumstances leading to the onset of the extremity pain provide the Paramedic with important clues as to the likely cause of the pain. Sudden pain suggests an acute origin, such as a vascular occlusion or trauma. Following the OPQRST mnemonic, the Paramedic should obtain the time of onset; events preceding the onset of pain; the location, quality, recurrence, radiation, and relieving factors; and severity of the pain. A history of fever, night sweats, or chills suggests an infectious cause of the patient's extremity pain. The presence of a rash, redness, or swelling of the skin also suggests a cellulitis or other soft tissue infection. Swelling may indicate a venous occlusion or soft tissue infection, while coolness compared to the other leg may indicate an arterial occlusion. Joint swelling may indicate one of the many arthritic conditions discussed earlier. Proximal muscle aches with a recent history of overexertion or physical restraint, especially when combined with dark urination, may indicate rhabdomyolysis. In adolescent children with insidious onset of hip or knee pain, the Paramedic

Femoral popliteal bypass

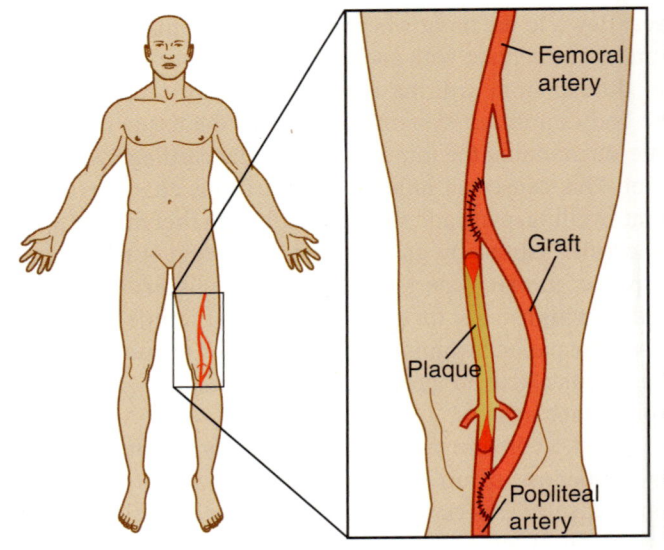

Figure 22-11 An example of femoral-popliteal vascular bypass in a lower extremity for atherosclerosis of the femoral artery.

should consider SCFE as a possible cause. Finally, pain that is worse with movement suggests the cause is a joint, bursa, or tendon.

The past medical and surgical histories also provide the Paramedic with key information. Patients who have diabetes are at higher risk for developing infections, vascular issues, and nerve pain, also known as neuropathic pain. Patients who are on chronic steroids for respiratory or inflammatory conditions are at higher risk for stress fractures from osteoporosis. A history of osteoporosis increases the risk of fracture from minor trauma. A history of atrial fibrillation suggests the possibility of an acute arterial occlusion if the atrial fibrillation is poorly controlled. A past surgical history of a hip fracture in an elderly individual also suggests the possibility of a pathologic fracture. A history of a **vascular bypass** in an extremity, where a vascular surgeon takes a blood vessel and bypasses a blocked artery in the lower extremity (Figure 22-11), alerts the Paramedic to a past history of vascular issues and an increased chance of vascular occlusion.

CASE STUDY (CONTINUED)

During the initial assessment, Mr. McCarthy's airway, breathing, and circulation are intact. During the detailed exam, the Paramedics obtain a set of vitals that includes a pulse rate between 92 and 108 and irregularly irregular, respiratory rate of 16 and easy, a blood pressure of 156/88, and a room air oxygen saturation of 98%. An inspection of Mr. McCarthy's right leg shows no bruising, open skin, erythema, or ulcers. The skin on the right leg is paler and cooler than that of the left. The lower leg and foot is tender to the touch, causing Mr. McCarthy to jump. There is no swelling noted in the right leg. The Paramedic is unable to palpate the dorsalis pedis or posterior tibial pulse in the right foot. Those pulses are present in the left foot, but are weak. Mr. McCarthy's abdomen is soft, non-tender, and without masses on palpation.

Mrs. McCarthy mentions that her husband had a history of an irregular heartbeat and was supposed to take a medication for it. Mr. McCarthy states that is true; he was taking Coumadin, but stopped because he kept bruising his legs.

CRITICAL THINKING QUESTIONS

1. What are the elements of the physical examination of a patient with suspected deep vein thrombus?
2. Why is a 12-lead ECG a critical element in this examination?

Examination

As with all patients, the Paramedic rapidly performs a primary assessment, identifying and managing any immediate life-threatening conditions. Once the life-threatening conditions have been addressed, the Paramedic should move on to a detailed physical examination. In many cases, the physical exam leads to additional questions.

Examination of the painful extremity involves inspection and palpation of the extremity. First, the Paramedic should inspect the extremity for any obvious injury, deformity, areas of edema or erythema, or other skin changes. The Paramedic should palpate the extremity for skin temperature compared with the opposite extremity; palpate the extremity for bony and soft tissue tenderness; and assess the distal pulses, sensation, and muscle strength on each affected extremity, comparing it with the opposite side.

Absent distal pulses combined with cold skin raise the Paramedic's suspicion for an acute arterial occlusion.[17,18] Edema and erythema on one extremity with good distal pulses may be indicative of either cellulitis or a DVT. A cutaneous abscess is often noted by localized swelling in a circular or oval area that is raised and tender, and is often associated with surrounding erythema. Flexor tenosynovitis has four classic physical examination findings that include swelling of the entire digit, finger held in a flexed position, severe pain with passive extension, and tenderness and swelling localized along the tendon sheath. The patient's range of motion should be assessed for painful atraumatic joints. The skin color and temperature over painful joints is also compared with the same joint on the opposite extremity.

CASE STUDY (CONTINUED)

The Paramedics assist Mr. McCarthy to a standing position, but the pain is too great for him to bear weight on his right leg. The Paramedics move Mr. McCarthy out of the house using a stair chair. While moving Mr. McCarty into the ambulance, the two Paramedics quickly review the history and physical examination findings and develop the paramedical diagnosis.

CRITICAL THINKING QUESTIONS

1. What is the significance of atrial fibrillation related to Mr. McCarthy's leg pain?
2. What potential diagnoses are considered in Mr. McCarthy's case?

Assessment

As the Paramedic proceeds through the history and physical, he narrows down his list of paramedical differential diagnoses to the most likely cause for the patient's complaint. As determined by a history of sudden worsening of leg pain, known vascular problems, and absence of trauma, the Paramedic should suspect acute arterial occlusion. An absence of an infective cause would support that diagnosis.

Assessment of a borderline tachycardic and irregularly irregular rhythm, suggests a history of atrial fibrillation. A history of atrial fibrillation, past vascular issues, diabetes, and hypertension would put any patient at risk for an acute arterial occlusion.

A physical examination might reveal distal pulses are absent and that the skin below the knee is cold to the touch compared to the contralateral limb. These findings confirm the likelihood an acute arterial occlusion.

CASE STUDY (CONTINUED)

After loading Mr. McCarthy into the ambulance, the Paramedic starts an intravenous line, draws blood, and administers analgesia. The Paramedic also attaches Mr. McCarthy to a cardiac monitor and runs a 12-lead ECG. Both the monitor strip and 12-lead ECG demonstrate atrial fibrillation and no acute ST or T wave changes.

CRITICAL THINKING QUESTIONS

1. What is the standard of care of patients with suspected acute arterial occlusion?
2. What are some of the patient-specific concerns and considerations that the Paramedic should consider when applying this plan of care that is intended to treat a broad patient population presenting with acute arterial occlusion?

Treatment

In most instances, treatment of acute extremity pain consists of support and comfort. The Paramedic should consider applying ice to the painful area if either an injury is suspected or the patient is suffering from an exacerbation of one of the chronic causes of extremity pain. The Paramedic should place the extremity in a position of comfort. If marked edema is present, she should consider elevating the extremity. For patients in severe pain, the Paramedic should consider administering appropriate analgesic medications.[19,20] If the history and physical exam suggest other acute conditions, the Paramedic should perform appropriate treatments for those conditions.

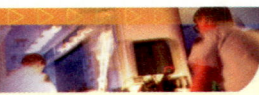

PROFESSIONAL PARAMEDIC

Treatment with fibrinolytics to lyse a clot has been controversial. Initially expense, complications, and high reocclusion rates limited the use of this treatment. With the FDA rescinding approval for the use of urokinase, streptokinase remained the only drug approved for extremity clot lysis. However, with the advent of catheter-directed systems in which the systemic concentration of the drug is low and total dose needed for clot lysis is low, some physicians have again begun treatment with fibrinolytics.

The Paramedic reassesses Mr. McCarthy's vital signs, including pain level, a few minutes after administering analgesia. The Paramedic also reassesses Mr. McCarthy's leg to ensure there have not been any changes in his examination. Mr. McCarthy's vitals remain constant, his cardiac rhythm remains in atrial fibrillation at a rate of between 90 and 100, and his pain level decreases from an 8:10 to a 5:10 after analgesia.

CRITICAL THINKING QUESTIONS

1. What are some of the predictable complications associated with acute arterial occlusion?
2. What are some of the predictable complications associated with the treatments for acute arterial occlusion?

Evaluation

During transport, the patient's vital signs are reassessed at least once, and perhaps additional times depending on the length of the transport. This includes assessing the patient's level of pain. The Paramedic should address any changes in the patient's vital signs, including hypotension and tachycardia that may develop as part of worsening sepsis or dysrhythmias that produce hypotension.

CASE STUDY CONCLUSION

The ambulance pulls into St. Maria's emergency department and the Paramedics transfer Mr. McCarthy over to the stretcher in room 7. The attending physician then obtains a history and examines Mr. McCarthy. She is unable to obtain distal pulses on Mr. McCarthy's right leg either by palpation or with a handheld Doppler. Suspecting an acute arterial occlusion, the attending physician pages the vascular surgeon. Mr. McCarthy is then placed on heparin in the emergency department and taken a short time later for an emergent vascular bypass of his lower extremity. Several days later, Mr. McCarthy is released from the hospital to a rehabilitation facility to improve the strength in his weakened leg.

CRITICAL THINKING QUESTIONS

1. What is the most appropriate transport decision that will get the patient to definitive care?
2. What are the advantages of transporting a patient with suspected acute arterial occlusion to these hospitals, even if that means bypassing other hospitals in the process?

Disposition

Patients with unstable vital signs should be transported to the nearest emergency department for stabilization. Most hospitals will not have a concern with handling all of these patients who present with a complaint of extremity pain. If the Paramedic suspects the patient may require surgical intervention by an orthopedist, general surgeon, or vascular surgeon, he should make reasonable attempts to bring the patient directly to an appropriate emergency department. If there is any question, the Paramedic should not hesitate to call for an on-line medical consult to ensure the appropriateness of the destination.

CONCLUSION

The underlying cause of extremity pain can range from the benign and bothersome to limb- or life-threatening conditions. Early identification of limb-threatening conditions by the Paramedic speeds treatment for the patient, improving the chances of saving the patient's limb.

KEY POINTS:

- Paramedic assessment in the case of extremity pain involves identifying those patients who have an emergent problem and directing those patients to the ED staff.

- An acute vascular occlusion occurs when a vessel is occluded or the vessel's diameter decreases, limiting blood flow.

- The two likely causes of an embolus are peripheral vascular disease with decreased blood flow or atrial fibrillations with ejection of a part of a clot from the heart.

- Venous occlusions occur due to blood pooling in the extremity or the placement of a catheter, which allows clots to form around it.

- Risk factors for lower extremity venous occlusions include immobility of any type, use of oral contraceptives, pregnancy or obesity, and genetic conditions which affect blood clotting.

- Risk factors for upper extremity occlusions include placement of central lines.

- Fractures that occur in the absence of trauma are termed pathologic fractures.

- Children and adolescents are at risk for damage to the growth plate of the femur even with little to no trauma.

- Soft tissue infections called cellulitis can occur in the superficial layers of the skin.

- Soft tissue infections can affect tendons, bones, and joints.

- Breakdown of muscle can lead to rhabdomyolysis, in which crush, electrical shock, some medications, and overexertion causes muscles to release proteins into the blood, causing renal failure.

- Chronic causes of extremity pain include arthritis, bursitis, and tendonitis.

- Onset of the pain, events leading to the pain, and quality of the pain are important clues. Past medical history also suggests which patients may be at greater risk for emergent or chronic conditions.

- Swelling, discolorations, temperature, and the presence and quality of pulses are important examination points.

- Treatment for vascular disorders is supportive and comforting.

REVIEW QUESTIONS:

1. In an arterial occlusion, what blocks the artery? How does it occur?

2. In deep vein thrombosis of the legs, what is blocking blood flow? How do they develop?

3. What is the outcome of an arterial occlusion if no medical intervention is performed? What if no venous occlusion is performed?

4. What can cause a fracture of an extremity in the absence of any trauma?

5. What is a slipped capital femoral epiphysis? Who is at risk for it?

6. How is cellulitis different from fasciitis?

7. What patients are at risk for developing rhabdomyolysis?

CASE STUDY QUESTIONS:

Please refer to the Case Study in this chapter, and answer the questions below:

1. What clues exist for the paramedical diagnosis of acute arterial occlusion?

2. List at least four factors that Mr. McCarthy has that place him at risk for a vascular occlusion.

3. Should the Paramedics have given Mr. McCarthy additional analgesia? Why or why not?

REFERENCES:

1. Henke PK. Approach to the patient with acute limb ischemia: diagnosis and therapeutic modalities. *Cardiol Clin.* 2002;22(4):513–522.

2. Sontheimer DL. Peripheral vascular disease: diagnosis and treatment. *Am Fam Physician.* 2006;73(11):1971–1976.

3. Wells PS. Integrated strategies for the diagnosis of venous thromboembolism. *J Thromb Haemost.* 2007;5 Suppl 1:41–50.

4. Scarvelis D, Wells PS. Diagnosis and treatment of deep-vein thrombosis. *CMAJ.* 2006;175(9):1087–1092.

5. Race TK, Collier PE. The hidden risk of deep vein thrombosis—the need for risk factor assessment: case reviews. *Crit Care Nurs Q.* 2007;30(3):245–254.

6. Selby R, Geerts W, et al. Hypercoagulability after trauma: Hemostatic changes and relationship to venous thromboembolism. *Thromb Res.* 2009;124(3):281–287.

7. Herrera-Soto JA, Duffy MF, et al. Increased intracapsular pressures after unstable slipped capital femoral epiphysis. *J Pediatr Orthop.* 2008;28(7):723–728.

8. Clark DC. Common acute hand infections. *Am Fam Physician.* 2003;68(11):2167–2176.

9. Boles SD, Schmidt CC. Pyogenic flexor tenosynovitis. *Hand Clin.* 1998;14(4):567–578.

10. Rigopoulos D, Larios G, et al. Acute and chronic paronychia. *Am Fam Physician.* 2008;77(3):339–346.

11. Phillips PS, Haas RH. Statin myopathy as a metabolic muscle disease. *Expert Rev Cardiovasc Ther.* 2008;6(7):971–978.

12. Klopstock T. Drug-induced myopathies. *Curr Opin Neurol.* 2008;21(5):590–595.

13. Harper CR, Jacobson TA. The broad spectrum of statin myopathy: from myalgia to rhabdomyolysis. *Curr Opin Lipidol.* 2007;18(4):401–408.

14. Ordog GJ, Wasserberger J, et al. Electronic gun (taser) injuries. *Ann Emerg Med.* 1987;16(1):73–78.

15. O'Brien DJ. Electronic weaponry—a question of safety. *Ann Emerg Med.* 1991;22(5):583–587.

16. Schlesinger N. Diagnosis of gout. *Minerva Med.* 2007;98(6):759–767.

17. Ouriel K. Thrombolytic therapy for acute arterial occlusion. *J Am Coll Surg.* 2002;194(1 Suppl):S32–S39.

18. Strandness DE, Jr. Acute arterial occlusion. *Heart Dis Stroke.* 1993;2(4):322–324.

19. Rogovik AL, Goldman RD. Prehospital use of analgesics at home or en route to the hospital in children with extremity injuries. *Am J Emerg Med.* 2007;25(4):400–405.

20. Abbuhl FB, Reed DB. Time to analgesia for patients with painful extremity injuries transported to the emergency department by ambulance. *Prehosp Emerg Care.* 2003;7(4):445–447.

CHAPTER 23

BLEEDING DISORDERS

KEY CONCEPTS:

Upon completion of this chapter, it is expected that the reader will understand these following concepts:

- That hematologic disorders vary in nature and severity but affect the entire organism
- That hemostasis includes primary and secondary methods to stop bleeding and then stabilize the clot
- How hematological disorders may be subtle and require a good history to support a suspicion of bleeding disorders

ANATOMY CONCEPTS:

Prior to reading this chapter the Paramedic student should be familiar with the following anatomy and physiology concepts:

- Gastrointestinal anatomy
- Mesenteric blood system

Paramedic 12 is dispatched to 132 Figby Street, upper right apartment, for a 32-year-old male complaining of back and leg pain. MedComm states the patient told the call taker there was no recent trauma. The Paramedics discuss the possible causes of nontraumatic pain in such a relatively young patient.

CRITICAL THINKING QUESTIONS

1. What are some of the possible causes of leg pain?
2. How is the absence of trauma related to the leg pain?

OVERVIEW

Hematological disorders can occur in a variety of forms that affect many different aspects of the circulatory system, including clotting factors, platelets, and red blood cells. For the purposes of this discussion, these disorders are divided into hereditary coagulation disorders, acquired coagulation disorders, anemias, and other red blood cell disorders. Although a detailed knowledge of the coagulation cascade and the key components of blood are prerequisite objectives to this chapter, it is important to first provide a brief review of the coagulation cascade and the fibrinolytic system.

Chief Concern

Coagulopathy is a term used to describe any bleeding disorder due to problems with the coagulation cascade. The management of patients with hematological disorders can be challenging for the Paramedic. Although some conditions are relatively common, others are encountered much less frequently and sometimes only in a critical care transport setting. Knowledge of these disorders, however, can provide the Paramedic with the tools needed to appropriately manage patients with hematological disorders.

Coagulation System Review

The body uses a series of mechanisms to maintain **hemostasis**, an adequate blood volume, by preventing the loss of blood from bleeding. In the initial actions, termed primary hemostasis, the objective is to rapidly form a clot to provide initial control of blood vessel damage. Secondary hemostasis activates shortly after initiation of primary hemostasis, with the objective of stabilizing the blood clot to prevent dislodgement and allowing the body's repair mechanisms to kick in and make repairs to the damaged tissue.

Primary Hemostasis

The process of primary hemostasis depends on the interaction between the innermost layer of cells in the lining of the blood vessel and circulating platelets in the blood. When damage occurs to the blood vessel wall, a clotting factor called von Willebrand factor (vWf) is released from the damaged cells. vWf attracts platelets that are flowing past the damaged area and attaches them to the wall of the blood vessel. Initially, collagen (i.e., connective tissue), vWf, and platelets begin to form a plug in the damaged blood vessel. Fibrinogen, also known as factor I or fI, then begins to attract more platelets to the forming clot. Fibrinogen produces a link between the platelets closest to the damaged blood vessel and to the additional platelets attracted to the site of injury. Therefore, the four elements required for primary hemostasis to occur include normal collagen in the inner layers of the blood vessel, circulating platelets that function normally, an adequate amount of vWf, and an adequate amount of fibrinogen.

Secondary Hemostasis

The goal of secondary hemostasis is to strengthen the clot plug in the damaged vessel to ensure that it is not dislodged. This process involves attracting additional platelets to the clot and using the clotting factor fibrin to provide a firm and insoluble matrix of fibers in the clot. Secondary hemostasis is achieved through activation of the **coagulation cascade**, a series of clotting factors or proteins that change form (e.g., XII changes to XIIa), thereby activating the next step in the cascade (Figure 23-1). The final product in this cascade is the cross-linked fibrin that forms the solid matrix which stabilizes the clot.

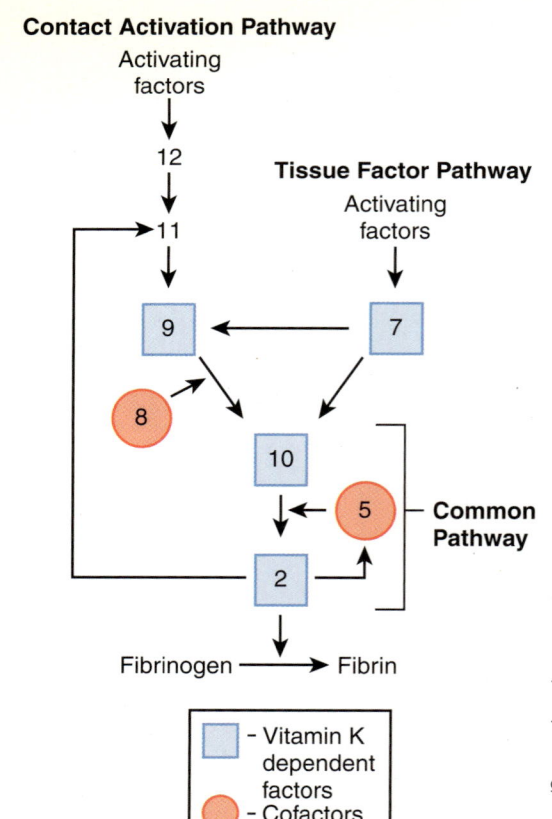

Figure 23-1 The coagulation cascade.

The upper part of Figure 23-1 shows the two pathways that initiate the cascade. The tissue factor pathway on the right is activated by the release of tissue factor from the damaged blood vessel and rapidly produces thrombin to provide an initial layer of clot over the damaged vessel. The pathway on the left is the contact activation pathway and is activated by contact with the damaged blood vessel. This pathway activates more slowly than the tissue factor pathway. Both pathways cause the reaction that transforms factor X to factor Xa at the start of the common pathway. The clotting factors are all produced in the liver. Several of the clotting factors—specifically factors II, VII, IX, and X—utilize vitamin K in the production of the clotting factors, making vitamin K an essential nutrient for the coagulation system.

If left unchecked, the coagulation cascade would run until a clot forms that occludes the blood vessel. The cross-linked fibrin matrix is purposely not dissolvable, and would remain in place permanently. Fortunately, the fibrinolytic pathway (Figure 23-2) exists which allows the body to keep the coagulation cascade in check. It will not allow the clot to propagate past a reasonable size and will break down the clot as the vessel is repaired. The protein plasminogen is degraded by tissue plasminogen activator (tPA) into plasmin. tPA is released from the blood vessel lining when it is damaged. Plasmin then breaks down the cross-linked fibrin in the clot, producing fibrin degradation products and another protein fragment, a product of clot breakdown called D-dimer.

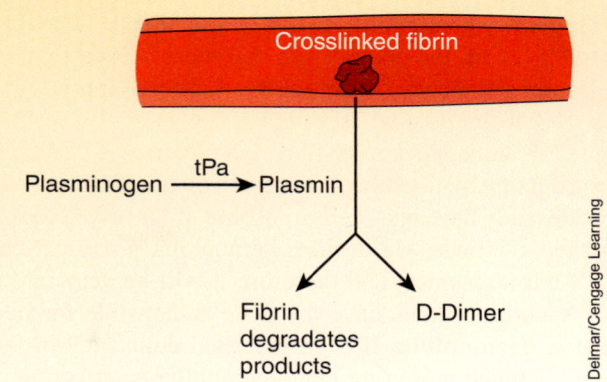

Figure 23-2 The fibrinolytic pathway.

STREET SMART

Naturally occurring streptokinase and tPa serve as the basis for the class of medications called fibrinolytics. These drugs are used to dissolve blood clots in the setting of myocardial infarction, thrombotic stroke, and hemodynamically unstable pulmonary embolism. Streptokinase is a toxin produced by the streptococcus bacteria and was the first medication in this class, followed by tPa.[1,2] Currently, synthetic versions of these naturally occurring compounds are often used in fibrinolysis.

In addition to dissolving existing clots, the **fibrinolytic system** also slows down the activation of several of the proteins in the coagulation system. Antithrombin III attaches itself to factors XIIa, XIa, IXa, and thrombin and decreases their function, effectively putting the breaks on the coagulation cascade. Two other proteins—protein C and protein S—that are produced in the liver will bind to each other and then bind to factors Va and VIIIa, thereby also inhibiting the coagulation cascade. Two common anticoagulant medications—heparin and warfarin—act by these mechanisms to provide

STREET SMART

The D-dimer is often measured as a nonspecific indication of clotting. Most often, it is used to assist in determining if the patient developed a venothromboembolus in the form of a deep vein thrombosis (DVT) or pulmonary embolism (PE). The D-dimer is very nonspecific, meaning that if the value is elevated, it does not necessarily mean that the patient has either a DVT or PE.[3-6] The same is true if the D-dimer is low—a practitioner cannot say with 100% certainty that the patient does not have a DVT or PE.

system anticoagulation to patients with a variety of conditions. Deficiencies in these three proteins can produce a hypercoagulable state in which a person is prone to clotting and developing a VTE.

The coagulation and fibrinolytic mechanisms act in a balance to both provide essential functions for the coagulation system. The coagulation cascade activates rapidly to help stabilize the clot formed by primary hemostasis, whereas the fibrinolytic cascade acts slowly to provide a check on the coagulation cascade as well as to break down the clot as the body repairs the damaged vessel.

Hereditary Coagulation Disorders

A hereditary coagulation disorder is caused by an inherited deficiency in the coagulation system. People with a hereditary coagulation disorder are more prone to develop life-threatening hemorrhage with a less-significant trauma than a person without the coagulation disorder. Although there are numerous specific disorders, this discussion concerns the three that most commonly occur: hemophilia A, hemophilia B, and von Willebrand disease.

Together, hemophilia A and hemophilia B account for over 99% of all the coagulation disorders caused by a clotting factor deficiency.[7] **Hemophilia A** affects approximately 1 in 10,000 males and is a deficiency in factor VIII (see Figure 23-1). Females rarely develop the disease because the gene affecting hemophilia A is located on the X chromosome. As males only have one X chromosome, if the affected gene is inherited, the male will develop hemophilia A. Females have two X chromosomes, and therefore it will be very rare that both X chromosomes have the gene responsible for hemophilia A. **Hemophilia B** is an inherited deficiency in factor IX and is much more rare than hemophilia A, affecting only 1 in 35,000 males. The gene responsible for hemophilia B is also located on the X chromosome; therefore, males are affected by the condition.

The severity of hemophilia is measured as a percent of normal function. A person without hemophilia has clotting factors which function at 100%. A person with less than 1% activity of the affected factor is considered to have severe hemophilia. These patients may develop spontaneous bleeding and, in the setting of injury, may have difficult-to-control hemorrhage. People with moderate disease have a level between 1% and 5% of normal clotting factor function. These individuals also may have spontaneous bleeding; however, this is far less frequent than in those with severe disease. Again, trauma may produce difficult-to-control bleeding. People with mild disease have between 5% and 25% of factor activity and will only bleed in the setting of trauma. Patients with over 25% of factor activity may never know they have hemophilia unless they experience heavy bleeding during surgery, trauma, or other procedures in which the bleeding is more severe than expected. Testing these individuals often reveals a mild hereditary coagulation disorder. Fortunately, most people with hemophilia do not have an issue with minor cuts or abrasions; however, the more significant the trauma the more chance there is for severe bleeding.

People who have hemophilia often experience easy bruising or bruising out of proportion to the injury. People with hemophilia may also develop a **hemarthrosis**, or bleeding into their larger joints (most commonly the knee). People with hemophilia may also less commonly develop a cerebral bleed with minor head injury or an epidural hematoma.[8]

Von Willebrand disease is a hereditary coagulation disorder that results in a lack of von Willebrand factor (vWf) in the inner lining of the blood vessels. As discussed previously, vWf is essential for primary hemostasis. vWf also acts as a carrier protein for factor VIII and helps to increase factor VIII's half-life in the blood, thus playing a role in secondary hemostasis. Estimates suggest von Willebrand disease affects approximately 1% of the population, both male and female, and affects people to a varying degree.[9] There are three subtypes of the disease. Type I, the most common type, affects almost 80% of the people who have von Willebrand disease. Most often patients with von Willebrand disease will have bleeding that affects the skin, mucous membranes (especially epistaxis), and the gastrointestinal tract. Rarely will patients with von Willebrand disease develop a hemarthrosis as do people with hemophilia.

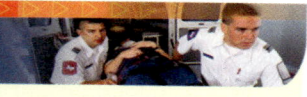

STREET SMART

Intramuscular injections should be avoided in patients with a hereditary coagulation disorder as a significant muscular hematoma may develop as a result of the injection. The patient is at risk for developing a compartment syndrome in that extremity from the intramuscular injection.

STREET SMART

Patients with a history of hemophilia who sustained minor head or spinal trauma should always be transported to an appropriate emergency department for evaluation regardless of the minor mechanism of injury and should be strongly urged not to refuse care. Patients with a history of hemophilia who complain of a new headache or a focal neurological deficit on physical examination are also considered to have an intracranial hemorrhage until proven otherwise by an emergent head CT at the emergency department regardless of their level of consciousness.

Acquired Coagulation Disorders

In contrast to hereditary coagulation disorders, acquired coagulation disorders develop secondarily as a result of another disease process or condition. They may develop acutely as a result of an acute condition, or they may develop slowly as a result of chronic diseases. Acquired coagulation disorders can be divided into conditions that cause **thrombocytopenia** (a decreased level of circulating platelets) and conditions that cause dysfunctional platelets (in which the platelet level may be normal but the platelets do not function properly). The person may experience an out-of-control coagulation system in the setting of severe sepsis or trauma, and conditions that produce a hypercoagulable state may occur.

Thrombocytopenia

Platelets are produced in the bone marrow along with red and white blood cells. These platelets normally live for approximately 10 days until they have outlived their usefulness and are destroyed and recycled by the body. The body's normal platelet count is between 150,000 and 450,000 platelets per microliter of blood. Thrombocytopenia can develop as a result of decreased platelet production or through destruction of circulating platelets which occurs faster than platelets can be produced. Platelet production can be slowed in the setting of chronic malnutrition, certain medications (e.g., Histamine-2 blockers), chronic alcoholism, and diseases that affect the person's bone marrow.[10]

Increased destruction of platelets may occur in the setting of an autoimmune condition called idiopathic thrombocytopenic purpura. In **idiopathic thrombocytopenic purpura (ITP)**, the body's immune system is triggered to develop an antibody to its own platelets, usually through infection or some other attack on the immune system. The antibodies attach themselves to the person's platelets and the white blood cells destroy the platelets. In this condition, the remaining platelets continue to function properly, which reduces the risk of spontaneous bleeding until the platelet count drops dangerously low. The purpura in ITP develops as small amounts of bleeding occur in the capillary bed (producing scattered petechiae) or small hemorrhages develop (Figure 23-3).

Another common immune-related cause of thrombocytopenia is **heparin-induced thrombocytopenia (HIT)**. HIT occurs when a patient taking the anticoagulant heparin develops antibodies to heparin. These antibodies, in turn, activate platelets and encourage thrombosis.[11] This platelet activation is global and will decrease the circulating platelet level faster than the body can produce new platelets. HIT can occur in patients receiving a low molecular weight heparin, or one of several medications derived from heparin that are also used as anticoagulants. HIT may occur as early as one to five days

after starting heparin or may occur as late as 12 days after, which may be a time period after a patient has been discharged from the hospital.[12] The platelet count will return to normal on its own several days after stopping heparin. However, repeated exposures to heparin will worsen the condition. Patients who develop HIT are more prone to develop acute arterial occlusion or VTE.

Several other conditions may develop that also cause an increase in platelet destruction but which are not immune-related conditions. One condition occurs when the spleen sequesters platelets, or holds them (and often other blood cells) within the spleen and does not release them back into the circulation. One of the spleen's functions is to destroy and recycle blood cells that are old and no longer functioning. When the spleen sequesters blood cells, the cells are forced together in a small space to the point at which the blood cells can become damaged and destroyed. Other conditions include several that cause an increased use of platelets, therefore significantly decreasing the platelet count. Three of these conditions will be discussed in more detail in the section on hemolytic anemia. A fourth condition, disseminated intravascular coagulation, will be discussed later in this section.

Dysfunctional Platelets

Not only is it important to have a sufficient amount of platelets circulating in the blood, but those platelets must function properly. Chronic diseases can disrupt the platelets' ability to function properly. Uremia, or a buildup of urea and other waste products normally filtered out by the kidney, alter the configuration of the surface proteins on platelets and decrease their ability to attach to vWf and to each other. Regular hemodialysis typically filters enough waste products to allow the platelets to function normally. If the patient is not compliant with scheduled dialysis, however, the patient is prone to more significant bleeding even with a normal platelet count. Unfortunately, transfusion of platelets into a uremic environment will also damage the transfused platelets, negating the transfusion.

Patients who have chronic liver disease will not be able to produce a sufficient amount of the clotting factors and the regulatory proteins required for the coagulation system

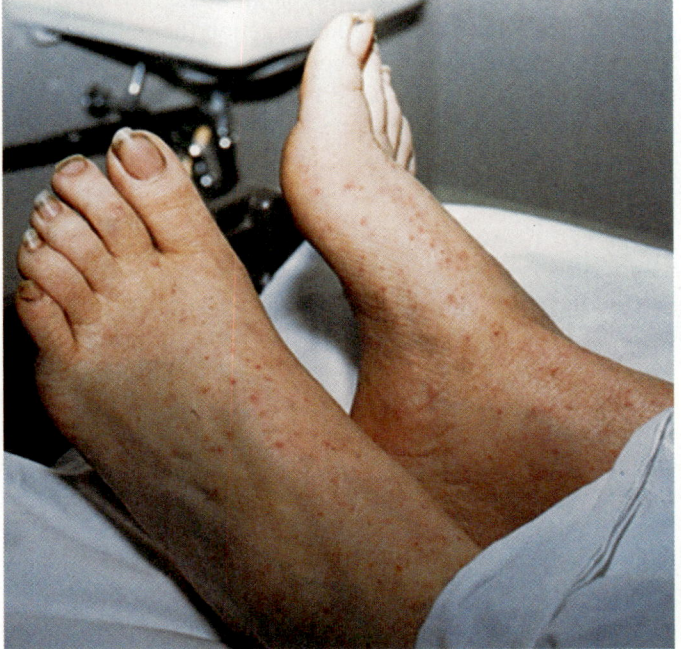

Delmar/Cengage Learning

Figure 23-3 Petechiae.

to work properly. Severe liver disease increases the ammonia level, which also affects the platelets' ability to clump together to form a clot. Patients with severe liver disease may also have more of a tendency to activate their fibrinolytic system than people without liver disease, further increasing the risk of bleeding.

Disseminated Intravascular Coagulation

Disseminated intravascular coagulation (DIC) is a condition in which there is an overactivation of both the coagulation and fibrinolytic systems. The overactivation of the coagulation system produces significant amounts of fibrin which clot the smaller blood vessels and capillaries, thereby consuming platelets and clotting factors. The overactivation of the fibrinolytic system causes breakdown of larger clots and promotes bleeding. Often the smaller clots that occlude the smaller blood vessels are not affected. DIC becomes a paradoxical condition in which the patient is both clotting and bleeding at the same time.[13] DIC occurs most often in sepsis, but can also occur in trauma, pregnancy, after delivery, and in other conditions that cause a widespread inflammatory response.

The small clots that occlude the smaller vessels limit blood flow to the organs and can produce end-organ damage, especially to the kidneys, the brain, and the heart. Occluded vessels in the skin at the fingertips and toes can cause gangrene as the tissue becomes ischemic. Bleeding often occurs from mucosal tissues in the mouth, nose, and gastrointestinal tract as these surfaces are most likely to be damaged. Bleeding also occurs from surgical sites, intravenous catheter insertion sites, and sites of other procedures that break the surface of the skin. **Purpura fulminans** is a term used to describe widespread arterial and venous thrombosis and occlusion producing a purplish discoloration of the affected areas. Purpura fulminans is most often associated with sepsis.

In addition to bleeding from the activation of the fibrinolytic system, bleeding also occurs due to the consumption of coagulation factors and platelets. The overactivation of the coagulation system quickly uses up all available coagulation factors. Since the body cannot keep up with this consumption, bleeding may occur with the slightest injury. Although DIC involves both the fibrinolytic and coagulation systems, patients will often clinically present with more of one than the other.

Circulating Anticoagulants

The term "circulating anticoagulants" is actually a misnomer. Circulating anticoagulants are a group of proteins that actually shift the balance of the coagulation–fibrinolysis system more toward clotting. Patients who have circulating anticoagulants are more prone to develop thrombus and have a higher risk of developing a VTE. These proteins are acquired and often the result of antibodies developed against the fibrinolytic pathway. Common circulating anticoagulants include antiphospholipid antibody, lupus anticoagulant, and anticardiolipin antibody. These often develop in patients who have an underlying autoimmune condition (e.g., lupus), reaction to certain medications, malignancy, pregnancy, or HIV. These circulating anticoagulants inhibit, or slow, the reactions in the fibrinolytic pathway, resulting in increased clotting.

Anemias

Anemia is defined as decreased hemoglobin and can be either acute or chronic in nature. Chronic anemia can be due to a variety of causes, with nutrient deficiency, chronic gastrointestinal bleeding, and heavy menses as three common causes. Vitamin B12, folate, and iron are essential vitamins and minerals used in the production of red blood cells and hemoglobin. Deficiency in these compounds, either due to poor intake or malabsorption in the small intestine, decreases the amount of hemoglobin and red blood cells produced. Chronic gastrointestinal bleeding may be insidious and go unrecognized until the stool is tested for occult blood. Many younger females are chronically anemic from heavy menses. In these two situations, blood loss occurs faster than it can be replaced, resulting in a chronic anemia. Many patients acclimate to the anemia if it occurrs gradually, allowing the body to compensate. In these situations, the hemoglobin level will decrease to a very low level before the patient develops symptoms.

Acute anemia occurs as a result of either acute blood loss or acute red blood cell destruction. Anemia due to blood loss is seen in the setting of trauma, acute gastrointestinal bleeding, heavy vaginal bleeding, or bleeding in patients with a coagulopathy. Red blood cell destruction can occur for a variety of reasons that will be discussed in the following sections.

Congenital Hemolytic Anemias

Congenital hemolytic anemias are caused by a genetic condition that, when active, may result in an acute hemolytic anemia. An acute hemolytic anemia is an acute anemia that is caused by rapid red blood cell destruction (hemolysis) when the condition is active. Two common congenital hemolytic anemias that will be discussed in this section are sickle cell disease and G6PD deficiency.

Sickle Cell Disease

Sickle cell disease is an inherited condition that predominantly affects people of African descent and—to a lesser extent—people of Middle Eastern, Indian, and Mediterranean descent. In sickle cell disease, a percentage of the normal hemoglobin in the red blood cells is replaced by a different form of hemoglobin. When this form of hemoglobin, called HbS, is deoxygenated, it deforms the red blood cell into the characteristic sickle shape (Figure 23-4), hence providing the name of the condition.

There are actually several different forms of the hemoglobin molecule. The hemoglobin in a normal red blood cell is made up of four hemoglobin molecules. The configuration that makes up 96% to 98% of hemoglobin is two α molecules and two β molecules. Another form, the δ molecule, replaces the β molecule in 2% to 3% of hemoglobin. Fetal hemoglobin

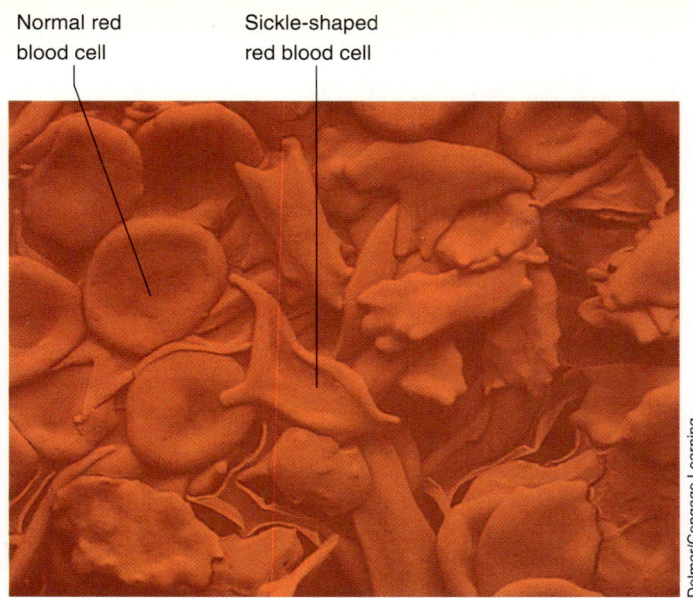

Normal red blood cell

Sickle-shaped red blood cell

Delmar/Cengage Learning

Figure 23-4 Sickle cell anemia.

is the predominant molecule in place of the β molecule during the first four months of life and composes a very small percentage of hemoglobin in the normal adult. In sickle cell disease, the S form of the hemoglobin molecule replaces the β molecule in the red blood cell. In order to have sickle cell disease, a person must inherit the sickle cell gene from both parents. People with sickle cell trait only inherited one gene and do not have issues with sickle cell disease.

When the person with sickle cell disease undergoes a stressor on the body, the red blood cells that contain HbS become deoxygenated more rapidly and change into the sickle shape shown in Figure 23-4. Normally, the red blood cells are flexible and can navigate the capillaries without a problem. However, these sickle-shaped red blood cells are not flexible enough to navigate smaller blood vessels. The sickled red blood cells occlude the smaller blood vessels, causing both local ischemia and hemolysis, or destruction of red blood cells. The sickling can be reversible with supplemental oxygen; however, red blood cells eventually become nonfunctional and are destroyed by the spleen.

The pain crisis caused by small vessel occlusion often produces diffuse pain in the extremities, the back, and in the joints. Bone pain can also be severe. Occlusions can cause enough ischemia to develop infarction of the affected tissues.[14-16] Frequently the spleen loses its ability to function in filtering out old blood cells because of the constant congestion and may require surgical removal. Infection is a significant concern with patients who have sickle cell disease and repeated sickle cell vaso-occlusive crisis due to the spleen's inability to function properly.

Two significant conditions that can occur as part of a sickle cell crisis are chest crisis (also known as chest abdominal) and abdominal crisis. A patient with **chest crisis** often complains of chest pain that is sharp and may change with

inspiration and expiration, fever, a productive cough, and other signs of pneumonia. Chest crisis can be serious when lung tissue becomes necrotic and bleeds. Pneumonia and pulmonary infarction are often involved. Acute chest syndrome is a leading cause of death among patients with sickle cell disease.[17] **Abdominal crisis** occurs when there is infarction of portions of the abdominal organs. In addition, jaundice may develop from liver infarction.

Other complications of sickle cell disease include renal infections, stroke, ischemic heart disease and heart failure, and poorly healing skin ulcers. These all occur from occlusion of the smaller blood vessels and the resulting infarction of these organs. **Aplastic crisis** can occur when there is massive red blood cell hemolysis and is often precipitated by a viral illness. The hemoglobin can drop rapidly and the patient may require blood transfusion. The overall life expectancy for patients with severe sickle cell disease is very poor, with very few people surviving into their late forties.

CULTURAL/REGIONAL DIFFERENCES

Healthcare providers may be reticent to provide analgesia, especially narcotics, to some patients based on concern for drug addiction/drug seeking behaviors. The pain of sickle cell crisis results from occlusion of blood vessels and can be related to the pain of angina or myocardial infarction. The pain may be severe and should be managed with the same level of professional care offered to the MI patient.

G6PD Deficiency

Glucose-6-phosphate dehydrogenase (G6PD) is an enzyme required for one pathway of energy production within cells. Red blood cells are completely dependent on this particular pathway because other biochemical methods of creating energy would damage hemoglobin. People who have G6PD deficiency have a genetically decreased amount of this enzyme present. When certain medications (Table 23-1)

Table 23-1 Medications and Other Substances That Should Be Avoided with People Who Have G6PD Deficiency

- Antimicrobials
  - Sulfonamides
  - Antimalarials
  - Fluoroquinolones
- Moth balls
- Fava beans

or foods are given to people with G6PD deficiency, the red blood cells are stressed and may undergo hemolysis and destruction, thus decreasing circulating hemoglobin.[18,19] An acute hemolytic anemia can develop in people who are given these substances.

Immune-Mediated Hemolytic Anemia

As with the hereditary hemolytic anemia, **immune-mediated hemolytic anemias** involve the destruction of red blood cells. In contrast, however, this is usually due to antibodies that develop against either the red blood cells or platelets, with the end result being red blood cell destruction.

Autoimmune Hemolytic Anemia

In **autoimmune hemolytic anemia**, the patient develops antibodies that work against the patient's own red blood cells. In other words, the immune system attacks and destroys the patient's own red blood cells. This may occur for an unknown reason or as a result of a systemic autoimmune disease. Autoimmune hemolytic anemia is also sometimes seen in sepsis, HIV, and lymphoma.

Alloimmune Hemolytic Anemia

An **alloimmune hemolytic anemia** occurs when the person develops antibodies to red blood cells after an exposure to another individual's red blood cells. This mechanism also causes immune system destruction of red blood cells. A hemolytic transfusion reaction caused by a mismatch of blood typing is one example of an alloimmune hemolytic anemia. In this case, the blood being transfused is of a type different than the patient's blood type. The patient's antibodies attach to the new red blood cells, causing the immune system to attack and destroy the transfused red blood cells.

Another common example occurs when there is mixing of maternal and fetal blood that are each of a different Rh factor. If the mother's Rh– blood mixes with the fetus' Rh+ blood, the mother will develop antibodies against the Rh+ fetal red blood cells. Maternal–fetal blood mixing can occur during delivery or in the setting of prenatal trauma. Although this may not be an issue during the current pregnancy, in subsequent pregnancies the maternal antibodies can attack and destroy the fetal red blood cells, causing a potentially fatal hemolytic anemia of the newborn. Fortunately, a product called RhoGam administered to the Rh– mother will prevent the formation of these antibodies.

Thrombotic Thrombocytopenic Purpura

Thrombotic thrombocytopenic purpura (TTP) is a condition in adults in which platelets clump together and partially occlude the small blood vessels. When this occurs, the red blood cells are damaged and break apart, producing the hemolytic anemia. It was recently discovered that TTP is caused by either a congenital or acquired deficiency in an enzyme that is responsible for breaking von Willebrand factor down to its normal size. The process for manufacturing von Willebrand

factor includes a step at the end which uses a specific enzyme to make the von Willebrand factor physically smaller. This larger-than-normal von Willebrand factor molecule adheres to the wall of the smaller blood vessel and sets off the clumping of platelets as they travel through the smaller blood vessels. The red blood cells have difficulty getting through the partially occluded blood vessels and often break up, causing a **microangiopathic** (meaning affecting the smaller blood vessels) hemolytic anemia (abbreviated MAHA). Ischemia can develop in the organs supplied by the occluded blood vessels. The organs most often affected include the brain, kidneys, heart, pancreas, spleen, and adrenal glands.[20] One hallmark feature of TTP is altered mental status.

TTP can either be congenital or acquired. In congenital TTP, a genetic defect causes the decreased levels of the enzymes that produce normal-sized von Willebrand factor. In acquired TTP, antibodies are developed against the enzyme, decreasing the amount of the enzyme available, ultimately setting the stage for TTP. Some of the causes of acquired TTP include existing autoimmune disease (for example, lupus), cancer, pregnancy, certain infections, and certain medications. Pregnancy is the most common cause of acquired TTP, and occurs early in pregnancy.

Hemolytic Uremic Syndrome

Hemolytic uremic syndrome (HUS) is similar to TTP in that platelets clumping in the small blood vessels in the kidney cause localized ischemia within the kidney as well as a hemolytic anemia as the red blood cells have difficulty passing through the smaller blood vessels. HUS typically affects small children age 6 months to 4 years old and is often associated with an infectious cause.[21] Although the end result of platelet clumping in the small blood vessels associated with a hemolytic anemia is similar to TTP, the pathophysiology is different than that of TTP. In HUS, there is damage to the inner lining of the small blood vessels in the kidneys, which sets off the platelet clumping and coagulation cascade within the kidney. As opposed to TTP, the enzyme deficiency in the production of von Willebrand factor is not present.

The microvessel damage in the kidneys is most often caused by the toxin produced by many bacteria or viruses. A specific strain of the E. coli bacteria that can be found in unclean water or poorly cooked meats is most often responsible for HUS in children.[22] Several other specific bacterium are also responsible as well as several viruses. HUS can also be associated with pregnancy, presenting with hypertension and a hemolytic anemia after a normal delivery. AIDS and malignancies can also cause HUS. The most common preceding complaint is diarrhea.

Hemolytic, Elevated Liver Enzymes and Low Platelets (HELLP)

Hemolytic, Elevated Liver enzymes, and Low Platelets (HEELP) is a syndrome that is associated with pre-eclampsia, a complication of pregnancy that is discussed further in Chapter 36. Although described more completely later, this syndrome is mentioned here because of the hemolytic anemia associated with the syndrome.

Toxic Causes of Hemolytic Anemia

Several infections and toxins can cause a hemolytic anemia by directly causing breakdown of red blood cells. Malaria, a parasitic infection that affects the red blood cells, is the most common infection-related hemolytic anemia in the world. In many cases, the bacteria attaches to the red blood cell during the infection. The body's immune system identifies the bacteria as something that is foreign and requires its destruction. Instead of just attacking the bacteria, the white blood cells also destroy the red blood cells that are attached to the bacteria. Several toxins, especially those from certain toxic spiders and poisonous snakes, can also cause a hemolytic anemia. The toxin injected directly attacks the red blood cells, producing the hemolytic anemia.

Mechanical Damage

A patient can develop a hemolytic anemia as a result of mechanical damage to the red blood cells. This often occurs during extreme exercise on a hard surface (e.g., soldiers who are marching and long distance runners). This is generally not clinically significant as only a small amount of red blood cells are actually damaged and the patient's hemoglobin does not drop significantly.

Other Red Blood Cell Disorders

Two other red blood cell disorders that do not produce bleeding are methemoglobinemia and polycythemia. **Methemoglobinemia** is a form of hemoglobin that is not able to carry oxygen. The condition often occurs after there has been a stressor on the red blood cells from medications, toxins, or chemicals.

Polycythemia is defined as an increased amount of circulating solid blood components. This includes increased white blood cell count or platelet count, but is sometimes used to describe elevated red blood cell count. Polycythemia is a compensatory mechanism in chronic obstructive pulmonary disease (COPD). It attempts to increase oxygen delivery by increasing the number of red blood cells available to transport oxygen.[23,24] Relative polycythemia can occur if the patient is dehydrated. Polycythemia can also be caused by an overproduction of blood cells in the bone marrow and may be related to malignancy.

The problem with polycythemia is the viscosity, or thickness, of the blood is increased, becoming more like a jelly or syrup. The thicker blood does not flow as well through the smaller blood vessels. The slower the blood flows, the more likely it is to coagulate and form clots in the smaller blood vessels. As in the other conditions discussed previously, the limited blood flow can cause ischemia in the organs or skin supplied by those blood vessels.

CASE STUDY (CONTINUED)

When the Paramedics arrive on scene, they find an African American male seated on the stoop in front of 132 Figby Street, leaning against the railing, in obvious discomfort.

"Hello, did you call for an ambulance?"

"Yes, I did," Reginold Harrison replies.

"How can we help you today?"

Mr. Harrison goes on to explain that he has sickle cell disease and he began having pain about four hours ago, which steadily became worse and did not get better with the analgesics that were prescribed by his primary doctor.

One Paramedic assists Mr. Harrison to the ambulance while the other obtains a more detailed history. He finds out Mr. Harrison gets five or six pain crises per year, with the last one occurring two months ago. This pain is typical for his pain crises, but is more severe. Mr. Harrison denies having trouble breathing, abdominal pain, or fever. His last transfusion and admission to the hospital were both approximately a year ago. Mr. Harrison has a history of hypertension in addition to sickle cell disease.

CRITICAL THINKING QUESTIONS

1. What are the important elements of the history that a Paramedic should obtain?
2. What is the symptom pattern for acute sickle cell crisis?

History

Obtaining an accurate history may be the Paramedic's key to suspecting a bleeding disorder. Many patients will know that they have a bleeding disorder. However, if this is the first time the patient has had a problem or developed an acquired disorder, the patient may not be aware of the condition.

History of Present Illness

The specific direction of the interview may take a different pathway based on the patient's chief concern. The Paramedic should use the OPQRST mnemonic to help explore complaints related to pain. For non-pain-related complaints, the OPQRST mnemonic can still be helpful in determining when the patient's symptoms started, associated symptoms, and factors that improve the symptoms or make them worse.

Several specific historical features help the Paramedic explore the possibility that a patient has a bleeding disorder (Table 23-2). In the setting of trauma, even minor trauma, the Paramedic should ask the patient who has a known bleeding disorder, or who is at risk for developing a bleeding disorder, if he struck his head or lost consciousness. Individuals who are on dialysis, have liver disease, and who are alcoholic are at risk for a bleeding disorder.

If the patient relates a history of sickle cell disease and pain related to a sickle cell crisis, it is important for the Paramedic to determine if this crisis is similar to past crises. This is so even if the patient has chest or abdominal pain, neurological complaints, or a fever. It is also helpful to know how frequently the patient experiences pain crises, hospital admissions, and transfusions. These features may indicate a more serious pain crisis.

Table 23-2 Historical Factors Suggestive of a Bleeding Disorder

- Easy bruising
- Purple-colored punctuate rash (petechiae)
- Bleeding from gums when brushing teeth
- Heavy menstrual periods
- Frequent epistaxis (nosebleeds)

If the patient complains of a rash or bruising, the Paramedic should determine if the patient was recently admitted to the hospital or a nursing home, or was recently immobile. Patients who were on either heparin or a low molecular weight heparin medication may have developed delayed heparin-induced thrombocytopenia.

Past Medical History

Patients who have a past medical history of a bleeding disorder will often know about their disorder and can provide that history to the Paramedic, especially in the setting of trauma. Many patients who have hemophilia or von Willebrand disease will seek care for minor trauma as a preventative measure so they can obtain treatment before bleeding becomes severe. Patients who have a history of sickle cell disease will also often relate that history when seeking care of a vaso-occlusive crisis. A patient history of having bleeding during surgery or during minor procedures may also indicate the presence of a bleeding disorder.

CASE STUDY (CONTINUED)

The Paramedic obtains a set of vital signs on Mr. Harrison while his partner completes a physical examination. Mr. Harrison's skin is warm, flushed, and moist, there is no palpable extremity edema or tenderness, his lungs are clear with wheezes at both bases, and his heart is regular. Mr. Harrison has no abdominal, back, or spinal tenderness. The Paramedic records the first set of vitals as blood pressure of 160/100, pulse of 120 beats per minute, a pulse oximetry reading of 92% on room air, and a respiratory rate of 22.

CRITICAL THINKING QUESTIONS

1. What are the elements of the physical examination of a patient with suspected sickle cell crisis?
2. Why is a neurological assessment a critical element in this examination?

Examination

As with the history, the physical examination will depend on the patient's chief concern. The Paramedic should start with the primary assessment and rapidly identify and immediately correct issues related to the patient's airway, breathing, or circulation. A rapid neurological assessment will also uncover gross disabilities.

Once the primary assessment is completed, the Paramedic can move on to a focused assessment based on the patient's chief concern. The Paramedic should examine the patient's head for evidence of cranial nerve dysfunction including pupil size, equality, and reaction. The Paramedic should examine the patient's chest for abnormal lung sounds and murmurs. She should also examine the abdomen for signs of internal bleeding, including tenderness, firm distention, or bruising on the flanks. The Paramedic then examines for painful extremities to determine distal function, including pulses, sensation and motor function, and bony tenderness. She should examine swollen joints for tenderness and stability. Finally, the Paramedic should examine the patient's skin for color, temperature, moisture, petechiae, and bruising.

CASE STUDY (CONTINUED)

Based on the history, the Paramedics conclude that Mr. Harrison is having a sickle cell vaso-occlusive crisis. The Paramedics are concerned about Mr. Harrison's abnormal vital signs even though he does not complain of pain in his chest or trouble breathing. They encourage the ambulance crew to quickly package the patient and prepare for immediate departure.

CRITICAL THINKING QUESTIONS

1. What is the significance of the atraumatic leg pain?
2. What diagnosis did the Paramedic announce to the patient?

Assessment

Many bleeding disorders may be difficult to detect. Certainly in critical patients with impaired airway, breathing, or circulation status, it may be difficult to determine the red flags in the history that would cause the Paramedic to suspect a bleeding disorder. In some cases, however, the patient provides the past history of a bleeding disorder or provides an indication of the development of one. For patients with known bleeding disorders, the Paramedic should attempt to detect red flags that indicate a potentially serious complication.

CASE STUDY (CONTINUED)

The first Paramedic starts an intravenous line on Mr. Harrison while another Paramedic applies nasal cannula oxygen at 4 liters per minute. Mr. Harrison receives 100 cc of normal saline and 10 mg of morphine in divided doses until he expresses relief from the pain.

CRITICAL THINKING QUESTIONS

1. What is the standard of care of patients with suspected sickle cell crisis?
2. What are some of the patient-specific concerns and considerations that the Paramedic should consider when applying this plan of care that is intended to treat a broad patient population presenting with sickle cell crisis?

Treatment

The treatment of most bleeding disorders is usually supportive, focusing on optimizing oxygen delivery by maintaining an adequate airway, breathing, and circulation. The Paramedic should perform the usual bleeding control measures on external bleeding. Hemarthrosis may be treated using an ace wrap around the affected joint to assist in applying compression and limit bleeding. Supplemental oxygen may assist in improving oxygen delivery, even in the setting of anemia.

Paramedics may be exposed to patients who have active bleeding with a history of hemophilia or von Willebrand disease during interfacility transfer situations. Often the patient is being treated with either cryoprecipitate or fresh frozen plasma, two blood products that are used to replace factor deficiencies. DDAVP, a medication that is administered either as an infusion or as a nasal spray, is also used to treat patients who have hemophilia A or von Willebrand disease. DDAVP helps release extra von Willebrand factor into circulation and may be enough to slow or stop bleeding.[25] Since von Willebrand factor is a carrier for factor VIII, DDAVP also increases factor VIII levels. These patients may also require blood transfusions during transfer.

Patients who call with sickle cell disease-related pain are treated with oxygen, fluids, and analgesia. Supplemental oxygen increases the blood's oxygen-carrying capacity and will sometimes reverse red blood cell sickling, improving pain. Fluids will ensure adequate hydration and decrease the viscosity of the blood, helping the sickled red blood cells to flow through the smaller vessels. Although fluids may be administered intravenously, patients who have frequent sickle cell crises may have poor venous access from repeated attempts at intravenous access. Oral fluids are just as effective as intravenous fluids during the sickle cell crisis in rehydrating the patient. Analgesia may be administered orally, subcutaneously, or intravenously. The Paramedic should be aware that patients who are on chronic opioid medications may have developed a high tolerance and therefore require a significantly higher dose of analgesia. These patients typically know what works for them during their pain crisis. Some patients supplement opioid analgesia with nonsteroidal anti-inflammatory medications (NSAIDs) or acetaminophen. Patients who develop chest crisis may require mechanical ventilation.

Patients who develop ITP are typically treated by stopping the inciting medication or trigger. If a transfusion of platelets is required, the Paramedic administers intravenous steroids before the transfusion so the transfused platelets are not attacked by the patient's immune system. On the other hand, patients who have TTP often need to be transferred to a tertiary care center to undergo plasmapheresis, a procedure in which the blood is removed and run through a machine similar to that used for hemodialysis. The machine removes the blood cells from the patient's plasma and infuses them back with fresh donated plasma or saline. This removes the antibodies that caused the immune reaction. Paramedics may treat patients with hereditary TTP by administering fresh frozen plasma.[26] Patients with TTP and HUS may also require blood transfusion in order to compensate for the hemolytic anemia. The Paramedic will often encounter these patients in an interfacility transfer situation in which a patient with one of these conditions is being transferred to a tertiary care facility with the resources to care for these patients. Many community hospitals do not have the equipment or expertise to care for these patients.

Patients who develop DIC are truly critically ill patients who have a very poor prognosis. Excellent supportive care with airway and ventilatory management, fluid resuscitation, and bleeding control measures are key to providing care. Again, Paramedics may encounter these patients in an interfacility transfer setting. The Paramedic may also encounter patients who are treated with blood product transfusions if there is a significant amount of bleeding. Intravenous heparin also may be used in situations where clotting is the predominant component.

CASE STUDY (CONTINUED)

Just before arrival, the Paramedic notes that Mr. Harrison's respiratory rate and work of breathing has increased and he complains of shortness of breath. The Paramedic auscultates Mr. Harrison's lungs, which shows coarse rhonchi bilaterally with some wheezing on the right. Mr. Harrison is placed on a cardiac monitor and continuous pulse oximetry. His pulse oximetry on the 4 liters per minute by nasal cannula oxygen has dropped from 98% to 88% and his respiratory rate has increased from 22 per minute to 28 per minute. The Paramedic is concerned that Mr. Harrison has developed an acute chest crisis. He is switched from supplemental oxygen by nasal cannula over to a nonrebreather mask. The intubation roll is opened, and the emergency department is notified by radio report of Mr. Harrison's deteriorating condition.

CRITICAL THINKING QUESTIONS

1. What are some of the predictable complications associated with sickle cell crisis?
2. What are some of the predictable complications associated with the treatments for sickle cell crisis?

Evaluation

Through vigilant patient monitoring and continual reassessment, the Paramedic is alerted early on to changes in the patient's condition. Patients with a known or suspected bleeding disorder may develop bleeding during transport. Patients who suffered a head injury may also have a rapid decline in mental status. The Paramedic should always be ready to take action should the patient rapidly decline.

Mr. Harrison's respiratory status deteriorates at the emergency department driveway. The Paramedic starts providing ventilatory assistance with the bag-valve mask. Mr. Harrison's gag reflex is still intact and he does not tolerate an oral airway. Since they are at the emergency department, the Paramedic elects to place two nasopharyngeal airways and continue ventilation with the bag-valve mask rather than initiating RSI on the ramp to the emergency department. Mr. Harrison is brought directly into the resuscitation room where he undergoes RSI by the emergency physician. An X-ray of the chest confirms the Paramedic's suspicion that Mr. Harrison has developed an acute chest crisis. Despite the excellent prehospital and hospital care, Mr. Harrison develops a bilateral pneumonia with acute respiratory distress syndrome and dies four days later.

CRITICAL THINKING QUESTIONS

1. What is the most appropriate transport decision that will get the patient to definitive care?
2. Was the decision to perform ventilation with a bag-valve mask assembly instead of intubating the patient prudent?

Disposition

Most patients can be well cared for at the local community hospital. Unless the patient has a known bleeding disorder, it would be prudent for the Paramedic to transport the patient with a suspected bleeding disorder to the community hospital to confirm a disorder is present. Patients with a history of a bleeding disorder may specifically request transport to the tertiary care center or hospital where they receive their care. Patients who have a history of hemophilia or von Willebrand disease and sustain minor trauma should be transported to a trauma center unless the distance is prohibitive. Patients requiring specific treatments may be transferred from a community hospital to a tertiary care center for specialty care not available at the community hospital.

CONCLUSION

Bleeding disorders include a wide range of conditions that can affect all of the cell lines in the blood. Some of these disorders are hereditary, whereas many are acquired disorders, often due to viral infections or unknown causes. Bleeding disorders can include conditions that affect the platelets, causing either bleeding or overactive clotting. Red blood cell disorders also provide a wide range of conditions. The coagulation system can also run into overdrive as a result of multisystem trauma or sepsis. The Paramedic, as the first healthcare provider to encounter the patient, has the opportunity to identify these issues early in care and positively impact patient outcome.

KEY POINTS:

- Coagulopathy describes bleeding problems that develop from the coagulation cascade.

- Hemostasis is a series of mechanisms designed to prevent blood loss.

- Primary hemostasis is the development of a plug to stop bleeding.

- Primary hemostasis depends on
  - Normal collagen
  - Normal circulating platelets
  - Adequate von Willebrand factor
  - Adequate fibrinogen

- Secondary hemostasis depends upon the coagulation system.

- The coagulation cascade includes a step to dissolve or lyse the formed clot via fibrinolysis.

- The fibrinolytic system also slows down coagulation.

- Coagulation disorders can be hereditary or acquired.

- The most common hereditary disorders include
  - Hemophilia A
  - Hemophilia B
  - Von Willebrand disease

- Acquired disorders develop secondary to another disease process or medication. These include
  - Thrombocytopenia and thrombocytopenia purpura

  - Dysfunctional platelets secondary to kidney or liver disease
  - Disseminated intravascular coagulation
  - Circulating anticoagulants from lupus, malignancy, pregnancy, or HIV
  - Hemolytic uremic syndrome
  - Hemolysis, elevated liver enzymes, and low platelets (HELLP)

- Anemia is a condition in which there is a decrease in hemoglobin.

- Acute anemia results from blood loss or red cell destruction.

- Chronic anemia results from heavy menses, nutritional abnormalities, or chronic gastrointestinal bleeds.

- Polycythemia causes an excess of red blood cells, leading to an increased blood viscosity.

- An accurate history is essential, especially in the face of potential trauma.

- Treatment of most bleeding disorders is supportive.

- Continued monitoring is important.

REVIEW QUESTIONS:

1. Differentiate primary hemostasis from secondary hemostasis.
2. Describe the interaction of the fibrinolytic system with coagulation.
3. List three hereditary coagulation disorders. How do they differ from each other? How would a history of each of them alter your care of patients?
4. Explain the mechanism of disseminated intravascular coagulation.
5. How does polycythemia differ from anemia? Name at least two complications of polycythemia.

CASE STUDY QUESTIONS:

Please refer to the Case Study in this chapter, and answer the questions below:

1. What is the most important piece of history that the Paramedics received from Mr. Harrison?
2. Name at least three other complications that should concern the Paramedics in light of Mr. Harrison's history.
3. How does the addition of supplemental oxygen assist in the care and treatment of Mr. Harrison?

REFERENCES:

1. Kellett J, Clarke J. Comparison of "accelerated" tissue plasminogen activator with streptokinase for treatment of suspected myocardial infarction. *Med Decis Making*. 1995;15(4):297–310.
2. White HD. Selecting a thrombolytic agent. *Cardiol Clin*. 1995;13(3):347–354.
3. Marill KA. Serum D-dimer is a sensitive test for the detection of acute aortic dissection: a pooled meta-analysis. *J Emerg Med*. 2008;34(4):367–376.
4. Soderberg M, Brohult J, et al. The use of D-dimer testing and Wells score in patients with high probability for acute pulmonary embolism. *J Eval Clin Pract*. 2008 15(1):129–133.
5. Kabrhel C. Outcomes of high pretest probability patients undergoing D-dimer testing for pulmonary embolism: a pilot study. *J Emerg Med*. 2008;35(4):373–377.
6. Kline JA, Runyon MS, et al. Prospective study of the diagnostic accuracy of the Simplify D-dimer assay for pulmonary embolism in emergency department patients. *Chest*. 2006;129(6):1417–1423.
7. Agaliotisl DP, MD. Available at: **http://www.emedicine.com/med/TOPIC3528.HTM**. Accessed July 28, 2009.
8. Mishra P, Naithani R, et al. Intracranial haemorrhage in patients with congenital haemostatic defects. *Haemophilia*. 2008;14(5):952–955.
9. Pollak ES, MD. Available at: **http://www.emedicine.com/MED/topic2392.htm**. Accessed July 28, 2009.
10. Nachman RL, Rafii S. Platelets, petechiae, and preservation of the vascular wall. *N Engl J Med*. 2008;359(12):1261–1270.
11. Alberio L. Heparin-induced thrombocytopenia: some working hypotheses on pathogenesis, diagnostic strategies and treatment. *Curr Opin Hematol*. 2008;15(5):456–464.
12. Arepally G, Cines DB. Pathogenesis of heparin-induced thrombocytopenia and thrombosis. *Autoimmun Rev*. 2002;1(3):125–132.
13. Bick RL, Arun B, et al. Disseminated intravascular coagulation. Clinical and pathophysiological mechanisms and manifestations. *Haemostasis* 1999;29(2–3):111–134.
14. Adams RJ. Big strokes in small persons. *Arch Neurol*. 2007;64(11):1567–1574.
15. Tsironi M, Aessopos A. The heart in sickle cell disease. *Acta Cardiol*. 2005;60(6):589–598.
16. Ahmed S, Shahid RK, et al. Unusual causes of abdominal pain: sickle cell anemia. *Best Pract Res Clin Gastroenterol*. 2005;19(2):297–310.
17. Melton CW, Haynes, J, Jr. Sickle acute lung injury: role of prevention and early aggressive intervention strategies on outcome. *Clin Chest Med*. 2006;27(3):487–502, vii.
18. Frank JE. Diagnosis and management of G6PD deficiency. *Am Fam Physician*. 2005;72(7):1277–1282.
19. Dalal BI, Kollmannsberger C. Drug-induced haemolysis and methaemoglobinaemia in glucose 6-phosphate dehydrogenase deficiency. *Br J Haematol*. 2005;129(3):291.
20. Symonette D, MD, MPH. Available at: **http://www.emedicine.com/emerg/TOPIC579.HTM**. Accessed July 28, 2009.
21. Michael M, Elliott EJ, et al. Interventions for hemolytic uremic syndrome and thrombotic thrombocytopenic purpura: a systematic

review of randomized controlled trials. *Am J Kidney Dis.* 2009:53(2):259–272.

22. Panos GZ, Betsi GI, et al. Systematic review: are antibiotics detrimental or beneficial for the treatment of patients with Escherichia coli O157:H7 infection? *Aliment Pharmacol Ther.* 2006;24(5):731–742.

23. Chambellan A, Chailleux E, et al. Prognostic value of the hematocrit in patients with severe COPD receiving long-term oxygen therapy. *Chest.* 2005;128(3):1201–1208.

24. Similowski T, Agusti A, et al. The potential impact of anaemia of chronic disease in COPD. *Eur Respir J.* 2006;27(2):390–396.

25. Vande Walle J, Stockner M, et al. Desmopressin 30 years in clinical use: a safety review. *Curr Drug Saf.* 2007;2(3):232–238.

26. Ellis J, Theodossiou C, et al. Treatment of thrombotic thrombocytopenic purpura with the cryosupernatant fraction of plasma: a case report and review of the literature. *Am J Med Sci.* 1999;318(3):190–193.

CHAPTER 24

BACK PAIN

KEY CONCEPTS:

Upon completion of this chapter, it is expected that the reader will understand these following concepts:

- The causes of nontraumatic back pain: musculoskeletal abnormalities, infections, cancers, or pathologic fractures
- The importance of recognizing the history and physical red flags that indicate a serious medical or surgical emergency
- The ways to manage the patient's pain through positioning and medication

ANATOMY CONCEPTS:

Prior to reading this chapter the Paramedic student should be familiar with the following anatomy and physiology concepts:

- Neuroanatomy of the spinal cord
- Musculoskeletal system

Northern Ambulance is dispatched priority one to a call at 90 Woodlake Road for a 45-year-old male complaining of back pain and weakness in both legs. EMS has been to that location many times before and it is always the same complaint—back pain. En route, the Paramedics consider several conditions that may cause the EMD dispatcher to dispatch this as a high priority call. "Could this be potentially life-threatening?" thought the Paramedic. "After all, it's just a back ache!"

CRITICAL THINKING QUESTIONS

1. What are some of the possible causes of back pain?
2. How is the leg weakness related to back pain?

OVERVIEW

Nontraumatic back pain is a common patient complaint. Lumbar pain affects an estimated 85% of adults under the age of 50 years old, and approximately 20% of Americans suffer from lower back pain annually.[1] Although most episodes of low back pain are troublesome but non-life-threatening, others are symptoms of a serious illness, especially in children. Nontraumatic back pain occurs in the absence of a traumatic injury (e.g., from a fall or from a motor vehicle crash). Instead, most often nontraumatic back pain occurs as a result of muscle strain (e.g., from improper lifting technique while moving a patient to the stretcher).[2,3] However, lower back pain can also occur as the result of a serious medical illness. The Paramedic needs to be able to identify the patients who have symptoms or signs suggestive of a serious medical condition and identify those patients as a higher priority to the emergency department staff.

Anatomy Review

The spinal column (Figure 24-1) is made up of 33 vertebrae that both support the human while walking upright and protect the spinal cord. The spinal cord begins at the base of the brain and runs down the spinal canal just behind the vertebral body. Pairs of spinal nerves exit the spinal column through holes created by the joining of two adjacent vertebrae (Figure 24-2) and travel either to muscles or to sensory organs within the body. These nerves start in the spinal cord. At approximately the level of the second lumbar vertebrae, the spinal cord separates into individual spinal nerves. This gives the spinal cord the appearance of a horse's tail, thus leading to its name: cauda equina.

Between each pair of vertebrae are thick disks made up of a firm and fibrous outer layer and a smaller, more fluid inner core (Figure 24-3). The disks provide flexibility and shock absorption for the loads produced by walking, bending, and lifting. As the patient ages, the more fluid-like center portion becomes stiffer and the disk decreases in height. When the spinal column is hyperflexed or hyperextended, the disk can bulge through the ligamentous fibers that hold the spinal column together, providing one potential source of pain.[4,5] At certain levels in the spinal column, the disk can provide pressure on a section of the spinal cord or the spinal nerve root. This may cause pain at that level of the back, shooting pain down the distribution of the nerve, numbness in the area covered by the nerve, or muscle weakness, depending on which portion of the cord or the spinal nerve is affected.

It is important to note that as humans age, many people will develop minor disk **herniation**, commonly known as bulging disks, that often do not cause pain. It is also important

to note that just because a patient may have a history of disk herniations, the pain the patient is currently experiencing is not necessarily due to that condition.

Chief Concern

If a patient complains of back pain, the Paramedic must consider several conditions as its cause. Musculoskeletal back pain, by far the most common cause for back pain, often develops from lifting, stretching, or moving in a way that puts additional stress on the muscles or ligaments that make up the spinal column. This can happen from the occiput down to the coccyx, and can involve pain in the upper or lower extremities.

Muscle strain, which often causes microscopic tears and swelling in the muscles, results in stiffness and pain. Injury to the ligaments that connect the vertebrae to each other, to the ribs, and in the pelvis can also become sprained and produce pain. There does not necessarily need to be a single inciting event that produces the back pain.

Back pain can occur from repetitive use (e.g., the stiffness one feels after moving several heavy patients during a busy ambulance shift). This type of pain often appears some period of time after the inciting event occurs and is accompanied by a lot of stiffness. In a small number of cases, an acute disk herniation can occur and be the source of the patient's back pain. In these cases, there tends to be an identifiable event that occurred, with the onset of pain immediately following the incident. The pain caused by disk rupture is believed to come from tearing in the ligaments that help hold the disks

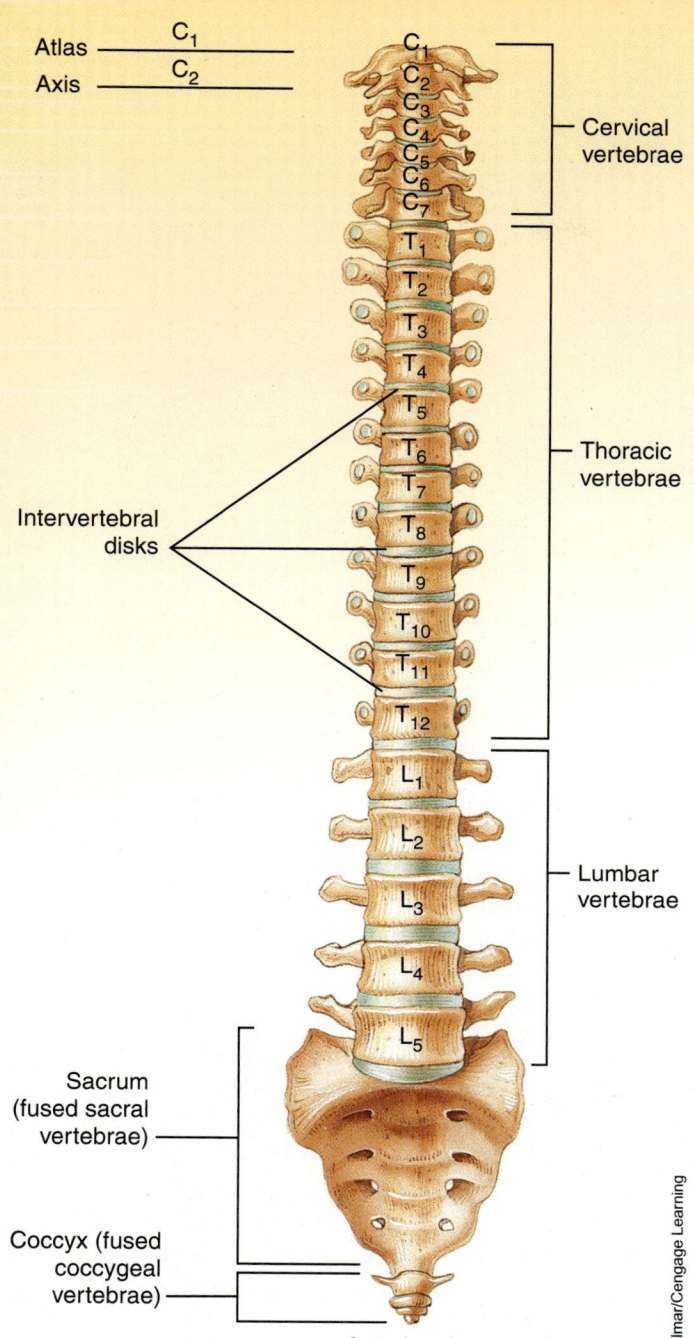

Atlas — C₁
Axis — C₂

C₁
C₂
C₃
C₄
C₅
C₆
C₇
— Cervical vertebrae

T₁
T₂
T₃
T₄
T₅
T₆
T₇
T₈
T₉
T₁₀
T₁₁
T₁₂
— Thoracic vertebrae

Intervertebral disks

L₁
L₂
L₃
L₄
L₅
— Lumbar vertebrae

Sacrum (fused sacral vertebrae)

Coccyx (fused coccygeal vertebrae)

Anterior view

Delmar/Cengage Learning

Figure 24-1   The spinal column.

There is little room between the bony surface of the vertebral canal and the spinal cord. Any condition that causes compression of the spinal cord can become dangerous and cause permanent nerve damage or paralysis. In a severe vertebral disk herniation, the disk can cause enough compression on the cord to produce permanent nerve damage. This is most often seen in the setting of trauma. However, it can occur in rare cases of atraumatic back pain.

Degeneration of the disks and the vertebral joints as people age can cause **spinal stenosis**, a narrowing of the spinal canal. Over time, this can produce pain and apply pressure to the cord or the spinal nerve roots.

Infections can occur in the disk (**diskitis**) or within the spinal canal (epidural abscess) and produce pain or compression of the spinal cord.[6,7] These infections are most often due to bacteria that have travelled in the bloodstream from another location in the body to the disk or around the spinal cord. Bleeding can also occur from the veins and arteries that supply the disk or the spinal cord and cause an epidural hematoma within the spinal canal.

Many types of cancer can spread or metastasize to the spine and cause either nontraumatic fractures of the vertebrae or compression of the spinal cord. Osteoporosis, a condition often associated with elderly women although men can be affected as well, is a change in the structure of the bones that makes them more brittle. These changes can cause fractures to occur with minimal stress on the bone.

Any of these conditions can cause a collection of signs and symptoms that indicate the patient has an acute spinal cord compression (Figure 24-5). As this is a surgical emergency, the patient experiencing an acute spinal cord compression should be taken to a facility with the capability to perform spinal surgery to relieve the pressure on the spinal cord.[8] When this spinal cord compression occurs in the lumbar spine, it is called **cauda equina syndrome**.

Other nonmusculoskeletal causes of nontraumatic back pain include rupture of an abdominal aortic aneurysm, kidney stones, and pyelonephritis (Table 24-1).

The abdominal aorta runs down the left side of the vertebral column from the diaphragm down to approximately the level of the second or third lumbar vertebrae before it divides into the iliac arteries which continue to the legs. As discussed in a previous chapter, this blood vessel is at risk of rupture in patients with longstanding hypertension. Although abdominal aortic aneurysm ruptures more frequently cause abdominal pain, if the aorta dissects or ruptures posteriorly, the patient will often complain of back pain rather than abdominal pain. Other symptoms associated with back pain from a rupture of an abdominal aortic aneurysm include syncope or near syncope, either unilateral or bilateral cold leg, or neurologic symptoms.

Kidney stones, also known as renal calculi, typically occur from calcium that builds up in the kidney over time. This calcium forms small collections or stones which produce pain when they move into the ureter and travel down

in place between the vertebrae. If a spinal nerve or a part of the spinal cord is compressed, the patient may complain of pain that shoots down into an extremity, or may complain of a sensation of numbness in that extremity (Figure 24-4). This is almost always unilateral. In rare circumstances, the disk protrudes in the center, providing significant pressure on the spinal cord, producing bilateral symptoms.

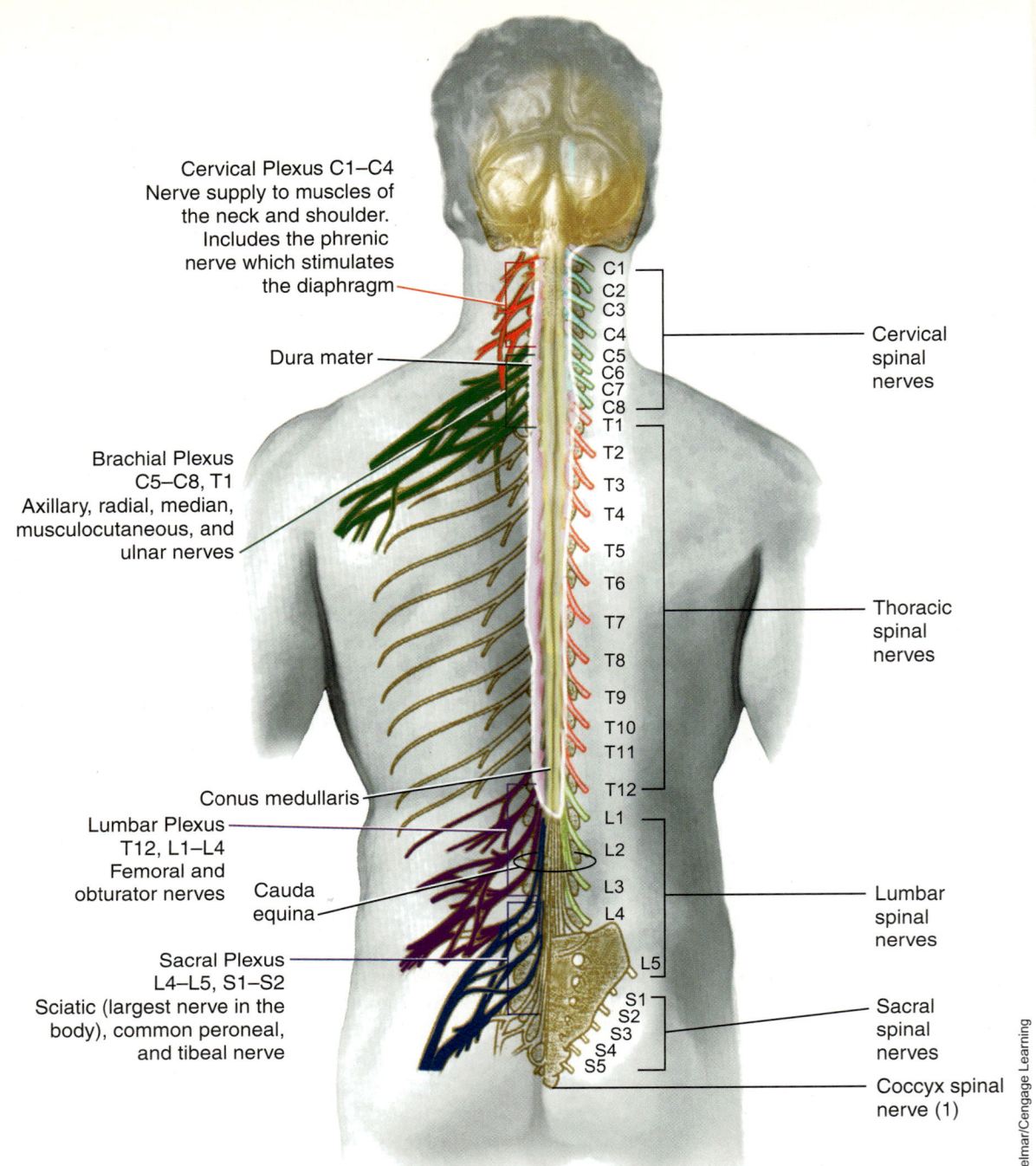

Cervical Plexus C1–C4
Nerve supply to muscles of
the neck and shoulder.
Includes the phrenic
nerve which stimulates
the diaphragm

Dura mater

Brachial Plexus
C5–C8, T1
Axillary, radial, median,
musculocutaneous, and
ulnar nerves

Conus medullaris

Lumbar Plexus
T12, L1–L4
Femoral and
obturator nerves

Cauda
equina

Sacral Plexus
L4–L5, S1–S2
Sciatic (largest nerve in the
body), common peroneal,
and tibeal nerve

C1
C2
C3
C4
C5
C6
C7
C8
T1
T2
T3
T4
T5
T6
T7
T8
T9
T10
T11
T12
L1
L2
L3
L4
L5
S1
S2
S3
S4
S5

Cervical
spinal
nerves

Thoracic
spinal
nerves

Lumbar
spinal
nerves

Sacral
spinal
nerves

Coccyx spinal
nerve (1)

Delmar/Cengage Learning

Figure 24-2 The spinal nerves.

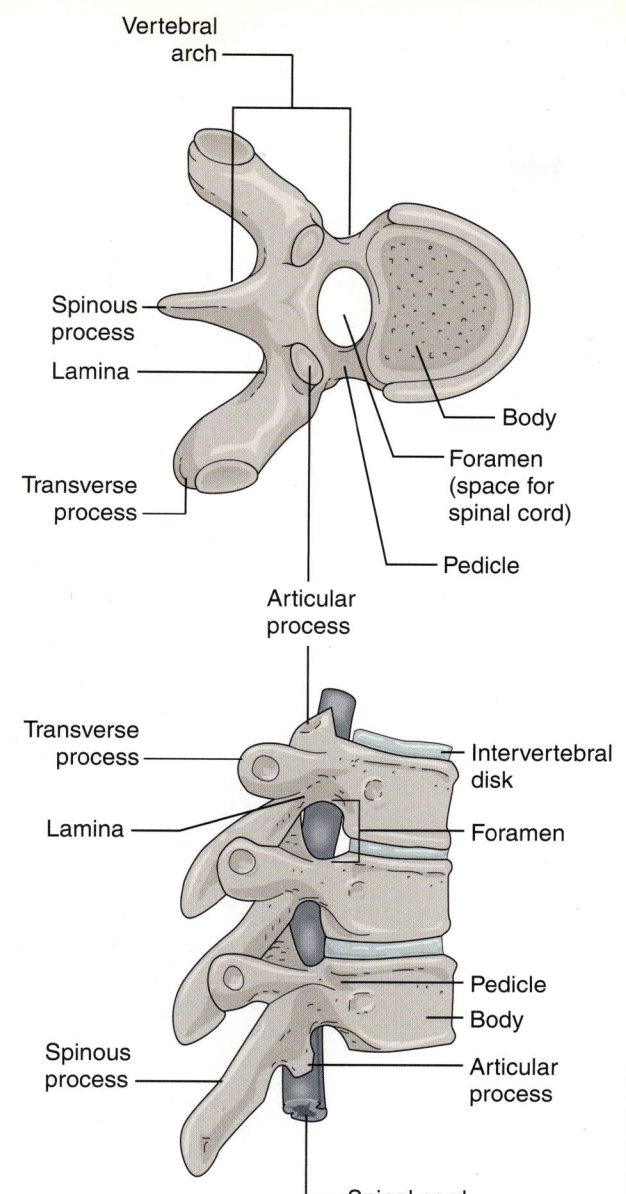

Figure 24-3 The vertebral disks are located between adjacent vertebrae.

Delmar/Cengage Learning

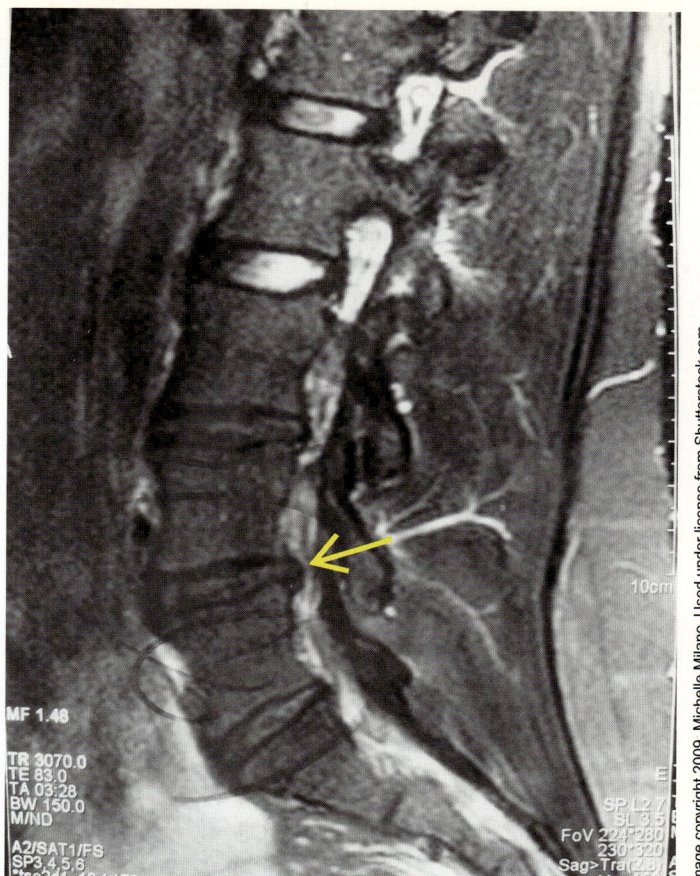

Figure 24-4 Disk herniation.

Table 24-1 Causes of Lower Back Pain

- Musculoskeletal pain
  - Muscle strain
    - Ligament injury
  - Disk herniation
    - Degeneration of disks
    - Spinal stenosis
  - Infection
    - Diskitis
    - Epidural abscess
  - Epidural hematoma
  - Cancer
    - Bone cancer
    - Metastasis
  - Osteoporosis

- Nonmusculoskeletal
  - Rupture of abdominal aortic aneurysm
  - Kidney stones
  - Pyelonephritis

toward the urinary bladder, causing the typical colicy (on and off) flank pain that radiates to the groin. However, larger kidney stones that are lodged in the renal pelvis can produce pain that is just to the left or right of the midline at the level of the lower ribs.

In the same way, **pyelonephritis**, or infection of the kidney, can produce back pain. Pyelonephritis is more common in women and is usually the result of a urinary tract infection that has spread up the ureter to the kidney. Patients who have pyelonephritis will often be febrile and appear ill.

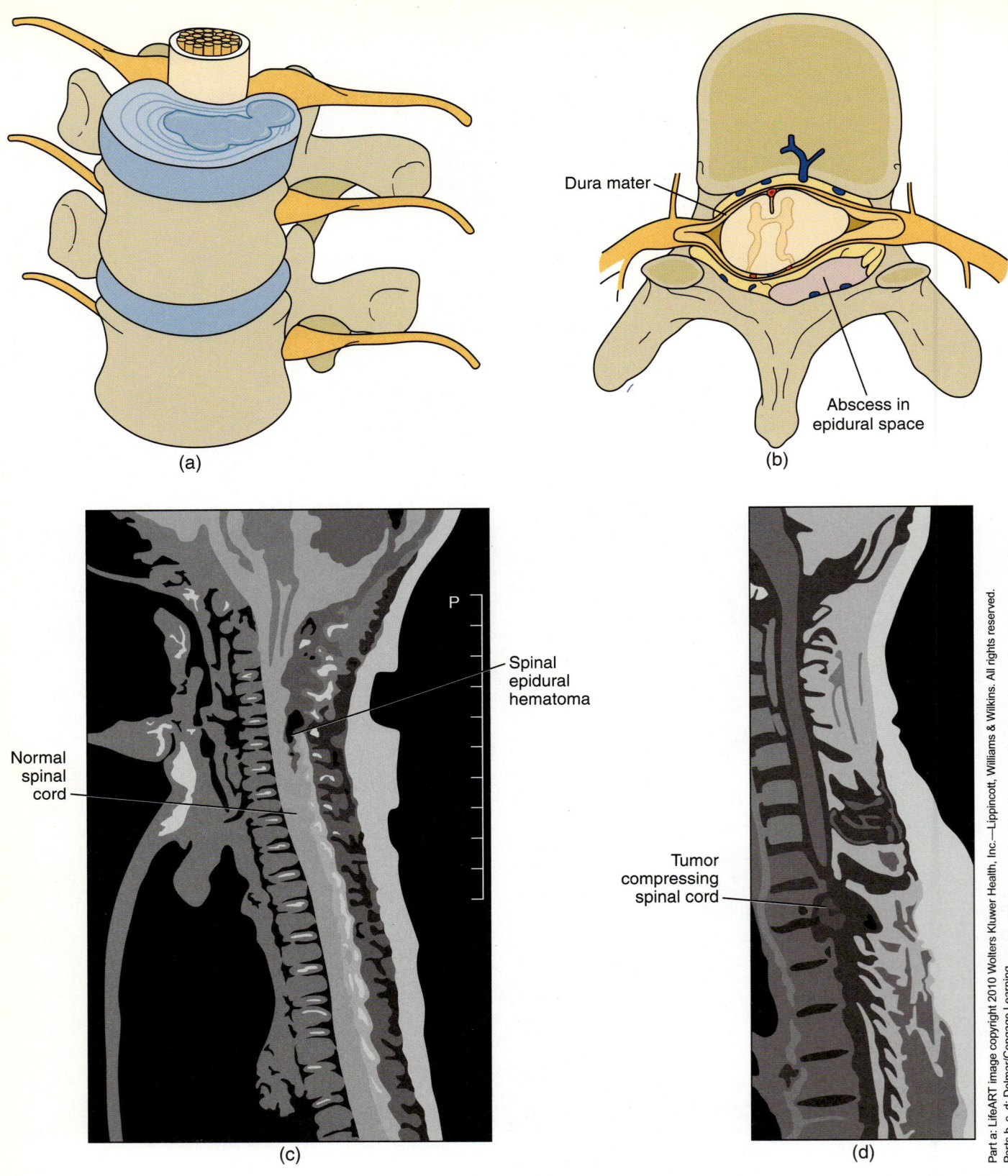

(a)

(b)

Dura mater

Abscess in
epidural space

P

Spinal
epidural
hematoma

Normal
spinal
cord

(c)

Tumor
compressing
spinal cord

(d)

Figure 24-5   Causes of acute spinal cord compression: (a) central disk herniation, (b) epidural abscess, (c) spinal epidural hematoma, and (d) cancer.

The Paramedics ring the doorbell. They are met by Sally Jones, who says, "My boyfriend, Steve Johnson, hurt his back again but this time he can't get up."

Sally directs the Paramedics into the living room, where Steve is lying on the couch in obvious distress. Steve states that he was lifting a heavy box in the garage about four hours ago when the pain started. He complains of pain in the lower back, more around the midline, with numbness between his legs and shooting pain down his thighs. He was helped to the couch by Sally because his legs felt weak. While lying on the couch, he feels like he needs to urinate. However, he tried and had difficulty urinating, which is new. His past medical history is unremarkable except for a back injury at work 10 years ago. He does not have night sweats or fevers and does not complain of abdominal pain. Steve denies taking any regular medications.

CRITICAL THINKING QUESTIONS

1. What are the important elements of the history that a Paramedic should obtain?
2. What is the symptom pattern for acute spinal cord compression?

History

Obtaining a thorough directed patient history is an important aspect of determining whether a medical or surgical emergency exists in a patient who complains of back pain. The Paramedic first asks an open-ended question to attempt to determine the history of present illness, and then asks more focused questions to narrow down the paramedical differential diagnosis. It is important to determine whether the immediate cause of the back pain is related to direct trauma to the spine in the recent past. If direct trauma to the spine is found during the history, then the patient will likely require immobilization.

There are a number of red flags in the history that could suggest a medical or surgical emergency (Table 24-2).[9–11] After the Paramedic obtains a history of what happened from the open-ended questions following the OPQRST mnemonic, the Paramedic should ask about the presence or absence of these red flags in every patient who complains of nontraumatic back pain. These factors should be reported as both pertinent positives if the patient has experienced them in recent history and as pertinent negatives if the patient has not experienced them.

Table 24-2 Historical Red Flags

- Saddle anesthesia
- Loss of control of bowel/bladder function
- Night sweats
- Night fevers
- Unintended weight loss
- Abdominal pain

Saddle anesthesia is a numbness or "pins and needles" sensation located in the skin territory of the perineum between the legs, the external genitalia, and the anus. Sensation to this area of the skin is covered by the S4 and S5 nerves, which are the most distal nerves in the spinal cord (Figure 24-6). A significant compression of the spinal cord at any level should produce saddle anesthesia.

Change in bowel and bladder control—either incontinence or retention of stool or urine—is another red flag, as cord compression affects the nerves that control both the anal sphincter and the urinary bladder sphincter. Most commonly, a patient with a cord compression will be incontinent of stool but will develop urinary retention. This occurs because the urinary bladder sphincter does not open to allow the patient to urinate. Eventually the urinary bladder becomes distended enough that urine will dribble out, giving the appearance of incontinence.

Stool incontinence occurs as the control of the anal sphincter is lost and the sphincter relaxes, allowing stool to

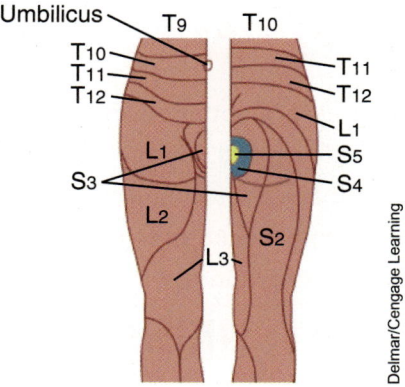

Figure 24-6 The S4 and S5 dermatomes cover the skin in the perineum.

ooze from the anus. The Paramedic should question every patient who has back pain as a primary complaint about bowel and bladder incontinence and retention. For patients who have difficulty walking and moving as a result of their back pain, it is important to clarify whether their incontinence is because they could not get to the bathroom in time due to the difficulty walking as a result of the pain or whether they simply were not able to control their bowel or bladder.

Night sweats and fevers (which occur while the patient is sleeping) are nonspecific signs that are often associated with infectious diseases. However, these can also be symptoms associated with cancers. Generalized muscle aches often occur with fever from a variety of infectious diseases, and tend to be worse with an elevated temperature. In the context of a patient with back pain as the primary complaint, these symptoms raise the concern for an infectious disease or cancer as a source of the back pain. When coupled with saddle anesthesia or new bowel or bladder dysfunction, it raises the concern about an epidural abscess or tumor producing spinal cord compression as the source of the patient's pain.

Unintended weight loss is considered loss of a few pounds without intentional dietary or exercise changes. Again, this is a nonspecific symptom which can alert the Paramedic to a more serious underlying cause of her patient's back pain. The Paramedic should start with the question of whether there was any recent weight loss and then follow that up with whether the weight loss was intentional (e.g., intentional decreased oral intake) or unintentional. When coupled with other red flags, unintended weight loss makes the Paramedic suspicious for cancer as the source of the patient's back pain.

Another red flag is abdominal pain associated with the back pain. Although a benign cause of both abdominal and back pain is constipation, the Paramedic should be concerned about the presence of an aortic aneurysm rupture. Individuals who have longstanding and poorly controlled hypertension and who are older are at risk for developing an aortic aneurysm. Associated historical information that would increase the suspicion of an abdominal aortic rupture includes syncope, lightheadedness, or lightheadedness with change from lying to sitting or sitting to standing position.

Past Medical History

The patient's past medical history also plays an important role in reaching the paramedical diagnosis. For the patient complaining of back pain, it is important for the Paramedic to note prior injuries and any long-term deficits from those injuries (e.g., chronic pain, weakness, or numbness). It is often helpful for the Paramedic to ask the patient how the current pain is different from the past episodes of pain. A past history of hypertension, cancer, and aortic aneurysm are also important and related to the historical red flags discussed previously. For example, a history of osteoporosis may lead the Paramedic to consider the possibility of a stress or compression fracture of the spine in the paramedical differential diagnosis.

Past surgical history may provide some important information. For example, if the Paramedic discovers that the patient recently had spinal surgery and was doing well up until recently, the Paramedic may consider a postsurgical complication (e.g., an abscess) as a potential source of the patient's pain. Likewise, a history of spinal surgery may also indicate to the Paramedic that the patient has had a past injury and may be at increased risk for further injury.

Medications the patient takes on a regular or occasional basis may also provide some clues. For example, the patient may not provide a history of a past back injury or prior episodes of back pain. When the Paramedic reviews the patient's medications and she discovers that the patient takes analgesics, it provides a prompt for the Paramedic to ask what pain the patient is treating with the analgesic. This is also true with antihypertensives and many other medications.

Finally, the Paramedic should ask the patient about medication allergies or sensitivities he may have that would change what medications the Paramedic may be able to administer to the patient.

CASE STUDY (CONTINUED)

A full set of vitals are obtained from Mr. Johnson. They are slightly elevated but within the normal range for an adult. A brief focused physical examination shows that Mr. Johnson does not have any localized spinal tenderness, but has a lot of muscle spasm around the spinal column in the lower lumbar area. Mr. Johnson's pants appear moist from a small amount of urinary incontinence. His leg movement does increase the pain. Sensation and strength in the legs seem to be decreased.

CRITICAL THINKING QUESTIONS

1. What are the elements of the physical examination of a patient with back pain?
2. Why is a peripheral neurological examination a critical element in this examination?

Examination

The Paramedic should obtain a complete set of vital signs from the patient and closely investigate any abnormalities. When performing the physical examination, there are several red flags that can indicate the presence of one of the life-threatening conditions that cause back pain (Table 24-3). The order of the examination may vary depending on the position in which the patient is found and the patient's ability to ambulate. The focused exam should incorporate the following features.

The Paramedic palpates the spine to determine if midline spinal tenderness is present. Depending upon the clinical information and the Paramedic's suspicion of recent trauma, the presence of tenderness may be an indication for spinal motion restriction. The Paramedic may also be able to detect muscle spasm in the muscles adjacent to the spine. The Paramedic should palpate the abdomen for tenderness and the presence of a tender midline abdominal mass that may suggest the presence of an aortic aneurysm. In moving toward the lower extremities, the Paramedic should look at the groin/lower abdomen area for evidence of incontinence. The Paramedic should evaluate pulses at the femoral artery and the dorsalis pedis for equal strength. Pulses that are not equal may indicate aortic rupture.

The muscle strength in the lower extremities is also assessed for equality. It may be difficult for the patient to move the upper legs if there is significant pain as upper leg movement can worsen the pain. It is important to look for differences in strength between the two legs that may indicate nerve compression. Symmetric but weak muscle strength may also indicate nerve or central cord compression.

The Paramedic should assess the patient's lower extremity sensation along the inner (medial) and outer (lateral) aspects of both legs, the dorsum (top) of the foot, and the plantar surface (bottom) of the foot while asking the patient if the touch feels the same on both sides. New deficits may indicate a nerve compression. Patients who have had a prior injury may have residual deficits from that injury—either weakness, numbness, or both a sensory and a motor deficit. If a difference is found during the examination and the patient has had a prior injury, the Paramedic should ask the patient if there was weakness or numbness remaining from that previous injury.

Table 24-3 Physical Exam Red Flags for a Patient Who Complains of Back Pain

- Unequal strength
- Unequal sensation
- Evidence of incontinence
- Abdominal mass
- Unequal pulses
- Fever

CASE STUDY (CONTINUED)

Mentally reviewing the symptom complex, the Paramedic remembers that Mr. Johnson had an onset of severe lumbar pain while lifting a heavy object a few hours ago. The pain goes down both legs and now he has paresthesias between his legs. There is no abdominal pain. Mr. Johnson has had difficulty in urinating, but has signs on the physical examination of slight urinary incontinence. The physical examination also reveals that Mr. Johnson has very little motor strength or sensation in both of his lower legs. His lower extremity pulses are equal, and his abdominal exam reveals no tenderness.

In working through the paramedical diagnosis, the Paramedic can probably exclude a ruptured aortic aneurysm as there is no abdominal pain, tenderness, masses, or circulation issue in the lower extremities. Mr. Johnson does not have any fever or weight loss, which makes cancer or an infection less likely. He does not have any signs or symptoms consistent with a kidney stone. What Mr. Johnson does have are several serious signs and symptoms that are consistent with an acute cord compression. The muscle weakness and decreased sensation combined with the saddle paresthesia and urinary retention all point toward an acute cord compression.

CRITICAL THINKING QUESTIONS

1. What is the significance of the saddle paresthesia?
2. What diagnosis did the Paramedic announce to the patient?

Assessment

After the patient assessment, the Paramedic should consider the possible conditions and try to narrow the list down to a most likely paramedical diagnosis. This involves reflecting on the pertinent positive and negative findings from the history and physical examination and comparing those findings to the potential conditions. As potential paramedical diagnoses are eliminated, the two or three most likely paramedical diagnoses will become apparent. Although other minor syndromes may exist, the worst case scenario is acute cord compression.

CASE STUDY (CONTINUED)

The Paramedic places an 18 gauge IV catheter into Mr. Johnson's left hand and attaches a saline lock. Mr. Johnson receives morphine before he is moved into the ambulance stretcher. Although Mr. Johnson is anxious to get to the hospital, the Paramedic reassures him it would be best if he allowed the morphine to start to work. Within a few minutes Mr. Johnson's facial expression softens and the patient appears visibly more relaxed. This signal indicates to the Paramedic that it is time to carefully transfer Mr. Johnson to the ambulance gurney. Although the idea of using a backboard to minimize movement of the spine has merit, the idea of the patient riding to the hospital on a rigid backboard seems more like punishment than treatment. Instead, the Paramedic elects to use the split (scoop) stretcher.

CRITICAL THINKING QUESTIONS

1. What is the national standard of care of patients with suspected acute cord compression?
2. What are some of the patient-specific concerns and considerations that the Paramedic should consider when applying this plan of care that is intended to treat a broad patient population presenting with acute cord compression?

Treatment

As with every patient, the Paramedic should address any airway, breathing, or circulation issues as the first priority of treatment. Circulatory collapse can occur both in a ruptured abdominal aortic aneurysm and sepsis from a severe infection. The Paramedic should initially support the patient with IV fluids. If an abdominal aortic aneurysm rupture is suspected, the Paramedic should administer normal saline or lactated Ringer's intravenously in boluses of 250 mL at a time, reassessing the blood pressure between boluses. The target blood pressure is a systolic blood pressure of 90 to 100 mmHg systolic. Raising the blood pressure above that level can increase the pressures around the ruptured area, dislodging any clot that may have formed in an attempt to stabilize the rupture. For a patient who is believed to be septic, the blood pressure should be supported with up to 2 liters of normal saline as a means of resuscitating the patient.

Providing analgesia is another important treatment which the Paramedic can provide, especially if the patient's pain is worse with movement. Depending upon the specific medications available within the system, several intravenous, subcutaneous, and oral agents can be used. Oral agents include medications that are opioid and acetaminophen combination medications (e.g., hydrocodone/acetaminophen), nonsteroidal medications (e.g., ibuprofen), and acetaminophen alone. Due to the slow onset of action of these oral medications, they may not be effective as a first-line agent in a patient complaining of moderate to severe pain.

Several medications are available for either intravenous or subcutaneous delivery that may be a better choice in patients with moderate to severe pain. Opioid agents (e.g., morphine and fentanyl) are stronger medications that can be administered intravenously, intramuscularly, or subcutaneously to provide analgesia. Ketorolac is a nonsteroidal medication that can also be administered intravenously or intramuscularly.

Regardless of the route of administration chosen by the Paramedic, there is evidence that administering both types of analgesia in cases of acute pain provides a synergistic effect with a larger decrease in pain level than either medication alone.[12-14] The Paramedic should assess the patient's pain both before and after administration of analgesia and document the pain levels on the patient care report. When administering opioid medications, the Paramedic should assess the patient for hypotension and respiratory depression, which are both potential side effects of those medications. The patient may require a second dose of analgesia depending upon the response to analgesia, the transport time, and road conditions during transport.

In general, patients who have nontraumatic back pain do not require spinal motion restriction with a cervical collar or a long spine board. Although the long spine board may be used as a lifting and moving device if it will allow minimal patient discomfort, it should be removed from the stretcher at the first opportunity and certainly not used for long transport. If there is any concern about direct trauma to the patient's spine, then the patient should undergo spinal motion restriction precautions.

En route to the hospital, the Paramedic finds the patient's vital signs have remained unchanged and his pain level is decreased to a 6/10 from a 9/10. She repeats the neurologic and motor examination on the lower extremities and finds little lower extremity movement, a change from her earlier examination. Based on Mr. Johnson's continued pain, he receives another dose of morphine at 0.05 mg/kg, reducing his pain to a level of 2/10.

CRITICAL THINKING QUESTIONS

1. What are some of the predictable complications associated with acute cord compression?
2. What are some of the predictable complications associated with the treatments for acute cord compression?

Evaluation

The Paramedic should reassess the patient during transport, including checks of the patient's pain levels and vital signs. Increasing pain may occur from the transport itself or may indicate a change in the patient's condition. Increased heart rate may indicate increased pain or may be a sign of early shock, especially when coupled with a decreased diastolic blood pressure. The Paramedic should immediately address any abnormal vital signs.

If spinal cord compression is suspected, the Paramedic should reevaluate the neurologic and motor examination to detect any change in condition. If an abdominal aneurysm rupture is suspected, the Paramedic should closely follow the blood pressure and heart rate.

CASE STUDY CONCLUSION

At the hospital, report is given to the medical and nursing staff. The physician confirms the history and physical examination findings, orders a stat MRI, and calls the neurosurgeon on call. The MRI shows an acute cord compression from a central disk herniation between L4 and L5 vertebrae.

Mr. Johnson undergoes emergency surgery an hour later to decompress his spinal cord. A week later, Mr. Johnson is transferred to an acute rehabilitation facility after regaining some strength in his legs. However, he still has residual problems with his ability to control his bladder.

CRITICAL THINKING QUESTIONS

1. What is the most appropriate transport decision that will get the patient to definitive care?
2. What are the advantages of transporting a patient with suspected acute cord compression to hospitals with orthopedic surgery, even if that means bypassing other hospitals in the process?

Disposition

The vast majority of patients who present to EMS with non-traumatic back pain can be taken to any emergency department for care. The Paramedic should consider transport to a specialty center if she is highly suspicious of a ruptured aortic aneurysm or an acute spinal cord compression as the source of the patient's back pain. A patient who has a ruptured aortic aneurysm needs to be in a facility with vascular surgery services that can repair the aorta. Likewise, a patient who has a spinal cord compression needs to be in a facility where a spine surgeon can operate to relieve the pressure on the spinal cord. If the patient's vital signs are unstable, then the patient should be taken to the nearest hospital for stabilization and then transferred to another facility. If a specialized facility is a significant distance away or the paramedical diagnosis is not as clear, then the patient should be taken to the closest hospital. The Paramedic should follow local or regional protocols and policies on patient transport.

CONCLUSION

Although the majority of the patients who access the emergency medical system with a concern of back pain have a painful but non-life-threatening condition, some patients actually have a serious underlying disease. Whether the patient has an abdominal aneurysm, an acute cord compressive syndrome, or musculoskeletal back pain, the Paramedic must dive sufficiently into the patient's history and perform a thorough enough physical examination to identify those patients with these life- and limb-threatening disorders.

KEY POINTS:

- Separating the spinal vertebrae are thick discs that serve as shock absorbers.

- Musculoskeletal back pain is the most common cause of back pain.

- Acute disc herniation can cause the disc to bulge from between the vertebrae and put pressure on the spinal nerves.

- Narrowing of the spinal canal can place pressure on the spinal nerves.

- Infections or metastatic disease can cause pain in the back.

- Fractures can occur with little to no trauma in the face of osteoporosis.

- Causes of nonmusculoskeletal pain include kidney infection and stones or a ruptured abdominal aortic aneurysm.

- Signs and symptoms of a surgical emergency for nontraumatic back pain include:
  - Pins and needles in the lower back and perineum
  - Altered bowel or bladder habits, most commonly with stool incontinence and urinary retention
  - Night sweats
  - Night fever
  - Unintended weight loss
  - Abdominal pain

- The patient's history should include any prior injuries and any deficits from those injuries.

- The patient's exam should include a side-to-side comparison of strength, movement, and sensation.

- The Paramedic must manage the patient's pain.

REVIEW QUESTIONS:

1. Describe the composition and function of the discs between vertebrae.
2. Name at least six causes of musculoskeletal back pain. Which is the most common?
3. How would the history of a patient with kidney stones vary from one with musculoskeletal back pain?
4. Define saddle anesthesia.
5. Describe how a Paramedic would test for leg strength and sensation.

CASE STUDY QUESTIONS:

Please refer to the Case Study in this chapter, and answer the questions below:

1. What is the significance of the patient's prior back injury without chronic back pain?

2. Would you have immobilized Mr. Johnson's spine? Explain your answer.

3. Would you have administered a second dose of morphine? Why or why not?

4. What are the significant clues in Mr. Johnson's history and exam that support the Paramedic's diagnosis of acute cord compression?

REFERENCES:

1. Perina D. Mechanical back pain. **Available at: http://www .emedicine.com/emerg/topic50.htm**. Accessed March 3, 2008.

2. Kinkade S. Evaluation and treatment of acute low back pain. *Am Fam Physician*. 2007;75(8):1181–1188.

3. Chou R, Qaseem A, et al. Diagnosis and treatment of low back pain: a joint clinical practice guideline from the American College of Physicians and the American Pain Society. *Ann Intern Med*. 2007;147(7):478–491.

4. Borenstein D. Epidemiology, etiology, diagnostic evaluation, and treatment of low back pain. *Curr Opin Rheumatol*. 1995;7(2):141–146.

5. Costello RF, Beall DP. Nomenclature and standard reporting terminology of intervertebral disk herniation. *Magn Reson Imaging Clin N Am*. 2007;15(2):167–174, v–vi.

6. Davis DP, Wold RM, et al. The clinical presentation and impact of diagnostic delays on emergency department patients with spinal epidural abscess. *J Emerg Med*. 2004;26(3):285–291.

7. Curry WT, Jr., Hoh BL, et al. Spinal epidural abscess: clinical presentation, management, and outcome. *Surg Neurol*. 2005;63(4):364–371; discussion 371.

8. Broos PL, Janzing HM, et al. Life saving surgery in polytrauma patients. *Przegl Lek*. 2000;57 Suppl 5:118–119.

9. Braddom RL. Perils and pointers in the evaluation and management of back pain. *Semin Neurol* 1998;18(2):197–210.

10. Winters ME, Kluetz P, et al. Back pain emergencies. *Med Clin North Am*. 2006;90(3):505–523.

11. McCarthy CJ, Gittins M, et al. The reliability of the clinical tests and questions recommended in international guidelines for low back pain. *Spine*. 2007;32(8):921–926.

12. Munro HM, Walton SR, et al. Low-dose ketorolac improves analgesia and reduces morphine requirements following posterior spinal fusion in adolescents. *Can J Anaesth*. 2002;49(5):461–416.

13. Reuben SS, Connelly NR, et al. Ketorolac as an adjunct to patient-controlled morphine in postoperative spine surgery patients. *Reg Anesth*. 1997;24(4):343–346.

14. Sevarino FB, Sinatra RS, et al. The efficacy of intramuscular ketorolac in combination with intravenous PCA morphine for postoperative pain relief. *J Clin Anesth*. 1992;4(4): 285–288.

CHAPTER 25

DISORDERS OF CENTRAL CIRCULATION

KEY CONCEPTS:

Upon completion of this chapter, it is expected that the reader will understand these following concepts:

- How hypertension places a patient at significant risk for myocardial infarction, heart failure, stroke, and renal failure
- The recognition that most EMS calls result from a patient's inability to take medications regularly or from poorly controlled hypertension
- That field treatment is most often directed at the complications of hypertension, not at reducing the pressure

ANATOMY CONCEPTS:

Prior to reading this chapter the Paramedic student should be familiar with the following anatomy and physiology concepts:

- Major blood vessels

"Starr Ambulance Medic 14, respond to 43 Broadway, upper floor, for a 35-year-old male with high blood pressure and a nosebleed that can't be controlled," dispatch crackles. As they travel the five minutes to 43 Broadway, the Paramedics discuss what might cause a severe nosebleed. They remember the hemophilic kid that was bumped in the nose by his dog and how that started a nosebleed. Then there was the old woman who had cardiac syncope, fell face first in a "dead man's fall" onto her face, and suffered a broken nose and a severe nosebleed. These two experienced Paramedics know enough to not dismiss a nosebleed as simply a minor inconvenience.

CRITICAL THINKING QUESTIONS

1. What are some of the possible causes of epistaxis?
2. How is the hypertension related to the epistaxis?

OVERVIEW

According to the Centers for Disease Control National Center for Health Statistics, approximately 45 million people visited a primary care office with hypertension and nearly 4 million visited the emergency department with hypertension as a primary diagnosis.[1] Hypertension was also the primary cause of death for approximately 25,000 people, and was a contributing factor in up to 300,000 deaths.[2] Hypertension is a risk factor in developing cardiovascular disease (including heart failure and myocardial infarction), stroke, and renal failure. In many individuals, the exact cause of their hypertension is unknown. However, regardless of the cause, hypertension is easily detectable and treatable.

Chief Concern

Hypertension is divided into three different classes (Table 25-1).[3] Initially, hypertension is silent, causing no signs or symptoms. A patient may have hypertension for several years before he becomes symptomatic or the hypertension is discovered during a routine physical examination. In general, blood pressure does not need to be lowered acutely in the prehospital or emergency department environment. However, the EMS assessment can provide some clues as to the effects of the patient's elevated blood pressure on the body.

Hypertension can cause lasting effects on the brain, the heart, the kidneys, and the peripheral blood vessels (Figure 25-1). In the brain, the cerebral perfusion pressure (CPP) is dependent on the mean arterial pressure (MAP). If the MAP increases, as it does with hypertension, the CPP also increases. The increase in CPP causes microscopic damage to the blood vessels in the brain which ultimately result in narrowing of these vessels and ischemic disease. This ultimately manifests as a transient ischemic attack (TIA) or stroke when a vessel supplying a portion of the brain is blocked by a clot. Lack of blood flow can also occur in a portion of the brain if the demand for oxygenated blood exceeds the supply, just as angina produces chest pain. Longstanding hypertension can cause the smaller blood vessels in the brain to rupture or leak, causing intracranial hemorrhages and hemorrhagic strokes.

In the heart, systemic hypertension increases the pressure the left ventricle needs to overcome in order to maintain blood flow to the body. The extra force required will increase the size of the heart muscle much in the same way that a weightlifter increases muscle mass by lifting increasingly heavier weights. In contrast to the strengthening of the heart that occurs with exercise, this bulking up of the heart

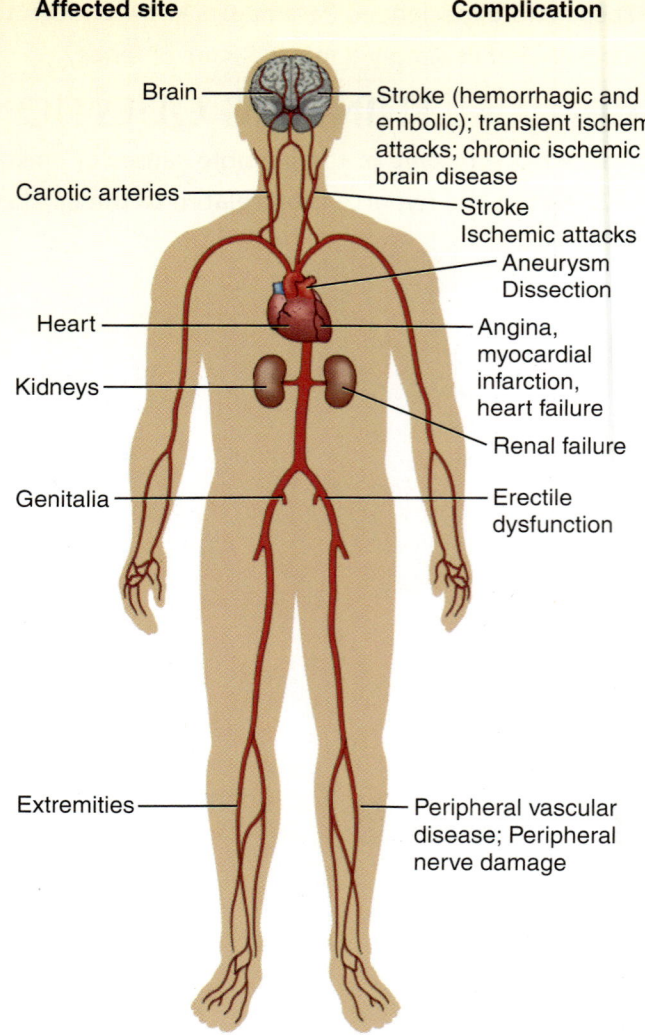

Affected site	Complication
Brain	Stroke (hemorrhagic and embolic); transient ischemic attacks; chronic ischemic brain disease
Carotic arteries	Stroke Ischemic attacks
	Aneurysm Dissection
Heart	Angina, myocardial infarction, heart failure
Kidneys	Renal failure
Genitalia	Erectile dysfunction
Extremities	Peripheral vascular disease; Peripheral nerve damage

Figure 25-1 The effects of hypertension on the body.

Table 25-1 The Joint National Committee Classifications of Hypertension

Prehypertension	Systolic Blood Pressure (SBP) 120 to 130 mmHg or Diastolic Blood Pressure (DBP) 80 to 89 mmHg
Stage I Hypertension	SBP 140 to 159 mmHg or DBP 90 to 99 mmHg
Stage II Hypertension	SBP > 160 mmHg or DBP > 100 mmHg

continues on a gradual basis. Eventually, the left ventricle is significantly larger. The negative effects of this left ventricular hypertrophy (LVH) include weakening of the muscular wall of the heart and dysrhythmias. The weakening of the heart muscle results in heart failure and, in rare cases, can lead to myocardial rupture. Hypertension also accelerates the formation of plaques on the walls of the coronary blood vessels, decreasing blood flow to the myocardium and increasing the risk for myocardial infarction.

Hypertension affects the kidneys by decreasing the diameter of the blood vessels within the kidney, limiting blood flow to the kidney and impairing the kidney's filtering function. In the setting of hypertension, the limited blood flow to the kidney sets off a cascade of the renin–angiotensin–aldosterone system (RAA). This causes a further increase in blood pressure. The end result of this process is kidney failure and dependence on dialysis, which can occur at a young age in patients who develop hypertension in their late teens or early twenties.

The damage to blood vessels is not limited to the brain, the heart, and the kidneys, however. All of the smaller peripheral blood vessels are also affected. The results of peripheral blood vessel damage include development of an aortic aneurysm, peripheral vascular disease, peripheral nerve damage, and erectile dysfunction. Peripheral vascular disease can significantly compromise blood flow to the extremities, causing pain, difficult-to-heal infections, and ultimately amputation of the extremity.

When called for hypertension-related complaints, the Paramedic will most often encounter a patient who has not been able to take his antihypertensive medications or a patient who is having an issue with poorly controlled hypertension. In addition to those calls, the Paramedic will encounter many patients who have hypertensive blood pressure readings based upon the definitions in Table 25-1. Some of these patients will be hypertensive due to pain, anxiety, or other factors related to the reason they called for Paramedic assistance, whereas some patients will truly be hypertensive. Taking a moment to briefly educate the stable patient about the effects and risks of hypertension can serve as the motivation for that patient to seek medical assistance in controlling his blood pressure.

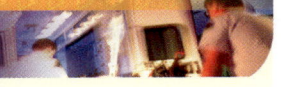

PROFESSIONAL PARAMEDIC

Approximately 80% of Paramedics believe that education of patients should be part of their responsibilities. However, only 25% say they have actually educated their patients about their condition and about the means to care for themselves.

A patient presenting with an elevated blood pressure can fall into one of three categories.[4] A **hypertensive emergency** is defined as severe hypertension that results in acute impairment of an organ system (e.g., the brain, heart, lungs, or kidneys).[5] An **acute hypertensive episode** is the opposite end of the spectrum, where a patient presents with Stage II hypertension as defined in Table 25-1, but without signs or symptoms of end-organ damage. The middle gray zone is **hypertensive urgency**, which is defined as an acute hypertensive episode without evidence of end-organ damage, even though the patient has risk factors to develop acute end-organ damage. In the field, it is impossible to distinguish between these last two categories. Therefore, hypertensive emergency will be examined.

An abrupt increase in a patient's blood pressure can cause a lack of blood flow through these narrowed cerebral blood vessels, increase damage to those vessels, and cause cerebral edema. This manifests itself as altered mental status, seizures, or visual disturbances from the hypertension. The term for this condition is **hypertensive encephalopathy**.[6] It is difficult to definitively define hypertensive encephalopathy in the prehospital setting as a CT scan of the brain is required to exclude hemorrhage or stroke as a cause for the altered mental status or seizures. Many patients report that they can feel that their blood pressure is elevated or they may develop a mild headache when their blood pressure is elevated above baseline. The relationship between an elevated blood pressure and development of a headache is controversial in the literature.

Cardiopulmonary manifestations of a hypertensive emergency includes chest pain, chest pressure, or myocardial infarction. The sudden increase in hypertension is greater than the heart's ability to overcome the patient's afterload, and the heart begins to fail. This form of left-sided heart failure often presents as an acute pulmonary edema with severe dyspnea and may occur without chest pain or pressure. The increase in blood pressure may also produce myocardial ischemia if coronary blood flow is reduced. In extreme cases, the patient may have an ST-elevation myocardial infarction, although a non-ST-elevation myocardial infarction (NSTEMI) is much more common. Ruptures of an aortic aneurysm, both thoracic and abdominal, are less common manifestations of a hypertensive emergency. Both can occur with significant acute blood pressure elevation in a patient with an existing aneurysm. The sudden rise in blood pressure increases the shear forces that occur as blood is pumped through the dilated, thinned, and irregular vessel lumen, developing a small tear in the wall. The longer the pressure remains elevated, the more likely the tear will extend, and eventually the wall will rupture. Rupture of an aortic aneurysm must be considered in patients who complain of posterior or sharp chest pain, abdominal pain, or back pain and are significantly hypertensive.

Renal manifestations of a hypertensive emergency are also difficult to detect without access to blood tests available in the emergency department. Uremic patients may complain of generalized itching or also present with altered mental status. This is due to the loss of the kidneys' filtering ability and buildup of nitrogen in the blood.

The discussion of the various causes and complications of hypertension would not be complete without briefly discussing the spectrum of conditions of pregnancy-induced hypertension, pre-eclampsia, and eclampsia. These conditions typically occur in pregnant women during the late part of the second trimester or in the third trimester. In rare cases, it can occur earlier in the second trimester or within the two weeks after delivery. The Paramedic should always consider these conditions for child-bearing age women who present with neurologic symptoms or new seizures coupled with hypertension.

CASE STUDY (CONTINUED)

The ambulance arrives at 43 Broadway. The Paramedics grab the first-in bag and head up the stairs to the second floor. As they reach the top of the stairs, they hear Joe Wilson call out to come in through the open apartment door. The two Paramedics cautiously approach, survey the scene, and ensure the scene is safe to enter.

The Paramedics find Mr. Wilson sitting in a kitchen chair clutching his head. The Paramedics introduce themselves as Paramedics with Starr Ambulance and ask Mr. Wilson what they can do for him.

"My head is killing me!" Mr. Wilson exclaims. "I ran out of my blood pressure medications a week ago. I always get a headache when my blood pressure goes up! And my nose is bleeding and I can't stop it!"

CRITICAL THINKING QUESTIONS

1. What are the important elements of the history that a Paramedic should obtain?
2. What is the symptom pattern for hypertensive crisis?

History

The history of present illness in this situation may vary depending upon the patient's complaint. Regardless of the patient's chief concern, the Paramedic needs to gather information that will help determine if the hypertensive episode is producing end-organ damage. After the general discussion of the events leading up to the call for EMS, the Paramedic should ask directed questions specifically related to the neurologic, cardiovascular, and renal systems.

From a neurologic standpoint, the Paramedic should ask about headaches, double vision or vision loss, numbness, and weakness. If the patient has an altered mental status or is unconscious, this information may need to be obtained from bystanders. The presence of seizures is also important. For the unconscious patient, asking bystanders about preceding complaints may also provide a clue as to the cause of the altered mental status.

From a cardiovascular standpoint, the Paramedic should question the patient about cardiac-related symptoms. This includes asking about both chest pain and pressure, as some patients do not associate pressure with pain. Dyspnea may indicate heart failure or an angina equivalent in the patient with past cardiac disease. Any abdominal or back pain should alert the Paramedic to assess the patient for a ruptured abdominal aneurysm.

From a renal standpoint, the Paramedic should ask the patient questions about generalized itching, skin color change, decrease in urination, and confusion. Although the renal effects of hypertension are difficult to assess without access to a blood chemistry analyzer, subtle clinical signs may be present to alert the Paramedic to end-organ issues secondary to hypertension.

Finally, the Paramedic should question child-bearing age females of the possibility of pregnancy or recent delivery. If the female patient is pregnant, the Paramedic should determine how far along she is in the pregnancy and if she has had hypertension during the pregnancy. For the female patient who delivered a child within the last few weeks, the Paramedic should ask about hypertension during her pregnancy.

In the past medical history, it is important for the Paramedic to focus on the presence or absence of a prior history of hypertension, diabetes, cardiovascular disease, renal insufficiency or failure, known thoracic or abdominal aneurysm, and prior embolic or hemorrhagic stroke. These are conditions that may indicate the patient has had an issue with past hypertension, alert the Paramedic to patients who already have had end-organ damage from longstanding hypertension, and may highlight those asymptomatic patients who require blood pressure treatment at the emergency department.

The Paramedic obtains a blood pressure of 240/140, a pulse rate of 96 beats per minute, and a respiratory rate of 18 breaths per minute. His SaO$_2$ is 92% on room air. She finds the pupils are reactive and equal. Mr. Wilson winces when she shines her penlight into his eyes. The Paramedic performs a complete neurologic examination on Mr. Wilson and does not notice any deficits, except that Mr. Wilson cannot see her finger when she moves it into the lower left of his visual field. During the cardiopulmonary examination, the Paramedic notes that Mr. Wilson has fine rales at both lung bases.

CRITICAL THINKING QUESTIONS

1. What are the elements of the physical examination of a patient with suspected hypertensive crisis?
2. Why is a cardiopulmonary examination a critical element in this examination?

Examination

The Paramedic should rapidly perform a primary assessment and correct any immediate life-threatening conditions. In regard to patients with a potential diagnosis of hypertensive emergency, the Paramedic will need to closely assess the patient's airway for adequate protection and breathing for adequate ventilations, intervening as needed. The Paramedic should also determine the patient's blood glucose level if the patient has an altered mental status. Once the primary assessment is completed, the Paramedic's physical exam should focus on detecting subtle clues to end-organ damage that may not have been apparent during the history. This focused examination is also divided into neurological, cardiovascular, and renal components.

From a neurological standpoint, the Paramedic should conduct a complete neurologic examination to detect any problems with either the brain or neurologic function. From a cardiopulmonary standpoint, the Paramedic should auscultate the heart for murmurs and the lungs for rales. In addition, the Paramedic should assess the patient for signs of an aortic aneurysm by evaluating pulses for equality and strength. The Paramedic should palpate the abdomen for the presence of a pulsating mass. From a renal standpoint, the Paramedic should examine the patient's skin for color and evidence of scratching. These signs may not be present even in those with advanced disease because renal failure does not normally produce a defined set of physical examination findings.

STREET SMART

Patients with a history of Marfan syndrome are at greater risk for an abdominal aortic aneurysm and may experience it at an earlier age.

The Paramedic places an intravenous line, fills several blood tubes, and reviews the 12-lead ECG that the other Paramedic acquired. The 12-lead ECG reveals tall R waves in the precordial leads, which are indicative of left ventricular hypertrophy, and inverted T-waves throughout the precordial leads. The Paramedic considers her paramedical differential diagnosis while they move Mr. Wilson down the stairs to the stretcher waiting one story below.

CRITICAL THINKING QUESTIONS

1. What is the significance of the inverted T waves in the precordial leads?
2. What diagnosis did the Paramedic announce to the patient?

Assessment

The history of a headache with some vision loss is frequently suggestive of an acute neurological process. These patients often have a longstanding history of hypertension, which puts them at greater risk for chronic end-organ damage. This symptoms complex suggests that the severe elevation in blood pressure is causing issues with the brain and the heart, and defines this episode as a hypertensive emergency.

As one Paramedic continues with the neurological component of the exam, Mr. Wilson shows no deficits except an inability to see an object held off to his left side. He also has fine rales at both lung bases.

CRITICAL THINKING QUESTIONS

1. What is the standard of care of patients with suspected hypertensive emergency?
2. What is the difference between a hypertensive emergency and a hypertensive urgency?

Treatment

Treatment of hypertension in the prehospital setting has long been controversial. At one point in the past, Paramedics aggressively lowered patients' blood pressures. However, this was found to be harmful to patients, especially those with cerebral hemorrhage or those who had an underlying condition that produced the patient's hypertension.[7] Asymptomatic patients with an elevated blood pressure do not require treatment in the prehospital setting.

Starting with the primary assessment for a patient with a hypertensive emergency, the patient's airway may need to be suctioned or secured to protect it from aspiration if the patient presents with a seizure or significantly decreased level of consciousness. Ventilatory support may be required if the patient is unconscious or presents with acute pulmonary edema. At a minimum, supplemental oxygen should be administered to help the delivery of oxygen to potentially ischemic tissues. Circulatory support with intravenous fluids is generally not necessary in patients who present with hypertension. Administration of glucose to a hypoglycemic patient may improve altered mental status if it is caused by the hypoglycemia.

Patients exhibiting symptoms and signs of heart failure should be treated with nitrates. Nitrates can be administered either sublingually by tablet or spray, topically with paste, or intravenously. Nitrates cause venodilation, which may decrease the patient's blood pressure. Supplemental oxygen can improve the sensation of dyspnea and improve the delivery of oxygen to the heart.

From a neurological standpoint, supplying supplemental oxygen may again provide additional oxygen to potentially ischemic tissues. Acute decrease in the patient's blood pressure may unintentionally decrease the cerebral perfusion pressure below the point required for blood flow to the brain, worsening cerebral ischemia and edema that may be present. Some medical control authorities may direct their Paramedics to utilize either nitrates or beta-adrenergic blocking medications (e.g., metoprolol or labetalol) to slowly decrease the patient's blood pressure. Although this will achieve the objective of lowering the patient's blood pressure, treating the blood pressure in this situation is controversial and is not performed in most EMS systems.

If the patient presents with a hypertensive urgency, defined as elevated blood pressure and risk factors for end-organ damage, there is no role for acute treatment of the blood pressure in the prehospital setting. The Paramedic should treat the primary medical condition if appropriate, and offer transportation to the emergency department for a more detailed assessment of the patient's health.

If pre-eclampsia or eclampsia are present, the patient should be given an infusion of 4 grams of magnesium sulfate over 10 to 15 minutes to treat the effects of these conditions.

The Paramedic reassesses Mr. Wilson during transport. His blood pressure after the administration of three sublingual nitroglycerine tablets is 200/120. His headache is unchanged; however, his chest pressure has resolved. A repeat 12-lead ECG shows that the precordial R waves remain tall; however, the inverted T waves in the anterolateral leads have resolved and are now upright. This heightens the Paramedic's suspicion of cardiovascular disease. A lingering concern about a cerebral hemorrhage prompts the Paramedic not to administer aspirin. The rationale is documented in the patient care record.

CRITICAL THINKING QUESTIONS

1. What are some of the predictable complications associated with hypertensive emergency?
2. What are some of the predictable complications associated with the treatments for hypertensive emergency?

Evaluation

During transport, the Paramedic should continually monitor and reassess the patient. A sudden drop in the patient's blood pressure may indicate a rupture of the thoracic aorta. For patients with altered mental status, the Paramedic should continually monitor the airway and ventilation, intervening when appropriate to protect the airway or support ventilation. Intubated patients should be monitored during transport with waveform capnography to ensure correct placement of the endotracheal tube and serve as another means of monitoring the patient's ventilation and perfusion. The vital signs should be reassessed after treatments, paying close attention to the patient's blood pressure. If there is any concern that the blood pressure requires treatment, it is suggested that on-line medical control is consulted to develop an appropriate treatment plan.

CASE STUDY CONCLUSION

At the emergency department, report is given and the concern regarding the cerebral hemorrhage is shared with the nurse. When the Paramedics return later that day with another patient, they catch up with the emergency physician taking care of Mr. Wilson for follow-up. Mr. Wilson had a small cerebral hemorrhage in the occipital lobe of his brain, which accounted for the vision loss, and he had mild heart failure. This all occurred from the sudden increase in his blood pressure after he ran out of his antihypertensive medication. His blood pressure was lowered in the ED to a systolic blood pressure of between 180 and 190 mmHg, representing a 20% to 25% decrease which is the target for acute emergency department management of a hypertensive emergency.[8] He is in the process of admission to a telemetry floor bed for observation of both his heart and brain and will undergo an MRI of his brain the following day.

CRITICAL THINKING QUESTIONS

1. What is the most appropriate transport decision that will get the patient to definitive care?
2. What are the advantages of transporting a patient with hypertensive emergency to a stroke center, even if that means bypassing other hospitals in the process?

Disposition

Patients who have problems that require airway management or ventilatory support should be brought to the closest emergency department for stabilization and treatment. Patients who have a hypertensive emergency should also be brought to the nearest emergency department. If the Paramedic's evaluation determines that the patient has an ST-elevation myocardial infarction, the patient should be transported to a facility capable of treating that patient with angioplasty unless the transport distance is too great. In that case, the patient should be brought to the local hospital while preparations are made to transfer the patient to a tertiary care center. Patients exhibiting signs of a stroke should also be transported to a stroke center unless transport time is excessive. Patients with asymptomatic hypertension can be transported to any emergency department for evaluation and appropriate treatment.

CONCLUSION

Hypertension is a common condition that is insidious in onset. Although many of the complications of hypertension are preventable, most develop because patients do not suspect they have a problem with their blood pressure. Many patients access the emergency medical system when either their blood pressure is elevated or when they develop symptoms as discussed in the chapter. Although blood pressure control is a long-term goal, in the vast majority of patients, aggressive reduction in a patient's blood pressure, both in the ambulance and in the emergency department, has the potential to do more harm than good.

KEY POINTS:

- A significant number of people see a physician or visit an emergency department for hypertension-related conditions.

- Hypertension is a risk factor for cardiovascular disease, stroke, and renal disease.

- Hypertension alters the cerebral perfusion pressure, leading to ischemic disease of the brain.

- Systemic hypertension causes the left ventricle to hypertrophy, creating a risk for dysrhythmias, altered contractility, and rupture.

- Hypertension changes the blood flow within the kidney, reducing filtration.

- Other risk factors associated with hypertension include aortic aneurysms, peripheral vascular disease, peripheral nerve damage, and erectile dysfunction.

- Noncompliance with medications is often the basis for an EMS call.

- Three categories exist for hypertension calls:
  - Hypertensive emergency
  - Acute hypertensive episode
  - Hypertensive urgency

- An acute change in blood flow within the brain due to hypertension is termed hypertensive encephalopathy.

- Hypertension can lead to an MI, with Non-STEMI being more common.

- By creating an increased peripheral vascular resistance, left-sided heart failure is common, presenting with pulmonary edema but without chest pain or pressure.

- Shear forces increase in the face of elevated blood pressure, leading to aortic aneurysm rupture.

- Hypertension is implicated in three complications of pregnancy.

- History of the present illness should include questions regarding end-organ damage in the cardiovascular, neurologic, and renal systems.

- When gathering the patient's past medical history, the Paramedic should ask specifically about hypertension plus diabetes mellitus, cardiovascular disease, renal insufficiency, aneurysm, or stroke.

- As in taking a history, after the initial exam, further examinations should focus on the cardiovascular, neurological, and renal systems.

- Treatment of hypertensive calls focuses upon the patient's ABCs and conditions associated with the hypertension as opposed to reducing the pressure.

- The Paramedic should consult medical control for orders to treat the patient's blood pressure.

- Unless the patient presents with a STEMI or stroke, the patient can be transported to the closest emergency department.

REVIEW QUESTIONS:

1. How does hypertension place a patient at risk for cardiovascular disease? Stroke? Renal disease?

2. Differentiate hypertensive emergency from acute hypertensive episode from hypertensive urgency.

3. How does hypertensive encephalopathy manifest?

4. Regarding the history of the current complaint, what questions should the Paramedic ask about cardiac-related symptoms? Neurologic symptoms? Renal symptoms?

5. Describe exam clues of end-organ damage in the cardiovascular system, neurological system, and renal system.

CASE STUDY QUESTIONS:

Please refer to the Case Study in this chapter, and answer the questions below:

1. Name at least two reasons why Mr. Wilson may have been noncompliant with his medications.

2. What is the relationship of the visual change that Mr. Wilson exhibits and the treatment protocols common to his history and exam?

REFERENCES:

1. Center for Disease Control, National Center for Health Statistics web site. Available at: **http://www.cdc.gov/nchs/fastats/hyprtens.htm**. Accessed March 24, 2008.

2. American Heart Association. Statistical fact sheet: high blood pressure statistics. Available at: **http://www.americanheart.org/downloadable/heart/1199892787721FS14HBP08.pdf**. Accessed March 24, 2008.

3. Chobanian AV, Bakris GL, Black HR, et al. Seventh report of the Joint National Committee on Prevention, Detection, Evaluation, and Treatment of High Blood Pressure. *Hypertension*. 2003;42(6):1206–1252.

4. Wu M, Chanmugam A. Hypertension. In Tintinalli J, Kelen GD, and Stapczynski JS, eds. *Emergency Medicine a Comprehensive Study Guide,* sixth edition. New York: McGraw-Hill; 2004.

5. Hebert CJ, Vidt DG. Hypertensive crises. *Prim Care*. 2008;35(3):475–487, vi.

6. Gifford, RW, Jr., Westbrook E. Hypertensive encephalopathy: mechanisms, clinical features, and treatment. *Prog Cardiovasc Dis*. 1974;17(2):115–124.

7. American College of Emergency Physicians Clinical Policies Subcommittee on Asymptomatic Hypertension. Clinical policy: critical issues in the evaluation and management of adult patients with asymptomatic hypertension in the emergency department. *Ann Emerg Med*. 2006;47:237–249.

8. McCowan C. Hypertensive emergencies. Available at: **http://www.emedicine.com/emerg/topic267.htm**. Accessed March 24, 2008.

CHAPTER 26

DISORDERS OF THE HEAD, EYES, EARS, NOSE, AND THROAT

KEY CONCEPTS:

Upon completion of this chapter, it is expected that the reader will understand these following concepts:

- That abnormalities of the head, eyes, ears, nose, and throat may be traumatically induced or medically caused
- That careful questioning and assessment is necessary to determine if the patient's complaint indicates a serious underlying condition

ANATOMY CONCEPTS:

Prior to reading this chapter the Paramedic student should be familiar with the following anatomy and physiology concepts:

- Anatomy of the head, eyes, ears, nose, and throat
- Physiology of sight and hearing

CASE STUDY:

On a particularly busy Thursday afternoon, dispatch for City Ambulance Corporation simultaneously dispatches two ambulances to opposite sides of the city. The first is called to a city office building for a 36-year-old woman with dizziness. The second is requested at the home of a 63-year-old man with 20 minutes of uncontrolled heavy nosebleed. Unit 468 responds to the office building while Unit 476 travels to a residential neighborhood for the nosebleed.

CRITICAL THINKING QUESTIONS

1. What are some of the possible nonneurological causes of vertigo?
2. How is dizziness related to a nosebleed?

OVERVIEW

The Paramedic commonly encounters disorders of the head, eyes, ears, nose, and throat (further abbreviated HEENT), resulting either from trauma or from other medical causes. The presentation of a patient with an HEENT disorder can be related to a serious underlying medical condition or a new focal problem that is self-limited. The Paramedic serves an important role in providing initial stabilization and treatment, and is able to describe and manage early and evolving symptoms if and when they progress. Because of the potential for airway compromise, loss of sight or hearing, or brain injury, the Paramedic should undertake management of HEENT emergencies with great care and a high sense of urgency.

Chief Concern

The regions of the head and neck are anatomically and physiologically complex. In fact, they are so complex that at least six different medical specialties exist to care for specific areas of the head and neck. Although a complete review of this complex anatomy is beyond the scope of this chapter, it is important to be familiar with its basic anatomical terms and regions, as well as physical exam techniques for assessing the head, ears, eyes, nose, and throat. This chapter will highlight specific methods of evaluation as they pertain to individual disorders and diagnoses.

The various systems of the head and neck, while closely associated anatomically, are very different from each other functionally. However, there is significant overlap between symptoms (i.e., between the ear and throat, or between the eyes and cranium). Therefore, when a patient complains of a particular symptom or exhibits a specific sign, it is important for the Paramedic to carefully consider how those symptoms could be related to other systems within the head or neck.

Head

Headache is an extremely common complaint among emergency department patients, representing approximately 2% to 4% of all ED visits.[1] Since many of these patients use prehospital services as a means of access to the healthcare system, the Paramedic must be familiar with certain headache characteristics in order to appropriately treat and disposition the patient. A patient with a headache may be suffering from a condition as benign as a cluster or tension headache, but due consideration must be given to the potential that the patient is experiencing a catastrophic event such as a subarachnoid hemorrhage (SAH) or another significant intracranial disorder (tumor, infection, etc.). Certain historical clues, as will be discussed later in this chapter, may help differentiate these potentially life-threatening causes of headache from the benign causes.

Ear

Earache is a frequent complaint, especially in the pediatric population. Most commonly the cause of an earache is infection, either as **otitis media** (middle ear infection) or **otitis externa** (outer ear infection). However, the presence of a foreign body; rupture of the tympanic membrane from trauma, pressure, or infection; and the presence of a tumor can all lead to earache and should be considered by the Paramedic when infection is less likely. **Tinnitus** (ringing in the ears) may accompany an earache and may be a sign of trauma, medication overdose, or increased pressure from fluid in the middle ear.

Dizziness is another common complaint. Although it may not be a patient's chief concern, it may be associated with the chief concern. It is estimated that up to 30% of patients over the age of 65 will complain of dizziness at some time.[2] Dizziness can be very difficult to manage because the term "dizzy" is defined in different ways by different patients. One person may define dizziness as a sense of loss of balance, whereas another describes lightheadedness, and yet another senses the room spinning around (a condition known as vertigo). Because of the variety of definitions for a common term, it is important to elicit the precise meaning from the patient in order to form a correct differential diagnosis and initiate appropriate treatment.

To understand the origins of dizziness, the Paramedic must understand the neuroanatomy that pertains to balance. The vestibular system, which is part of cranial nerve VIII, is responsible for providing information to the brain on one's location in space and orientation. Disruption of this system, either from mechanical forces (e.g., a spinning amusement park ride) or from physiological causes (e.g., dehydration, vertigo, or infection), can give the patient the feeling of spinning.

Vertigo is the term used to describe an abnormal sense of motion, often but not always of a spinning nature. A typical scenario is a middle-aged patient who is unable to get out of bed because the room seems to be spinning around, causing the patient to become "motion sick" whenever he attempts to move.

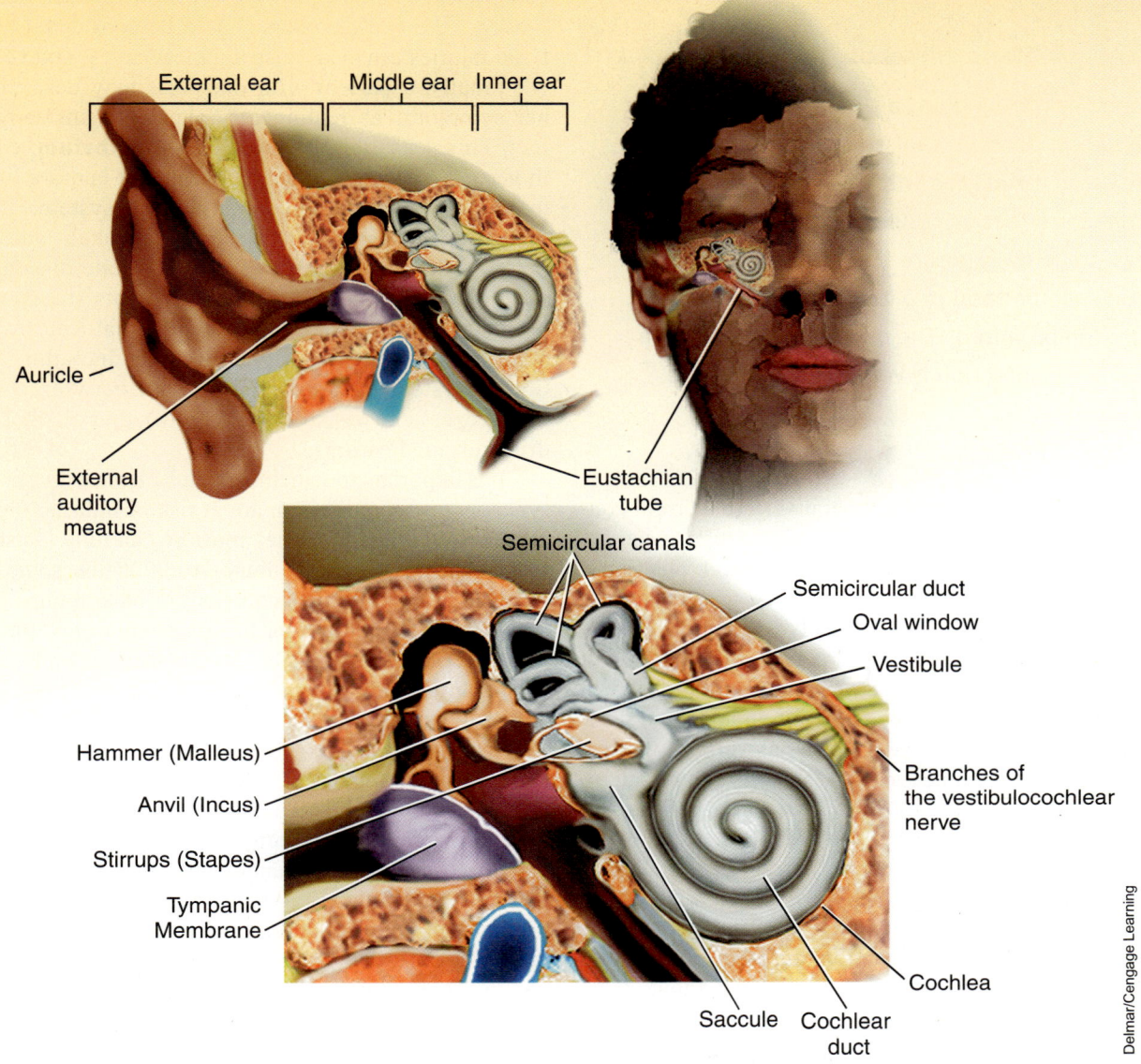

External ear   Middle ear   Inner ear

Auricle

External
auditory
meatus

Eustachian
tube

Semicircular canals

Semicircular duct

Oval window

Vestibule

Hammer (Malleus)

Anvil (Incus)

Stirrups (Stapes)

Tympanic
Membrane

Branches of
the vestibulocochlear
nerve

Cochlea

Saccule   Cochlear
duct

Delmar/Cengage Learning

Figure 26-1   The vestibular organs in the inner ear are responsible for balance.

Vertigo as a condition can be either benign or serious, depending on the origin and characteristics of the symptoms. Patients with **peripheral vertigo** have vertigo because of their vestibular organs located in the inner ear (Figure 26-1), whereas patients with **central vertigo** suffer from disorders of the central nervous system and tend to have a poorer prognosis.

The distinction between the two types of vertigo can be difficult to ascertain. Certain historical questions, however, can give clues to the origin. Patients with peripheral vertigo typically complain of sudden onset of symptoms, usually quite severe and debilitating, and frequently associated with nausea, vomiting, and occasional hearing loss.[3] By contrast, central vertigo is generally gradual in onset, chronic and continuous, and usually not associated with nausea or vomiting.[4] Although these characteristics are by no means exclusive

enough to place a patient in one category or another, they do serve as guiding principles when triaging and treating a patient (Table 26-1).

Table 26-1   Peripheral versus Central Vertigo

	Peripheral	**Central**
Onset	Sudden	Gradual
Intensity	Moderate to intense	Usually less intense but poorly defined
Associated Symptoms	Occasional hearing loss/ tinnitus, nausea/vomiting	Varies; usually less associated symptoms
CNS Signs/ Symptoms	Absent	Usually present

Three specific causes of peripheral vertigo warrant consideration: benign paroxysmal positional vertigo, Ménière disease, and labyrinthitis. **Benign paroxysmal positional vertigo (BPPV)** is vertigo that occurs due to a change in head position. Although it usually resolves when the head is moved to a different position, it can persist after the motion ceases. As the name suggests, it is a benign condition but can cause extremely uncomfortable symptoms and may not seem benign to the patient. **Ménière disease** has vertigo, tinnitus (ringing in the ears), and hearing loss as a symptom pattern. This is due to an abnormality in the circulation of fluid in the inner ear, and may occur up to several times per week. **Labyrinthitis** is an inflammatory response in the inner ear which causes rapid onset of vertigo symptoms that slowly resolve within a few hours to days. It may follow an upper respiratory infection or may occur in an otherwise healthy adult. Symptoms typically resolve completely without recurrence. It is almost impossible to distinguish between most causes of vertigo in the early phases, and this distinction should be made by the treating physician in the receiving ED. However, any patient complaining of vertigo should be carefully observed by the Paramedic for signs of worsening symptoms or mental status changes.

Although vertigo is a specific complaint along the "dizziness" spectrum, there are multiple other potential causes of dizziness. Again, it is important for the Paramedic to adequately define the complaint of dizziness in order to understand these causes. Some patients may describe their symptoms as lightheadedness or feeling faint, as if they are going to pass out. Medically, this is called **pre-syncope** or **near-syncope**.[5] Although the patient may not actually pass out, there is an indication for the Paramedic to search for the cause in order to prevent a syncopal episode.

Cardiac dysrhythmias, dehydration, alcohol, certain medications (including aspirin, diuretics, antihypertensives, antidepressants, and hypoglycemic agents), and impaired blood flow as occurs with carotid artery narrowing are all potential sources of pre-syncopal or near-syncopal episodes, and as such should be considered in the patient complaining of lightheadedness. Since pre-syncope can deteriorate into syncope, the two disorders should be considered the same. Head injuries can also cause lightheadedness and vertigo.

Finally, a patient with dizziness may describe his or her symptoms as feeling off-balance or unsteady on the feet. This sensation, known as **disequilibrium**, can occur in vertigo or pre-syncopal episodes, but is more likely due to abnormalities in the central nervous system, especially the cerebellum. Tumor, ischemia (stroke), and hemorrhage in the cerebellum can all precipitate disequilibrium and should be considered in any patients stating they are unsteady on their feet. Other potential causes include abnormalities of the peripheral nerves including the vestibular system; lack of coordination between the visual input (eyes) and visual center (brain); and alcohol, certain drugs, or medications.[6]

It is important to remember that patients with vertigo, pre-syncope, or disequilibrium are at risk of injuring themselves or others, and therefore they must be carefully assisted so as to prevent a secondary injury. Additionally, some patients involved in motor vehicle collisions or other trauma may give a history of dizziness prior to loss of control of the vehicle. This information should be documented and relayed to the receiving ED staff.

Eye

Blurred vision, eye pain, foreign body presence, and redness are common concerns regarding the eye that can range in severity from simple **conjunctivitis** (also known as pink eye) to corneal abrasion and acute angle-closure glaucoma. It is not necessarily important for EMS personnel to make a diagnosis of these conditions, but it is important to recognize that many untreated ocular disorders can be sight-threatening and therefore must be taken seriously. Blunt or penetrating trauma to the eye is an obvious threat to one's vision, but other medical causes of vision impairment should be understood in the absence of trauma.

A complaint of blurred vision is very nonspecific. Foreign body presence, infection, glaucoma, retinal detachment, corneal abrasion, and stroke are all known causes of blurred vision. Because this differential is so wide, it is important for the Paramedic to determine when the visual changes began, if one or both eyes are involved, and whether there are any associated symptoms. These historical clues will aid in narrowing down the Paramedical diagnosis. For instance, a patient complaining of blurred vision in the right eye may also complain of a scratching sensation in that eye and increased tear production. In this case, foreign body presence and corneal abrasion should be considered. In contrast, a patient with sudden painless loss of vision of the right eye may have suffered an acute retinal detachment in that eye. These historical details are important since treatments for these conditions differ significantly, with one requiring antibiotics and the other surgical correction.

Time of onset is of particular importance. Blurred vision that has gradually commenced or worsened (days to weeks) is more frequently related to underlying medical problems and may be less urgent. Acute blurred or loss of vision suggests a more emergent condition. Retinal detachment is one condition that occurs suddenly and requires urgent specialist intervention. Another more common problem is acute angle-closure glaucoma.[7] In **acute angle-closure glaucoma**, the pressure within the eye increases rapidly and dramatically and can cause dysfunction of the optic nerve, leading to permanent loss of vision. This is not to be confused with chronic glaucoma in which the eye pressure is chronically elevated but does not cause sudden visual loss. Although the end result may be the same, a small chronic elevation in eye pressure is less threatening than a sudden increase in pressure. The patient who develops acute glaucoma typically complains of a painful, occasionally red eye with a "mid-dilated pupil." In other words, the pupil is neither constricted nor dilated and does not react to light (Figure 26-2). If this is suspected, the Paramedic should transport the patient in a supine position to the emergency department without patches or other covering over the eye.[8]

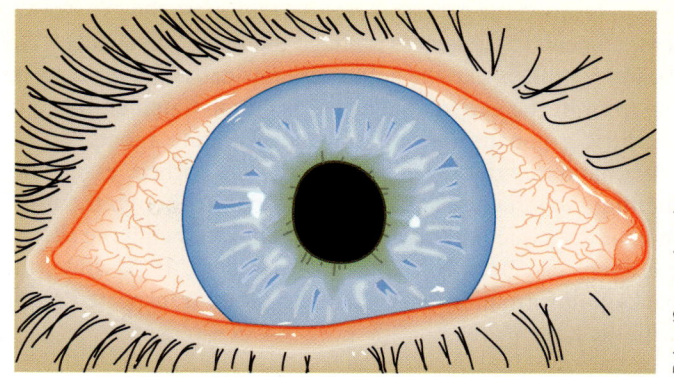
Figure 26-2 Mid-dilated pupil as seen in acute angle-closure glaucoma.

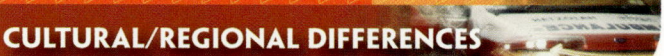
CULTURAL/REGIONAL DIFFERENCES

Glaucoma is the primary cause of blindness among African Americans.

Abrasion of the cornea can cause significant pain and irritation to the eye. Most patients with corneal abrasion can recall a sensation of a foreign body that may remain at the time the patient calls for service. Because the abrasion is a scratch on the outer layer of the eye, it distorts the way light travels through the cornea to reach the back of the eye, much like a scratch on a lens or glass. This distortion leads to a sense of blurred vision. Corneal abrasions are rarely emergent conditions unless there is the possibility that a foreign body is still embedded within the eye. Paramedics may be able to examine the eye using fluorescein dye and a Wood's lamp (ultraviolet light). An abrasion in the cornea will absorb the dye and appear green on examination under the ultraviolet light (Figure 26-3). If a foreign body is seen at that time, it should be left in place until ED personnel are able to remove it. These patients will require antibiotics.

Blurred vision may also be a sign of an underlying medical condition. When this is suspected, it is important for the Paramedic to ask the patient about other symptoms. Some patients with migraines may have a specific type called **ocular migraines**. These patients may experience intense headache, nausea, and vomiting along with blurred vision or even blindness. Most patients will be able to inform the Paramedic that these symptoms are typical of their migraines. Dizziness and blurred vision may be signs of dehydration or pre-syncope. Unilateral blurred vision

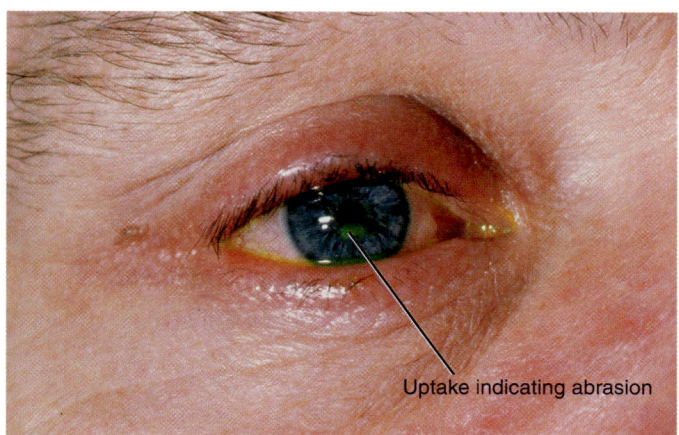
Uptake indicating abrasion

Figure 26-3 Corneal abrasion as seen under ultraviolet light (Wood's lamp) following fluorescein staining.

associated with facial weakness or other neurologic deficits may be an indicator of TIA or stroke and should be considered in the differential diagnosis in patients with risk factors. Hyperglycemia is another medical condition that may cause blurred vision.

Chemical irritation of the eyes can range from simple irritation to vision loss and even physical necrosis (decay) of the eye. Many people who use chemicals as part of their work or hobbies will wear protective goggles, but even these are imperfect in completely eliminating the risk of chemical exposure. Most of the time these patients will know the names of the chemicals involved and will be able to provide a material safety data sheet (MSDS) with relevant information regarding the treatment of eye injuries. This is not always the case, however, and is certainly not likely when the exposure occurs outside of a routine use of chemicals. In addition, household items and environmental agents are a common source of exposure and may not be readily identifiable at the time of injury.

In general, chemical irritants are classified as either alkali or acidic. This distinction is extremely important as it

Disorders of the Head, Eyes, Ears, Nose, and Throat **541**

will determine the potential extent of injury to the eye. Acidic irritants tend to cause less damage than alkaline agents.[9] The reason for this is that the acidic irritants cause the proteins on the front of the eye to coagulate, or clump together, preventing further penetration into the eye. Alkaline agents, on the other hand, rapidly penetrate through the cornea, essentially melting the structures as it burns deeper. Although the treatment is the same for both of these agents, knowing the chemical agent can help guide patient treatment. If possible, the package information or MSDS should be transported along with the patient.

Nose

Epistaxis, commonly referred to as nosebleed, can occur for a variety of reasons, and can range in severity from simple oozing of blood to heavy arterial hemorrhaging. Most people will experience nosebleed at some point in their lifetime, but the majority will have self-limited bleeding that does not require emergency services.[10] For those patients who do, however, it is important for the Paramedic to determine the severity of the bleeding, protect the airway, and control the bleeding.

The first distinction that must be made is whether the bleeding is due to trauma or nontrauma causes. In those patients who have epistaxis as a result of trauma, there is a high likelihood for other injuries, including facial fractures and head injuries. These patients may need immobilization and/or airway control, depending on the mechanism of injury. Most of the time a single direct blow to the nose causes the bleeding, but occasionally there are other significant facial injuries. Since blood in the nasal passages will drip posteriorly when a patient is supine, great care must be taken to ensure the patient does not aspirate the blood, especially if the patient's mental status is altered. Suction should be readily available and used frequently as needed.

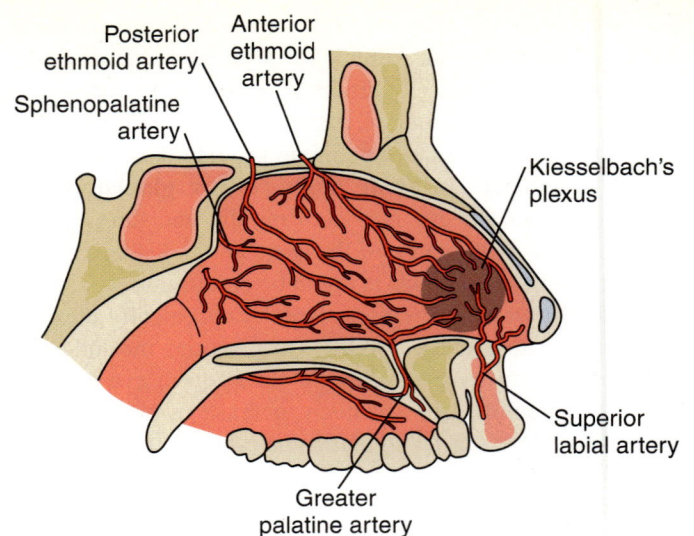

Figure 26-4 Cross-section of the nasal passage showing the location of Kiesselbach's plexus (anterior epistaxis) and the sphenopalatine artery (posterior epistaxis).

Spontaneous epistaxis is usually divided into two categories: anterior nasal bleeding and posterior nasal bleeding, with the majority being anterior. The most common causes of bleeding in spontaneous epistaxis are nose-picking, infection, and dried nasal passages.[11,12] The source of the bleeding may be difficult to determine without direct visualization inside the nasal passages. However, although it may be permissible to gently look inside the nose to evaluate the source of bleeding, it is preferable in the prehospital setting to attempt to control the bleeding without searching deeply for the source.

Anterior nosebleeds are usually going to occur as a result of bleeding at a specific vascular plexus (collection of small blood vessels) called Kiesselbach's plexus (Figure 26-4). The source of bleeding in this case is usually under low pressure, even though the bleeding may be heavy.

Posterior bleeding, on the other hand, is usually the result of bleeding from the sphenopalatine artery in the posterior nasal passage. Posterior bleeding may be under high pressure and very difficult to control in the prehospital setting. These patients are at risk of airway compromise and significant hemorrhaging, potentially resulting in shock.[13]

Throat

Throat pain is not as common as other issues in the prehospital setting. Causes of sore throat can range in severity from simple viral or bacterial infections to more severe conditions including peritonsillar abscess, Ludwig's angina, retropharyngeal abscesses, and epiglottitis. Ludwig's angina and retropharyngeal abscess are potentially fatal and

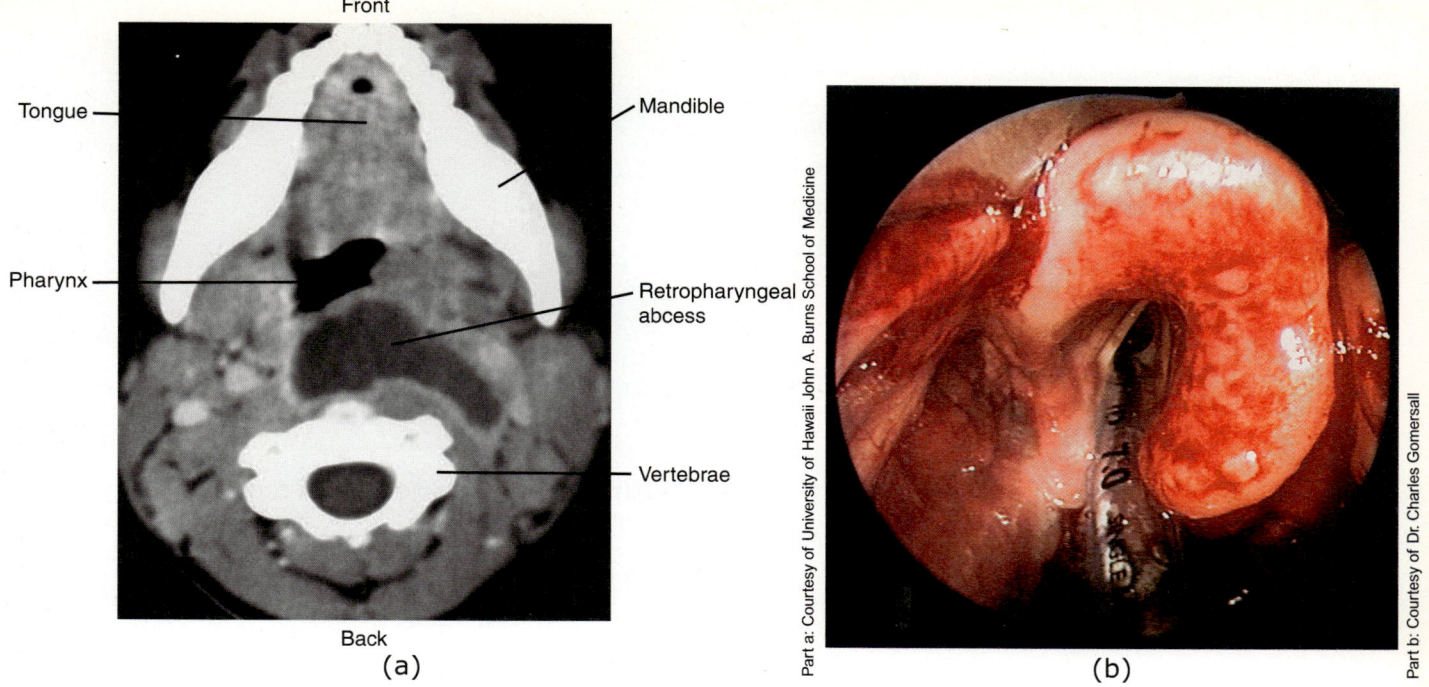

Front

Tongue

Pharynx

Back

(a)

Mandible

Retropharyngeal abcess

Vertebrae

Part a: Courtesy of University of Hawaii John A. Burns School of Medicine

Part b: Courtesy of Dr. Charles Gomersall

(b)

Figure 26-5 (a) Retropharyngeal abscess (b) epiglottitis.

may cause rapid airway compromise. What may seem like a routine sore throat could become an airway emergency in a very short period of time, so the Paramedic must be familiar with these symptoms in order to act quickly and accurately to establish airway control.

A **peritonsillar abscess** forms in the posterior tissues of the mouth around the tonsil and occurs as an extension of a bacterial infection involving the tonsil. The abscess can be seen during examination of the mouth as fullness in the 2 o'clock or 10 o'clock position that protrudes into the mouth, moving the uvula to the opposite side and displacing the tonsil downward.

A **retropharyngeal abscess** is a bacterial infection located in the soft tissue between the pharynx and vertebrae (Figure 26-5a). Since it is behind the pharyngeal wall, it is not visible on routine examination of the pharynx.[14] Although it has traditionally been a disease of children, there have recently been increasing cases of retropharyngeal abscess in adult patients. The hallmark symptoms are sore throat, fever, trouble swallowing, muffled voice, and stiff neck. This latter symptom is due to the fact that the pocket of infection is located directly in front of the cervical spine, and movement of the neck stretches and moves the prevertebral tissue, causing pain. Patients therefore attempt to avoid exacerbating their symptoms by holding their head and neck in slight flexion and as still as possible. A rare complication of retropharyngeal abscess is

extension into the pharynx or even erosion into the nearby spine or carotid arteries.

Epiglottitis, like retropharyngeal abscess, was once a disease seen almost exclusively in children, but now occurs much less frequently in children and more frequently in adults. It has become exceptionally rare in recent years, owing to the widespread use of certain vaccines in children. The primary pathophysiology involves infection and inflammation of the epiglottis, leading to swelling and potential obstruction of the airway (Figure 26-5b). The classic triad of symptoms described in children are drooling, dysphagia (trouble swallowing), and respiratory distress. Additional symptoms may include fever and sore throat. These may or may not be seen in adult patients presenting with epiglottitis, and a muffled voice accompanying sore throat may be the only clue to the diagnosis.

Ludwig's angina is a severe complication of dental infections that causes swelling of the floor of the mouth and neck and potential airway compromise. This condition involves the spread of bacteria from the infected tooth or teeth along the tissue planes in the floor of the mouth (Figure 26-6). Patients usually complain of swelling, pain, difficulty swallowing, and difficulty breathing. In addition, the tongue may be elevated on physical exam owing to the swollen tissues at the base. Ludwig's angina can rapidly progress and occlude the airway within a matter of several hours.

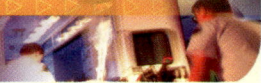
Maintenance of the airway is important in throat complaints. The Paramedic should intubate the patient only when absolutely necessary to avoid an increase in swelling or cause bleeding into the airway that cannot be controlled.

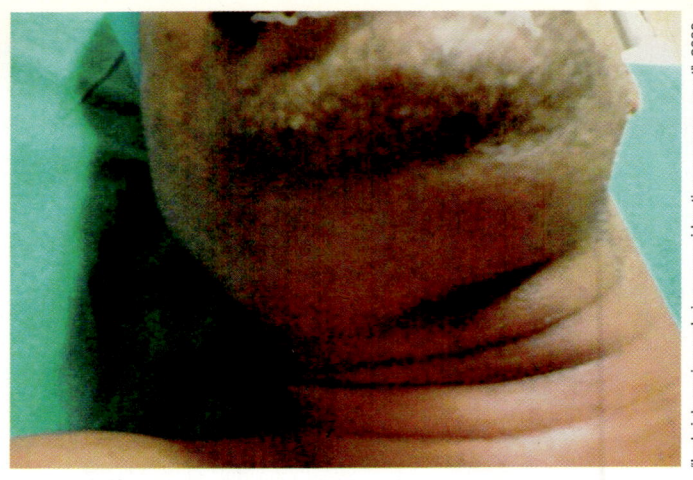

"Ludwig's angina and airway considerations: a case report", 2008 Kulkarni et al; licensee BioMed Central Ltd. Used under a

Figure 26-6 Photograph of a patient with Ludwig's angina.

CASE STUDY (CONTINUED)

City Ambulance 468 arrives on-scene at the office building and is greeted by security. "Hello, I'm Officer Smith. Come with me, please." The Paramedics proceed down the hall behind the security officer. They arrive in a room and find a middle-aged Caucasian woman seated in a chair with a moist towel on her head and surrounded by coworkers. They introduce themselves to the patient, who then responds, "Oh, thank you so much for coming. I'm Angela Peabody and I've got this awful dizzy feeling. It feels as though the room is just spinning around me."

The Paramedics learn from Mrs. Peabody that her symptoms began that morning and have included the spinning sensation and nausea. She has never had these symptoms before and doesn't know how to make them go away, although they are worse when she moves and better when she keeps her head perfectly still. She wishes to go to a hospital for evaluation.

Meanwhile, across the city, the other Paramedics from Ambulance 476 arrive at their location and find a middle-aged Asian man seated in a lawn chair by the side of the road holding his nose.

"Hello there. We are with the ambulance and we understand you have a nosebleed."

"As a matter of fact, I do," replies Mr. Wang. "It started almost a half hour ago, and I can't seem to get it to stop. I've tried tilting my head back, leaning forward, and pinching my nose and it still seems to be oozing out of me whenever I let up pressure."

"Have you had any injury to your nose lately?" inquires the Paramedic.

"Not that I can recall. This just seemed to start out of the blue."

CRITICAL THINKING QUESTIONS

1. What are the important elements of the history that a Paramedic should obtain?
2. What is the symptom pattern for labyrinthitis?

History

Obtaining a good history of present illness in patients is important for patients with complaints regarding the head, ears, eyes, nose, and throat. Sometimes a patient will be forthcoming with information regarding the present condition. Other times, the Paramedic will have to direct the questioning in order to obtain the proper information. Using the OPQRST mnemonic helps the Paramedic avoid missing important details and historical clues about a patient's symptoms. Because disorders of the head, eyes, ears, nose, and throat are varied, specific historical clues have been discussed in the context of each of these disorders. However, there are some general principles that apply for all of these disorders.

Time and nature of onset are important for the Paramedic to determine early in the course of evaluation. Did the symptoms start suddenly or did they have a gradual onset? Have these symptoms persisted for several hours or are these symptoms that have been ongoing for days? These types of questions are important because the sudden onset of symptoms is frequently associated with conditions that have high morbidity and mortality.

For instance, subarachnoid hemorrhages frequently present with a sudden onset "thunderclap headache," and acute angle-closure glaucoma usually presents with sudden eye pain. In contrast, a sudden onset of vertigo is usually indicative of a benign peripheral cause as opposed to central causes (such as brain tumors or bleeds) that develop more gradually. Similarly, the duration of symptoms is important to know. A patient with a sore throat and trouble swallowing for a week, or a patient with blurred vision of one month's duration, are unlikely to have conditions that will rapidly deteriorate during transport.

Likewise, it is important to understand what the patient was doing at the time of symptom onset. Was the patient grinding metal when he noticed sharp pain in his eye? Was the patient blowing her nose when it began to bleed heavily? Knowing the context in which the symptoms began can provide important diagnostic information and can help direct early treatment.

Lastly, the Paramedic should determine whether or not a patient has had similar symptoms in the past, and what has been done for these symptoms. Many patients have chronic conditions that recur throughout their lifetimes; although the conditions are chronic, the patients still need to seek medical care. Simply asking the patient whether he or she has had any similar symptoms previously and how this episode compares to prior episodes can provide the Paramedic with insight into the nature of the condition and the methods of treatment. This is not to say that a recurrent condition should not be taken seriously. A patient may have recurrent tonsillitis that is usually managed with antibiotics, but in the present episode the patient may have developed a retropharyngeal abscess.

Past Medical History

A patient's past medical history is extremely important in managing the medical conditions. Although a patient's mental status or critical medical illness may prohibit the Paramedic from gathering the past medical history, this should be obtained as thoroughly as possible from family members and/or friends present at the scene. This is one area in which the prehospital professionals have an extremely important and

unique role. Many patients keep medication lists at home, either on the refrigerator, in a desk, or with their purses or wallets. The Paramedic should attempt to locate and transport a medication list—or the medications themselves—with the patient. This opportunity to be present in a patient's home and physically transport medications or a list is something that cannot be done once the patient has arrived in the emergency department.

A medication history and current medication list should be obtained from every patient, if possible. This would include not only the medications the patient is currently taking, but also any recent changes in medications. Changes in the type or dosing of a medication can cause changes in a patient's hemodynamic status or mental status, so these medication changes should be noted. For instance, a patient who presents with near syncope and has recently had an increase in metoprolol may be suffering from orthostatic hypotension related to a dose that is too high for that patient.

A patient with "dizziness" who has recently been taken off insulin may be hyperglycemic due to a medication change. A patient with altered mental status and pinpoint pupils who takes narcotic pain medications may have taken too many. Knowing the current medications is also important in patients with epistaxis. Patients who take anticoagulation (such as warfarin) or antiplatelet medications (such as aspirin or Plavix®), or who have a hereditary bleeding disorder such as hemophilia, are at greater risk of bleeding. Therefore, knowing that a patient is taking one or more of these medications or suffers from such a chronic condition can help the Paramedic understand why a particular bleeding event will not stop, and will help guide management once the patient has arrived at the emergency department.[15]

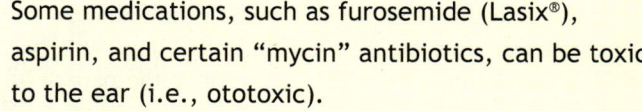

STREET SMART

Some medications, such as furosemide (Lasix®), aspirin, and certain "mycin" antibiotics, can be toxic to the ear (i.e., ototoxic).

Although acute allergic reactions and anaphylaxis are discussed in Chapter 30, it is important to note that airway obstruction and compromise from anaphylaxis or angioedema can occur as a result of medications. The ACE inhibitors are notorious for causing angioedema, and certain antibiotics are common sources of allergic anaphylaxis. Knowing whether or not a patient is taking these medications can help a Paramedic determine why a patient has a particular reaction and how it can be reversed.

The Paramedic asks Mrs. Peabody about other medical problems. "I don't have any medical problems, other than high cholesterol, and that has been controlled for years with diet and exercise. I don't take any medications right now. I did have tubes put in my ears as a child, but that was years ago."

Meanwhile, the other Paramedics are controlling Mr. Wang's nosebleed with direct pressure as they prepare to place him in their ambulance. Once they are situated and start driving to the hospital, the Paramedic asks Mr. Wang about his past medical history.

"I have a history of atrial fibrillation and I take Coumadin for that. I also have high blood pressure, for which I take a water pill, and metoprolol."

Mrs. Peabody is en route to City Hospital aboard Ambulance 468. While en route, the Paramedic examines her pupils and finds them to be reactive and equal. He tests her external ocular muscles and notes them to be equal bilaterally. He performs a brief neuro exam with no focal deficits elicited. Mrs. Peabody's blood sugar is 85 mg/dL.

The other Paramedic across town is examining Mr. Wang on Ambulance 476 by looking in both nostrils as best she can with a penlight. She notes bleeding in the right nare that seems to be oozing from the upper part of the nasal septum. She examines the pharynx to find a little blood dripping down the back of the patient's throat, but not causing any airway compromise.

CRITICAL THINKING QUESTIONS

1. What are the elements of the physical examination of a patient with labyrinthitis?
2. What are the elements of the physical examination of a patient with epistaxis?

Examination

Even though the conditions discussed in this chapter are isolated to the neck and above, it is imperative for the Paramedic to perform an adequate physical examination on all patients. This would include not only the pertinent systems involved, but also the heart and lungs on all patients.

As in all emergency exams, attention should be given first to airway, breathing, and circulation. There is nothing more important in caring for emergency patients than a patent airway, and this must be determined immediately upon the patient examination. For the majority of patients with HEENT complaints, this will be easy since the patient will usually be able to speak to the Paramedic and describe details of the conditions. If a patient is able to do this, then it can be accurately determined that—at present—the airway is patent. However, since many of these conditions, including epistaxis, retropharyngeal abscess, and Ludwig's angina, can rapidly deteriorate and cause airway obstruction, the airway must be constantly yet gently reassessed in order to be sure there is no decline in patency. In children with epiglottitis, there should be no attempt to visualize inside the mouth unless the child is in severe respiratory distress or not breathing. Otherwise, upsetting a child too much can cause the child to cry, which could lead to further swelling of the epiglottis and obstruction.[16]

Breathing and circulation are the next priority in examinations. These have been discussed previously in the chapter in regard to their specific conditions, and the reader should refer to them as necessary. A patient who is at risk for C-spine precautions should have them taken early in the course of management.

The patient's mental status should also be taken into consideration when evaluating patients with potential head trauma or other HEENT disorders. Again, the majority of patients will have normal mental status, but underlying medical conditions and serious complications of HEENT disorders such as infection, injury, medications, and shock can predispose a patient to having an altered mental status. Awareness of vital signs and continued vigilance for airway compromise should be maintained throughout transport in a patient with altered mental status.

The major focus of the Paramedic's exam for most HEENT conditions will involve assessing for symmetry. Since the structures on the head and face are usually roughly symmetrical in most patients, evaluating for a specific complaint should include an assessment of symmetry between the two sides. Any deviation from symmetry should be documented and should be considered in context of the patient's symptoms. For example, a patient complaining of right eye pain who has redness of the sclera and sluggish or absent pupillary response on penlight exam should raise suspicion for acute angle-closure glaucoma. Even patients with more general symptoms like weakness and "dizziness" should have a careful assessment for symmetry, as abnormal facial features may be a clue to an underlying TIA or stroke. Check the blood sugar on patients who complain of dizziness or blurred vision as these may indicate hypo- or hyperglycemia.[17–19]

Specific components of the physical exam pertaining to HEENT exams include examination of the ears using an otoscope and of the eyes using an ophthalmoscope and fluorescein staining.

An **otoscope** is an instrument used to evaluate the inside of the ear canal (Figure 26-7). It is usually outfitted with a battery-powered light source and magnifier through which one may examine the canal. A disposable plastic speculum is placed on the end to allow a closer look inside. The examiner must be extremely cautious not to push in too far, as careless examining could lead to trauma to the external or even middle ear canal.

The **ophthalmoscope**, used to examine the posterior wall of the eye, contains a series of different magnifying lenses on a disc through which the examiner can view the retina at different degrees of focus (Figure 26-8a). In particular, the Paramedic is looking for crisp margins of the optic disc and normal color of the retina—usually a yellow/orange (Figure 26-8b). The ophthalmoscopic exam can be very difficult unless the patient's pupils are dilated, and care should not be delayed pending an exam in the ambulance. Few ophthalmic emergencies will require a prehospital funduscopic examination. In contrast, inspecting for corneal abrasions using fluorescein staining of the eye may be useful in the prehospital setting.

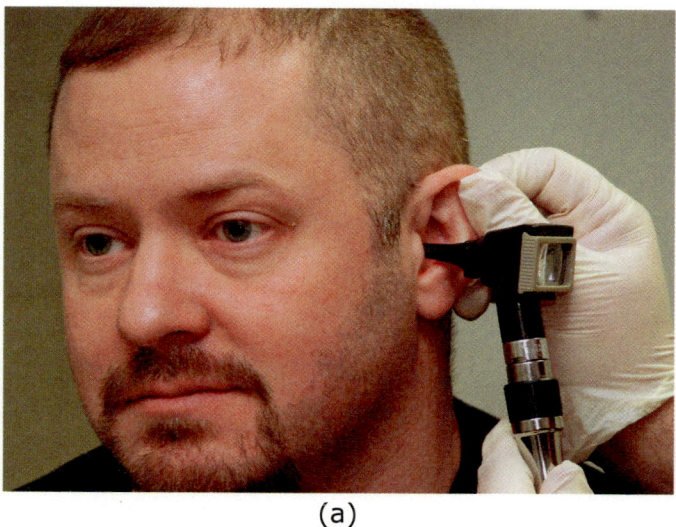
(a)

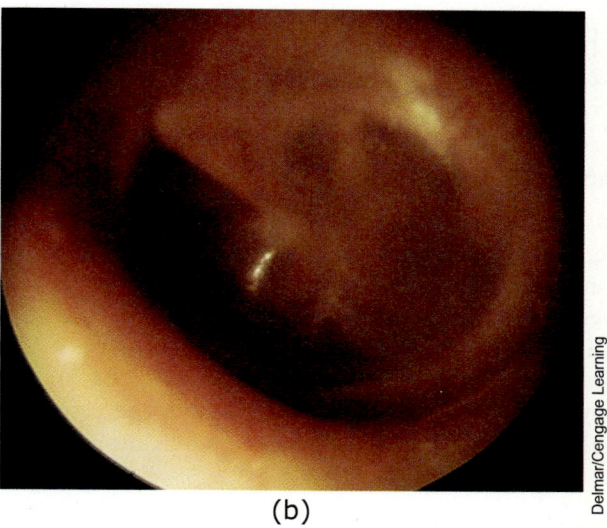
(b)

Delmar/Cengage Learning

Figure 26-7 (a) The otoscope is used to examine the patient's ear canal. (b) Appearance of a healthy tympanic membrane.

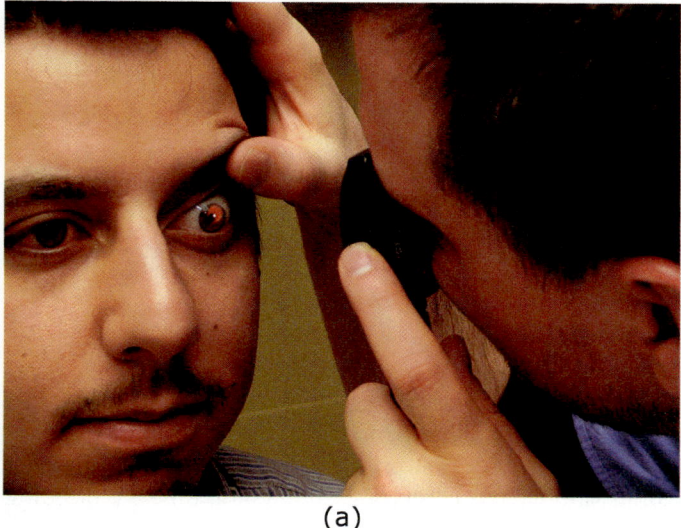
(a)

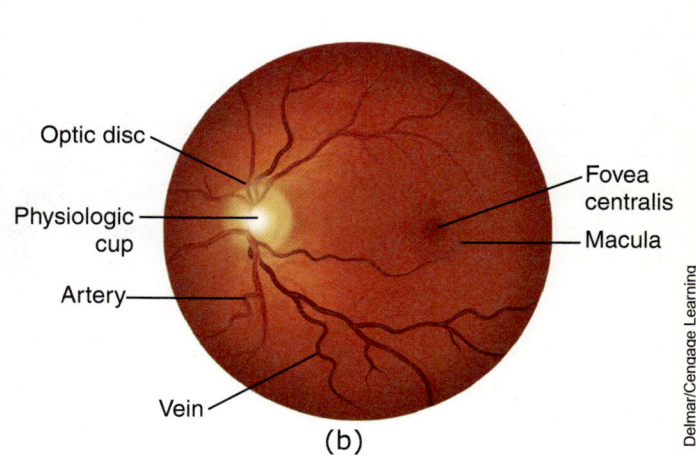
(b)

Optic disc
Physiologic cup
Artery
Vein
Fovea centralis
Macula

Delmar/Cengage Learning

Figure 26-8 (a) An ophthalmoscope is used for the funduscopic exam. (b) View through an ophthalmoscope of a normal retina. This view is difficult to obtain unless the patient's pupils have been dilated.

In the case of Mrs. Peabody, her symptoms of dizziness appear to be more indicative of vertigo than lightheadedness. They developed suddenly, are worse with movement to the point where she cannot walk, and get better when she keeps her head still. Her blood sugar is normal. These factors all point toward benign vertigo as a possible cause for Mrs. Peabody's chief concern and not other systemic conditions, such as a cardiac event, glucose problems, or stroke.

Mr. Wang's condition is more straightforward. On examination, his epistaxis appears to be an anterior epistaxis. Although the Paramedic notices a small amount of blood dripping down into the pharynx during his exam, the bleeding is oozing in nature and appears to be coming from an anterior source on examination. The duration of the nosebleed is likely related to the patient taking warfarin (Coumadin) for his atrial fibrillation.

CRITICAL THINKING QUESTIONS

1. What is the significance of the dizziness going away when the patient holds her head still?
2. What are other causes of an anterior epistaxis?

Assessment

As the Paramedic listens to a patient's history, examines the patient, and prepares for transport, he should be able to narrow the paramedical differential diagnosis to form an overall assessment of the patient. Unlike chest pain or back pain, which are frequently vague complaints, most HEENT conditions are specific to one body part and are usually easy to narrow down. However, one must be careful not to exclude potential causes of illness too quickly, since drawing conclusions about a diagnosis too soon can lead to mismanagement of the patient's medical condition.

The symptoms of vertigo include lightheadedness. The symptoms develop suddenly, are worse with movement to the point where the patient cannot walk, and get better when the patient keeps the head still.

An epistaxis is a small amount of blood dripping down into the pharynx seen on exam. The bleeding is oozing in nature and appears to be coming from an anterior source.

Mrs. Peabody is en route to City Hospital aboard Ambulance 468 and has started to vomit violently. Road sickness coupled with vertigo has made her feel very nauseous.

The cross-town Paramedic examines Mr. Wang on Ambulance 476 and examines his pharynx to find the bleeding is becoming more steady again. She elects to pack the nose using a commercially available device that the medical director just authorized for service.

CRITICAL THINKING QUESTIONS

1. What is the standard of care of patients with nausea and vomiting?
2. What is the procedure for packing an anterior nosebleed?

Treatment

The treatment for conditions involving the head, eyes, ears, nose, and throat is usually specific to the condition, but the basic general principles of emergency management still apply. Since this anatomic region includes components of the airway, the ABCs (airway, breathing, and circulation) are heavily stressed when treating HEENT emergencies. Airway management, including assessing for patency of the airway and the patient's ability to maintain that patency, must always be the Paramedic's first priority. In any condition in which the airway may be compromised, including heavy bleeding into the pharynx or soft tissue swelling, a patent and secure airway should be attained as soon as possible using either airway maneuvers such as jaw thrust or chin lift, and/or orotracheal intubation. For those Paramedics with rapid sequence intubation (RSI) as part of their intubation skills, this may be performed if indicated to ensure the patient's airway does not contribute to further hemodynamic compromise.

In some patients, even if airway collapse may be imminent, intubation should be deferred, if possible, until the patient arrives in the emergency department. Epiglottitis and Ludwig's angina may expand rapidly, causing obstruction. However, unless the patient is in respiratory extremis, the Paramedic should not manipulate the region by laryngoscope. These conditions can worsen immediately if the patient is upset or the airway is touched, so these patients should be intubated in a controlled environment by an anesthesiologist, ENT, or highly trained emergency physician. Occasionally, some patients may have complete airway obstruction; if so, a cricothyrotomy is required to secure the airway. However, cricothyrotomy may be difficult in these circumstances due to airway distortion by the rapidly expanding mass.

Once the airway has been secured, the patient's breathing and circulation should be assessed. Most patients with HEENT conditions will have no breathing difficulty as long as their airway is patent. Assessment of the circulation, however, may reveal evidence of circulatory compromise. Patients with vertigo or syncope may be suffering from dehydration and may benefit from IV fluids while en route to the emergency department. Patients with significant epistaxis will need control of their bleeding as part of their primary survey and treatment. Aside from these few occasions, most patients in this category will need only a cursory primary survey before moving onto treatment of their specific conditions.

Patients with headache and dizziness should be transported comfortably with frequent reassessment of vital signs and mental status. Rarely are pain medications or antiemetics indicated, and these medications should only be administered with permission from on-line medical control. Any change in mental status should prompt a reassessment of the ABCs and may be an indication for cardiac monitoring and IV access. Patients with intractable vomiting related to these conditions may benefit from an IV or IM antiemetic.[20]

Patients with ocular foreign bodies or chemical exposure should have immediate and continuous irrigation of their eye(s) with tap water or normal saline, if available. All industrial or educational sites where chemicals are in use are required by OSHA to have eye wash stations in close proximity, and the patient should begin irrigation there prior to the arrival of EMS personnel.[21,22] Once the patient is in the Paramedic's care, irrigation should continue with normal saline for at least 20 minutes of total irrigation time. Commercial devices such as the Morgan® Lens (Figure 26-9) are particularly useful as they contain a plastic shield that sits on the eye and permits a constant stream of sterile saline to irrigate the eye. If a Morgan® Lens or eye wash cup is not available, IV tubing can be held to the eye to allow copious irrigation. The eye should be irrigated from medial to lateral to avoid cross-contamination of the opposite eye.

Visible ocular foreign bodies should not be removed in the prehospital setting.[23] Instead, the eye should be protected

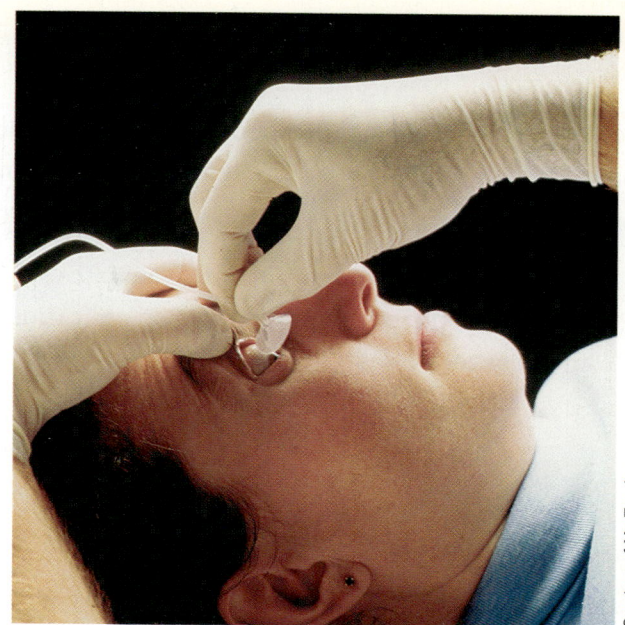

Courtesy of MorTan, Inc.

Figure 26-9 After anesthetizing the affected eye with tetracaine, the Morgan® Lens is placed between the cornea and eyelids and attached to a liter bag of normal saline for irrigation.

to avoid further injury and the patient transported in a supine position.

Management of epistaxis involves protecting the airway and stopping the bleeding. In most cases, simple pressure on either side of the bridge of the nose is enough to stop bleeding. Since Kiesselbach's plexus lies in this location, direct pressure should be enough to tamponade the bleeding. Pressure should be held continuously for at least 15 minutes, either by the EMS personnel or by the patient. If the bleeding is posterior, there is little that can be done in the prehospital setting to control the bleeding. In these cases, pressure should still be maintained over Kiesselbach's plexus since the source may not be immediately certain. However, if that fails to control hemorrhaging, supportive care including airway control and IV fluids should be initiated. Packing of the nasal passages is generally not performed in the field.

STREET SMART

Blood in the stomach can cause nausea and vomiting. The Paramedic should keep the patient with epistaxis seated upright and leaning slightly forward (if appropriate for the patient's condition) to prevent blood from running down the throat. The Paramedic should allow the patient to use suction or provide a basin to catch the blood.

The Paramedic treats Mrs. Peabody with IV fluids and ondansetron for her nausea. During the 30-minute transport time, the Paramedic notes improvement in her symptoms.

CRITICAL THINKING QUESTIONS

1. What are some of the predictable complications associated with epitaxis? Vertigo?
2. What are some of the predictable complications associated with the treatments for epitaxis and vertigo?

Evaluation

Nausea is a common complication associated with both vertigo and epitaxis. In the case of the patient with an epitaxis, swallowed blood can lead to nausea and subsequent vomiting, which in turn raises the blood pressure and can increase epitaxis in a posterior nosebleed.

A common symptom of increased intracranial pressure, and central neurogenic pathology in general, is nausea. This nausea can lead to vomiting that in turn, raises intracranial pressure.

> **CASE STUDY CONCLUSION**

Ambulances 468 and 476 arrive within five minutes of each other. Since the emergency department is busy, both patients are taken to triage and assessed by the triage nurse. Mrs. Peabody, still feeling a sense of spinning, is sent to a room in the emergency department. Mr. Wang, whose nosebleed continues to ooze, is triaged urgent, but will wait in the hallway until a new bed opens up.

Mrs. Peabody is discharged home later that evening with a prescription for meclizine and a diagnosis of benign paroxysmal positional vertigo.

Mr. Wang is found to have an anterior epistaxis at Kisselbach's plexus and undergoes nasal packing by the emergency physician. He is discharged with instructions to follow-up at the emergency department in two days for packing removal.

CRITICAL THINKING QUESTIONS

1. What is the most appropriate transport decision that will get these patients to definitive care?
2. What if the patients refused transportation to the emergency department following prehospital treatment?

Disposition

The appropriate disposition for almost all HEENT complaints is the emergency department. Occasionally a patient may sign off if the symptoms completely resolve and the patient is willing to accept the risk of not undergoing medical evaluation. However, in most instances the patient should be encouraged to accept transport to a hospital for assessment. The Paramedic who responds quickly, accurately, and appropriately can have a significant impact on the outcome of patients with HEENT disorders, and a careful assessment with consideration of the paramedical differential diagnosis can prevent further complications both during transport and during the patient's recovery period.

CONCLUSION

Disorders of the head, eyes, ears, nose, and throat range from the troublesome to the life-threatening. A thorough understanding of the pathophysiology of these conditions will assist the Paramedic in identifying the patients who have life-threatening conditions.

▶ KEY POINTS:

- Since a headache may be either benign or life-threatening, the Paramedic must ask about the presentation and effects.

- Complaints regarding the ear may be in terms of the external ear and ear canal, the middle ear and hearing, or the inner ear with hearing and balance.

- Peripheral vertigo results from disruption of the vestibular system, is usually sudden in onset, and is accompanied by hearing changes.

- Ménière disease, benign paroxysmal positional vertigo, and labyrinthitis are forms of peripheral vertigo.

- Central vertigo results from damage within the central nervous system, is more gradual in onset, and is accompanied by nausea.

- Time of onset is important in differentiating emergent conditions in the eye from benign ones that have gradual onset coupling with less severe conditions.

- Alkali burns to the eye cause greater tissue damage than acidic burns.

- Spontaneous anterior epistaxis is generally less severe due to environmental causes and low pressure vessels than posterior epistaxis, which usually involves an arterial bleed.

- Abscesses and swelling in the pharynx endanger the airway.

- OPQRST is a useful mnemonic in assessing the current history of HEENT complaints.

- Medications or changes in a medication regimen may cause changes in the patient's fluid balance or mental status and show as complaints of the HEENT systems.

- The otoscope is used for ear examinations.

- The ophthalmoscope is used for a funduscopic eye exam.

- Eye irrigation should be from medial to lateral, take at least 20 minutes, and have repeated administration of a topical anesthetic such as tetracaine.

- Treatments for HEENT complaints stress the concern for airway coupled with complaint specifics.

▶ REVIEW QUESTIONS:

1. How would the Paramedic differentiate otitis media from otitis externa?
2. What are the differences between vertigo, syncope, and disequilibrium?
3. What causes blurred vision?
4. Which location of spontaneous epistaxis is more severe? Why?

5. What emergent concern should the Paramedic have for a patient with peritonsillar abscess, retropharyngeal abscess, or Ludwig's angina?
6. How should the Paramedic treat a patient with an alkali burn?

CASE STUDY QUESTIONS:

Please refer to the Case Study in this chapter, and answer the questions below:

1. What concerns exist for a 36-year-old woman with a complaint of dizziness?

2. What field tests should be performed for someone with dizziness?

3. What initial concerns do you have for a person with epistaxis?

4. What conditions in a past medical history are indicators that epistaxis may be prolonged or severe?

REFERENCES:

1. Edlow JA. Headache. *Harwood-Nuss' Clinical Practice of Emergency Medicine*. fourth edition. Philadelphia: Lippincott Williams & Wilkins; 2005.

2. Krajicek ME, Decker WW. Dizziness. *Harwood-Nuss' Clinical Practice of Emergency Medicine*. fourth edition. Philadelphia: Lippincott Williams & Wilkins; 2005.

3. Macleod D, McAuley D. Vertigo: clinical assessment and diagnosis. *Br J Hosp Med (Lond)*. 2008;69(6):330–334.

4. Seemungal BM. Neuro-otological emergencies. *Curr Opin Neurol*. 2007;20(1):32–39.

5. Hainsworth R. Pathophysiology of syncope. *Clin Auton Res*. 2004;14 Suppl 1:18–24.

6. Anderson DC, Yolton RL, et al. The dizzy patient: a review of etiology, differential diagnosis, and management. *J Am Optom Assoc*. 1995;66(9):545–558.

7. Hodge C, Lawless M. Ocular emergencies. *Aust Fam Physician*. 2008;37(7):506–509.

8. Darkeh AK. Glaucoma, acute angle-closure. Available at: **http://www.emedicine.com/emerg/topic752.htm**. Accessed July 28, 2009.

9. Melsaether CN. Burns, ocular. Available at: **http://www.emedicine.com/emerg/topic736.htm**. Accessed July 28, 2009.

10. Kucik CJ, Clenney T. Management of epistaxis. *Am Fam Physician*. 2005;71:305–311, 312.

11. Gifford TO, Orlandi RR. Epistaxis. *Otolaryngol Clin North Am*. 2008;41(3):525–536, viii.

12. Alvi A, Joyner-Triplett N. Acute epistaxis. How to spot the source and stop the flow. *Postgrad Med*. 1996;99(5):83–90, 94–96.

13. Reaven D, Kharasch M, et al. Management of posterior epistaxis. *Acad Emerg Med*. 2008;15(6):585.

14. Brito-Mutunayagam S, Chew YK, et al. Parapharyngeal and retropharyngeal abscess: anatomical complexity and etiology. *Med J Malaysia*. 2007;62(5):413–415.

15. Srinivasan V, Patel H, et al. Warfarin and epistaxis: should warfarin always be discontinued? *Clin Otolaryngol Allied Sci*. 1997;22(6):542–544.

16. McEwan J, Giridharan W, et al. Paediatric acute epiglottitis: not a disappearing entity. *Int J Pediatr Otorhinolaryngol*. 2003;67(4):317–321.

17. Abarbanell NR. Is prehospital blood glucose measurement necessary in suspected cerebrovascular accident patients? *Am J Emerg Med*. 2005:23(7):823–827.

18. Adams J, Aldag G, et al. Does the level of prehospital care influence the outcome of patients with altered levels of consciousness? *Prehosp Disaster Med*. 1996;11(2):101–104.

19. Ng CL. Diagnostic challenge—is this really a stroke? *Aust Fam Physician*. 2006;35(10):805–808.

20. Jaslow D, Klimke A. Prehospital pharmacology: anti-emetics. *Emerg Med Serv*. 2007;36(11):56–61.

21. Lusk PG. Chemical eye injuries in the workplace. Prevention and management. *AAOHN J*. 1999;47(2):80–87; quiz 88–89.

22. Spector J, Fernandez WG. Chemical, thermal, and biological ocular exposures. *Emerg Med Clin North Am*. 2008;26(1): 125–136, vii.

23. Bledsoe BE, Ho B. Sight-threatening eye injuries: prehospital management of ophthalmological emergencies. *JEMS*. 2004;29(10):94–106; quiz 108–109.

The ambulance service is dispatched to Great Oaks Nursing Home for a 79-year-old man with shortness of breath. The call, originally a routine transfer for evaluation, has been upgraded because the patient is unstable. The nursing home indicates that the patient's shortness of breath may be related to an infection. With those words, the Paramedics prepare their personal protective equipment.

CRITICAL THINKING QUESTIONS

1. What are some of the possible causes of infection-related shortness of breath?

2. Why would a patient with an infection become unstable?

OVERVIEW

The changes of aging combine to make the elderly patient more prone to infection. Thus, the elderly frequently have a reason to call for Paramedic help. Paramedics should have a general understanding of the pathogens which cause infection and need to know how to treat the consequences of infection.

Chief Concern

Although an infection can occur anywhere in the body, most infections in the elderly can be linked to one of three sources, represented by the mnemonic PUS: **P**neumonia, **U**rinary tract infections, and **S**kin breakdown.[1] This triad of infections can progress to cause systemic inflammatory response syndrome and shock.

An **infection** is an attack of microorganisms, called **microbes**, upon the body that results in disease. There are six general classifications of microbes—worms, fungus, protozoa, bacteria, viruses, or prions—all of which cause disease. Some microbes have an interdependent and mutually beneficial (symbiotic) relationship with their host. For example, the presence of a benign microbe may prevent an infection from another microbe through **competitive inhibition**.

The Paramedic is most concerned about those microbes that produce disease, called **pathogens** (from the Greek for "that which produces suffering"). Worms (the scientific term is **helminthes**) are parasites that live inside the body and feed off the host. In contrast, although fleas, lice, and ticks feed off the host as well, they live outside the body. Although some worms exist in the skin, the pathogenic helminthes are generally found in the intestinal tract. These intestinal worms are usually ingested by the unsuspecting patient through undercooked meats—such as pork, beef, or fish—or via contaminated water. Once in the body's digestive tract, the worm sheds its egg shell and infects the host.

Fungi are like helminthes in that they are both eukaryotes, a group of microorganisms that contain a nucleus. However, a fungus reproduces by means of **spores**. Spores differ from seeds in that, although they both germinate, seeds have a nutrient store which permits independent growth, whereas spores must have a host that provides nutrition in order to grow. Spores tend to survive for long periods of time, even under unfavorable conditions, until they germinate.

Protozoa, fungus, and bacteria all absorb and decompose organic matter. **Protozoa** have an advantage over these other life forms because they are mobile, typically via amoeboid action or with a tail (flagella) to propel them. Protozoa, like the fungus, have an ability to form a protective layer (called a **cyst**) to protect them from harsh conditions. A protozoan cyst is capable of surviving for prolonged periods of time without food and can withstand disinfecting chemicals.

A **bacterium**, a single unicellular life form, can be the source of many diseases. These metabolically active life forms are abundant inside the human body; in fact, there may be 10 times more bacteria than cells in the body. Bacteria are described by their shapes. Some bacteria are spherical, or cocci (Greek for grain); others are rod-shaped bacilli (Latin for stick); and still others are spiral shaped (spirilla). When bacteria are linked to one another, they can be diploid (paired), in chains, or in clusters.

The Gram stain helps distinguish and describe bacteria based on their cell walls. The cell walls of those bacteria that are Gram positive stain purple, whereas those that stain pink are considered Gram negative. Gram-negative bacteria generally cause more disease because the cell wall, the outermost membrane, contains endotoxins, which are released when the cell is destroyed. Often it is the endotoxins, not the bacteria specifically, that lead to **sepsis**, a state of systemic inflammation.

The **virus**, unlike the fungus and bacterium, is not an independent life form and requires a host in order to be able to grow and reproduce. To survive, each single virion (entire virus particle) injects its genetic material into a cell, reprogramming the cell so that it produces the materials it needs. Because the virus is not an independent life form but rather exists inside the body's cells, anti-infective treatments (such as antibiotics) do not work as well.

The smallest infective agent may be the proteinaceous infectious particle, or prion. The **prion** consists of a protein which infects cells in a manner similar to virion and tends to affect nerve cells. Prions differ from virions because they do not contain nucleic acids, found in DNA, and because the pathology of prions differs. Prions form groups or aggregates that are called plaques. These neural plaques, called amyloids, form holes in the tissue and disrupt the neural structure. The resulting disruption of neural structure can lead to convulsions, ataxia, a gait analogous to the drunkard's stagger, and behavioral changes (Figure 27-1).

Infection

Chain of Infection

A series of events, called the **chain of infection**, must occur between a source and host before an infection occurs. First, there must be a disease-producing infectious agent that is **contagious** (capable of being passed) either directly or indirectly. These infectious agents, or pathogens, include protozoa, fungi, bacterium, virion, and prion (Figure 27-2).

These infectious agents must exist in a reservoir. These reservoirs include water, food, and natural animal reservoirs (called **zoonoses**), such as cattle, sheep, dogs, and birds.

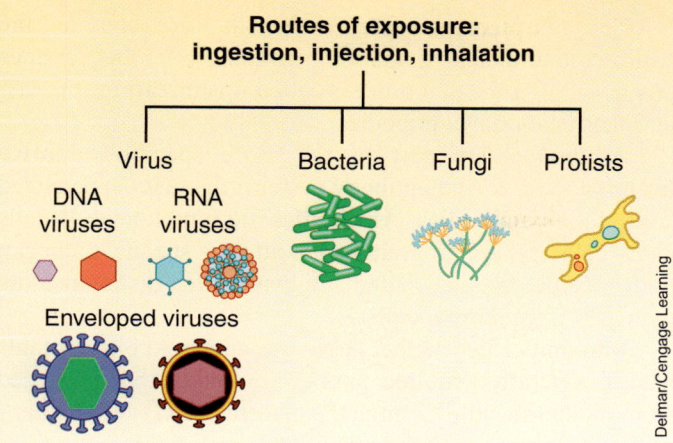

Routes of exposure:
ingestion, injection, inhalation

Virus   Bacteria   Fungi   Protists

DNA viruses   RNA viruses

Enveloped viruses

Delmar/Cengage Learning

Figure 27-1   Microorganisms.

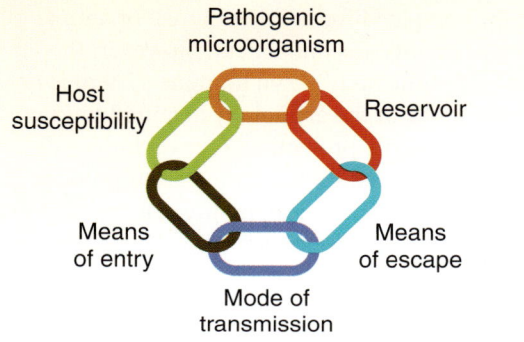

Pathogenic microorganism

Host susceptibility

Reservoir

Means of entry

Means of escape

Mode of transmission

Delmar/Cengage Learning

Figure 27-2   Chain of infection.

In some cases the **carrier** is asymptomatic (i.e., without signs of infection) and is unaware of being the reservoir for the disease. An example of a famous carrier is "typhoid Mary," who in her capacity as a cook infected at least 47 people in the New York City area with typhoid. Typhoid Mary is an interesting case of public health officials using epidemiological study and being able to track the source of the infection to one individual.

Next, there has to be an exit, a route of escape for the pathogen to leave the reservoir. That exit can be direct (e.g., via stool or mucous secretions) or indirect (e.g., via an intermediary such as the mosquito). If the pathogen is transmitted indirectly from the reservoir to another person by using another organism who is not infected but acts as a carrier, that organism is called a **vector**. For example, the flea (a vector) transmits the zoonotic disease of the plague from black rats to humans during a flea bite.

In some instances, the vector transfers the infectious material (e.g., stool) passively and mechanically, without becoming infected themselves. An example of a mechanical transfer of a pathogen would be when the common house fly has contamination on its legs and then lands on food. Filth-spreading house flies have been known to spread conjunctivitis, poliomyelitis, typhoid fever, tuberculosis, and cholera.

A number of direct means exist that are routes a pathogen can take to be transmitted to a potential host. The most common route of transmission may be the airborne droplet. These droplets, in the sneeze of the infected individual, contain the pathogen along with mucus. The droplets can range in size from 5 microns to 0.5 microns. People who are in close proximity to the infected person (generally within three feet) may inhale these droplets and become infected.

Alternatively, these airborne droplets can fall, or rain out, onto an inanimate surface, called a **fomite** (Latin for tinder, used to start a fire), where they remain until some unsuspecting person touches the surface and then transfers the pathogen from hand to mouth or other mucous membrane. Fomites are generally smooth, nonporous surfaces. The pathogens' resiliency is a major determinant of transmissibility. For example, the virus responsible for hepatitis B has been known to survive in a dried drop of blood on a fomite for weeks. However, the human immunodeficiency virus (HIV), the virus responsible for acquired immunodeficiency syndrome (AIDS), is very fragile and only survives for minutes outside of the body.

▷▷▷▷▷▷▷▷▷▷▷▷▷▷▷

STREET SMART

In some cases, hotels and restaurants are changing hardware over from stainless steel to copper because copper, as a fomite, is less likely to transmit disease.

Disease can also be transmitted by direct contact between the infected individual and the potential host. Examples of direct contact could be as simple as a handshake or ingestion of contaminated foods. Direct contact can also occur during sexual intercourse.

In some unfortunate cases, the disease is spread from healthcare provider to an unsuspecting patient, thus causing **iatrogenic disease**. In some other cases, disease is transmitted from mother to child, called vertical transmission. Examples of vertically transmitted diseases include syphilis and human immunodeficiency virus.

Infectivity

Several factors impact the disease's **infectivity**, the pathogen's ability to cause an infection. These factors include the dose, virulence, and the host's resistance to disease. Of these, the host's resistance may be most important.

The patient has several defenses—some specific and some nonspecific—that prevent infection. The nonspecific defenses include the skin and the mucous membranes. They generally exclude microbes. Covering the external body, the skin provides an impenetrable layer of dead cells (a barrier) which deprives microbes of the nutrients necessary for their survival. Furthermore, the skin secretes an antimicrobial substance called sebum from the sebaceous glands. These sebaceous glands are found on any hair-covered surface and are connected to the hair follicles.

Mucous membranes cover the remaining exposed surfaces of the body which are not covered by skin, as well as the internal surfaces of the digestive, genitourinary, and respiratory organs. The respiratory mucous membranes secrete a watery fluid called mucus. Mucus traps microbes for external expectoration or internal ingestion where stomach acid neutralizes the microbes.

Similar to the lungs, the genitourinary system also produces copious amounts of mucus that trap bacteria and flush it out during urination. Typically, urine is a clear and copious yellow liquid. **Turbidity** in urine, a sign of urinary tract infection, is caused by bacteria suspended in the urine, making the urine cloudy or hazy.

The intestinal mucosa forms a physical, or intrinsic, barrier between the capillary-rich intestinal wall and the contents within the lumen of the intestine. This intestinal wall is made up of cells that are closely joined together, in tight junctions that seal the space between and around the cells. Without this single layer of tightly joined epithelial cells, microbes could easily enter into the systemic circulation.

The mucosa of the intestine also forms an extrinsic barrier of mucous secretions. The first secretion that bacteria encounter is the acid secreted by the stomach's goblet cells. The acid, consisting primarily of hydrochloric acid (HCl), denatures proteins and breaks down lipids, physically destroying microbes in the process of digestion.

Bacteria surviving the stomach's hostile environment are ejected into the intestine. These bacteria are attracted to the carbohydrates in the mucin, a key element of mucus, and bind with the mucin. They are then expelled in the stool.

Despite the constant turnover of the lining of the intestines, some bacteria manage to flourish. These benign bacteria struggle with pathogenic bacteria for limited nutrient resources. This competitive inhibition prevents the pathogenic bacteria from getting a foothold in the intestine and causing an infection.

If a pathogen manages to overcome the body's non-specific defenses, the body has a second defense called **immunity**. Immunity can be either innate or adaptive. The innate immune system has cells that respond to all pathogens. The innate immune system responds to chemical mediators called **cytokines**, such as histamine and leukotrienes, which are released by injured cells in a process called **inflammation**. Phagocytes such as neutrophils of the innate immune system begin to absorb, via phagocytosis (literally meaning cell eating), the offending microbes. However, the innate immune system has a limited capacity to respond to infection. To continue the defense, the neutrophils attract leukocytes and lymphocytes.

Leukocytes (white blood cells) are single-celled organisms which work independently of any other cells to clear cellular debris and microbes. Leukocytes include mast cells, eosinophils, basophils, and neutrophils, all of which identify and destroy disease-causing pathogens.

The **complement system** helps the body continue the antimicrobial attack by marking invading microbes. It does this by coating them, a process called **opsonization**, for easier identification by antibodies.

Antibodies are part of the more specific **adaptive immune system** (the antibody system) that uses specialized cells, called antibodies. **Antibodies** are lymphocyte B cells and T cells that are programmed to attack a specific pathogen with specific proteins, called antigens, which distinguish the pathogen from normal cells.

Immunity can be either passive or active. At birth, infants have a naturally acquired passive immunity that is passed from mother to child through the placenta (IgG) and mother's milk (IgA), protecting the infant from bacterial infection.

Taking a clue from the mother, physicians can also provide artificially acquired passive immunity in the form of immunoglobulin. Immunoglobulin is an immunization with antibodies obtained from either human or animal plasma that confers immunity for the patient. However, this immunity is short-lived as the body's own immune system is not triggered by the presence of the artificially acquired immunity.

For long-term protection (active immunity), the body has to be stimulated by the pathogen to produce antibodies. Naturally acquired active immunity is a result of the patient's exposure to the disease and the body's immune response to that challenge. Often other factors, such as dose and virulence (discussed shortly), combine to lower the threat created by the disease and permits the body to naturally form an acquired active immunity.

Perhaps the single greatest advance in medicine was the development of artificially acquired active immunity through inoculation, then by vaccination. After observing naturally acquired active immunity, it was logical to develop a way to weaken, or attenuate, the pathogen, or to use its inactivated toxin, thus allowing the body to respond to and develop an immunity for the pathogen without risk of infection.

The patient's ability to mount an immune response is partly predicated on the patient's health. Factors predicting a patient's health can be divided into either nature or nurture. A patient's nutritional status, a nurturance factor, has a great impact on a patient's ability to withstand an infection (**host resistance**). Patients in both extremes—cachexic and obese—are more prone to infections.

Some of the other variables that affect a patient's ability to withstand infection (host resistance) include extremes of age as well as comorbidities such as diabetes (Table 27-1).

A patient's nature can also have an impact on her ability to contract a disease. For example, the first Americans had little resistance to European diseases such as smallpox, which devastated these native populations. Recent research as a result of the genome project has suggested that there are a number of diseases that a person may be prone to, or resist, as a result of genetics.

The ability of a pathogen to cause an infection, called its **pathogenesis**, is based on a combination of virulence and dose. **Dose** is described as the physical number of microbes

Table 27-1   Variables That Affect Host Resistance

- Age
  - Infants (expired passive immunity)
  - Elderly (declining immune function)
- Alcoholism
  - Cirrhosis
- Gastric acidity
  - Antacids
- Immune compromise
  - Human immunodeficiency virus
  - Leukemia
- Metabolic disorders
  - Emphysema (chronic hypoxia)
  - Diabetes (hyperglycemia)
- Occupational risk
  - Healthcare provider
- Pregnancy
- Prescription medications
  - Antibiotics (competitive inhibition)
- Trauma
  - Burns

Table 27-2   Variables That Affect Pathogenesis

- Dose
- Virulence
- Gene expression
  - Immunity (influenza mutation)
- Susceptibility
  - Acid
- Infection
  - Competitive inhibition

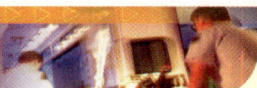

PROFESSIONAL PARAMEDIC

Rene and Jean Dubos, in their classic *The White Plague,* identified the principles of resistance to infection when they wrote, "In the final analysis, the fight against tuberculosis can be carried along two independent approaches, by preventing the spread of the bacilli through procedures of public health and by increasing the resistance of man through a proper way of life."

present. In some cases, a very small number of microbes are necessary in the **inoculums**, the microbe introduced into the body. For example, as few as 10 cells are needed for an Escherichia coli infection whereas, alternatively, it may take as many as 100 million vibrio cholerae cells to infect a patient. However, it is possible to ingest 100 million vibrio cholerae cells in one sip of contaminated water.

In addition to dose, **virulence** (Latin for "full of poison") is another factor in pathogenicity. Broadly, virulence speaks to several factors in pathogenesis, such as ease of entry, route of entry, dose, and host defense. More narrowly, virulence speaks to the fitness of the microbe to survive and thrive in the host. Spore formation and cyst formation are two mechanisms microbes use to evade host defenses and thrive in a host. A virus that has been weakened, or **attenuated**, is less virulent and more easily overcome by the host's defenses (Table 27-2).

Epidemiology—that branch of medicine that studies the causes, distribution, and control of disease—measures the virulence of infectious diseases in terms of **morbidity** (the number of infected individuals) and **mortality** (the number of deaths caused by an infection). The morbidity of a disease is typically measured in terms of the number of infected persons (number of cases reported) per population. The mortality of a disease is usually described in terms of percentage of infected persons who died.

Toxins

Pathogens can kill by one of two mechanisms: (1) exhaustion of the host or (2) poison. The latter, poison, is the result of either bacteria creating and secreting a destructive chemical compound—typically a protein called an **exotoxin**—or a destructive chemical compound that is released with the bacteria's destruction called an **endotoxin**.

An exotoxin can further be defined according to the tissues that are affected. Almost all toxins are cytotoxins, chemical compounds that disrupt cellular metabolism or destroy essential components of the cell such as the cell wall membrane. Neurotoxins affect the nervous system whereas enterotoxins affect the gastrointestinal system.

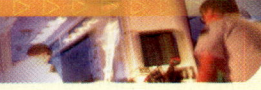

PROFESSIONAL PARAMEDIC

Certain strains of staphylococcus aureus and streptococcus pyogenes produce toxins called superantigens that cause an immense immunological response. This response creates an enormous amount of cytokines, leading to vasodilatation and the signs associated with toxic shock.

The majority of exotoxins are sensitive to heat, emphasizing the importance of properly cooking food. One bacterium, clostridium botulinum, produces a very potent neurotoxin called botulinum toxin (Latin for sausage poison) that blocks the release of acetylcholine. Botulinum works like other acetylcholine blockers, such as curare, and produces a paralysis of smooth muscles, including the diaphragm. The result of diaphragmatic paralysis is respiratory arrest and death.

Endotoxins are not secreted by bacteria but are released when the bacteria is destroyed (or lysed) by antibodies. The remains of the bacterial cell wall, containing endotoxins, then attach to macrophages which, in turn, trigger the release of cytokines, those signaling proteins that attract macrophages and lymphocytes. The resultant stimulation of the inflammatory system leads to the signs and symptoms associated with sepsis, further discussed in the next chapter.

Stages of Infection

There are four stages of infection: incubation, prodromal, infectious, and recovery. The **incubation period** is that time between contact with the infectious microbe and the appearance of the first symptoms. During the incubation period, the patient is subclinical (asymptomatic). Each pathogen has a different incubation period. The patient's resistance to the disease is a factor in the duration of the incubation period.

As the infection gets a footing, the patient starts to become symptomatic. These initial symptoms—such as aches, fever, headache, and **anorexia** (a lack of appetite)—are often nonspecific in the **prodromal phase**. If the patient's resistance is high—that is, the host's defenses are effective against the infection—the patient may never experience the full effects of the infection. If the patient's resistance is low, however, then the patient will proceed to the next stage. It should be noted that some diseases progress so rapidly, especially in patients with low resistance, that the prodromal phase is almost nonexistent.

Typically a patient is most contagious (able to transmit the infectious disease) during the incubation and/or the prodromal stages. During this larger **communicable period**, the patient is able to transfer the infection. Some diseases, such as diphtheria, are able to be transmitted from the first day of exposure. Other diseases, such as measles, are more contagious during the prodromal period than during the actual illness. Some diseases are intermittently contagious, such as tuberculosis and syphilis, and the communicable state may exist over a prolonged period of time for this reason.

At this point, the patient is grossly symptomatic and the disease runs its course. During the illness, the patient's immunological resistance is put to the test. As the infection comes to its zenith, called its **acme**, the full force of the patient's immunological defenses are brought to bear on the infection. If the patient's defenses fail, then the patient succumbs to the illness. If the patient's defenses bring the infection's progress to a halt, but cannot rid the body of the infection, then the patient may become a carrier. However,

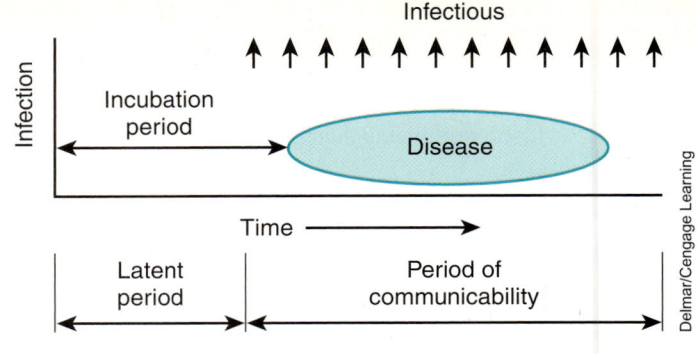

Figure 27-3 Infectious process.

if the patient's immune system (or medical intervention discussed in medical pharmacology) is successful, then the patient will recover.

During the recovery period, referred to as **convalescence**, the patient's body makes repairs to any damage. In some cases, the body is unable to return to normal and some remnants of the infection, called the **residuals**, remain. The pox mark, depressions on the surface of the skin, is an example of a residual. In other cases, the result of the infection leaves a **sequela**, a morbid condition of the disease. The paralysis of polio is an example of the sequela of the disease poliomyelitis (Figure 27-3).

Infectious Diseases

The diseases described in the following text (Table 27-3) are all capable of producing a rash. The Paramedics should be familiar with the most common infectious diseases that they may encounter. The mnemonic TEST—standing for **T**ransmission, **E**pidemiology, **S**ymptoms, and **T**reatment—is useful for learning these diseases.

Respiratory Diseases
Common Cold

The first respiratory disease to be discussed is the common cold. Precisely because it is common and because the symptom pattern of the common cold is characteristic of many other respiratory diseases, it merits attention.

The etiology, or causative agent, of the common cold is one of several hundred viruses in either the rhinovirus family or the coronavirus family. The common cold is a disease that can enter the nose via either inhalation of airborne droplets (i.e., from a sneeze) or by hand contact with a contaminated inanimate surface (fomite) that is then transferred to the nose. The ease of transmission of the common cold explains the three to four colds that an average adult will have each year.

The symptom pattern for the common cold includes **catarrhal signs**, discharge from a mucous membrane such as the runny nose (rhinorrhea) and a sore throat secondary to postnasal drip into the oropharynx. The focus of the infection is the key difference between the common cold and other respiratory diseases. The symptoms of the common cold are almost exclusively found above the shoulders.

Table 27-3   Common Infectious Diseases

- Pediculosis
  - Pediculus humanus capitis
  - Pthirus pubis
  - Sarcoptes scabiei
- Helminthes
  - Hymenolepiasis
  - Trichinosis
- Fungus
  - Aspergillosis
  - Candidiasis
  - Histoplasmosis
  - Tinea pedis
- Protozoa
  - Giardia lamblia
  - Toxoplasmosis
  - Trichomoniasis
- Bacteria
  - Borrelia burgdorferi
  - Clostridium botulinum
  - Staphylococcus aureus
  - Escherichia coli
  - Klebsiella
  - Enterobacter
  - Campylobacter
  - Cholera
  - Helicobacter pylori
  - Haemophilus influenzae
  - Salmonella
  - Shigellosis
  - Yersinia pestis
  - Streptococcus pneumoniae
  - Diphtheria
  - Pneumococcal pneumonia
  - Group A streptococcus
  - Tuberculosis
  - Syphilis
  - Gonorrhea
  - Chlamydia
  - Pertussis
  - Anthrax bacillus
  - Coxiella burnetii
  - Tularemia
  - Rickettsia
  - Typhus
- Viral
  - Human immunodeficiency virus
  - Hepatitis A
  - Hepatitis B
  - Hepatitis C
  - Hepatitis D
  - Herpes simplex
  - Human papilloma virus
  - Chickenpox
  - Measles
  - Mumps
  - Rubella
  - Poliomyelitis
  - Rhinovirus
  - Respiratory syncytial virus
  - Cytomegalovirus
  - Influenza
  - Ebola hemorrhagic fever
  - Smallpox
- Prion
  - Bovine spongiform encephalopathy

Treatment for the common cold is generally supportive, as the virus is self-limiting. The concern with the common cold is that it can weaken the patient's immune system, leading to the development of secondary bacterial infections.

Pediatric Respiratory Syncytial Virus

A respiratory infection that can mimic the common cold is the **respiratory syncytial virus (RSV)**. An RSV infection often starts with a low-grade fever, runny nose, and a cough. If left untreated, the RSV can progress to **bronchiolitis**, an infection of the bronchioles that typically presents with wheezing. The patient populations most at risk for RSV are infants less than one year of age, with the majority being hospitalized younger than six months.[2-4]

RSV is spread by airborne droplets and can contaminate inanimate surfaces (fomites). Fortunately, RSV is short-lived outside the body and can be inactivated by simple means, such as soap and water.

The peak period for RSV outbreaks are late fall to early spring and the diagnosis is made by antigen detection assays. Treatment for an RSV infection is supportive and, as needed, oxygen and beta-agonists.

Influenza

Influenza may be one of the oldest diseases known to man which still exists today. Described by Hippocrates, and called by such names as "le grippe" over the centuries, influenza originally was thought to be due to astrological influences or imbalances in the humors. Influenza is now known to be caused by an RNA virus of the orthomyxoviridae family and is a classic example of a zoonotic disease.

A **zoonotic disease** is any disease that is transmitted from an animal (a vector) to humans. The list of zoonoses (animal-borne diseases) is long and the sources (vectors) are almost as long (Table 27-4).

The transmission of influenza is similar to that of the common cold—inhalation of aerosol droplets and contact with contaminated fomites. Worldwide, influenza occurs in seasonal epidemics. To date, there have been three major **pandemics**, an infectious disease that is contagious (easily spread) and affects a large portion of the human population.

Table 27-4 Zoonosis

Zoonosis	Vector
Anthrax	Sheep
Bovine tuberculosis	Cows
Ebola fever	Monkeys
Distemper	Dogs
Influenza	Pigs
Malaria (not true zoonosis)	Mosquitoes
Rabies	Bats
Toxoplasmosis	Cats

Patients with influenza generally present with constitutional signs such as fever, muscle ache, headache, malaise, and fatigue.[5] These **constitutional signs**, signs that indicate general illness but are not specific to a certain disease, are coupled with a sore throat and paroxysms of coughing. If the influenza infection settles in the respiratory tract, as it often does, the patient may contract croup (laryngotracheobronchitis) or pneumonia. Although colds generally do not cause a fever, influenza does. A persistent low grade fever (<101°F) is a cardinal sign of influenza.

The diagnosis of influenza centers around identifying the means through which the body is trying to rid itself of the virus. Although sneezing and coughing are the most prominent signs, vomiting and diarrhea, as well as a fever, are other signs of influenza.

In general, treatment of the "flu" is supportive, including fluids, oxygen, and rest. If the patient develops a secondary bacterial infection, such as croup or pneumonia, then a physician may order antibiotics.

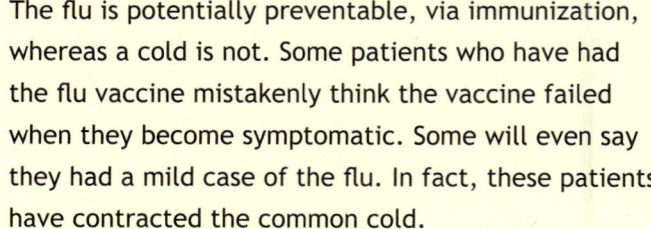

STREET SMART

The flu is potentially preventable, via immunization, whereas a cold is not. Some patients who have had the flu vaccine mistakenly think the vaccine failed when they become symptomatic. Some will even say they had a mild case of the flu. In fact, these patients have contracted the common cold.

STREET SMART

A single sneeze can release 40,000 disease-laden particles ranging in size from 0.5 to 5 microns in diameter. Although the large particles tend to fall, or "rain out," the smaller particles are inspirable and, when inhaled, can cause an infection. Therefore, it is important for a person to cover his mouth whenever he is sneezing.

The flu vaccine is recommended for Paramedics, to not only protect themselves but also because they come in contact with patients who are at risk for the flu. Otherwise, the Paramedic could be a carrier of the flu. The list of people for whom the vaccine is recommended (Table 27-5) can also be read to mean that these are the patient populations that the

Table 27-5 Patient Populations Recommended to Receive the Flu Vaccine

- Newborns to toddlers
- Elderly
- Concomitant conditions
  - Emphysema
  - Heart failure
  - Diabetes
  - AIDS
- Women who are pregnant
- Healthcare workers

Paramedic is at risk of infecting if the Paramedic does not get the flu vaccine.

Haemophilus Influenzae

Haemophilus influenza, a bacterial infection, is not the causative agent of the flu and should not be confused with influenza, the viral infection, as was originally supposed. H. influenzae is an opportunistic bacterium that lives in its host (humans) in the upper respiratory tract and only becomes problematic when a viral infection, like influenza, weakens the host. Because these two infections often occur simultaneously, many thought H. influenzae caused the flu.

H. influenzae occurs in two types: encapsulated or type B and non-encapsulated H. influenza, or type non-B. The haemophilus influenza (haemophilus is Greek for blood-loving) is a respiratory infection. When the amount of H. influenzae is great (the bacterial load), it will enter the bloodstream and disseminate to the joints, pleura, pericardium, alveoli, and the meninges to cause infection.

Up to 80% of patients have non-B haemophilus influenza in their nasopharynx. Non-B haemophilus influenza is responsible for a number of serious infections including otitis media (middle ear infection), sinusitis, conjunctivitis, and even pneumonia.

Infection of the nasopharynx with haemophilus influenza type B (HiB) is rare and is typically spread by inhalation of airborne droplets. If unimpeded, HiB causes cellulitis, epiglottitis, and bacterial meningitis.[6,7]

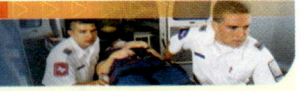

STREET SMART

Pediatric epiglottitis can be life-threatening, as it can potentially obstruct the airway and suffocate the child. Fortunately, the incidence of epiglottitis has dropped dramatically as a result of the H. influenzae type B (HiB) vaccine.[8]

Streptococcus

As the causative agent of strep throat, the term "streptococcus" immediately conjures the thought of a strep throat. However, streptococcus is also responsible for a number of other medical ailments from dental caries to meningitis. A problematic strain of streptococcus is streptococcus pyogenes, a group A streptococcus (GAS).

S. pyogenes infections start with a sore throat (strep throat), and can develop into rheumatic fever or scarlet fever. Rheumatic fever affects connective tissues and, if left untreated, can lead to damaged heart valves. It also tends to affect school-aged children.

Scarlet fever, another complication of the infection, is the result of the endotoxins of streptococcus pyogenes. Scarlet fever has been prevalent in the population for centuries and has gained widespread attention in such novels as *Little Women* and *The Velveteen Rabbit*. Scarlet fever is characterized by a sore throat, a "strawberry tongue," a bright red tip of the tongue, and a sandpaper-like rash over the upper body. The rash of scarlet fever can also produce a distinctive pattern that is described as "slapped cheek and white moustache." Slapped cheek syndrome is also seen in other common childhood diseases including measles and rubella.

Other symptoms associated with scarlet fever include a high fever (>101°F), constitutional signs, flushed face with circumoral pallor, and the rash. Typically the rash starts at the chest and/or axilla and spreads. The rash blanches under pressure (such as is seen in testing for capillary refill) and is worse in the folds of the skin.

Yersinia Pestis

Yersinia pestis, also known as the plague, is an airborne disease that was thought to potentially be the cause of the second of three plagues. This second plague, called the Black Plague, caused the death of one-third of Europe's population between 1347 and 1353.[9] Although less problematic today because of antibiotics such as streptomycin, Yersinia pestis is seen in the southwest United States as well as in Asia.

The plague, a zoonotic disease, is carried by the fleas on black rats which, in turn, bite unsuspecting humans if no other rodent host is available. Once infected, the patient may spread the plague by airborne droplets. The typical incubation period for pneumonic plague is two to four days, although it has been known to cause death in as little as 24 hours.

The symptoms associated with the pneumonic plague include headache, lethargy, and—perhaps most importantly—**hemoptysis**, which is bloody sputum. Hemoptysis is also a clinical sign seen with tuberculosis, another airborne disease, making the diagnosis more difficult.

The treatment of plague is largely supportive. Any patient with suspected plague should be encouraged to seek medical treatment. Untreated pneumonic plague can have a

95% mortality rate; however, simple antibiotic treatments, such as erythromycin, are effective as a treatment.

Tuberculosis

Another ancient respiratory disease, tuberculosis, has been found in the bones of Egyptian mummies, yet is still prevalent today. Previously called consumption, or the white plague, tuberculosis is a wasting disease that has a high mortality rate.

Caused by the aerobic mycobacterium tuberculosis, the oxygen-loving tuberculosis enters the lungs and typically becomes a lesion in the apex of the lungs, where the oxygen tension is highest (Figure 27-4).

Once in the lungs, the tuberculosis is surrounded by a mass of alveolar macrophages. This mass of tuberculosis and lymphocytes forms a nodule, called a tubercle. It remains dormant in the lungs until the host is weakened. Therefore, a person may contract tuberculosis but remain asymptomatic for years while the disease is in the latent phase.

Estimates suggest that as many as 10 million Americans are infected with tuberculosis. However, only 10% of those patients will have the active disease. It has further been estimated that over one-third of the world's population has been exposed to tuberculosis.[10] Legal immigrants with active tuberculosis are still banned from entry into the United States.[11,12]

Tuberculosis typically becomes active when the host (the patient) becomes weakened (e.g., by cancer, age, chemotherapy, or AIDS). Then the mycobacterium breaks down the scar tissue that has been surrounding it and starts to destroy more tissue. This destruction leads to characteristic cavities in the lungs.

Tuberculosis is an aggressive infection. Therefore, it takes much of the body's energy to combat the infection, causing the patient to lose weight (hence the origin of the disorder's old name, consumption). As the tuberculosis progresses, it breaks down capillaries and alveoli alike, causing blood to enter into the bronchioles. Blood in the bronchioles is an irritant and causes the patient to cough blood (hemoptysis), which is a characteristic sign of tuberculosis.

Active tuberculosis is also associated with **night sweats**, a drenching diaphoresis thought to be due to the body's immune response to the infection. Other associated symptoms—such as fever, chills, and generalized weakness—are all associated with the body's immune system response to the invading infection.

Because of its location in the lungs, tuberculosis can also cause chest pain, secondary to pleuritis. The disease can spread, via the lymphatic system, to the neck. Once there, the tuberculosis enlarges the lymph nodes of the cervical chains, a condition called **lymphadenopathy**. It then forms into a painless mass that is cold to the touch and cyanotic in appearance. The tuberculosis, once in the lymphatic system, can spread like cancer to all parts of the body. For example, tuberculosis in the bones of the thoracic spine is called Pott's disease.

Treatment for tuberculosis typically consists of the antibiotics isoniazid, rifampin, and pyrazinamide, or some combination of these and other antibiotics, for several months.

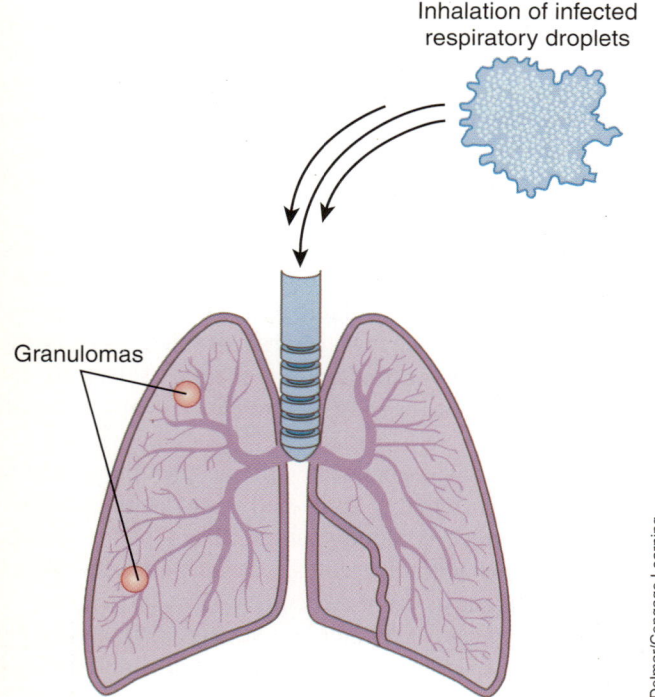

Inhalation of infected respiratory droplets

Granulomas

Delmar/Cengage Learning

Figure 27-4 Tuberculosis.

Although 10 tuberculosis drugs have been developed since the 1940s, isoniazid and rifampin still remain first line.

Paramedics should first focus on protective measures such as applying a high-efficiency particulate air (HEPA) mask. Although the patient may be a risk to the Paramedic, it generally takes a prolonged period of exposure in a confined space to become infected. Often the Paramedic is more of a risk to the patient. The patient's tuberculosis is active because the patient is weakened by some other condition, such as cancer, chemotherapy, or HIV, and in that weakened state is at risk for infections brought by the Paramedic. The Paramedic should also place a mask on the patient to help further decrease the likelihood of spread of the disease, especially while moving the patient from the ambulance to a negative pressure room in the emergency department.

Bacillus Calmette—Guerin (BCG), a vaccine used against tuberculosis, was created by weakening, or attenuating, tuberculosis. The well spring for this concept was the success that scientists had vaccinating against smallpox with cowpox, a similar disease. Albert Calmette and Camille Guerin, working in the Pasteur Institute, created the vaccine in 1919. Interestingly, the United States does not routinely vaccinate the public, preferring testing for exposure instead. This is, in part, because of the limited efficiency of vaccination (85%) and the limited duration of protection (15 to 20 years).

The diagnostic test for tuberculosis is the Mantoux test using purified protein derivative (PPD) derived from sterile tuberculosis cultures. Created by French physician Charles Mantoux, the PPD, at a dose of 5 tuberculin units, is injected intradermally. The site is then observed for a reaction 48 to 72 hours later. A positive reaction is a raised area, called an induration, measured in millimeters. A minor reaction is approximately 5 mm and is considered positive if the patient has concomitant illness or recent exposure to a patient with active tuberculosis. A moderate reaction of 10 mm is considered positive for immigrants and high risk individuals (e.g., diabetics). A 15 mm induration is considered positive for persons with no known risk factors for tuberculosis.[13,14] It should be noted that vaccination with the BCG vaccine may cause the PPD to read positive but is not necessarily a contraindication for PPD testing.[15]

Multi-drug resistant tuberculosis, which is resistant to the two main tuberculosis first-line drugs (isoniazid and rifampin), resulted in a 70% to 90% mortality rate in the 1990s. This occurred primarily in the HIV population. Extensively drug-resistant tuberculosis (XR–TB) was seen in an outbreak that occurred in South Africa, but was not restricted to South Africa. XR–TB is resistant to three of the second-line drugs as well as all of the first-line drugs.

Pediatric Respiratory Disease
Croup

Perhaps the most common pediatric respiratory disease is croup. Croup is actually not a separate disease but a syndrome of symptoms associated with laryngotracheobronchitis, an infection starting from the throat and ending in the lungs (the upper airway). There are multiple causative agents for croup including the parainfluenza virus and common bacterial infections.

Croup is a syndrome that occurs most commonly in children from three months to three years and presents as difficulty in breathing. Often occurring in the fall months, the patient with croup presents with a characteristic raspy or brassy cough, often described as being like a seal bark, as well as an often audible inspiratory stridor that is aggravated by the cough. This stridor and cough is the result of swelling of the vocal cords and the throat.

The traditional treatment for croup is inhalation of warm mist. Parents have been known to take their child into the bathroom and turn on a hot shower to produce steam or use a humidifier. Children usually tolerate mild cases of croup without further intervention and the disease resolves spontaneously in less than one week.

In moderate cases of croup, it may be necessary to administer inhaled beta-agonists to help relieve the bronchospasm and the laryngospasm, as well as administer oxygen, usually by blow-by apparatus.

In severe cases of croup, probably less than 1% of cases, it may be necessary for the Paramedic to intubate the child to provide an airway as well as administer anti-inflammatory steroids intravenously. Intubation should be considered when oxygen, provided by positive pressure ventilation, fails to raise the child's oxygen saturation and the child appears exhausted.[16]

Pertussis

Another pediatric respiratory disease that has seen a recent resurgence is pertussis, also known as whooping cough. Pertussis, caused by inhalation of airborne droplets containing the bacterium bordetella pertussis, is another disease of the upper airway and is highly contagious.

Whooping cough, like croup, presents as a syndrome with three distinct phases. The first phase, the catarrhal stage, presents with cough, sneezing, and a runny nose, illustrating its upper respiratory origin. It has the appearance of the common cold. The next stage is marked by the classic whooping cough that gave pertussis its name. During the paroxysmal stage, fits of coughing can be so severe that some patients vomit. The whooping sound of the cough is created by a prolonged active inspiratory phase and is followed by a hacking cough during exhalation. During the paroxysmal phase, the patient may also present with an inspiratory wheeze, which is different from the expiratory wheeze of asthma.

Finally, during the convalescent phase, the patient begins to recover. This recovery may be complicated by aspiration pneumonias, secondary bacterial or superinfections, and malnutrition.

Pertussis is a relatively rare disease in the United States because of mass public vaccination programs of children with the diphtheria, tetanus, and pertussis (DTaP) vaccine. However, periodic outbreaks are reported each year. Treatment of pertussis consists of the administration of macrolide antibiotics, such as erythromycin, and rest.[17] Persons in close contact with the patient, including Paramedics, may be prophylactically treated for one to three weeks with the same macrolide antibiotics.

Epiglottitis

Epiglottitis, a childhood disease of great concern in the past, is another pediatric respiratory syndrome with multiple etiologies including haemophilus influenza, streptococcus pneumonia, and streptococcus pyogenes. Epiglottitis is a focused infection of the epiglottis. When infected and inflamed, it swells and can cause an airway obstruction.

Like pertussis, epiglottitis proceeds through three phases. In the first phase, the emergent phase, the symptoms of epiglottitis are vocal changes, sore throat, and fever. As the condition progresses to the second phase, or urgent phase, the airway becomes more occluded and the patient will lean forward in a classic "sniffing" position and be observed "pulling to breathe" (using the sternocleidomastoid or strap muscles to breathe).

In the third phase, or the premorbid phase, the patient will have difficulty swallowing, coupled with the high pitched whistling of inspiratory stridor and fever. This triad of symptoms is cause for concern for the Paramedic because, if left untreated, epiglottitis can lead to complete obstruction of the airway and respiratory arrest. Although possible, the quintessential sign of epiglottitis, drooling, is seen in only about 10% of cases.

During the premorbid phase of epiglottitis, the Paramedic should focus on maintaining the patient's airway with manual methods. Mechanical manipulation of the airway (e.g., to intubate) may cause complete airway obstruction.[18] If the airway does become occluded, or the Paramedic is unable to maintain adequate ventilation and oxygenation with positive pressure ventilation, then a surgical airway might be considered. Otherwise, the care of the patient with suspected epiglottitis consists of placing the patient in the position of comfort, providing humidified oxygen (by small volume nebulizer, if needed), and transporting the patient to definitive care. If the airway should become occluded en route, then the Paramedic should divert to the closest emergency department with emergency airway capabilities while attempting positive pressure ventilation and a surgical airway. Fortunately, the incidence of pediatric epiglottitis has declined since the introduction of the HiB vaccine, making these emergencies less common.

Gastrointestinal Diseases

Abdominal cramping and diarrhea are frequent patient complaints and may be the prologue to an impending gastrointestinal infection. The cramps and frequent watery bowel movements are the result of hyperperistalsis, the body's way of ridding itself of viruses, bacteria, and parasites. Such infectious etiologies may be the result of poor food handling or contaminated water. Other etiologies of diarrhea include allergy and food intolerance.

The symptom complex associated with these gastrointestinal infections is called gastroenteritis, and commonly includes anorexia (loss of appetite), nausea (with or without vomiting), and dehydration. The last sign, dehydration, is perhaps the most problematic. If left unresolved, severe dehydration from gastroenteritis can lead to hypovolemia and shock.

Cholera

Cholera is a classic example of an infection that leads to massive diarrhea. Cholera, caused by the bacterium vibrio cholera, was first discovered by Robert Koch. Along with cholera, Koch discovered the microbes responsible for tuberculosis and anthrax, and he created "Koch's postulates," the basis for modern microbiological study.

Cholera is endemic to parts of India, where the Ganges River is used as a source of water. The disease is spread through the contaminated feces of the victim and can rapidly become an epidemic. Within two to three days of ingestion of feces-contaminated water, the next patient starts to experience "explosive" diarrhea and rice water stools.

The movement of water into the small intestine, caused by an enterotoxin, or pore-forming toxins, is so rapid that shock may occur within hours. A patient with cholera may lose as much as 20% of body weight from this massive diarrhea. Patients with untreated cholera can have mortality rates of 50% or more.[19]

Patients at particular risk include those on antacids and those who are receiving acid reducers, such as proton pump inhibitors (PPI), for the treatment for peptic ulcer disease (PUD) as well as gastroesophageal reflux disease (GERD). Stomach acid plays a major role in reducing both the dose and the virulence of ingested cholera.

Cholera is a major concern whenever water treatment facilities are overwhelmed or incapacitated, such as during a major flood or hurricane. Simple boiling or chlorination of drinking water and washing bedding and night clothing with chlorine can prevent the spread of the disease. To date, there have been seven major cholera pandemics in history, starting in the 1800s and continuing to the 1970s. A cholera outbreak was reported in Iraq in 2007.

Treatment of cholera consists of supportive measures including intravenous hydration and basic antibiotics. With treatment, mortality from cholera can be reduced to less than 1%. However, there has been an increasing concern about a multiple drug-resistant strain of cholera that current therapies may be ineffective in treating.

Dysentery

Although diarrhea can be distressing, blood in the diarrhea, called **dysentery**, can be even more alarming. Dysentery represents a higher level of intestinal wall involvement and is often associated with severe cramps and **tenesmus**, a persistent need for a bowel movement, which may be painful.

The etiology of dysentery is typically either bacterial or amoebic. The common causative agent of bacteria dysentery is the bacilli shigella. **Amoebic dysentery**, also known as traveler's dysentery, is caused by ingestion of contaminated water which contains protozoa, unicellular life forms that consume bacteria. It should be noted that not all protozoa produce disease. Many protozoa exist in the intestinal tract in a **symbiotic relationship**, a mutually beneficial association, with their human hosts.

Shigellosis

The etiology of bacillary dysentery is shigella, a pathogen that is transmitted by the fecal–oral route, via the hand to mouth. Foods contaminated with fecal material—such as potatoes, raw vegetables, meat, and milk—can also transmit shigella.

The onset of **shigellosis**, an infection with shigella, is usually within 12 to 24 hours. It may be initially dismissed as gastroenteritis because of the mild cramping, until the arrival of bloody stools signaling dysentery. The symptom pattern associated with shigellosis includes cramping, vomiting, dysentery, and tenesmus. One of the other distinguishing characteristics of shigellosis is the accompanying fever.

Amoebic Dysentery

The most common etiology of amoebic dysentery is the protozoa, entamoeba histolytica (Greek for tissue dividing).The cysts of the E. histolytica are found in soils and then ingested by their human hosts on improperly prepared foods. Like shigella, the E. histolytica causes abdominal cramping and dysentery. Unlike the shigellosis, it does not tend to cause fever. The treatment for E. histolytica is supportive, intravenous infusions, and the drug metronidazole (Flagyl®).

Clostridium Difficile

Clostridium difficile, more commonly known as C. dif, is a bacterial infection of the intestinal tract that creates colitis-like conditions. Part of the normal intestinal flora in some individuals, C. dif is kept in check by competitive inhibition from other bacteria. Therefore, when a patient is treated by an antibiotic, particularly cephalosporins or the "mycins," for an infection, the resulting "sanitization" of the bowel allows the C. dif to proliferate. C. dif is resistant to most antibiotics and causes antibiotic-associated diarrhea.

Cross-contamination of C. dif from patient to provider is possible. Under harsh conditions, C. dif forms a hardy spore which is capable of existence outside of the body. If fecal-contaminated bedding, for example, comes in contact with a surface (fomite), the potentially infectious spores remain. Then incidental contact made by an unsuspecting person can transmit the C. dif by the fecal–oral route. The acid-resistant

C. dif spore passes through the stomach and into the colon. Simple decontamination methods using hypochlorite (bleach) can inactivate the spores of C. dif.

One of the characteristics which differentiates C. dif diarrhea from other diarrhea is the foul smell. The presence of foul smelling stools, use of antibiotics, abdominal pain, and persistent diarrhea is highly predictive of clostridium difficile.

C. dif causes its symptoms via two mechanisms: enterotoxin (toxin A) and cytotoxin (toxin B). These two toxins combine to cause both diarrhea and inflammation of the intestine. The standard treatment of C. dif includes metronidazole (Flagyl©), anti-inflammatory medication, and supportive care such as intravenous fluids.

An alternative treatment approach has been suggested to control C. dif. Physicians are ordering **probiotics** (competitive bacteria, such as lactobacillus found in active culture yogurt) that help to restore the intestinal flora and create a competitive inhibition of C. dif.[20]

Giardia Lamblia

Perhaps one of the first pathological microbes discovered, **giardia lamblia** is a protozoan parasite that is barely visible to the naked eye. It was discovered by the inventor of the microscope, Antoni van Leeuwenhoek, in 1681 when he examined his own diarrhea. Giardia lamblia is a common parasite in dogs, cats, cows, sheep, deer, and beavers.

The last carrier of this parasite mentioned, the beaver, is responsible for a wilderness condition called "beaver fever." Hikers taking a drink from a mountain stream may be unaware of the beaver dam upstream, or the fact the water is contaminated with beaver feces containing giardia cysts. Because of the cyst formation, giardia is resistant to chlorination and other simple sanitation measures.

Once inside the gastrointestinal tract, the flagellated protozoa move to the walls of the small intestine and start to colonize there. In some cases, the patient becomes infected and symptomatic while others, about 50%, become carriers of giardia, continuing to spread the protozoa in their feces.

The symptom pattern associated with giardia is similar to other gastrointestinal diseases but is notable for the presence of flatulence. The flatulence, a foul sulphuric smell similar to rotten eggs, is accompanied by **steatorrhea**, fatty stools with a notable odor. The treatment for giardia lamblia, like E. histolytica, is supportive, intravenous infusions, and the drug metronidazole (Flagyl®).

Flagyl

The medication metronidazole (Flagyl®) has an interaction with alcohol that causes a disulfiram-like reaction. Disulfiram (Antabuse®) is used under a limited number of conditions to treat alcoholism.[21] In the normal metabolic pathway, alcohol is acted upon by the enzyme alcohol dehydrogenase, which converts the alcohol to acetaldehyde. Then the enzyme acetaldehyde dehydrogenase, in turn, breaks acetaldehyde into acetic acid, which is then harmlessly excreted into the urine.

Disulfiram interferes with the enzyme acetaldehyde dehydrogenase, which results in elevated levels of acetaldehyde. Acetaldehyde causes tachycardia (secondary to elevated dopamine levels), flushing of the skin, and shortness of breath, but most notably disulfiram causes profound nausea and violent vomiting. These obnoxious side effects of toxic levels of acetaldehyde in the body are intended to dissuade the patient from drinking alcohol. Interestingly, disulfiram was originally developed as a treatment for parasitic protozoan infections. Metronidazole, when taken for a protozoan infection, acts like disulfiram and the patient becomes nauseous when ingesting alcohol.

Cryptosporidium

Cryptosporidium, a protozoan parasite, is another source of diarrheal infection and is transmitted in contaminated water (i.e., fecal–oral route). The protozoan is notable because the spore (oocyst) can survive for prolonged periods and is resistant to disinfectants such as chlorine.

The initial symptoms occur between 2 and 10 weeks and the resulting abdominal cramps and diarrhea, accompanied by a low grade fever, can last up to two weeks. Once the symptoms subside, the patient is now a carrier capable of transmitting the disease to others. Paramedic care focuses on replenishing the volume lost and other supportive care and transporting the patient to an emergency department for a definitive diagnosis.

Borreliosis

Although borreliosis (i.e., Lyme disease) is not an amoebic disease, it is another woodland disease, and perhaps more importantly an emerging infectious disease. First identified in Lyme, Connecticut, in 1975, borreliosis is caused by borrelia burgdorferi, a Gram A negative bacterium that is a spirochete like syphilis.

Spread by the common deer tick, Lyme disease has become one of the most common tick-borne diseases in the United States and is found in almost all 50 states, although it is endemic to the northeast seaboard and the Midwest. Occurring most frequently in the spring and summer, the infection usually takes one to two weeks before the initial onset of symptoms, although it can take months for the infection to develop in some people.

The infection following a deer tick bite, and subsequent borreliosis, leaves a bull's eye-shaped skin infection, or erythema migrans (EM), that is pathognomonic of Lyme disease and is seen in approximately 80% of Lyme disease cases.[22,23] Flu-like symptoms—such as fever, myalgia, and malaise—are also associated with Lyme disease.

Untreated Lyme disease tends to affect the heart and the musculoskeletal system. During the acute phase, patients may experience heart blocks or palpitations and, over time, develop myocarditis. However, the typical sequela for Lyme disease includes joint pain (arthralgia), arthritis, and peripheral paresthesia.

The apparent lack of a tick bite (often difficult to see under the best of conditions) or the absence of EM, in combination with nonspecific flu-like symptoms, makes the diagnosis difficult. Therefore, some people assume that they have either chronic fatigue syndrome or fibromyalgia. This is unfortunate because the treatment of Lyme disease is curable with a number of antibiotics.

Food-Borne Illness

Not unexpectedly, food-borne illness is the result of ingesting foods that cause disease. Food-borne illness can be broken down into three categories: food infection, food intoxication, and food poisoning. Food infection is the presence of bacteria such as E. coli, salmonella, or campylobacter on the food stuff. Food intoxication is the production of endotoxins from bacteria such as staphylococcus or clostridium botulinum.

Finally, food poisoning occurs when (1) food is improperly stored, thus permitting decay; (2) decayed materials, such as soil, are not removed during processing; or (3) foods are properly prepared and properly cooked to remove pathogens, but the food itself is poisonous, such as wild mushrooms.

The symptoms of food-borne illness generally include nausea, with vomiting, diarrhea, and abdominal cramps. After the body purges itself of the offending substance, the patient generally recovers in several hours. Patients particularly vulnerable to food-borne illness are the very young (infants and toddlers) and the very old, as well as those with debilitating illnesses.

Food Infection
Escherichia Coli

Only certain strains of **Escherichia coli (E. coli)**, a bacteria commonly found in the large intestine, can be pathogenic. In fact, the nonpathogenic strains of E. coli, in a symbiotic relationship, are responsible for producing vitamin K for the body and for competitive inhibition of more pathogenic bacteria.

The primary source, or reservoir, for pathogenic E. coli is beef or dairy cows. Manure from these cows is used to fertilize vegetables, such as spinach, and can contaminate groundwater with E. coli. These strains of pathogenic E. coli can cause abdominal cramping. The associated diarrhea which follows is generally self-limiting, but can be life-threatening to the volume-sensitive elderly and infants. E. coli escaping the confines of the intestine (e.g., via a ruptured appendix) can progress to peritonitis.

Typically, E. coli responds well to antibiotics of the mycin classification. However, continual mutation creates drug-resistant strains of E. coli. Paramedic care focuses on providing supportive care, such intravenous infusions, and transportation to definitive care for antibiotic treatment. E. coli is also responsible for the majority of urinary tract infections (UTI) and can lead to life-threatening hemolytic uremic syndrome (HUS).[24,25]

Salmonella

Salmonella, most famous for causing typhoid fever (Salmonella typhi), can also cause food-borne illness. Salmonellosis, caused by salmonella enterica, is famously transmitted by raw eggs and uncooked chicken but can also be transmitted in egg-based foods, such as mayonnaise-laced potato or egg salad. Although freezing and refrigeration slow its growth, it does not destroy the salmonella bacteria; only cooking at temperatures above 165°F will destroy salmonella.

Along with diarrhea, salmonella can cause fever, chills, nausea with vomiting, and headaches within 12 to 24 hours of ingestion of contaminated foodstuffs. Salmonellosis can be prevented by simple infection control methods such as sanitizing food preparation surfaces with isopropyl alcohol or bleach and complete cooking of foodstuffs containing raw eggs.

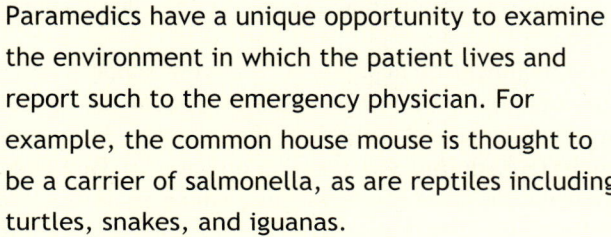

STREET SMART

Paramedics have a unique opportunity to examine the environment in which the patient lives and report such to the emergency physician. For example, the common house mouse is thought to be a carrier of salmonella, as are reptiles including turtles, snakes, and iguanas.

Food Intoxication

Food intoxication, as the name implies, is caused by toxins. Food poisoning can also be caused by toxins. However, food intoxication is the result of overproliferation of naturally occurring bacteria, as a result of poor food storage, whereas food poisoning is the result of the contamination of foods with poor food preparation. Often food intoxication does not substantially change the flavor of the food, leaving the patient unaware of the source of her illness.

Staphylococcus Aureus

Staphylococcus aureus is normally an innocuous bacterium that is found over most surfaces of the human body but is kept in check by the normal flora. However, when staphylococcus aureus contaminates food it tends to flourish, creating enterotoxin in the process. If the enterotoxin-rich foodstuff is ingested, then the patient may experience abdominal cramping and diarrhea.

The Paramedic should note that the enterotoxin does not have a particular odor or alter the taste of the food, making it nearly undetectable to the unsuspecting patient. A classic example of a by-product of "spoiled food," the enterotoxin exists despite the elimination of the bacteria by cooking, as enterotoxin is heat-resistant. Foods that tend to support staphylococcus aureus include processed meats; any protein including hams, tuna, and chicken; and milk and milk products.

Botulism

Botulism, caused by the bacterium clostridium botulinum, is a food-borne disease that was more common before modern food processing. Modern food canning uses a quick cook process (121°C for three minutes) to neutralize any botulinum before the food is canned. Amateur home canners, however, may not take the necessary steps in the canning process to prevent botulism. Certain home-canned foods, particularly low acid foods such as corn and green beans, are more likely to grow clostridium botulinum. When clostridium botulinum develops in the culture-like medium of canned foods, it creates gas which causes both aluminum and steel cans to bulge. Therefore, any can with a bulge on the end is suspect and should be discarded.

The patient with botulism intoxication can be symptomatic in as little as 12 hours. However, the symptoms usually occur 24 to 36 hours later, long after the suspect meal was ingested. This span of time from intoxication to symptom presentation reinforces the importance of an accurate and complete meal history.

The typical symptom pattern for botulism includes a dry mouth, slurred speech, and difficulty in speaking, mimicking the symptoms of a stroke. Other symptoms that lead the Paramedic away from the diagnosis of stroke include bilateral **ptosis** (drooping eyelids), vomiting, and diarrhea. If left untreated, botulism can lead to eventual paralysis of respiratory muscles and respiratory arrest. Part of the differential diagnosis of botulism are Guillain–Barré and myasthenia gravis, both of which can mimic the symptom pattern of botulism.

Treatment for botulism is supportive, with emphasis on airway control and respiratory support, particularly in advanced cases. The key to the diagnosis of botulism is a high index of suspicion that canned foods are the culprit. The Paramedic is in the unique position of investigating the home environment for the offending canned food and bringing the product to the emergency department for further analysis.

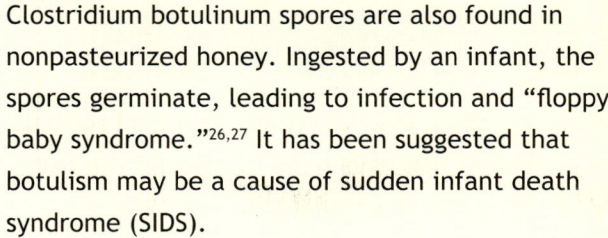

STREET SMART

Clostridium botulinum spores are also found in nonpasteurized honey. Ingested by an infant, the spores germinate, leading to infection and "floppy baby syndrome."[26,27] It has been suggested that botulism may be a cause of sudden infant death syndrome (SIDS).

Food Poisoning

Food poisoning is the contamination of foodstuffs. Typical food processing practices, such as pasteurization and hand washing, usually prevent food poisoning. Another major source of food poisoning is improper cooking. Major contributors to food poisoning include campylobacter jejunum and infectious hepatitis.

Campylobacter Jejunum

Campylobacteriosis is the result of gut contamination with the bacteria campylobacter jejuni (e.g., from ingestion of raw milk, hamburger, or shellfish), a ubiquitous bacteria found in most farm animals, particularly chickens. It is responsible for almost three times more outbreaks of food poisoning than salmonella in the United States.

Campylobacter is usually neutralized by stomach acid, as it is sensitive to hydrochloric acid. Individuals with gastroesophageal reflux disease (GERD), also known as heart burn, may be taking acid-reducing medications which leave them more predisposed to campylobacteriosis.

The **prodrome**, that period of incubation preceding an infection, for campylobacteriosis includes a diffuse and nonspecific symptom complex such as fever, headache, and muscle aches (myalgia), and then proceeds to the typical symptom pattern of campylobacteriosis.

The bacterium campylobacter jejuni settles in the jejunum of the small intestine, leading to watery loose bowel movements. Campylobacteriosis symptom complex includes abdominal cramps and diarrhea for a prolonged time, often two to five days post ingestion.

In some advanced cases, the infection can lead to bloody diarrhea and systemic complications. In other cases, the campylobacteriosis can lead to a condition called **toxic megacolon**. An enormously distended and dilated colon becomes dysfunctional and causes abdominal distention and systemic infection.

Simple infection control measures such as pasteurization and cooking of foodstuffs can prevent campylobacteriosis. Treatment is focused on supportive care, as the disease is generally self-limiting.

In some cases, following a bout of campylobacter-induced diarrhea, patients have progressed to the disease Gullain-Barré, an autoimmune disorder of the peripheral nervous system, which leads to weakness and flaccid paralysis.

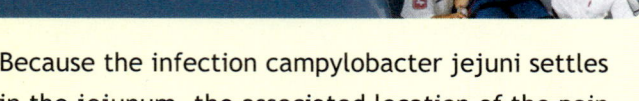

STREET SMART

Because the infection campylobacter jejuni settles in the jejunum, the associated location of the pain can be suggestive of appendicitis.

Acute Hepatitis

Hepatitis, as a series of diseases labeled A, B, C, and so on, is actually the result of a number of separate viral infections that have a similar impact on the liver, leading to the label

hepatitis. It should be noted that there are a number of other causes of hepatitis including toxins and drugs, Epstein–Barr virus, and yellow fever, as well as alcohol abuse.

During the early stage of hepatitis, the symptoms are nonspecific and include low grade fevers, diarrhea, and headache. As the disease progresses, the patient may experience anorexia, abdominal tenderness, and the characteristic **jaundice**, a yellowing of the skin and the sclera of the eyes.

Hepatitis A

Hepatitis A (i.e., infectious hepatitis) is caused by the hepatovirus hepatitis A (HAV). Found around the world, hepatitis A is most prevalent in developing countries with poor sanitation and wastewater treatment. However, cases are still being reported in the United States, primarily as a result of food service employees who are infected handling foodstuffs.

Transmitted via the fecal–oral route, the infection presents with nonspecific flu-like symptoms approximately two to six weeks after exposure. Over time, approximately six to nine months, the patient may experience the classic signs of hepatitis.

The treatment of hepatitis A is largely supportive during the course of the infection and most patients do not have lasting liver damage as a result of the infection. In high risk situations (e.g., during disaster relief operations), Paramedics may receive the hepatitis A vaccine, which should provide adults immunity for approximately 25 years and children immunity for 15 to 20 years.

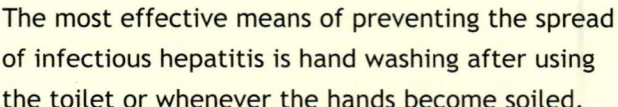

STREET SMART

The most effective means of preventing the spread of infectious hepatitis is hand washing after using the toilet or whenever the hands become soiled.

Hepatitis B

Hepatitis B (HBV), originally called serum hepatitis, is transmitted via either blood or bodily fluids, making it a cause of concern for Paramedics. Although HBV can be transmitted directly via sex or vertically from mother to child, HBV is easily transmitted via contaminated needles, particularly hollow bore needles such as the type used in injections and intravenous access.[28]

The DNA virus that causes HBV is found worldwide but is endemic to Africa and Far East Asia, where horizontal transmission is more common. The pathogenesis of HBV is owed to its interference with the liver cell reproduction.

Once infected, there is an approximately two-week to three-month incubation period followed by a three- to six-month infectious period. During the latter half of the infectious period, the patient may become symptomatic. During the symptomatic phase of HBV, the patient progresses through the usual symptom pattern of hepatitis and an unfortunate few patients may progress to fulminate hepatic failure (including toxic buildup of ammonia levels) with resulting cerebral edema and cerebral encephalopathy.

Although the immune system of most patients can effectively combat the HBV infection, prevention remains the cornerstone of medical therapeutics. There are several HBV vaccines available that use recombinant DNA technology. OSHA actually requires that the HBV vaccine be made available to healthcare workers, including Paramedics, without charge.

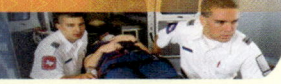

STREET SMART

HBV is thought to be the leading cause of liver cancer. It is hoped that the vaccination of school-aged children with HBV vaccine will eliminate liver cancer in the next generation.

Hepatitis C

Hepatitis C, originally known as non-A, non-B hepatitis, is another bloodborne viral infection. Similar to HBV, hepatitis C virus is passed along via blood-to-blood contact. Unlike HBV, the symptoms of hepatitis C virus are mild and the majority of patients have no symptoms during the acute phase.

The diagnosis of hepatitis C virus is usually made after elevated liver enzymes are returned, leading credence to the importance of annual physical examinations. At present, hepatitis C virus is the leading cause of liver transplants. Unlike hepatitis B, hepatitis C is not eliminated from the patient without medical therapies including antiviral drugs and interferon.

Hepatitis D

Hepatitis D is caused by another virus, an RNA virus (unlike hepatitis B and C, which are caused by a DNA virus), which is active only in the presence of HBV. Therefore, hepatitis D is either a coinfection or a superinfection and complicates the care of the patient with HBV. Because of its status as a coinfection or superinfection, the patient is more likely to experience fulminate liver failure and has a subsequent higher mortality rate.

Drug-Resistant Strains

The discovery of penicillin, a modern miracle that was first mass produced in 1943, was shortly followed by the discovery of the first penicillin-resistant microbe, streptococcus pneumoniae, in 1967. Since that time, multiple strains of drug-resistant bacteria have been discovered and each time pose a threat as another emerging disease.

Although complacency and overutilization of antibiotics has been blamed for the creation of these drug-resistant strains of bacteria, they continue to mutate and overcome the obstacles that antibiotics pose to their survival.

One such bacteria that is commonly known to Paramedics is **multiple–resistant Staphylococcus aureus (MRSA)**. This was formerly known as methicillin-resistant Staphylococcus, reinforcing the evolving nature of this bacterial threat.

MRSA, referred to in the common press as the superbug, is found in the hospital setting, and as such is a nosocomial infection. Within that community, MRSA colonizes the nostrils, open wounds, intravenous sites, and urinary catheters and is easily transmitted, by contact, from person to person. It must be treated with intravenous antibiotics.

Another drug-resistant bacteria that Paramedics should be familiar with is multi-drug resistant tuberculosis (MDR-TB).[29] This bacterium is resistant to the two standard antibiotic therapies for TB: isoniazid and rifampin. A newer, more pathogenic tuberculosis bacterium has developed, called extensively drug-resistant tuberculosis (XDR–TB). This condition, which is particularly problematic among the HIV-positive patient population; they have a 70% to 90% mortality from XDR-TB.

Acute Inflammatory Response

Whenever the body is being harmed, inflammation will occur. For example, inflammation can occur when a patient is burned, has suffered frostbite, or is exposed to toxins, poisons, and chemicals. However, the majority of cases of inflammation are due to infection (Figure 27-5).

Wherever the invading pathogen enters the body, mast cells in the area respond to the attack. Mast cells are located at the typical portals of entry (i.e., the skin, respiratory tract, and digestive tract) and destroy the invading pathogens through a process called **phagocytosis**. The name "mast" comes from the German "mastzellen" which translates to feeding cells. This is appropriate, because mast cells literally engulf (eat) the offending pathogen. Once the pathogen is within the mast cell, it is destroyed by the cell's lysosomes.

Mast cells are also alarm cells that secrete heparin and histamine that trigger the inflammatory process. The heparin and histamine are contained within the mast cells in granules. When the mast cell is stimulated it degranulates (i.e., it releases the heparin and histamine). Mast cells will also degranulate when triggered by a physical (i.e., trauma) or chemical stimulus.

The results of the release of heparin and histamine are vasodilation, increased vascular permeability, and a migration of leukocytes to the site of the infection. The increased local perfusion (i.e., vasodilation caused by histamine) permits an increase in the leukocytes carrying blood into the area. Histamine also opens up the space between the endothelial cells that line the capillaries, permitting migration of the leukocytes into the tissues. The capillaries, which are now "leaky," also allow intravascular fluid to leak into

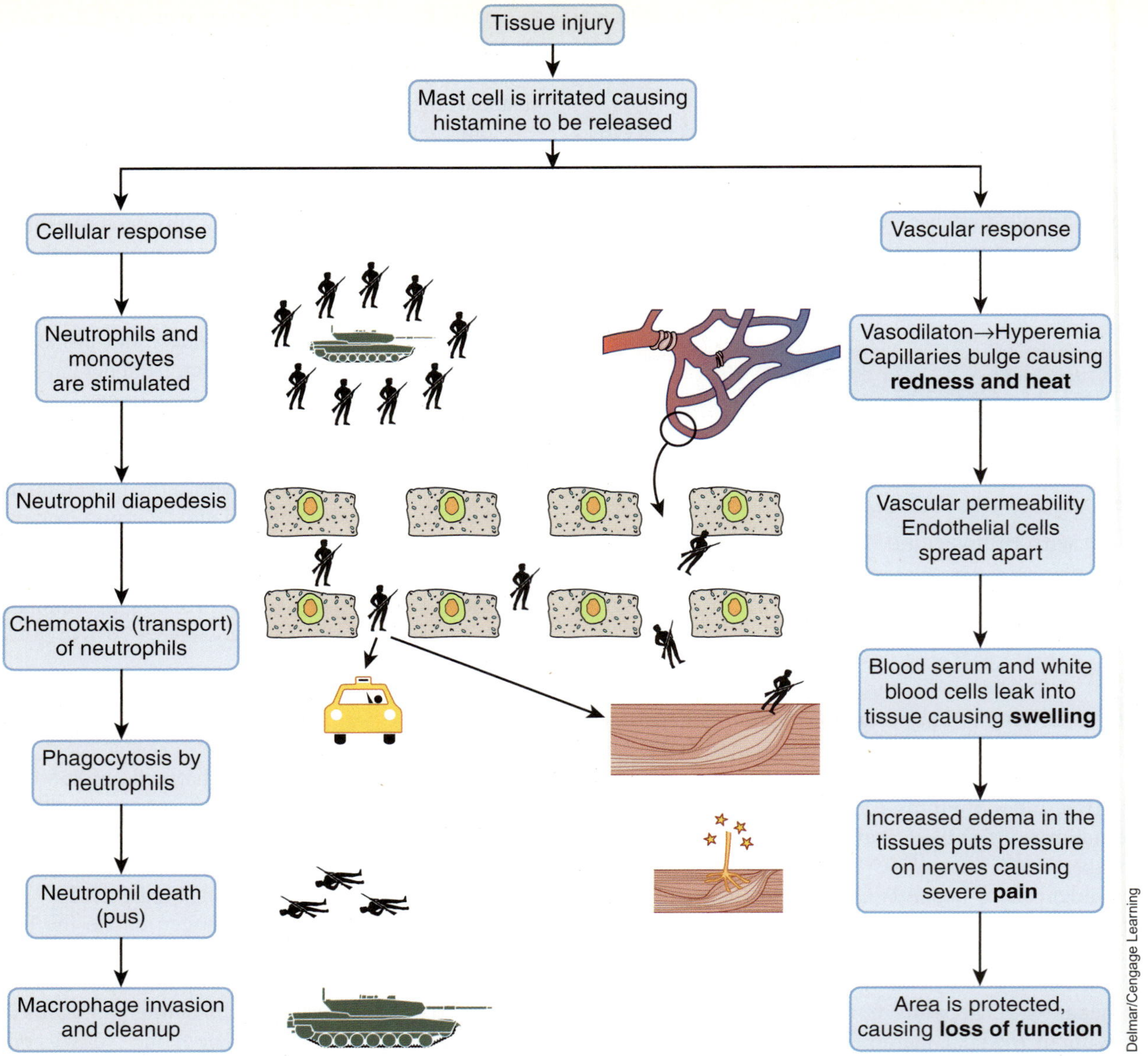

Figure flowchart

Tissue injury

↓

Mast cell is irritated causing histamine to be released

↓ (splits to two branches)

Cellular response (left branch)

↓

Neutrophils and monocytes are stimulated

↓

Neutrophil diapedesis

↓

Chemotaxis (transport) of neutrophils

↓

Phagocytosis by neutrophils

↓

Neutrophil death (pus)

↓

Macrophage invasion and cleanup

Vascular response (right branch)

↓

Vasodilaton→Hyperemia Capillaries bulge causing **redness and heat**

↓

Vascular permeability Endothelial cells spread apart

↓

Blood serum and white blood cells leak into tissue causing **swelling**

↓

Increased edema in the tissues puts pressure on nerves causing severe **pain**

↓

Area is protected, causing **loss of function**

Delmar/Cengage Learning

Figure 27-5   Process of inflammation.

the interstitial space, or the third space. This leakage results in localized edema.

The cardinal signs of an infection are caused by the inflammatory response. Inflammation (Greek for flame) causes the symptoms of calor (warm to the touch), rubor (redness), tumor or swelling, dolar (pain), and loss of function. These symptoms are the result of vasoactive mediators, such as histamine released from mast cells, which cause localized vasodilation and open the junctions between the cells to allow the white blood cells (leukocytes) into the area.[30] Mast cells also release prostaglandins that can cause further vasodilation as well as fever and pain.

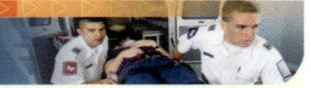

STREET SMART

Antipyretics and analgesics inhibit prostaglandins that are released by the mast cells and cause fever and pain.

Once in the area, these leukocytes attempt to remove the offending infection via opsonization and phagocytosis. Opsonization is a process that binds and coats the pathogen for a targeted attack by leukocytes that in turn engulf and destroy the pathogen. Leukocytes use digestive chemicals within the lysosomes, in a process called phagocytosis, to destroy the opsonized pathogen.

This movement of protein and antibody-containing plasma fluid, or **exudates**, into the area will cause localized swelling (i.e., edema) and point tenderness to the injury. Eventually, the inflammation will lead to the formation of yellow-tinged white pus or purulence. If the purulence is on the surface of the skin, then macules filled with the purulence can form into small pimples, larger boils, or interconnected boils called **carbuncles**. If the infection is within the body, then it will form an abscess. An abscess forms its own cavity; however, if the purulence collects in an existing cavity (e.g., the pleural cavity), it may be called an **empyema**.

As the infection intensifies, two types of leukocytes (i.e., white blood cells) from the immune system are recruited: the granulocytes and agranulocytes. The granulocytes have three classifications: neutrophils, basophils, and eosinophils. Neutrophils make up the majority of granulocytes and phagocitize, using lysosomes, both bacterial and fungal infections. If the infection is parasitic in nature, then eosinophils—rather than neutrophils—phagocitize the infection. Finally, basophils, making up less than 1% of granulocytes, assist the mast cells by releasing histamine and maintaining vasodilation.

By and large, the granulocytes are responsible for a generalized immune response to parasites, bacteria, and fungus. The agranulocytes are responsible for what is more traditionally thought of as the immune response by attacking viruses.

As the term implies, agranulocytes do not have the lysosomes (i.e., granules) for digestion of phagocitized microbes and work by an antibody–antigen mechanism instead. However, like granulocytes, agranulocytes have three classifications: lymphocytes, monocytes, and macrophages.

The first category, lymphocytes, can be further divided into B cells, T cells, and natural killer cells. B cells and T cells work to make antibodies and kill viruses. T cells also release a chemical called interferon, originally called macrophage-activating factors, that phagocitize infected cells.

Natural killer cells, the third lymphocyte, kill all unnatural cells (i.e., cancerous, infected, and old dysfunctional cells) by releasing proteins that connect to cells that are missing receptors that mark the cell as native, and force a process called **apoptosis** (i.e., programmed cell death).

The monocytes, the second classification of granulocyte, migrate from the bloodstream to the tissues, where they become macrophages and aid neutrophils in the attack by phagocitizing bacteria. However, monocytes have a further advantage in that they can kill via antibody-mediated cellular cytotoxicity (discussed further in a moment).

Macrophages are also capable of releasing nitric oxide, the active chemical in nitroglycerine. Nitric oxide helps to maintain vasodilation through direct smooth muscle relaxation. One of the major roles of macrophages is to introduce foreign proteins found on the microbe, called an **antigen**, to helper T cells who make antibodies.

The T cells then release the antibodies that attach to the bacteria's surface antigen in a key and lock fashion. These antibody–antigen complexes make it easier for the macrophages to attach to and attack the bacteria.

Macrophages also release cytokines, a signaling protein compound that communicates (i.e., signals) to other immune cells. These cytokines cause macrophages to migrate to the source of the infection (i.e., chemotaxis), and cause the classic systemic effects of an infection (i.e., anorexia, fever, and tachycardia). These cytokines also activate three more systems.

Systemic Inflammatory Response

When a localized infection spreads beyond the confines of the abscess, and the inflammation with it, the infection activates three other systems: the complement system, the kinin system, and the coagulation system. These three systems combine with the inflammation to create a systemic response to the pathogen.

As the name suggests, the complement system works together with the immune system to attack infections. However, the complement system does not act alone and must be activated by cytokines or antigen–antibody complex. These antibodies—immunoglobins found in the blood and named immunoglobin G (IgG), immunoglobin M (IgM), and so on—coat the bacteria for phagocytosis through opsonization. The complement system also releases a number of cytokines that increase the intensity of the immune system's response.

The **kinin system** further continues the inflammatory response by maintaining the vasodilation, specifically the polypeptide bradykinin, a potent vasodilator.

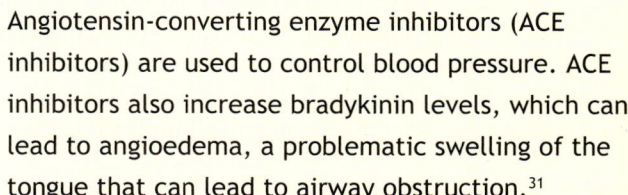

STREET SMART

Angiotensin-converting enzyme inhibitors (ACE inhibitors) are used to control blood pressure. ACE inhibitors also increase bradykinin levels, which can lead to angioedema, a problematic swelling of the tongue that can lead to airway obstruction.[31]

The inflammatory system is also aided by the coagulation system. Using fibrin, stimulated by cytokines and other prothrombus proteins (such as prostaglandins), the coagulation system forms a net over the infection site, confining the infection to a certain area.

When an infection becomes systemic, cytokines signal immune cells to respond to the assault. These cytokines are also responsible for the patient's high fever as well as the malaise, anorexia, and nausea that often accompanies a systemic infection.

Upon arriving, the Paramedics are directed to Room 27C for a Mr. Kenyon. They ask what brought Mr. Kenyon into the nursing home. The nurse says that, in addition to his diabetes, he had been falling at home and originally came for rehabilitation just two weeks ago. Shortly after arriving, he developed an open wound along his shin, which became infected. His treatment with a course of antibiotics led to diarrhea and now he has irritation and an open wound on the buttocks as well.

Today he presents with fever, tachypnea, and hypotension. The physician is notified and orders a transfer to the hospital for further evaluation.

CRITICAL THINKING QUESTIONS

1. What are the important elements of the history that a Paramedic should obtain?
2. What is the symptom pattern for acute inflammatory response?

History

One of the greatest hazards of aging is immobility. The human body is intended to function best when standing upright, thereby using gravity to facilitate bodily functions. For example, a person naturally uses gravity to suspend and expand the lungs to help facilitate breathing. The patient lying flat has decreased rib cage expansion and an increased residual capacity in the lungs. The stagnant air left in the lungs leads to reduced oxygen tension and increased risk of hypoxia. Furthermore, without the ability to breathe deeply or cough effectively, fluids such as phlegm tend to pool in the lungs, leading to pneumonia.

To compound the problem, the cilia within the airways would normally help to move pathogen-laden mucus out of the airway (i.e., the mucous elevator). The elderly have both fewer cilia and goblet cells, leading to decreased mucous production, and the mucous elevator quickly becomes dysfunctional. Add a weaker diaphragm and stiffer, less compliant lungs that prevent the patient from coughing up these secretions, and you have a situation where secretions cannot be cleared completely, leaving a perfect medium for infection.

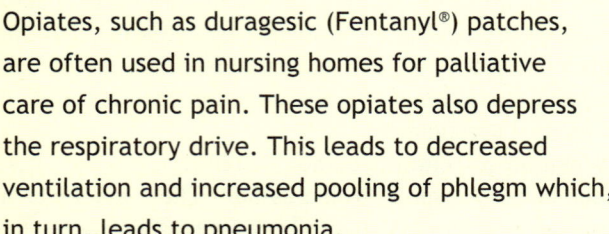

STREET SMART

Opiates, such as duragesic (Fentanyl®) patches, are often used in nursing homes for palliative care of chronic pain. These opiates also depress the respiratory drive. This leads to decreased ventilation and increased pooling of phlegm which, in turn, leads to pneumonia.

Similarly, a review of the kidney's gross anatomy reveals that the kidneys drain downward, assisted by gravity. When a patient is supine, urine tends to collect in the renal pelvis and remain stagnant. Encroaching infections from the urethra, aided by instrumentation of the urethra by catheters, can settle into the kidneys. This causes **pyelonephritis**, an ascending urinary tract infection.

Finally, the combination of thinner skin (a natural consequence of aging), decreased peripheral blood flow (from declining cardiovascular function), and bed rest can lead to the development of bed sores. Bed sores are open wounds found over bony areas such as the hips, elbows, knees, and especially the bony sacrum. These wounds are breeding grounds for infection, especially if the wound is contaminated with feces and/or stale urine.

With an understanding of the dangers of immobility, the Paramedic should focus the history on recent events. Has the patient been recently discharged from the hospital and did the patient have a nosocomial infection, such as MRSA, while in the hospital? There has been an increase in the number of patients placed in long-term healthcare facilities because of dementia. A patient with dementia may behave in a manner that is dangerous and subsequently may need to be either physically or chemically restrained for his own protection. The Paramedic should ask if the patient has been restrained and for how long.

However, the most common reason for enforced bed rest may be fractures, particularly hip fractures. The Paramedic should inquire if the patient has recently fallen or if the patient has had surgery for a long bone fracture.

In some instances, the history is difficult to obtain from the elderly patient. Common alternative sources for the medical history are caregivers and the patient's chart. A history of any of these events should cause the Paramedic to be suspicious of infection.

When the Paramedics arrive in Mr. Kenyon's room, they find him lying in a semi-Fowler's position on his bed with the side rails up. He doesn't take notice of their arrival and only moans when his name is called. The nurse tells the crew that usually Mr. Kenyon has a great sense of humor and likes to discuss politics with the staff. The Paramedics ask when Mr. Kenyon was last out of bed and what his last vital signs and blood sugar were.

The nurse reports that, per the chart, Mr. Kenyon was seated in the chair yesterday morning but required more than the usual assistance to get out of bed. His last set of vital signs, taken approximately 45 minutes ago, were temp of 97.8°F rectally, pulse 115 and slightly irregular, respirations of 28 and shallow, with a blood pressure of 94/64 and a glucose of 104.

CRITICAL THINKING QUESTIONS

1. What are the elements of the physical examination of a patient with suspected acute inflammatory response?
2. Why is the temperature a critical element in this examination?

Examination

The typical sign of an infection is a fever of unknown origin (FUO). Often the elderly are unable to mount a febrile response to an infection, taking away this vital sign for infection. In the case of the elderly, the Paramedic should focus on the alternative sign of an infection, the sudden onset of confusion or delirium. **Delirium** is an acute alteration of mental status secondary to a physiologic imbalance. After ruling out hypoxia and hypoglycemia as potential causes of delirium, the Paramedic should suspect infection as the source of delirium in the elderly.

Delirium, unlike dementia, is not a progressive deterioration of mental function but rather an acute decline that has a specific set of symptoms. This set of symptoms makes delirium a clinical syndrome. Delirium is manifest by psychological impairment, loss of awareness of time or place marked by confusion, and general agitation. Key to the diagnosis of delirium is the time of onset. Delirium occurs in hours to days whereas dementia is a constant and progressive deterioration over weeks to months. For an elderly patient, delirium might manifest by restlessness, pulling at catheter tubing, and sleeplessness at night, as well as an inability to focus attention during conversation.

The patient starts to become increasingly agitated and uncooperative with care. Based on the patient's presentation and the symptom complex, the Paramedic makes a diagnosis of acute inflammatory response. In light of the patient's advanced age and comorbidities, the Paramedic decides to transport the patient emergently to the general hospital.

CRITICAL THINKING QUESTIONS

1. What is the significance of the hypotension and fever?
2. What diagnosis did the Paramedic announce to the nursing staff?

Assessment

Although confusion, hallucinations, and agitation are also common signs with psychological conditions, the Paramedic should assume that any elderly patient with these symptoms is manifesting delirium, and not dementia or mental illness. Almost by definition, delirium is a temporary condition that is potentially reversible. Failure to identify and treat these conditions can result in permanent injury to the patient.

The Paramedics provide high-flow, high-concentration oxygen, despite a satisfactory pulse oximeter reading, since the Paramedics understand the impact of fever upon the oxyhemoglobin curve. Next, the Paramedics focus on restoring Mr. Kenyon's blood pressure, via intravenous infusions, and check his blood glucose levels. Next, the Paramedics, unwisely, try to stand Mr. Kenyon up to transfer him to the stretcher, whereby the patient immediately passes out and collapses to the floor.

CRITICAL THINKING QUESTIONS

1. What is the standard of care of patients with acute inflammatory response?
2. What are some of the patient-specific concerns and considerations that the Paramedic should consider when applying this plan of care that is intended to treat a broad patient population presenting with acute inflammatory response?

Treatment

The brain needs a constant supply of oxygen and blood glucose to function. Initial treatment of the patient who is mentally dysfunctional (i.e., confusion) should be focused on eliminating hypoxia and hypoglycemia as potential causes.

At its core, infection in general causes a problem of oxygen delivery at the cellular level. Tissues have an inability to extract oxygen from the blood as a result of the peripheral edema that interferes with the diffusion of oxygen to the cells. As a consequence of the imbalance between tissue oxygen demands and oxygen delivery, cells revert to anaerobic respiration with the resulting production of lactic acid. The acidemia-induced rightward shift of the oxyhemoglobin dissociation curve results in decreased affinity of hemoglobin to bind with oxygen, thus requiring a higher partial pressure of oxygen to attain the same oxygen saturation (see the Bohr effect for more details).

Some Paramedics depend on pulse oximetry to titrate their oxygen therapy to optimal effect. However, pulse oximeters depend on adequate peripheral perfusion for a reading, and many elderly patients have poor peripheral perfusion. For this reason, the use of pulse oximetry with the elderly may result in erroneous readings. If the pulse oximeter reading is dubious, and the patient appears delirious, then high-flow, high-concentration oxygen via mask is in order.

Although stress-induced hyperglycemia is common in patients with an infection, the elderly patient should be monitored for hypoglycemia. The brain of the elderly patient has poor tolerance for the hypoglycemia that can occur when the patient is hypermetabolic due to infection. The Paramedic should consider administering glucose to any patient with a blood glucose under 70 to 80 mg/dL.

Although studies have shown a decrease in mortality after stroke when glucose is normalized, other studies have shown that callous administration of high-concentration glucose, a hyperosmolar solution, can be devastating to the fragile cells of the elderly patient's brain. Paramedics should consider dividing the dose of glucose and/or diluting the glucose in order to decrease the osmolarity shift.

Transportation

The Paramedic should be cautious about asking an elderly patient who has been on bed rest to stand or walk to a stretcher, since blood pools in the chest of the supine patient. This increased venous pooling is sensed by venous volume receptors which, in turn, cause a reduction of antidiuretic hormone secretion. The resulting diuresis can decrease blood plasma volumes by approximately 500 mL in the first 24 to 48 hours of bed rest.

Typically a patient who is asked to stand also holds her breath (i.e., the Valsalva maneuver) as she attempts to stand. This momentary breath holding results in increased intrathoracic pressures and a decreased venous return. The normal heart, sensing the decreased venous return, compensates by increasing the heart rate (within 5 to 15 seconds), and the sympathetic nervous system constricts to raise pressure (within 15 to 20 seconds). The elderly patient is often unable to mount this compensatory tachycardia, due to medications such as beta blockers or vascular disease.

As a result of the combination of decreased blood volume and diminished cardiac responsiveness, coupled with use of the Valsalva maneuver, the patient's blood pressure drops precipitously, cerebral perfusion is compromised, and the patient experiences syncope.

While en route to the hospital, Mr. Kenyon remains unstable and unresponsive to the fluid challenges. The patient is intubated with an end-tidal carbon dioxide reading of less than 32 mmHg and a sustained tachypnea. Despite a persistent tachycardia greater than 120 bpm and a two liter normal saline fluid infusion, the patient remains hypotensive. The Paramedic with Mr. Kenyon elects to start a dopamine infusion and prepares a second intravenous access for the dopamine. Once the IV is established, the Paramedic starts to quickly titrate the dopamine infusion, every 5 to 10 minutes, until a satisfactory mean arterial pressure (65 mmHg) is obtained.

CRITICAL THINKING QUESTIONS

1. What are some of the predictable complications associated with acute inflammatory response?
2. What are some of the predictable complications associated with the treatments for acute inflammatory response?

Evaluation

One of the most serious complications of a systemic infection is the development of **systemic inflammatory response syndrome (SIRS)**, a pathological condition that arises when cytokine levels become so elevated (e.g., during a cytokine storm, because of unchecked T cell and macrophage activity) that the cytokines have a negative effect on the body. A cytokine storm, as a result of a positive feedback loop with the immune system, is analogous to the inappropriate immune response seen with anaphylaxis.

Cytokines are proinflammatory chemical mediators that signal immune cells—such as T cells and macrophages—to respond to the infection. These cells, in turn, secrete more cytokines, which results in more immune cells becoming drawn into the attack. This is a classic example of a positive feedback loop.

However, in cases of an overwhelming infection the levels of cytokines can raise to dangerous levels, creating unique problems associated only with the presence of elevated cytokines, and can lead to complications such as **acute respiratory distress syndrome (ARDS)**.[32]

For example, one cytokine, tumor necrosis factor, is responsible for apoptotic cell death, the natural death of an aged cell. During a cytokine storm, elevated levels of tumor necrosis factor can lead to the premature death of cells, particularly immature immune cells, with devastating results. Elevated cytokine levels also increase the release of nitric oxide, the chemical in nitroglycerin that causes vasodilation. Finally, elevated levels of cytokines cause the release of proteases, protein-dividing enzymes that damage endothelial cells that line the capillary beds, increasing the fluid lost to the third space and causing intravascular hypovolemia.

Table 27-6 SIRS Criteria

- Elevated heart rate (>90 bpm)
- Alteration in body temperature (>38°C or <36°C)
- Sustained tachypnea (>20 bpm)
- Low end-tidal carbon dioxide (EtCO$_2$ <32 mmHg)
- Elevated white cell count (leukocytosis)

The clinical syndrome, systemic inflammatory response syndrome, is the result of these various cytokines and is defined as having a fever, tachycardia, tachypnea, and a low end-tidal carbon dioxide level (Table 27-6).

If untreated, SIRS will progress to profound hypotension and hypoperfusion as a result of hypovolemia from third spacing. Leaky capillaries in the lungs result in pulmonary edema that results in ventilation–perfusion mismatch and adult respiratory distress syndrome. In some cases, the patient may experience disseminated intravascular coagulation (DIC). DIC is a result of an imbalance between coagulation and fibrinolysis that results in inappropriate clot formation, vascular blockage, and consequential ischemia and end-organ damage. Paradoxically, the loss of clotting factors—to inappropriate clotting and thrombocytopenia associated with DIC—results in hemorrhage and shock.

Like anaphylaxis or severe traumatic shock, the Paramedic must act quickly to restore hemodynamic stability. As the prototypical distributive shock, this is accomplished by a combination of aggressive fluid resuscitation and use of vasopressors. The drug of choice in the case of SIRS is dopamine. As a vasopressor, dopamine can increase blood pressure through vasoconstriction. As an inotropic agent, dopamine can also increase the myocardial force of contraction.[33] Typically dopamine is in a standard concentration and infused at 5 to 20 micrograms per kilogram of patient's weight per minute if the patient remains unresponsive to fluid bolus.

If the patient remains unresponsive to dopamine (i.e., the systolic pressure remains 40 mmHg less than baseline), then the Paramedic could consider an epinephrine drip. Epinephrine is a powerful vasoconstrictor and is typically mixed as one milligram in 270 cc of solution, yielding a solution of 4 micrograms per mL, and then the infusion is started at 1 to 2 micrograms per minute to a maximum of 10 micrograms per minute.

CASE STUDY CONCLUSION

Mr. Kenyon's vital signs are essentially unchanged from the earlier report given to the emergency department by the nurse: blood glucose is 110 and pulse oximetry with a good waveform showed 89% even after the oxygen was applied. Most importantly, the patient remained unconscious and hypotensive.

Upon their return to the emergency department later that day, both Paramedics inquire about Mr. Kenyon. The physician tells them that he likely had clostridium difficile complicated by a local infection of the open wound on his shin.

CRITICAL THINKING QUESTIONS

1. What is the most appropriate transport decision that will get the patient to definitive care?
2. What is the long-term prognosis for the patient?

Disposition

The rapid development of SIRS, and the subsequent need for rapid medical intervention, could be compared to the golden hour of trauma care. Volume infusions and vasopressors are but a stopgap measure in the treatment of the patient with SIRS. The definitive treatment is aggressive antibiotic therapy while in a critical care unit. Rapid transportation to a receiving facility capable of providing these services is imperative.

CONCLUSION

Infectious diseases strike patients of all ages, with very young and elderly patients at risk for developing systemic inflammatory response syndrome. The Paramedic must not only effectively treat the patient but also remember to use appropriate infection control procedures to protect herself from the spread of disease. With more of a public health focus on pandemic flu preparation, Paramedics will become an integral part of first-line care.

KEY POINTS:

- An infection is an attack by microbes that results in disease.

- Pathogens include
  - Bacteria
  - Viruses
  - Funguses
  - Protozoa
  - Helminthes (worms)
  - Prions

- Some bacteria can release exotoxins as they grow or endotoxins as they die. Both toxins are capable of causing disease.

- In order for infectious disease to result, the chain of infection between source and host must exist.

- Components of the chain of infection are
  - Reservoir
  - Exit from reservoir
  - Route of transmission
  - Host

- Infectivity is based on dose, virulence, and host resistance.

- The host resistance results from barriers, inflammation, and immunity.

- Dose is the actual number of microbes whereas virulence is the capacity of the microbe to survive.

- Infectious diseases are tracked by morbidity (the number of people who develop the disease) and mortality (the number of people who die from the disease).

- There are four stages of infection:
  - Incubation
  - Prodrome
  - Infectious
  - Recovery

- Common respiratory diseases include
  - Common cold
  - Respiratory syncytial virus
  - Influenza
  - Haemophilus influenzae
  - Streptococcus
  - Yersinia pestis
  - Tuberculosis
  - Croup
  - Laryngotracheobronchitis
  - Pertussis
  - Epiglottitis

- Common gastrointestinal diseases include
  - Gastroenteritis
  - Dysentary
  - Shigellosis
  - Clostridium difficile
  - Amoebic dysentery
  - Giardia lamblia
  - Cryptosporidium

- Food-borne diseases include
  - Escherichia coli
  - Salmonella
  - Food intoxication
  - Botulism
  - Campylobacter jejunum
  - Hepatitis A

- Bloodborne diseases include
  - Hepatitis B, C, and D

- Drug-resistant strains of known infections are emerging due to the use of antibiotics.

- Systemic inflammatory response syndrome (SIRS) results from spread of a localized infection with activiation of complement, kinin, and coagulation systems. The inflammatory response continues, harming healthy tissues well beyond that which was necessary to halt the original infection. Signs include

- Elevated heart rate
- Above or below normal temperature
- Tachypnea
- Low EtCO$_2$
- Elevated white blood cell count

- A history of immobility is cause for the Paramedic to consider an infection.

- Although a fever is a common indicator of infection, the elderly patient may be unable to produce a fever.

- Delirium is an indicator for infection in the elderly patient.

REVIEW QUESTIONS:

1. Define an infection.
2. Name six pathogens.
3. How do exotoxins differ from endotoxins?
4. Describe the components of the chain of infection.
5. What is the likely cause of drug-resistant strains of known infections?
6. What causes SIRS? Give at least four signs.
7. Explain why an elderly patient with an infection may present with a subnormal temperature and a change in mental status.

CASE STUDY QUESTIONS:

Please refer to the Case Study in this chapter, and answer the questions below:

1. Name at least three risks that Mr. Kenyon has for a potential infectious process.
2. Is Mr. Kenyon likely to have delirium or dementia? Support your answer.
3. What do Mr. Kenyon's vital signs and repeat vital signs suggest about the likely cause of his mental status?

REFERENCES:

1. Richards CL, Jr. Preventing antimicrobial-resistant bacterial infections among older adults in long-term care facilities. *J Am Med Dir Assoc*. 2005;6(2):144–151.
2. Smyth RL, Openshaw PJ. Bronchiolitis. *Lancet*. 2006;368(9532):312–322.
3. Kimpen JL. Management of respiratory syncytial virus infection. *Curr Opin Infect Dis*. 2001;14(3):323–328.
4. Van Woensel JB, Kimpen JL, et al. Respiratory tract infections caused by respiratory syncytial virus in children. Diagnosis and treatment. *Minerva Pediatr*. 2001;53(2):99–106.
5. Kelly H, Birch C. The causes and diagnosis of influenza-like illness. *Aust Fam Physician*. 2004;33(5):305–309.
6. Prasad K, Karlupia N. Prevention of bacterial meningitis: an overview of Cochrane systematic reviews. *Respir Med*. 2007;101(10):2037–2043.
7. Swingler G, Fransman D, et al. Conjugate vaccines for preventing Haemophilus influenzae type B infections. *Cochrane Database Syst Rev*. 2007;2:CD001729.
8. Morris SK, Moss WJ, et al. Haemophilus influenzae type b conjugate vaccine use and effectiveness. *Lancet Infect Dis*. 2008;8(7):435–443.
9. Nohl J. *The Black Death: A Chronicle of the Plague*. Yardley, PA: Westholme Publishing; 2006.

10. Cain KP, Benoit SR, et al. Tuberculosis among foreign-born persons in the United States. *JAMA*. 2008;300(4):405–412.

11. Ailinger RL, Moore JB, et al. Adherence to latent tuberculosis infection therapy among Latino immigrants. *Public Health Nurs*. 2006;23(4):307–313.

12. Gittler J. Controlling resurgent tuberculosis: public health agencies, public policy, and law. *J Health Polit Policy Law*. 1994;19(1):107–147.

13. King AB. Accurately interpreting PPD skin test results. *Nurse Pract*. 1999;24(5):144–147.

14. Long CO, Holmes NJ, et al. The tuberculin skin test. Administration and interpretation. *Home Healthc Nurse*. 1993;11(3):13–18.

15. Ciesielski SD. BCG vaccination and the PPD test: what the clinician needs to know. *J Fam Pract*. 1995;40(1):76–80.

16. Levy RJ, Helfaer MA. Pediatric airway issues. *Crit Care Clin*. 2000;16(3):489–504.

17. Altunaiji S, Kukuruzovic R, et al. Antibiotics for whooping cough (pertussis). *Cochrane Database Syst Rev*. 2007;3:CD004404.

18. Repasky TM. Emergency! epiglottitis. *Am J Nurs*. 1995;95(9):52.

19. Zuckerman JN, Rombo L, et al. The true burden and risk of cholera: implications for prevention and control. *Lancet Infect Dis*. 2007;7(8):521–530.

20. Surawicz CM. Role of probiotics in antibiotic-associated diarrhea, Clostridium difficile-associated diarrhea, and recurrent Clostridium difficile-associated diarrhea. *J Clin Gastroenterol*. 2008;42 Suppl 2:S64–S70.

21. Suh JJ, Pettinati HM, et al. The status of disulfiram: a half of a century later. *J Clin Psychopharmacol*. 2006;27(3):290–302.

22. Dandache P, Nadelman RB. Erythema migrans. *Infect Dis Clin North Am*. 2008;22(2):235–260, vi.

23. Bratton RL, Whiteside JW, et al. Diagnosis and treatment of Lyme disease. *Mayo Clin Proc*. 2008;83(5):566–571.

24. Copelovitch L, Kaplan BS. The thrombotic microangiopathies. *Pediatr Nephrol*. 2008;23(10):1761–1767.

25. Zakarija A, Bennett C. Drug-induced thrombotic microangiopathy. *Semin Thromb Hemost*. 2005;31(6):681–690.

26. Brook I. Botulism: the challenge of diagnosis and treatment. *Rev Neurol Dis*. 2006;3(4):182–189.

27. Zellweger H. The floppy infant: a practical approach. *Helv Paediatr Acta*. 1983;38(4):301–306.

28. West DJ. The risk of hepatitis B infection among health professionals in the United States: a review. *Am J Med Sci*. 1984;287(2):27–33.

29. Drobniewski F, Balabanova Y, et al. Clinical features, diagnosis, and management of multiple drug-resistant tuberculosis since 2002. *Curr Opin Pulm Med*. 2004;10(3):211–217.

30. Marino P. *ICU Book, The,* second edition. Philadelphia: Lippincott Williams & Wilkins; 1997.

31. Israili ZH, Hall WD. Cough and angioneurotic edema associated with angiotensin-converting enzyme inhibitor therapy. A review of the literature and pathophysiology. *Ann Intern Med*. 1992;117(3):234–242.

32. Deja M, Hommel M, et al. Evidence-based therapy of severe acute respiratory distress syndrome: an algorithm-guided approach. *J Int Med Res*. 2008;36(2):211–221.

33. Beal AL, Cerra FB. Multiple organ failure syndrome in the 1990s. Systemic inflammatory response and organ dysfunction. *JAMA,* 1994;271(3):227–233.

CHAPTER 28

INFECTIOUS DISEASES: RASH

KEY CONCEPTS:

Upon completion of this chapter, it is expected that the reader will understand these following concepts:

- That rashes may indicate a benign or life-threatening condition, so finding a rash is an important clinical sign
- The importance of including a patient's vaccination history as part of the past medical history
- The importance of surveillance and early detection of infectious diseases as public health measures that involve Paramedics

ANATOMY CONCEPTS:

Prior to reading this chapter the Paramedic student should be familiar with the following anatomy and physiology concepts:

- Inflammatory response
- Immunology

The ambulance squad is called to the Student Health Clinic at the State University for an 18-year-old male patient who has come in with a rash, fever, and severe headache. As they grab their personal protective equipment, the Paramedic talks to the EMT about possible causes for this combination of signs and symptoms.

CRITICAL THINKING QUESTIONS

1. What are some of the possible causes of rash?
2. How are fever and headache related to the rash?

OVERVIEW

A rash, fever, and severe headache are the classic signs of an infection, and a patient with these symptoms should seek immediate medical attention. Although many infections are benign (not harmful), some infections are potentially life-threatening. The challenge for the Paramedic is to try to distinguish between the two extremes of an infection and make the correct clinical decision regarding the patient's care.

Chief Concern

The diseases described in the following paragraph are all capable of producing a rash. While tedious to learn, Paramedics should be familiar with the most common infectious diseases that they may encounter. The mnemonic TEST, standing for **T**ransmission, **E**pidemiology, **S**ymptoms, and **T**reatment, is useful for learning these diseases. The Paramedic should be aware of the various transmission vectors for these diseases so spread to both the Paramedic and other individuals can be prevented (Table 28-1).

Childhood Diseases

During childhood, children are exposed to many diseases. Each time a child's immune system responds to and overcomes a disease, that child develops a greater resistance

Table 28-1 Diseases and Modes of Transmission

- Droplet
  - Chickenpox (varicella)
  - Common cold (rhinovirus)
  - Influenza
  - Whooping cough (pertussis)
  - Tuberculosis
  - Mumps
  - Measles
  - Rubella (German measles)
- Fecal–oral
  - Cholera
  - Hepatitis A (infectious hepatitis)
  - Polio (poliomyelitis)
  - Salmonella
- Sexual
  - Human immunodeficiency virus
  - Chlamydia
  - Gonorrhea
  - Syphilis

to the disease. Five of these typical infectious diseases of childhood—measles, mumps, rubella, roseola, and chickenpox—manifest with a widespread rash, called an **exanthema** (Figure 28-1).[1]

Chickenpox

Chickenpox, caused by the **varicella zoster virus (VZV)**, is transmitted by either airborne droplet via a cough, or by physical contact with a contaminated fomite. In the past, chickenpox was seen as a common childhood disease and more of a nuisance than a danger. However, since the introduction of the varicella vaccine in the mid-1990s, chickenpox has become a rarity. However, the varicella vaccine does not offer life-long immunity and is only thought to be effective for 10 years. Therefore, introduction of chickenpox, via immigration from countries that do not vaccinate, can cause sporadic outbreaks.

Chickenpox has an incubation period of 10 to 20 days. The patient is most contagious in the two days before the first pox (a small, itchy, irregularly shaped blister) appears. The patient with chickenpox proceeds with classic catarrhal signs (inflammation of the mucous membranes) with or without conjunctivitis (inflammation of the outer eye). The appearance of the classic pox appears a day or two later and covers

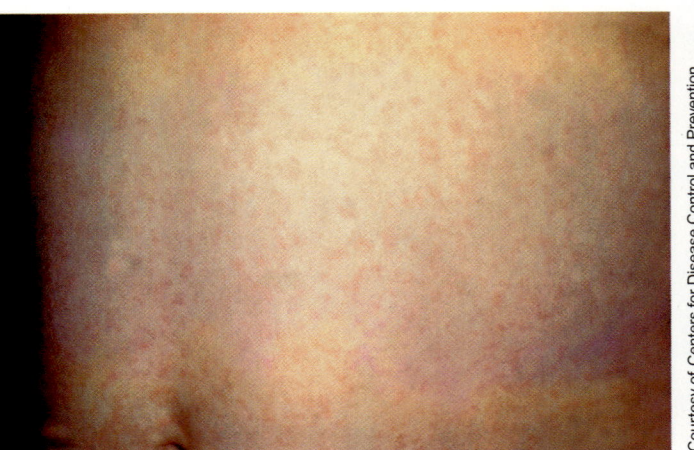

Figure 28-1 Exanthema.

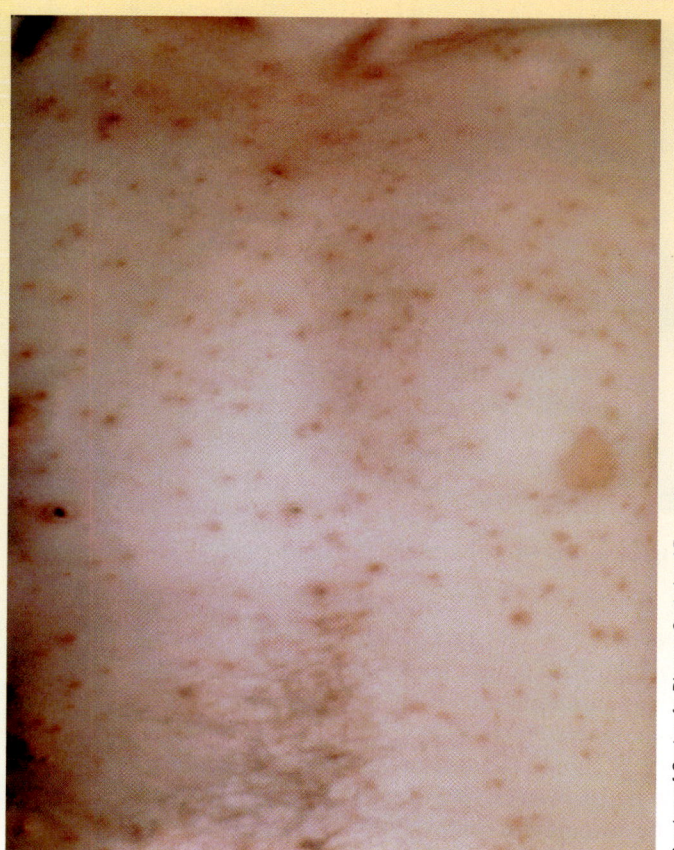

Figure 28-2 Chickenpox.

the central body, sparing the hands (Figure 28-2). The fluid within the pox is highly contagious, containing thousands of varicella viruses. The patient remains contagious until the pox ruptures and dries up (scabs over). The complete cycle of pox may take days to a week to resolve, coming in waves of outbreaks.

Chickenpox has been positively linked to congenital birth defects including microcephaly (small head), hydrocephaly (water on the brain), damage to the eye (causing blindness), and other neurological disorders.

As chickenpox is generally self-limiting, treatment is largely supportive. Perhaps the most disconcerting symptom of chickenpox is the pruritus, or itching, which can be somewhat relieved with antihistamines like diphenhydramine (Benadryl®). In some instances, the patient may have self-applied calamine lotion, a topical preparation that contains zinc oxide and has a distinctive pink–salmon color; however, studies have never shown a therapeutic effect to calamine lotion's use.

Any associated low grade fever can be treated with acetaminophen. Patients should avoid taking aspirin, as aspirin administered during viral infections has been associated with Reye's syndrome, a rare but potentially fatal disease that affects the brain and the liver.[2-4]

The Paramedic's concern with any viral infection is a secondary bacterial infection that develops because of the weakened immune system. Open lesions on the skin, called pox marks, permit entry of opportunistic bacteria into the body, which often leads to pus formation and secondary scarring.

STREET SMART

An outbreak of chickenpox in later years can lead to a condition called **shingles**. Shingles (**herpes zoster**) is caused by varicella zoster virus (VZV), the same virus which causes chickenpox. VZV, also called human herpes 3 (HHV-3), is one of the eight herpes viruses that afflict man. Zostavax®, a concentrated form of the chickenpox vaccine, can be given to the elderly to prevent shingles.

Roseola

Roseola is another childhood infection caused by the herpes virus. Like chickenpox, roseola is transmitted by airborne droplet or physical contact and is highly contagious. Typically affecting children between the ages of 6 months and 3 years, roseola starts as an unexplained fever.[5] The high fever (greater than 101°F) can rise so rapidly that the child has a febrile seizure.

After the fever subsides in approximately one to two days, a truncal rash appears, spreading outward to the patient's extremities but sparing the face. Unlike chickenpox, roseola does not cause catarrhal symptoms. The disease is treated with hydration and fever reducers (antipyretics).

Rubeola (Measles)

Measles is an ancient disease caused by the paramyxovirus **rubeola**. Reports of people having measles have appeared as early as 900 B.C. Like chickenpox, measles is transmitted by inhalation of airborne droplets or contact with infectious fluids. Measles is most contagious during the three to five days after the patient's rash appears.

Although the disease occurs worldwide, measles is only occasionally seen in the United States because of children's vaccination with the mumps, measles, and rubella vaccine. Unvaccinated individuals, particularly those between the ages of 2 and 12 years of age, are 90% at risk of infection with exposure.

Following an approximately two-week incubation period, the patient with measles will start to experience the prodromal symptoms (early warning signs) of measles which can be summed up with the three Cs: cough, **coryza** (head cold with runny nose), and conjunctivitis (eye

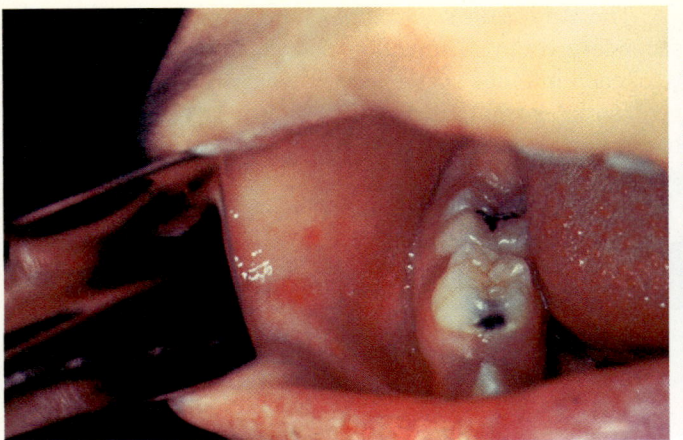

Figure 28-3 Koplik's spots.

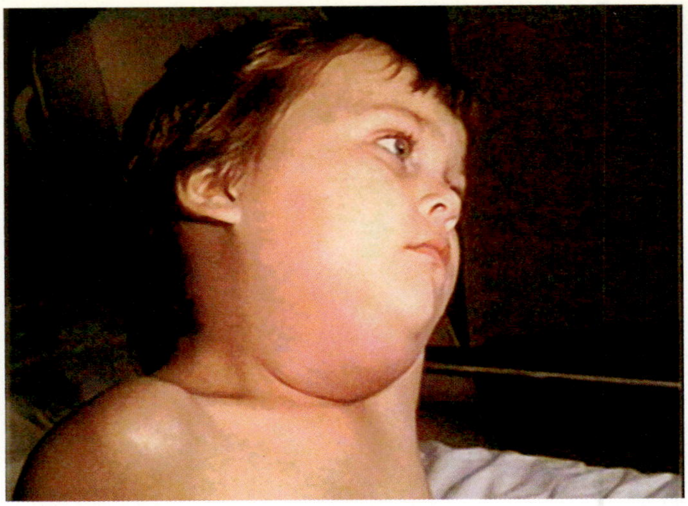

Courtesy of Centers for Disease Control and Prevention

Figure 28-4 Swollen parotid glands of mumps.

Courtesy of CDC/NIP/Barbara Rice

irritation). Following the prodrome, a raised flat (maculopapular) rash that starts at the head and proceeds in a cephalic-to-caudal fashion (head to toe) will emerge. Measles is distinguishable from other rash-producing diseases by the appearance of **Koplik's spots**, irregularly shaped red spots with white centers that resemble a bull's eye, inside the oropharynx along the buccal and lingual mucosa (Figure 28-3).

Along with antipyretics for the high fever and antipruritics for the rash, the treatment of measles usually involves quarantine and rest. Complications from measles range from diarrhea to encephalitis. Immunocompromised patients are at greatest risk of life-threatening complications. Mortality is one per thousand cases in developed countries.[6,7]

Rubula (Mumps)

Painful swollen salivary glands are a distinctive clinical marker for the paramyxovirus that causes mumps. **Mumps**, like measles (rubeola), is spread by inhalation of airborne particles of spittle or contact with saliva-coated clothing. It is a highly contagious disease, particularly among unvaccinated children between 2 and 12 years of age.

The typical prodromal symptoms for mumps include fever, headache, sore throat, and the distinctive swollen parotid glands in about 50% of cases (Figure 28-4). In particular, the patient may complain of point tenderness with palpation at the temporomandibular junction. Accompanying fever with vomiting and a headache may herald the onset of meningitis or encephalitis, a rare but dangerous development. In post-pubescent patients, mumps can infect the patient's testes (orchitis) or ovaries (oophoritis) and can, in rare cases, lead to sterility.

As in the other viral illnesses mentioned, treatment for the mumps is symptomatic. The greatest concern the patient may voice is jaw pain, especially with chewing. This pain, coupled with a high fever, may lead to anorexia. Both these symptoms should be treated with antipyretics, such as acetaminophen. As with every viral infection in children, the patient should avoid taking aspirin. The application of ice to the patient's neck, proximal to the parotid glands, may help relieve some discomfort.

Rubella (German measles)

Originally confused with measles and scarlet fever, **rubella** (from the Latin meaning "little red") is characterized by a distinctive red rash. Originally described by a number of German physicians, rubella has also been called **German measles**. Rubella is transmitted via airborne droplets but, uncharacteristically for a childhood viral disease, can also be passed in the urine and feces.

Despite a relatively long incubation period (two to three weeks), rubella is a mild, short-lived infection, averaging three days, leading some to call it the "three day measles." Besides the characteristic red rash that spreads centrifugally (from the core to the extremities), the patient may also experience a low grade fever and swollen glands (Figure 28-5). Some patients—particularly women—may develop joint pain, or **arthralgia**.

Although rubella is relatively benign when compared to other childhood viral diseases, it can be particularly problematic for the pregnant patient. The unborn child whose mother contracts rubella, particularly in the first trimester, is at risk of **congenital rubella syndrome**. The newborn with congenital rubella syndrome is at risk for a number of congenital birth defects of the heart (patent ductus arteriosus), hearing impairment, cataracts, and mental retardation.

As a consequence of the widespread use of the triple vaccine for mumps, measles, and rubella (MMR), the

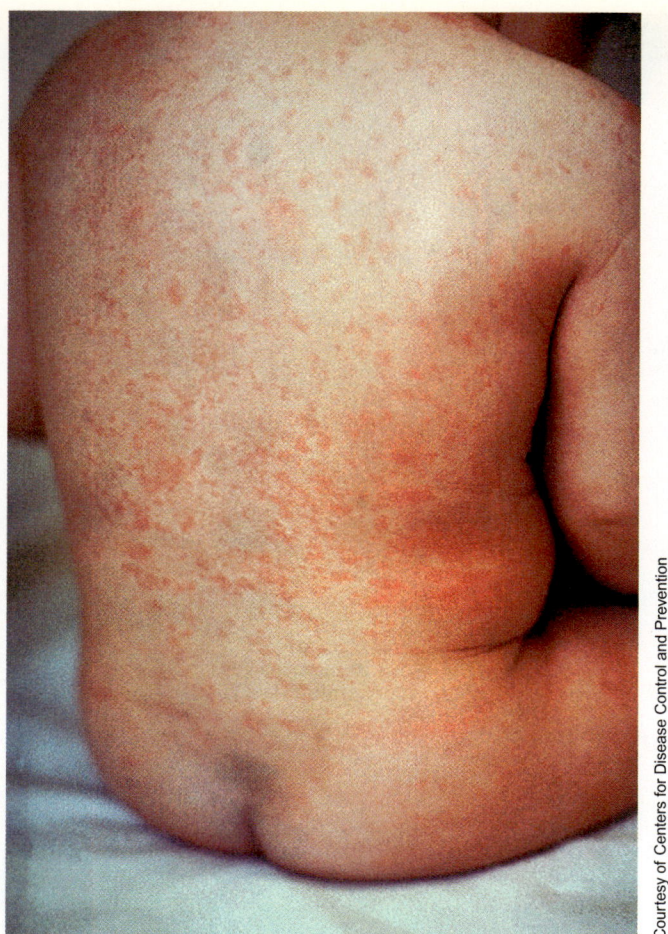

Figure 28-5 Rubella.

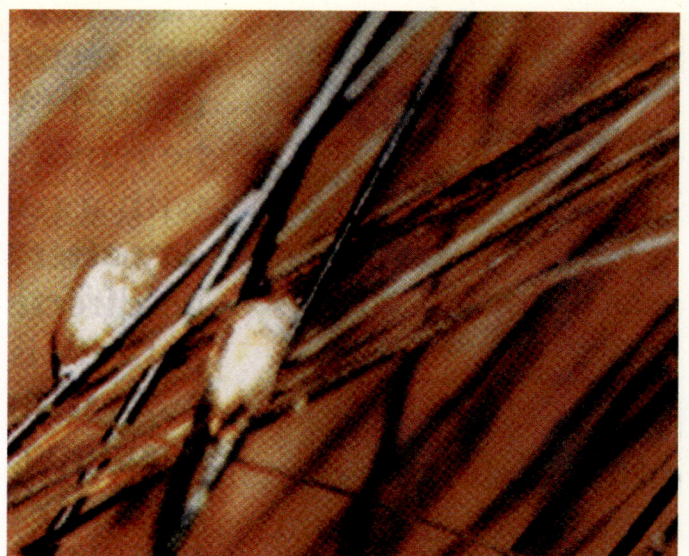

Figure 28-6 Lice nits.

incidence of these three childhood diseases has dropped dramatically to approximately one case for every three-quarter million population. The vaccine for mumps, measles, and rubella is recommended for all children at ages 1 to 1 1/2 years and again between the ages of 4 and 6. However, the vaccination only provides about 80% of the population with immunity and may need to be repeated between the ages of 11 and 12.

Pediculosis

Although lice is not a microbial infection, no discussion of childhood diseases would be complete without mentioning them. The common louse can be found on the head (**pediculosis capitis**), on the body (**pediculosis corporis**), and/or on the genitals (**pediculosis pubis** or **pthirus pubis** [crabs]) (Figure 28-6).

Lice spare no economic group and is endemic in some regions of the United States. Lice infest either clothing or hair, laying eggs (called nits) which mature into blood-sucking lice. Lice serve as a natural reservoir for the disease typhus and are capable of spreading it to those infested with the parasite.

At the size of a sesame seed, lice can move rapidly and spread both dung (as black specks) and nits (as white pearls) with the appearance of a small grain of rice. The treatment of lice includes permethrin (Nix®) or malathion (Ovide®), although the primary efforts should be focused on preventing the spread of the lice. For example, lice can be transferred via clothing, such as in a coat room. All the patient's clothing with suspected lice infestation should be laundered in hot water at temperatures greater than 131°F.

STREET SMART

The blood in the gut of a louse can be used to identify a rapist through DNA testing. For this reason, the clothing of a rape victim should be placed in a brown paper bag, without shaking or folding.

Scabies

Scabies are mites, not lice, and are barely visible on the skin. Unlike lice, scabies burrow under the skin, causing pruritis. Caused by the mite sarcoptes scabiei, scabies are transmitted from person to person through direct contact; for this reason, scabies is sometimes classified as a sexually transmitted disease.

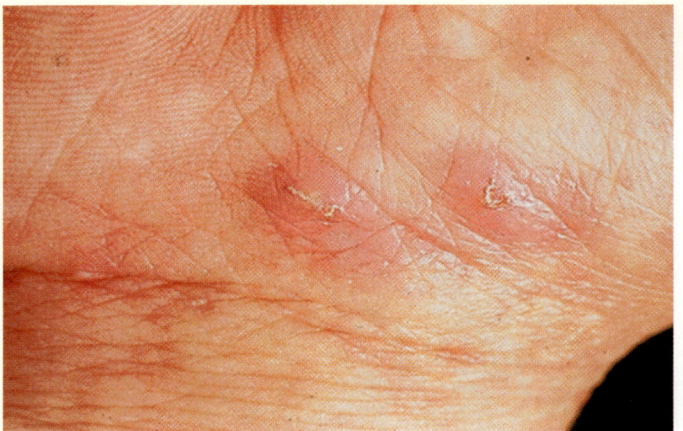

Figure 28-7 Scabies.

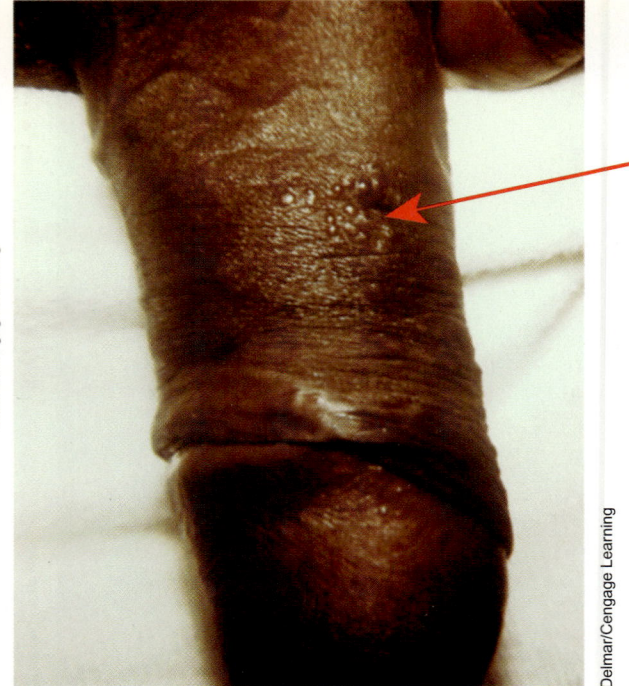

Figure 28-8 Syphilitic chancre.

As the pregnant mite tunnels under the dead layer of the patient's skin (the stratum corneum), she lays eggs. These eggs are responsible for the pruritus that can cause an allergic reaction, raising wheals (hives) that can resemble a rash (Figure 28-7). These symptoms may develop four to six weeks after the initial infestation, leading to concerns that the patient may have transferred the scabies to other intimate partners during that time.

Scabies tend to burrow into the webs of fingers, large joints (such as elbows and armpits), and the nipples (areola) of the breast. Scabies can also be found, as evidenced by their burrows, in the genitals as well as along the belt line.

Patients with scabies are treated with products containing permethrin or lindane (Kwell®). As with lice, prevention is the key to the treatment of scabies. Daily washing of the patient's clothing in hot water, vacuuming floors, and so on, as well as placing contaminated articles that cannot be washed into a plastic bag for a period not less than two weeks, will all help to limit the spread of scabies.

Sexually Transmitted Diseases

Some sexually transmitted diseases are capable of producing the prodromal symptoms of a rash, headache, and viral symptoms. **Sexually transmitted diseases (STD)**, formerly known as venereal disease (VD), are passed person to person through intimate contact. Some STDs, such as Chlamydia, are becoming endemic among youth. It is important to make a distinction between a sexually transmitted disease, where the patient is symptomatic, and a **sexually transmitted infection (STI)**, where the patient remains asymptomatic. A classic example is the case of the human immunodeficiency virus. It is possible to be infected with HIV (an STI) without being symptomatic, whereas acquired immunodeficiency syndrome (AIDS) would be considered an STD. Therefore, the Paramedic should be aware that a patient can have an STI but still need medical attention.

Syphilis

Syphilis may be the only disease to pass from the new world to the old world. Variously named for the different localities that had endemics caused by the disease (for example, "the disease of Naples"), syphilis is Latin for the French disease.

The causative agent of syphilis is the spirochete Treponema pallidum, transmitted by direct contact with lesions (called **chancres**) during sexual activity or by contact with blood (Figure 28-8).

As a bloodborne disease, syphilis is transmitted by microtears that occur during intercourse on the genital mucosa of each partner. Syphilis, like rubella (German measles), can also be passed horizontally from mother to child. Despite articles written by such notables as Professor William Allen Pusey, who wrote "The Principles and Practice of Dermatology 1917," syphilis cannot be contracted from inanimate surfaces such as a toilet seat, doorknobs, or drinking fountains.

From its early origins, and as a testament to the interconnectedness of people, syphilis is found in every human population, with an approximate rate of 2.1 cases of syphilis per 100,000 population in the United States.[8]

Syphilis has three described stages: primary, secondary, and tertiary. During the primary stage, a hard red nodule is raised on the skin surface (penis, vagina, or anus) and then ulcerates, leaving a depression filled with Treponema pallidum. These chancres are usually painless and develop between 10 and 90 days post-exposure and last from one to five weeks before spontaneously resolving.

Without antibiotic treatment, the syphilis progresses to the secondary stage. During the secondary stage, there are no chancres but the patient may develop a rash on the hands as well as generalized signs of infection including malaise, fever, and swollen lymph glands. During this period of about 10 weeks, the patient remains contagious.

The syphilis then goes into the tertiary stage. This latency phase may last months to years in duration while the bacteria infects the eyes, brain, heart, nerves, and bones, with neurological or cardiac involvement most common. During the tertiary stage, syphilis forms **gummas**, a form of granulomas, as well as infects the brain. Now referred to as **neurosyphilis**, the central nervous system's involvement causes headaches, meningeal signs such as nuchal rigidity, and cranial nerve involvement. Perhaps the most telling sign of neurosyphilis is the psychotic features including personality changes, insomnia, and paranoia, which might lead to the conclusion that the patient has "gone mad." However, the resulting insanity of neurosyphilis is generally more akin to dementia, which involves memory loss and personality changes.

The spirochete that causes syphilis is capable of crossing the placental barrier during a pregnancy. If the pregnancy occurred while the mother was in the primary or secondary stage of syphilis, then the infant is at risk of being stillborn. If the mother is in the third, or tertiary, stage, then the child may be born with an innocent infection of syphilis.

▷▷▷▷▷▷▷▷▷▷▷▷▷▷▷

STREET SMART

The pupils of the patient with tertiary syphilis are bilateral small pupils which are not able to constrict in bright light but will constrict with accommodation. Accommodation occurs when the patient focuses on an object and the object is brought closer to the patient, resulting in papillary reaction. The phenomenon has been known as prostitute's eyes or Argyll Robertson pupils.[9]

During the Wasserman test, an older test for syphilis, human blood serum from the patient was combined with sheep's blood containing cardiolipin to see if the blood would lyse from the sheep's antibodies. In contrast, existing tests for syphilis use monoclonal antibodies and fluorescence or polymerase chain reaction (PCR) testing.

The earliest treatments for syphilis used toxic mercury rubs, which riddled the bones and sometimes led to madness, or an arsenic compound called Salvarsan or Dr. Ehrlich's magic bullet. Contemporary treatment of syphilis uses antibiotics such as penicillin. Although sufferers of this STI seldom seek Paramedic care, those that do would receive supportive care.

Gonorrhea

Gonorrhea was originally thought to be leakage of semen from the penis (*gono*—Greek for seed and—*rrhea* from the Greek for flow; i.e., flow of seed). Gonorrhea may have received its more famous moniker ("the clap") from the old French "clapier," which means brothel. Regardless of the origin of its slang term, gonorrhea is a serious public health concern. Typically an STI, the causative agent for gonorrhea is the bacterium Neisseria gonorrhoeae, Gram-negative gonococci bacteria. Gonorrhea is capable of being transmitted by contact with an infection to the penis, the vagina (specifically the cervix), and the anus. Gonorrhea can also be transmitted horizontally to a newborn during passage through the birth canal. The resulting conjunctivitis, if untreated, can lead to permanent blindness. Silver nitrate drops placed in the infant's eyes prevent this from occurring.

Gonorrhea, although one of the most common STIs, has seen a decline in incidence since the public health initiatives of the 1970s. However, a newer strain of penicillin-resistant gonorrhea has been cause for concern, which could lead to an increase in cases of gonorrhea in the future.

Even if treated, gonorrhea can lead to chronic pelvic pain secondary to pelvic inflammatory disease (PID) in women and infertility secondary to fallopian tube scarring. This tubal scarring may also lead to an increase in life-threatening ectopic pregnancy.

Following mucosal inoculation, an odorous purulent discharge from the penis, anus, or vagina occurs within two days to two weeks and is associated with dysuria or difficulty with urination. Males may also note scrotal swelling and tenderness. If the patient has an oropharyngeal infection, then the patient may experience a mild pharyngitis (sore throat). On occasion, autoinoculation of the eye, by unwashed hands, can lead to purulent ocular discharge and conjunctivitis. Some women may be subclinical and/or asymptomatic because of the endocervical involvement, which leaves no outward manifestation of the infection.

As the untreated infection progresses, the disseminated gonococcal infection (DGI) can cause low grade fevers, arthralgia or pain in the joints, and a rash that can be seen on all body surfaces (including the palms and soles of the feet) except the head. The gonorrheal infection can then progress to the meninges, causing bacterial meningitis.

The classic treatment of gonorrhea was penicillin. However, other broad spectrum antibiotics, such as fluoroquinolones like Ciprofloxacin® from the "floxacin" group, and cephalosporins such as ceftriaxone (Rocephin®), are more effective.

Chlamydia

Chlamydia is the most commonly transmitted STI in the United States and has reached epidemic proportions. Chlamydia is caused by the Gram-negative bacterium Chlamydia trachomatis (not to be confused with the trichomonas vaginalis or "trich" infection.)

Chlamydia is estimated to cause as many as four million infections annually and may be present in as many as 10% of sexually active teenagers.[10,11] Although a genital Chlamydia infection has almost no associated mortality, the consequences of infection can be devastating. Chlamydia is a leading cause of pelvic inflammatory disease and infertility.

Known as the "silent" disease, Chlamydia starts as a mild urethritis (inflammation of the urethra), with or without painful urination. The infection then resolves and leaves the patient, particularly males, in the carrier state. The infected woman is at particular risk for infertility (as a result of mucosal changes), ectopic pregnancy, and (if pregnancy does occur) miscarriage, premature rupture of membranes (PROM), and preterm labor. Newborns of women with Chlamydia tend to have low birth weight, and risk neonatal pneumonia and conjunctivitis. As in other diseases, treatment for Paramedics is supportive and the patient should be transported to a medical facility for definitive treatment with antibiotics.

Human Immunodeficiency Virus (HIV)

Although **human immunodeficiency virus (HIV)** is not an infection which generally causes a rash, it is included in this discussion of sexually transmitted infections because of its close relationship with other STI. HIV is a retrovirus that is transmitted in blood, semen, vaginal fluids, and breast milk, but is generally not transmitted in saliva, urine, feces, or tears.

The typical route of transmission for HIV is sexual intercourse. In the past, HIV was thought to be a "gay man's" disease, transmitted primarily in same-sex relationships. However, HIV is also transmitted between heterosexual couples and is the dominant mode of transmission worldwide. HIV can also be transmitted via shared needles, by drug addicts, and horizontally from mother to child during childbirth. In the past, HIV could also be transmitted via blood transfusion. However, modern blood screening techniques can identify and eliminate this potential route of transmission. HIV infection has become a pandemic, particularly in third world countries.

Once a cell, typically a macrophage, is infected with HIV, the virus will invade a cell and either become dormant or proliferate. Some individuals are "nonconverters": although

exposed to the virus, their individual genetic makeup makes them resistant to the infection.

If the virus proliferates, and the viral load increases, there is a corresponding decrease in the T cell numbers (count) and an acute viremia occurs. During the initial infection, the patient's immune system responds, decreasing the viral load, and the patient experiences a mild flu-like syndrome including (in order of occurrence) fever, malaise, myalgia or muscle pain, rash, headache, and night sweats. This mixed initial presentation is often either ignored by the patient, dismissed as the flu, or may be misdiagnosed because of its presentation, which is similar to a number of other viral illnesses.

With the patient's viral load reduced by the immune system, HIV enters into a clinical latency period that can last anywhere between 2 weeks to 20 years. During the clinical latency period, the patient remains contagious.

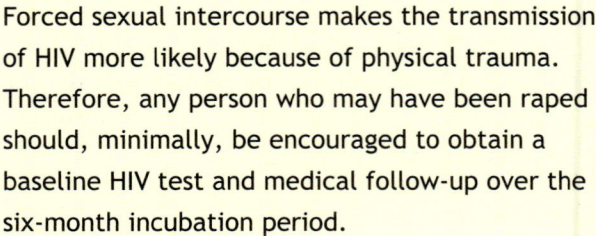

STREET SMART

Forced sexual intercourse makes the transmission of HIV more likely because of physical trauma. Therefore, any person who may have been raped should, minimally, be encouraged to obtain a baseline HIV test and medical follow-up over the six-month incubation period.

The third stage is collectively referred to as **acquired immune deficiency syndrome (AIDS)** and includes a number of clinical conditions and diseases. During this later phase of the HIV infection, the patient's declining immune system response, specifically the CD4 T cell count, leaves him vulnerable to a number of opportunistic infections (such as candidiasis) and cancers such as Kaposi's sarcoma. This loss of cellular immunity can also lead to flare-ups in tuberculosis and recurrent upper respiratory infections (URI).

Patients with AIDS are likely to present with fever, swollen glands, weakness, and weight loss. Two symptoms—night sweats and chills—are also suggestive of AIDS and its major pulmonary diseases, tuberculosis (TB) and pneumocystis carinii pneumonia (PCP). The patient may also present with persistent diarrhea secondary to salmonella, shigella, campylobacter, and Escherichia coli. However, the diarrhea may be a side effect of the HIV drugs, the antibiotics used to treat other infections, or both.

Patients with AIDS may also experience AIDS dementia complex (ADC). ADC presents with cognitive, motor, and behavioral impairments that can be easily confused with psychotic disorders or toxic syndromes.[12]

The cancers associated with AIDS are thought to be the result of co-infection with an oncogenic (i.e., cancer causing) virus. For example, Kaposi's sarcoma (KS), a cancer of the connective tissues and skin, is thought to be the result of infection by the Kaposi's sarcoma-associated herpes virus (KSHV) and cervical cancer is thought to be caused by human papilloma virus (HPV).

There is no cure for AIDS. Therefore, all care of the patient with AIDS is supportive. With highly active antiretroviral therapy (HAART) it is thought that the progression of HIV to AIDS can be halted and that HIV in the future will be more like a chronic infection.

Emerging Infectious Disease

Disease and pestilence have accompanied humans since the beginning of recorded time, and quite possibly before that as well. During that time, physicians have tried various remedies to either cure these diseases or ameliorate the suffering they caused. However, in the last 100 years medicine has substantially decreased the morbidity and mortality due to disease. What change occurred that had a significant impact on the incidence of infectious disease? Improved sanitation clearly had the greatest impact on the epidemiology of disease. Starting with the achievements of the Romans, clean water and sanitary sewers have long been recognized as an important public health measure to decrease disease among a population sharing communal resources. Concurrent development of vaccines and antibiotics has also had a tremendous impact on reduction of disease, resulting in an increase in the longevity of life. In addition, improvements in medical detection and treatment have certainly had an impact.

Yet, there has recently been a dramatic increase (58%) in the number of deaths blamed on infectious diseases in the United States. The reemergence of infectious disease as a major cause of mortality and morbidity has been independently attributed to increased urbanization, modern transportation, and lack of universal health care. Perhaps the most important factor may be microbial adaption and the creation of drug-resistant strains of infection.

Emerging infectious diseases can be classified into three categories: new diseases (e.g., SARS), re-emerging diseases (e.g., the West Nile virus), and the newest classification, drug-resistant infections. Methicillin-resistant Staphylococcus aureus (MRSA), discovered in England in 1961, is an example of a drug-resistant strain of infection. MRSA has mutated to become resistant to the beta-lactam antibiotics such as penicillin and methicillin as well as cephalosporins.[13–16]

Infection Control

To stem the impact of these emerging diseases, the public health system, including Paramedics, must take certain measures early in a disease's history. The first step in controlling these emerging infections is surveillance and early detection.

A vigilant program of surveillance at the local, county, state, and national level will help identify disease outbreaks early. This is accomplished through reports of symptom **clusters**, events such as multiple cases of diarrhea or flu-like symptoms. These events are compared against the expected incidence of those symptoms within a given population in order to identify variation.

Epidemiological information of disease prevalence, incidence of reportable diseases, and so on, is shared with others in a **Morbidity and Mortality Weekly Report (MMWR)**. Paramedics, from their unique position sitting between the public and the hospital, can help with the identification of cases. This advantage is amplified when one considers that Paramedics transport many patients to many hospitals across a region. Seeing "the big picture" may bring the total number of reportable cases to a critical mass, whereas each individual hospital may not appreciate the magnitude of an outbreak.

Once a potential outbreak has been identified (e.g., an epidemic curve is noted on a histogram of cases), then public health measures shift from surveillance to containment and vaccination in order to control the outbreak. The three containment strategies are isolation, quarantine, and restrictions.

Isolation is the movement of infected and ill patients to a facility separate from the population. In single cases of disease, an outbreak can be isolated in a hospital. In community-wide outbreaks, however, it may be necessary to isolate the infected patients in alternative locations, such as hotels, in order to protect the vulnerable non-infected patients in the hospital. Considering that most hospitals are staffed for routine operations, and do not have a **surge capacity** large enough to care for the influx of new patients at both facilities, it may be necessary to enlist additional auxiliary healthcare professionals, such as dentists, veterinarians, and Paramedics.

Simultaneously, those people who are infected but not ill will need to be placed in quarantine. Quarantine was originally used to hold ships in harbor for 40 days (quarantine is from the Latin *quaranta giorni* or 40 days), as people believed that the Black Plague would manifest within a crew in that time. Quarantine can be brief (e.g., for the period of time for decontamination), or may persist for a longer time period. The length of quarantine is a function of the disease and the effectiveness of containment of the contamination.

Quarantine can be performed on a case-by-case basis, using house arrest. To actualize those quarantines, people or industries might permit a liberal leave policy. Quarantine can also involve entire communities. Examples of community quarantine include the quarantine of Chinatown within San Francisco in 1900 (to contain the plague) and the 1972 outbreak of smallpox in Yugoslavia.

Another effective containment strategy is movement restriction. Using powers of martial law, the government can prevent people from traveling. In the United States, citizens have certain freedoms which prevent the government and its law enforcement agents from restricting that freedom. If a person believes his liberty has been abridged, he can bring a lawsuit (called a writ of *habeas corpus*) to the courts and demand release from the unlawful imprisonment. However, the United States Constitution, Article 1 Section 9, allows the government to suspend *habeas corpus* if the "public safety may require it."

A less noxious, but also less effective, method of movement restriction is social distancing. **Social distancing**, while not a strict quarantine, prevents the spread of communicable disease by banning public gatherings (i.e., limiting access to places where groups of people congregate, such as theaters and schools).

EMS and Infection Control

Paramedics practice standard precautions for infection control—specifically wearing gloves and hand washing—whenever they are in routine contact with a patient. However, during an outbreak Paramedics may need to take special precautions.

Airborne transmission is a common denominator in many of these contagious diseases. Droplets of less than 5 microns, which can be inhaled by the Paramedic, may contain the diseases tuberculosis, smallpox, SARS, and even measles. To prevent infection, the Paramedic should wear a suitable mask, such as an N95 mask (Figure 28-9).

For droplets greater than 5 microns that "rain out," thus contaminating exposed surfaces, the Paramedic should consider wearing a gown and/or placing a mask over the patient's mouth to prevent the spread of disease.[17] Contaminated surfaces should be thoroughly cleaned between patient contacts to further prevent the spread of disease.

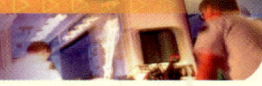

PROFESSIONAL PARAMEDIC

Since a Paramedic does not want to bring an infection home to his family, it might be wise for him to have a supply of disposable masks on hand for personal use in case of an outbreak.

The number of Paramedics having contact with the patient should be minimized if an outbreak of a contagious disease is suspected. Although it may be the existing practice for one Paramedic to switch duties (such as driving) with another Paramedic, Paramedics should remain with one role during a suspected disease outbreak in order to decrease the number of persons exposed. If possible, the opening between the driver's compartment and the patient compartment should be closed and the door sealed.

To further decrease the number of persons exposed to the contagion, the Paramedic should discourage the family from riding in the ambulance and encourage them to use private transportation.

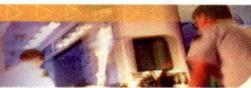

PROFESSIONAL PARAMEDIC

A low grade fever is a classic sign during the prodrome of many diseases. To detect SARS, airport officials have used temperature sensors and thermal imagers to identify suspected cases. Current technologies, such as temporal artery thermometers and noncontact digital infrared thermometers, can provide Paramedics with critical information for infection control.

Public Vaccination Program

During the process of containment, microbiologists, pharmacists, and physicians will be working on an effective vaccine to prevent further spread of the disease. The process of discovering and using vaccination began early in human history. For example, the ancient Chinese (200 B.C.) were known to snort the powdered scabs of smallpox victims. Arabian physicians were known to inject a small, nonlethal dose of the disease (called an inoculant), into a distal site such as the back of the hand, in a process called **inoculation**. Inoculation against smallpox became standard practice in the Western

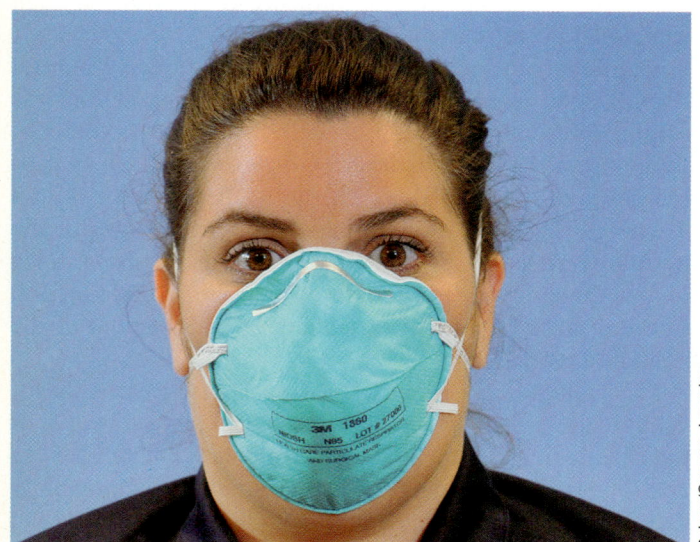

Figure 28-9 Wearing a mask for droplet protection.

Delmar/Cengage Learning

world after Lady Montagu had her children inoculated by an Arabian physician while she was stationed with her husband, Sir Edward Montagu, in Turkey.

Inoculation, also called variolation (Latin—smallpox), fell out of favor because inoculation still carried a risk of causing the disease. Therefore, vaccination was implemented. A vaccine is created by one of three common mechanisms. The first and classic mechanism is to inactivate the pathogen, killing it by heat or by chemical sterilization. Formaldehyde was a chemical commonly used for this task. The "dead" virus would then be injected into the body and the body's immune system, sensing a foreign protein, would mount an immune response.

In some cases, the dead virus was not sufficient to stimulate the immune system. In those cases, a weakened, or attenuated, virus would be used. Unfortunately, like inoculation, individuals with a weakened immune system—such as the elderly and those with cancer or AIDS—could contract the disease from the vaccine.

The last method of vaccination involved purifying a subunit of the virus. It was then attached to another benign virus to create a vaccination for the individual. The benign virus acted as a Trojan horse to carry the intended virus protein.

In the first case of vaccination, Dr. Edward Jenner administered cowpox virus, which has a antigen similar to smallpox, to patients to provide immunization against smallpox. The term "vaccine" (which stems from the Latin *vacca*, meaning cow) owes its origins from this original discovery, which helped launch the field of immunology.

In all cases, vaccination is the administration of the pathogenic proteins, also called immunogens (immune generator), to produce an antigenic–antibody response in a process of artificial immunity in order to protect the person from disease. These immunogens have a tendency to stimulate the immune system faster than the actual disease, thereby providing protection when the person is exposed to the disease.

Although prophylactic vaccination of the entire population would be ideal, such as occurs with the routine immunizations that children receive against known infectious diseases, emerging diseases prevent this. Instead, public health officials depend on three alternative strategies: ring vaccination, targeted vaccination, and mass vaccination.

With **ring vaccination**, the persons immediately at risk due to their proximity with the infected or ill people (the "ring" around the infected population), even if they haven't had direct contact with them, are vaccinated. This procedure works like a fire break and, like a fire break, needs to be instituted early, during the disease's incubation period.

With the disease contained, the remaining population in the affected area receives a **targeted vaccination**. Targeted vaccinations are effective at preventing epidemics in some cases, but the effectiveness of these vaccination campaigns are limited by mobility and mass transit.

Contact tracing is the identification of the person or persons with the infection. If the origin of the disease cannot be found, then **mass vaccination** of the potential population at risk is in order. The problem with mass vaccination is that it is expensive in terms of human resources and medical resources. Hospitals and schools, among other organizations, must have an outbreak plan to deal with emerging diseases (Table 28-2).

Table 28-2 Elements of an Outbreak Plan

- Planning and response committee
  - Multidisciplinary
    - Public health department
    - Local hospitals
    - Public safety
      - Emergency medical services
      - Law enforcement
      - Fire service
  - Response coordinator
- Preparedness and response plan (preplan)
  - Written policies regarding work practices
    - Movement restrictions
    - Liberal leave policy
    - Essential personnel
- System preparedness
  - Identify criteria for adequate response
  - Test response capabilities
  - Develop alternative strategies for deficits
- System surveillance
  - Education regarding disease epidemiology
  - Screening tools
  - Detection of clusters
  - List of health department contacts
- System response
  - Procedures for rapid containment
    - Isolation
    - Quarantine
    - Movement restrictions
  - Community healthcare delivery
    - Protect in place
    - Commandeered facilities
  - Community vaccination
    - Ring vaccination
    - Targeted vaccination
    - Mass vaccination

The nurse meets the arriving ambulance at the door to the clinic. Their patient, Stefan, who was originally from Lithuania, became ill with a headache and fever yesterday evening and had tried to self-treat with aspirin and fruit juices. He came to the clinic today because he didn't feel better and now has a rash. The nurse adds that Stefan had received all required immunizations for entrance into the school including vaccinations for meningitis and pneumonia.

The Paramedics don PPE before entering the exam room. Stefan is sitting on an exam table looking miserable. He has a blotchy rash with some areas of swelling. He states that it is quite itchy and he has scratched many areas. He tries to smile at the crew and says this is one lesson he hadn't intended to learn while in the United States.

CRITICAL THINKING QUESTIONS

1. What are the important elements of the history that a Paramedic should obtain?
2. What is the symptom pattern for meningitis?

History

When confronted with a patient with a possible infection, the history of the present illness can sometimes be more valuable in identifying the offending pathogen than laboratory tests. After proper introductions have been made, the Paramedic should ascertain the patient's chief concern, being careful to note it in the patient's own words if possible.

Next, the Paramedic should focus on asking systemic questions that might suggest the incubation and prodrome of the infection. In a head-to-toe fashion, the Paramedic should ask the patient if she had any headaches, or loss of visual or auditory acuity, that would suggest central nervous system involvement. The Paramedic should also inquire if the patient has a stiff neck (**nuchal rigidity**), which is a sign of meningeal involvement.

Next, the Paramedic should ask the patient if she has any breathlessness, wheezing, or has noticed the presence of a productive cough. If the cough is productive, the Paramedic should also ask about the color and volume of the sputum.

As the gastrointestinal system is the portal of entry for many infections, the Paramedic should ask the patient about gastrointestinal symptomology, such as nausea, vomiting, and diarrhea, as well as loss of appetite (i.e., anorexia). Continuing in the cephalocaudal fashion, the Paramedic should inquire if the patient has had any difficulty or pain with urination as well as hematuria (visible blood in the urine). Lastly, the Paramedic should ask the patient if she is experiencing joint pain or arthritic-like symptoms.

Although a drug history is routine during a Paramedic's history taking, the Paramedic should specifically inquire if the patient is taking part in any intravenous drug use as this is another potential portal of entry for infection.

If the patient presents with a fever, it is appropriate for the Paramedic to ask when the fever started, how high the fever has gotten, and if the patient has taken any antipyretics (such as acetaminophen) to lower the fever. If the patient has symptoms suggestive of liver involvement or cerebral involvement, such as headache or delirium, it is appropriate to ask if the patient mistakenly took aspirin. These symptoms are suggestive of Reye's syndrome, a potentially fatal complication following aspirin ingestion during viral illness.

Some patients complain of pruritus, an itching sensation that originates in the nerve endings of the skin and is thought to be induced by the release of histamine from mast cells during an inflammatory response from serotonin. These irritated nerve endings tend to cause a spinal reflex action called a scratch.

Past Medical History

Germane to any history of a patient suspected of having contracted an infectious disease is the patient's immunization history. Most students entering into school in the United States must have proof of immunization for certain diseases (Table 28-3). However, alien residents and illegal immigrants may not have had the complete battery of immunizations typically required. In those cases, the Paramedic should ask for proof of immunizations, which is frequently found with the patient's "traveling papers."

The Paramedic should note the patient's last meal, as anorexia is a common prodromal sign, as well as any associated nausea with or without vomiting. Exotoxins, such as those like botulinum produced by bacteria, can cause these gastrointestinal symptoms.

Table 28-3 School Immunizations[18]

- Diphtheria, tetanus, and pertussis (DTaP)
- Human papilloma virus*
- Meningococcal
- Pneumococcal**
- Influenza**
- Measles, mumps, rubella (MMR)
- Inactivated poliovirus
- Hepatitis A**
- Hepatitis B*
- Varicella

Not listed by common childhood immunizations

- Polio (TOPV)
- Haemophilus influenzae (HiB)

Notes:

*Not universally required

**Certain high risk groups

Source: Centers for Disease Control and Prevention Advisory Committee on Immunization Practices, the American Academy of Pediatrics and the American Academy of Family Physicians.

Finally, when discussing events preceding the current event, it is appropriate for the Paramedic to ask the patient if there has been any recent foreign travel. Often outbreaks of contagions occur after a traveler has left a country and the traveler is unaware that she may be a carrier.

Contact Tracing

When an infectious disease breaks out, particularly a newly emerged disease without a previous history, it is important to find out who also may have been exposed to the contagion (i.e., those who were in contact with the patient). This investigation, called **contact tracing**, can help prevent secondary cases of infection from occurring among these exposed individuals. Although contact tracing may seem like common sense, by its nature contact tracing requires the patient to reveal her acquaintances and breaches her right to privacy. However, and under limited circumstances, the public good (i.e., prevention of outbreak and infection control) outweighs the individual's right to privacy. In those cases, the patient may be compelled to name her associates. This is often the case when the disease is a **reportable disease**, diseases of public health importance. The classic examples of reportable diseases are sexually transmitted diseases.

Reportable diseases are reported, in writing or by telephone, to local and/or state health departments and/or the federal Centers for Disease Control and Prevention (CDC). When there is a potential for epidemic spread, the health department or the CDC may use their powers to quarantine individuals (i.e., contacts and/or isolate infected individuals).

Although a Paramedic does not usually perform contact tracing, concise notes on address and location as well as the identity of others on-scene can be very helpful to health department investigators. This information can be invaluable for certain time-sensitive investigations, such as those surrounding bacterial meningitis.

CASE STUDY (CONTINUED)

After the primary assessment, the Paramedic proceeds to physically examine Stefan in a head-to-toe fashion. Before the brief exam of Stefan, the Paramedic covers him with a blanket, places a mask on him, and brings him by stretcher to the ambulance.

Stefan's airway is open, and he is tachypneic and tachycardic at 110. He has a generalized rash consisting of non-fluid-filled raised areas. Although he can touch his chin to his chest, he complains of increased pain in doing so.

CRITICAL THINKING QUESTIONS

1. What are the elements of the physical examination of a patient with suspected meningitis?
2. Why is a head and neck examination a critical element in this examination?

Examination

Just like when taking the history of present illness, the physical examination of the patient with a suspected contagious disease should proceed from a head-to-toe, or cephalocaudal, fashion. The Paramedic should examine the patient's airway for reddened areas suggestive of pharyngitis as well as exudates (i.e., pus) in the throat. The oropharynx and nasopharynx are common portals of entry for infection. The presence of small red spots with a white center found on the mucosa may be Koplik's spots, which are suggestive of measles.

The patient's eyes and nose should also be examined for rhinorrhea (fluid from the nose) and conjunctivitis (reddening of the eye), both signs of irritation. Although nonspecific, these two signs are often associated with measles as well.

Preceding posterior to the throat, the Paramedic should palpate the temporomandibular junction (TMJ) for point tenderness that is intensified with chewing (a symptom suggestive of the mumps). Next, the Paramedic should gently palpate the anterior neck, immediately inferior to the earlobe, for signs that the parotid glands are inflamed. The parotid glands, the largest of the salivary glands, also become inflamed during the mumps.

The Paramedic should observe the patient's anterior neck and palpate for signs of swollen lymph nodes proximal to the length of the carotid groove. Swollen lymph nodes, called **lymphadenopathy**, are often seen in several infectious diseases of the throat.

Next, the Paramedic should palpate the posterior neck for pain on palpation and ask the patient to place her chin on her chest. The presence of neck pain (i.e., nuchal rigidity) with flexion is one of the **meningeal signs**, along with photophobia and headaches. This triad of signs is characteristic of meningitis, an irritation of the meninges that surround the brain that can be caused by an infection.

Exanthema

A rash on the skin, the largest organ of the body, can be the most visible manifestation of a systemic infection. These whole body rashes, called an exanthema, are the result of the body's immune response to the pathogen. Although a Paramedic is not expected to identify each pathogen by its rash, the Paramedic should be able to accurately describe the rash to an emergency department. With this information, the physician or nurse can then make an informed decision about the need for and type of isolation that may be necessary.

First, the Paramedic should note the appearance of the rash. A raised lesion is called a papule, whereas one that is flat and cannot be felt is called a macule. While examining the appearance of the rash, the Paramedic should note its color. Rashes may range in color from brown (more likely a freckle) to red. Papules, on the other hand, are raised lesions that can be palpated. Papules, unlike pustules, do not contain white blood cells in viscous fluid called pus.

However, some raised lesions appear like a tiny blister and contain a clear, serous fluid that is loaded with virus; these are called **vesicles**. When observing a vesicle, the Paramedic should immediately use barrier protections to prevent accidental cross-contamination.

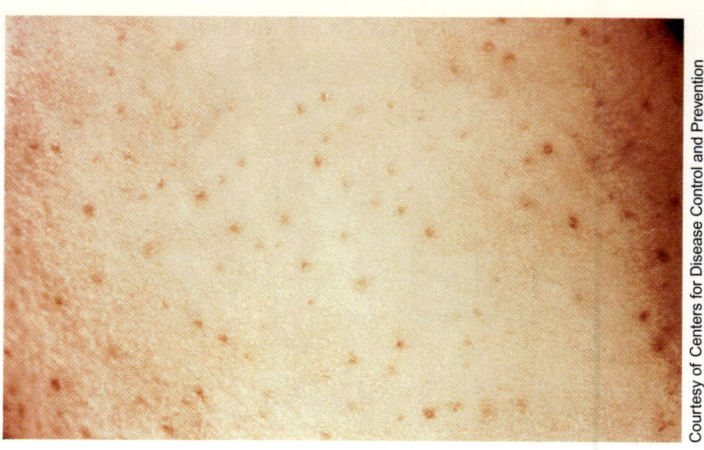

Courtesy of Centers for Disease Control and Prevention

Figure 28-10 Petechiae and purpura.

Purple or maroon-colored lesions may be called **purpura**. The appearance of purpura is due to microvascular bleeding under the skin secondary to endotoxins and may be representative of a systemic blood infection or **septicemia**. Pinpoint lesions with the same discoloration are called **petechiae**. A pattern of these lesions may raise the Paramedic's suspicion for typhus and may also be seen in cases of meningitis (Figure 28-10).

Many rashes are accompanied by **erythema**, reddened areas that appear like flushing and blanch under finger pressure, like capillary refill. These are due to capillary congestion secondary to an inflammatory response.

Next, the Paramedic should note the distribution of the rash. A rash may only be seen on the extremities, or may be a centrifugal rash that starts at the core and migrates to the extremities. A larger number of lesions may also be seen in the hollows of the body (e.g., as happens with chickenpox) or along creases on the body (e.g., as happens with scarlet fever). Few infections affect the palms of the hand, with notable exceptions like syphilis and the rickettsia that causes Rocky Mountain spotted fever.

A limited distribution of lesions in a certain location, such as around the patient's wrist or waist, without the accompanying systemic signs (such as fever) is suggestive of contact dermatitis of a noninfectious origin. Finally, the Paramedic should ask the patient about the progression of the rash. For example, the rash from measles migrates in a cephalocaudal fashion.

CASE STUDY (CONTINUED)

When the Paramedic flashes the penlight into Stefan's eyes, he flinches. "Did that hurt your eyes?" the Paramedic asks. Stefan nods yes.

CRITICAL THINKING QUESTIONS

1. What is the significance of the elevated ST segment?
2. What diagnosis did the Paramedic announce to the patient?

Assessment

Meningitis can be divided into either bacterial meningitis or viral meningitis. Viral meningitis, also called aseptic meningitis, is probably the most common form of meningitis. Many patients contract viral meningitis and dismiss the symptoms as being the "flu." Most commonly, viral meningitis is caused by an enterovirus that enters the body through the oral mucosa and travels to the brain. Other viruses that have been identified as causative agents include the chickenpox virus (i.e., varicella zoster), mumps, herpes simplex type 2, and influenza.

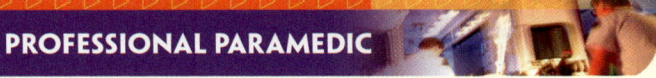

PROFESSIONAL PARAMEDIC

Meningitis can also be the result of drug reaction and inflammatory diseases such as lupus erythematosus and even some types of cancer.

Although rare, bacterial meningitis is potentially lethal, as bacteria entering the bloodstream via the upper respiratory tract travel to the brain. Several causative bacteria have been implicated in bacterial meningitis: pneumococcal, meningoccal, and haemophilus. Although haemophilus influenzae b (the term "influenzae" is not related to the flu) was once the most common cause of bacterial meningitis, the development of the HiB vaccine has dramatically decreased its incidence.

A highly contagious form of meningitis is meningococcal meningitis. As many as 10% to 15% of cases of meningococcal meningitis are fatal. Populations at risk include those who are immunosuppressed, travelers to or from endemic areas of the world, and populations living in close proximity, such as college dorms and prisons.

The last etiologic agent, pneumococcal meningitis, may be the most serious. Caused by the bacteria Streptococcus pneumonia (the same infection that can cause pneumonia), it can quickly spread to the brain, causing permanent neurological damage and even death.

CASE STUDY (CONTINUED)

Stefan agrees to transportation to the hospital for further medical evaluation. He asks, "What are you going to do to me?" while being loaded in the ambulance. Stefan expresses concern that he does not want to get anyone else sick.

CRITICAL THINKING QUESTIONS

1. What is the standard of care of patients with suspected meningitis?
2. What are some of the patient concerns specific to meningitis?

Treatment

The general care of the patient with a suspected infection starts with the Paramedic's personal self-protection, protection of others involved in care, and protection of the public from a potential contagion. By utilizing standard precautions, including barrier devices like a mask, the Paramedic provides supportive care.

Supportive care for the patient generally revolves around providing rest, reducing fever, and relieving discomfort. The first item, rest, includes keeping stimulation, such as loud noises, to a minimum as well as utilizing dim lighting. Although antipyretics such as acetaminophen or ibuprofen are rarely given in the prehospital setting, even a cool washcloth applied to the forehead can help reduce the fever. The last treatment, relief of discomfort, generally refers to the headache that accompanies meningitis. Prehospital treatments are limited; however, patients who complain of nausea can be treated with antiemetics.

The Paramedic should try to obtain intravenous access. Dehydration is often associated with the accompanying fever and a fluid bolus may be in order.

CASE STUDY (CONTINUED)

While inbound to the hospital, with lights dimmed and a washcloth across the patient's forehead, the Paramedic tries to obtain more specific information about the patient's immunizations. Suddenly the patient seizes.

CRITICAL THINKING QUESTIONS

1. What are some of the predictable complications associated with acute meningitis?
2. What are some of the predictable complications associated with the treatments for acute meningitis?

Evaluation

Some patients may present with the classic triad of meningeal signs (nuchal rigidity, photophobia, and headache), indicating they are at risk for generalized seizures and status epilepticus. The following discussion identifies some of the more common causes of meningitis as well as what must be included when identifying other nonmeningeal etiologies of convulsions.

Neisseria

Another potential etiology of a meningitis-induced seizure is the Gram-negative bacterium called **Neisseria meningitidis** (i.e., meningococcus). As with other diseases, the incidence of meningococcus meningitis has decreased in the United States because of the vaccination of school-aged children.

Meningococcus is a rapidly developing infection that starts with a prodrome that includes fatigue and fever, and then progresses to the classic triad of meningeal signs. However, meningococcus can progress so rapidly that the classic triad of meningeal signs does not have time to develop and the only evidence of the systemic infection is the nonblanching rashes called purpura and accompanying petechiae.

If left untreated, the infection can lead to seizures, coma, and death in as little as 24 hours. The risk of death is so great that doctors may treat **empirically** (i.e., based on the clinical presentation without a diagnosis), knowing full well that the antibiotic may eliminate any chance for a laboratory confirmation. For this reason, any person with a nonblanching rash should be seen in the emergency department immediately and respiratory precautions observed during transport.

Rabies

Rabies can also produce a convulsive state. Transmitted by the saliva in the bite of an infected mammal—such as a dog, raccoon, or bat—the causative agent of rabies (Latin for rage), the lyssavirus, starts to attack the central nervous system.

Although rabies is found throughout most of the world, the combination of mass vaccination of animals and the use of rabies vaccine, in conjunction with immunoglobulin for post-exposure prophylaxis within two weeks of exposure, has almost eliminated rabies as a cause of death in developed countries. Initially, rabies presents with flu-like symptoms after a 3- to 12-week incubation period. The disease then progresses into an acute infection of the brain (i.e., an **encephalitis**) that is manifest with confusion, agitation, and delirium.

The creation of large quantities of saliva and difficulty swallowing, as a result of the infection, are the quintessential signs of rabies. Thereafter, the patient cannot drink for fear of choking, a condition called **hydrophobia**, and the disease rapidly progresses to cause brain damage, coma, and death.

Tetanus

Although tetanus is relatively rare in the United States because of immunizations, the causative agent of tetanus (Clostridium tetani) is found worldwide, including in the United States. Typically it appears in soil, particularly soil contaminated with manure.

Tetanus can cause a symptom complex that can appear like a convulsion. Signs of tetanus include spasms of the skeletal muscles, secondary to the neurotoxin called tetanospasmin which is produced by the Clostridium tetani. The neurotoxin works by decreasing the level of the inhibitory neurotransmitter gamma-aminobutyric acid (GABA) in the brain. As a result, the slightest stimulation (such as lifting the patient) can cause skeletal muscle contraction. Starting at the small muscles, the first sign of tetanus is the classic lockjaw, a tightening of the jaw muscles (**trismus**), making airway control difficult.

Tetanus can also cause **risus sardonicus**, a contortion of the face, with raised eyebrows and a twisted grimace, likened to an evil sneer. The "Joker" in the Batman series evidenced the smile of risus sardonicus. Finally, tetanus can cause a massive skeletal muscle contraction that causes the entire body to arch, a condition called **opisthotonus**, whenever the body is touched. This contraction has been strong enough to break long bones.

Poliomyelitis

Previously one of the major causes of paralysis worldwide, particularly among children (it's sometimes referred to as infantile paralysis), poliomyelitis may now be eradicated worldwide due to mass vaccination programs. The vaccine, developed as a result of the pioneering works of Dr. Sabin and Dr. Salk, and with the help of the March of Dimes, is one of the childhood immunizations.

Polio's rise to the public's consciousness may have come as a result of the invention of the iron lung. Previously, when the virus entered the central nervous system, it would impact motor neurons. This would lead to a flaccid paralysis of skeletal muscles, including the diaphragm, which in turn led to respiratory arrest and death. With the advent of the negative pressure ventilator (i.e., iron lung), patients could be supported until they recovered from the effects of the virus.

An enterovirus, poliomyelitis is transferred from person to person via the fecal–oral route and is extremely virulent. Polio infection starts with a one- to three-week incubation period. During that time, the patient (usually unaware of the infection) is capable of transmitting the highly contagious virus to others. The symptoms of polio can be divided into three phases. In the first phase, the patient experiences the classic prodrome of any viral infection (i.e., low grade fever, headache, sore throat, and/or nausea and vomiting). This phase tends to last less than three or four days and over 90% of the population recover from the infection without knowing that they contracted polio.

During the next phase, the patient presents with classic meningeal signs (i.e., severe headache, nuchal rigidity, as well as muscle pain and high fever). If the patient's resistance is low, then the patient may progress to the final phase which includes muscle weakness and muscle paralysis. During the final phase, the patient may have difficulty breathing as a result of muscle paralysis and may need assisted ventilation. Less than 1% of patients progress to the final phase.

A trivalent oral polio vaccine (TOPV), which contains three serotypes of polio, is typically administered to children under 5 years of age. There is no cure for polio contracted by the unimmunized patient. Treatment in those cases is largely supportive, including analgesia for muscle pain, antipyretics for fever, and respiratory support as needed.

CASE STUDY CONCLUSION

Stefan's seizure is short-lived and self-limiting, and his postictal period is short and uneventful. Once in the ambulance, the Paramedic places oxygen on Stefan, starts an IV line, and draws blood. He advises Stefan that a more complete set of bloods, including blood cultures, will be drawn at the hospital. The Health Clinic has notified the ED of Stefan's condition and reason for transport. Just before arriving at the ED, the Paramedic confirms that the ED is aware of Stefan and updates his condition.

Several weeks later, Stefan stops by the ambulance garage to thank the crew and ask some questions about prehospital care. He tells them he had viral meningitis that fortunately ran its course without any complications.

CRITICAL THINKING QUESTIONS

1. What is the most appropriate transport decision that will get the patient to definitive care?
2. Why is it important to alert the emergency department of an impending arrival of suspected meningitis?

Disposition

Although individual cases of infectious diseases can be handled routinely, using barrier devices and isolation rooms, epidemics of these contagions may require some modifications of existing infrastructure as well as advanced planning.

For example, the typical ambulance is a positive pressure environment (i.e., air pressure is greater inside the patient compartment to prevent gasses, such as carbon monoxide fumes, from entering). The problem is that the air is exhausted to the ambient environment and many of these infectious diseases are airborne. The alternative is a negative pressure ambulance, similar to an isolation room that causes air to flow into the patient compartment. This is achieved by mechanically exhausting air while decreasing the air intake. To be effective, negative pressure rooms must be sealed, including the driver's compartment.

Alternatively, if this type of conversion is unavailable or impractical, then the air within the patient compartment should be recirculated through high-efficiency particulate air filters (HEPA).

In every case, the Paramedics must notify the receiving facility of their patient's condition prior to arrival so appropriate precautions, such as isolation, can be taken to prevent further spread of the infection.

CONCLUSION

Infectious diseases are commonly encountered by the Paramedic in routine practice. The importance of adequate infection control procedures cannot be overemphasized in order to appropriately protect the Paramedic from the spread of infectious diseases.

KEY POINTS:

- Many diseases may produce a rash. The Paramedic can use the mnemonic TEST to learn these diseases.

- There are five common childhood infections that produce an exanthema:
  - Chickenpox
  - Roseola
  - Rubeola
  - Rubella
  - Pediculosis and scabies

- Sexually transmitted diseases capable of producing a prodrome (which may include a rash, viral symptoms, and headache) include
  - Syphilis
  - Gonorrhea
  - Chlamydia
  - HIV/AIDS

- Emerging infectious diseases are classified into three categories:
  - New diseases
  - Re-emerging diseases
  - Drug-resistant diseases

- Infection control begins with surveillance and early detection.

- Expected symptoms per population are compared with actual reports of symptoms to identify any variations from the norm.

- Containment and vaccination are employed to control an outbreak.

- Isolation is part of containment and is designed to move ill patients away from the non-ill population.

- A sudden influx of patients, called a surge, may tax a healthcare facility's resources, requiring the use of auxiliary personnel for patient care.

- Quarantine is a method of keeping infected but not yet ill people from moving around in the general public.

- Social distancing is a less onerous method of keeping potentially infected but not ill people from exposing others. Examples of social distancing include closing schools or theaters.

- Modes of transmission of disease include droplet, fecal-oral, and sexual.

- Vaccination may occur through use of dead virus, weakened or attenuated virus, or purifying a component of the virus.

- Vaccination programs can be aimed at those persons immediately at risk due to proximity to the infected persons (ring), a population in the same geographic area as the infected persons (targeted), or the entire potential population (mass).

- Hospitals, schools, and so on, must have outbreak plans.

- The patient's past medical history should include an immunization history.

- The patient's physical exam should proceed in a head-to-toe fashion.

- A skin exam must include the description of any rashes.

- The patient with an infectious disease is often at risk for convulsions.

REVIEW QUESTIONS:

1. Name the components of the mnemonic TEST.
2. Name five childhood diseases capable of producing a generalized body rash.
3. List the three classifications for emerging infections.
4. How does isolation differ from quarantine?
5. Define social distancing.
6. Differentiate attenuated virus vaccination from vaccinations using inactivated or purified viruses.
7. List the components of an outbreak plan.

CASE STUDY QUESTIONS:

Please refer to the Case Study in this chapter, and answer the questions below:

1. What PPE should the crew be using for this patient? Explain your answer.
2. Name at least three causes of the rash that this patient has developed.
3. What is the value to the Paramedic of identifying the appearance of the rash?
4. Explain the importance of notifying the ED of the patient's condition even though the Health Clinic had already called.

REFERENCES:

1. Hogan PA. Viral exanthemas in childhood. *Australas J Dermatol*. 1996;37 Suppl 1:S14–S16.
2. Glasgow JF. Reye's syndrome: the case for a causal link with aspirin. *Drug Saf*. 2006;29(12):1111–1121.
3. Orlowski JP, Hanhan UA, et al. Is aspirin a cause of Reye's syndrome? A case against. *Drug Saf*. 2002;28(4):228–231.
4. Belay ED, Bresee JS, et al. Reye's syndrome in the United States from 1981 through 1997. *N Engl J Med*. 1999;340(18):1377–1382.
5. Meade RH, 3rd. Exanthem subitum (roseola infantum). *Clin Dermatol*. 1989;7(1):92–96.
6. Zimmerman RK, Middleton DB. Vaccines for persons at high risk, 2007. *J Fam Pract*. 2007;56(2 Suppl Vaccines):S38–S46, C4-5.
7. Griffin DE, Pan CH, et al. Measles vaccines. *Front Biosci*. 2008;13:1352–1370.
8. Aral SO, O'Leary A, et al. Sexually transmitted infections and HIV in the southern United States: an overview. *Sex Transm Dis*. 2006;33(7 Suppl):S1–S5.
9. Thompson HS, Kardon RH. The Argyll Robertson pupil. *J Neuroophthalmol*. 2006;26(2):134–138.
10. Tarr ME, Gilliam ML. Sexually transmitted infections in adolescent women. *Clin Obstet Gynecol*. 2008;51(2):306–318.
11. Ginige S, Fairley CK, et al. Interventions for increasing Chlamydia screening in primary care: a review. *BMC Public Health*. 2007;7:95.
12. Uthman OA, Abdulmalik JO. Adjunctive therapies for AIDS dementia complex. *Cochrane Database Syst Rev*. 2008;3:CD006496.
13. Powell JP, Wenzel RP. Antibiotic options for treating community-acquired MRSA. *Expert Rev Anti Infect Ther*. 2008;6(3):299–307.
14. Sakoulas G, Moellering RC, Jr. Increasing antibiotic resistance among methicillin-resistant Staphylococcus aureus strains. *Clin Infect Dis*. 2008;46 Suppl 5:S360–S367.
15. Chastre J. Evolving problems with resistant pathogens. *Clin Microbiol Infect*. 2008;14 Suppl 3:3–14.
16. Naber,CK. Future strategies for treating Staphylococcus aureus bloodstream infections. *Clin Microbiol Infect*. 2008;14 Suppl 2:26–34.
17. Lateef F, Lim SH, et al. New paradigm for protection: the emergency ambulance services in the time of severe acute respiratory syndrome. *Prehosp Emerg Care*. 2004;8(3):304–307.
18. Centers for Disease Control and Prevention. Recommended immunization schedules for persons aged 0–18 years old. United States, 2008. *MMWR*. 2007;56(51&52):Q1–Q4.

CHAPTER 29

DISORDERS OF THE IMMUNE SYSTEM

KEY CONCEPTS:

Upon completion of this chapter, it is expected that the reader will understand these following concepts:

- The interconnectedness of the immune system with all body systems
- How overstimulation or hyper-responsiveness of the immune system leads to allergy, anaphylaxis, or organ transplant rejection
- Why immune deficiency leaves the body unprotected
- How the body can develop antibodies against itself

ANATOMY CONCEPTS:

Prior to reading this chapter the Paramedic student should be familiar with the following anatomy and physiology concepts:

- Immune system

Rural Ambulance 10 is dispatched to a home on County Route 1 for the report of a 12-year-old girl with fever and abdominal pain. The dispatch relates that the child is "medically fragile" and had a recent kidney transplant. As the Paramedics quickly respond, they discuss how "kids" make them nervous and how they know next to nothing about kidney transplants.

CRITICAL THINKING QUESTIONS

1. What are some of the possible causes of fever and abdominal pain related to a recent kidney transplant?
2. What does it mean to be medically fragile?

OVERVIEW

The human immune system is the body's natural defense system against disease. Physical barriers such as skin and mucous membranes prevent the entrance of various organisms into the body, whereas chemical responses generated by the body's immune cells act to deactivate or kill those that gain entry. When functioning properly, the body is able to defend itself against the thousands of pathogens it encounters on a daily basis. However, alterations in the immune system's normal activity—either resulting in underactivity (as seen in immunosuppression) or overactivity (as in autoimmune diseases)—can lead to significant morbidity and mortality. The Paramedic's ability to recognize and respond to such situations is critical; therefore, he must have a basic understanding of the immune system and its associated disorders.

Before discussing immune system disorders, it is important to review normal immune system function. Immune system disorders can then be broadly divided into conditions where the immune system is overactive and conditions where the immune system is underactive or deficient.

Normal Immune System Function

The first line of defense against the invasion of organisms such as bacteria, viruses, and fungi are the natural physical barriers. The skin, often considered the largest organ of the body, provides a boundary between the environment and the body's underlying tissues and organs. In addition to resisting physical penetration of organisms, various skin secretions such as oil and sweat create a hostile environment in which these microorganisms cannot survive. Although it is easy to take the function of the skin for granted, consider that even a small breach in skin integrity (such as an abrasion, small laceration, etc.) can render the body susceptible to disease and infection.[1,2] Even more devastating for the body's immune system is the patient who has suffered severe burns on large surfaces of the body.[3]

Mucous membranes provide an important barrier for the various openings in the body. These membranes are able to slow and trap organisms as they attempt to enter the body through the nose, mouth, anus, vagina, or urethra. The pH of the mucus provides unfavorable conditions for bacterial or viral survival, and the physical texture and thickness of these secretions allows the body to trap them and eventually eliminate them from the body (through processes like sneezing or coughing/expectorating). In some cases, these membranes extend far into the body's internal organs, such as down the trachea to the lungs or into the stomach from the esophagus. Cilia in the nose and respiratory tract also aids in trapping foreign particles and preventing them from entering the lungs, whereas stomach acids kill the majority of pathogens entering through the digestive tract (Figure 29-1).

Although the physical barriers protect the body from the majority of potential invaders, some organisms are able to evade these defenses and stimulate the immune system from

Allergic reactions

Skin contact | Injection | Ingestion | Inhalation

Poison plants | Bee sting | Medication | Pollen
Animal scratches | | Nuts and shellfish | Dust
Pollen | | | Mold and mildew
Latex | | | Animal dander

Delmar/Cengage Learning

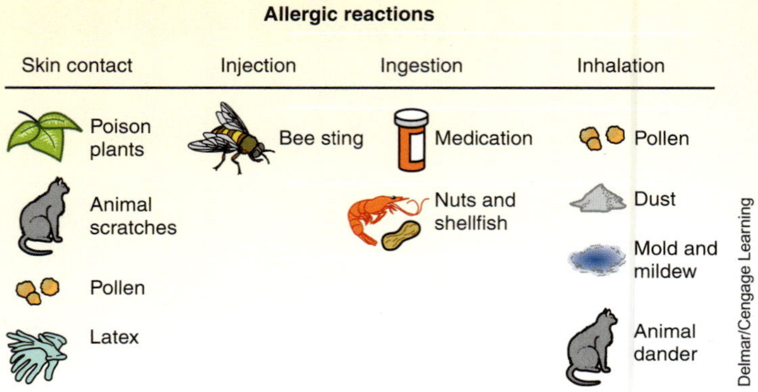

Figure 29-1 Sources of allergens and modes of entry into the body.

within. When this occurs, the body releases chemical factors that act to target and kill the offending organism. In order to understand even the basics of the immune system, however, one must have a working knowledge of the key components and reactions.

Antigens are particles or organisms that stimulate an immune response (Figure 29-2). These can include dust, pollens, bacteria, fungi, viruses, antibiotics, or other medications.

White blood cells (lymphocytes) are produced in the bone marrow and mature in other organs of the body, including the

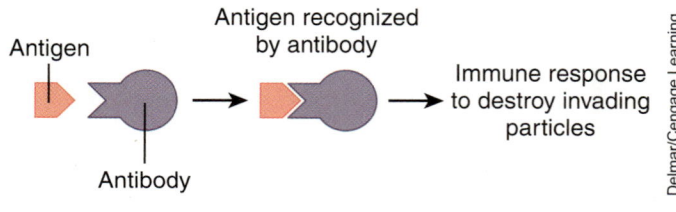

Antigen | Antigen recognized by antibody | Immune response to destroy invading particles

Antibody

Delmar/Cengage Learning

Figure 29-2 Antigen.

thymus and spleen. They can be divided into two major categories: T cells and B cells. The T cells are the primary surveillance cells that circulate throughout the blood searching for antigens. When encountered, they secrete various chemicals that recruit other components of the immune system. A lack of T cells (as seen in HIV/AIDS) will cause a deficient immune reaction when provoked. B cells are lymphocytes that generate plasma cells that, in turn, secrete antibodies when stimulated. These cells require prior exposure to—and sensitization by—the offending antigen. The antibodies produced are specific to a particular antigen, and when released will target and bind to the antigen to promote its deactivation and elimination from the body.[4] The sensitization of B cells is the primary function of immunization.

Mast cells (mastocytes) are immune cells stimulated by antigen–antibody complexes. Once stimulated, they release a variety of granules and chemicals, including histamine, heparin, and other **cytokines** (immune chemicals) that are responsible for the body's reaction to immune stimulation (Figure 29-3). The results of these chemical releases include vascular leaking, smooth muscle stimulation, and increased secretions from nasal, bronchial, or gastric cells. Mast cells play a particularly important role in hypersensitivity and allergic reactions.[5]

Once the immune system has been engaged, the chemicals released stimulate multiple other responses throughout the body. In the case of stimulation by bacteria and viruses, the body may begin by trying to purge the offending organism. Coughing, vomiting, and diarrhea are all natural responses to certain types of pathogens. Some immunologic chemicals will cause the body temperature to rise, generating fever that kills the bacteria or virus by raising the body's temperature too high for their survival. When stimulated by other objects such as foods, medications, or environmental agents, the response may include increased respiratory secretions, resulting in runny nose, cough, watery eyes, and skin reactions such as rashes. Occasionally this reaction may be so severe as to compromise the patient's airway, as seen in anaphylactic reactions.

Obviously a dysfunction in any one of these areas of immune response will limit the body's ability to fight off disease, but the overstimulation of these components can be equally as disastrous. Therefore, when encountering patients with immune system disorders, the Paramedic must carefully consider whether the patient is responding appropriately, or whether she is responding too much or too little.

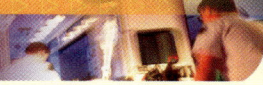

Anaphylaxis is IgE mediated. Anaphylactoid reactions are not IgE mediated. However, the signs and symptoms of both may be the same (i.e., puritus and urticaria).

Chief Concern

Since the immune system is interconnected with the rest of the body organ systems, it may be difficult for the Paramedic to recognize its role in the presenting chief concern. Allergic and anaphylactic reactions are usually straightforward and easy to identify, but conditions such as fevers, infections, and even common complaints of headache and chest pain may all have immunologic etiologies. Therefore, the Paramedic must keep an open mind when treating patients, and must at least consider immune conditions in almost any presenting complaint.

Allergic reactions are the result of an inappropriately excessive response to an antigenic exposure.[6–9] When stimulated by a particular antigen, the body's natural response of antibody release and mast cell activation is augmented. Excessive release of mast cell granules and chemicals—in particular histamine—results in a disproportionate response of vascular permeability, inflammatory mediator secretion, respiratory secretions, and/or smooth muscle contraction. The end result is a reaction that can be as simple and benign as a rash, or as complex and life-threatening as anaphylaxis.

The body's reaction to poison ivy is an example of a simple allergic response. Although this type of response may take several days to develop, it illustrates a localized reaction to a localized stimulation. At the site of exposure, the antigen (oil from the poison ivy leaf) stimulates release of inflammatory chemicals, resulting in the redness seen in a rash, vascular permeability (resulting in localized swelling at the site of exposure), and histamine release (resulting in itching). In most cases, this response is self-limited to the site of contact and does not create a full systemic response.

In some cases, a patient may have previously been sensitized to an antigen, and subsequent exposure can trigger a severe response. When this occurs, the patient is said to have an **anaphylactic reaction**. Anaphylaxis is a true medical emergency; if not recognized and treated swiftly, it can cause airway collapse and death.[10] Certain medications, foods, or chemicals can cause localized reactions, specifically angioedema.

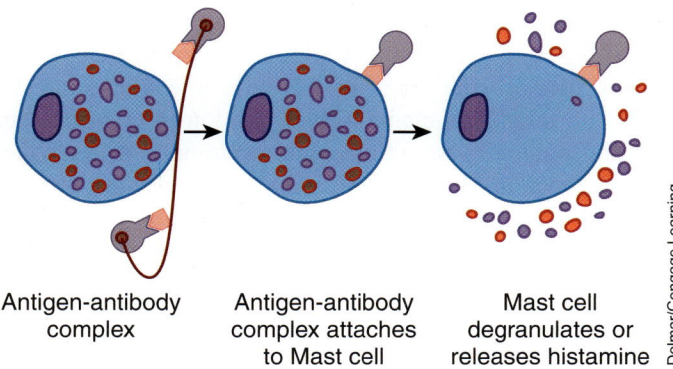

Antigen-antibody complex → Antigen-antibody complex attaches to Mast cell → Mast cell degranulates or releases histamine

Delmar/Cengage Learning

Figure 29-3   Mast cell releasing histamine.

Angioedema is a localized swelling of the lips, tongue, or upper airway in response to specific antigenic stimuli.

Some people develop antibodies to their own body cells, a condition known as **autoimmunity**. This immunity disorder is usually genetic in nature and results in immune responses to a person's own cells. Virtually all cells can act as antigenic stimulants, with the exception of certain cells in the brain, eye, testicles, and uterus. Most patients have autoimmunity to only one type of cell in the body, and therefore the response is generally localized to that type of tissue. Sjøgren's disease, for example, results from autoantibodies to exocrine glands of the face, which manifests most commonly as dry eyes and dry mouth.[11]

Autoimmune disease can range in severity from occasional flare-ups to chronic unrelenting painful responses. Among the autoimmune diseases are systemic lupus erythematosus (SLE or lupus), rheumatoid arthritis (RA), dermatomyositis, polymyositis, ankylosing spondylitis, and inclusion-body myositis. Although each of these syndromes is rare, systemic lupus erythematosus and rheumatoid arthritis are two of the more common diseases. As such, Paramedics should be familiar with them.

Systemic lupus erythematosus is a disease that predominantly affects women between the ages of 15 and 40. The cause of this disorder is unknown, but genetic and environmental factors, including UV light exposure, have been implicated as potential causes. Systemic lupus erythematosus affects virtually all tissues in the body, and therefore may have a variety of effects. The most common manifestation is joint pain and swelling, which affects approximately 95% of patients. This is the most common reason why the patient seeks medical attention, and is responsible for the greatest number of lost workdays in patients with systemic lupus erythematosus.[12] Although joint pain is the most common manifestation of lupus, the most commonly recognized sign is a malar or butterfly rash on the face. This characteristic rash spares the nasolabial folds, and may range in appearance from subtle to deep red (see Figure 29-4). Other possible consequences of systemic lupus erythematosus include oral ulcers, kidney disorders (lupus glomerulonephritis), pericarditis, and occasionally aortic or mitral insufficiency. In addition, a severe vasculitis (inflammatory response of the blood vessels) is common.

Rheumatoid arthritis affects approximately 1% of the U.S. population and occurs due to the presence of rheumatoid factor in the patient's blood. The rheumatoid factor, which consists of multiple types of autoantibodies, usually targets synovial joints in the body. The end result is painful deterioration of joints, particularly in the hands. The common characteristic of rheumatoid arthritis is joint stiffness on wakening that gradually improves throughout the day (as opposed to osteoarthritis which worsens as the day progresses).[13,14] When rheumatoid factor targets the joints of the neck, progressive degeneration of the C-spine may ensue, predisposing a patient to certain types of spinal cord injuries.

Patients who receive transplanted organs stimulate the immune system to attack the transplanted organ. Although

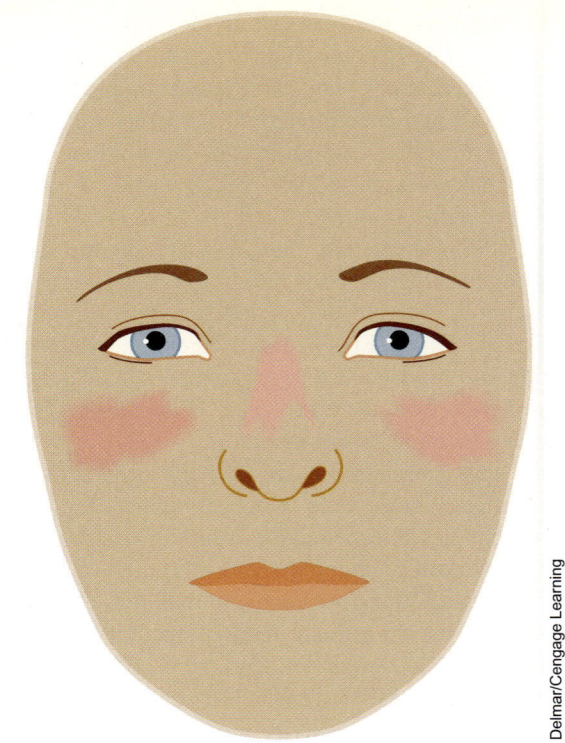

Delmar/Cengage Learning

Figure 29-4 The characteristic malar rash of SLE. Note how the nasolabial folds are spared.

organs are matched as best as possible to the recipient, the match is never exact. In transplant rejection, the recipient's immune system attacks the transplanted organ. **Hyperacute transplant rejection** occurs at the time of transplantation and usually is a result of a mismatch of the major antigens, similar to administering the incorrect blood type to a patient.[15] This life-threatening rejection occurs during or immediately after the operation and, as a result, the transplanted organ must be removed. **Acute transplant rejection** occurs as early as a week after transplant but can occur months to years after transplant as well. In acute rejection, the immune system attacks the transplanted organ and causes symptoms that are related to the failure of that organ. For example, if a patient is rejecting a kidney, the patient may notice a decrease in urinary output, mild edema, or pain over the site of the transplanted kidney. If a transplanted heart is rejected, the patient may present with signs and symptoms consistent with heart failure. In general, patients who have received transplants are educated on the signs of rejection and communicate early with their physicians. Acute rejection is often treated in the hospital with several medications to help suppress the immune reaction. By doing this, the patient often avoids permanent damage. In contrast, **chronic transplant rejection** can occur from repeated episodes of acute rejection or due to a low level immune attack on the transplanted organ.[16] In chronic transplant rejection, the organ becomes permanently damaged and eventually is unable to function. The only treatment for chronic transplant rejection is to transplant a replacement organ.

Immunodeficiencies

Although it is clear that overactivity of the immune system can lead to significant disease and disorder, the lack of immune response is an entirely different problem with potentially devastating consequences. Known as **immunodeficiency**, the lack of immunologic response to stimulating antigens has several potential causes.

Perhaps the most commonly recognized source of immunodeficiency in the world is the human immunodeficiency virus/acquired immune deficiency syndrome (HIV/AIDS). At the time of this writing, an estimated 33 million people are living with HIV, with over 22 million of them in sub-Saharan Africa.[17] Approximately 1.1 million people are infected with HIV in the United States.[18] This global public health crisis is responsible for hundreds of deaths daily throughout the world, with tens of thousands of new infections arising each year. As the name implies, this disease is responsible for creating immune deficiency, and particularly targets the body's T cells. Since T cells are responsible for the initial stimulation of an immune response, a deficiency in the number of circulating T cells will ultimately result in a diminished immune response. People infected with HIV are susceptible to a wide variety of disease, ranging from the simple colds that affect everyone else, to the opportunistic infections of Kaposi's sarcoma, thrush, cytomegalovirus, and various fungal infections. Although great strides have been made in disease surveillance and prevention, a cure has not yet been discovered. This disease continues to be responsible for thousands of deaths annually.

Certain medications can render one's immune system impotent. Most of the time, this is the desired effect of these medications. Steroids and other immunomodulating drugs are designed to blunt the immune response by blocking the inflammatory cytokines released by immune cells. Many patients with autoimmune disorders are on chronic steroids or other immunomodulating medications in order to blunt their inappropriate autoimmune response. Steroids and other immunomodulators are given to transplant recipients in order to prevent their own immune system from mounting a response to the foreign tissue transplanted into their body. Although in both cases the immunosuppression is protective and in many cases life-saving, it does render the patient susceptible to foreign antigens since the natural immunity is blocked. Therefore, patients receiving immunosuppressive medications, including steroids, may present with signs of infection and even sepsis.[19]

Immunosuppression may also be an undesired side effect of certain medications. In particular, the chemotherapy agents used in many cancer patients may diminish a patient's immune response. These medications are designed to kill the fast growing tumor or cancer cells, but unfortunately also kill other fast growing or fast reproducing cells, including white blood cells. Therefore, a patient receiving chemotherapy may be neutropenic (low neutrophils—a type of white blood cell), and therefore susceptible to similar types of diseases as patients with HIV or transplant recipients.[20]

CASE STUDY (CONTINUED)

The Paramedics arrive on-scene, directed to the house by local volunteer fire police who arrived a few minutes earlier. As they enter the house, they encounter the patient, a 12-year-old girl named Michelle who appears in moderate discomfort. Her mother begins to explain the situation to the Paramedics.

"I don't know what is happening. Michelle had a little stomach upset yesterday. This morning she was in a lot of pain and had a fever of 103°F when I took her temperature. I called her doctor and she said to bring Michelle to the emergency department."

"Michelle had a kidney transplant last year because she developed kidney failure after an infection," Michelle's mother continues. "She is taking a bunch of medications for that, but otherwise she is healthy." Michelle sheepishly admits that she has forgotten to take her immunosuppressant medications the last few days.

"Does Michelle have any allergies that you're aware of?"

"No. She's never been allergic to anything in the past."

"Has she taken anything for the fever or pain?"

Michelle's mother answers, "I gave her some Tylenol a half hour ago after I spoke with Michelle's doctor."

CRITICAL THINKING QUESTIONS

1. What are the important elements of the history that a Paramedic should obtain?
2. What is the symptom pattern for acute organ rejection?

History

When treating a patient with an autoimmune flare-up, the Paramedic should ask the patient about the time course of current symptoms, the usual progression of the disease process, any triggers that have been identified in the past or present, and the usual associated symptoms. Most patients will know this information, and since most autoimmune disorders involve systems other than the airway, the patient is usually the best source to answer these questions. However, old records or family members may serve as additional resources. Most patients with autoimmune disorders will have a complaint of pain, so the Paramedic should inquire whether their current pain is typical of their usual symptoms. Pain that is different than usual may be a clue that there is a disorder other than the autoimmune disease causing the pain.

Fever, cough, chills, rash, dysuria, shortness of breath, chest pain, or headache may all be presenting signs and symptoms of complications related to immunosuppression. In patients susceptible to typical and opportunistic infections, the Paramedic must use information from patients, family, and even old medical records (if available) to determine the underlying cause of immunosuppression and the potential source of infection. Determining whether or not the patient has had contact with sick persons or recent hospitalizations may help the Paramedic narrow the source and type of infection and aid the receiving facility in antibiotic choice.

Past Medical History

The past medical history is perhaps the most important information that can be obtained other than the history of present illness in a patient suffering from an immune reaction. The AMPLE mnemonic can be used, with careful attention given to allergies, medications, and previous history.

Information about allergies must be elicited any time a patient is thought to have an acute allergic reaction, including hives (urticaria), angioedema, or anaphylaxis. Items that bring about these reactions would include medications, foods, environmental stimuli (pollens, bee stings, etc.), animal dander, detergents, soaps, or even certain fabrics. In addition to eliciting the source of allergy, it is important for the Paramedic to determine the type of allergic response. Some patients have a minimal rash as the manifestation of the allergy. Other patients develop full anaphylaxis. This is seen most frequently with the use of certain antibiotics. It is crucial for the Paramedic to determine what happens to a patient when she is exposed to the antigenic source. Some patients may confuse allergies and intolerances. Vomiting after eating certain foods such as milk products is usually an intolerance to the sugars in the milk, but is not a true allergy. A swollen throat following ingestion of peanuts, however, is likely a true allergic response.

The Paramedic should obtain a full medication list if at all possible. Patients and family members should be asked about medicines being taken, and when possible should bring them along to the hospital. In particular, the Paramedic should ask whether there are any new medications being taken or any changes in medication doses or frequency. Antibiotics and ACE inhibitors are especially important to identify because of their high allergenic potential.[21,22] In addition, steroids, immunosuppressant medications, and HIV drugs may help to determine an underlying medical condition, which is useful in guiding diagnostic planning and treatment. Most patients undergoing chemotherapy will not have their medications readily available at home, and therefore may not know the names or types of medicines they are receiving. If this occurs, the Paramedic should at least document that the patient is receiving chemotherapy in order to facilitate further investigation by the emergency department staff.

New and existing medical conditions should be documented and communicated to the hospital staff. Autoimmune disorders such as systemic lupus erythematosus and rheumatoid arthritis may present with typical symptoms, but Paramedics may require information regarding unusual manifestations of common complaints such as headache and chest pain to make a correct diagnosis. A history of organ or tissue transplantation, cancer, or immunodeficiency syndromes should clue the provider into looking closely at the medication list to see which types of medicines the patient is taking. Previous surgeries—especially splenectomy or, in rare cases, thymectomy—should be documented since loss of both glands results in impaired immunity. Patients who have had kidney, pancreas, lung, and heart transplants are placed on immunosuppressive medications that predispose them to infection. Patients who underwent surgical procedures related to cancer should be questioned about current chemotherapy for a similar reason.

Whether interacting with children or adults, the Paramedic should obtain a vaccination history. Although most infants and children in the United States are vaccinated according to particular schedules, these may vary from state to state. In addition, not all parents choose to vaccinate their children.[23–26] Therefore, the Paramedic should ask the patient about his history of vaccination, or about any recent vaccination (as they can elicit immune responses), as this is an important component of the past medical history.

Social and Family History

Finally, the Paramedic should take a brief social and family history. Although most autoimmune diseases do not run in families, the genetic predisposition and a family history may be clues to the diagnosis when the patient presents with the disease for the first time.[27] A social history is particularly important in terms of establishing disease transmission. Patients who are active or former IV drug abusers are at high risk for HIV infection. Although a history of sexual activity may be another important piece of information regarding HIV risk, this type of questioning is not appropriate for the Paramedic to ask.

As the Paramedic gathers more information, an EMT on-scene retrieves the medications Michelle is taking. The Paramedic finds out that Michelle's abdominal pain is in the lower left part of her abdomen, does not radiate, and is constant. Michelle admits she developed some burning while urinating two days ago and has been urinating less frequently than normal, but didn't say anything to her mother.

CRITICAL THINKING QUESTIONS

1. What are the elements of the physical examination of a patient with suspected acute organ rejection?
2. Why is an abdominal examination a critical element in this examination?

Examination

Performing a thorough physical exam begins with the basics. Airway, breathing, and circulation are always the starting point of any examination, and are especially important when examining and treating a patient with a potential for airway and/or circulatory collapse. Although physical exam techniques have been discussed in previous chapters, several important key elements of the exam are important to the patient suffering from allergic-type reactions.

The Paramedic must constantly reassess the patient's airway during transport because of the potential for rapid deterioration due to facial, pharyngeal, or laryngeal edema. Signs such as facial swelling, tongue swelling, uvular or tonsillar swelling, stridor, and wheezes are all indicators that the airway is potentially unstable and should be closely monitored. Evidence of tachycardia frequently accompanies allergic or anaphylactic responses, and a decline in blood pressure secondary to a developing shock state may lead to thready, weak pulses. The patient's skin should be examined for any rashes developing, and for the presence of mottling and cyanosis, as seen in hypoperfusion or hypoxia.

If the patient is not suffering from an allergic response, the exam is the same, but emphasis shifts to other components. Skin temperature may be an indicator of fever in the immunocompromised patient. Various rashes may develop that could indicate underlying viral infections (such as shingles) or bacterial infections (such as MRSA). Track marks on the extremities may indicate that a patient is an IV drug abuser and potentially immunocompromised from HIV.

The Paramedic assessment shows a macular rash along the abdomen as well as a reddened area at the costovertebral angle. Not needing any more convincing, the Paramedic asks the EMT to help package the patient for immediate transport while he speaks to the mother, who is anxiously standing to the side watching everything.

CRITICAL THINKING QUESTIONS

1. What is the significance of the patient's rash?
2. What diagnosis did the Paramedic announce to the patient's mother?

Assessment

In cases of patients with known immune system conditions, the Paramedic will be directed toward issues with those conditions by the patient's history. For other patients, the presence of urticaria and other signs of an allergic reaction will indicate an allergic exposure. Worsening of joint pain or the presence of the typical rash in systemic lupus erythematosus may indicate a flare-up of those conditions. Patients who have a history of immunosuppression—whether due to medications, chemotherapy, or infection (e.g., with HIV)—are at risk for infection and may rapidly become septic. Transplant rejection should also be considered in patients who have received a transplant even if not all the signs and symptoms of rejection for that organ are present.

The Paramedic is concerned that Michelle either has a urinary infection that traveled to her kidney, because of the burning with urination and fever, or may be rejecting her transplanted kidney because she did not take her medications over the last few days.

The Paramedic obtains intravenous access on Michelle and places her on the non-invasive blood pressure monitor, the pulse oximeter, and the ECG.

CRITICAL THINKING QUESTIONS

1. What is the standard of care of patients with suspected organ rejection?
2. What are some of the patient-specific concerns and considerations that the Paramedic should consider when treating the patient with organ rejection?

Treatment

The Paramedic's initial treatment priorities focus on aggressively managing the patient's airway, breathing, and circulation. Once airway and breathing have been secured and stabilized, the Paramedic's attention turns to the patient's circulatory status. Mottled or cyanotic skin may reflect hypoxia, or may be caused by hypoperfusion from anaphylactic shock. In immunosuppressed patients suffering from possible infection, skin mottling can represent hypoperfusion from septic shock. Although the long-term management of these shock states is different, the initial treatment should include IV crystalloid fluids (LR or 0.9% NS).[28] Intravenous access is critical in these patients, so the Paramedic should quickly attempt to start an IV.

Drug choices in the prehospital setting usually include antihistamines and steroids for the allergic patient. Occasionally an autoimmune response is so severe that the patient requires pain medication while en route to the receiving facility. Some medical professionals advocate for early pain control with parenteral pain medications (such as IV morphine).

While the ambulance begins to pull back onto County Route 1 en route to the hospital, the Paramedic reexamines Michelle. She has present abdominal sounds and her abdomen is tender in the left lower quadrant which is directly over her transplanted kidney. Her skin is warm to the touch and flushed.

The Paramedic records a set of vital signs as a blood pressure of 90/40, pulse of 112, respiratory rate of 18, a temperature of 103.5°F, and room air pulse oximetry of 98%.

CRITICAL THINKING QUESTIONS

1. What are some of the predictable complications associated with a superimposed infection in a patient with an organ transplant who is on immunosuppressant medications?
2. What are some of the predictable complications associated with the treatments for hypotension secondary to kidney failure?

Evaluation

Medical conditions are dynamic, and the patient's status may change during transport. The Paramedic must maintain constant vigilance to assess for changes in the patient, including improvement or deterioration. In the setting of hypotension and intravenous fluid administration, monitoring the respiratory status is important in ensuring the patient does not become fluid overloaded. Airway and ventilation status should be constantly monitored to ensure the patient's airway remains patent and ventilation is adequate.

STREET SMART

Although epinephrine auto-injectors (EpiPens) are common, some patients also carry preloaded syringes of diphenhydramine and dexamethasone.

The Paramedics are on their way to Women and Children's Hospital where Michelle had her kidney transplant. Although the trip is about 20 minutes longer than the trip to General Hospital, the Paramedic feels that Michelle requires the specialty services at Women and Children's Hospital, especially if it is determined that Michelle is rejecting her kidney.

About a half an hour after leaving the scene, the crew arrives with Michelle and her mother at the emergency department at Women and Children's Hospital. The Paramedic reports to the triage nurse that Michelle may have either pyelonephritis or transplant rejection and that her vitals stabilized with gentle fluid resuscitation.

CRITICAL THINKING QUESTIONS

1. What is the most appropriate transport decision that will get the patient to definitive care?
2. What are the advantages of transporting a patient with suspected organ rejection to these hospitals, even if that means bypassing other hospitals in the process?

Disposition

In almost all cases, patients encountered for immune-related concerns should be transported to the appropriate emergency department for further evaluation and treatment. Even benign-appearing allergic reactions can progress to more serious responses, and therefore the patient should be evaluated by an emergency physician. Any unstable patient should be taken to the closest facility as soon as possible. Some patients may be receiving treatments at specialty centers, and it may be appropriate to bypass the closest facility to transport a patient to her usual center for continuity of care. This can only be done, however, if the patient is hemodynamically stable enough to bypass a closer hospital.

Disorders of the immune system can present a significant challenge to the Paramedic and even to the emergency medical staff at a receiving hospital. It is important for the Paramedic to gather as much information as possible on the patient's past medical history and medications and communicate this information to the receiving hospital in a clear and succinct manner. Whether the immune response is too great or too small, or even appropriate, the response to an immunological emergency must be swift and decisive. Attention to the basics in assessment and treatment may be the difference between the patient's life and death.

CONCLUSION

The immune system serves to provide the body with a comprehensive defense against attacking organisms. Although this defense system is essential, in some cases the body can turn on itself, overreact to an external stimulus, or attack transplanted tissue. With a good understanding of the immune system, the Paramedic will be able to effectively support patients with immune system disorders.

KEY POINTS:

- The immune system is the body's natural defense against disease.

- The body's first line of defense is natural barriers: skin and mucous membranes.

- Antigens stimulate an immune response.

- Lymphocytes are divided into two major categories:
  - B cells generate plasma cells which will secrete antibodies.
  - T cells survey the body and recruit other parts of the immune system.

- Antibodies are specific to a certain antigen and require prior sensitization.

- Mast cells release histamine, heparin, and cytokines when stimulated.

- Allergic reactions are an excessive response to an antigen exposure.

- Subsequent exposures to an antigen may cause an exaggerated response that can be life-threatening.

- Autoimmunity occurs when the patient develops antibodies to his own cells.

- Well-known autoimmune diseases include:
  - Systemic lupus erythematosus
  - Rheumatoid arthritis
  - Dermamyositis
  - Polymyositis
  - Ankylosing spondylitis

- The body's immune system is stimulated when tissue is transplanted into the body.
  - Hyperacute transplant rejection occurs at the time of transplantation.
  - Acute transplant rejection occurs weeks to months after transplant.
  - Chronic transplant rejection occurs secondary to repeated acute attacks.

- Immunodeficiency may occur secondary to viral infections such as HIV, medications such as steroids or immune modulators, or as a result of chemotherapy.

- For autoimmune flare-ups, the Paramedic should ask the patient about the timing of signs/symptoms, usual progression of a flare-up, triggers, and usual associated signs/symptoms.

- For a potential allergic reaction, the Paramedic should inquire about the patient's allergies, medications, and previous history. Regarding the current episode, the Paramedic should determine the patient's exposure history and usual reactions.

- Initial treatment of immune disorders includes aggressively managing the patient's airway, breathing, and circulation.

REVIEW QUESTIONS:

1. Name two components of the barrier portion of the immune system.
2. Differentiate B cells from T cells.
3. How do antigens differ from antibodies?
4. What is the role of mast cells in an allergic response?
5. Describe the cause of an autoimmune disease.
6. How is an acute transplant rejection treated at the hospital?
7. Is a patient who is immunodeficient from chemotherapy at greater risk from you as a healthcare provider or to you as a provider? Explain your answer.

CASE STUDY QUESTIONS:

Please refer to the Case Study in this chapter, and answer the questions below:

1. Michelle is prescribed immunosuppressant drugs. Is she at greater risk of contracting an infection than other children of the same age? Why or why not?
2. Would you have transported Michelle to the closer hospital or to the one where she had the transplant performed? What is the rationale for your answer?

REFERENCES:

1. Biedermann T. Dissecting the role of infections in atopic dermatitis. *Acta Derm Venereol*. 2006;86(2):99–109.
2. Singer AJ, Dagum AB. Current management of acute cutaneous wounds. *N Engl J Med*. 2008;359(10):1037–1046.
3. White CE, Renz EM. Advances in surgical care: management of severe burn injury. *Crit Care Med*. 2008;36(7 Suppl): S318–S324.
4. Sompayrac LM. *How the Immune System Works*. Malden, MA: Wiley-Blackwell; 2008.
5. Kalesnikoff J, Galli SJ. New developments in mast cell biology. *Nat Immunol*. 2008;9(11):1215–1223.
6. Hubert P, Jacobs N, et al. The cross-talk between dendritic and regulatory T cells: good or evil? *J Leukoc Biol*. 2007;82(4): 781–794.
7. Berend N, Salome CM, et al. Mechanisms of airway hyperresponsiveness in asthma. *Respirology*. 2008;13(5): 624–631.
8. Romagnani S. Regulation of the T cell response. *Clin Exp Allergy*. 2006;36(11):1357–1366.
9. Katz HR. Inhibitory receptors and allergy. *Curr Opin Immunol*. 2002;14(6):698–704.
10. Lieberman P, Camargo CA, Jr., et al. Epidemiology of anaphylaxis: findings of the American College of Allergy, Asthma and Immunology Epidemiology of Anaphylaxis Working Group. *Ann Allergy Asthma Immunol*. 2006;97(5):596–602.
11. Venables PJ. Management of patients presenting with Sjogren's syndrome. *Best Pract Res Clin Rheumatol*. 2006;20(4):791–807.
12. Pipili C, Sfritzeri A, et al. Deforming arthropathy in systemic lupus erythematosus. *Eur J Intern Med*. 2008;19(7):482–487.
13. Pincus T. Clinical evidence for osteoarthritis as an inflammatory disease. *Curr Rheumatol Rep*. 2001;3(6):524–534.
14. Hammond A. Rehabilitation in musculoskeletal diseases. *Best Pract Res Clin Rheumatol*. 2008;22(3):435–449.
15. Rose AG. Understanding the pathogenesis and the pathology of hyperacute cardiac rejection. *Cardiovasc Pathol*. 2002;11(3):171–176.
16. Matas AJ. Impact of acute rejection on development of chronic rejection in pediatric renal transplant recipients. *Pediatr Transplant*. 2000;4(2):92–99.
17. World Health Organization. AIDS Update 2009. Available at: **http://data.unaids.org/pub/Report/2009/2009_epidemic_ update_en.pdf**. Accessed December 26, 2009.
18. Centers for Disease Control and Prevention. HIV prevalence estimates—United States, 2006. *Morbidity and Mortality Weekly Report* 2008;57(39):1073–1076..
19. Bertoni E, Zanazzi M, et al. Long-term steroid side effects in renal transplantation need a safe steroid withdrawal: a single-center experience. *Transplant Proc*. 1998;30(4):1303–1304.
20. Bodey GP. Unusual presentations of infection in neutropenic patients. *Int J Antimicrob Agents*. 2000:16(2):93–95.
21. Nikpoor B, Duan QL, et al. Acute adverse reactions associated with angiotensin-converting enzyme inhibitors: genetic factors and therapeutic implications. *Expert Opin Pharmacother*. 2005;6(11):1851–1856.

22. Cunha BA. Antibiotic side effects. *Med Clin North Am*. 2001;85(1):149–185.

23. Hamlin J, Senthilnathan S, et al. Update on universal childhood immunizations. *Curr Opin Pediatr*. 2008;20(4):483–489.

24. O'Brien J. Vaccine Research—11th Annual Conference: cutaneous formulations, universal vaccinations and recently licensed vaccines. *IDrugs*. 2008;11(7):471–474.

25. Zimmerman RK, Middleton DB, et al. Routine vaccines across the life span, 2007. *J Fam Pract*. 2007;56(2 Suppl Vaccines):S18–S37, C1-3.

26. Falagas ME, Zarkadoulia E. Factors associated with suboptimal compliance to vaccinations in children in developed countries: a systematic review. *Curr Med Res Opin*. 2008;24(6):1719–1741.

27. Ebo DG, Stevens WJ. Hereditary angioneurotic edema: review of the literature. *Acta Clin Belg*. 2000;55(1):22–29.

28. Brown SG. Cardiovascular aspects of anaphylaxis: implications for treatment and diagnosis. *Curr Opin Allergy Clin Immunol*. 2005;5(4):359–364.

CHAPTER 30

ANAPHYLAXIS

KEY CONCEPTS:

Upon completion of this chapter, it is expected that the reader will understand these following concepts:

- That anaphylaxis is the most severe form of an allergic reaction
- How the anaphylaxis is mediated by the immune and the complement system to cause the inflammatory response
- The emergency medications that support the blood pressure, promote bronchodilation, and decrease capillary permeability

ANATOMY CONCEPTS:

Prior to reading this chapter the Paramedic student should be familiar with the following anatomy and physiology concepts:

- Immune system

Sac County EMS is dispatched to a call, along with Ida Grove Fire Department first responders, for a 27-year-old female complaining of shortness of breath, which is a possible allergic reaction to a bee sting. En route, the Paramedics consider the possible presentation of allergic reactions and the other potential conditions which can present in similar ways.

CRITICAL THINKING QUESTIONS

1. What are some of the possible causes of anaphylaxis?
2. How is trouble breathing related to anaphylaxis?

OVERVIEW

Allergic reactions range in severity from mild reactions that cause pruritus (itching) to severe reactions of anaphylaxis (anaphylactic shock) that can result in respiratory distress, hypotension, and altered mental status. Although most allergic reactions are non-life-threatening, anaphylaxis can quickly result in death. Anaphylaxis results in between 500 to 1,000 deaths per year in the United States.[1]

Chief Concern

Allergic reactions occur after the patient is exposed to an inciting agent known as an allergen. Common agents that can cause allergic reactions include medications (such as antibiotics), insect bites and stings, and certain foods such as peanuts and eggs.

The body's immune system plays a key role in allergies and anaphylaxis. The immune response is composed of a complex cascade of events designed to destroy pathogens and foreign substances that enter the body. The immune response begins with the exposure of the body to an **antigen**, which is any foreign substance that can induce an immune response. Specialized white blood cells called B lymphocytes make antibodies that are known as immunoglobulins. The human body makes five general types of immunoglobulins: IgA, IgD, IgG, IgE, and IgM. One of them, immunoglobulin E (IgE), plays a key role in allergic reactions.[2] When an **allergen** (antigen) enters the body, a massive amount of IgE is released and binds to the antigen, forming an antigen–antibody complex. This complex triggers the release of histamine from mast cells, a type of immune system cell that is present in tissues. This release of histamine and other substances into the tissues causes vasodilation and leaky blood vessels, producing the signs and symptoms associated with an allergic reaction: a pruritic (itchy), red, raised rash called **urticaria** (Figure 30-1); throat swelling; limb and facial swelling; and wheezing. In severe allergic reactions, hypotension develops as the patient goes into anaphylactic shock.

Many other conditions can present with signs and symptoms similar to allergic reactions, so it is important that the Paramedic consider these conditions as part of the differential diagnosis. A few conditions with similar signs and symptoms to an allergic reaction are chronic obstructive pulmonary disease (COPD), asthma, aspiration, airway obstruction, and **angioedema** (rapid swelling of the dermis). It is important to note that patients with moderate to severe asthma tend to be more susceptible to allergens and may be more likely to develop an allergic reaction.

Angioedema, an **anaphylactoid**, (i.e., allergic-like) reaction that is not an IgE-mediated reaction like anaphylaxis, usually involves significant swelling of the lips, face, upper airway, and tongue (Figure 30-2) but may also include the digestive tract. Angioedema can either be hereditary or acquired and often occurs due to a problem with the complement system, a cascade of proteins and reactions that occur as part of the

immune system with the end result being destruction of foreign cells. One of the products of the complement system pathway is a chemical called **bradykinin** that serves various functions; however, its most important function is as a potent

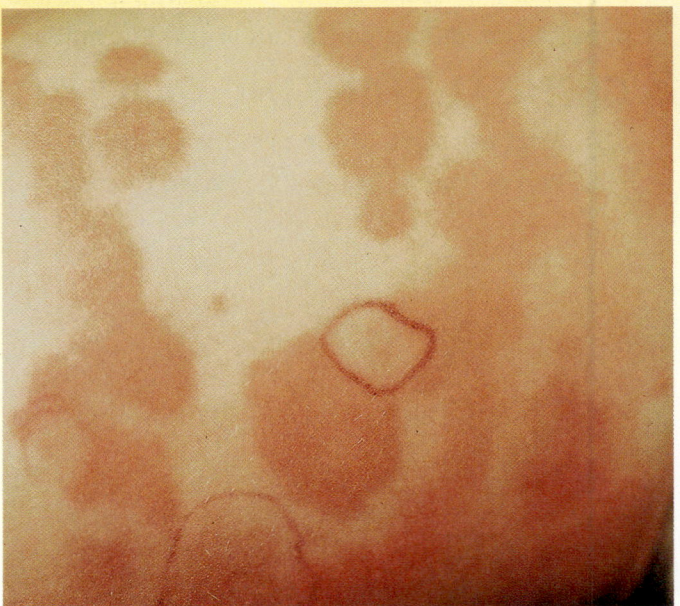

Figure 30-1 Urticaria. As more plaques develop, the entire surface of the affected skin becomes diffusely erythematous.

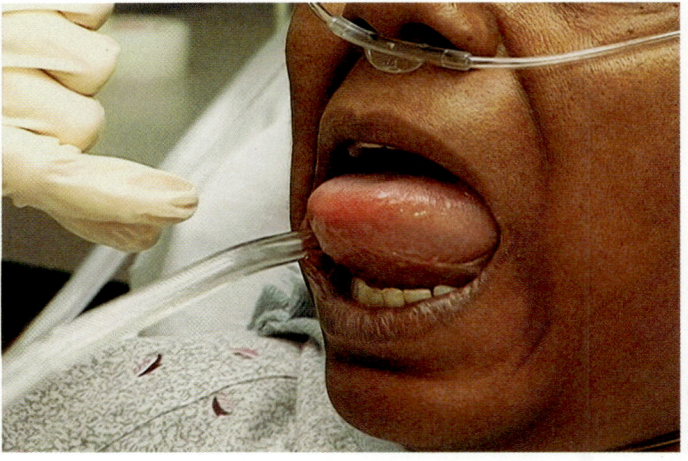

Figure 30-2 A patient demonstrating the signs of severe angioedema.

vasodilator. When present, bradykinin causes the capillaries to leak, allowing fluid to shift into the tissues in an action similar to—but more impressive than—the action of histamine. In hereditary angioedema, there is usually either a deficiency or a functional problem in one of the proteins that slows down the complement pathway.[3] Any activation of the pathway, often by an allergen, can produce significant edema. In many cases, the exact cause or trigger is unknown. A class of drugs called angiotensin-converting enzyme inhibitors (ACE inhibitors), used to treat high blood pressure, has been shown to be a cause of angioedema, which may develop even if a patient has been on the medication for several years. This occurs because ACE also breaks down bradykinin; therefore, if ACE is inhibited, bradykinin won't be broken down as fast and will build up. This explains why some patients can be on their ACE inhibitor for several years before developing angioedema.

Angiotensin receptor blocker medications, another class of antihypertensive mediations, may also cause milder forms of angioedema.[4,5] Finally, autoimmune conditions can develop where antibodies are formed against the protein that slows the complement system, producing a deficiency and setting the stage for the patient developing angioedema.

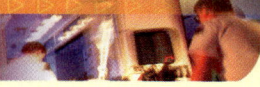

PROFESSIONAL PARAMEDIC

The number of cases of patients who have had an allergic reaction to eggs, wheat products, and peanuts has increased in the United States in the last several decades.

CASE STUDY (CONTINUED)

The Paramedics are met at the front door by a firefighter first responder who leads them down the hall to the kitchen, where they are introduced to Jack and Linda Smith.

Jack states, "My wife Linda said that she can't breathe so I called 9-1-1." Linda is sitting on a chair in obvious respiratory distress.

One Paramedic elicits a history from Jack and Linda while the other gets a set of vitals and places a nonrebreather oxygen mask on Linda. Linda had just finished eating a sandwich with the kids when she started to complain of itching all over and Jack noticed that she had developed a red rash. She then started to complain of trouble breathing and that her throat was closing up. She also got very sweaty. Her past medical history is unremarkable; she has no history of asthma or previous difficulty breathing. She does not take any medications except for birth control pills. She is not allergic to any medications. She does not smoke. When asked if she ever had an allergic reaction in the past she says no, but then adds that a week ago she had some itching after eating some cookies with nuts in them. Jack then states that today he made peanut butter and jelly for the kids and did not wash the knife before he cut Linda's turkey sandwich.

CRITICAL THINKING QUESTIONS

1. What are the important elements of the history that a Paramedic should obtain?
2. What is the symptom pattern for acute anaphylactic reaction?

History

In patients who appear to be in distress, it is important for the Paramedic to begin treatment during the history taking and to use family members to help obtain a thorough, directed patient history. The Paramedic first asks an open-ended question in hopes of determining the history of present illness, and then asks more focused questions to narrow down the differential diagnosis. The Paramedic should determine whether the patient has **pruritus** (itching), urticaria (hives), shortness of breath, throat swelling, or voice changes. Pruritus and urticaria suggest a hypersensitivity reaction which can rapidly progress to anaphylaxis. In addition, throat swelling and voice changes that include hoarseness may indicate swelling in the airway that may require aggressive treatment to avoid airway compromise.

The Paramedic should ask the patient about exposures to new medications, foods, or insect stings to help narrow the differential diagnosis. The Paramedic should use the AMPLE mnemonic to help obtain a detailed history. Does the patient have allergies to any medications and, if so, what is the nature of the reactions? Common medications that cause anaphylaxis include penicillin, cephalosporins, tetracycline, and nonsteroidal anti-inflammatory drugs.[6] Patients with a history of asthma may have more severe bronchospasm with anaphylaxis. The Paramedic should also ask the patient about taking antihypertensive medications, specifically those in the angiotensin-converting enzyme and angiotensin receptor blocker classes which are most associated with angioedema.

CASE STUDY (CONTINUED)

The Paramedic is very concerned about Linda. She is seated in a tripod position in obvious respiratory distress. She has an audible stridor that can be heard without a stethoscope. When placing his stethoscope on Linda's supraclavicular fossa, he notes the urticaria that is starting to rise. Appreciating wheezes at the apex of the lungs, he moves to get some medications out of the drug box. From his peripheral vision, he notices Linda scratching her neck.

CRITICAL THINKING QUESTIONS

1. What are the elements of the physical examination of a patient with suspected anaphylaxis?
2. Why is a pulmonary examination a critical element in this examination?

Examination

Initial airway evaluation is very important, so a Paramedic must look for signs of airway obstruction or potential obstruction. These can include stridor, tongue edema, or inability to speak. Moving on to assessment of breathing, the Paramedic should note the patient's respiratory rate, work of breathing, use of accessory muscles, and breath sounds. Circulatory compromise can also occur, resulting in tachycardia and hypotension. The Paramedic should obtain a complete set of vital signs and closely investigate any abnormalities. When obtaining the vital signs, there are several red flags that can indicate to the Paramedic the presence of life-threatening anaphylaxis. Tachycardia, tachypnea, and hypotension indicate shock.

Cutaneous manifestations of allergic reactions include **erythema** (redness), urticaria (hives), and edema (swelling) of the face, neck, hands, and/or feet. Lesions are red and raised with irregular borders and vary in size and shape. Lesions may become confluent and the entire skin surface can be involved with diffuse erythema and edema.

Signs of poor perfusion include altered mental status, diaphoresis (sweating), cool skin, and delayed capillary refill.

In anaphylaxis, the patient's immune system is activated and there is a massive release of histamine into the bloodstream. Histamine is a substance that binds to receptors in the body, resulting in bronchoconstriction, vasodilatation, increased vascular permeability, and gastric acid secretions.[2] Bronchoconstriction presents as shortness of breath and wheezing. As his airway narrows, the patient will attempt to compensate by breathing faster and using accessory muscles in addition to the diaphragm, resulting in visible retractions. Vasodilatation causes a relative hypovolemia, resulting in tachycardia. This is exacerbated by the increased vascular permeability that causes the blood vessels to become leaky and for the serum to move from the vasculature into the surrounding tissues, causing edema and worsening the hypovolemia. The combination of vasodilatation and increased vascular permeability results in shock, along with tachycardia, hypotension, and altered mental status.

In angioedema, the patient will develop the typical swelling in the face, lips, and tongue. Occasionally, the swelling may also include the periorbital areas of the face and extend down the neck past the thyroid cartilage.

CASE STUDY (CONTINUED)

Linda has an onset of an itchy red rash after being exposed to peanuts, and her symptoms have rapidly progressed to include the feeling of her throat closing and shortness of breath. The physical examination also reveals that Linda is retracting and has bilateral wheezing. Her vital signs, skin color, and condition indicate that she is in shock.

CRITICAL THINKING QUESTIONS

1. What is the significance of urticaria?
2. What diagnosis did the Paramedic announce to the patient?

Assessment

In working through the potential paramedical diagnoses, the Paramedic should exclude chronic obstructive airway disease. In addition to asthma, airway obstruction from foreign body aspiration is also possible. A comparison of the symptom pattern to symptom complexes for different etiologies for both wheezing and urticaria narrows the differential to the most likely Paramedic diagnosis: anaphylaxis.

CASE STUDY (CONTINUED)

Linda is awake and able to speak. She has bilateral wheezing with good air movement and is breathing quickly and is retracting. Her skin is cool and clammy; her pulse weak and rapid. Vital signs are a pulse of 110, blood pressure of 76/54, and a respiratory rate of 30, with a pulse oximetry of 92%. Realizing that the ABCs are not stable, the Paramedics instruct the firefighters to get the stretcher.

An 18 gauge IV catheter is placed into Linda's left arm and a 1 liter bag of normal saline is run wide to give her a bolus of fluids. A rhythm strip is identified as sinus tachycardia. Linda then receives epinephrine 0.5 mg of 1:10,000 solution through the IV. The Paramedics then move Linda to the ambulance stretcher. They package Linda with her legs elevated and move her to the ambulance. Linda also receives Benadryl 50 mg IV and Solu-Medrol 125 mg IV.

CRITICAL THINKING QUESTIONS

1. What is the standard of care of patients with suspected anaphylaxis?
2. What are some of the patient-specific concerns and considerations that the Paramedic should consider when applying this plan of care that is intended to treat a broad patient population presenting with acute coronary syndrome?

Treatment

The Paramedic must address any airway, breathing, or circulation issues as the first priority of treatment. In the case of a patient with severe anaphylaxis, the soft tissues of the patient's upper airway can become edematous and can rapidly result in occlusion of the airway. All patients with anaphylaxis should be placed on high-flow, high-concentration oxygen via a nonrebreather face mask.[7] The Paramedic should consider endotracheal intubation if airway edema is present and progressing. In severe anaphylaxis, intubation can be very difficult due to the edema. If so, a surgical airway may be needed.

If the patient is hemodynamically unstable, the Paramedic should rapidly establish IV access, administer IV fluid boluses, and position the patient supine with legs elevated.

Epinephrine is the drug of choice for the treatment of anaphylaxis. Epinephrine is a sympathomimetic medication that causes bronchodilation and peripheral vasoconstriction, increasing blood pressure. The dose of epinephrine for moderate allergic reactions is 0.3 to 0.5 mg (0.3 to 0.5 mL) of a 1:1,000 solution administered intramuscularly.

Comparisons of epinephrine administered subcutaneously versus epinephrine administered intramuscularly showed the time to therapeutic serum concentration was significantly shorter with intramuscular injection (5 minutes intramuscular versus 20 minutes subcutaneous). The Paramedic should administer epinephrine early during the course of treatment if anaphylaxis is suspected. Studies have shown that even the correct dose of epinephrine will not effectively reverse anaphylaxis once shock is established. If epinephrine is given intramuscularly while the patient is in shock, the Paramedic should also concurrently provide aggressive fluid resuscitation.

In profound cases of anaphylaxis, as manifested by severe hypotension and unconsciousness, the dose of epinephrine is 0.3 to 0.5 mg (3 to 5 mL) of a 1:10,000 solution slowly administered intravenously.[8-11] This dose may be repeated every five minutes.

The Paramedic should use caution when administering epinephrine to the elderly and those with heart disease due to the added stress that the resultant tachycardia can have on the patient's heart. Intravenous epinephrine infusion is an acceptable alternative administration method in those cases.

STREET SMART

Patients who are taking beta blockers may not respond to epinephrine. Alternatively, glucagon may be considered in those cases.

Antihistamines are another class of medications that are useful in the treatment of allergic reactions and anaphylaxis. Antihistamines block the histamine receptors in the body, limiting the body's natural response to histamine.

Diphenhydramine is the most common antihistamine used. The dose of diphenhydramine is 25 to 50 mg administered intravenously or intramuscularly. A side effect of diphenhydramine is sedation.

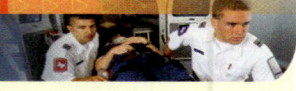

STREET SMART

Although antihistamines stop the effects of histamine from worsening, they do not reverse the response that has already occurred.

Albuterol is another medication that is useful in treating the bronchoconstriction and laryngeal edema associated with allergic reactions and anaphylaxis. Albuterol, an inhaled beta agonist that results in bronchodilation, should be used if the patient is wheezing. The dose is 2.5 mg in 3 mL of saline administered in a nebulizer.

Corticosteroids such as methylprednisolone (Solu-Medrol) are also effective in treating allergic reactions and anaphylaxis. Corticosteroids act to suppress the patient's immune response, resulting in decreased inflammation. Although corticosteroids are effective in the treatment of anaphylaxis, their use is controversial in the prehospital setting as the onset of action is one to two hours, and thus there is no short-term benefit to using these medications.[12] The dose of methylprednisolone is 125 to 250 mg administered intravenously or intramuscularly.

Although angioedema is not a true anaphylactic reaction and does not respond in the same way to the medications discussed previously, some sources nonetheless advocate using those medications to treat angioedema. Airway management is of key importance. In rapidly developing angioedema, the Paramedic should consider early intubation either orally or nasally in order to prevent complete airway obstruction. Standard oral intubation may be extremely difficult, and the Paramedic may have to use a blind nasotracheal approach or a cricothyroidotomy in order to secure the airway.

CASE STUDY (CONTINUED)

During the one-hour transport to Sac City Hospital, Linda seems to improve. Then she suddenly seems to decompensate again. At first the Paramedic thinks there might be some peanut-related substance in the albuterol that they had given earlier, but then he remembered that the medical director reassured them that this was no longer a problem. The Paramedic continues reassessing the patient.

CRITICAL THINKING QUESTIONS

1. What are some of the predictable complications associated with anaphylaxis?
2. What are some of the predictable complications associated with the treatments for anaphylaxis?

Evaluation

The Paramedic should reassess the patient during transport, including a review of the airway, breathing, and circulation, as well as vital signs. After administering a medication, it is important for the Paramedic to note the patient's response to treatment to determine what needs to be done next. Patients with anaphylaxis can deteriorate rapidly even with appropriate and timely management. The Paramedic should continue to closely monitor the airway in patients who have an allergic reaction or angioedema, as the swelling associated with both conditions can progress rapidly and require aggressive airway management.

CASE STUDY CONCLUSION

After transferring Linda over to the hospital gurney in room 1, the Paramedic provides a brief report to the attending emergency physician. The physician confirms the history and physical examination findings and orders another dose of epinephrine and another liter of IV fluids.

Linda improves over the next few hours. She is admitted to the hospital overnight for observation and is discharged home the next day. She is given a prescription for an EpiPen and told to avoid contact with peanuts. She makes an appointment to see an immunologist for allergy testing.

CRITICAL THINKING QUESTIONS

1. What is the most appropriate transport decision that will get the patient to definitive care?
2. What are the advantages of transporting a patient with suspected anaphylaxis after she has self-medicated with an EpiPen?

Disposition

All patients with allergic reactions or anaphylaxis should be transported to the hospital. Patients who have a potential airway problem or who are hemodynamically unstable need to be quickly transported to the closest appropriate medical facility.

CONCLUSION

An allergic reaction is an example of the immune system overreacting to an allergen, whether it is a food, a smell, or contact with another substance. Allergic reactions can range from a non-life-threatening but bothersome rash to anaphylaxis, or shock. Death may be averted if the Paramedic responds aggressively to the severe allergic reactions.

KEY POINTS:

- Allergic reactions range from mild to life-threatening.

- Allergens are the causative agents of allergic reactions.

- The allergic response relies on the action of the patient's immune system.

- The immune response results in histamine release from mast cells, causing vasodilation and increasing capillary permeability.

- Some signs and symptoms of an allergic reaction include an itchy rash; throat, limb, and facial swelling; and wheezing.

- COPD, asthma, aspiration, foreign body airway obstruction, and angioedema can mimic the signs and symptoms of an allergic reaction.

- Angioedema is an anaphylactoid reaction that occurs secondary to the action of bradykinin.

- The Paramedic should obtain a patient history that includes exposure to new medications, foods, or environmental substances.

- Patients who have a history of asthma may suffer more severe bronchospasm during an allergic reaction.

- ACE inhibitors may cause an anaphylactoid reaction, resulting in airway swelling.

- Patients with anaphylaxis need high-flow, high-concentration oxygen. The Paramedic should consider endotracheal intubation if airway edema is present and worsening.

- Epinephrine is the drug of choice for the bronchoconstriction and hypotension resulting from anaphylaxis.

- Antihistamines limit the body's response to histamine release.

- Inhaled beta agonists work with epinephrine to promote bronchodilation.

REVIEW QUESTIONS:

1. Describe the severity of allergic reactions.
2. Which cells release histamine? What is the role of histamine in the allergic reaction?
3. Name at least three signs or symptoms of an allergic reaction.
4. Name at least four imitators of an allergic reaction.
5. What class of drugs is often implicated in angioedema reactions?
6. How does the history of asthma affect a patient suffering an allergic reaction?
7. Describe the action of epinephrine, antihistamines, and inhaled beta agonists in the treatment of anaphylaxis.

CASE STUDY QUESTIONS:

Please refer to the Case Study in this chapter, and answer the questions below:

1. What clue exists in Linda's history that suggests she may be suffering an allergic reaction?
2. What presenting signs and symptoms are consistent with an allergic reaction?
3. Name the drug classification for each of the following medications. State how each medication is used in the treatment of an allergic reaction.
   a. Epinephrine
   b. Diphenhydramine
   c. Methylprednisolone
   d. Albuterol

REFERENCES:

1. Krause R. Anaphylaxis. E-medicine online Emergency Medicine Textbook. Available at: **http://www.emedicine.com/emerg/ TOPIC25.htm**. Accessed December 7, 2008.
2. Murphy K, Janeway C, et al. *Janeway's Immunobiology 7e*. New York: Garland Science; 2008.
3. Zuraw BL. Clinical practice. Hereditary angioedema. *N Engl J Med*. 2008;359(10):1027–1036.
4. Pillans PI, Coulter DM, et al. Angioedema and urticaria with angiotensin converting enzyme inhibitors. *Eur J Clin Pharmacol*. 1996;51(2):123–126.
5. Jain M, Armstrong L, et al. Predisposition to and late onset of upper airway obstruction following angiotensin-converting enzyme inhibitor therapy. *Chest*. 1992;102(3):871–874.
6. Tintinalli J, Kelen G, et al. *Emergency Medicine*. New York: McGraw-Hill, Medical Pub. Division; 2004.
7. Stafford CT. Life-threatening allergic reactions. Anticipating and preparing are the best defenses. *Postgrad Med*. 1989;86(1):235–242, 245.
8. Simons FE. Epinephrine (adrenaline) in the first-aid, out-of-hospital treatment of anaphylaxis. *Novartis Found Symp*. 2004;257:228–243; discussion 243–247, 276–285.
9. Pongracic JA, Kim JS. Update on epinephrine for the treatment of anaphylaxis. *Curr Opin Pediatr*. 2007;19(1):94–98.
10. Pumphrey RS. Lessons for management of anaphylaxis from a study of fatal reactions. *Clin Exp Allergy*. 2000;30(8): 1144–1150.
11. Sheikh A, Shehata YA, et al. Adrenaline (epinephrine) for the treatment of anaphylaxis with and without shock. *Cochrane Database Syst Rev*. 2008;4: CD006312.
12. Knapp B, Wood C. The prehospital administration of intravenous methylprednisolone lowers hospital admission rates for moderate to severe asthma. *Prehosp Emerg Care*. 2003;7(4):423–426.

CHAPTER 31

BARIATRIC MEDICINE

KEY CONCEPTS:

Upon completion of this chapter, it is expected that the reader will understand these following concepts:

- The common health risks associated with obesity
- The pathophysiology of obesity
- The difficulties of BLS and ALS treatment plus the transport of obese patients

ANATOMY CONCEPTS:

Prior to reading this chapter the Paramedic student should be familiar with the following anatomy and physiology concepts:

- Cardiovascular anatomy
- Respiratory physiology
- Endocrine physiology

The Paramedics receive an emergency call from Jennifer Kreschen. She states that she just found her mother lying on the floor of their second story apartment. Her mother, Joan Balogi, had tripped over her small dog and fallen. She hadn't been able to get up and was on the floor for more than two hours.

Mrs. Balogi is well known to the crews. She has frequent episodes of difficulty breathing and never fails to send a thank you note and plenty of her home-baked pastries after each call. She is also a very large woman, so moving her safely takes some planning.

CRITICAL THINKING QUESTIONS

1. What are some of the possible medical conditions common to bariatric patients that could be exacerbated by a fall?
2. How is trouble breathing related to the patient's obesity?

OVERVIEW

Obesity has become a national epidemic. Over 54% of the population of the United States is overweight and approximately 100 million Americans are clinically obese.[1] Furthermore, these numbers are growing. As a clinical syndrome, obesity has seen a large increase (over 30%) in just the last four decades. Obesity has become the second leading cause of preventable death in the United States, superseded only by tobacco smoking.

Chief Concern

The Metropolitan Life Insurance tables may have been the earliest efforts to describe normal and abnormal weights for a person, adjusted for height. First published in 1959, and revised again in 1983, the Metropolitan Life Insurance tables tied weight to longevity for the purposes of assigning risk to life insurance.[2,3] The tables would suggest that there is a direct link between being either overweight or underweight and to life expectancy. Obesity was defined as being greater than 10% over the ideal weight projected for an individual's sex and height. Morbid obesity was defined as being greater than 100% over the projected ideal weight.

Due to concerns about the validity of the methods used to create the Metropolitan Life Insurance tables, and in an effort to find a better description of obesity, physicians have resorted to the **body mass index (BMI)** (Figure 31-1). The BMI is a calculation which starts with the patient's weight in kilograms and divides it by the patient's height, in meters, squared. The resulting number represents the BMI.

A normal BMI is between 20 and 25. Individuals with a BMI less than 20 are considered underweight and therefore are at risk for certain conditions. Those patients with a BMI over 25 but less than 28 are considered overweight but are still considered healthy. When the patient's BMI exceeds 28, then the patient is termed **obese**.

As there is a wide range of weights that people can attain, obesity has been divided into four classifications according to statistical health risk. Those patients with a BMI between 28 and 35, or class I obesity, have a number of health risks which occur because of their obesity. Those patients with a BMI between 35 and 40, or class II obesity, have malignant obesity. By definition, malignant obesity suggests that the patient, who is at least 60% over ideal weight, has twice the risk of all causes of mortality than a patient with a healthy weight.

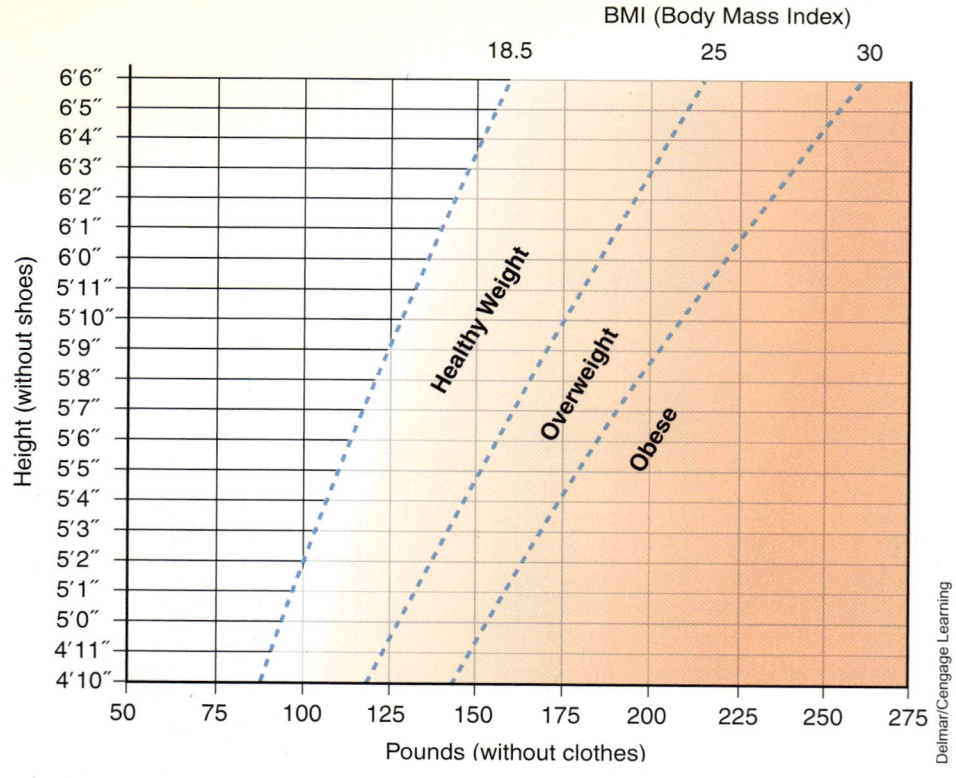

Figure 31-1 BMI chart.

The third class, the morbidly obese patient, has a BMI greater than 40 and is at least 100% over **ideal body weight**, which is defined as a weight at which a person is most healthful for the person, and is at great risk for the complications associated with obesity. Finally, the newest classification of obesity is class IV or super morbid obesity. These patients, with a BMI greater than 60, have attendant complications of obesity specific to their condition.

Although these indices of weight are helpful in assigning populations to risk pools and perhaps treatment pathways, they are only gross estimates of body fat. An NFL football player may be heavy but is actually "over lean," meaning the person has a large amount of muscle rather than fat. Overweight lean men have actually been shown to have lower blood pressures, lower lipid levels, and better glucose tolerance.

A useful working definition of obesity may be excessive body fat that results in an impairment of health. This definition speaks to the consequences of obesity and not to the patient's actual weight.

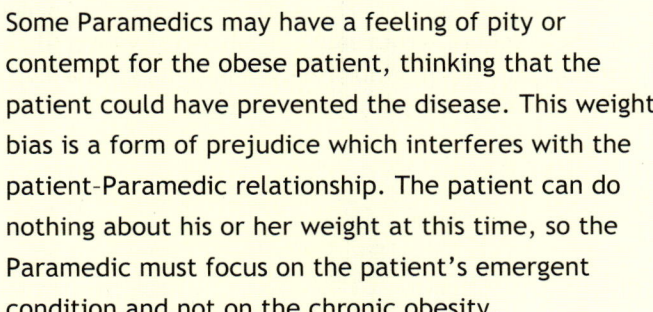

PROFESSIONAL PARAMEDIC

Some Paramedics may have a feeling of pity or contempt for the obese patient, thinking that the patient could have prevented the disease. This weight bias is a form of prejudice which interferes with the patient-Paramedic relationship. The patient can do nothing about his or her weight at this time, so the Paramedic must focus on the patient's emergent condition and not on the chronic obesity.

Health Risks Associated with Obesity

The health risks for patients with obesity are numerous: cancer, diabetes, hypertension, stroke, coronary artery disease, nonalcoholic steatohepatitis, and osteoarthritis.[4–7] The patient who is 20% above ideal weight has a 25% increased risk of coronary artery disease whereas the patient who is 40% above ideal weight (BMI greater than 30) has a 70% increase of risk of coronary artery disease.

Diabetes

There is a close correlation between obesity and diabetes. The patient with obesity has a threefold risk of developing type 2 diabetes. Approximately 90% of patients with diabetes have type 2 diabetes and approximately two-thirds of patients with type 2 diabetes are obese (BMI greater than 27). The close correlation between obesity and type 2 diabetes is reflected in the increase in type 2 diabetics (25%) in the last 10 years alone, which mirrors the increase in the number of patients with obesity.

The hallmark of type 2 diabetes is the development of insulin resistance. Insulin resistance occurs when pyruvate dehydrogenase, the enzyme that directs metabolism of lipids or glucose, causes an increase in the amount of free fatty acids. The increased free fatty acids, used in lipid formation, inhibit glucose utilization in the muscle (**insulin resistance**) (Figure 31-2). Without adequate glucose, the muscles call for the liver to release more glucose through chemical mediators. This increased hepatic glucose output leads to hyperglycemia. Increased glucose levels in the bloodstream stimulate the pancreas to produce more insulin to lower the blood sugar. The increased insulin demand leads to **hyperinsulinemia**. The pancreas, which is not intended to produce these quantities of insulin, starts to falter and the ensuing pancreatic failure leads to type 2 diabetes.

Cardiovascular Complications

Although some think that adipose tissue is stored energy, it is still metabolically active. As such, adipose tissue needs oxygen, glucose, hormones, and so on, from blood, just like any other tissue. To meet that demand, the body has to create new blood vessels (angiogenesis). For every kilogram (2.2 pounds) of body weight, it is estimated that the body creates approximately 25 miles of new blood vessels.

The increase in the number of blood vessels increases the systemic vascular resistance (SVR) which the heart has

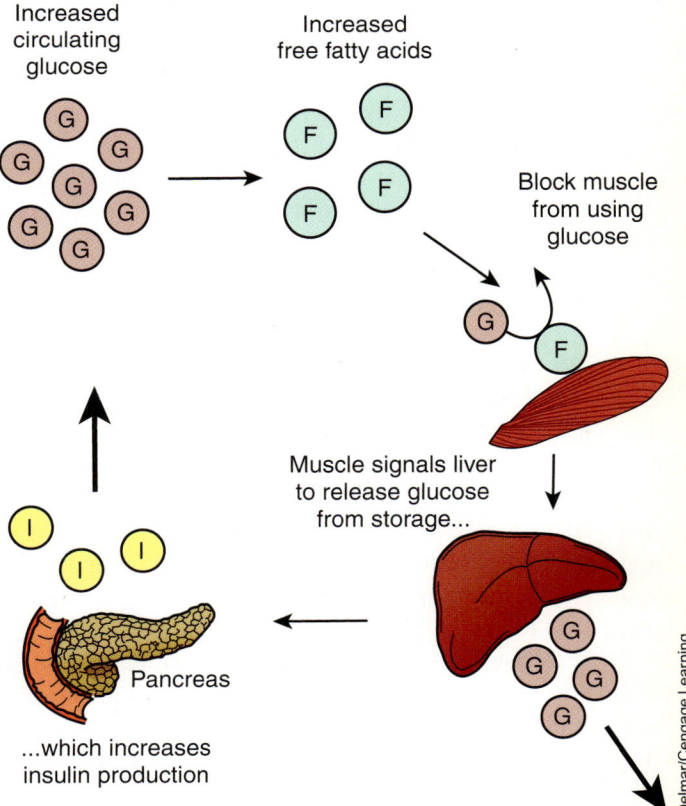

Figure 31-2 Mechanism of insulin resistance.

to overcome to sustain perfusion in those tissues. An analogy can be made to a fire engine pumper trying to supply an increased number of hoses. To keep water flowing under adequate pressure, the pump must overcome the friction loss, the resistance created by the walls of the hose.

Compounding the problem of increased systemic vascular resistance is the increased blood volume needed to fill those blood vessels. To overcome increased systemic vascular resistance and the augmented blood volume, the heart has to increase both its stroke volume as well as its heart rate. In other words, heart rate times stroke volume equals cardiac output ($SV \times HR = CO$).

To accomplish this dual task, the body secretes adrenaline (epinephrine). Adrenaline increases both the force and the rate of cardiac contraction, through stimulation of the beta sympathetic receptors, to increase cardiac output. Adrenaline also stimulates alpha sympathetic receptors in the systemic vasculature. This stimulation leads to peripheral vasoconstriction. Increased peripheral vasoconstriction, coupled with increased systemic vascular resistance and an augmented blood volume, leads to systemic hypertension. By definition, systemic hypertension is a diastolic pressure greater than 90 mmHg.

The heart of the patient who is obese now has to overcome hypertension. To do so, it must beat harder and faster. As a result, the hyperdynamic, or forcefully beating, heart starts to hypertrophy, resulting in increased muscle mass. This hypertrophy changes the shape and volume of the ventricular chambers, a process called remodeling. The remodeled ventricle is no longer able to accept the same quantity of blood as a normal left ventricle. Therefore, there is a decreased cardiac output, which in turn leads to more tachycardia, ventricular remodeling, and so on. In other words, there is a positive feedback loop with negative consequences.

When the blood fails to enter the heart, and backs up into the lungs, the patient starts to experience pulmonary edema and other signs of backward failure. As there is also less blood in the ventricles to be ejected, the patient's blood pressure falls and the patient experiences forward failure.

Pulmonary Complications

The lungs, like the heart, must meet the increased needs of the excessive metabolically active adipose tissues. These oxygen demands of the adipose tissue are coupled with the increased oxygen demands of the underlying muscles that support the adipose tissue. These tissues, both adipose and muscle, also create greater quantities of carbon dioxide which need to be expired.

In response to the increased pulmonary demands, the patient's respiratory rate and depth increase. Unfortunately, the large abdominal mass (**panniculus**) creates a functional physical barrier to a deep breath. Obesity can cause as much as a 35% loss of the patient's functional residual capacity as a result of this restrictive lung defect.[8,9] The impact of this loss can be two-fold.

First, the patient is prone to transient hypoxia, particularly when lying flat. This hypoxia can be most pronounced at night when the patient is sleeping and can result in sleep apnea. Because of the recurrent hypoxia, the hormone erythropoietin (EPO) is secreted by the kidneys, which in turn stimulates the bone marrow to produce erythrocytes, or red blood cells. The resulting increase in red blood cells, as measured by hematocrit, creates a condition called polycythemia. **Physiologic polycythemia** is a condition most often seen in patients with chronic obstructive pulmonary diseases (such as emphysema) that increases the viscosity of the patient's blood. This increased viscosity makes it more difficult for the patient's heart to pump the blood, resulting in further deterioration of the patient's cardiac function.

The patient with obesity also retains carbon dioxide as a result of the restrictive lung defect. Increasing carbon dioxide levels (hypercarbia) lead to lethargy (called CO_2 narcosis) and somnolence. The excessive daytime sleepiness (somnolence) and sleep apnea result in physiologic polycythemia, thus reinforcing the positive feedback loop.

Approximately 10% of the population of morbidly obese patients may develop Pickwickian syndrome, named after the character Fat Boy Joe in the *Pickwick Papers* written by Charles Dickens. The symptom pattern associated with **Pickwickian syndrome**, or obesity hypoventilation syndrome, includes morbid obesity, transient hypoxia, hypercarbia, and often obstructive sleep apnea.

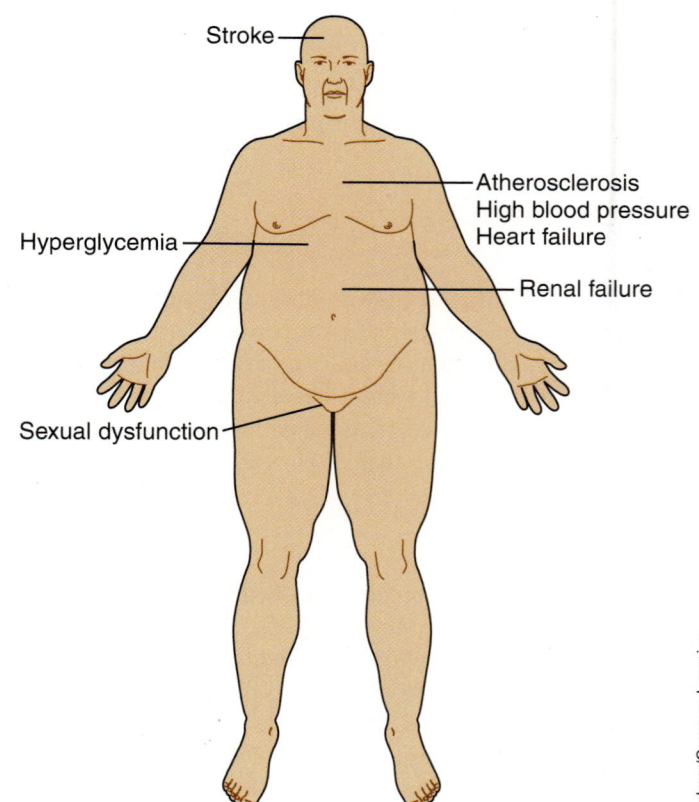

Stroke

Atherosclerosis
High blood pressure
Heart failure

Hyperglycemia

Renal failure

Sexual dysfunction

Delmar/Cengage Learning

Figure 31-3 Complications of obesity.

Persistent hypoxia observed in obesity hypoventilation syndrome causes pulmonary vasoconstriction as the body redirects blood to better aerated portions of the lung. This pulmonary vasoconstriction (pulmonary hypertension) increases the resistance that the right ventricle has to pump against. The right ventricle, being a volume pump and not a pressure pump, starts to fail against this pulmonary hypertension and leads to a condition called cor pulmonale (right ventricular failure). Clearly, obesity can lead to a variety of complications (Figure 31-3).

CASE STUDY (CONTINUED)

Arriving at Mrs. Balogi's side, the crew notes that she is conscious and able to answer their questions. She went to take a step backward and stepped onto the dog, which upset her balance. She fell into the wall and then slid down onto the floor. With nothing to grab hold of, she couldn't get up.

Mrs. Balogi has two complaints at the moment. Her right shoulder hurts and she feels very short of breath. Her daughter, Jennifer, notes that she doesn't seem as awake as usual. Jennifer also mentions that the last time her mother was in the hospital, she weighed 420 pounds and hadn't lost any weight since then.

CRITICAL THINKING QUESTIONS

1. What are the important elements of the history that a Paramedic should obtain?
2. What is the symptom pattern for post-obstructive pulmonary edema?

History

The patient's increasing shortness of breath can be attributed to several causes including backward heart failure, cor pulmonale, or restrictive lung defect. Regardless of the etiology, the Paramedic should obtain a standard history for shortness of breath, with a specific focus on signs of heart failure.

The Paramedic should ask if the patient has **paroxysmal nocturnal dyspnea (PND)** (shortness of breath at night) and **orthopnea** (need to sit upright to breath properly). Some patients with obesity cannot sleep lying flat and prefer to sleep with many pillows or in a lounge recliner chair.

The patient's weight may be a particularly sensitive portion of the history. Although some patients may become defensive when asked about their weight, the Paramedic should explain that it is important information needed for patient care.

CASE STUDY (CONTINUED)

The Paramedic proceeds to the physical examination, although obtaining vital signs seems like a daunting task. For example, the thigh blood pressure cuff is too small for the patient's arms. The patient's shortness of breath is becoming increasingly worse despite the administration of high-flow, high-concentration oxygen. Auscultation of breath sounds reveals rales (crackles) bilaterally that extend into the apices from the base of the lungs and the patient's pulse oximetry is low despite the high-flow, high-concentration oxygen.

CRITICAL THINKING QUESTIONS

1. What confounds the physical examination of the obese patient with suspected acute pulmonary edema?
2. Why is creative thinking important in this examination?

Examination

While forming a general impression of the patient, the Paramedic might be struck by the patient's body habitus. The **body habitus** implies a physique that, when observed, would cause the Paramedic to suspect certain medical conditions may coexist. For example, a barrel chest suggests that the patient may have emphysema, a condition in which barrel chest is common. The morbidly obese patient is prone to metabolic syndrome (the triad of hypertension, hyperglycemia, and hyperlipidemia), cancer, stroke, and cardiac disease.

Cardiac disease, particularly heart failure due to left ventricular failure or cor pulmonale, is seen as a significant contributing factor in the death of all morbidly obese patients. The six **cardinal signs** typically seen in a patient with heart failure are a jugular venous distention, ventricular gallop, pulmonary edema manifested by rales, hepatojugular reflex, dependent peripheral edema, and peripheral cyanosis. However, these signs may be obscured in the morbidly obese patient.

The Paramedic's difficulty in assessing the morbidly obese patient for heart failure lies in the patient's body habitus. The patient's body shape prohibits the proper assessment for heart failure. The first cardinal sign of heart failure is jugular venous distention. The jugular veins of the morbidly obese patient are difficult to observe. Next, rales are commonly heard at the base of the lungs of the patient in heart failure. Due to the panniculus, morbidly obese patients have chronic rales. These rales are due to the atelectasis that occurs when the lungs cannot expand completely and the alveoli collapse. Although many patients experience atelectatic rales, these rales clear with deep inspiration whereas the rales of the morbidly obese patient are chronic.

The Paramedic will further have difficulty when auscultating for a ventricular gallop, the split heart sound that signals heart failure. The depth of the patient's chest wall, particularly along the fifth intercostal space, only permits a muffled heart sound to be appreciated.

As the patient's heart continues to fail backward, and the blood backs up, the liver typically becomes engorged. The morbidly obese patient's liver may already be enlarged (hepatomegaly) secondary to nonalcoholic steatohepatitis (fatty liver); thus, this sign is unreliable.

Next, patients with chronic heart failure will develop peripheral dependent edema as a result of changing fluid dynamics. The morbidly obese patient has chronic peripheral edema, largely owed to peripheral vascular insufficiency. As a result of this poor peripheral circulation, the morbidly obese patient will develop venous stasis and lymphedema. These two conditions leave the legs of the morbidly obese patient edematous.

Finally, and due to peripheral vascular insufficiency, the morbidly obese patient often experiences peripheral cyanosis, making this last sign of heart failure questionable for the morbidly obese patient.

Vital Signs

As a result of the increased demands upon the heart, and the subsequent adrenaline secretion, the morbidly obese patient is chronically hyperdynamic. The Paramedic can expect persistent tachycardia, without evidence of hemorrhagic loss, and hypertension. However, the body habitus of the morbidly obese patient makes it difficult to obtain vital signs.

The classic pulse point to obtain a patient's heart rate is the lateral wrist. In some instances, the patient may have a hanging fold of skin that covers the pulse point, making assessment difficult. The traditional alternative pulse site is the brachial pulse in the antecubital fossa. In the obese patient, this site is also buried under layers of flesh, making palpation difficult. Finally, the Paramedic can resort to the carotid pulse, only to find that the patient's adipose tissue which is covering the patient's shoulders makes the neck appear nonexistent. In the worst case scenario, and assuming the Paramedic cannot find the first three pulse points, the Paramedic can attempt to auscultate an apical pulse. Lifting the pendulous breasts, the Paramedic would place the stethoscope at the fifth intercostal space at the midclavicular line. As the heart of the morbidly obese patient may have hypertrophy, it may be necessary to move the stethoscope laterally until the point of maximal intensity is appreciated.

Like the heart, which is hyperdynamic, the combination of hypercarbia, hypoxia, and a functional restrictive lung defect induces chronic tachypnea in the morbidly obese patient. The assessment of the respirations of the morbidly obese can be a challenge. Although rapid, the respirations tend to be shallow and thus the chest wall movement is barely perceptible. Because the patient must enlist accessory muscles, such as the abdominal muscles, the Paramedic should focus on the rise and fall of the abdominal wall, particularly the epigastric region.

Auscultation of the lungs of the morbidly obese patient can also be a challenge inasmuch as the flesh tends to obscure many auscultation sites. However, the Paramedic can appreciate tracheal breath sounds at the suprasternal notch, an area that is notably absent of adipose tissue. Bronchial breath sounds can be auscultated at the angle of Louis, apical breath sounds at the supraclavicular space at the midclavicular line or at the intrascapular space at the posterior, and alveolar sounds at either the infrascapular space or under the breasts at the midclavicular line.

Obtaining a reliable blood pressure is also a daunting task for the Paramedic. Traditional blood pressure cuffs will not fit around the patient's upper arm. In some cases, it is necessary to use a thigh cuff on the upper arm to obtain a blood pressure. Alternatively, a large adult cuff can be placed on the forearm and the stethoscope placed over the radial pulse. The morbidly obese patient is often hypertensive; however, using too small a blood pressure cuff can lead to erroneously high readings.

CASE STUDY (CONTINUED)

The patient's lung sounds, although difficult to auscultate, show rales midway up each side. Mrs. Balogi's abdomen is tender without evidence of trauma and sacral edema is noted. The Paramedics are unable to assess for jugular venous distention or hepatojugular reflex due to Mrs. Balogi's weight. A 12-lead ECG reveals no acute processes, but the complexes are very small and hard to distinguish. There is a reddened area on her right shoulder but no deformity and pulses. Movement and sensation are present in the right arm.

CRITICAL THINKING QUESTIONS

1. What is the significance of the small ECG complexes?
2. What diagnosis did the Paramedic announce to the patient's daughter?

Assessment

The Paramedic assessment for this patient would be heart failure secondary to obesity. The Paramedic's first focus should be on treating any hypoxia that is present and then focusing on problems of ventilation.

CASE STUDY (CONTINUED)

Mrs. Balogi is obviously struggling to breath, and first responders have already started her on high-flow, high-concentration oxygen. The Paramedic knows that it is going to take some time for the needed resources and personnel to assemble and he is starting to become concerned. He wonders, "Can she wait that long?" and then considers, "What can I do to help stabilize the situation in the interim?"

CRITICAL THINKING QUESTIONS

1. What are some of the patient-specific concerns and considerations that the Paramedic should consider when applying a plan of care that is intended to treat an obese patient?

Treatment

If the patient is somnolent, secondary to carbon dioxide narcosis, then the Paramedic should consider the use of a nasopharyngeal airway (NPA). The NPA, or nasal trumpet, slides behind the redundant folds of tissue in the morbidly obese patient's oropharynx, providing a patent airway and an improvement in ventilation.

Any patient with difficulty breathing should be placed in the upright, or high-Fowler's, position to improve lung expansion by suspending the lungs within the thoracic cage. The Paramedic should not depend on pulse oximetry to provide an oxygen saturation reading (SpO_2), since it is not uncommon for the light sources in the pulse oximeter's probe to be unable to penetrate the layers of skin. If the patient has an altered mental status, then the Paramedic should administer high-flow, high-concentration oxygen to the patient.

If the patient's breathing appears inadequate, or the patient's mental status does not improve with high-flow, high-concentration oxygen, then the Paramedic should consider manually ventilating the patient with the bag–mask assembly.

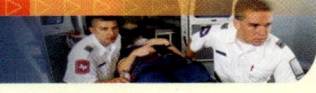

STREET SMART

The use of continuous positive airway pressure ventilation (CPAP) can improve the patient's oxygenation, thus avoiding the necessity of intubation. Some morbidly obese patients who have sleep apnea are familiar with CPAP and will readily accept its use.

Advanced Airway Modalities

With a patient in extremis (i.e., decompensating), the Paramedic may ordinarily be inclined to intubate the patient to control the airway. However, this decision should be seriously considered in the case of the morbidly obese patient. Obese patients have increased acidity of stomach acid, as well as an increased volume of stomach acid.[10] These conditions, coupled with increased intra-abdominal pressure (particularly when lying flat), cause these patients to be at greater risk of aspiration.[11]

If the patient is somnolent or unconscious and not breathing, the Paramedic should control the patient's airway. The body habitus of the morbidly obese patient includes a short thick neck, making alignment of the three axes difficult. A large tongue, plus redundant folds of oropharyngeal tissue, makes visualization of the patient's glottis difficult. The key to a successful intubation is positioning.

To prepare for intubation of the morbidly obese patient, the Paramedic may remember the mnemonic SOAP (Suction, Oximeter, Airways, and Pharmacology at standby). Next, the Paramedic should elevate the patient to about a 45-degree angle. The objective is to be able to create an imaginary line from the external auditory meatus and the sternum (Figure 31-4). Frequently, large amounts of padding are needed behind the patient's shoulders (use foam wedges or blankets) to raise the chest to that position.

Alternatively, the Paramedic can elect to intubate while the patient is on the stretcher with the head elevated. If the patient is on the ground, no padding is immediately available, and speed is essential to the patient's survival, then another person can stand in front of the patient, straddle and face the patient, and grasp the patient's wrists. In this position, the Paramedic (who is behind the patient's head) would instruct the other provider to a semi-seated position (Figure 31-5). This method is physically taxing to the other provider. In some cases, two providers (one on each wrist) are needed.

The next step in preparation for intubation is oxygenation. Several minutes of high-flow, high-concentration oxygen will create nitrogen wash out and permit the Paramedic more time to intubate. Although an average patient, who has achieved nitrogen wash out, may tolerate five or six minutes of apnea before hypoxia, the morbidly obese patient will only be able to tolerate two or three minutes under the same conditions.[12,13] Therefore, it is imperative that the Paramedic have all the necessary equipment assembled before attempting the intubation.

Due to the large tongue and redundant folds of flesh in the patient's oropharnyx, the Paramedic should consider the use of a large Macintosh (#4) blade to intubate. The Z–flange permits the Paramedic to control the patient's tongue and improve visualization by trapping the tongue to the side. Alternatively, a Robert–Shaw blade, a crossover between a Miller and Macintosh laryngoscope blade, can be considered. The Robert–Shaw blade has both the length of a Miller as well as the large flange characteristic of a Macintosh. The longer reach and flatter blade permits better compression of the tongue while enabling the Paramedic to hold the floppy epiglottis out of the way.

With the help of an assistant, who can use a large oropharyngeal airway as a hook to perform a cheek pull to clear the view, the Paramedic inserts the laryngoscope blade and attempts intubation. Although the use of external laryngeal manipulation (ELM) may be desirable, it is difficult to identify landmarks. However, if the laryngeal cartilage can be appreciated, then the assistant should be directed to apply backward, upward, rightward pressure (BURP) to improve visualization of the glottis opening.

Once the endotracheal tube has been inserted, the Paramedic should use secondary confirmation methods to ensure proper placement. Because auscultation may be difficult in that the patient's large abdomen obscures epigastric sounds and breath sounds may be muffled, the Paramedic should utilize end-tidal capnography.

If unable to intubate, the Paramedic should consider the use of a subglottic airway device such as the laryngeal mask

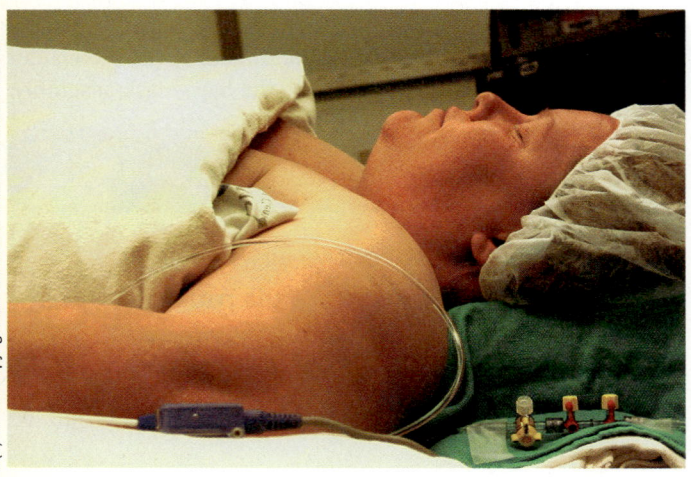

Figure 31-4 Improper positioning of the obese patient for intubation.

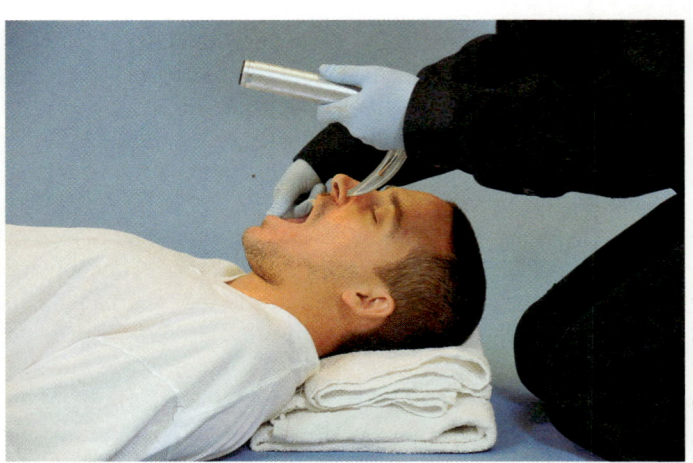

Figure 31-5 Head elevated laryngoscopy position.

airway (LMA) or the King LT airway device. Although obesity is listed as a relative contraindication for the use of the LMA, its use may be acceptable under certain circumstances.[14]

If it is not possible to elevate the patient's head (e.g., because of concerns for hypotension), the Paramedic should consider placing the patient in the left lateral decubitus position. In this position, the patient's tongue and redundant folds of tissue fall to the side. It also helps to keep any vomitus or secretions from the right mainstem bronchus, potentially preventing an aspiration.

Medication Administration

The Paramedic's first step in medication administration is to choose the route. Obtaining intravenous access in the morbidly obese patient is problematic. To distend these veins, it may take an extra long tourniquet; a two- or three-foot length of Penrose drain can be used. Since surface veins which are normally visible are buried within the skin, standard length angiocatheters will not reach them. As a minimum, a two-inch catheter should be utilized to attempt intravenous access.

In some emergent cases, it may be necessary for the Paramedic to consider the use of an intraosseous (IO) needle. Unfortunately, most IO needles are too short to reach the tibia or femoral sites. The only possible alternative is the use of a sternal IO, as the flesh overlying the sternum is generally thin.

When considering medication administration, the Paramedic should keep in mind that the patient with obesity will have altered pharmacodynamics. As a result of an increased blood volume and interstitial fluids, there will be an increased volume distribution. The implication is that when a drug reaches its therapeutic effect at a larger-than-normal dose, the half–life elimination will be increased.

In addition, there is likely to be a decreased clearance of fat-soluble medications (lipophilic drugs) such as diazepam. For this reason, many of these medications are dosed at the patient's estimated lean weight or the patient's ideal body weight.

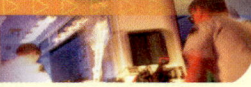

PROFESSIONAL PARAMEDIC

The Paramedic should explain to the patient the need for—and use of—extra manpower and equipment and emphasize its importance for the patient's safety and comfort, as well as the Paramedic's safety.

Transportation

Paramedics should encourage a culture of safety in patient care, especially in caring for and transporting morbidly obese patients. Policies, equipment, and teamwork should focus, first, upon the Paramedic's safety.

Some Paramedic agencies have established no lift policies for carrying morbidly obese patients. A no lift policy means that no patient shall be manually lifted when there are mechanical devices to assist the Paramedic with lifting. A no lift policy supports the Paramedic who encourages the patient to self-lift (stand and pivot) and bans the use of cradle lifts and shoulder lifts (hook and toss methods).

An example of a mechanical device which can assist the Paramedic with lifting is hover pads, a pneumatic lift device that brings a patient from the floor to the level of the stretcher where the patient can then be slid across and onto the stretcher. Other assistive devices that can be used to lift the morbidly obese patient include friction reducing sheets (specially coated sheets) and transfer boards. Another lifting device which can be used to transfer the obese patient from bed to stretcher is the Hoyer® lift, a sling system that suspends a patient for transfer. Currently there are portable sling systems available which can support over 350 pounds and can be operated by one person.

As the EMS industry continues to focus on reducing back injuries, and the Occupational Safety and Health Administration (OSHA) monitors Paramedic injury rates and encourages the use of ergonomic devices, newer lifting technologies will become available.[15–17] For example, a new "standing and raising aid (SARA)" device is being used in hospitals to help patients weighing up to 420 pounds stand and pivot. Its use may be adapted to the prehospital environment as well.

Some Paramedics have also formed patient lift teams that are called for when the patient is morbidly obese. These lift teams have trained together to prevent uncoordinated lifts, which lead to back injury. These lift teams are also fitted for back belts which help stiffen the spine and decrease internal spinal forces. In one study, there was a 95% reduction in lift-related injuries as a result of using lift teams within a hospital.

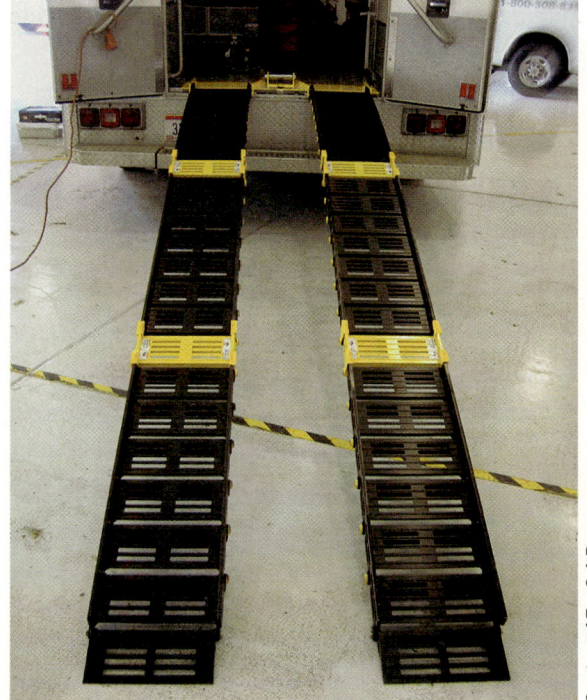

Courtesy of TranSafeRamps.com

Figure 31-6 Transfer ramps.

Special Provisions for Transportation

The continuing trend toward obesity will mandate that Paramedics retool to accommodate these patients. Paramedics will need, and should use, special heavy-duty reinforced stretchers and special aluminum ramps which are capable of holding a patient weighing over 1,000 pounds. Some EMS systems have created special bariatric ambulances that include these reinforced stretchers, ramps, and electric winch systems that can be used to load the patient into the ambulance (Figure 31-6).

CASE STUDY (CONTINUED)

The Paramedic crew explains to Mrs. Balogi that they are going to call for additional manpower to help move her as safely and comfortably as possible. Four additional team members arrive with specialized bariatric equipment rated for Mrs. Balogi's size. She is moved to a basket stretcher for transport down the backstairs but becomes very agitated. Reassessment shows that she is tachycardic and tachypneic with pulse oximetry dropping to 84% while on a nonrebreather mask. Rales are noted over the apices. The crew moves quickly to reposition Mrs. Balogi and treat her with positive pressure ventilation.

CRITICAL THINKING QUESTIONS

1. What are some of the predictable complications associated with having a bariatric patient lie flat?
2. What are some treatments that could help prevent post-obstructive pulmonary edema?

Evaluation

The patient's agitation, tachypnea, and hypoxia in this case is highly suggestive of **post-obstructive pulmonary edema (POPE)**. POPE can occur when the patient breath-holds while being laid flat, after which the airway suddenly becomes occluded. The resulting increase in blood flowing back into the lungs causes an increase in pulmonary capillary pressures. The increased pulmonary capillary pressure causes fluids to leak into the alveolar space and pulmonary edema to form almost instantly.

The patient with POPE should immediately be raised to the seated position. The Paramedic should treat this type of flash pulmonary edema aggressively with high-flow, high-concentration oxygen and continuous positive airway pressure (CPAP).

CASE STUDY CONCLUSION

Mrs. Balogi is transferred up the ramps at the rear of the ambulance and transported to the county hospital which has a bariatric service. This hospital is especially prepared to care for bariatric patients and is already familiar with Mrs. Balogi.

CRITICAL THINKING QUESTIONS

1. What is the most appropriate transport decision that will get the patient to definitive care?
2. What are the advantages of transporting a bariatric patient to these hospitals, even if that means bypassing other hospitals in the process?

Disposition

When considering the destination hospital for a patient with obesity, the Paramedic should be familiar with the capabilities of hospitals within the jurisdiction. In many EMS systems, certain hospitals have invested in equipment capable of caring for a large patient, including bariatric wheelchairs, heavy-duty Hoyer® lifts, and open CAT scans.

CONCLUSION

Obesity has become a significant public health issue in the United States, and is linked as a primary cause of several chronic medical conditions. The assessment and treatment of obese patients presents a challenge to the Paramedic. Therefore, the Paramedic must employ several tools at his disposal to help safely care for obese patients.

KEY POINTS:

- Obesity has become the second leading cause of preventable death in the United States, surpassed only by tobacco smoking.

- Obesity may be defined as excessive body fat that results in an impairment of health.

- Health risks for patients with obesity include cancer, diabetes, hypertension, stroke, coronary artery disease, nonalcoholic steatohepatitis, and osteoarthritis.

- Obtaining a history and exam of the obese patient may be difficult due to the patient's embarrassment over weight and body changes obscuring landmarks.

- Expected alterations in vital signs include tachycardia, tachypnea, and hypertension.

- Signs of heart failure are likely present in the obese patient.

- The Paramedic should use positioning to facilitate adequate ventilation.

- The Paramedic should adjust positioning and equipment when intubating the bariatric patient to adjust for patient anatomy.

- When treating the bariatric patient, the Paramedic should consider medication route, dose, and readministration times.

- Paramedics should be aware of the bariatric equipment available in their region.

- Paramedics should remain vigilant in assessing for post-obstructive pulmonary edema (POPE).

REVIEW QUESTIONS:

1. How does obesity complicate the patient's history?

2. What modifications might the Paramedic need to make when assessing for
   - Lung sounds
   - Heart sounds and apical pulses
   - Vital signs

3. What alterations are necessary when intubating an obese patient?

4. What considerations should the Paramedic take in moving the patient from bed to stretcher, floor to stretcher, down a flight of stairs, into the ambulance?

5. How does a patient's increased weight affect medication administration?

CASE STUDY QUESTIONS:

Please refer to the Case Study in this chapter, and answer the questions below:

1. What complications are likely to exist for Mrs. Balogi after having lain on the floor for two hours?

2. How would CPAP assist Mrs. Balogi in breathing better? How would it help improve her oxygen saturation?

REFERENCES:

1. Wang Y, Beydoun MA. The obesity epidemic in the United States—gender, age, socioeconomic, racial/ethnic, and geographic characteristics: a systematic review and meta-regression analysis. *Epidemiol Rev*. 2007;29:6–28.

2. Kushner RF. Body weight and mortality. *Nutr Rev*. 1993;51(5):127–136.

3. Williamson DF. Descriptive epidemiology of body weight and weight change in U.S. adults. *Ann Intern Med*. 1993;119 (7 Pt 2):646–649.

4. Bullo M, Casas-Agustench P, et al. Inflammation, obesity and comorbidities: the role of diet. *Public Health Nutr*. 2007;10(10A):1164–1172.

5. Segura J, Ruilope LM. Obesity, essential hypertension and renin-angiotensin system. *Public Health Nutr*. 2007;10(10A): 1151–1155.

6. Sampsel S, May J. Assessment and management of obesity and comorbid conditions. *Dis Manag*. 2007;10(5):252–265.

7. Poobalan AS, Aucott LS, et al. Long-term weight loss effects on all cause mortality in overweight/obese populations. *Obes Rev*. 2007;8(6):503–513.

8. Parameswaran K, Todd DC, et al. Altered respiratory physiology in obesity. *Can Respir J*. 2006;13(4):203–210.

9. Marchiondo K. Pickwickian syndrome: the challenge of severe sleep apnea. *Medsurg Nurs*. 2000;9(4):183–188.

10. Harter RL, Kelly WB, et al. A comparison of the volume and pH of gastric contents of obese and lean surgical patients. *Anesth Analg*. 1998;86(1):147–152.

11. Chang KK, Jawan B, et al. Effect of preoperative fasting time on gastric volume and pH. *Ma Zui Xue Za Zhi*. 1989;27(2): 149–152.

12. Walls R. *Manual of Emergency Airway Management*. Philadelphia: Lippincott Williams & Wilkins; 2008.

13. Levitan RM, Chudnofsky C, et al. Emergency airway management in a morbidly obese, noncooperative, rapidly deteriorating patient. *Am J Emerg Med*. 2006;24(7):894–896.

14. Frappier J, Guenoun T, et al. Airway management using the intubating laryngeal mask airway for the morbidly obese patient. *Anesth Analg*. 2003;96(5):1510–1515, table of contents.

15. Patient lift teams: effective strategy to reduce back injuries and related costs. *Healthc Hazard Manage Monit*. 2005;18(9):1–6.

16. Safety pros: lift teams, transfer devices reduce costly back injuries. *Hosp Secur Saf Manage*. 1998;19(3):8–10.

17. Charney W, Simmons B, et al. Zero lift programs in small rural hospitals in Washington state: reducing back injuries among health care workers. *Aaohn J*. 2006;54(8):355–358.

CHAPTER 32

DISORDERS OF UNEXPLAINED WEIGHT LOSS

KEY CONCEPTS:

Upon completion of this chapter, it is expected that the reader will understand these following concepts:

- How medical care shifts from curative care to comfort care in the terminal stage of disease
- How signs and symptoms common to the terminally ill patient may not indicate the terminal event and should be assessed and treated as appropriate
- That management of pain is a key component of end of life care
- How care extends to the family

ANATOMY CONCEPTS:

Prior to reading this chapter the Paramedic student should be familiar with the following anatomy and physiology concepts:

- Cellular physiology
- Immune system physiology

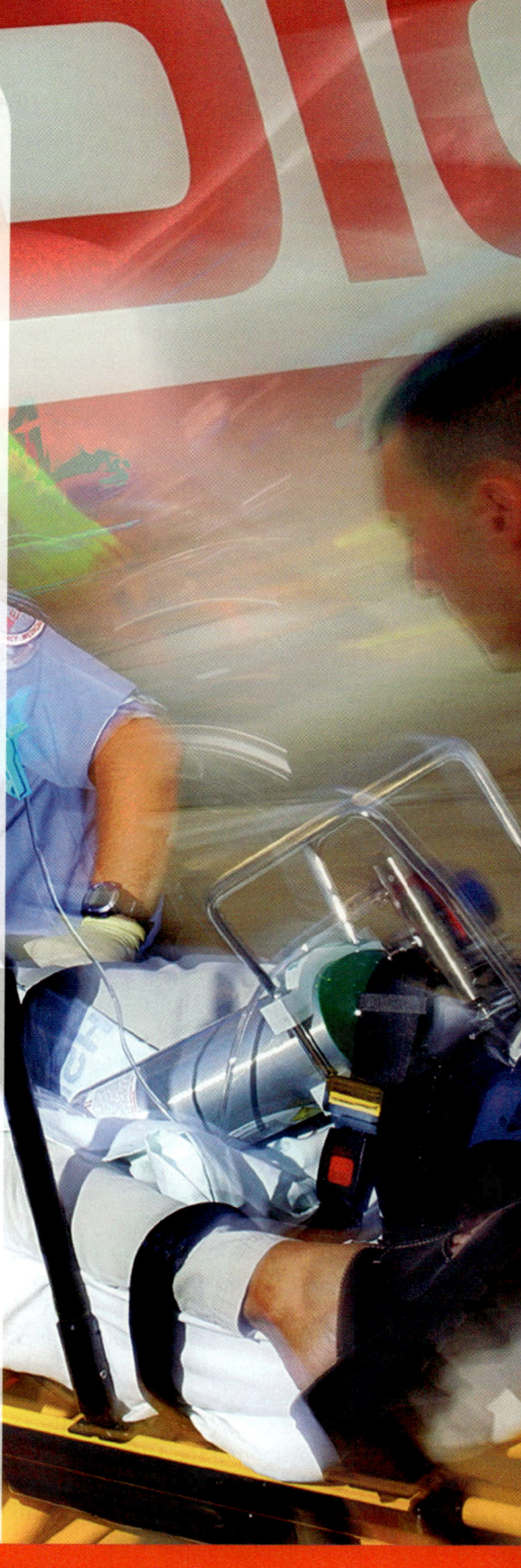

A call comes in for an 83-year-old man, Mr. Serafini, who is no longer able to walk. His wife has been caring for him at home and she is worried that he may have had a stroke. While en route, the Paramedics consider the possibility of a stroke but also discuss other possible causes of a change in a patient's mobility.

Upon arrival, the Paramedics are greeted at the door by Mrs. Serafini. She says that her husband has prostate cancer and his treatments are no longer effective. He hasn't been eating well and has lost a lot of weight. Today, he is no longer able to get up from the bed and she is worried that he has had a stroke.

CRITICAL THINKING QUESTIONS

1. What are some of the possible causes of sudden onset of weakness?
2. How is stroke related to cancer?

OVERVIEW

Despite the advances of medicine, a number of diseases continue to vex physicians. Although the symptoms of these diseases can be made more tolerable, the diseases continue to progress, ultimately ending in the patient's death. As a caregiver, the Paramedic's role is to support the patient during the advanced stages of the disease and provide palliative care (comfort measures).

Chief Concern

Generalized weakness and unexplained weight loss is suggestive of the end stage of several diseases including tuberculosis (consumption), AIDS, and cancer. The care of these diseases, when in the terminal stage, focuses less on the cure of the patient and more on the care of the patient.

Tuberculosis

Although the incidence of tuberculosis has markedly declined in the United States, tuberculosis is still a major cause of mortality in both AIDS-ridden and war-ravaged countries.[1,2] As an opportunistic infection, the mycobacterium tuberculosis seeds the lungs of the AIDS-infected patient and waits for the patient's immune system to weaken. Once the patient is weak, tuberculosis lives up to its old name (consumption) and starts to compete with the body for its energy. The patient then begins to waste away (unexplained weight loss).

Tuberculosis can also spread to other organs beyond the lungs (extrapulmonary tuberculosis). For example, tuberculosis can spread to the skeletal system and cause tuberculosis osteomyelitis. Formerly known as Pott's disease, tuberculosis riddles bones, particularly the thoracic and lumbar vertebrae, leading to bony destruction and nontraumatic compression fractures.

Renal tuberculosis occurs when disseminated tuberculosis enters the kidneys and progressively destroys the renal parenchyma until the kidney fails. Renal tuberculosis can also spread to the adrenal glands just superior to the kidneys, leading to destruction of the adrenal cortex and the development of Addison's disease.

Acquired Immunodeficiency Syndrome

The human immunodeficiency virus (HIV) eventually can develop into **acquired immunodeficiency syndrome (AIDS)**. After an initial self-limited acute retroviral syndrome of several days, followed by a prolonged latent period that is sometimes as long as eight to ten years, the HIV virus starts to manifest clinically. A specific symptom pattern, also known as AIDS-related complex, is frequently seen in early AIDS (Table 32-1). Although the HIV virus itself does not lead to the patient's death, the destruction of the patient's immune system permits opportunistic infections, like tuberculosis, to

Table 32-1 Clinical Findings of AIDS-Related Complex

- Unexplained weight loss
- Generalized fatigue (i.e., malaise)
- High fever, either intermittent or continuous
- Persistent diarrhea with unknown cause
- Night sweats

Table 32-2 Pathology Associated with Stage IV AIDS

- HIV-wasting syndrome
- Opportunistic infection (examples)
  - Pneumocystis jiroveci (carinii) pneumonia (PCP)
  - Toxoplasmosis
  - Cytomegalovirus (CMV)
  - Extrapulmonary tuberculosis (TB)
- Cancers
  - Lymphoma
  - Kaposi's sarcoma (KS)

infect the patient in end-stage, or class IV, AIDS (Table 32-2). The AIDS patient with HIV-wasting syndrome can present similarly to the patient with end-stage cancer.

CULTURAL/REGIONAL DIFFERENCES

Although the diagnosis of tuberculosis generally carries no stigma, many families are embarrassed or stigmatized by a diagnosis of AIDS or cancer. The Paramedic should be sensitive to the family's concerns and use the terminology favored by the family.

Cancer

Hippocrates described the appearance of breast cancer (an outwardly visible cancer) as crab-like and named it cancer (Latin for crab). Cancer can be found in every organ and tissue of the body. Perhaps that's why many cancers owe their name to their origin. Like hepatitis, the term "cancer" does not describe a single disease but is an umbrella term that describes a number of disorders that have a common root—disorganized cell growth.

Under normal circumstances, cell growth and death is controlled by the cell's DNA. Cells naturally die from apoptosis, a programmed cell death, rather than necrosis or damage from injury. On any given day, approximately 20 to 32 billion cells naturally dissemble and their contents are reabsorbed during the process of apoptosis. Through a balance of natural cell division and regeneration (mitosis) and cell dissolution (apoptosis), the body is able to maintain homeostasis.

In the case of cancer, there is an uncontrolled division of cells and loss of control of cell apoptosis by the DNA, usually due to damaged (mutated) DNA. There are many causes of DNA mutation: exposure to radiation such as the ultraviolet light in sunlight, exposure to chemicals such as tobacco smoke, exposure to toxins such as heavy metals, and exposure to microbes, such as hepatitis B (the leading cause of liver cancer) or the human papilloma virus (venereal warts), the leading cause of cervical cancer.[3]

A number of cancers seem to have a genetic link. For example, women with the BRCA (breast cancer) inherited gene mutation have a increased risk for breast cancer.[4] The number of sources of cancer, chemical carcinogens, ionizing radiations, infectious diseases, and the patient's heredity reinforce that cancer is not a single disease but rather an umbrella term for a number of disorders.

As the number of mutated cells grows, a mass starts to appear. Galen, a Greek anatomist considered the father of medicine, called this mass a tumor or *oncos* (Greek for swelling). This term persists with the study of cancer assuming the name oncology. To lend perspective to the concept of a tumor, a million cancer cells can occupy a space on the head of a pin and one billion cancer cells would only produce a lump about one-half inch in diameter.

The initial uncontrolled cell growth is called the primary tumor. The cancer is typically labeled for the location in which it originates (e.g., a sarcoma is a tumor within connective tissue) or by its appearance (e.g., one type of lung cancer is called oat cell cancer).

Cancerous growths can also spread via several mechanisms to other parts of the body (**metastasis**) where the cells can become a secondary tumor. For example, breast cancer often metastasizes to the bone. Cancer metastasizes by either infiltration (using lytic enzymes), active movement (via the lymphatics or bloodstream), or by physical invasion of the tumor into other cavities or organs. Cancer can affect epithelial, connective, and embryonic tissues (Table 32-3).

Cancer Staging

Cancer is often graded by stages. Staging a cancer allows the patient to be placed into treatment groups with similar treatment strategies. A stage of cancer is a description of the cancer's extent of involvement in the body. The exception to staging is leukemia because leukemia is systemic by nature.

Stage I cancer is typically a small area of cancer that is limited to one organ and is generally curable by simple therapeutic techniques. Each successive stage of cancer is more advanced and tends to metastasize. The final stage of cancer, stage IV, is advanced metastatic disease and is generally inoperable.

Cancer may further be staged according to the TNM (tumors, nodes, and metastasis) staging system (Table 32-4).[5–7] The TNM staging system is only used for cancers that produce a solid tumor. For example, if a

Table 32-3 Cancer Terminology

- Carcinoma (epithelial cells)
  - Breast [+]
  - Prostate*
  - Lung** [++]
  - Colorectal
  - Ovarian
  - Bladder
  - Pancreatic
  - Endometrial
- Sarcoma (connective tissue)
  - Lymphoma
  - Leukemia [#]
  - Melanoma
- Blastic (embryo)
  - Neuroblastoma

Notes:

*Most common cancer in men

**Most common cause of cancer mortality in men

[+] Most common cancer in women

[++] Most common cause of cancer mortality in women

[#] Most common childhood cancer

Table 32-4 TNM Cancer Staging System

- Tumor
  - T0 – localized (i.e., in situ)
  - T4 – large primary tumor—generally inoperable
- Nodes
  - N0 – no lymph node involvement
  - N4 – extensive dissemination
- Metastasis
  - M0 – none present
  - M1 – metastasis present

woman had a lump in her breast that was positive and her axillary node had cancer cells, then she would be graded T2N1M0.

Cancer Treatments

Traditionally the treatment of cancer consists of three general modalities: surgery, chemotherapy, and radiation. The goal of surgery is simple: to remove (excise) the tumor. Some of the first successful breast cancer treatments, dating back to the Middle Ages, involved surgery. However, since these surgeries often involved removal of large amounts of tissue, with the attendant risks of infection, alternative treatments were pursued.

In the early 1900s, Madame Marie Curie was the first to use radiation to treat cancer, a discovery that won her the Nobel Prize and led to a new branch of medical therapeutics called radiotherapy. **Radiotherapy** uses focused energy to kill cancer cells in a specific area (target tissue) while sparing the rest of the body. Radiotherapy can be used alone (as a curative treatment), in conjunction with other treatments (as an adjunctive treatment), or for symptomatic relief (or palliative care). However, there are risks associated with radiation therapy: acute side effects (such as radiation burns, mucosal ulcerations, and edema) and long-term side effects (such as infertility).

The treatment of disease by chemicals (medications) is called **chemotherapy**. Chemotherapy is a specialized branch of pharmacology, as the treatment of cancer with medications is a narrow practice. The potential of chemotherapy was first suspected when patients, with accidental exposure to mustard gas, were found to have a low white blood cell count. Physicians, seeing the advantage in this side effect, began to treat lymphoma patients with mustard gas, giving rise to the era of modern chemotherapy. Some chemotherapeutic drugs are antibiotics which have been successfully used to treat cancer. The classes of chemotherapeutic agents are (1) alkylating antineoplastic agents that attach to the DNA and destroy the rapidly dividing cancer cells, (2) antimetabolites that eliminate essential elements needed to create DNA, and (3) plant alkaloids that prevent certain cell functions.

However, other therapeutic approaches also exist, such as complementary medicine and alternative medicine. Alternative medicines are nontraditional medical approaches such as megavitamins and herbal remedies. The claims of some alternative cancer treatments have been met with ridicule from the medical community as being unsupported by science. However, the medical community has been accepting of some nontraditional medical therapies. These treatments, such as acupuncture and massage, are considered supplementary to standard medical treatment (Table 32-5). This approach,

Table 32-5 Complementary Medicine

- Anxiety
  - Massage
  - Hypnosis
- Nausea
  - Aromatherapy
  - Acupuncture
- Fatigue
  - Physical therapy
  - Massage
- Pain
  - Acupuncture
  - Biofeedback

a blending of traditional and complementary medicine, is referred to as **integrative medicine**.

Following treatment, cancer may go into **remission**, a disease-free state in which there is a possibility that the cancer may return at a later time. The therapeutic goal of cancer care is to have the cancer go into remission. The patient's **prognosis**, the predicted outcome of the disease, and chance for remission is multifactorial. The patient's current state of health, the state of medical therapeutics, and the type of cancer are several dynamics that are factored into a patient's statistical chance of survival (prognosis). If a patient has been cancer free for five years, then the patient is generally considered to be cured of cancer.[8] Unfortunately, this is not always the case; a recurrence of cancer can return and devastate the patient.

End of Life Care

Although the focus of Paramedics has traditionally been curative, there are circumstances in which a cure is not possible. In these situations, the Paramedic must refocus and provide care which reduces suffering and improves the quality of life without prolonging life.[9–11] This type of care, **palliative care**, is provided to patients who have a terminal illness regardless of the proximity of death.

Hospice, a traditional place of rest for weary travelers, has become a place of rest for terminally ill patients. Hospice care, whether provided at home or in the hospital, provides care for both the patient and the family through a multidisciplinary team of nurses, doctors, social workers, clergy, and counselors. Hospice care encompasses physical, mental, and spiritual care to manage the patient's distress and to decrease her suffering.

Mrs. Serafini indicates that Mr. Serafini is having increasing difficulty managing to get out of bed, and today he simply felt too weak and uncomfortable to do so. She also says that he thought he was going to die soon but didn't want to spend his last days in a hospital.

CRITICAL THINKING QUESTIONS

1. What are the important elements of the history that a Paramedic should obtain?
2. What is the importance of the patient's statement, "I don't want to die in the hospital?"

History

The triad of symptoms for a patient with overwhelming cancer is made up of anorexia, weight loss, and malaise. **Anorexia** is an eating disorder characterized by a lack of desire to eat. Unlike the psychiatric disorder anorexia nervosa, anorexia is the medical symptom for decreased appetite that owes its origins to a metabolic disturbance, such as cancer. One of the characteristics of anorexia is early satiation, a feeling of fullness after eating very little.

Anorexia, in combination with the hypermetabolic cancer, quickly results in significant weight loss and malaise. **Malaise** can be described as a generalized discomfort that is associated with being unwell. Although not specific for cancer, malaise is an indication of serious illness.

Patients with cancer often also complain of nausea, with or without vomiting, that may be due to chemotherapy or radiotherapy. **Night sweats**, or sleep hyperhidrosis,

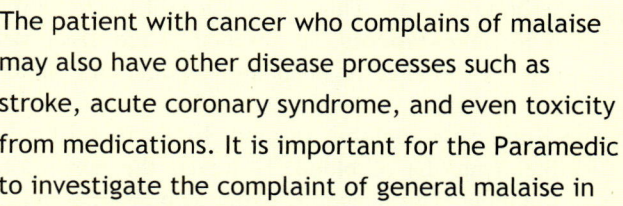

STREET SMART

The patient with cancer who complains of malaise may also have other disease processes such as stroke, acute coronary syndrome, and even toxicity from medications. It is important for the Paramedic to investigate the complaint of general malaise in order to ascertain its origins.

is a common complaint of drenching sweat that wets the patient's bedclothes. Night sweats can be seen in pathologic conditions (such as cancer or tuberculosis), as well as in benign conditions (such as menopause) or due to use of certain medications.

CASE STUDY (CONTINUED)

Mrs. Serafini brings the Paramedics to her husband's bedside. His face has a skeletal appearance and his eyes appear sunken. His bed linens are clean and dry and pillows are available to help prop up Mr. Serafini. Primary assessment shows that he has a patent airway, breathing is adequate although slightly labored, and distal pulses are present. A quick Cincinnati stroke scale shows clear but quiet speech. There is no pronator drift, although it requires great effort for Mr. Serafini to elevate his hands. He has a symmetrical smile. Blood glucose is 98.

CRITICAL THINKING QUESTIONS

1. What are the elements of the physical examination of a patient with end-stage cancer?
2. Why is the Cincinnati stroke scale a critical element in this examination?

Examination

The patient with terminal cancer may have an unmistakable appearance secondary to **paraneoplastic syndrome**, physical signs that are the result of the cancer's effect on the nervous system. The first sign of paraneoplastic syndrome is that the patient is gaunt and emaciated in appearance. The eyes appear sunken into the orbits and the skin, now paper thin, is prone to skin tears. The emaciation is due to loss of muscle as a result of the combination of anorexia and the wasting of muscles to supply the hypermetabolic cancer with energy (Table 32-6).

Other signs associated with cancer that the Paramedic may also note include large ecchymotic areas or purpura. The purpura, caused by bleeding under the skin, is secondary to the anemia which often accompanies terminal cancer. The combination of cancer therapies, such as radiation and chemotherapy, and the metabolic demands of the cancer impair the bone marrow. This suppression of the bone marrow leads to **pancytopenia**, an absence of red blood cells (anemia), white blood cells, or leukocytopenia and platelets (thrombocytopenia).

The normal hemoglobin level is 14 to 16 milligrams per deciliter (mg/dL) of blood. However, the hemoglobin level of a patient with cancer is likely to be 8 or 9 mg/dL. As a result, the patient will appear to have pallor and may have occult blood loss in the urine and/or stool. This occult loss of blood is secondary to concomitant platelet deficit (thrombocytopenia).

Along with anemia and thrombocytopenia, the patient may also experience leukocytopenia. **Leukocytopenia** is a decline in the number of circulating white blood cells. As a result, the patient with cancer who has leukocytopenia is unable to effectively combat infection.[12] In many cases, pneumonia or another infection is ultimately the cause of the patient's death.

Table 32-6 Signs of Paraneoplastic Syndrome

- Tremors secondary to loss of fine motor control
- Difficulty walking secondary to loss of muscle tone
- Wasting of limbs
- Neurological signs (many suggestive of stroke)
  - Slurred speech
  - Difficulty swallowing
  - Memory loss
  - Visual problems
  - Sleep disturbances
  - Dementia
  - Seizures

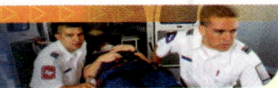

STREET SMART

The patient with end-stage cancer may still be hypoxic despite a SpO_2 reading of 100%. Although the available hemoglobin may be saturated, there is insufficient hemoglobin to meet the patient's metabolic or—in the case of a patient with cancer—hypermetabolic needs.[13]

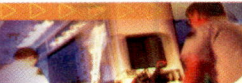

PROFESSIONAL PARAMEDIC

The Paramedic will often choose to wear a mask to protect the patient who is immune deficient, called **reverse or protective isolation**, as opposed to the usual self-protection.

CASE STUDY (CONTINUED)

The Paramedic is very concerned that, despite the patient's wishes to remain home and not die in the hospital, Mrs. Serafini may be unable to provide the care that is needed to comfort Mr. Serafini.

CRITICAL THINKING QUESTIONS

1. What is the significance of the patient's weight loss and loss of muscle?
2. What diagnosis did the Paramedic announce to the patient?

Assessment

The patient with cancer who has the classic triad of symptoms (loss of appetite, loss of weight, and malaise) may have cachexia. **Cachexia** is a wasting syndrome that is thought to be induced by inflammatory cytokines such as tumor necrosis factor (TNF) (cachexin). Upwards of 80% of patients with terminal cancer may develop cachexia as a premorbid sign. Cachexia is more common in solid tumor cancers, with the exception of breast cancer. Associated signs of cachexia include a swollen belly secondary to ascites (accumulation of fluid in the peritoneal cavity). Ascites form due to insufficient proper protein production, leading to increased vascular permeability and edema.

Patients with cachexia are unable to make proteins, including immunoglobins. Without immunoglobins, the patient is unable to mount an effective immunological response to any invading infection. Decreased immunoglobins (antibodies) and leukocytopenia combine to leave the patient immunocompromised and at risk for systemic infections. Furthermore, protective vaccinations, such as the flu vaccine, are infective in this patient population.

CASE STUDY (CONTINUED)

The Paramedic is able to convince both Mr. and Mrs. Serafini that transportation to the hospital will enable them to obtain help with the care of Mr. Serafini.

CRITICAL THINKING QUESTIONS

1. What is the standard of care of patients with end-stage cancer?
2. What services might be available to the Serafini family?

Treatment

Treatment of the patient with cachexia is largely supportive. The Paramedic should treat the patient's shortness of breath with oxygen and treat other conditions as they present. Nausea, a common complaint, should be treated with antiemetic medications. Pain should be treated with an appropriate analgesic.

CASE STUDY (CONTINUED)

Mr. Serafini motions to the Paramedic to come closer. He says he does not want to burden his wife but he is having considerable pelvic pain. He wants to know if there is anything that the Paramedic can do to help relieve some of his discomfort.

CRITICAL THINKING QUESTIONS

1. What are some of the predictable complications associated with end-stage cancer?
2. What are some of the predictable complications associated with the treatments for end-stage cancer?

Evaluation

Often, upon evaluation, the patient may complain of pain, either due to the cancer or the patient's handling during transportation. The pain of cancer is thought to be due to either blockage of blood vessels (leading to ischemic pain), space-occupying lesions putting pressure on nerves and creating pain, or from inflammation. Pain can also occur because of nontraumatic fractures and/or skin tears. The Paramedic should carefully investigate the patient's pain history, inquiring if the patient has a pain plan and if any analgesia has been prescribed.

Since the pain associated with cancer is so common (60% to 80% of patients with cancer are estimated to have pain), physicians frequently have a pain management plan. Most pain plans are three tiered.

The first tier is non-narcotic, anti-inflammatory medications such as ibuprofen. To increase the efficiency of these NSAIDs, the physician may order the coadministration of antidepressants, anticonvulsants, antiemetics, and anxiolytics. Because of the potential of untoward effects from polypharmacology, the Paramedic should take a careful medication history and carefully consider the concomitant administration of other medications.

The second tier pain medications are opiate combinations with NSAIDs. Examples of second tier pain medications include synthetic narcotics (such as propoxyphene) and methylmorphine, a natural opioid alkaloid that is also synthesized. Methylmorphine is actually a pro-drug that requires hepatic transformation. In some cases, cancer metastasis or declining cardiovascular function impairs liver function, leaving the patient without analgesia. The patient then proceeds to tier three.

The third tier drugs are opiates. There has been some resistance to prescribing opiates to patients with cancer for fear that they will develop an addiction. The difference between addictive behavior and proper prescribing practice is the objective. The patient addicted to opiates is seeking the euphoric feeling, whereas the patient with cancer is seeking to manage the pain so that he can attend to the activities of daily living (ADL). Others are concerned that opiates may hasten the onset of death. The cancer, and its associated complications, is the cause of death for these patients; opiates only help assure a painless passage.

Although it would be unusual for the Paramedic to provide routine pain medications, the Paramedic may be called upon to treat breakthrough pain. **Breakthrough pain** is a severe episode of pain that requires more than the regular analgesia prescribed for the patient. The pain can occur either spontaneously or from a number of causes, such as transferring the patient from a bed to a stretcher. It is estimated that one-half to one-third of cancer patients experience breakthrough pain.

Patients with breakthrough pain may be suddenly unable to walk, have difficulty sleeping, and may be visibly upset and crying about the pain. The ideal analgesia for breakthrough pain should be easy to administer, quick acting, and of a short duration, so that it does not interfere with the routine pain management plan. Opiates are commonly used for this purpose. Concurrent use of relaxation techniques—such as imagery, distraction techniques, and breathing exercises—can improve the efficiency of the opiates.

CASE STUDY CONCLUSION

Mr. Serafini is transported nonemergently to the local hospital with a hospice service. His signs of respiratory effort are treated with oxygen and proper positioning. The Paramedics convey his wishes to die at home to the receiving nurse.

Three weeks after caring for Mr. Serafini, the two Paramedics receive a card from his wife. She tells them that he had been referred to hospice, came home from the hospital with nursing support, and was able to die at home as he had wished. She thanked the Paramedics for being there when they needed them and in treating Mr. Serafini with kindness and respect.

CRITICAL THINKING QUESTIONS

1. What is the most appropriate transport decision that will get the patient to definitive care?
2. What are the advantages of transporting a patient with end-stage cancer to a hospital with a hospice service, even if that means bypassing other hospitals in the process?

Disposition

Although many patients with cancer are routinely transferred to a local hospital, many request transportation to a hospital with a palliative care unit.[14] These hospitals have special palliative care teams that are familiar with the care of patients with cancer. Currently, 55% of the hospitals in the United States with over 100 beds have a palliative care unit available.

CONCLUSION

Cancer and infectious diseases like HIV and tuberculosis are conditions that cause several generalized symptoms (e.g., weight loss and night sweats). The immune system becomes depressed from the chronic disease, opening the door for opportunistic infections to take hold and complicate the patient's care. In some instances, the Paramedic will be called upon to assist with end of life care for a patient suffering from cancer. Compassionate care by the Paramedic will help provide comfort for the patient and family.

KEY POINTS:

- The end stage of several diseases—such as tuberculosis (consumption), AIDS, and cancer—present with similar signs and symptoms. Treatment is focused on comfort care of the patient.

- Tuberculosis, although primarily a lung disease, can also affect other organs.

- Acquired immune deficiency syndrome destroys the patient's immune system, permitting opportunistic infections to take hold. The opportunistic infections generally lead to the patient's death.

- Cancer describes a number of disorders that have a common root: disorganized cell growth.

- Cancers can affect epithelial, connective, and embryonic tissues.

- Cancer staging allows for effective treatment planning.

- Cancer treatments consist of chemotherapy, radiation, and surgery.

- Pain management is key to a patient's comfort. Increasing opiate use is not an indicator of addiction but rather of unmanaged pain.

- Palliative care, which is noncurative in nature, is indicated for anyone with a terminal disease regardless of proximity of death.

- Hospice care, whether provided at home or in the hospital, provides care for both the patient and the family through a multidisciplinary team of nurses, doctors, social workers, clergy, and counselors. It is viewed as end of life care.

REVIEW QUESTIONS:

1. What signs and symptoms are common to the terminally ill patient with TB, AIDS, or cancer?
2. Besides the lungs, what other organs can be affected by tuberculosis? How do each of these manifest?
3. How do opportunistic infections lead to the death of a patient with AIDS?
4. How does staging allow for effective treatments?
5. What three general categories or treatments exist for patients with cancer?
6. What is breakthrough pain?
7. How does palliative care differ from hospice care?

CASE STUDY QUESTIONS:

Please refer to the Case Study in this chapter, and answer the questions below:

1. What are some causes of a sudden change in mobility in an elderly patient? How would you assess for each?

2. What causes exist for weight loss in an elderly patient?

3. What social concerns should you have regarding the Serafini family?

REFERENCES:

1. Ducati RG, Ruffino-Netto A, et al. The resumption of consumption—a review on tuberculosis. *Mem Inst Oswaldo Cruz.* 2006;101(7):697–714.

2. Small PM, Fujiwara PI. Management of tuberculosis in the United States. *N Engl J Med.* 2001;345(3):189–200.

3. Bertram JS. The molecular biology of cancer. *Mol Aspects Med.* 2000;21(6):167–223.

4. Taylor MR. Genetic testing for inherited breast and ovarian cancer syndromes: important concepts for the primary care physician. *Postgrad Med J.* 2001;77(903):11–15.

5. Sobin LH. TNM: principles, history, and relation to other prognostic factors. *Cancer.* 2001;91(8 Suppl):1589–1592.

6. Sobin LH. TNM: evolution and relation to other prognostic factors. *Semin Surg Oncol.* 2003;21(1):3–7.

7. Sobin LH. TNM, sixth edition: new developments in general concepts and rules. *Semin Surg Oncol.* 2003;21(1):19–22.

8. Flechtner H, Bottomley A. Fatigue and quality of life: lessons from the real world. *Oncologist.* 2003;8 Suppl 1:5–9.

9. Tapsfield A. Improving the care of dying patients in the community. *Nurs Times.* 2006;102(35):28–32.

10. Eues SK. End-of-life care: improving quality of life at the end of life. *Prof Case Manag.* 2007;12(6):339–344.

11. Kutner JS, Blake M, et al. Predictors of live hospice discharge: data from the National Home and Hospice Care Survey (NHHCS). *Am J Hosp Palliat Care.* 2002;19(5):331–337.

12. Gafter-Gvili A, Fraser A, et al. Meta-analysis: antibiotic prophylaxis reduces mortality in neutropenic patients. *Ann Intern Med.* 2005;142(12 Pt 1):979–995.

13. Rajkumar A, Karmarkar A, et al. Pulse oximetry: an overview. *J Perioper Pract.* 2006;16(10):502–504.

14. Desai MJ, Kim A, et al. Optimizing quality of life through palliative care. *J Am Osteopath Assoc.* 2007;107 (12 Suppl 7):ES9–ES14.

CHAPTER 33

MEDICAL RESUSCITATION

KEY CONCEPTS:

Upon completion of this chapter, it is expected that the reader will understand these following concepts:

- That adequate delivery of oxygen to the tissues is the primary goal of medical resuscitation
- That Paramedics develop the skill needed to distinguish a sick patient from a non-sick patient
- The importance of using an algorithmic approach to rapidly identify goals, since multiple medical conditions can lead to a change in oxygenation at the tissue level

ANATOMY CONCEPTS:

Prior to reading this chapter the Paramedic student should be familiar with the following anatomy and physiology concepts:

- Electrophysiology
- Cardiac conduction

The EMS call requesting Paramedics to Brotherhood Lodge is for Mrs. Switzer, an 85-year-old female who is not responding appropriately. Her family reports that her blood sugar is 142 but she is delayed in answering questions and seems to look right through them. As the Paramedics enter the lodge looking for their patient, the more experienced Paramedic utters, "Uh-oh."

CRITICAL THINKING QUESTIONS

1. What are some key concerns that a Paramedic should address when confronted with a critically ill patient?
2. What is the "order of resuscitation"?

OVERVIEW

The word "resuscitate" derives from a Latin word that means "to reawaken." Thus, resuscitation is defined as "to revive from apparent death or from unconsciousness."[1] One focus is attempting resuscitation on a patient who is already near death. Given the varied but low rates of survival, a lot of resources are spent on individuals with a very poor chance of survival. A more broad application of resuscitation, however, is to the patient who is critically ill but in a pre-arrest state, or not quite dead yet. Aggressive management of this group of patients often can provide enough support for the patient's condition to stabilize and then improve. The earlier a critical illness is identified and treated, the more likely a patient will survive. This chapter reviews the identification and management of patients who are critically ill due to medical causes and discusses the decision-making processes and general principles that are applicable to resuscitation of the medical patient.

Chief Concern

In order to generalize **resuscitation** of a critically ill patient across multiple different conditions, the Paramedic must keep in mind that the primary goal of resuscitation is to ensure the adequate delivery of oxygen to the patient's organs and tissues. If the Paramedic optimizes oxygen delivery using the principles discussed in this chapter, then the delivery of other substrates required by the body for proper function—as well as the removal of waste products—is assured. Although all of the body's tissues are important, the tissues most important from the respect of oxygen delivery are the heart and the brain (the vital organs). These two organs are highly sensitive to decreases in oxygen delivery. In fact, death of brain cells begins within four minutes of cessation of blood flow to the brain.[2] Paramedics must be alert for signs of altered mental status, as this is often the first sign of hypoxia.

The adequate delivery of oxygen is based on four main components. The first component is a clear and unobstructed airway. Multiple reasons exist for airway obstruction and impaired pathway. In order to oxygenate patients, a patent pathway must be present for oxygen to enter through the mouth or nose down to the alveoli in the lungs.

The second component is adequate oxygenation of the patient. Oxygenation refers to the movement of oxygen into the lungs, across the alveoli membrane, and into the blood. In addition to the clear and unobstructed airway, supplemental oxygen is often required to improve the patient's oxygenation. This serves several purposes. First, supplemental oxygen ensures that all the patient's hemoglobin is saturated with oxygen molecules.[3] Second, a small amount of oxygen molecules are transported in the blood as a dissolved gas. This is helpful when the critically ill patient is severely anemic, whether from acute blood loss or from a chronic disease. Although the total amount of increased oxygen delivery using these two methods is relatively small, in critically ill patients the goal is to optimize oxygen delivery. A third advantage of supplemental oxygen is that, after several deep breaths or two to five minutes of high-flow, high-concentration oxygen, the nitrogen that comprises most of the air in the lungs is replaced by oxygen (i.e., nitrogen washout). This creates a large oxygen reservoir that can help prevent hypoxia during airway procedures.[3]

The third key component is adequate ventilation. Ventilation is the movement of air in and out of the lungs. In order for oxygen to diffuse into the blood and carbon dioxide to diffuse out of the blood, the lungs must be adequately ventilated. Diffusion of oxygen and carbon dioxide across the alveolar membrane is based on the concentration of these gasses on either side of the interface. Ventilation is the key to moving a sufficient amount of oxygen into the alveoli to diffuse across into the blood as well as the key to removing carbon dioxide from the alveoli. The removal of carbon dioxide is more dependent on the patient's ventilation than the movement of oxygen into the lungs, especially when supplemental oxygen is administered to the patient. Ventilation can occur due to the patient's own ventilatory effort or be augmented by the Paramedic.

The final key component is adequate tissue perfusion. Adequate tissue perfusion occurs when there is an adequate nutrient supply to the body's cells. Adequate blood circulation is essential in the transportation of oxygen, glucose, and other substrates required for cell function. The cells require these compounds to produce the energy needed to carry out their functions, whether the cell is part of the brain, skin, or other organs. In the absence of oxygen, glucose, and the other substrates, cellular metabolism switches from aerobic metabolism (which uses oxygen) to anaerobic metabolism (which is without oxygen). However, anaerobic metabolism is less efficient than aerobic metabolism. More importantly, the by-products of anaerobic metabolism are very acidic. The buildup of these acidic by-products due to inadequate circulation

Table 33-1 The Four Key Elements in Achieving the Goal of Ensuring Adequate Oxygen Delivery

1. Clear and unobstructed airway
2. Adequate oxygenation
3. Adequate ventilation
4. Adequate circulation

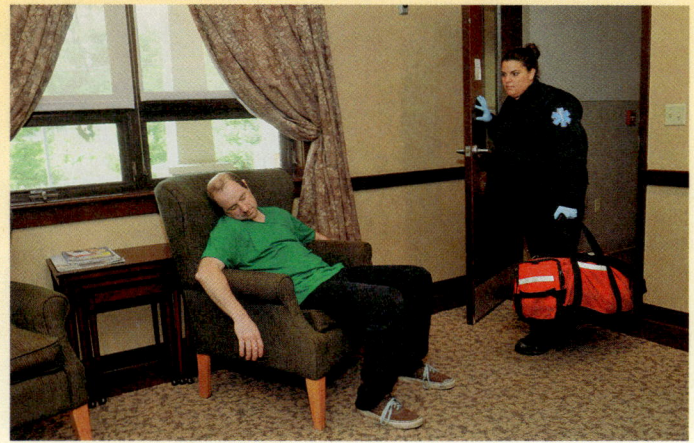

Figure 33-1 Seasoned Paramedics can often decide whether a patient is sick or not sick from the doorway.

produces a local environment in the body that is very acidic. This further reduces the ability of oxygen, glucose, and other substrates to move from the blood into the cells. Acidity shifts the oxyhemoglobin curve to the right and affects the ability of oxygen to bind to hemoglobin. It also affects the function of hormones and neurotransmitters.[4] In the extreme situation (when the patient is in shock), the patient becomes globally acidic, affecting medications administered by the Paramedic (e.g., epinephrine and other epinephrine derivatives including the vasopressors).

The three components of the circulatory system that affect adequate tissue perfusion are the vessels (pipes), the heart (pump), and the amount of fluid in the circulatory system (fluid volume). Each of these three components can often compensate for minor deficiencies in the other components. However, if one component has a moderate deficiency, beyond the other organ's ability to compensate, the body may start to decompensate.

Tissue perfusion may also be affected by other chemicals and toxic substances that impair cellular respiration (the movement of and use of oxygen, glucose, and other substrates by the cell). Just as inadequate circulation can cause a localized acidosis, some toxic substances also produce the same acidic environment. Some of these toxic substances have specific antidotes whereas others are treated purely with supportive care. In order to successfully resuscitate a critically ill patient, the Paramedic must be able to identify and manage the four key elements (Table 33-1) of ensuring adequate oxygen delivery.

Initial Patient Contact: Sick vs. Not Sick

Seasoned Paramedics often can determine if their patient is critically ill at the moment of initial patient contact (Figure 33-1). There are many names for this ability, including the look test, sick vs. not sick, and doorway diagnosis. What allows these Paramedics to identify a critically ill patient from the moment they first lay eyes on the patient? Although experience plays a role in this ability, observation skills and honing in on the things that flag an ill patient are also important. This is why the more hands-on experience the Paramedic student has during his clinical experience, the better she will be at making these observations accurately. When the Paramedic observes common features in these patients, it helps build a personal database of the appearance of sick patients.

Table 33-2 Paramedical Differential Diagnosis for the Patient with Altered Mental Status

- Hypoxia
- Hypoglycemia
- Infection
- Toxicological (including alcohol and recreational drugs)
- Hypotension

For example, a patient's normal behavior upon a Paramedic entering a scene would be for the patient to attempt to make eye contact, regardless of the patient's age. Patients who do not attempt to make eye contact with the Paramedic, even after introductions, likely have mental status changes. This is especially true in children, as their natural curiosity causes them to examine new individuals. Alterations in mental status from the patient's baseline require immediate evaluation by the Paramedic in an effort to determine the cause of the altered mental status (Table 33-2).

A rapid doorway observation of the patient's airway provides an indication of its patency. At times, foreign material (e.g., blood or saliva) can be observed during the initial look. Bubbling in the airway indicates that the airway needs to be quickly suctioned and reevaluated. Stridor appreciated from the doorway is also a sign that an upper airway obstruction may be present. In addition, snoring respirations heard from the doorway may indicate a partial airway obstruction and should raise questions as to whether the patient is able to protect his own airway.

The patient's position may indicate the presence of significant respiratory distress as well. The tripod position, in which the patient is leaning forward with hands resting on his knees (Figure 33-2), is an indicator of severe respiratory distress and impending respiratory failure.[5] Agonal, gasping

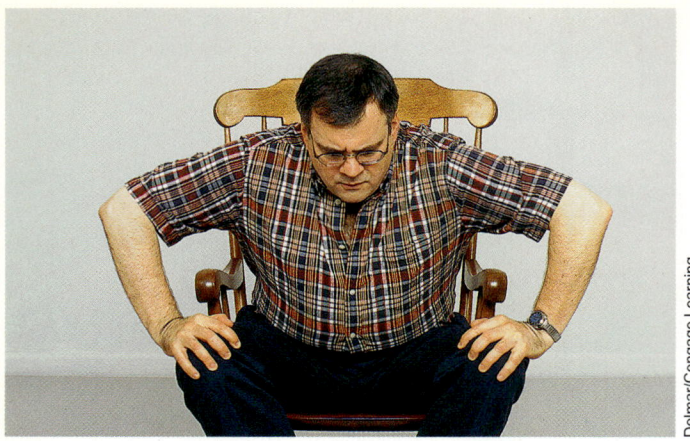

Figure 33-2 A patient in respiratory distress in the tripod position.

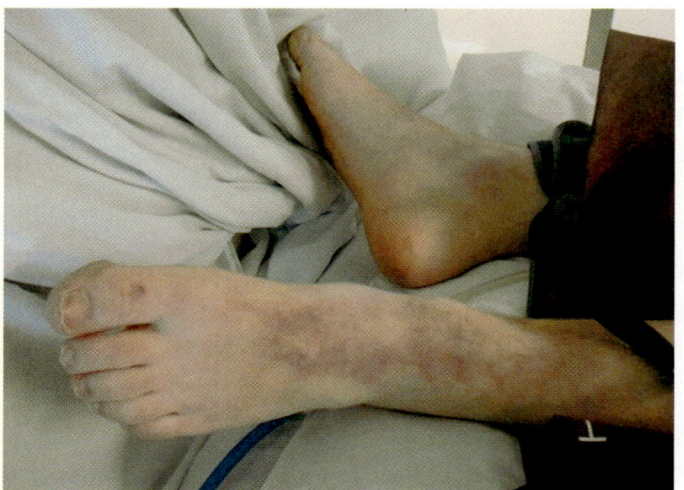

Figure 33-3 Mottled skin indicating poor perfusion.

Table 33-3 Observations from the Initial Contact Which Indicates a Patient Is Sick

- Patient does not make eye contact
- Bubbling or gurgling in the airway
- Snoring respirations
- Tripod position
- Agonal respirations
- Cyanosis
- Pale, gray, or mottled skin

respirations are also a sign of respiratory failure; patients with these often progress rapidly to apnea. Cyanotic mucous membranes and skin are also an indicator that the patient is hypoxic with impending respiratory failure.

The patient's skin color during the Paramedic's initial look upon the scene also provides a visual indication of the patient's perfusion status. A patient with pink-colored or normal skin tone is well perfused and not likely in shock. As a patient becomes hypotensive for any reason, the body compensates by shunting blood away from the skin and toward the core organs, producing pallor, grey-toned skin, or mottled skin (Figure 33-3). Patients with darker complexions will also develop a lighter shade of skin tone. The palms of the hands, soles of the feet, and lips also provide an indication of perfusion status in darker complexioned patients.

The factors discussed in this section (Table 33-3) all help the Paramedic determine from the doorway that a patient is critically ill and requires immediate intervention. By taking the time to look for these features in every patient encounter during clinical experience and in clinical practice, the Paramedic student will gain the experience needed to rapidly identify critically ill patients.

Clear and Unobstructed Airway

The first key factor in achieving the goal of oxygen delivery is ensuring the patient has a clear and unobstructed airway.

Assessment

As discussed previously, during the Paramedic's initial look it may be apparent that the patient's airway is in jeopardy. Snoring or gurgling in the patient's airway during inspiration or expiration is a sign that the airway is either partially obstructed by some foreign material or is obstructed by extra airway tissues.[6] Patients who are deeply unconscious will relax their airway muscles, causing the extra airway tissue present in most people to partially obstruct the airway. In addition, patients with snoring respirations who do not respond to stimulus may not be able to adequately protect their own airway.

The Paramedic should inspect the patient's mouth and nose for foreign material that can be easily suctioned and cleared, then open the airway with either a jaw thrust or head-tilt, chin-lift maneuver. The Paramedic may only need to suction and open the airway to maintain a clear and unobstructed path. In addition, the Paramedic can use a tongue depressor or oral airway to assess the patient for a gag reflex (Figure 33-4). If the patient accepts the oral airway without gagging, that provides an indication for immediate airway management as the patient has lost his ability to protect his airway.

Management Plan

Patients who are unable to protect their airway require management to ensure a clear and unobstructed airway. This can be achieved using a variety of methods. For patients who have a gag reflex, medication-facilitated intubation may be an appropriate option. Prior to administering sedative or paralytic medications, the Paramedic should assess the patient's airway for the signs of a difficult airway and ensure the patient is adequately preoxygenated. If features of a difficult airway are present, two reasonable options for

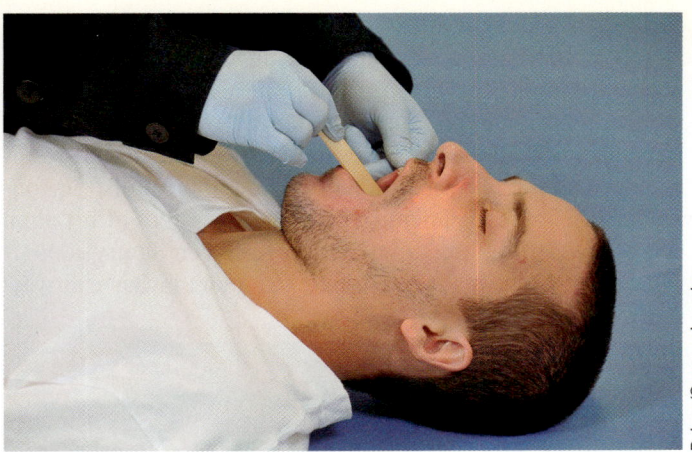

Figure 33-4 A Paramedic assessing the patient for the presence of a gag reflex using a tongue depressor.

the Paramedic are to attempt intubation using sedation only or proceeding with sedation and paralysis using a supraglottic airway instead of an endotracheal tube. However, several studies have concluded that intubation with sedation only, as opposed to sedation and paralysis, often does not provide for adequate visualization of the airway.[7,8] Therefore, the number of attempts at intubation are increased before success is achieved. Based on this research, intubation using sedation only is not recommended in most circumstances.

Clear consequences that result from multiple attempts at intubation not only include airway trauma and hypoxemia, but also a decreased likelihood of success that distracts the Paramedic from other management priorities.[1,9] Every time the Paramedic attempts an intubation, the risk of airway trauma increases. For example, airway trauma can produce bleeding which obstructs visualization. Airway trauma also produces edema in the airway structures (which may affect visualization of the vocal cords), affects the ability of the endotracheal tube to pass through the cords into the trachea, and distorts airway anatomy.

Hypoxia is often prevented by adequate preoxygenation of the patient prior to intubation. Repeated intubation

attempts without adequate oxygenation increases the likelihood of hypoxia. Even one episode of hypoxia in a patient with a traumatic brain injury significantly increases mortality and morbidity.[10]

Distraction from treatment priorities is a real concern in the limited resource environment during prehospital care. Multiple intubation attempts in effect put blinders on the Paramedic as he focuses all of his efforts at successfully intubating the patient. Critically ill patients often have multiple problems across multiple body systems requiring multiple interventions. In a situation where there are multiple Paramedics, there may be adequate resources to care for all of these needs. However, most Paramedics will practice in a situation in which she is the only Paramedic attending to and directing patient care. In this situation, the Paramedic cannot put on blinders and lose sight of overall patient management. The Paramedic may make a judgment to place a supraglottic airway after the first missed attempt rather than making multiple attempts at intubation.[11–14] Another reasonable approach when confronted with difficult visualization would be to go directly to placing a supraglottic airway device without attempting intubation. In this way, the airway is rapidly secured and the Paramedic can continue assessing and treating the critically ill patient.

Adequate Oxygenation

The second key element to achieving the goal of adequate oxygen delivery is ensuring the patient has adequate oxygenation. Although this may sound somewhat redundant, without an adequate amount of oxygen diffusing into the blood from the alveoli, the tissues will not receive enough oxygen. Normally, room air FiO_2 of 21% provides more than enough oxygen to well oxygenate all of the body's cells even under extreme physical stress. However, the critically ill patient will exhaust his reserve capacity even before the Paramedic is summoned to the scene. The body's reserve includes additional oxygen, nutrients, and glucose that is stored and released when the body is under stress and requires additional resources. Critically ill patients invariably require supplemental oxygen because oxygen delivery is impaired in some way.

Assessment

Patients who are cyanotic are in impending respiratory failure and need immediate attention. One early indicator of an issue with oxygenation is agitation and altered mental status. The brain is sensitive to changes in the blood PaO_2, with moderate hypoxia causing agitation.[15] As discussed earlier, many critically ill patients have alterations in their blood oxygen-carrying capacity. In these cases, supplemental oxygen helps maximize oxygen saturation and improves oxygen delivery.

Management Plan

All critically ill patients should receive high-flow, high-concentration oxygen until stabilized, including patients with a history of chronic obstructive pulmonary disease. Critically ill patients with a history of COPD often need increased oxygen, even if their baseline SaO_2 is in the 80s to low 90s. Once the patient is stabilized, the FiO_2 can be titrated to ensure adequate oxygenation.

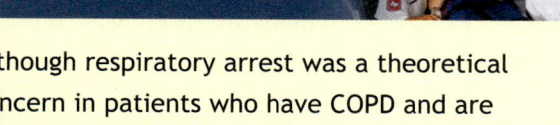
The Paramedic may deliver supplemental oxygen by nonrebreather mask, a continuous positive airway pressure (CPAP) device, a bag–valve mask, or by an invasive airway technique (e.g., endotracheal intubation). The key point to remember is that the Paramedic should select the device that will most appropriately accomplish the objective of maximizing oxygen delivery to the cells. In some cases, this may mean endotracheal intubation, while in other cases a less invasive method or a supraglottic airway device (e.g., the King™ airway) may be the best choice.[17–19]

Adequate Ventilation

The third key element to achieving the goal of adequate oxygen delivery is ensuring the patient has adequate ventilation. Without adequate movement of air into and out of the lungs, diffusion of oxygen into the bloodstream and diffusion of carbon dioxide out of the bloodstream will not occur.

Assessment

Patients who exhibit increased work of breathing, those who are sitting in a tripod position, and those with agonal respirations or abnormal respiratory patterns are in impending respiratory failure and need immediate attention. Patients assume the tripod position in order to physiologically maximize the size of their thoracic cavity. The accessory muscles of respiration are recruited to also assist in both the inspiratory and expiratory phases of respiration.

Signs of increased work of breathing include increased chest wall excursion, inability to talk due to respiratory distress, sternal retractions, rib retractions, use of abdominal muscles, and use of the anterior neck muscles with inspiration.[20]

Management Plan

Patients who exhibit increased work of breathing may require ventilatory assistance. For patients who are conscious and can be calmed by the Paramedic, CPAP may be an excellent choice. Although used primarily for patients in acute pulmonary edema, evidence suggests CPAP may also be helpful for other causes of respiratory distress.[21] CPAP helps improve the patient's work of breathing by splinting open the alveoli. Much of the energy expended during inspiration goes into reopening collapsed alveoli. With the alveoli splinted open by the continuous pressure, the patient's work of breathing decreases and allows therapies directed at the cause of respiratory distress to work, thus avoiding intubation. Unconscious or obtunded patients with poor respiratory effort or an increased work of breathing often require ventilatory support with a bag–valve mask as a bridge to a more invasive airway.

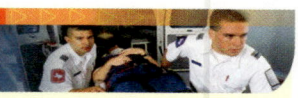
As previously discussed, the Paramedic must keep the entire clinical picture in mind when choosing appropriate interventions. The patient who has overdosed on opiates and has depressed respiratory drive can often be managed by assisting ventilations with a bag–valve mask until an appropriate dose of naloxone can be administered to reverse the opiates, returning adequate ventilations. By endotracheally intubating patients with an opiate overdose prior to administering naxolone, the Paramedic puts the patient at risk during the intubation process as well as increases the risk of vomiting and aspiration once the patient is extubated. A more appropriate approach would be for the Paramedic to assist ventilations while administering naloxone either intravenously, intramuscularly, or via nasal aerosolization. The patient is then reassessed, and the Paramedic may consider an advanced airway procedure if the patient does not respond appropriately to adequate naloxone.

The Paramedic also needs to consider other tasks involved in the resuscitation. If only one body system is involved with the critical illness, then the time to perform endotracheal intubation may be reasonable. For patients who have multiple acute issues, however, it may be more appropriate for the Paramedic to utilize an alternative invasive airway technique that is inserted more rapidly. Again, the end goal is to provide the patient with adequate ventilation to support oxygen diffusion into the blood and adequate removal of carbon dioxide.

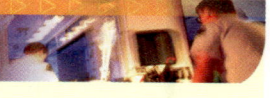

Adequate Circulation

The final key element to achieving the goal of adequate oxygen delivery is ensuring the patient has adequate circulation. This goal is a little more challenging than the other three in that the management of circulation depends more heavily on the pathophysiology of the patient's underlying critical illness. Although there are decision-making processes involved in the management of the other three key elements, the management of circulation is more straightforward. The three components which affect adequate perfusion include vascular tone (pipes), the heart (pump), circulating blood volume, ultimately improving acidosis at the cellular level.

Assessment

A patient who exhibits an ashen gray or pale skin color, or mottling of the skin, is likely suffering from inadequate perfusion. Regardless of the cause of hypotension or poor perfusion, blood is first shunted from the skin to improve perfusion to the brain and heart. The poor skin color is a visual clue for Paramedics that circulation has been diverted from the skin to the core organs. Another means of assessing perfusion is skin temperature. Patients who have inadequate perfusion will also have cool and sometimes clammy skin. Altered mental status with agitation and delayed capillary refill are other indications of poor perfusion.[22]

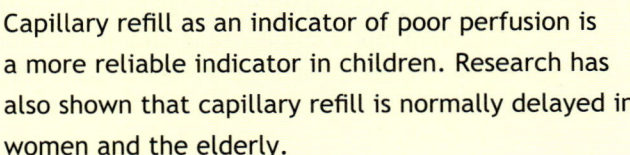

STREET SMART

Capillary refill as an indicator of poor perfusion is a more reliable indicator in children. Research has also shown that capillary refill is normally delayed in women and the elderly.

The pulse oximeter may also be helpful in detecting inadequate perfusion. In addition to assessing the SpO_2, the Paramedic should assess the quality of the oximeter waveform. A good waveform (Figure 33-5a) generally indicates peripheral blood flow, whereas a poor waveform (Figure 33-5b) indicates inadequate peripheral perfusion.

All of the signs described previously may occur in a patient with relatively normal vital signs. In young, healthy individuals, the body has an amazing capability to compensate and maintain near normal vital signs. Subtle clues in the vital signs which indicate inadequate perfusion include a widened pulse pressure (in which the systolic blood pressure is normal or slightly elevated while the diastolic blood pressure is decreased) and tachycardia. Again, the Paramedic must keep the entire clinical picture in mind when developing a treatment plan as tachycardia may result from pain, anxiety, or respiratory distress.

The Paramedic should obtain a 12-lead electrocardiogram on all critically ill patients to determine if the cause

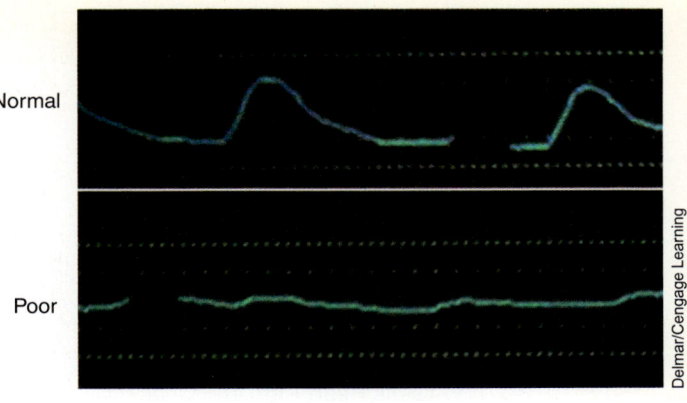

Delmar/Cengage Learning

Figure 33-5 (a) Normal pulse oximetry waveform. (b) Poor pulse oximetry waveform indicating poor peripheral perfusion.

of inadequate perfusion is from a myocardial infarction. Continuous cardiac monitoring should also be used to detect dysrhythmias that may be the primary cause of inadequate perfusion.

Management Plan

The three components to consider in the management of inadequate perfusion include the heart (pump), circulating blood volume (fluids), and vascular tone (pipes). The Paramedic can use an algorithmic approach to manage inadequate perfusion (Figure 33-6).

Pump

The heart is the first component for the Paramedic to address when managing inadequate perfusion. First, the Paramedic should assess the patient's heart rate and rhythm. If the patient is bradycardic with signs of inadequate perfusion, the Paramedic should attempt to increase the patient's heart rate either pharmacologically or with transcutaneous pacing. If the patient is severely tachycardic, generally with a rate above 160 beats per minute, the Paramedic should attempt to slow the patient's heart rate, again either pharmacologically or with synchronized cardioversion. In general, if the patient is hypotensive, electrical treatment is more rapid and definitive.[23] If the patient's systolic blood pressure is above 90 mmHg, then pharmacologic treatments can be attempted prior to moving to electrical treatments. Treating the patient's heart rate and rhythm may resolve perfusion issues if the primary cause of poor perfusion is the rhythm. Tachycardia below a rate of 160 rarely causes inadequate perfusion unless the patient has multiple underlying medical issues.

The other component of the heart is contractility. Primary cardiogenic shock results when there is inadequate forward blood flow due to inadequate contractility. The two main reasons for inadequate contractility are an exacerbation of heart failure or stunned myocardium from a myocardial infarction. Hypotension in both cases requires support with vasopressor medications to maintain adequate forward blood

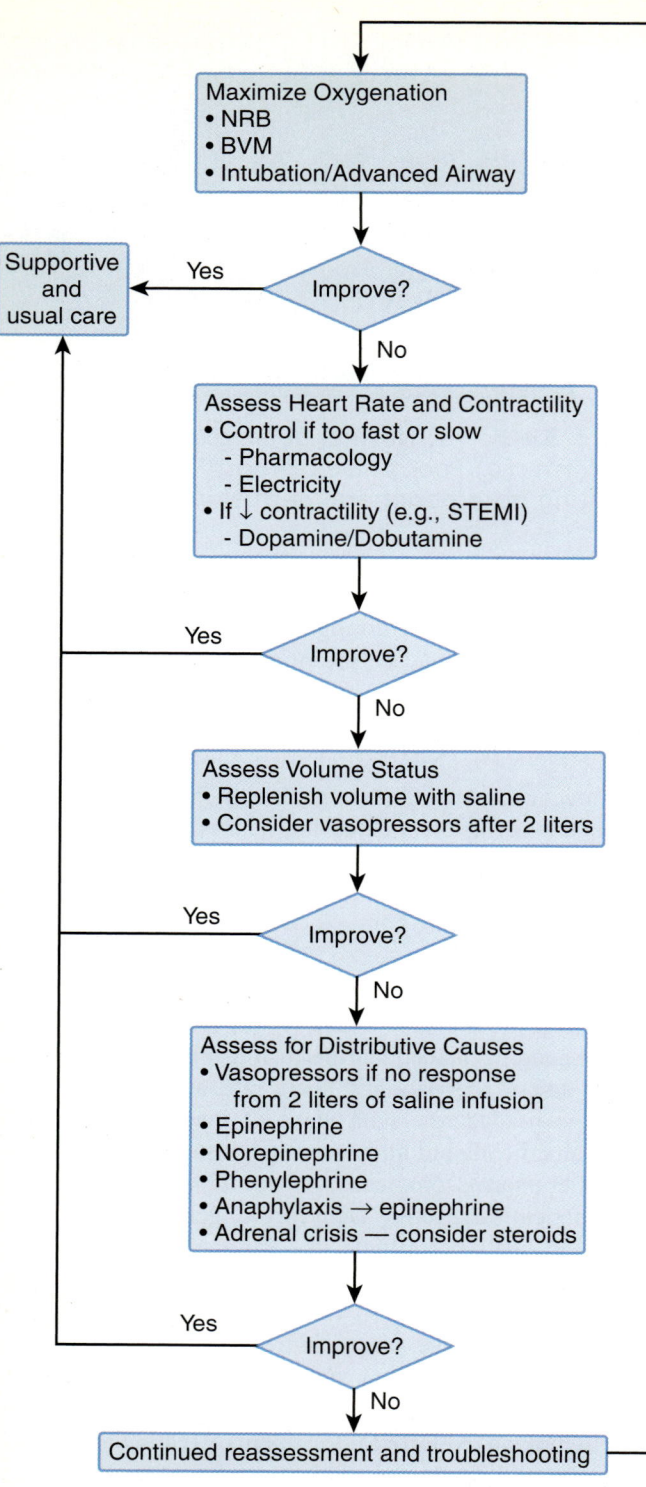

Figure 33-6 Algorithmic approach to the management of inadequate circulatory status.

emergent transport to the emergency department to reopen occluded coronary arteries. Depending upon regional resources, this may involve direct transport by ground or by air to a hospital capable of performing primary angioplasty. Alternatively, it may involve transport to the nearest emergency department for administration of fibrinolytic medication. Paramedics in some EMS systems can also administer fibrinolytic medications to selected patients with a STEMI. Patients who develop primary cardiogenic shock may require placement of a **balloon pump** at the hospital, which is inserted by a cardiologist or cardiothoracic surgeon to mechanically augment blood flow from the heart. The Paramedic may encounter a balloon pump in a critical care transfer setting.

Volume

Circulating blood volume is the next component for the Paramedic to address when managing inadequate perfusion. As long as the heart has adequate pumping power, the patient should be able to tolerate large boluses of intravenous fluid to replace lost circulating blood volume. In the elderly patient, pediatric patient, and patients with underlying cardiovascular or renal disease, however, fluid boluses should be administered at smaller volumes with frequent reassessment to ensure the patient does not develop heart failure from fluid overload.

Lack of circulating blood volume can occur in one of two ways, either through fluid loss or through blood loss. Acute severe blood loss from a medical standpoint most often occurs from gastrointestinal bleeding. Blood loss from an acute upper or lower gastrointestinal bleed can be devastating, with the patient rapidly progressing into hypovolemic shock. As discussed in previous chapters, upper gastrointestinal bleeding originates in the stomach or lower esophagus and can present with either hematemesis (bloody emesis or vomit), melena (black stool that represents significant blood in the stool), or hematochezia (bright red or maroon bloody stools). The presence of massive amounts of blood in the gastrointestinal tract speeds up the transit time of material to the point where severe rectal bleeding may actually originate in the stomach. Lower gastrointestinal bleeding can originate from a number of different sites, but most often from diverticulum located in the sigmoid colon.[26] Lower gastrointestinal bleeding can also occur from colon tumors that invade into the colon wall and expose the blood supply. The treatment for acute blood loss includes administering up to 2 liters of normal saline intravenously with a target systolic blood pressure of between 90 and 100.[27] Overresuscitation with intravenous fluids may worsen bleeding in situations where the bleeding cannot be easily controlled. Not only does overresuscitation dilute hemoglobin and coagulation factors, prolonging bleeding time, but rapidly raising the blood pressure may dislodge any clots that have formed to provide hemostasis.

Severe dehydration can be caused by a variety of reasons including infection from increased insensible water losses, fluid loss as in the case of diabetic ketoacidosis, or poor oral

flow. Although dopamine, a mixed α and β agonist, is often used as a first-line vasopressor, dobutamine may provide more β stimulation, thus increasing contractility with less of an increase in heart rate.[24,25]

Patients who have evidence of an acute ST-elevation myocardial infarction (STEMI) on the 12-lead ECG require intake of fluids. In most cases, the total amount of fluid loss is significant with some patients requiring 4 liters of intravenous fluid in order to adequately fluid resuscitate. Most patients, even those with poor cardiac function, can handle fluid replacement. The only difference in treatment in patients with poor cardiac function is that fluid resuscitation should occur in small frequent boluses so as not to overload cardiac function with too rapid infusion of intravenous fluids.

Blood Vessels

The next key component to address relating to perfusion is the vascular system, specifically the blood vessels or "pipes." The common end result in septic shock, anaphylaxis, and adrenal crisis is systemic vasodilation. The patient becomes hypotensive not from a loss of circulating volume but because the volume of the vessels (the pipes) has become significantly larger than the circulating volume (Figure 33-7). In sepsis, this occurs due to the systemic inflammatory response of the immune system as it fights the infection. In some cases, endotoxins released by the bacteria that caused the infection directly affect the size and permeability of the blood vessels, causing them to relax. This increases the volume of the vessels, and they become leaky. In anaphylaxis, massive histamine response produces vasodilation and leaky blood vessels.

Vascular tone is also affected by natural steroid production. Much like the other conditions, adrenal crisis causes hypotension through the loss of vascular tone. However, in the case of adrenal crisis, the hypotension does not respond to intravenous fluids.[28]

In following **early goal-directed therapy (EGDT)**, a standardized treatment algorithm used to treat sepsis to ensure adequate perfusion, the Paramedic should administer up to 2 liters of normal saline intravenously.[29] If the patient's perfusion is still poor after the 2 liters of normal saline are administered, the Paramedic should start the patient on a vasopressor. The vasopressor of choice in the case of sepsis is norepinephrine, which is almost a pure alpha adrenergic medication and will decrease blood vessel diameter, thus increasing the blood pressure without increasing the patient's heart rate.[30,31] Alternative vasopressors include phenylephrine (another alpha adrenergic medication) and dopamine (a mixed alpha and beta adrenergic vasopressor). One disadvantage of using dopamine in this situation is the increased contractility and heart rate, both of which increase myocardial oxygen demand and may produce ischemia.

In anaphylaxis with hypotension or poor perfusion, the Paramedic should administer epinephrine to the patient intramuscularly as an initial agent to counteract the massive histamine release and to rapidly improve vessel tone. In suspected adrenal crisis, administering high dose intravenous steroids will restore vascular tone.

The commonality in treatment in all patients who develop issues with systemic vasodilation and leaky blood vessels is to administer medications that help increase vascular tone. The blood vessel diameter is thereby reduced, in effect shrinking the container size (Figure 33-7) down to meet the circulating volume present in the body. In most cases, it is reasonable to provide up to 2 liters of intravenous normal saline before starting on vasoactive medications.

Cellular Respiration

As previously stated, the goal of the circulatory system is to deliver oxygen and nutrients to the cells. Many toxins often act at the cellular level, disrupting the transport of materials into the cell or affecting the processes within the cell. Some toxins have antidotes (Table 33-4) that can be administered to reverse the processes. Others require aggressive supportive care of the airway, oxygenation, ventilation, and circulatory system until the body is able to correct the problem. Whether the toxin is an unknown toxin, or is a known toxin with an antidote that is not available to the Paramedic, the best care is aggressively maintaining a clear and open airway and ensuring adequate oxygenation, ventilation, and circulation.

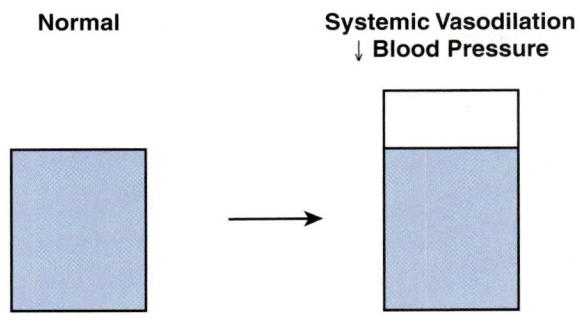

Normal

Systemic Vasodilation ↓ Blood Pressure

Delmar/Cengage Learning

If blood volume stays the same,
the pressure decreases if vessel volume increases.

Figure 33-7 Systemic vasodilation causes a drop in blood pressure because the circulating volume is not sufficient to fill the volume of the blood vessels.

Table 33-4 Common Toxins with Antidotes

Toxin	Antidote
Calcium channel blocker	Calcium
Beta blocker	Glucagon
Opioid	Naloxone
Tricyclic antidepressants	Sodium bicarbonate
Aspirin	Sodium bicarbonate
Acetaminophen	N-acetylcysteine
Toxic alcohols	Fomepizole
Organophosphates/nerve agents	Atropine, pralidoxime
Cyanide	Amyl nitrite, sodium thiosulfate
Digoxin	Digi-bind

Acidosis affects the patient at the cellular level by disrupting the action of natural catecholamines, and also affects any medications that have been administered to the patient. Acidosis often forms due to inadequate perfusion at the tissues. The best method of managing acidosis is to aggressively support the airway, oxygenation, ventilation, and circulatory system. As the acidosis is corrected, the patient's tissue perfusion will improve.

CASE STUDY CONCLUSION

Mrs. Switzer had a blood sugar of 142, her oxygen saturation was 92% with a good waveform and her heart rate was 134. She was warm to touch and pulses were thready at the wrist. Her family stated that she had had a productive cough but insisted on attending the annual memorial service at the Lodge. In addition to transport and oxygenation, the Paramedic continued to monitor Mrs. Switzer's ventilatory effort, mental status and vital signs and she also received a fluid bolus.

CRITICAL THINKING QUESTIONS

1. What is the most appropriate transport decision that will get the patient to definitive care?
2. What is the minimum standard of care for an ALS-worthy patient?

CONCLUSION

This chapter discussed an algorithmic approach to the care of the critically ill medical patient. By focusing on identification and aggressive management of the critically ill patient early in the encounter, the Paramedic will improve the patient's outcome. Reviewing this algorithmic approach and understanding the pathophysiology surrounding this approach will assist the Paramedic in making appropriate choices in caring for these patients. The end goal in caring for all critically ill patients regardless of their underlying condition is to deliver oxygen to the organs and the tissues. Maintaining a focus on this goal will help the Paramedic be successful in treating the sickest of medical patients.

KEY POINTS:

- Adequate delivery of oxygen to the tissues depends on
  - Clear airway
  - Adequate oxygenation
  - Adequate ventilation
  - Adequate perfusion

- Adequate delivery of oxygen permits the cell to use aerobic metabolism for energy production.

- Less efficient anaerobic metabolism yields acids as a by-product.

- Components of the circulatory system that affect perfusion are the heart, vessels, and fluid volume.

- In a rapid doorway observation, the Paramedic will assess for normal response to the provider, indicating mental status.

- Hypoxia, hypoglycemia, hypotension, infection, and toxicological abnormalities are immediately treatable causes of altered mental status.

- When observing airway patency and breathing effectiveness, the Paramedic should check patient posture, rate and rhythm of breathing, effort, and skin color. The Paramedic should manage any abnormalities in the patient's oxygen delivery.

- Derangements in perfusion require attention to the pumping ability of the heart, the integrity of the vessels, and blood volume.

REVIEW QUESTIONS:

1. Name the four components of adequate oxygen delivery.
2. Differentiate aerobic metabolism from anaerobic metabolism in terms of efficiency and by-products.
3. What components of the circulatory system affect perfusion?
4. What indicator represents mental status in the "from the doorway" observation?
5. Name at least five immediately treatable causes of altered mental status.
6. Name five assessments of airway and breathing.

CASE STUDY QUESTIONS:

Please refer to the Case Study in this chapter, and answer the questions below:

1. What is the significance of Mrs. Switzer's response coupled with her blood sugar result?

2. What common features are immediately assessed in a "from the doorway" exam?

3. Describe your initial impression of Mrs. Switzer.

4. What management techniques should you consider?

5. If Mrs. Switzer's blood pressure remains low, what management techniques do you have as a Paramedic that can assist her?

REFERENCES:

1. Stephens SW, Brown T, Cofield SS. Value of multiple prehospital intubation attempts. *Prehosp Emerg Care*. 2007;11(1):123.

2. Lundy-Ekman L. *Neuroscience: Fundamentals for Rehabilitation*. St. Louis: Saunders; 2007.

3. Ron W. *Manual of Emergency Airway Management*. Philadelphia: Lippincott Williams & Wilkins; 2008.

4. Siegel G. *Basic Neurochemistry, Seventh Edition: Molecular, Cellular and Medical Aspects (BASIC NEUROCHEMISTRY)*. Toronto: Academic Press; 2005.

5. Goldberg C. A practical guide to clinical medicine. Available at: **http://meded.ucsd.edu/clinicalmed/lung.htm.** Accessed September 28th, 2008.

6. Kim JW, Yoon IY, et al. Comparison between tongue base and soft palate obstruction in obstructive sleep apnea. *Acta Otolaryngol*. 2008;1–7.

7. Li J, Murphy-Lavoie H, et al. Complications of emergency intubation with and without paralysis. *Am J Emerg Med*. 1999;17(2):141–143.

8. Suprun C. Paralysis analysis: using succinylcholine to help, not harm. *JEMS*. 2008;33(10):78–82.

9. Wang H. Out of hospital endotracheal intubation—where are we now? *An Emer Med*. 2006;47(6):532–541.

10. Hoyt J. Debunking myths of chronic obstructive pulmonary disease. *Crit Care Med*. 1997;25(9):1450–1451.

11. Nolan JP, Soar J. Airway techniques and ventilation strategies. *Curr Opin Crit Care*. 2008;14(3):279–286.

12. Barata I. The laryngeal mask airway: prehospital and emergency department use. *Emerg Med Clin North Am*. 2008;26(4):1069–1083, xi.

13. Pollack CV, Jr. The laryngeal mask airway: a comprehensive review for the Emergency Physician. *J Emerg Med*. 2001;20(1):53–66.

14. Ho AM, Karmakar MK, et al. Choosing the correct laryngeal mask airway sizes and cuff inflation volumes in pediatric patients. *J Emerg Med*. 2008;35(3):299–300.

15. Miller MO. Evaluation and management of delirium in hospitalized older patients. *Am Fam Physician*. 2008;78(11):1265–1270.

16. New A. Oxygen: kill or cure? Prehospital hyperoxia in the COPD patient. *Emerg Med J*. 2006;23(2):144–146.

17. Lutes M, Worman DJ. Failure of the King LT to act as a conduit to the trachea for a gum elastic bougie. *J Emerg Med*. 2009. epub ahead of print.

18. Russi CS, Wilcox CL, et al. The laryngeal tube device: a simple and timely adjunct to airway management. *Am J Emerg Med*. 2007;25(3):263–267.

19. Russi CS, Miller L, et al. A comparison of the King-LT to endotracheal intubation and Combitube in a simulated difficult airway. *Prehosp Emerg Care*. 2008;12(1):35–41.

20. Kallet RH, Diaz JV. The physiologic effects of noninvasive ventilation. *Respir Care*. 2009;54(1):102–115.

21. Marchetta M, Sheldon RL, Resanovich M. Prehospital use of CPAP: a study of intubation rates up to 12 hours after hospitalization. *Prehosp Emerg Care*. 2007;11(1):124.

22. Pamba A, Maitland K. Capillary refill: prognostic value in Kenyan children. *Arch Dis Child*. 2004;89(10):950–955.

23. Tintanelli J. *Emergency Medicine: A Comprehensive Study Guide*, sixth edition. New York: McGraw-Hill Professional; 2003.

24. Petersen JW, Felker GM. Inotropes in the management of acute heart failure. *Crit Care Med*. 2008;36(1 Suppl):S106–S111.

25. El Mokhtari NE, Arlt A, et al. Inotropic therapy for cardiac low output syndrome: comparison of hemodynamic effects of dopamine/dobutamine versus dopamine/dopexamine. *Eur J Med Res*. 2008;13(10):459–463.

26. Zuccaro G. Epidemiology of lower gastrointestinal bleeding. *Best Pract Res Clin Gastroenterol*. 2008;22(2):225–232.

27. Weldon DT, Burke SJ, et al. Interventional management of lower gastrointestinal bleeding. *Eur Radiol*. 2008;18(5):857–867.

28. Picolos MK, Nooka A, et al. Bilateral adrenal hemorrhage: an overlooked cause of hypotension. *J Emerg Med*. 2007;32(2):167–169.

29. Rivers EP, Coba V, Whitmill M. Early goal directed therapy in severe sepsis and septic shock: a contemporary review of the literature. *Curr Opin Anesthes*. 2008;21(2):128–140.

30. Farand P, Hamel M, et al. Review article: organ perfusion/permeability-related effects of norepinephrine and vasopressin in sepsis. *Can J Anaesth*. 2006;53(9):934–946.

31. Sharma VK, Dellinger RP. The International Sepsis Forum's controversies in sepsis: my initial vasopressor agent in septic shock is norepinephrine rather than dopamine. *Crit Care*. 2003;7(1):3–5.

SECTION 11

MATERNAL HEALTH AND THE NEWLY BORN

This section focuses the discussion on women's health issues that the Paramedic will encounter. This section covers conditions that can occur in the non-pregnant female as well as the pregnant female. The Paramedic is guided through the normal delivery process, the complicated childbirth, and, finally, newborn resuscitation.

34

GYNECOLOGICAL DISORDERS

KEY CONCEPTS:

Upon completion of this chapter, it is expected that the reader will understand these following concepts:

- How abnormal conditions in the gynecologic system can cause pain, bleeding, or both
- Pelvic pain as an indicator of gynecological, obstetrical, genital, urinary, or gastrointestinal conditions
- The importance of a patient's history, including the sexual history, in developing the differential diagnosis

ANATOMY CONCEPTS:

Prior to reading this chapter the Paramedic student should be familiar with the following anatomy and physiology concepts:

- Female reproductive system

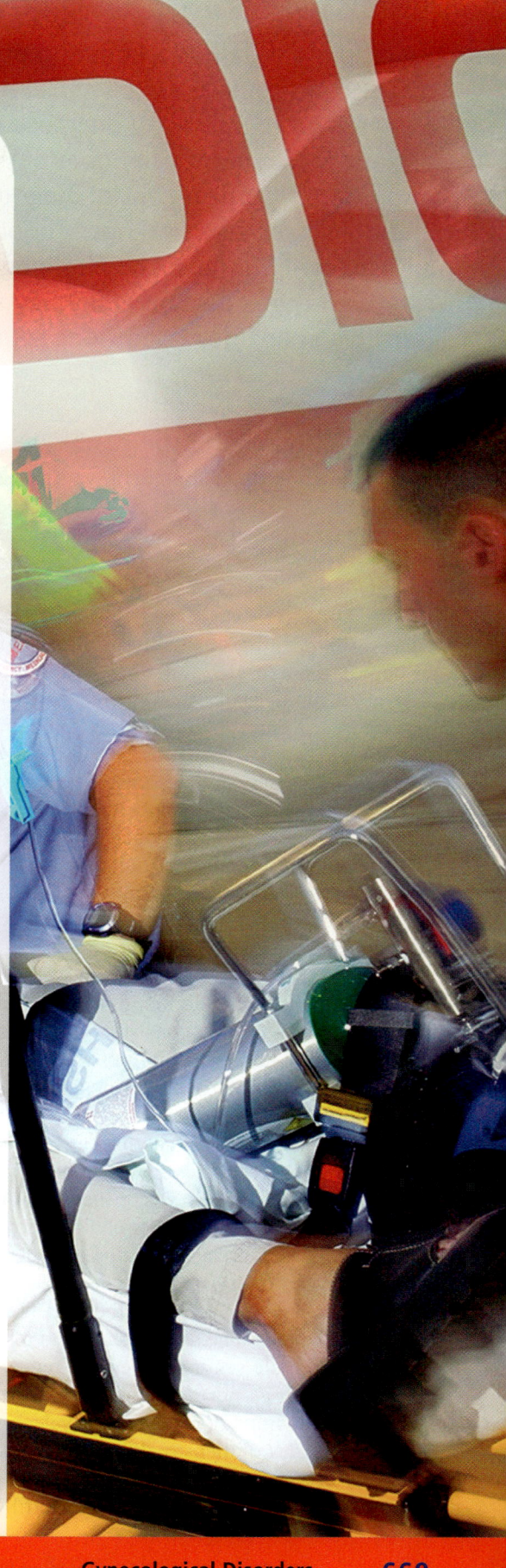

CASE STUDY:

Taos County EMS Medic 27 is dispatched priority one to a call for a 29-year-old female complaining of lower abdominal pain. A Paramedic and an EMT respond to the call. En route, they discuss several conditions which may cause abdominal pain in women of childbearing age, ranging from menses to menarche.

"Dispatch, Taos County EMS on the scene," declares the EMT. The Paramedic grabs the first-in bag and they walk to the front door together. They are met by a young man who states, "Please hurry, my girlfriend is in a lot of pain." He leads them down the hall to the bedroom, where they see a young woman who appears to be in pain, curled up in a fetal position on the bed.

"Hello, I'm a Paramedic with Taos County EMS. How can we help you?"

"My belly hurts really badly, worse than ever before," the patient, Sarah, replies.

CRITICAL THINKING QUESTIONS

1. What are some of the possible causes of lower abdominal pain in women of childbearing age?
2. What is the implication of the comment, "My belly hurts really badly, worse than ever before?"

OVERVIEW

Abdominal pain is a common prehospital patient complaint. Due to the wide range of conditions that can cause abdominal pain, it presents the Paramedic with a challenge to correctly diagnose and treat the cause of the abdominal pain. The patient's complaint of abdominal pain requires the Paramedic to consider a broad list of paramedical differential diagnoses and narrow them down based on the history and physical exam findings. Abdominal pain in women of childbearing age presents an especially unique and challenging problem for a Paramedic to diagnose and treat. Although these patients may have abdominal pain from other conditions, the Paramedic must also consider conditions related to the female reproductive system.

Anatomy Review

The female reproductive system is located in the pelvic cavity and consists of the vulva, vagina, uterus, fallopian tubes, and the ovaries (Figure 34-1) The external female genitalia are called the vulva and consist of the labia majora, labia minora, clitoris, accessory glands which provide lubrication, and the **introitus**, or vaginal opening (Figure 34-2). The vagina extends from the introitus to the cervix, the opening of the uterus. The vagina is the organ of copulation and also functions as the birth canal during delivery. The uterus, a pear-shaped muscular organ, is the site where the embryo implants and the fetus develops during pregnancy.

The inner lining of the uterus, the endometrium, becomes thicker and rich in blood supply during the menstrual cycle in preparation for implantation of an embryo. If an embryo does not implant, the endometrial lining sluffs off and is expelled during menses. Although the cycle is typically regular with menses occurring every 28 days, many women have a history of irregular menses and may have either shorter or, more commonly, longer cycles. Menstrual cycles are measured from the first day of menses to the first day of the following menses. Menses are also usually consistent in regard to the duration and amount of flow. Irregularities in flow and duration can occur due to a variety of conditions, such as pregnancy and hormones (both those ingested and those from imbalances in the body).[1] As the woman approaches menopause, menstrual cycles often become irregular and the amount of flow can vary. Heavy menstrual flow is termed **menorrhagia** whereas irregular menstrual bleeding is called **metrorrhagia**.[2] Often women will describe a combination of both conditions, which is termed **metromenorrhagia**.

The ovaries, two walnut-sized organs in the pelvis, are the female gonads. The ovaries store and release eggs as well as produce female sex hormones that regulate the menstrual cycle. The ovaries normally take turns releasing an egg at about the midpoint of the menstrual cycle, or roughly 14 days after the first day of menstrual flow. Once the egg is released, it travels down one of the two fallopian tubes to the uterus. The fallopian tube is the usual site of fertilization where the ovum and spermatozoa combine to form an embryo. The embryo then implants in the uterus to begin the process of growth and development.

Chief Concern

Pelvic pain in a female can be caused by urinary, gastrointestinal, gynecologic, and obstetric conditions. For any female patient complaining of pelvic or lower abdominal pain, the Paramedic should consider several conditions specifically related to the female reproductive system. Gastrointestinal and urinary tract conditions that can cause pelvic pain include appendicitis, diverticulitis, urinary tract infections, and kidney stones. The pelvic disorders discussed in this chapter can be divided into those that cause pain and those that cause bleeding.

Pelvic Pain

Common disorders that cause pelvic pain in females include problems with the ovaries, uterus, vagina, and the external genitalia. These common disorders can also be divided into conditions related to an infection and conditions related to only pain. These conditions will be reviewed by anatomic location, starting internally and moving externally.

Ovarian cysts are fluid-filled sacs that develop on the ovaries (Figure 34-3). As part of the normal expulsion of a mature egg cell from the ovary, a follicular cyst develops and then ruptures, expelling the egg toward the fallopian tube. Upon rupture, these cysts may cause short-lived sharp pain related to ovulation. Larger ovarian cysts can also develop over several cycles. These cysts are usually painless as they grow but can cause severe pain if they begin to leak or rupture. The cyst can rupture spontaneously or as a result of sexual intercourse, exercise, or trauma. Often there is a small amount of bleeding associated with the cyst. On rare occasions, bleeding can be severe enough to cause abnormal vital signs. Occasionally, what are thought to be larger ovarian cysts are actually benign tumors filled with material that developed from stem cells (e.g., hair and teeth). These tumors must be surgically removed.

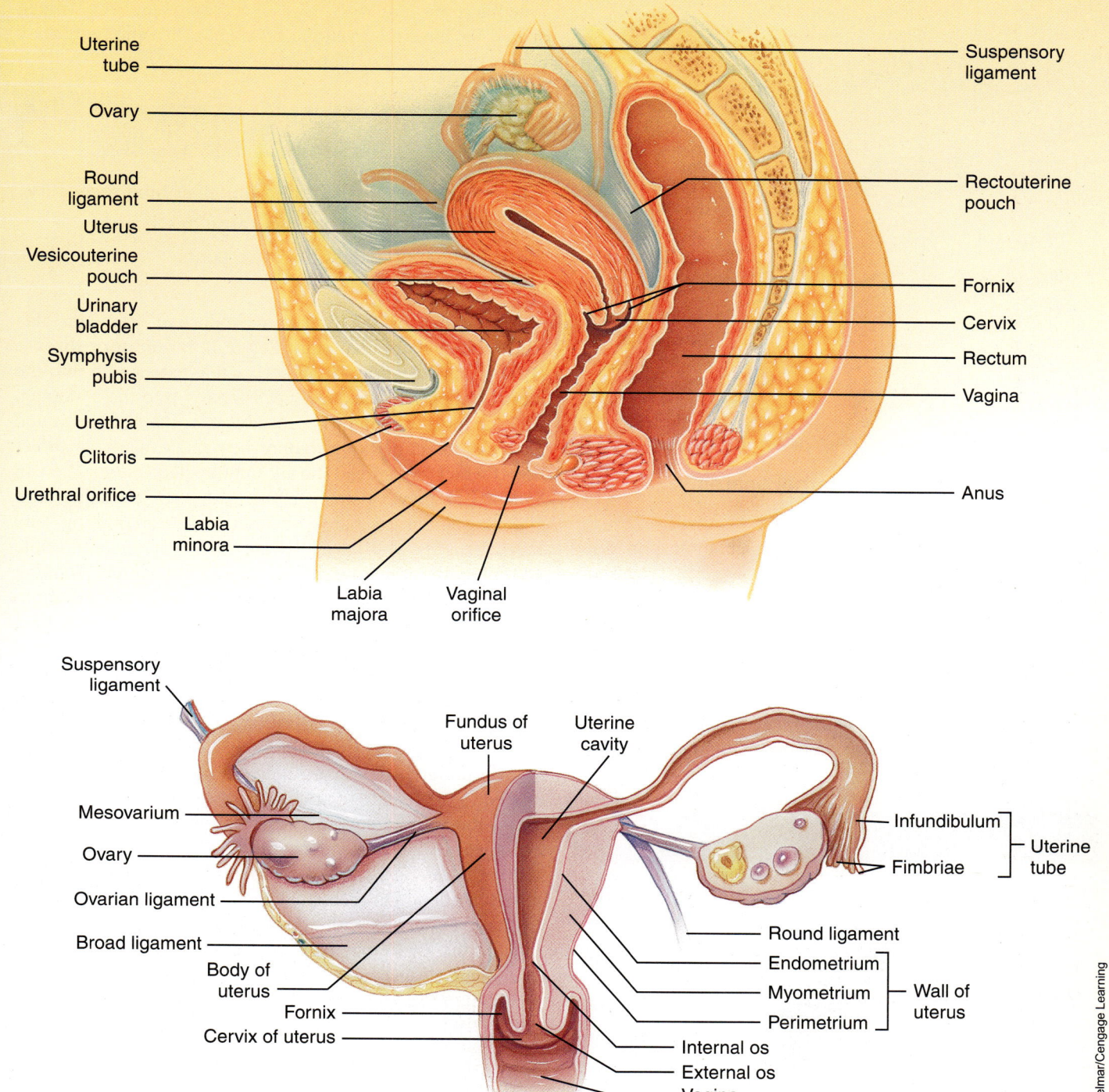

Figure 34-1 Internal female pelvic anatomy.

Another cause of lower abdominal pain originating from the ovary is ovarian torsion. **Ovarian torsion** is an uncommon but serious medical condition that occurs when the ovary twists on the ovarian ligament attaching the ovary to the uterus.[3,4] The blood supply for the ovary follows the ovarian ligament. When the ovary twists around the ligament, the blood supply is greatly reduced or completely cut off (Figure 34-4). The ovary becomes ischemic, producing

the pain. If the blood supply is cut off for more than several hours, the ovary can become necrotic, affecting the ovary's viability. Ovarian torsion results in severe lower abdominal pain sometimes associated with nausea and vomiting. Undiagnosed ovarian torsion can result in the death of the ovary and thus cause infertility.

Ectopic pregnancy (Figure 34-5) occurs when an embryo implants anywhere outside the uterus. Although

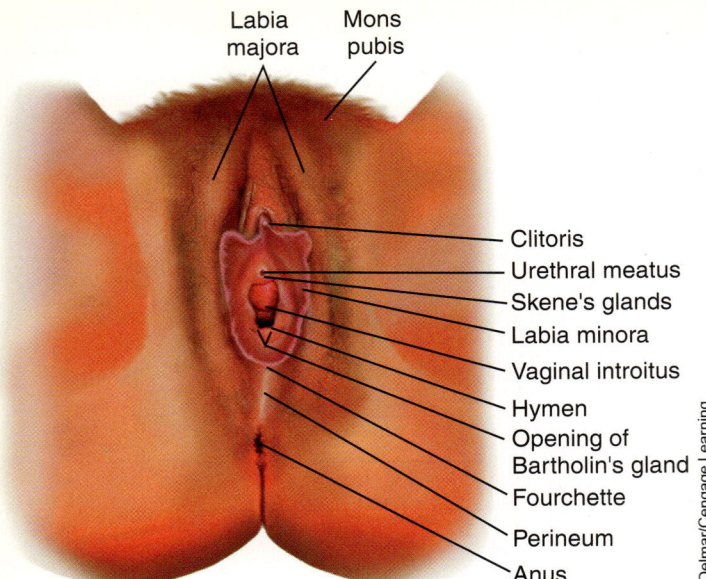

Figure 34-2 Female external anatomy.

Labia majora
Mons pubis
Clitoris
Urethral meatus
Skene's glands
Labia minora
Vaginal introitus
Hymen
Opening of Bartholin's gland
Fourchette
Perineum
Anus

the most common site for ectopic implantation is in a fallopian tube, the embryo can implant anywhere in the abdomen or in the upper, nonstretchable portion of the uterus.[5] As the embryo grows, it stretches the fallopian tube, causing the patient pain. As the embryo continues to grow, it can rupture the fallopian tube and cause uncontrolled bleeding, resulting in hemorrhagic shock.[6] Embryos which implant elsewhere often rupture and cause bleeding. A past history of pelvic inflammatory disease, previous ectopic pregnancy, or

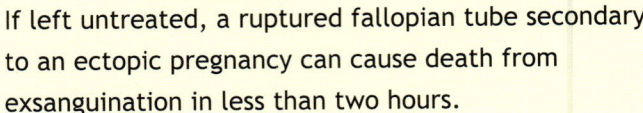

STREET SMART

Abdominal pain and a positive pregnancy test are red flags for ectopic pregnancy. Certain forms of birth control such as an intrauterine device (IUD) increase the risk for ectopic pregnancy.

fallopian tube surgery (such as a tubal ligation) put women at risk for having an ectopic pregnancy. Ectopic pregnancy occurs in up to 2% of all pregnancies.[7]

STREET SMART

If left untreated, a ruptured fallopian tube secondary to an ectopic pregnancy can cause death from exsanguination in less than two hours.

Infections of the female reproductive tract can also cause lower abdominal pain. **Pelvic inflammatory disease (PID)** is an infection of the cervix that extends up into the uterus, fallopian tubes, and occasionally into the abdomen. PID is most commonly caused by sexually transmitted bacterial infections (e.g., gonorrhea and Chlamydia infections) which are spread during unprotected intercourse.[8] In addition to pelvic pain, patients with PID may also have a thick vaginal discharge, dysuria, nausea, vomiting, and fever. Patients who have PID are markedly uncomfortable and often are only comfortable in a fetal position. Walking produces severe pain, and patients with PID often demonstrate a hunched forward gait. In severe cases, the patient can develop sepsis as pus fills the pelvis. An abscess occasionally will form in the fallopian tube as a result of severe infection (Figure 34-6). Both severe PID and tubo-ovarian abscesses require hospitalization, intravenous antibiotics, and often surgery as treatments.

Endometriosis is another painful pelvic condition related to the female reproductive system. Although it is not clear what causes endometriosis, the thinking is that some endometrial tissue from the lining of the uterus migrates into the pelvis. This tissue continues to respond to the hormones during the menstrual cycle, potentially producing the pain associated with endometriosis. More recently, it is thought that there may be some immune or hormonal cause of endometriosis that is different than the classic view of the condition.[9,10] Some of the other signs and symptoms include

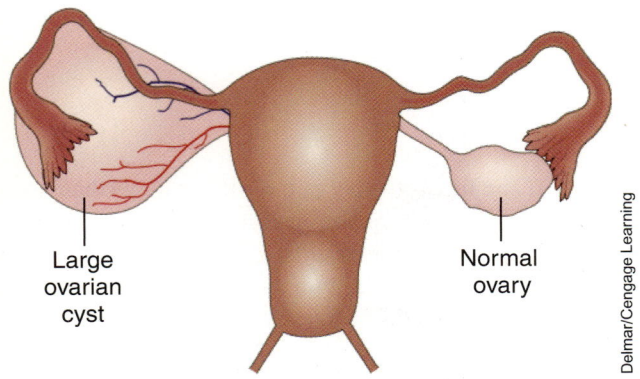

Large ovarian cyst

Normal ovary

Figure 34-3 Ovarian cysts develop on the ovary.

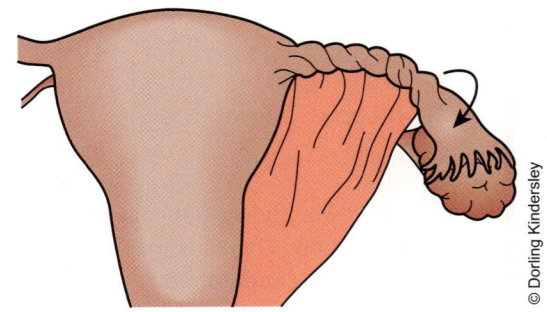

Figure 34-4 The blood supply to the ovary is threatened in an ovarian torsion because it is often cut off when the ovary twists around its ligament.

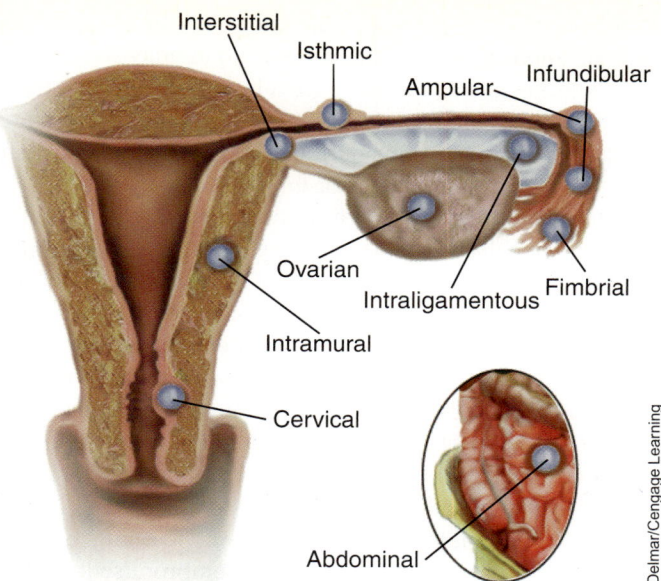

Figure 34-5 An ectopic pregnancy most often implants in the fallopian tube, which ruptures and bleeds as the embryo grows. Other potential sites of implantation are also shown.

painful menses (**dysmenorrhea**), menorrhagia, or metrorrhagia; lower abdominal, pelvic, or back pain; pain during intercourse; bloating; nausea; vomiting; pain during urination; or pain during exercise.

Uterine prolapse is another condition that can range from troublesome to painful. Uterine prolapse occurs when the cervix and part of the uterus protrude from the vaginal opening (Figure 34-7). This is often caused by stretching of the pelvic floor muscles, which occurs during normal childbirth. These muscles sometimes do not regain the muscle tone which existed prior to delivery. As the woman ages, the muscles and connective tissue continue to weaken. The severity

of a uterine prolapse can range from descent of the cervix and uterus into the vagina to protruding out of the vaginal opening. A prolapse in which the uterus protrudes from the vaginal opening predisposes the reproductive organs to both trauma and infection.

Vulvovaginitis is an inflammation of the vulva and vagina. It is primarily caused by infections but can also result from an irritant, allergic response, or from insertion of a foreign body into the vagina. Vulvovaginitis usually presents with vaginal discharge associated with itching or pain. Infections may be caused by a bacterial or fungal source.

Patients call EMS when **vaginal foreign bodies** become lodged and/or cannot be retrieved. Examples of foreign bodies include tampons, sexual gratification objects, and many other objects. These foreign bodies cause a wide range of complaints from mild discomfort to severe pain. Foreign bodies that have been lodged for a period of time are prone to cause infection and may be a source of sepsis in an otherwise young and healthy woman.[11] The Paramedic should not attempt to remove the foreign body as it is difficult to determine if internal injury occurred without further testing at the emergency department. Stabilization and transport are indicated instead.

External infections can cause the patient mild to severe pain. Bartholin gland abscess occurs when the Bartholin gland duct becomes obstructed and infected. The resulting abscess that forms can produce a painful mass at the entrance to the vagina (Figure 34-8). Another painful infection of the external genitalia is herpes. During an outbreak, the herpes lesions produce a significant amount of painful swelling and may render the patient unable to urinate (Figure 34-9). This most often occurs during the first outbreak but can also occur during subsequent outbreaks.

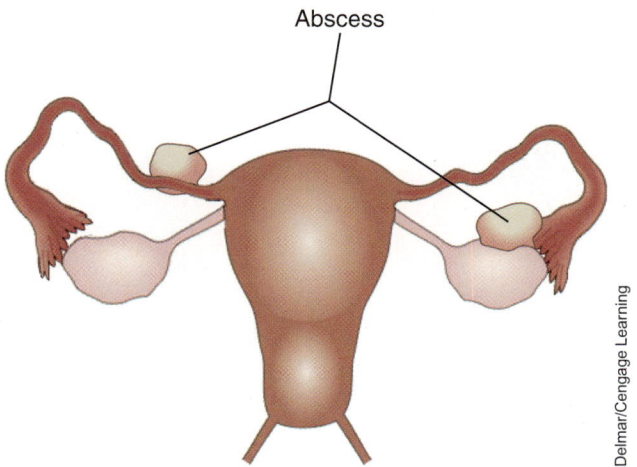

Figure 34-6 A tubo-ovarian abscess may develop in the fallopian tube of a patient who has PID.

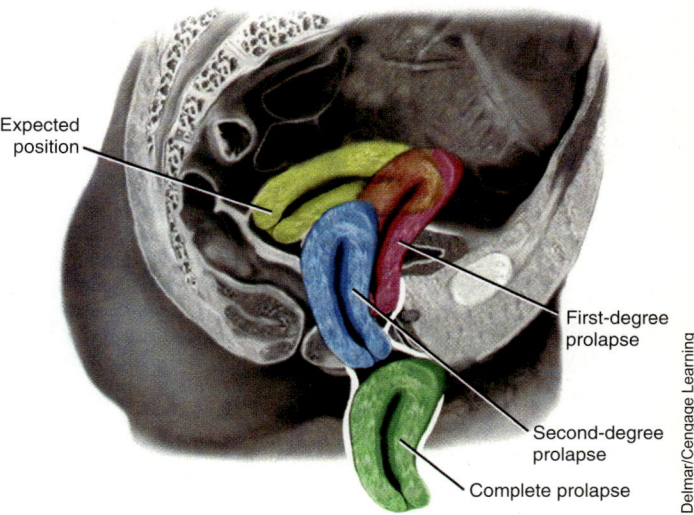

Figure 34-7 In a uterine prolapse, the cervix and uterus descend into the vagina and occasionally will protrude from the vaginal opening.

Gynecological Disorders **673**

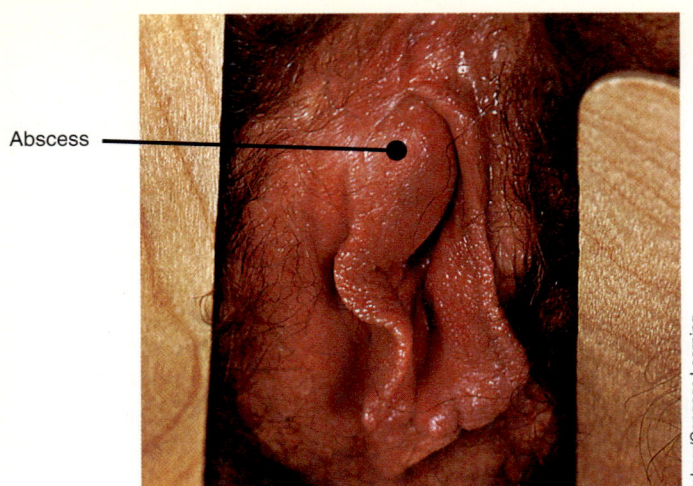

Abscess

Figure 34-8 A Bartholin gland abscess can become painful and obstruct the vaginal opening.

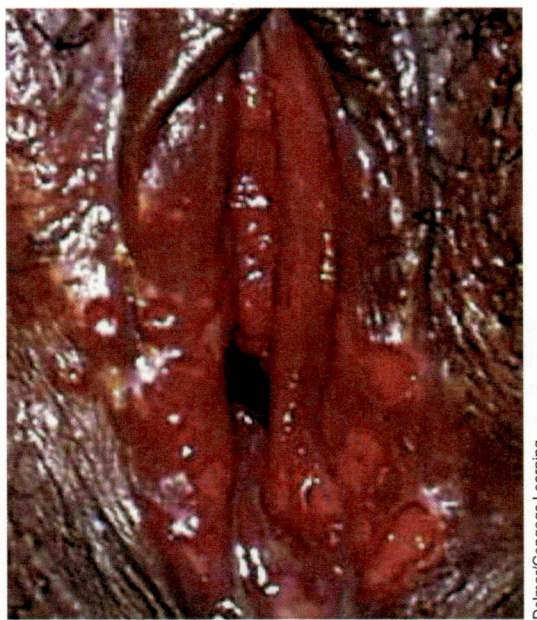

Figure 34-9 A herpes outbreak can be extremely painful and obstruct urination.

Vaginal Bleeding

As discussed in the previous section, vaginal bleeding normally occurs on a cyclic basis approximately every 28 days. Most often the flow is regular, not very heavy, and lasts three to five days in duration. In contrast, heavy menstrual flow can occur at irregular times or with a prolonged duration and may be severe enough to cause severe anemia and hypotension. The generic term used to describe abnormal menses related to bleeding is **dysfunctional uterine bleeding**.

Vaginal bleeding that occurs in a pregnant female is always concerning to the patient and may be indicative of several conditions. Although patients with ectopic pregnancies most often present with a complaint of pain, in a small

number of patients, vaginal bleeding may be the only indication. Spotting, or small drops of blood, may occur during implantation and be mistaken for a lighter than usual menses. In addition, some women will spot throughout their pregnancy. Heavier bleeding during early to middle pregnancy may indicate a spontaneous or threatened abortion.

In a **spontaneous abortion**, the pregnancy terminates on its own, often due to a genetic issue with the fetus.[12] The patient may report passing a large amount of clots in addition to blood. If the patient was further along in the pregnancy, the fetus may be visible in the products passed. A **threatened abortion** is heavy vaginal bleeding in a pregnant patient who has not yet passed the fetus, but may spontaneously terminate the pregnancy. It is important to remember that a small amount of early pregnancy bleeding is normal in up to 25% of pregnancies, with only half of those actually undergoing a spontaneous abortion.[13]

Bleeding in late pregnancy is very concerning as the survivability of the viable fetus may be compromised. Painless, bright red vaginal bleeding in the third trimester of pregnancy may be associated with a **placenta previa** (Figure 34-10a), a condition in which the placenta covers part of the cervix rather than being completely implanted along the inner uterine wall. Painful bright red vaginal bleeding associated with abdominal cramps or contractions in late pregnancy may signal a **placental abruption**, premature separation of the placenta from the uterus (Figure 34-10b). Both conditions can be emergencies for the mother and child.[14]

PROFESSIONAL PARAMEDIC

Although the medical term "abortion" means the ending of a pregnancy before 20 weeks' gestation regardless of cause, it may carry moral implications. The Paramedic should be prepared to use the layman's term of miscarriage when appropriate.

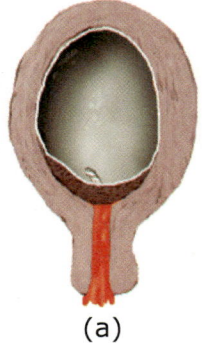
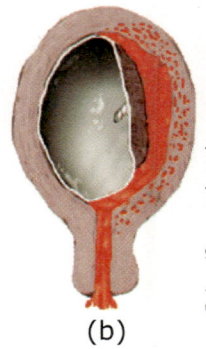

(a)   (b)

Figure 34-10 Bleeding in late pregnancy is concerning for either (a) placenta previa or (b) placental abruption.

The Paramedic elicits a history from Sarah while the EMT gets a set of vitals. Sarah has been having severe abdominal pain mostly in the left lower quadrant for a little over three hours. The pain is constant and she rates it as 10 out of 10, it does not radiate, and nothing she does seems to make the pain better. She also states that she feels weak and dizzy and like she is going to throw up. She denies having diarrhea, fever, chest pain, shortness of breath, and urinary symptoms. She is not allergic to any medications, and she takes no medications except for a multivitamin. She last ate four hours ago.

When asked, Sarah states that she is sexually active with her boyfriend and occasionally uses condoms. She had a sexually transmitted disease a few years ago but was told she was cured. Her last menstrual cycle started seven weeks ago and she had a small amount of vaginal bleeding today. She has never been pregnant.

CRITICAL THINKING QUESTIONS

1. What are the important elements of the history that a Paramedic should obtain?
2. What is the potential significance of the patient's earlier sexually transmitted disease?

History

The Paramedic first asks the patient an open-ended question to attempt to determine the history of present illness, and then asks more focused questions to narrow down the differential diagnoses. It is important to determine the location, severity, and characteristic of the abdominal pain as well as the associated symptoms. The Paramedic should use the OPQRST and AMPLE mnemonics to help obtain a detailed medical history.

In cases of females with lower abdominal pain, the key to narrowing the differential diagnosis may be obtained in the sexual history. Although obtaining a quick and detailed sexual history from a patient may be uncomfortable for the Paramedic, it is very important. The Paramedic should accomplish this with discretion and privacy as even close family members may not be aware of some aspects of the patient's sexual history. Is the patient sexually active? Is the patient utilizing methods to prevent STDs or pregnancy (e.g., condoms or birth control pills)? When did the last menstrual period occur and are menstrual periods usually regular? If the patient is complaining of vaginal bleeding, how does this compare to her normal menses? Missed, irregular, or late menses can indicate pregnancy; therefore, the Paramedic needs to consider pregnancy-related causes of the abdominal pain. The amount of vaginal bleeding is often measured by the number of pads the woman uses over a period of time. If the patient describes using one pad every two hours, she is

likely having more bleeding than if she used one pad every four hours. Patients who use one pad or more per hour are having severe bleeding and are at risk for developing hemorrhagic shock.

Patients with vulvovaginitis or pelvic inflammatory disease may report vaginal itching or pain. The pain of both conditions may increase with urination or sexual intercourse. Vaginal discharge is often described as being thick and having a foul odor. A history of a fever is concerning for a deeper pelvic infection or tubo-ovarian abscess.

Patients with an ectopic pregnancy may complain of abdominal pain, vaginal bleeding, or both. Although some patients will know that they are pregnant, many will not know at the onset of symptoms. It is important for the Paramedic to consider ectopic pregnancy in any young woman of childbearing age who complains of lower abdominal pain and/or vaginal bleeding. Since a woman can lose a large quantity of blood into the pelvis with a ruptured ectopic pregnancy, the Paramedic needs to recognize the symptoms of shock including altered mental status.

The patient's past medical history is also important and may provide clues to the current complaint. A history of ovarian cysts, past ectopic pregnancy, or PID may serve as a comparison for the patient's current concern.[5] Past surgical history may also help to exclude certain conditions. For example, a Paramedic can rule out ectopic pregnancy for a woman who has had a total hysterectomy (including removal of her ovaries).

The EMT obtains a full set of vitals while the Paramedic performs a brief focused physical examination. Sarah is awake and able to speak, and her airway is patent. She has clear bilateral breath sounds with good air movement. Her skin is cool and clammy, her pulse is weak and rapid, and her capillary refill is four seconds. Vital signs are a pulse of 120 and weak, blood pressure of 80/54, and a respiratory rate of 12, nonlabored.

The EMT prepares the stretcher and obtains the materials necessary for an intravenous line. The Paramedic inspects Sarah's abdomen and palpates all four quadrants. She is most tender in the left lower quadrant and she has involuntary guarding. There are no signs of trauma and no back tenderness on palpation.

CRITICAL THINKING QUESTIONS

1. What are the elements of the physical examination of a patient with suspected ectopic pregnancy?
2. Why is an abdominal examination a critical element in this examination?

Examination

The abdominal exam is very important and can provide valuable clues to help the Paramedic narrow down the paramedical differential diagnoses. The Paramedic should first inspect the patient's abdomen, looking for areas of bruising or ecchymosis (skin discoloration from loss of blood as a result of ruptured blood vessels) that indicate trauma, protrusions that indicate masses, and distention that indicates poor GI motility. After inspection, the Paramedic auscultates the abdomen for the presence of bowel sounds. In order to declare a patient as having absent bowel sounds, the Paramedic typically needs to listen to the abdomen for at least five minutes per quadrant. However, the Paramedic usually can very quickly determine if bowel sounds are present. The Paramedic then palpates all areas of the abdomen to determine the area of maximal tenderness, starting distant from where the patient complains of pain. Patients with peritonitis, or irritation of the inner lining of the abdomen, will have guarding (abdominal muscle contraction upon palpation of the abdomen) and rebound tenderness (increased pain when the pressure from palpation is released and the abdominal wall returns to its normal position). Patients with peritonitis may also walk with a wide-based shuffling gait.

When assessing shock, the Paramedic cannot rely solely on vital signs, especially blood pressure, as low blood pressure is a late sign of shock. The Paramedic must also look for signs of poor perfusion including altered mental status, diaphoresis, cool skin, and delayed capillary refill.

Sarah admits that she may be "late." She had some "spotting" recently but just thought she might be having a light period. Sarah also relates that her periods are very irregular and that being "late" never was a cause of concern in the past, since her period always came eventually.

CRITICAL THINKING QUESTIONS

1. What is the significance of the "spotting"?
2. What diagnosis did the Paramedic announce to the patient?

Assessment

An acute onset of lower abdominal pain with vaginal spotting and an irregular menstrual cycle can be signs of a medical emergency. A physical examination that reveals lower quadrant abdominal pain with rebound and guarding is of concern to the Paramedic and may indicate medical emergencies like ectopic pregnancy, hemorrhagic ruptured ovarian cyst, or pelvic inflammatory disease. Although hypotension may reflect blood loss, in the setting of an infection it may reflect septic shock.

CASE STUDY (CONTINUED)

The Paramedic places a 16 gauge venous catheter into Sarah's left arm and attaches a 1 liter bag of normal saline wide open to give her a bolus of fluids. Sarah is placed on a nonrebreather oxygen mask and is packaged with her legs elevated and a blanket to prevent heat loss.

CRITICAL THINKING QUESTIONS

1. What is the standard of care of patients with suspected ectopic pregnancy?
2. What are some of the patient-specific concerns and considerations that the Paramedic should consider when applying this plan of care that is intended to treat a broad patient population presenting with suspected ectopic pregnancy?

Treatment

It is critical for the Paramedic to address any airway, breathing, or circulation issues as the first priority of treatment. If the patient is hemodynamically unstable, the Paramedic should place the patient on high-flow, high-concentration oxygen; rapidly establish IV access; administer IV fluid boluses; and position the patient supine with legs elevated. Vaginal bleeding may be addressed by placing either a sanitary pad or an abdominal dressing between the patient's legs to absorb the vaginal bleeding. The Paramedic should avoid placing any material into the patient's vagina in an effort to stop the bleeding.

The treatment of abdominal pain by Paramedics is primarily supportive. Monitoring the airway, breathing, and circulation during transport is important as well as recognizing and treating shock, if present. The Paramedic should consider providing appropriate analgesia based on local and regional practices.

CASE STUDY (CONTINUED)

During the course of the transportation, Sarah suddenly becomes unresponsive. Although she has a palpable carotid pulse, the Paramedic cannot obtain a radial pulse and reaches over to open the saline solution to infuse wide open. The Paramedic then calls the hospital to advise them of the pending arrival of a patient with a possible ectopic pregnancy, and then starts a second intravenous line.

CRITICAL THINKING QUESTIONS

1. What are some of the predictable complications associated with a ruptured ectopic pregnancy?
2. Why did the Paramedic elect to contact the hospital before starting the second IV access?

Evaluation

The Paramedic should reassess the patient during transport, including the airway, breathing, circulation, and vital signs. Patients with hemorrhagic shock can deteriorate rapidly even with appropriate and timely management.

Patients may require additional intravenous fluid boluses to maintain an adequate blood pressure. Patients who develop altered or depressed mental status from shock may require airway management to ensure a patent airway.

CASE STUDY CONCLUSION

The intravenous fluids help to temporarily stabilize Sarah. After transferring Sarah over to the hospital gurney in room 17, the Paramedic provides a brief report to the attending emergency physician. The physician confirms Sarah's history and physical examination findings, and orders a urine pregnancy test. He then performs a bedside abdominal and pelvic ultrasound. The emergency physician points out to a significant amount of blood in the pelvis and what appears to be an ectopic pregnancy near her left ovary.

Sarah's blood is typed and cross-matched and she is transfused with two units of blood as she is taken to the operating room.

CRITICAL THINKING QUESTIONS

1. What is the most appropriate transport decision that will get the patient to definitive care?
2. What are the advantages of transporting a patient with suspected ruptured ectopic pregnancy to a hospital with emergency surgical capabilities, even if that means bypassing other hospitals in the process?

Disposition

Unstable patients should be taken to the closest appropriate emergency department while the Paramedic resuscitates the patient en route to the hospital. Although the paramedical differential diagnosis of pelvic pain in the female is broad, the Paramedic should consider taking a woman who may be pregnant to an emergency department with gynecological specialists available, provided that it is within a reasonable distance and the patient's condition can support the longer trip.

CONCLUSION

The diagnosis of a female patient who complains of pelvic pain or vaginal bleeding is challenging in the prehospital environment. When encountering patients with these chief concerns, the Paramedic needs to rapidly assess for signs of shock, hemorrhage, and sepsis and respond accordingly. Often the Paramedic can gather enough clues from the history and physical exam to greatly narrow down the list of possibilities, and in some cases arrive at the answer prior to arrival at the emergency department.

KEY POINTS:

- Internal female anatomical structures include the vagina, uterus, fallopian tubes, and ovaries.

- The vulva consists of the labia majora, labia minora, clitoris, accessory glands, and the introitus, which are collectively the external anatomical structures.

- Causes of female pelvic pain include urinary problems and diseases, gastrointestinal problems, gynecological disorders, and obstetrical disorders.

- Disorders can be divided into those that cause pain and those that cause bleeding.

- Painful pelvic conditions include
  - Ovarian cysts
  - Ectopic pregnancy

- Endometriosis
  - Uterine prolapse
  - Vulvovaginitis
  - Foreign bodies
  - External infections

- Conditions that cause bleeding include
  - Spontaneous abortion
  - Threatened abortion
  - Placenta previa
  - Placental abruption

- The patient's history is important in narrowing the differential diagnosis.

- Gynecological conditions can lead to hypoperfusion.

REVIEW QUESTIONS:

1. List the internal components of the female reproductive system. List the external components.
2. Female pelvic pain may result from conditions in which body systems?
3. Name the two signs/symptoms common to female abdominal pain and bleeding?
4. What is the difference between an ovarian cyst and ovarian torsion?
5. How can an ectopic pregnancy lead to the death of the female?
6. How does a spontaneous abortion differ from a threatened abortion?

CASE STUDY QUESTIONS:

Please refer to the Case Study in this chapter, and answer the questions below:

1. What conditions can lead to a complaint of lower abdominal pain in a 29-year-old woman?

2. What aspects of the patient's history are key to developing the differential diagnosis?

3. Name the physiological condition that the Paramedics are treating in the case study.

REFERENCES:

1. Abdel-Aleem H, d'Arcangues C, et al. Treatment of vaginal bleeding irregularities induced by progestin only contraceptives. *Cochrane Database Syst Rev*. 2007;2:CD003449.

2. Strickler RC. Dysfunctional uterine bleeding in ovulatory women. *Postgrad Med*. 1985;77(1):235–237, 240–243, 246.

3. McWilliams GD, Hill MJ, et al. Gynecologic emergencies. *Surg Clin North Am*. 2008;88(2):265–283, vi.

4. Hasiakos D, Papakonstantinou K, et al. Adnexal torsion during pregnancy: report of four cases and review of the literature. *J Obstet Gynaecol Res*. 2008;34(4 Pt 2):683–687.

5. Tintinalli J. *Emergency Medicine: A Comprehensive Study Guide*, sixth edition. New York: McGraw-Hill Professional; 2003.

6. Leach RE, Ory SJ. Modern management of ectopic pregnancy. *J Reprod Med*. 1989;34(5):324–338.

7. Bourgon D, MD. Ectopic pregnancy. Available at: **http://emedicine.medscape.com/article/403062-overview**. Accessed 2008.

8. Lareau SM, Beigi RH. Pelvic inflammatory disease and tubo-ovarian abscess. *Infect Dis Clin North Am*. 2008;22(4):693–708, vii.

9. Christodoulakos G, Augoulea A, et al. Pathogenesis of endometriosis: the role of defective "immunosurveillance." *Eur J Contracept Reprod Health Care*. 2007;12(3):194–202.

10. Lebovic DI, Mueller MD, et al. Immunobiology of endometriosis. *Fertil Steril*. 2001;75(1):1–10.

11. Herzer CM. Toxic shock syndrome: broadening the differential diagnosis. *J Am Board Fam Pract*. 2001;14(2):131–136.

12. Decherney A, Goodwin T, Nathan L. *CURRENT Obstetric & Gynecologic Diagnosis & Treatment* 10e. Columbus, OH. McGraw-Hill Medical; 2006.

13. Behera MA, MD. Threatened abortion. Available at: **http://emedicine.medscape.com/article/266110-overview**. Accessed 2008.

14. Sakornbut E, Leeman L, et al. Late pregnancy bleeding. *Am Fam Physician*. 2007;75(8):1199–1206.

CHAPTER 35

NORMAL PREGNANCY

KEY CONCEPTS:

Upon completion of this chapter, it is expected that the reader will understand these following concepts:

- The normal changes of pregnancy that can lead to medical consequences or exacerbate preexisting conditions
- The three time frames, called trimesters, pregnancy is divided into, each lasting approximately 13 weeks
- The differing health problems that may present during each trimester and their differing effects on mother and fetus

ANATOMY CONCEPTS:

Prior to reading this chapter the Paramedic student should be familiar with the following anatomy and physiology concepts:

- Physical anatomy of the female reproductive system
- The menstrual cycle and associated hormonal changes

It is July 4th, a sweltering, hot, humid day. The Paramedics receive a dispatch from the local parade ground where a woman, apparently pregnant, has collapsed after standing in the open field for two hours listening to political speeches.

Even on a regular summer day, that field is hot and unshaded. Water fountains are located just north of the field, about a five-minute walk off an empty field. Today, the field is not empty as a national candidate has made a campaign stop. The field is also surrounded with red and white bunting plus aluminum reflective banners. En route, the Paramedics consider the possibilities of the patient's condition.

CRITICAL THINKING QUESTIONS

1. What are some of the possible causes of syncope?
2. How might syncope be related to the patient's pregnancy?

OVERVIEW

If a pregnant woman falls as a result of syncope, it could be just a simple faint, secondary to the anemia of pregnancy. However, it could also be the start of a more ominous condition, such as eclampsia. In every case, the Paramedic must take a careful history and perform a physical examination to determine the likely diagnosis, treat the patient, and prevent further harm to the mother and her unborn child.

Chief Concern

When dealing with a pregnant patient with syncope, the Paramedic will want to know whether the patient is early or late in her pregnancy, and whether she is a healthy person or one with a lengthy medical history. Indeed, a patient's syncope may have nothing to do with her pregnancy but may instead relate to some preexisting medical condition. Women who are pregnant are prone to hypoglycemia. In addition, if it is a hot summer day, the woman may be dehydrated.

As a condition of pregnancy, venous stasis occurs, and pooling of blood occurs in her lower extremities. This all contributes to an episode of syncope. Compression of the veins in the legs by the enlarged uterus places women at risk of venous pooling by decreasing venous return after long periods of standing. These are just some of the issues surrounding pregnancy that might influence a Paramedic's care decisions for the pregnant woman presenting with syncope. The many physiologic changes of pregnancy can complicate the clinical picture. Therefore, the Paramedic should understand the changes that occur during pregnancy.

First Trimester Concerns

For women with regular menstrual cycles (normal is considered every 21 days to every 37 days), the absence of menstruation, or **amenorrhea**, is an indication of possible pregnancy. The Paramedic should keep in mind that there are many causes for amenorrhea other than pregnancy, such as hormonal imbalances. However, unless pregnancy is excluded as a possible cause of amenorrhea, it is safest to assume pregnancy in a woman of childbearing age.

The Paramedic should also bear in mind that many women are unaware that they are pregnant in the early stages, because there are no specific symptoms associated with fertilization of the egg and the start of pregnancy. In fact, some women still experience abdominal cramping as well as **spotting** (breakthrough vaginal bleeding) as their hormonal levels adjust to the pregnancy. Spotting may be an early sign of miscarriage, ectopic pregnancy, and even intercourse. It is estimated that up to 25% of women have some spotting in the first trimester.[1]

Pregnancy is divided into three time frames, called trimesters, lasting approximately 13 weeks each. The first trimester, which includes the earliest weeks of pregnancy, are defining for the developing fetus. As the ovum implants itself in the uterine wall and becomes an embryo, the outer layers of the embryo form to become the placenta while the inner layers form the fetus. Exposure to toxic substances during this period of development may be lethal to the fetus, or—if the fetus survives—the child may have life-long implications because of them. Exposure to specific toxins (teratogens) can affect the fetus's DNA and result in birth defects.[2]

By the seventh week of development, the embryonic period is completed. All the essential internal and external structures are present at this time. In the first trimester, high levels of estrogen and progesterone, produced by the developing placenta, cause breast enlargement and tenderness, pigmentary skin changes, and uterine enlargement in the mother. Increased circulating blood volume, coupled with vasodilation from high levels of circulating progesterone, may contribute to the common complaint of headaches in pregnant women.

Nausea and vomiting (morning sickness) is common (>70%) in the first trimester, and is thought to be hormonally mediated as well. Nausea and vomiting usually resolves by about the fifteenth week of pregnancy, as does the fatigue of early pregnancy.

By the end of the first trimester, the uterus can no longer be contained within the pelvis and the woman begins to show; that is, the abdomen is distended. Indeed, by term, the uterus has increased its capacity over 500-fold.

Placental Development

The placenta forms very early in the first trimester, and both the fetus and the mother contribute to its development. The placenta has two separate circulations—maternal and fetal—which exchange across the placental membrane.

The fetal circulation to the placenta is via two umbilical arteries, which remove deoxygenated blood and waste products from the fetus to the maternal circulation. Oxygen and nutrient-enriched blood enter the fetus from the mother through the single umbilical vein. The placenta is a vital organ with three main functions: metabolism, transfer of nutrients and waste, and endocrine functions (synthesis and secretion of hormones) (Figure 35-1). Issues with placental development and function have a significant impact on the health and well-being of the mother and fetus, which is discussed in Chapter 36 on complications of pregnancy.

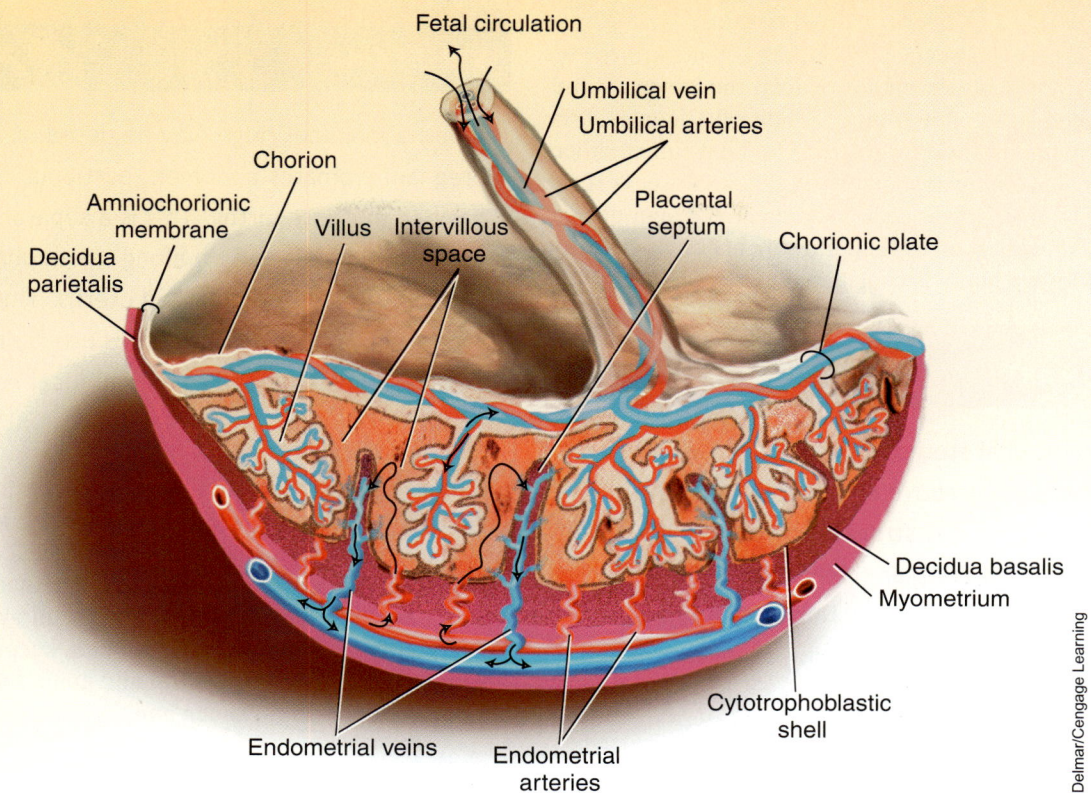

Figure 35-1 Placental functions. Oxygen, nutrients, and fetal waste products are exchanged via the placenta.

Second Trimester Concerns

The second trimester starts at the fourth month and continues to the end of the sixth month. As morning sickness and the fatigue associated with the beginning of pregnancy subside, the woman may feel energized. She will start to gain weight as the fetus grows, causing the abdomen to distend.

Uterine enlargement contributes to abdominal enlargement. By 20 weeks of pregnancy, the uterus may be palpable at the level of the umbilicus.[3] Each week thereafter, the height of the uterine fundus is roughly equivalent to the measurement of the top of the symphysis pubis to the top of the uterine fundus, measured in centimeters. Fetal growth is considered to be within normal limits if the fundal height measurement agrees with the number of weeks' gestation within 2 centimeters. For example, at 27 weeks, the uterus normally measures anywhere from 25 to 29 centimeters in a normally progressing singleton pregnancy.

Braxton–Hicks Contractions

Braxton–Hicks contractions—which are nonrhythmic, sporadic, and generally not painful—may also start in the second trimester. These contractions, also called "false labor," increase in frequency, intensity, duration, and regularity starting at the midpoint in the second trimester. They may continue throughout the third trimester, and are often falsely identified as labor contractions.

Braxton–Hicks contractions may be the result of dehydration, as volume replacement often causes the contractions to subside. Braxton–Hicks contractions may also be the result of uterine irritability, as both exercise and bladder emptying ease the contractions.

> **STREET SMART**
>
> Some women, particularly first-time mothers, have difficulty distinguishing Braxton-Hicks contractions from real labor. Others have been instructed by their primary caregiver to seek medical attention if the contractions occur more than four times in one hour.

Quickening

Although the fetal heart starts to beat at approximately the fourth week postfertilization, it is not detectable by auscultation with a Doppler stethoscope until approximately 12 weeks in an average weight woman, and not until approximately 18 to 20 weeks by a regular stethoscope.

This is also the time frame during which the woman will first start to appreciate fetal movement, called the **quickening**. Maternal perception of fetal movement, sometimes described as the fluttering of a butterfly, is one of the most useful methods of fetal surveillance. First-time mothers may feel the quickening at about 20 weeks or 18 weeks if she has previously given birth. Fetal movement is a sign of fetal well-being. Perception of 10 fetal movements or "kicks" in a period of up to two hours is considered to be reassuring.

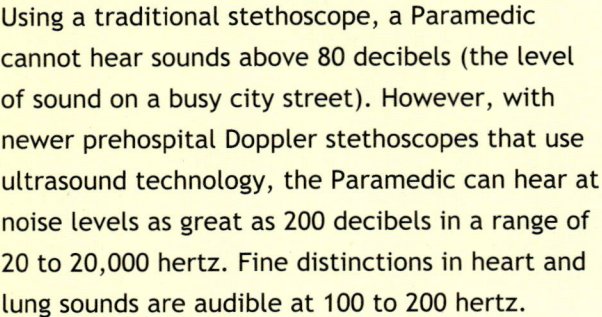

STREET SMART

Using a traditional stethoscope, a Paramedic cannot hear sounds above 80 decibels (the level of sound on a busy city street). However, with newer prehospital Doppler stethoscopes that use ultrasound technology, the Paramedic can hear at noise levels as great as 200 decibels in a range of 20 to 20,000 hertz. Fine distinctions in heart and lung sounds are audible at 100 to 200 hertz.

Third Trimester Concerns

During the third trimester, the fetus lays down subcutaneous fat and grows in weight and length. Correspondingly, the uterus also enlarges to accommodate the growing fetus. Women may complain of shortness of breath during this stage due to the enlarging uterus pressing against the abdominal organs and diaphragm, preventing full lung expansion.

Supine Hypotensive Syndrome

Supine hypotensive syndrome, also known as inferior vena cava syndrome, becomes more common in the third trimester.[4] This condition commonly occurs when a pregnant woman lies in the supine position. The weight of the uterus and its contents compresses the inferior vena cava and aorta, decreasing venous return to the heart, which in turn causes arterial hypotension.

The signs and symptoms of supine hypotensive syndrome include tachycardia, shortness of breath, a feeling of faintness or dizziness, sudden weakness, and cool clammy skin. If the mother rolls slightly to one side—usually the left side—the symptoms will resolve spontaneously.

Psychological Adaptations

Over half the pregnancies in the United States are unplanned. There are many reasons why a woman may be unaware that she is pregnant, or in denial that this is the case. Some women must hide a pregnancy because of issues related to employment, intimate partner violence (estimates are that up to 23% of pregnant women seeking routine prenatal care are subject

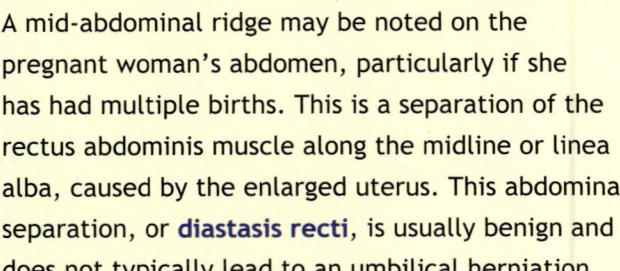

STREET SMART

A mid-abdominal ridge may be noted on the pregnant woman's abdomen, particularly if she has had multiple births. This is a separation of the rectus abdominis muscle along the midline or linea alba, caused by the enlarged uterus. This abdominal separation, or **diastasis recti**, is usually benign and does not typically lead to an umbilical herniation.

to intimate partner violence, and incidence increases during pregnancy), or family unrest. There is often an initial period of denial, then ambivalence, and ultimately, for many women, acceptance. With this in mind, the Paramedic must avoid making assumptions and instead maintain awareness of the vulnerability of many pregnant women, keeping in mind the heightened need to be respectful and nonjudgmental in interactions with pregnant women and their families.

Special Case: Abdominal Pain and Pregnancy

Abdominal pain is common in pregnancy (Table 35-1). The discomfort can result from stretching ligaments and movement of abdominal contents. Constipation, for example, is common in pregnancy, particularly the third trimester, and abdominal cramps may occur secondary to the constipation. The Paramedic should determine the woman's primary concern (in this case, presentation of abdominal pain) and consider if the abdominal pain has implications for pregnancy, is pregnancy related, or if pregnancy will have implications for addressing the abdominal pain.

For example, appendicitis is the most common acute surgical condition of pregnancy with an incidence of

Table 35-1 Extrauterine Causes of Abdominal Pain

- Appendicitis
- Bowel perforation
- Common gastroenteritis
- Diabetic ketoacidosis
- Kidney stones
- Ovarian cyst rupture
- Pancreatitis
- Peptic ulcer disease
- Pneumonia
- Pulmonary embolism
- Sickle cell crisis
- Urinary tract infection (cystitis)

1/2000 births.[5] As it is often confused with round ligament pain (described below), the pregnant woman may dismiss the abdominal pain until the appendicitis becomes acute or ruptures, leading to peritonitis. The primary treatment for acute appendicitis is appendectomy.

Several obstetric concerns accompany appendicitis. For example, the infection predisposes the pregnant woman to preterm labor if the appendix has ruptured. Diagnosis of appendicitis is more difficult in pregnancy because nausea, vomiting, and abdominal discomfort associated with appendicitis are common with pregnancy. The physical examination for classic signs of appendicitis is further complicated by displacement of organs by the enlarged uterus and its contents.

Many women will experience round ligament pain, a type of short sharp pelvic pain that occurs with change in position and is caused by the stretching of the round ligament (this is more common on the right side). The round ligament helps to support the uterus and is stretched by the expanding uterus. Round ligament pain can also occur with coughing, or even when the patient is rolling over in bed. Some pregnant women also experience low back pain, pelvic pressure, and urinary frequency as a result of the enlarged uterus compressing adjoining structures.

Gallbladder disease (cholecystitis) and gallstones (cholelithiasis) is the second most common cause of an acute abdomen in pregnancy that requires surgical intervention. A combination of decreased contractility and increased viscosity of the bile make the likelihood of gallstones, or gallsludge, more common.[6] Following a meal which is high in fat content, the woman may experience anorexia, nausea and vomiting, acid reflux (dyspepsia), and severe right upper quadrant pain that may radiate to the right scapula. This pain, or "biliary colic," heralds the passage—or attempted passage—of the gallstones/sludge. The pain may last for minutes to hours and is often worse with deep inspiration. This pain with deep inspiration upon palpation is called Murphy's sign.

Anatomic and Physiologic Changes of Normal Pregnancy

Any discussion of the care of pregnant women starts with consideration of the many and varied hormonal anatomic and physiologic adaptations that take place during the antenatal period, which encompasses the time from the first day of the last menstrual period (LMP) to the start of true labor.

The antenatal period is subdivided into three sections, or **trimesters**, each consisting of a roughly three-month period. Conventionally, these are the first trimester (weeks 1 through 12), second trimester (weeks 13 to 27), and third trimester (weeks 28 to 40).

Cardiovascular

Many remarkable changes occur in the woman during pregnancy. For example, during a normal pregnancy the woman's blood volume increases markedly from about the sixth week of pregnancy until weeks 32 to 34, when it levels off. This increased blood volume is the result of an increased plasma volume (approximately 50%) and overall volume. Therefore, although the red blood cell number, called the hematocrit, does increase (approximately 25%), the percentage of red blood cells actually decreases secondary to hemodilution.[7] This imbalance of plasma volume to hematocrit is referred to as the **anemia of pregnancy**. This increased blood volume is necessary to support the growing fetus with oxygen and glucose, eliminate waste, and compensate for blood loss at delivery. During a normal delivery, typical blood losses can be as much as 250 to 500 mL of blood. During a Caesarean section surgery, those losses can climb to 1,000 mL of blood.

It should also be noted that clotting factors—such as factors VII, X, XII, fibrinogen and platelets—also rise. Although these elements of coagulation do not rise above the normal level, they make the blood "hypercoagulable" in anticipation of blood loss during delivery. This hypercoagulable state can become problematic for the new mother if it leads to pulmonary embolism or a deep vein thrombosis. As a result of this increased blood volume, the cardiac output of the pregnant woman increases 30- to 50-fold. Most of this increase takes place during the first trimester and peaks at 20 to 24 weeks, at which point it is maintained.

Despite the increased blood volume and the increased cardiac output, there is a decrease in arterial blood pressure. This drop in blood pressure occurs due to a decrease in systemic vascular resistance, causing a mild (10 mmHg) drop in both systolic and diastolic blood pressure in some women. Many pregnant women will have a blood pressure in the 90/50 range. However, if blood pressure is found to be less, perfusion may be compromised and the etiology of the low blood pressure should be investigated. Acute events such as anaphylaxis and hemorrhage should also be ruled out.

During pregnancy, the hypotension that naturally occurs can result in orthostatic changes in blood pressure and will often cause women to feel dizzy or lightheaded when standing suddenly.

A pregnant woman may also experience hypotension secondary to supine hypotensive syndrome, which was discussed earlier. Supine hypotensive syndrome can occur

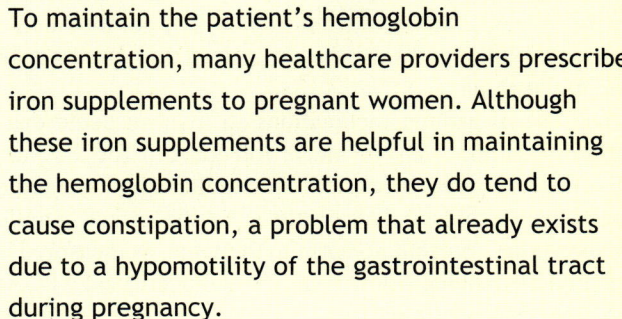

STREET SMART

To maintain the patient's hemoglobin concentration, many healthcare providers prescribe iron supplements to pregnant women. Although these iron supplements are helpful in maintaining the hemoglobin concentration, they do tend to cause constipation, a problem that already exists due to a hypomotility of the gastrointestinal tract during pregnancy.

when a woman lies on her back, so this position should be avoided after the middle of the second trimester. Treatment of maternal hypotension often simply involves changing the woman's position.

Maternal heart rate normally increases during pregnancy but tachydysrhythmia is rare. However, significant sustained tachycardia (above 100 beats per minute while resting) may be a sign of infection, anemia, or blood loss. A patient with this condition should be seen by a healthcare provider.

Pulmonary

Like the cardiovascular system, the patient's pulmonary system undergoes remarkable changes during pregnancy. The tidal volume increases 30% to 40% to accommodate the fetus's metabolic needs. Total lung capacity is reduced near term due to pressure of abdominal organs on the diaphragm. This reduces functional residual capacity by as much as 20%. The body compensates for this loss of excursion by increasing the anteroposterior and transverse diameters of the rib cage (the chest wall circumference) to accommodate the increased lung volume.

The pregnant woman's body also adjusts to the loss of lung capacity—and increased metabolic demands—by increasing the minute volume (the number of breaths in one minute). This increase in respiratory rate can be as much as 40% at term. Therefore, a woman in her third trimester who is breathing at a normal respiratory rate (i.e., the rate of a nonpregnant woman) is actually hypoventilating.

As a result of abdominal impingement on the lungs, dyspnea is a common patient complaint. About 60% of pregnant women complain of dyspnea on exertion.[8] However, such physiologic dyspnea is not to be confused with the pathologic dyspnea of diseases such as asthma.

Asthma in Pregnancy

In some cases, asthma can complicate the care of the pregnant woman. In about one-third of patients the asthma will remain stable, in another one-third the asthma will actually improve during pregnancy, and in the last one-third the patient's condition will worsen, particularly around midterm of the pregnancy.

Hormonal changes may be responsible for this worsened condition. Estrogen, for example, leads to tissue edema and bronchial swelling, increased capillary congestion, and an increase (hyperplasia) in mucous glands. The combination of increased swelling and secretions may lead to more bronchospasm and asthma.

The use of asthma medications to treat an acute exacerbation of asthma may be cause for concern for the Paramedic. The traditional bronchodilators utilized by Paramedics (inhaled beta/agonists) have little systemic effect. Studies have shown they present no harm to the fetus, as measured by congenital birth defects, low birth weight, decreased APGAR scores, and perinatal mortality.[9] Similarly, the use of ipratropium bromide has not been shown to harm the fetus.

Because of their smooth muscle relaxation properties, certain beta/agonists are used to slow labor, a procedure called **tocolysis**. Due to the combination of increased capillary permeability (secondary to hormones), intravenous fluid bolus, and use of beta/agonists leading to tachycardia, beta/agonists have been implicated in the production of tocolytic pulmonary edema. Any time a beta/agonist is administered to a pregnant woman, the Paramedic should carefully monitor her pulmonary status.

However, Paramedics should view the use of corticosteroids with more caution. Although several studies have shown no long term negative effects to the fetus from the administration of corticosteroids to the pregnant mother, use of steroids multiple times during pregnancy may cause maternal hyperglycemia, decreased fetal growth, and decreased neonatal birth weight.[10]

It is important to appropriately treat the asthma of a pregnant woman. Research suggests that infant outcomes may be worse if the asthma is permitted to persist. It may be necessary, in approximately 20% of women, to intervene with medications. These acute exacerbations of asthma are often due to either viral illness, such as the flu, and/or noncompliance with prescribed medications. Such noncompliance may be the result of the mother's concern for the effects (teratogenesis) on the fetus. Of greater concern for the mother, however, should be the significant risk of a low birth weight baby.

Gastrointestinal

To accommodate the increasing metabolic demands of both mother and fetus, the pregnant woman's gastrointestinal system undergoes changes as well. To facilitate absorption of needed nutrients, the hormone progesterone slows gastrointestinal motility, allowing for more time for absorption. This reduced motility also results in increased reabsorption of water, leading to harder stools and constipation (a common complaint among pregnant women).

Prolonged gastric emptying along with relaxation of the gastroesophageal sphincter contributes to heartburn and reflux during pregnancy. This acid reflux is exaggerated in the third trimester of pregnancy secondary to the elevation of the stomach by the growing uterus.

Perhaps the most alarming symptom of pregnancy is vomiting, or morning sickness. Hormonal changes contribute to nausea and vomiting in up to 70% to 85% of women in their first trimester of pregnancy.[11] Nausea and vomiting in pregnancy may be benign or it may be an indication of a larger problem, hyperemesis gravidarum.

Hyperemesis Gravidarum

Hyperemesis gravidarum literally means excessive vomiting of the pregnant woman. An alarming consequence of pregnancy, hyperemesis can be potentially life-threatening to mother and fetus alike.[12]

Thought to be caused by changes in hormonal levels during pregnancy (estrogen and progesterone have been implicated), hyperemesis can cause intractable nausea and vomiting leading to profound dehydration and a loss of as much as 20% of body weight. Unlike morning sickness that tends to abate around the start of the second trimester, hyperemesis is seen throughout the pregnancy.

Patients with hyperemesis gravidarum should be evaluated for orthostatic hypotension and treated with intravenous fluids accordingly. In advanced cases of hyperemesis (about 1% to 3%), the patient will need to be hospitalized for fluid and nutrient replacement. If left untreated, hyperemesis gravidarum can lead to ketosis, ketouria, convulsions, and coma.

Phenothiazines, like promethazine (Phenergan) at 12.5 to 25 mg IV, prochlorperazine (Compazine), and chlorpromazine (Thorazine) have been used successfully to control the woman's nausea. Another safe alternative may be diphenhydramine (Benadryl). Similarly, ondansetron (Zofran) has been used although its safety margin in pregnancy has not been established. For this reason, the Paramedic should consider contacting medical control for direction.

Renal

To accommodate the pregnant woman's increased blood volume, the kidneys must correspondingly increase the glomerular filtration rate, sometimes by as much as 50%. Along with an increase in the size of the kidneys, there is dilation of the ureters, which provides an easier route for urinary tract infections to move upwards and is thought to contribute to the increased incidence of pyelonephritis during pregnancy.

The urinary bladder, sharing the pelvis with the uterus, is typically displaced upwards and is flattened against the pubis bone. This results in a smaller capacity in the bladder and subsequent increased urinary frequency.

CASE STUDY (CONTINUED)

Upon arriving at the Parade Grounds, the Paramedics are directed to a knot of umbrellas just to the left of the stage. A number of women are shading the patient, who is lying unconscious on the grass. While one Paramedic begins assessing the patient, the other asks if anyone knows the patient and can answer some questions.

Two women say that they are cousins of the patient, whose name is Emilie. She is a 37-year-old woman having her first child and is due in about two weeks. Emilie has had several previous pregnancies that have ended in miscarriages, and she and her husband are thrilled about this pregnancy. The family is involved politically with the national candidate and are not from the local area. Other than being a little overweight (pleasantly plump, according to the cousin), Emilie is otherwise healthy.

CRITICAL THINKING QUESTIONS

1. What are the important elements of the history that a Paramedic should obtain?
2. Which medical conditions have special significance to the woman who is pregnant?

History

The history taking of a woman who is pregnant focuses on the mother's health, using the standard SAMPLE format, and then the history of the pregnancy. Conditions of concern include asthma, diabetes, and epilepsy, as these conditions can worsen during a pregnancy.

Present Pregnancy History

The Paramedic should ask the patient when her last period was and whether she experienced a complete cessation of menstruation. The Paramedic may also want to ask about nausea and vomiting, urinary frequency, fatigue, abdominal

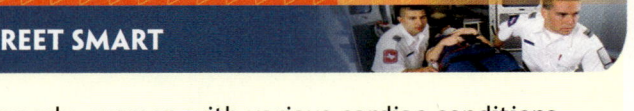

STREET SMART

Formerly, women with various cardiac conditions, such as valvular disorders, were advised to avoid pregnancy. With better prenatal care, many of these "at risk" women can now carry a pregnancy to term. However, the normal changes of pregnancy can cause increased stress on the heart, so these patients should have close medical supervision.

growth, and quickening as these are signs and symptoms that may help in determining whether a woman may be pregnant.

If a woman's chief concern has nothing to do with pregnancy, it is still helpful for the Paramedic to determine whether she may be pregnant, as this may impact treatment.

It is important for the Paramedic to obtain a thorough history of the present pregnancy in order to detect complications. Asking whether the woman has seen a midwife or other healthcare provider for her pregnancy is a good starting point. If the woman has been receiving prenatal care, that means she has had prenatal exams, she is obtaining ongoing evaluation and screening for complications, and she will have been provided with information about her pregnancy.

In the absence of any prenatal care, there may be conditions affecting her pregnancy that have gone undetected and untreated, such as gestational diabetes or pregnancy-induced hypertension (this will be discussed in Chapter 36 on complications of pregnancy). Women who do not seek prenatal care may have limited financial resources or other socioeconomic risk factors, are more likely to be very young, or may be either in denial of the pregnancy or unaware that they are pregnant.[13,14] These patients need to be reassured that they will receive proper medical care regardless of their ability to pay.

PROFESSIONAL PARAMEDIC

The professional Paramedic must learn the basic aspects of the Emergency Medical Treatment and Labor Act (EMTALA), enacted in 1986, which guarantees assessment and stabilizing treatment of women who are pregnant regardless of their ability to pay. Section 1867 of the Social Security Act imposes specific obligations on Medicare-participating hospitals that offer emergency services to provide a medical screening examination (MSE) when a request is made for examination or treatment for an emergency medical condition (EMC), including active labor, regardless of an individual's ability to pay. Hospitals are then required to provide stabilizing treatment for patients with EMCs. If a hospital is unable to stabilize a patient within its capability, or if the patient requests, an appropriate transfer should be implemented.[15]

Simply asking, "Have you had any problems with the pregnancy thus far?" is a good starting point for establishing the history of the pregnancy. Asking the woman when she believes the baby is due will help the Paramedic to target the history and examination for her stage in pregnancy and focus the evaluation accordingly. Determination of the present number of weeks' gestation will also provide the Paramedic with a focal point for further inquiry and investigation.

A wide array of symptoms is common during pregnancy, none of which are pathologic. Symptoms commonly associated with pregnancy include nausea, ptyalism (excessive salivation), fatigue, leukorrhea (whitish vaginal discharge), urinary frequency, heartburn, constipation, hemorrhoids, abdominal and breast striae (stretch marks), breast tenderness and leakage, lower extremity edema, varicosities and spider veins, round ligament pain, leg cramps, lightheadedness, mild sensations of pelvic pressure, and joint instability, especially of the pelvis.[16]

The list of concerns for a woman who is pregnant can be exhaustive. The Paramedic need only be compassionate and provide supportive care in those cases while being alert for signs of more serious conditions.

Menstrual History

Obtaining an accurate menstrual history helps the Paramedic in calculating the patient's estimated date of delivery and the gestational age of the current pregnancy. Many women do not know when their last period was, but they can usually tell the Paramedic if their periods are regular, and asking well-considered questions can sometimes help to narrow down the possibilities. The Paramedic should use national holidays or the woman's birthday to try to target the information. For example, "Do you remember having your period around New Year's?" "Have you had a period since your birthday in June?"

The **estimated date of delivery (EDD)** or **estimated date of confinement (EDC),** used interchangeably in practice, both refer to the best estimate of the date at which the fetus will be 40 weeks' gestation. The EDD can be calculated by Naegle's rule (Table 35-2), which is based on the first day of the last menstrual period (LMP). Many obstetrics calculators are available on-line. The Paramedic can download to a PDA or smartphone.

Obstetric and Gynecologic History

When taking a pregnant woman's obstetric history, the Paramedic should note the number of pregnancies, deliveries, and miscarriages she has experienced. A shorthand system for

Table 35-2 Naegle's Rule

Naegle's rule	=	Add 7 days to the date of the LMP, and then subtract 3 months from that date.
	=	LMP + 7 days − 3 months = EDC
Example: LMP	=	June 1
Add 7 days	=	June 8
Subtract 3 months	=	March 8

documenting this obstetric and gynecologic history is GPA, which stands for **G**ravid, **P**ara and **A**bortus. **Gravida** refers to the number of times a woman has been pregnant. It does not matter if the pregnancy ended in an abortion, a miscarriage, or a living baby—each counts as one in the total number of pregnancies in this determination. **Para** refers to the number of pregnancies that ended in the birth of a baby that reached the point of viability, which is often defined as 26 weeks of age or 1,000 grams. **Abortus** refers to the patient's total number of spontaneous abortions (miscarriages) and induced abortions.

The terms "gravid" and "para" are also used in medical terminology as a root word. For example, a woman who has never been pregnant would be **nulligravida**. A woman who is pregnant for the first time would be **primigravida**, whereas a woman who delivered for the first time would be **primipara**. Women who are **multigravida** have been repeatedly pregnant.

An alternative system sometimes used for the obstetric history is TPAL. In TPAL the T stands for number of **T**erm deliveries the mother has had, the P stands for the number of **P**reterm births, the A stands for the number of **A**bortions (both spontaneous and therapeutic), and the L stands for **L**iving infants. Regardless of the system used, the Paramedic should carefully document the pregnant woman's history of pregnancy.

A previous history of cesarean birth is particularly relevant, due to the increased risk of placenta previa, placenta accreta, and uterine rupture in women with a prior cesarean section—particularly with a classical or vertical incision. A higher number of previous cesarean sections increases the mother's risk of uterine rupture as well.

The Paramedic should also inquire about a previous child with a congenital anomaly such as patent ductus arteriosus or patent foramen ovale. These occurrences may place the current pregnancy at higher risk for the same issue.

A history of preterm birth (prior to 37 completed weeks' gestation) in a previous pregnancy predisposes the mother to increased risk of prematurity in subsequent pregnancies.[17–19] The risk of preterm birth increases as the absolute number of previous preterm births increases. Recurrence risk also increases as the gestational age at which the previous preterm births took place decreases. For example, if a woman gave birth at 28 weeks in the past, her risk of preterm delivery with a later pregnancy is greater than that for a woman who gave birth at 35 weeks' gestation in the past.

The elements of the gynecologic history should include any past uterine surgery (such as myomectomy or removal of fibroids, which could increase the risk of placenta previa) or cervical surgery or biopsies (which may have implications for cervical incompetence and risk of preterm delivery).

The Paramedic should not assume that a woman could not be pregnant just because she has undergone a sterilization procedure. Women who have had a tubal ligation for sterilization still have a 1 in 300 to 500 risk of getting pregnant subsequently.

Any history of sexually transmitted infections, especially Chlamydia or pelvic inflammatory disease, suggests increased risk of ectopic pregnancy (a pregnancy located outside the uterus, usually in the fallopian tubes).

These elements of a history of pregnancy (Table 35-3) are some "conversation starters" that lead the Paramedic to more in-depth questions.

Obesity and Pregnancy

Obesity has reached epidemic proportions among Americans, including women who become pregnant. Pre-pregnancy maternal obesity increases the risk of pregnancy-induced hypertension (possibly leading to eclampsia), venous thromboembolism (leading to pulmonary embolism), and gestational diabetes (leading to large, or **macrosomia** [over 4,500 grams], babies). These complications of pregnancy are discussed in Chapter 36.

Substance Use

Tobacco, alcohol, and recreational drug use can all adversely affect pregnancy and perinatal morbidity and mortality. The Paramedic should explore specific questions about the patient's drug use—both prescription and over the counter—as well as illicit drug use.

Pregnant women who are cigarette smokers have a higher risk of spontaneous abortion, placental abruption, placenta previa, preterm labor, and growth-restricted babies than nonsmokers.[20,21] The patient's risk increases with the number of cigarettes smoked. Secondhand smoke is also implicated as resulting in higher risk.

Fetal Alcohol Syndrome

Alcohol abuse, particularly in the first trimester, is the cause of fetal alcohol syndrome. Infants born with **fetal alcohol syndrome** have permanent birth defects such as growth retardation, facial anomalies, and central nervous system damage. Rates of perinatal death are estimated to be up to eight times greater for offspring of alcoholic mothers.

As alcohol easily crosses the blood–brain barrier, it also crosses the placental barrier. The major impact of alcohol on the fetus is on the central nervous system, particularly the brain. The exposure of the brain's neurons to alcohol at this important developmental period creates cognitive disabilities (such as attention deficits), impulsive behavior, and poor memory. It is suggested that fetal alcohol exposure during pregnancy may be the leading cause of mental retardation in these children.

Children with fetal alcohol syndrome are recognizable by their distinctive pattern of craniofacial defects and growth deficiency.[22] Children with fetal alcohol syndrome are significantly below the average height and weight of their peers, typically in the tenth percentile on the growth charts. Children with fetal

Table 35-3 Elements of the History of Pregnancy

- SAMPLE
  - Asthma
  - Diabetes
  - Epilepsy
- Signs of pregnancy
  - Nausea and vomiting (morning sickness)
  - Urinary frequency
  - Fatigue
  - Abdominal growth
  - Quickening
- Prenatal care
  - Prenatal vitamins
  - Iron supplements
- Expected date of delivery
  - Cessation of menses
- Obstetric history
  - Term deliveries
  - Preterm births
  - Abortions
    - Spontaneous
    - Therapeutic
  - Living infants
- Gynecologic history
  - Ovarian surgery
    - Oophorectomy
      - Ectopic pregnancy
    - Tubal ligation
  - Uterine surgery
    - Caesarian sections
    - Myomectomy
    - Hysterectomy
  - Cervical surgery
    - Biopsy
  - Sexually transmitted diseases
    - Chlamydia
      - Pelvic inflammatory disease
    - Genital herpes

Cocaine Use

Cocaine, as a sympathomimetic, can induce profound hypertension, leading to placental insufficiency and secondarily spontaneous abortion and placental abruption. Cocaine use is associated with many risks to the mother and fetus including stillbirth, preterm labor, preterm birth, growth retardation, developmental disabilities, and hemorrhage. However, determining which risks are attributable to cocaine and which are due to the presence of concomitant risk status of the cocaine user is difficult.

Exposure to Substances with Potential for Teratogenicity

A **teratogen** is any substance, agent, or environmental factor that has an adverse effect on the fetus, and may include alcohol, occupational exposures, cytomegalovirus, prescribed medications, and toxoplasmosis. Toxoplasmosis is a parasitic disease whose primary host is the common house cat. Initial exposure leads to a mild flu-like illness that often passes without notice. Congenital toxoplasmosis can lead to central nervous system damage, including congenital blindness. Since the protozoa that causes the disease is found in the cat's feces, pregnant women are advised to not handle cat litter.

Family History

The Paramedic should consider obtaining a family history as well, time permitting. A family history of a disorder, such as pregnancy-induced hypertension, diabetes, or hematologic or clotting disorders, places the woman at increased risk of developing that disorder.

Two final questions that are often very helpful in eliciting a patient history are: "What else about you do I need to know?" "Is there anything I should have asked that I haven't?"

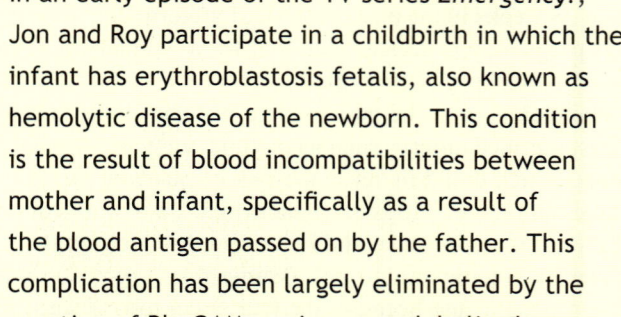

STREET SMART

In an early episode of the TV series *Emergency!*, Jon and Roy participate in a childbirth in which the infant has erythroblastosis fetalis, also known as hemolytic disease of the newborn. This condition is the result of blood incompatibilities between mother and infant, specifically as a result of the blood antigen passed on by the father. This complication has been largely eliminated by the creation of RhoGAM, an immune globulin that prevents the reaction.

alcohol syndrome also have three characteristic facial features. The first is a smooth philtrum (a flattened groove between the nose and upper lip), a thin vermilion (thin lips), and a small palpebral fissure (the separation between the upper and lower eyelids or the opening of the eyes), which leads to a wide and flattened bridge of the nose and epicanthal folds.

Emilie's exam shows an overweight woman who is obviously pregnant. Presently Emilie is verbal, has an open airway, and is breathing rapidly and shallowly. Her skin is warm and moist and her pulses are rapid and thready. While taking her pulse, the Paramedic notes that her rings have been removed, she is not wearing a watch (although her tan shows she did in the recent past), and her extremities are slightly swollen.

CRITICAL THINKING QUESTIONS

1. What are the elements of the physical examination of the pregnant patient?
2. Why is an abdominal assessment a critical element in this examination?

Examination

In addition to the primary assessment a Paramedic performs for any patient, the following elements should be considered when examining the pregnant woman. The Paramedic's assessment of the pregnant woman proceeds in a head-to-toe fashion and then returns to the gravid uterus.

Although most physical examinations are performed with the patient in the supine position, laying the pregnant patient supine creates a risk of the patient developing supine hypotensive syndrome (discussed earlier). Furthermore, a pregnant woman lying flat may feel short of breath from the weight of the gravid uterus on her diaphragm. For these reasons, the pregnant woman should be allowed to lie in a semi-reclined position. If it is necessary to have the patient supine (e.g., the patient is on a long backboard), then a pillow should be placed under the patient's right hip to slightly incline the pelvis to the left, displacing the uterus from the vena cava.

After introductions, the Paramedic should obtain a set of vital signs. Particular concern should be focused on the patient's blood pressure. Hypertension at any time during pregnancy is abnormal (the implications of pregnancy-induced hypertension (PIH) are discussed further in Chapter 36). Although classic definitions of hypertension are sufficient for use by the Paramedic (i.e., diastolic greater than 90 mmHg), the better definition is a systolic pressure 30 mmHg greater than baseline and/or diastolic pressure 20 mmHg greater than baseline.

There are many changes to the patient's skin during pregnancy. The Paramedic may note the patient has the **prurigo** of pregnancy (pruritis and soft papular lesions found on the hands and feet). The Paramedic should examine the patient's chest and thorax with caution. The breasts of the pregnant woman are tender and sensitive to touch. However, this should not deter the Paramedic from performing the routine cardiothoracic examination. For example, an innocent murmur may be appreciated upon auscultation. This murmur is secondary to the increased blood volume and strain upon the heart to maintain the cardiac output.

An examination of the limbs may reveal edema. Peripheral edema may be normal or it may be a sign of preeclampsia (discussed in Chapter 36). The Paramedic should note the level of the edema as per routine.

Examination of the Pregnant Abdomen

The Paramedic should examine the abdomen of a pregnant woman using a "look, listen, and feel" approach. First, the Paramedic should observe the abdomen for bruising, which can occur because of falls. The pregnant woman's distended abdomen changes her center of gravity and makes her unsteady and more prone to falls. Bruising can also occur because of domestic violence. The Paramedic should tactfully ask the patient how the bruises occurred and proceed accordingly.

Next, the Paramedic should observe for any scarring; for example, a previous classical caesarean section scar will have an obvious vertical scar along the midline of the abdomen from above the umbilicus. A low transverse "bikini" or **Pfannenstiel incision** would be found above the mons pubis (Figure 35-2).

Next, the Paramedic should observe for fetal movement. Fetal movement is indicative—but not absolutely

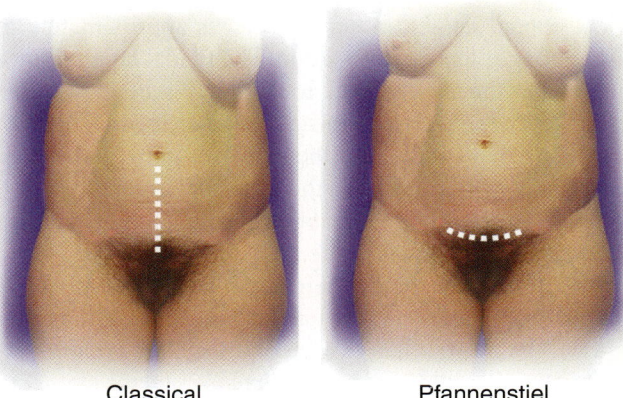

Classical   Pfannenstiel

Delmar/Cengage Learning

Figure 35-2 Prior surgical delivery with either classical or Pfannenstiel approach.

indicative—of fetal health. While observing for fetal movement, the Paramedic should ask the patient if she has experienced the quickening, the first sensations of fetal life. If the patient has experienced the quickening, then it may be possible to hear fetal heart tones. During the second trimester, it is often necessary to use a Doppler/ultrasonic stethoscope to hear fetal heart sounds. For the more advanced pregnancy, a regular stethoscope may be sufficient.

To improve the quality of the sound transmission, the Paramedic should auscultate in a quiet environment and use a conductive medium, such as water-soluble gel. Auscultation of fetal heart sounds is part practice and part luck. If the patient is heavy, then it may be difficult for the Paramedic to hear the heart sounds. The head of the stethoscope has to be angled precisely into the path of the sound as it projects from the abdomen.

The fetal heart sounds should be "too fast to count" and are usually between 120 beats per minute and 160 beats per minute. Sometimes two sets of heart sounds are heard. The second set is the mother's heart, appreciated in the abdomen because of the hyperdynamic state of the cardiovascular system. The heart sounds of mother and child are distinctly different and with practice can be separated. A second set of fetal heart tones could also be a twin's heart sounds. Fetal heart sounds are usually appreciated in specific locations (Figure 35-3).

Typically, it is easiest to hear the fetal heart tones over the fetus's back. The back can be appreciated by palpating the pregnant abdomen for the ridge that indicates the spine and then placing the stethoscope's bell next to the spine.

If the Paramedic cannot hear fetal heart tones, as is often the case, the Paramedic should not alarm the mother. The absence of fetal heart tones is more likely a function of operator error than fetal distress. However, any fetal heart rate less than 100 beats per minute is cause for concern and the patient needs further medical evaluation.

Next, the Paramedic should estimate the fundal height. This estimation is the number of centimeters above the symphysis pubis to the top of the fundus. The top of the fundus is palpated by cupping the hand of the firm portion of the abdomen from above.[23]

The fundal height, in centimeters, is approximately the same number of weeks of gestation. The fundal height is more accurate after the twelfth week to the thirty-second week as a rule. However, there are circumstances when the fundal height is inaccurate. For example, if the baby has started to descend during labor, or has dropped, then the fundal height will be inaccurate. Likewise, if the patient is anticipating twins, the fundal height will be inaccurate.

Determining the fundal height can be helpful in certain situations. For example, if the baby is breech, then the fundal height will be greater than expected. If the baby is side-lying, then the fundal height will be less than expected.

An alternative method to estimate gestational age is to measure the top of the fundus from the umbilicus. If the fundus is at the level of the umbilicus, then the fetus is at about

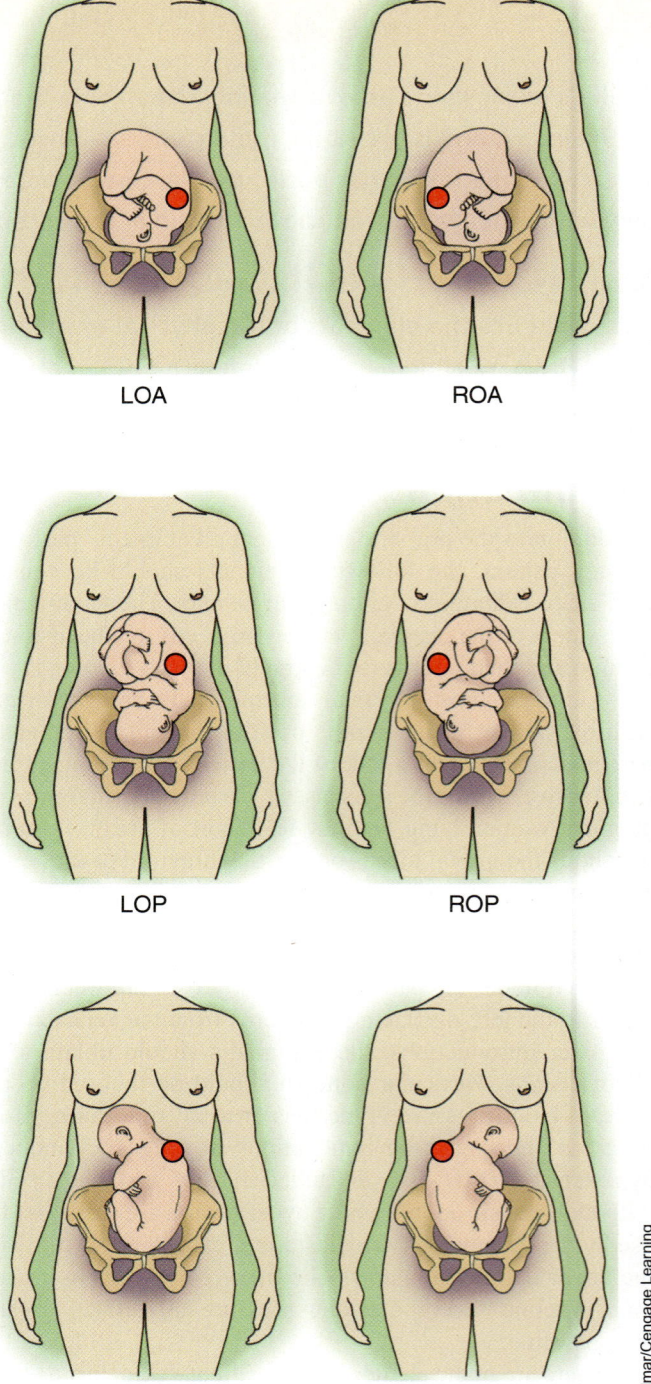

Figure 35-3 Points of auscultation of fetal heart sounds. The red dot indicates the best place to auscultate fetal heart sounds for that fetal position.

20 weeks. At 20 weeks, the Paramedic should appreciate fetal movement and fetal heart sounds. For every finger width the fundus is above the umbilicus, the Paramedic adds a week to 20. If the estimated gestational age is 20 or greater, then the fetus has a greater chance of survival if born prematurely.

While palpating for fundal height, the Paramedic may appreciate fetal movement, a sign of good fetal health, or the rigid abdomen of labor. The Paramedic may also be able to obtain the fetal outline, which helps the Paramedic understand if the fetus has rotated into a head-down position in preparation for delivery. The Paramedic should consider palpating for the fetal outline if the patient is at least 36 weeks' pregnant and birth may be imminent.

To determine the fetal position and presentation, using Leopold's four maneuvers, the Paramedic would stand next to the patient and face her. The Paramedic would first palpate the upper portions of the abdomen, proximal to the costal margin, and palpate downward, bilaterally, until the height of the fundus is felt.

The Paramedic would then, in the second maneuver, place the hands bilaterally at the mid-abdomen and, using the left hand to stabilize, push against the fetus with the right hand against the left hand. The Paramedic should be able to feel the fetus's back. Then the Paramedic repeats the maneuver using the right hand to stabilize.

The third move in Leopold's maneuver is to place one hand above the symphysis pubis and try to cup the infant's head with one hand. If legs are palpated, then the fetus is a breech presentation.

In the fourth maneuver, the Paramedic turns, faces the patient's feet, and palpates the lower abdomen bilaterally. The Paramedic is trying to locate the fetus's forehead. With this maneuver, the Paramedic can ascertain the **fetal lie**, the long axis of the fetus in line with the long axis of the mother, and the **fetal attitude**, the position of the head as either flexed or extended.

CASE STUDY (CONTINUED)

Although an episode of syncope can be ominous, in this case Emilie appears to not have suffered any harm from her syncope. Despite Emilie's protests that she would prefer to see her own obstetrician when she gets home, the Paramedic insists that she be at least "checked out." Her cousin, seeing the sense in being cautious, agrees and Emilie eventually decides that it cannot hurt to be evaluated.

CRITICAL THINKING QUESTIONS

1. What is the significance of the changes of pregnancy in relation to syncope?
2. What diagnosis did the Paramedic announce to the patient?

Assessment

Differentiation between common discomforts of pregnancy and potential complications of pregnancy is difficult since normal discomforts and physiologic adaptations of pregnancy often mimic more serious issues. Women with preterm labor, for example, may report pelvic pressure, increased vaginal discharge, backache, and menstrual-like cramps, all of which may occur in normal pregnancy.

Whenever pregnancy is suspected, the Paramedic's assessment of the woman should include determination of whether the issues concerning the woman are pregnancy related. Treatment considerations should take into account any implications they might have on the pregnancy and the developing fetus.

In this case, the Paramedic would consider a field diagnosis of syncope secondary to the changes of pregnancy and treat accordingly, ever mindful of other complications of pregnancy.

CASE STUDY (CONTINUED)

As Emilie appears stable for the moment, the Paramedic elects to move her to the air-conditioned comfort of the ambulance before starting anything more than basic treatments. Once on board, the Paramedic requests and gets Emilie's consent to start a precautionary intravenous access.

CRITICAL THINKING QUESTIONS

1. What is the standard of care of patients with syncope?
2. What are some of the patient-specific concerns and considerations that the Paramedic should consider when caring for a pregnant patient who has had an episode of syncope?

Treatment

The Paramedic should undertake emergency interventions to stabilize the mother as needed and based upon the field diagnosis.[24] To treat the mother is to treat the fetus; therefore, the mother's welfare is most important for the fetus's survival.

If the primary concern is related to a normal or common pregnancy complaint, such as hyperemesis or syncope, treatment involves supportive care. If a woman presents with syncope after standing in the hot sun the Paramedic would move her to a cooler location, evaluate her vital signs, provide hydration (either oral or intravenously as is appropriate), and examine her for any signs of trauma.

▶ CASE STUDY (CONTINUED)

Emilie relates to the Paramedic that her physician told her she had pre-eclampsia but that everything was under control. The Paramedic reassures Emilie that she is in good hands and that everything is under control. Emilie relaxes on the stretcher and closes her eyes. At that point, the Paramedic notices the start of a convulsion.

CRITICAL THINKING QUESTIONS

1. What are some of the predictable complications associated with pre-eclampsia?
2. What are some of the predictable complications associated with the treatments for pre-eclampsia?

Evaluation

Seizures can occur for many reasons. Eclampsia, a pathological condition of pregnancy, can cause seizures, as can epilepsy. In addition, a pregnant woman can be hypoglycemic, hypoxic, or have sustained a head injury due to a fall, all of which may lead to a seizure. Therefore, any time a pregnant woman seizes, the Paramedic must keep an open mind to the many possible causes of seizures.

Eclampsia

Eclampsia is a pregnancy-induced convulsion that complicates about 2% of pregnancies.[25] Typically, but not in every case, eclampsia is preceded by pre-eclampsia and/ or pregnancy-induced hypertension. The eclamptic seizure can have four phases, similar to an epileptic seizure. The first phase is aura-like with facial twitching, after which the patient enters into unconsciousness. This phase is almost immediately followed by the tonic phase, manifested by a stiffening of the body starting at the jaw. Finally, in the clonic phase, a rhythmic contraction and relaxation of the body occurs.

Although the majority of seizures (50%) take place during labor, convulsions can take place postpartum. The risk for seizures remains elevated for several weeks after delivery. In women with pregnancy-induced hypertension, convulsions take place prepartum.

The anticonvulsant of choice for the eclamptic patient is magnesium sulfate, whereas the anticonvulsant of choice for epilepsy is diazepam.[26,27] Therefore, it is important that the Paramedic carefully review the patient's medical history for signs of pre-eclampsia and pregnancy-induced hypertension or epilepsy. In every case, the patient should be evaluated and treated for hypoxia and hypoglycemia first.

If eclampsia is suspected, then four grams of magnesium sulfate should be administered intravenously. Magnesium sulfate is successful in treating 95% of convulsions secondary to eclampsia. If the patient continues to seize, then a trial of diazepam should be considered. Since diazepam has a class D indication for use in pregnancy, medical consultation is advised before its use.

Magnesium sulfate should be administered cautiously as it causes vasodilation, which can lead to hypotension. The Paramedic should first consider the patient's position (supine) and act accordingly.

Although magnesium sulfate can be administered intramuscularly, it is painful and its uptake can be erratic. Therefore, intravenous/intraosseous administration of magnesium sulfate is preferable. If IV/IO routes are not available, then the Paramedic may consider administering 10 grams deep intramuscularly in a divided dose, typically using the gluteal site. The magnesium sulfate can be mixed with 1 mL of 2% lidocaine for comfort.

As magnesium sulfate acts upon acetylcholine at the motor endplate, the patient's respirations should be monitored and the Paramedic should be prepared to slow the infusion and to assist the patient's ventilations.

The Paramedic immediately administers the magnesium sulfate and instructs the EMT to help him roll Emilie onto her left side. The convulsion seems to stop with the administration of magnesium sulfate, although Emilie remains unconscious. While the EMT performs basic airway maneuvers, including suctioning the airway and placing an oral airway, the Paramedic alerts the emergency department of their impending arrival. The receiving nurse tells the Paramedic that they will notify the birthing center and that the Paramedic should proceed to the birthing center with the patient immediately upon arrival.

CRITICAL THINKING QUESTIONS

1. What is the most appropriate transport decision that will get the patient to definitive care?
2. What are the advantages of transporting a patient with suspected eclampsia to the birthing center, even if that means bypassing the emergency department in the process?

Disposition

The patient should be transported in a left lateral position whenever possible in order to avoid supine hypotensive syndrome, to maximize blood flow to the uterus, and for the woman's comfort. The patient should be given oxygen by face mask to provide oxygen to the baby whenever there is concern about blood loss or other injury or any issues related to maternal oxygenation.

The decision regarding which facility to transport the pregnant woman to depends on the situation. After trauma, a trauma center may be indicated. If a high-risk situation such as preterm labor is suspected, transport to a facility with a neonatal intensive care unit is optimal. Another consideration is to take the woman, if possible, to the hospital where she receives prenatal care, or where her midwife or physician is affiliated, as this will promote continuity of care.

CONCLUSION

Normal pregnancy is a natural process that starts with fertilization and ends with the delivery of a baby. An understanding of this process will help the Paramedic effectively care for the pregnant patient.

KEY POINTS:

- Pregnancy is roughly divided into three 13-week periods called trimesters. Fetal development varies by trimester.

- During the first trimester
  - Placenta develops
  - Embryo grows/develops into fetus
  - Organs form

- During the second trimester
  - Fetus enlarges with perception of movement by mother

- During the third trimester
  - Fetal growth continues

- As the fetus enlarges during the third trimester, it can put pressure on the vena cava, decreasing blood return to the heart and causing hypotension when the mother lies flat.

- Morning sickness generally subsides by the second trimester whereas hyperemesis continues and can be a life threat.

- Patient history includes obstetrical and gynecological history
  - Last menstrual period
  - Number of pregnancies (gravid)
  - Number of deliveries (para)
  - Number of abortions (miscarriages) (abortus)

- Additional history can include
  - Cesarean sections
  - Congenital anomalies
  - Preterm deliveries
  - Gynecological surgeries

- Obesity in the mother can lead to pregnancy-induced hypertension (PIH), pre-eclampsia or eclampsia, thromboembolism, gestational diabetes mellitus, or large babies.

- Substances the woman may abuse during pregnancy can include tobacco, alcohol, or recreational drugs.

- A teratogen is any substance that may have an adverse effect on the fetus.
  - May include chemicals, medications, or infections

- Examination of the pregnant woman begins with the initial assessment, then a head-to-toe exam, and finally completing the exam by assessing the gravid uterus.

- Exam of the pregnant woman follows a "look, listen, and feel" approach
  - Look for bruising, scarring, and obvious movement
  - Listen for fetal heart tones
  - Feel for fundal height and position of the fetus

- Treating the mother will provide optimal care to the fetus.

REVIEW QUESTIONS:

1. Describe the patient's development of the structures of pregnancy during the
   - First trimester
   - Second trimester
   - Third trimester
2. Explain the physiology of the supine hypotension syndrome.
3. What is the difference between morning sickness and hyperemesis? Which is more threatening to the mother/fetus? Explain your answer.
4. Define gravida, para, and abortus. How does each contribute to paramedical care?
5. List at least four additional obstetrical or gynecological points that should be obtained during a patient history.
6. Name at least two reasons for concern when bruising is noted during exam of the pregnant patient.
7. Describe the best location for assessing fetal heart tones by regular stethoscope.
8. What is the optimal way to provide care to the fetus?

CASE STUDY QUESTIONS:

Please refer to the Case Study in this chapter, and answer the questions below:

1. What medical conditions can cause a syncopal episode in a 37-year-old healthy female? Environmental conditions? Pregnancy-related conditions?

2. Describe the implications of swollen extremities in a pregnant woman.

REFERENCES:

1. Deterding R, Hay W, Levin M, Sondheimer J. *Current Pediatric Diagnosis and Treatment*. New York: McGraw-Hill Professional; 2008.
2. Brent RL. Environmental causes of human congenital malformations: the pediatrician's role in dealing with these complex clinical problems caused by a multiplicity of environmental and genetic factors. *Pediatrics*. 2004;113 (4 Suppl):957–968.
3. Rennie D, Simel D. *Rational Clinical Examination*. New York: McGraw-Hill Professional; 2008.
4. Kinsella SM, Lohmann G. Supine hypotensive syndrome. *Obstet Gynecol*. 1994;83(5 Pt 1):774–788.
5. Doherty G, Way L. *Current Surgical Diagnosis & Treatment Obstetrics & Gynecology,* tenth edition. Columbus, OH.: McGraw-Hill Medical; 2005.
6. Chloptsios C, Karanasiou V, et al. Cholecystitis during pregnancy. A case report and brief review of the literature. *Clin Exp Obstet Gynecol*. 2007;34(4):250–251.
7. ACOG Practice Bulletin No. 95: anemia in pregnancy. *Obstet Gynecol*. 2008;112(1):201–207.
8. Budev MM, Arroliga AC, et al. Exacerbation of underlying pulmonary disease in pregnancy. *Crit Care Med*. 2005;33 (10 Suppl):S313–S318.
9. Cazzola M, Matera MG. Treatment of asthma during pregnancy: more solid evidence needed. *Thorax*. 2008;63(11):944–945.
10. Mariotti V, Marconi AM, Pardi G. Undesired effects of steroids during pregnancy. *Journal of Maternal-Fetal and Neonatal Medicine*. 2004;16(Supplement 2):5–7.
11. Snell LH, Haughey BP, et al. Metabolic crisis: hyperemesis gravidarum. *J Perinat Neonatal Nurs*. 1998;12(2):26–37.

12. Philip B. Hyperemesis gravidarum: literature review. *WMJ.* 2003;102(3):46–51.

13. Daniels P, Noe GF, et al. Barriers to prenatal care among Black women of low socioeconomic status. *Am J Health Behav.* 2006;30(2):188–198.

14. Johnson JL, Primas PJ, et al. Factors that prevent women of low socioeconomic status from seeking prenatal care. *J Am Acad Nurse Pract.* 1994;6(3):105–111.

15. United States Law. Available from **http://www.cms.hhs.gov/ EMTALA/**. Accessed October 12, 2008.

16. Gabbe SG, Galan H, et al. *Obstetrics: Normal and Problem Pregnancies: Book with Online Access.* Philadelphia, PA: Churchill Livingstone; 2007.

17. Kwee A, Smink M, et al. Outcome of subsequent delivery after a previous early preterm cesarean section. *J Matern Fetal Neonatal Med.* 2007;20(1):33–37.

18. Smith GC, Shah I, et al. Previous preeclampsia, preterm delivery, and delivery of a small for gestational age infant and the risk of unexplained stillbirth in the second pregnancy: a retrospective cohort study, Scotland, 1992–2001. *Am J Epidemiol.* 2007;165(2):194–202.

19. Surkan PJ, Stephansson O, et al. Previous preterm and small-for-gestational-age births and the subsequent risk of stillbirth. *N Engl J Med.* 2004;350(8):777–785.

20. London S. Associations between smoking, poor pregnancy outcomes are cumulative. *Perspect Sex Reprod Health.* 2008;40(4):238–239.

21. Rore C, Brace V, et al. Smoking cessation in pregnancy. *Expert Opin Drug Saf.* 2008;7(6):727–737.

22. Floyd RL, O'Connor MJ, et al. Recognition and prevention of fetal alcohol syndrome. *Obstet Gynecol.* 2005;106(5 Pt 1): 1059–1064.

23. Indraccolo U, Chiocci L, et al. Usefulness of symphysis-fundal height in predicting fetal weight in healthy term pregnant women. *Clin Exp Obstet Gynecol.* 2008;35(3):205–207.

24. Lavin JP, Jr., Polsky SS. Abdominal trauma during pregnancy. *Clin Perinatol.* 1983;10(2):423–438.

25. Subramaniam V. Seasonal variation in the incidence of preeclampsia and eclampsia in tropical climatic conditions. *BMC Womens Health.* 2007;7:18.

26. Duley L, Henderson-Smart D. Magnesium sulphate versus diazepam for eclampsia. *Cochrane Database Syst Rev.* 2003;4:CD000127.

27. Eclampsia Trial Collaborative Group, ed. Which anticonvulsant for women with eclampsia? Evidence from the Collaborative Eclampsia Trial. *Lancet.* 1995;345(8963):1455–1463.

CHAPTER 36

COMPLICATIONS OF PREGNANCY

KEY CONCEPTS:

Upon completion of this chapter, it is expected that the reader will understand these following concepts:

- The differing implications carried by the results of a patient history and exam depending upon the trimester of pregnancy

ANATOMY CONCEPTS:

Prior to reading this chapter the Paramedic student should be familiar with the following anatomy and physiology concepts:

- Female reproductive system

The Paramedics receive dispatch information to an apartment in upscale housing adjacent to the university campus. A 27-year-old female states she is pregnant and has started with vaginal bleeding.

The Paramedics are concerned about how far along in her pregnancy the woman is. They also express concern about injuries from trauma. The dispatch information seems sketchy, which is odd since their dispatchers are usually very thorough in asking for information.

CRITICAL THINKING QUESTIONS

1. What are the important elements of the history that a Paramedic should obtain?
2. What are the implications of vaginal bleeding?

OVERVIEW

Complications of pregnancy are the exception—not the rule. However, they do occur. Complications of pregnancies will be discussed by trimester, with complications more commonly found in the first, second, and third trimesters delineated separately. For example, although vaginal bleeding can take place at any time in a pregnancy, its cause will likely be different depending on when it occurs in the course of the pregnancy. Understanding the symptoms in the context of the trimester of pregnancy will help the Paramedic to identify, assess, treat, and evaluate the patient appropriately.

Chief Concern

The leading cause of infant mortality (birth to one year of life) is congenital malformations, or birth defects, the large majority of which cannot be prevented.[1] These congenital abnormalities often result in preterm birth, which is the leading cause of both perinatal mortality and neonatal morbidity.[2,3] Unfortunately, more than half of spontaneous preterm births occur in women with no apparent risk factors. One of the leading indicators of imminent preterm birth is bleeding.

First Trimester Vaginal Bleeding

First trimester vaginal bleeding can be caused by a number of conditions. For example, postcoital (after intercourse) bleeding may occur at any time in pregnancy and may be related to cervicitis, cervical polyps, or other concerns that are not necessarily obstetrically related. First trimester bleeding, or spotting, may be due to infection, such as a yeast infection. All suspected bacterial vaginosis—and vaginitis in general—should be assessed by a healthcare provider. Some first trimester bleeding may be caused by implantation of the embryo into the uterine lining (so-called implantation bleeding). In these cases, the bleeding is minor. More problematic is the bleeding associated with spontaneous abortion.

Approximately 20% of pregnant women experience some vaginal bleeding, other than spotting, in the first trimester. More than half will go on to have normal, term babies. For others, however, vaginal bleeding is a symptom indicating that they are at risk for complications of pregnancy.

Spontaneous Abortion

The most common reason for vaginal bleeding in the first trimester is **spontaneous abortion**, referred to as a miscarriage in lay terms.[4] Spontaneous abortion is defined as a pregnancy that ends before 20 weeks' gestation. The incidence of spontaneous abortion is difficult to estimate, but most sources put the number at as many as one in four to five pregnancies.

It is believed that 60% to 80% of spontaneous abortions in the first trimester are due to chromosomal abnormalities.[4] **Complete abortion** is the expulsion of all products of conception. With **incomplete abortion** some, but not all, of the products of conception are passed. A **missed abortion** is the death of the embryo or fetus before 20 weeks' gestation with no loss of any of the products of conception.

Ectopic Pregnancy

A pregnancy that implants outside the uterus is called an ectopic pregnancy. Over 90% of the time, this takes place in the fallopian tubes, and many people thus refer to ectopic pregnancies as "tubal pregnancies." The incidence is as high as 1 in 100 pregnancies. Risk factors include a prior ectopic pregnancy, assisted fertility, infection such as pelvic inflammatory disease, and any other factor that may contribute to fallopian tube scarring.[5] If a pregnancy takes place after a woman has had a tubal ligation (female sterilization procedure), that pregnancy is more likely to be an ectopic pregnancy. Therefore, if a woman presents with signs and symptoms of ectopic pregnancy, even though she insists she had a tubal ligation, the Paramedic should assume pregnancy until this is ruled out.

Any woman who presents with first trimester vaginal bleeding, especially with lower abdominal or adnexal pain, should raise the Paramedic's suspicion for ectopic pregnancy. A ruptured ectopic pregnancy is a true medical emergency which can result in hemorrhage and shock.

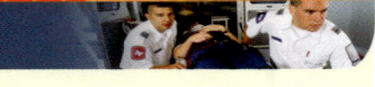

STREET SMART

The adage goes, "Any female, of childbearing age, who presents with lower abdominal pain is pregnant until proven otherwise."

Second Trimester Bleeding

Second trimester bleeding is less common than first trimester bleeding. Causes of second trimester bleeding include infection, incompetent cervix, and malformation of the uterus.[6] Of the three, infection is the most common cause. The changing environment in the vagina, secondary to hormonal changes, leads to bacterial and yeast infections.

Another cause of second trimester bleeding is an incompetent cervix. As the weight of the uterus increases and as the **fetus** grows, it presses down on the cervix. If the cervix is weakened, then bleeding may occur. Reasons that the cervix is weak and unable to contain the products of conception, also called an **incompetent cervix**, include damage to the cervix during a previous difficult birth; a congenitally malformed cervix; previous trauma to the cervix, such as from a dilation and curettage (D&C); or previous surgery to the cervix (e.g., secondary to cervical cancer).

Although an incompetent cervix only occurs in 1% to 2% of pregnancies, it may be responsible for 25% of miscarriages in the second trimester. When a woman bleeds in the second trimester, the physician may order her to go on bedrest, since laying supine takes pressure off the cervix. Alternatively, she may undergo a surgical procedure called **cerclage** wherein the cervix is sewn shut until the baby comes to term, which is roughly 36 to 38 weeks.[7–9]

The last reason why vaginal bleeding may occur in the second trimester is uterine malformation. Uterine malformation is thought to be a congenital anomaly that occurs in approximately 7% of the female population. In some extreme cases, the pelvis is completely devoid of a uterus. However, more common is the uterus **didelphys**, or double uterus. In some cases, the patient may even have a double vagina; in fact, cases exist of women sustaining multiple pregnancies in both uteruses. However, in many cases the uterus is "bicornate" (shaped like a heart), including a septum, and not like a pear as it is normally shaped. Since the smaller uterus is incapable of supporting pregnancy for the full term, a spontaneous abortion occurs.

Special Case of Molar Pregnancy

In some women, a mass (actually cysts) of grape-like tissue forms in the uterus instead of a placenta. Without the placenta, the fetus cannot survive. However, the tissue continues to grow. Called a **hydatidiform mole**, the tissue continues to stimulate all of the hormonal changes of pregnancy. A molar pregnancy, a degenerative process within the chorionic villi of the placenta, occurs in 1/1,000 pregnancies in the United States. The risk is increased among older gravidas (women 50 and over, who carry a risk of 1/500) and women with a previous history of molar pregnancy.

Symptoms of a hydatidiform mole include vaginal spotting, cramping, hyperemesis, uterine enlargement beyond what is expected for the gestational age of the pregnancy, hormonal levels that exceed expected levels for the gestational age of the pregnancy, or signs and symptoms of pregnancy-induced hypertension before 24 weeks' gestation. The most telling sign of a molar pregnancy is the vaginal discharge of grape-like tissue. Treatment for a molar pregnancy is

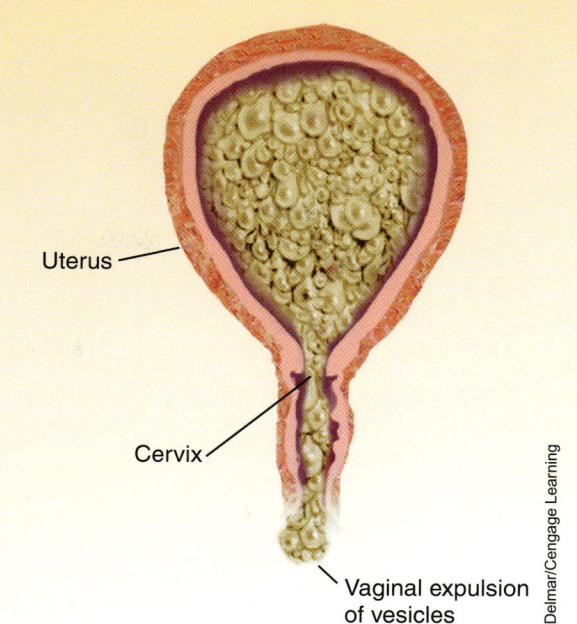

Figure 36-1 Molar pregnancy.

evacuation of the uterine contents, sometimes combined with chemotherapy (Figure 36-1).

Some women (about 15% to 20%) with a molar pregnancy go on to develop **gestational trophoblastic disease (GTD)** after the molar pregnancy is removed.[10] GTD can be thought of as an abnormal tissue growth that can develop into cancer.

Third Trimester Bleeding

Third trimester bleeding is relatively rare, occurring in only 3% to 4% of pregnancies. At this point, the pregnancy is well established. The most common causes of third trimester bleeding, other than the bloody show associated with normal labor, are placenta previa, placental abruption, and preterm labor. Although uterine rupture is a rare event, considering the rising incidence of cesarean section in the United States, this rare event is worthy of note.

Placenta Previa

One significant cause of third trimester bleeding is placenta previa. **Placenta previa** occurs when the placenta is implanted in the uterine wall such that it partially or completely covers the internal os, the opening of the uterus at the cervix. This abnormal implantation is a complete previa if it completely covers the os (Figure 36-2). Complete coverage of the os and cervix is problematic for childbirth and almost always necessitates a cesarean section.

If only a portion of the os is involved, it is called a partial placenta previa. The incidence of placenta previa is about 0.5% of pregnancies, or 1 in 200. Of the third trimester bleeding not associated with normal labor, 20% is due to placenta previa.

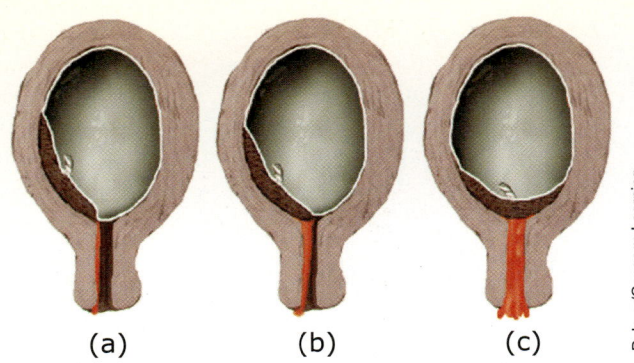

Figure 36-2 Placenta previa. (a) Low implantation (marginal). (b) Partial placenta previa. (c) Total placenta previa.

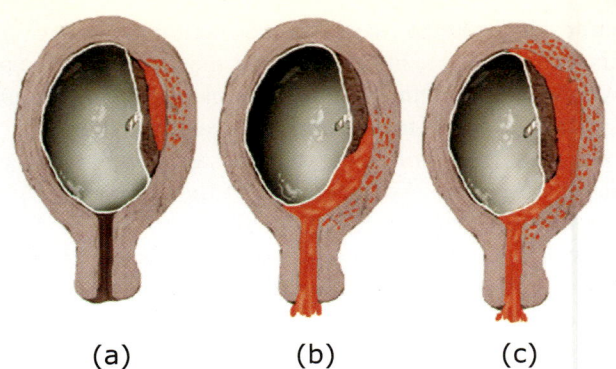

Figure 36-3 Placental abruption. (a) Central abruption, concealed hemorrhage. (b) Marginal abruption, external hemorrhage. (c) Complete abruption, external hemorrhage.

A patient with a previous cesarean section is at risk factor for placenta previa. Among women with a prior cesarean section, 1% to 4% experience placenta previa in a subsequent pregnancy.[11,12] This is a growing cause of concern in the United States, where some communities have cesarean section rates among patients as high as 30%. Other risk factors for placenta previa include tobacco smoking, multiple gestations, grand multiparity (more than seven previous pregnancies), and a history of placenta previa in a previous pregnancy.[13]

In addition to **antepartum hemorrhage** (i.e., bleeding before delivery), placenta previa can be associated with preterm labor, premature rupture of membranes, intrauterine growth restriction, and malpresentation. Pregnancies complicated by placenta previa are high risk, and many women are counseled to be on bedrest and pelvic rest.

Placental Abruption

Another cause of third trimester bleeding is placental abruption. **Placental abruption** refers to the premature separation of a normally implanted placenta from the uterine wall (Figure 36-3).

Hematoma formation occurs between the placenta and the decidua basalis of the uterine wall in placental abruption. This space-occupying lesion causes compression of the placenta and results in a decrease in oxygen-laden blood being transmitted to the fetus. Subsequently, the fetus becomes distressed. If the placental abruption is complete, then fetal death is inevitable unless an emergent cesarean section is performed.

The presenting symptoms of placental abruption, in order of occurrence, are vaginal bleeding, abdominal pain, fetal distress as manifest by relative bradycardia (heart rate less than 100 beats per minute), and premature labor.[14]

Not all cases of placental abruption present with vaginal bleeding, however. In fact, up to one-third of the cases of placental abruption do not present with vaginal bleeding. In those cases, the bleeding is sequestered behind the placenta as "hidden bleeding."

Placental abruption occurs in about 0.5% to 1.5% of pregnancies, but it is responsible for 30% of third trimester hemorrhages. Fetal mortality with clinically identified placental abruption is as high as 35%, whereas fetal mortality rates with severe abruption can reach 50% to 80%.[15] Maternal hypertension, trauma, and cocaine use with subsequent maternal hypertension, as well as previous incidence of abruption, are known to contribute to the risk of placental abruption. However, in most cases, the cause is not identifiable.

CULTURAL/REGIONAL DIFFERENCES

A cocaine-induced placental abruption that leads to a spontaneous abortion is referred to as a "street abortion" in some areas.

Uterine Rupture

Although rare, **uterine rupture** does occur in women who have had previous cesarean sections. With the occurrence of cesarean sections increasing in the United States, it is becoming more likely that a Paramedic may encounter a patient with a uterine rupture during his career.

Most uterine ruptures occur during labor, and over 90% are associated with a previous uterine scar, such as that from a prior cesarean section.[16–18] In women with a prior cesarean section, the risk of uterine rupture is about 0.05% to 0.1%. The risk of uterine rupture is even lower in women with no previous history of uterine surgery (one in 15,000), including cesarean section. Therefore, the absence of a history of cesarean section almost certainly eliminates the possibility of uterine rupture occurring during labor.

Other potential causes of uterine rupture include grand multiparity (a woman with a history of more than five childbirths) and forced labor with drugs such as oxytocin. Trauma may also cause uterine rupture in some rare cases, which are discussed shortly.

Signs and symptoms of uterine rupture vary and may include mild or severe third trimester vaginal bleeding, intense abdominal pain, or the complete cessation of pain after an intense period of pain. Other signs of uterine rupture may be dystonic uterine contractions (a series of involuntary sustained muscle contractions that do not progress the delivery) or complete cessation of uterine contractions. On exam, the patient's abdomen may be rigid (almost board-like) if there has been severe hemorrhage, and fetal remains may be easily palpated on the abdominal wall, as the fetus may be completely outside the uterine cavity.

A ruptured uterus is a surgical emergency for both mother and baby. In this situation, death is likely for the fetus unless an immediate perimortem cesarean section is performed. Death for the mother can occur as a result of severe hemorrhage and hypovolemic shock. Therefore, an emergency cesarean hysterectomy may need to be performed to save the mother.

Special Case of Trauma in Pregnancy

Trauma presents a special challenge to the Paramedic, as she is tasked with caring for not one but two patients. The Paramedic should focus on resuscitating the mother, since the most common cause of fetal death is maternal death. The most common cause of trauma-related fetal death is placental abruption.

About 7% of pregnancies are complicated by trauma.[19] The mechanism of injury in about 60% of blunt trauma cases in pregnancy is a motor vehicle collision. In some instances, the pregnant woman did not wear, or properly wear, a seat belt. Since seat belts are designed to be worn low over the pelvic girdle, they are uncomfortable to the pregnant woman.

Another 20% of blunt trauma in pregnancy can be attributed to falls. As the uterus grows, the woman's center of gravity shifts. Some women compensate for this shift by taking a wider stance; however, in some instances this correction is not sufficient. The woman becomes unsteady on her feet and falls forward onto the most prominent projection, the pregnant abdomen.

The final 20% of blunt trauma in pregnancy is related to assaults, in particular, domestic violence. Significant others, perhaps not pleased with the pregnancy, tend to strike the patient's protuberant abdomen with a blunt object, fist, or kick. In some circumstances, the perpetrator may shoot the abdomen. Although the pregnancy may be protective for the mother in these cases, since core organs are displaced away from the gravid uterus, fetal injury approaches 66%.

In many cases, there is placental abruption following the blunt force trauma, with vaginal bleeding in about 78% of cases, severe abdominal pain in about 60% of cases, and eventual fetal death in about 15% of cases. It should be noted that pelvic fractures often accompany placental abruption/uterine rupture secondary to blunt force trauma in motor vehicle collisions.

As the result of a trauma situation, an emergent cesarean section may be necessary to try to save the baby. However, this is not within the Paramedic's scope of practice. If the mother goes into cardiac arrest, cardiopulmonary resuscitation should begin immediately, the patient should be positioned with the pelvis rolled slightly to the left to move the uterus off the inferior vena cava and the patient should be quickly transported to the closest appropriate emergency department for a perimortem cesarean section. If the cesarean section can be performed within five minutes, there is a possible survival rate of 11% to 40%, provided the fetus is greater than 24 weeks' gestation.[20,21] It is important for the Paramedic to continue CPR throughout the cesarean section.

Maternal Complications of Pregnancy

There are three major maternal complications of pregnancy: pregnancy-induced hypertension, preeclampsia, and diabetes. Without proper medical care, any of these three complications of pregnancy can be life-threatening to the mother.

Pregnancy-Induced Hypertension

Chronic **pregnancy-induced hypertension (PIH)**, also called gestational-induced hypertension, complicates 5% of pregnancies. Pregnancy-induced hypertension is more common in first pregnancies, in patients who have a previous history of pregnancy-induced hypertension (up to 25% recurrence rate), teenagers, women over age 35, African-American women, women with diabetes, and women with chronic hypertension upon which pregnancy-induced hypertension may become superimposed.[22] Up to one-third of women with chronic hypertension will develop superimposed pregnancy-induced hypertension. Chronic hypertension is more common in older women, and may become more acute in pregnancy.

The exact cause of pregnancy-induced hypertension is unknown; however, vascular issues due to vasoconstriction, including decreased placental perfusion, are the main concerns with hypertension in pregnancy. In rare cases, seizures or eclampsia (which were discussed in Chapter 35) can occur.

High blood pressure in the second trimester, especially when combined with hyperemesis gravidarum (a severe form of nausea and vomiting of pregnancy), may be due to a molar pregnancy.

Symptoms sometimes associated with pregnancy-induced hypertension include headache, visual changes such as **scotomata** (a loss of an area of vision), and epigastric pain. These symptoms may be completely absent, or may present very late in the continuum of the disease, and should not be relied upon to gauge the disease's severity.

The treatment of pregnancy-induced hypertension depends on the severity of the illness and the fetus's gestational age. In severe pregnancy-induced hypertension, the treatment is to prevent eclampsia (seizure), control blood pressure, and deliver the baby.

A complication of pregnancy-induced hypertension can be placental abruption as well as poor progression of gestation, potentially leading to stillbirth. To control pregnancy-induced hypertension, some healthcare providers advocate the patient go on bedrest or hospitalization for fetal monitoring. In the acute setting, magnesium sulfate is often used to control the hypertension.[23,24] Corticosteroids prescribed to the mother are for the fetus. These corticosteroids encourage the development of the fetal lungs in the eventuality of premature birth.

Preeclampsia

Preeclampsia, formerly called toxemia of pregnancy, is based on a triad of nondependent edema (generalized or primarily including the hands and face), proteinuria (protein in the urine), and hypertension (blood pressure greater than 140/90 on two occasions at least four to six hours apart).[25] It usually presents in the third trimester.

Preeclampsia may originate from some substance released from the placenta which causes vascular dysfunction, including changes to the tissues of the liver and kidneys. The subsequent signs of preeclampsia—hypertension, edema, and protein in the urine—are secondary to changes within those organs. The cure for preeclampsia is birth, via delivery of the placenta during childbirth or therapeutic abortion.

Special Case of HELLP

In extreme cases, the patient may experience an obstetric emergency called the **HELLP syndrome**; HELLP stands for **H**emolytic anemia, **E**levated **L**iver enzymes, and **L**ow **P**latelet count syndrome. The onset of HELLP syndrome is characterized by malaise and circumferential upper abdominal pain. Some patients also experience headaches, blurred vision, and nausea with vomiting. Untreated HELLP syndrome can lead to widespread disseminated intravascular coagulation and acute renal failure. HELLP syndrome can occur anytime during pregnancy, usually after the twentieth week, and up to six to eight weeks following pregnancy.

Diabetes

Diabetes falls into two main categories when discussed in the context of pregnancy: pregestational diabetes (less than 1%) and gestational diabetes. **Gestational diabetes** is more akin to type 2 diabetes in which an insufficient amount of insulin is produced in relation to the body's demands. Gestational diabetes, which occurs because of the metabolic demands of pregnancy, is more common in obese women whose pancreases are already stressed. Due to increased obesity rates, gestational diabetes is on the rise in the United States, with an incidence of 1% to 12%, depending on the population studied.[26,27] In addition to obesity, risk factors for gestational diabetes include age, family history of gestational diabetes, a previous baby weighing more than 4,000 grams, or a previous stillbirth.

In the past, women with type 1 diabetes, or diabetes preceding pregnancy, were generally unable to conceive or continue pregnancy. Today, more women with preexisting diabetes are able to conceive and carry a baby to term. Similarly, women with gestational diabetes are also able to carry a baby to term. However, diabetes complicates the pregnancy. Diabetes contributes to increased risk of developing pregnancy-induced hypertension, **polyhydramnios** (excessive amniotic fluid), a large-for-gestational-age baby with associated risks for delivery complications, postpartum hemorrhage, infection, and first trimester spontaneous abortion. There is also an increased risk for the need for cesarean section delivery.

Generally speaking, acute complications of diabetes for pregnant women who are taking insulin are treated in the same fashion as those for women who are not pregnant, such as treatment of hypoglycemic shock or ketoacidosis.

CASE STUDY (CONTINUED)

The Paramedics are met at the door by a well-dressed young man who states that his girlfriend, who is 28 weeks' pregnant, began having some vaginal bleeding and abdominal pain this morning but didn't tell him anything until now (it is mid-afternoon). One Paramedic goes to assess the woman while the other Paramedic stays with her male companion to ask questions.

The woman states that she experienced some pain and vaginal bleeding this morning but hoped it would stop. The bleeding has now increased and she believes that she is having regular contractions. She denies any trauma but is otherwise vague at provocation of the pain and contractions.

Her boyfriend states that, before the pregnancy, both he and his girlfriend used crack cocaine regularly but he thought that she had quit when she discovered that she was pregnant.

CRITICAL THINKING QUESTIONS
1. What are the important elements of the history that a Paramedic should obtain?
2. What implication does the pain have along with vaginal bleeding in a woman who is 28 weeks' pregnant?

History

In addition to a standard history for pregnant women (discussed in Chapter 35), a focused history for the pregnant woman with complications will target a number of Paramedic concerns.

The first concern is the presence of bleeding. Bleeding in the first three months of pregnancy may signal spontaneous abortion. The Paramedic should ask the patient how severe the bleeding is, using a pad count as one measure.

The Paramedic should also ask if there is—or was—any associated cramping or unilateral pelvic pain. Placenta previa often presents as painless and sometimes with profuse vaginal bleeding. Alternatively, placental abruption may present with or without vaginal bleeding. It is often associated with severe abdominal pain and/or frequent or unremitting contractions, often lacking uterine relaxation between the contractions. The Paramedic should be particularly suspicious for abruption after trauma.

If the patient is having uterine contractions, then the Paramedic should ask about the time of onset, the frequency of contractions in minutes, the duration of contractions in minutes, and the intensity of the contractions. If the woman has delivered in the past, the Paramedic should inquire if the cramps or pain are similar to the labor contractions she experienced in the previous pregnancy. However, this symptom is not conclusive as many women experience each labor differently.

The Paramedic should also inquire if the woman has ruptured her membranes, which is usually characterized by a gush of liquid from the vagina. If she has, the Paramedic should ask if the fluid was clear, blood-tinged, or greenish in color. The Paramedic should also inquire about the time of the rupture and the amount of fluid present.

If the patient has a "**bloody show**," a small amount of pinkish or brown-tinged mucous discharge, it may be an indication of imminent delivery. A larger amount may indicate hemorrhage. In that case, the Paramedic should ask the patient about the amount, consistency, and color, as well as the presence of any clots.

The maternal sensation of fetal movement, called the quickening, is a sign of fetal health. The Paramedic should ask the patient about the last time she felt fetal movement.

CASE STUDY (CONTINUED)

The patient is found lying on her side in bed. Although she is hypotensive, the Paramedic recalls that this may be a normal blood pressure for a pregnant woman. However, he then notes that she is tachycardic, tachypneic, and that her skin is cool and clammy. With those findings, he corrects his earlier thoughts.

CRITICAL THINKING QUESTIONS

1. What are the elements of the physical examination of a patient with suspected hemorrhagic shock?
2. Why is a "pad count" a critical element in this examination?

Examination

The Paramedic's physical examination of the pregnant patient focuses on bleeding. The Paramedic should obtain a set of vital signs and assess for signs of shock. Recalling the physiologic changes of pregnancy, the Paramedic should recognize that the perimeters for hypotension and hypertension change.[28] Therefore, a pregnant woman with a blood pressure of 90/50 may not be in shock.[29] The Paramedic should look at the entire clinical picture, and in particular the patient's mental status, before making a prediction of shock.

The Paramedic should palpate the patient's abdomen carefully for signs of lower abdominal tenderness. A board-like abdomen may indicate uterine rupture, particularly in the presence of a cesarean section scar.

The Paramedic should only insert a gloved hand into the patient's vagina under extraordinary circumstances during delivery, which will be discussed in the next chapters.

Whenever possible, the Paramedic should auscultate for and monitor fetal heart tones for signs of decreased heart rate and relative bradycardia (i.e., heart rate less than 100 beats per minute).

CASE STUDY (CONTINUED)

The Paramedic elects to start intravenous access immediately. He remembers the saying, "To save the baby you have to save the mother." Although he is not sure of the exact cause of the patient's bleeding, he is sure that any bleeding in a woman who is 28 weeks' pregnant can be a problem.

CRITICAL THINKING QUESTIONS

1. What is the significance of the saying, "To save the baby you have to save the mother"?
2. What are the possible causes of bleeding in a pregnant woman at 28 weeks?

Assessment

The Paramedic's diagnosis is broad and all encompassing for the pathologies of bleeding related to pregnancy. The Paramedic should continue to assess for change in maternal status. With suspected placental abruption, deterioration in maternal and fetal status can be rapid.

CASE STUDY (CONTINUED)

The young woman is treated for hypoperfusion, likely caused by a placental abruption. She has two intravenous access lines in place; is given high-flow, high-concentration oxygen; and is transported on the stretcher in the left lateral recumbent position.

CRITICAL THINKING QUESTIONS

1. What is the standard of care of patients with bleeding during pregnancy?
2. Why was the patient transported in the left lateral recumbent position?

Treatment

The Paramedic's treatment revolves around supportive care such as providing oxygen for the mother and fetus as well as establishing intravenous access if bleeding is heavy or placenta previa, abruption, rupture, or trauma is suspected. A second intravenous access can be helpful if the Paramedic suspects hemorrhage and there may be possible transfusions of blood products.

CASE STUDY (CONTINUED)

While on board the ambulance, the patient states that she is experiencing abdominal pain, stating, "I think I am in labor." Not prepared to delivery a premature newly born in the ambulance, the Paramedic lets the saline infusion run free flow in order to bolus the patient and slow the labor, if possible.

CRITICAL THINKING QUESTIONS

1. What are some of the predictable complications associated with preterm labor?
2. What are some effective tocolytics?

Evaluation

The presence of preterm labor and rupture of the bag of waters suggests that birth is imminent. The combination of maternal hypertension, with bloody vaginal discharge, is suggestive of placental abruption. With a fetal mortality rate approaching 80% in cases of severe abruption, the Paramedic must make a rapid assessment for hypotension and treat the patient aggressively.

Preterm Labor

The definition of preterm labor is uterine contractions resulting in cervical change prior to 37 weeks' gestation. Preterm labor is the complication of pregnancy Paramedics are most likely to encounter.

Many women experience contractions—even regular, rhythmic contractions—in their third trimester that do not result in cervical change, and do not place the women at risk for preterm delivery. However, it is difficult for many women to differentiate between false labor and preterm labor as the symptoms are very similar. The only way to diagnose preterm labor is by cervical exam, a skill not performed by Paramedics.

Around 85% of preterm births take place between 32 and 36 weeks' gestation, resulting in minimal fetal or neonatal morbidity in most cases.[30] However, birth prior to 32 weeks may confer significant morbidity and mortality. This increased mortality is due to respiratory distress syndrome, intracranial hemorrhage, infection, necrotizing enterocolitis, and other factors. Infant mortality and morbidity increase significantly with decreasing gestational age. Although advances in the care of the preterm neonate have resulted in improved survival, life-long sequellae often accompany those very premature neonates who do survive.

The majority of causes of preterm labor are unknown. Risk factors include infection, multiple gestation, smoking, substance abuse (e.g., cocaine), previous preterm delivery, second trimester vaginal bleeding, and increased medical risks such as maternal hypertension and uterine anomalies. The Paramedic may identify any number of signs associated with preterm labor (Table 36-1).

To prevent premature delivery, the Paramedic may institute suppression of labor (**tocolysis**). Tocolytic agents include fluid bolus, magnesium sulfate, and specific beta/adrenergic agonists.[31] Treatment with tocolytic drugs has not been shown

Table 36-1 Signs Associated with Preterm Labor

- Abdominal cramps
- Blurred vision
- Fever greater than 101°F
- Lack of fetal movement
- Persistent vomiting
- Severe headaches
- Vaginal bleeding

to reduce preterm delivery; however, it can delay delivery for at least 48 hours.

The first therapy, a fluid bolus, is premised on the connection between antidiuretic hormone, oxytocin (the labor-inducing hormone), and the posterior pituitary gland. The posterior pituitary gland produces both but has limited production capabilities. Therefore, a fluid bolus challenges the posterior pituitary gland to produce antidiuretic hormone instead of oxytocin.

The other agents—magnesium sulfate and beta/adrenergic agonists—work to cause smooth muscle relaxation. As the uterus is made of smooth muscle, these agents suppress the contraction of the uterus and slow delivery.

The Paramedic's goal in using this therapy is to (1) sufficiently delay delivery until the mother may be transported to a facility with neonatal intensive care capability, (2) treat any underlying cause of the preterm labor, and (3) provide corticosteroid treatment for fetal lung maturation. Both maternal antepartal transport and steroids have been shown to decrease neonatal morbidity and mortality.[32]

Premature and Preterm Rupture of Membranes

Rupture of membranes before 37 weeks is considered **preterm rupture of membranes**. Up to 80% of these patients will go into labor within 24 hours of rupturing the membranes. Risk factors for preterm rupture of membranes include infection and multiple gestations.

Patients may describe a gush of fluid from the vagina or a constant trickle or sense of wetness. Patients often misinterpret the normal leukorrhea of pregnancy, a whitish mucous discharge from the vagina, or stress incontinence as the rupture of membranes.

The Paramedic elects to redirect the ambulance to a hospital with a high risk neonatal intensive care unit. Just after arrival at the emergency department, the patient's membranes rupture, followed by severe pain and a gush of bright red bleeding. She is rushed to the obstetrical surgical suite.

Several days later, the case comes up for review by the County Pediatric Death Assessment Committee. The Paramedics are complimented overall for their timely care of the mother and, by extension, her fetus. Unfortunately, the fetus died secondary to placental abruption, likely caused by cocaine use.

CRITICAL THINKING QUESTIONS

1. What is the most appropriate transport decision that will get the patient to definitive care?
2. What are the advantages of transporting a patient with suspected preterm labor to a hospital with a high risk neonatal intensive care unit, even if that means bypassing other hospitals in the process?

Disposition

The patient with suspected placental abruption should be placed in the left lateral position, to avoid supine hypotensive syndrome, and transported to a facility that provides both obstetrical services and neonatal intensive care whenever possible.

CONCLUSION

Although most pregnancies are uncomplicated, the Paramedic may be called to assist a woman with a complication of her pregnancy. As discussed in this chapter, the complications range from bleeding and the loss of the pregnancy to trauma. An understanding of the common complications of pregnancy will help the Paramedic take excellent care of the pregnant patient.

KEY POINTS:

- Vaginal bleeding is a key indicator of preterm delivery.

- Vaginal bleeding in the first trimester may result from non-pregnancy-related illness or injury, hormonal changes, implantation of the fertilized egg, spontaneous abortion, or ectopic pregnancy.

- Vaginal bleeding in the second trimester may be due to infection or the result of cervical abnormalities.

- Vaginal bleeding during the third trimester tends to result from placental derangements (abruption or previa) or uterine rupture and damage.

- Placenta previa results from placental implantation low in the uterus or partially or completely covering the cervix.

- Placental abruption results from a normally implanted placenta separating prematurely from the wall of the uterus.

- Uterine rupture is rare but may occur along the scar of a previous cesarean section.

- Trauma in pregnancy tends to occur from one or more of the following causes:
  - Motor vehicle collision
  - Falls
  - Assault

- Three complications of pregnancy that primarily affect the mother are
  - Pregnancy-induced hypertension
  - Preeclampsia
  - HELLP: Hemolytic anemia, elevated liver enzymes, and low platelet count
  - Diabetes

- The Paramedic should include questions about the following topics when gathering a history from a mother experiencing complications of pregnancy:
  - Bleeding
  - Cramping or pelvic pain
    - Document contractions
  - Membranes rupturing
  - Bloody show
  - Fetal movement

- The Paramedic should assess the mother with complications of pregnancy for signs of shock.

- The most likely complication of pregnancy the Paramedic may encounter is preterm labor.

- Tocolytic agents include fluids, magnesium sulfate, and beta/adrenergic agonists.

1. What concerns should the Paramedic have for a woman with vaginal bleeding in the first trimester? Second trimester? Third trimester?
2. How does placental previa differ from placental abruption?
3. What are the three likely causes of trauma in pregnancy? What is the likely explanation for each of these causes?
4. How is HELLP related to preeclampsia?
5. State at least four medical history questions that should be asked of a mother experiencing complications in her pregnancy.
6. Name three agents that work to suppress labor.

Please refer to the Case Study in this chapter, and answer the questions below:

1. What are the clues that help the Paramedics differentiate previa from abruption and uterine rupture?
2. Briefly explain the mechanism for placental abruption following cocaine use.

REFERENCES:

1. Deterding R, Hay W, et al. *Current Pediatric Diagnosis and Treatment*. New York: McGraw-Hill Professional; 2008.
2. Menon R. Spontaneous preterm birth, a clinical dilemma: etiologic, pathophysiologic and genetic heterogeneities and racial disparity. *Acta Obstet Gynecol Scand*. 2008;87(6):590–600.
3. Noguchi A. Lowering the premature birth rate: what the U.S. experience means for Japan. *Keio J Med*. 2008;57(1):45–49.
4. Dogra V, Paspulati RM, et al. First trimester bleeding evaluation. *Ultrasound Q*. 2005;21(2):69–85; quiz 149–150, 153–154.
5. Valley VT. Ectopic pregnancy. Available at: **http://emedicine.medscape.com/article/796451-overview**. Accessed September 22, 2008.
6. Koifman A, Levy A, et al. The clinical significance of bleeding during the second trimester of pregnancy. *Arch Gynecol Obstet*. 2008;278(1):47–51.
7. Fox NS, Chervenak FA. Cervical cerclage: a review of the evidence. *Obstet Gynecol Surv*. 2008;63(1):58–65.
8. Woodring TC, Klauser CK, et al. When is a cerclage indicated for cervical insufficiency? A literature review. *J Miss State Med Assoc*. 2006;47(9):264–266.
9. Simcox R, Shennan A. Cervical cerclage in the prevention of preterm birth. *Best Pract Res Clin Obstet Gynaecol*. 2007;21(5):831–842.
10. Garner EI, Goldstein DP, et al. Gestational trophoblastic disease. *Clin Obstet Gynecol*. 2007;50(1):112–122.
11. Abu-Heija AT, El-Jallad F, et al. Placenta previa: effect of age, gravidity, parity and previous cesarean section. *Gynecol Obstet Invest*. 199;47(1):6–8.
12. To WW, Leung WC. Placenta previa and previous cesarean section. *Int J Gynaecol Obstet*. 1995;51(1):25–31.
13. Miller DA, Chollet JA, et al. Clinical risk factors for placenta previa-placenta accreta. *Am J Obstet Gynecol*. 1997;177(1):210–214.
14. Oyelese Y, Ananth CV. Placental abruption. *Obstet Gynecol*. 108(4):1005–1016.
15. Hladky K, Yankowitz J, et al. Placental abruption. *Obstet Gynecol Surv*. 2002;57(5):299–305.
16. Turner MJ, Agnew G, et al. Uterine rupture and labour after a previous low transverse cesarean section. *BJOG*. 2006;113(6):729–732.
17. Guise JM, McDonagh MS, et al. Systematic review of the incidence and consequences of uterine rupture in women with previous cesarean section. *BMJ*. 2004;329(7456):19–25.
18. Guise JM, Berlin M, et al. Safety of vaginal birth after cesarean: a systematic review. *Obstet Gynecol*. 2004;103(3):420–429.
19. Chames MC, Pearlman MD. Trauma during pregnancy: outcomes and clinical management. *Clin Obstet Gynecol*. 2008;51(2):398–408.
20. Hauswald M, Kerr NL. Perimortem cesarean section. *Acad Emerg Med*. 2000;7(6):726.
21. Lanoix R, Akkapeddi V, et al. Perimortem cesarean section: case reports and recommendations. *Acad Emerg Med*. 1995;2(12):1063–1067.
22. Granger JP, Alexander BT, et al. Pathophysiology of pregnancy-induced hypertension. *Am J Hypertens*. 2001;14(6 Pt 2):178S–185S.

23. Moodley J. The management of hypertension in pregnancy: A review. *S Afr Med J.* 1980;58(3):103–109.

24. Rudnicki M, Frolich A, et al. The effect of magnesium on maternal blood pressure in pregnancy-induced hypertension. A randomized double-blind placebo-controlled trial. *Acta Obstet Gynecol Scand.* 1991;70(6):445–450.

25. Lyall F. (ed). *Pre-eclampsia: Etiology and Clinical Practice.* New York: Cambridge University Press; 2007.

26. Kim C, Newton KM, et al. Gestational diabetes and the incidence of type 2 diabetes: a systematic review. *Diabetes Care.* 2002;25(10):1862–1868.

27. Hadden DR. Geographic, ethnic, and racial variations in the incidence of gestational diabetes mellitus. *Diabetes.* 1985;34 Suppl 2:8–12.

28. Chancellor J, Thorp JM, Jr. Blood pressure measurement in pregnancy. *BJOG.* 2008;115(9):1076–1077.

29. Miller RS, Thompson ML, et al. Trimester-specific blood pressure levels in relation to maternal pre-pregnancy body mass index. *Paediatr Perinat Epidemiol.* 2007;21(6):487–494.

30. Decherney A, Nathan L. *CURRENT Obstetric & Gynecological Diagnosis & Treatment.* Columbus, OH.: McGraw-Hill Medical; 2002.

31. Hearne AE, Nagey DA. Therapeutic agents in preterm labor: tocolytic agents. *Clin Obstet Gynecol.* 2000;43(4):787–801.

32. Gabbe S, Galan H, et al. *Obstetrics: Normal and Problem Pregnancies: Book.* Philadelphia, PA: Churchill Livingstone; 2007.

CHAPTER 37

NORMAL CHILDBIRTH

KEY CONCEPTS:

Upon completion of this chapter, it is expected that the reader will understand these following concepts:

- Childbirth as a natural process
- Potential complications to mother and child from childbirth
- Stages of labor and anatomical changes in each stage

ANATOMY CONCEPTS:

Prior to reading this chapter the Paramedic student should be familiar with the following anatomy and physiology concepts:

- Female reproductive system

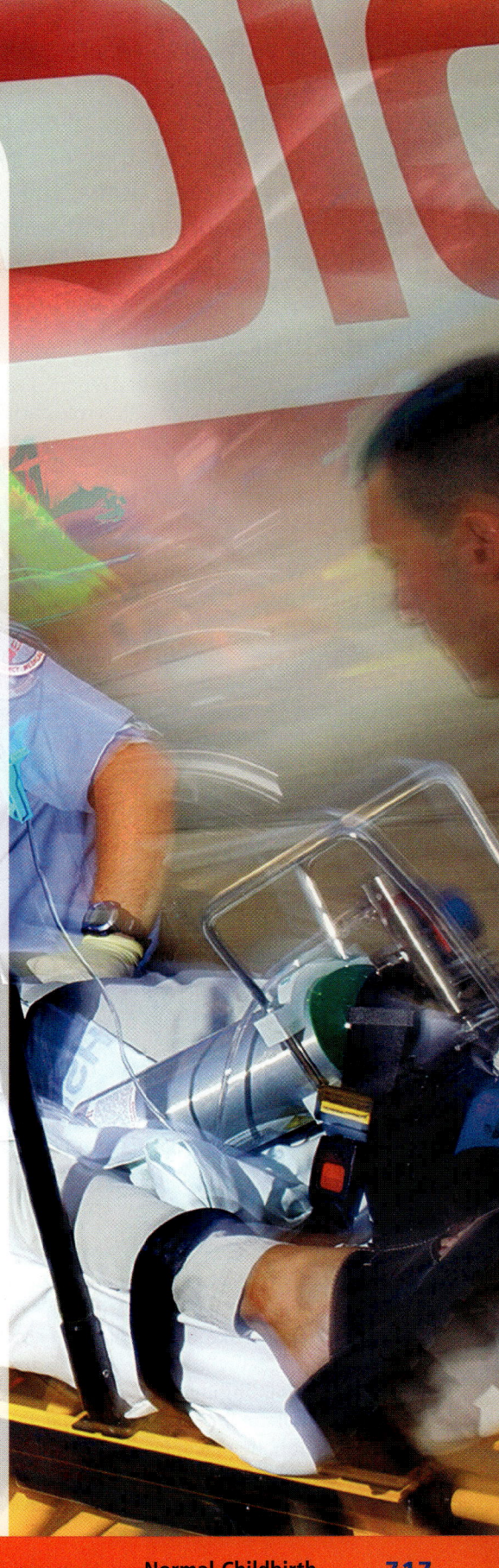

The Paramedics answer the phone and hear a woman screaming to the dispatchers. She is in her apartment with her 6-year-old son and 3-year-old daughter, and she has been having regular contractions for hours. Her boyfriend is unreachable by phone and her mother works an hour away. All her neighbors are at work and she can't leave the children to try to find anyone to take her to the birth center where she had planned to deliver the baby. While talking to the dispatcher, the woman can hardly get a full sentence out before another wave-like contraction peaks, and she is unable to speak. She states that her due date was the day before yesterday, and she thinks the baby is coming!

As the Paramedic drives to the address, her mind goes through the possible scenarios. Perhaps the patient is anxious because she is alone, and when the Paramedic arrives she can calm her down, assess the situation, and get her to the hospital. Hopefully, the Paramedic thinks, a neighbor or family member will also show up to take care of the other kids—best case scenario, maybe someone is already there. In any case, the Paramedic thinks that she should prepare to help the patient give birth because a third-time mother knows when a baby is coming, and she sounded convinced.

CRITICAL THINKING QUESTIONS

1. How do you assess a pregnant woman to see if she is ready to deliver?
2. How do you deliver in the field?

OVERVIEW

Although childbirth rarely happens in the field, the interest in home birth increases the likelihood that a Paramedic will be called upon to assist with a delivery.[1-3] Each home birth has a set of special circumstances that makes childbirth particularly challenging to the Paramedic. Fortunately, most childbirths require the Paramedic to do little more than assist and to be attentive to potential complications. If a complication occurs, the Paramedic should be prepared to intervene immediately for the sake of both mother and child.

Chief Concern

Childbirth is a natural process that requires very little intervention in most cases. The Paramedic's role during childbirth is to be aware of the normal childbirth processes and to intervene if a complication occurs. A review of the anatomy and physiology of pregnancy will precede the discussion of childbirth.

Anatomy and Physiology Review

During pregnancy, many organs change, and some new organs are created. Outwardly, the most obvious change in the body is the growing abdomen caused by an enlarging uterus. The uterus is a pear-shaped organ which has a top (fundus), a body, and the lower segment, which contains the cervix (a pair of openings or os). Early in the pregnancy, a mucous plug forms in the os and prevents infections from tracking from the vagina into the uterus. During labor, the cervix softens and thins (a process called effacement and dilation) so the infant may pass into the birth canal. At the onset of this process, the mucous plug is released and blood-tinged mucus, called the bloody show, flows.

The uterus is made up of three distinctive layers. The outermost layer, the **perimetrium**, is a serous membrane that envelops the uterus. The middle layer is a matrix of overlapping smooth muscles that allows forceful contraction during labor while the uterus shrinks, a process called **involution**. The innermost layer, the **endometrium**, provides nutrients to the fetus via the placenta. The opening of the uterus, the cervical os, leads to the vagina (the birth canal in lay terms). This muscular tube is distensible and capable of dilating to accommodate the infant during childbirth.

Organs Related to Pregnancy

Following ovulation and subsequent fertilization, which normally occurs in the distal one-third of the fallopian tube near the ampulla (a sac-like enlargement in the tube), the fertilized ovum (now called a zygote) travels to the uterus. In the uterus, the zygote implants, typically near the fundus of the uterus proximal to the entrance of the fallopian tube, and starts to develop the placenta.

The placenta serves three major functions. First, the placenta provides the nutrition for the developing fetus (the implanted zygote is now called a fetus). This transfer of oxygen and carbon dioxide, hormones and antibodies, electrolytes such as calcium, and by-products of metabolism (such as urea) is essential for fetal development.

The placenta also serves as an endocrine organ that secretes hormones. The first hormone secreted is beta human chorionic gonadotropin (beta-HCG), which stimulates placental growth. Next, the placenta secretes both progesterone (to support the pregnancy) and estrogen. Estrogen stimulates the growth of blood vessels (angiogenesis), particularly in the uterus and the milk glands, leading to breast enlargement. Toward the end of pregnancy, there is an imbalance in estrogen and progesterone. An increase in estrogen leads to labor. Conversely, a sudden decrease in progesterone may lead to premature labor as well as spontaneous abortion.[4]

Finally, the placenta acts as a barrier to potentially harmful substances. The placental barrier protects against infection by preventing microbes and some drugs from gaining access to the baby. However, the placental barrier does not prevent certain drugs, such as opiates, from crossing the placental barrier.

At full term, the placenta will weigh about one-sixth of the infant's weight and will appear as a disc-shaped mass of tissue with an umbilical stalk that emanates from approximately the midpoint. The umbilical cord typically has two smaller umbilical arteries and one large umbilical vein. The umbilical vein is responsible for carrying oxygenated, glucose-laden blood to the fetus. These three blood vessels, contained within a fibrous sheath, are surrounded by a protective gel called **Wharton's jelly**. At the time of childbirth, there may be as many as 40 twists in the umbilical cord but no knots. If a loop is formed and the fetus slips through the loop, then a knot would occur, essentially strangulating the fetus and causing a stillbirth.

The entire assembly—fetus, placenta, and umbilical cord—are contained within an **amniotic sac** (called the bag of waters in lay terms). Originating at the edges of the placenta, the amniotic sac contains about 1 liter of pressure-absorbing fluid. Excessive amniotic fluid causes a condition called **polyhydramnios**.[5] The amniotic fluid, which contains primarily water (98+%) as well as some fetal skin cells (used for analysis following an amniocentesis), is constantly replaced (about eight times a day) in order to maintain a hospitable environment for the fetus (Figure 37-1).

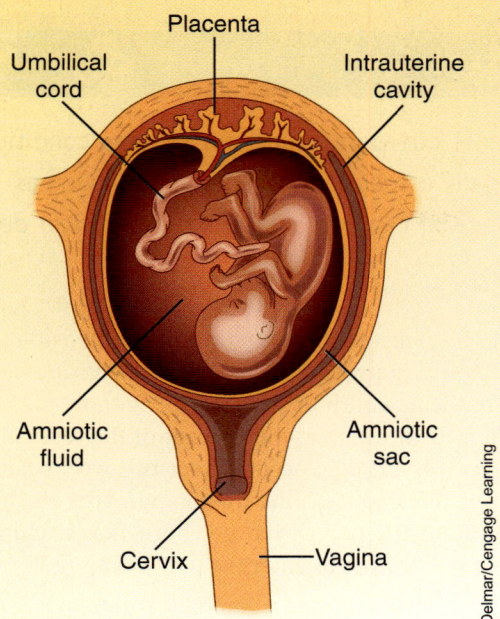

Figure 37-1 Organs of pregnancy.

Normal Childbirth

Childbirth is a normal physiologic process that most often requires little intervention by others beyond support of the laboring woman. Childbirth begins with labor, which is the result of the interplay of physiologic factors resulting in uterine contractions which cause cervical changes.

During the last four to eight weeks of pregnancy, most women will experience preparatory uterine contractions called **Braxton–Hicks contractions**. These are episodes of sporadic tightening of the abdomen or lower back that cause discomfort, but are usually tolerable for the woman. In labor, contractions intensify and become more frequent and more painful: They last longer and persist for hours. Generally, contractions have a beginning, a peak, and an end, with the resting tone of the uterus in between.

Labor is progressive, meaning that once regular contractions are established and cervical change has occurred, labor continues through several stages. These have been defined as first stage (which includes the latent and active phases), second stage, and third stage.

There are several signs of impending labor. The most noticeable may be **lightening**, the descent of the uterus deeper into the pelvis. Lightening usually occurs one to two weeks before the onset of labor in the first-time mother, and will happen sooner in the multigravida mother. Some women will note an increase in mucus-laden vaginal discharge, whereas others experience a burst of energy, colloquially referred to as the nesting syndrome, in anticipation of labor.

First Stage of Labor

Labor may start as the fetus settles into the pelvic outlet and the process of **effacement** (thinning of the cervix) and **dilation** (widening of the cervical os) occurs. This stage encompasses

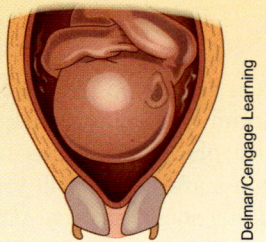

Figure 37-2 First stage of labor.

the time between the onset of progressive cervical change and complete dilation (often described as 10 centimeters). It is divided into a latent phase, which can last from several hours to several days, and an active phase, which is designated as the time from 4 centimeters dilation to complete dilation of the cervix (Figure 37-2).

The first sign of the latent phase that appears in the first stage of labor is the bloody show (secondary to discharge of the mucous plug) and the rupture of the bag of waters. It is important to remember that ruptured membranes are not universal. At this point, the woman starts to feel contractions—either regular or irregular—that signal the start of effacement and dilation. Contractions may last from 30 to 45 seconds in duration and may start out one-half minute apart and then increase in frequency. It is not uncommon for the woman to complain of lower back pain, abdominal cramps, and even experience diarrhea.

Figures most commonly used to define norms for the length of these designated stages of labor are controversial yet widely quoted. They are based on the work of Freidman, who described usual first stage labors as less than 20 hours for first-time mothers, and less than 14 hours for multiparas.[6] More recent data, however, places these estimates in question. Typical labors may be twice as long and still be considered within normal limits.

Second Stage of Labor

The second stage of labor extends from complete dilation of the cervix to birth of the baby. It is measured in terms of descent of the baby through the maternal pelvis, and depends on the strength of contractions, the position of the baby, and the expulsive, pushing efforts of the mother. The mother generally feels an urge to bear down and complains of pelvic pressure or the urge to defecate. This stage normally takes up to three hours for a first-time mother and 30 minutes to an hour in multiparas. However, there is great variability among women.

Third Stage of Labor

The third stage of labor lasts from the birth of the baby to birth of the placenta, which is discussed in detail shortly. The normal time interval of this stage is up to 30 minutes.[7] Signs of placental separation are bright red blood from the vagina, lengthening of the umbilical cord, and a change in the contour of the maternal abdomen. The mother delivers the placenta by pushing as she did for the baby, although the placenta generally requires less vigorous effort.

The Puerperium, or Fourth Stage of Labor

The **puerperium** is the period from the birth of the baby to six weeks postpartum. Critical physiological and psychological alterations take place during this time, most occurring within the first hours after childbirth for the mother and the newborn. During this stage maternal vital signs are checked regularly. Postpartum hemorrhage, one of the main causes of morbidity and mortality after childbirth, are most likely to happen within hours of the birth. Therefore, the mother is observed for blood loss and the firmness and size of the uterine fundus are watched carefully during this period.

The Cardinal Movements of Labor

The baby is an active participant in the birth process, maneuvering through what are called the **cardinal movements of labor** to achieve birth. These movements are engagement,

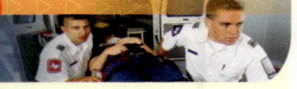

flexion, descent, internal rotation, and extension and external rotation (Figure 37-3). These movements are necessary in order for the newborn to be delivered without complication.

The first movement, the descent of the fetus, must occur before delivery. It may occur one or two weeks before delivery and is referred to as the lightening. After the baby drops into the mother's pelvis, the newborn flexes, chin to chest, allowing the occiput to enter the pelvic ring first.

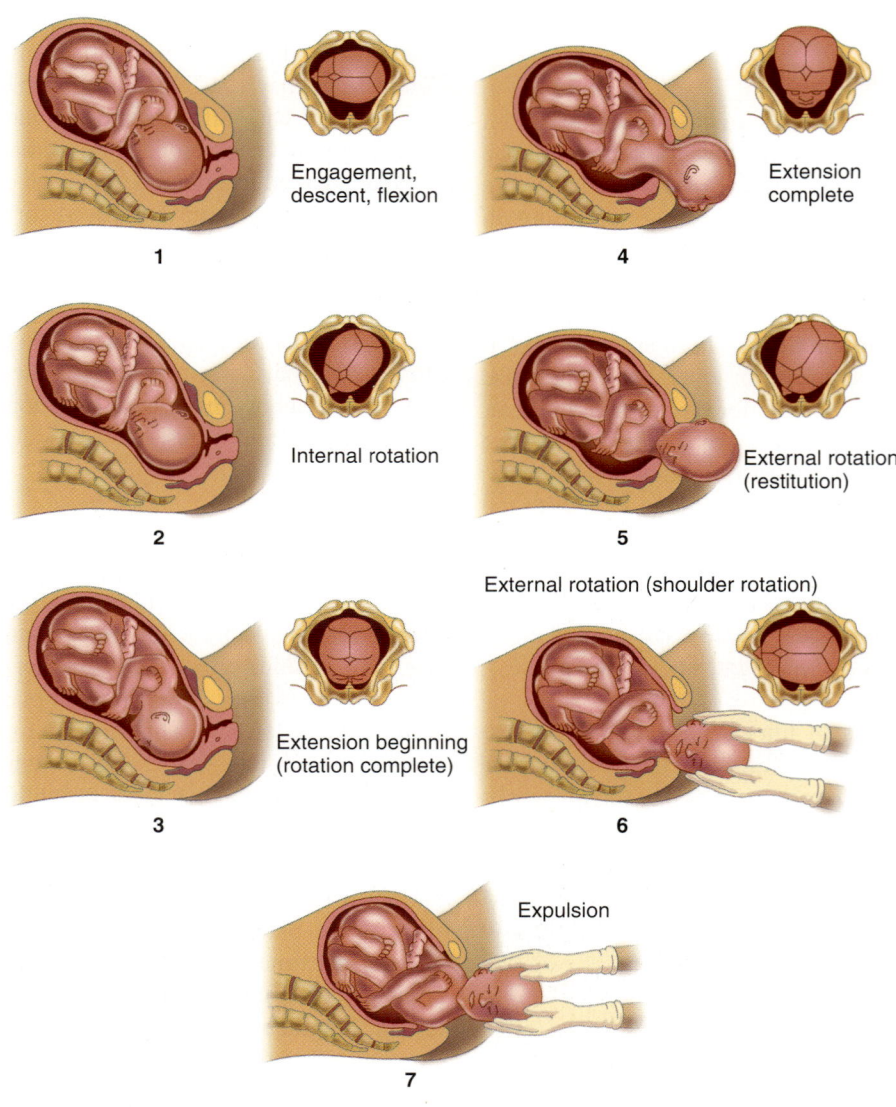

Figure 37-3 Cardinal movements of labor.

1 — Engagement, descent, flexion
2 — Internal rotation
3 — Extension beginning (rotation complete)
4 — Extension complete
5 — External rotation (restitution)
6 — External rotation (shoulder rotation)
7 — Expulsion

Delmar/Cengage Learning

Following flexion, the newborn's head is at the level of the ischial spine, referred to as zero station. At this point, the cervix is fully dilated and the birth is imminent. During this period of engagement, the fetus will rotate in an effort to pass the head through the pelvic opening. Most often the infant delivers with the occiput superior; however, if the newborn fails to rotate then the infant may be born face up, called occiput posterior.

Once the flexed head slips past the mother's pubic bone, the head naturally extends along the curvature of the birth canal and the head is delivered. With the head delivered, the last movement involves the newborn turning, called restitution, to deliver the shoulders under the pubic bone. Following external rotation, the newborn's body is delivered (i.e., expulsion), concluding the cardinal movements.

CASE STUDY (CONTINUED)

The Paramedic is met at the door by the caller's 6-year-old son who leads the Paramedic to the bedroom. The Paramedic finds the woman sitting on the edge of the bed, saying, "I think I just broke my water." The Paramedic, while donning gloves, asks if she can ask a few questions.

CRITICAL THINKING QUESTIONS

1. What are the important elements of the history that a Paramedic should obtain?
2. What are the important indicators of an impending delivery?

History

Following the primary assessment, the Paramedic should obtain a history of the pregnancy. On occasion, the Paramedic may need to obtain this history while performing the physical examination, owing to the urgency of the situation. Therefore, the Paramedic should be well practiced at obtaining a history of pregnancy.

History of Pregnancy and Labor

With a minor adaptation, the Paramedic can use the SAMPLE method of history gathering to obtain the history of the pregnancy. The first, and perhaps most natural, question is the estimated date of delivery (EDD). The EDD is useful in ascertaining if the infant will be premature, so the Paramedic may prepare accordingly.

The woman's chief concern is usually the labor, so the Paramedic's first question should regard when the labor started. Some women may be uncertain of when labor started, as the early symptoms can be nondescriptive flu-like symptoms instead of classic labor. The woman's degree of discomfort is highly variable, depending on cultural and psychological factors. The Paramedic should be accepting of the pain regardless of the pain level the woman describes.

The discomfort of labor is caused by a number of variables, each of which can be of differing intensity. A combination of cervical stretching; pressure on the nerve plexuses of the cervix; pressure on the muscles of the pelvic floor; pressure on the urethra, bladder, and rectum; as well as downward forces applying traction to the abdominal ligaments, all contrive to produce discomfort. It has been suggested that

one of the primary causes of labor pain is hypoxia of uterine muscles, secondary to muscular contractions.

The pain of labor is often described as a backache or menstrual-like cramps. However, back pain that does not change with position is suggestive of labor, not a backache, and is often accompanied by gastrointestinal cramping, nausea, and increased indigestion. Eventually the discomfort will radiate around to the abdomen, at which point the patient may recognize the onset of "true" labor.

The Paramedic should next determine the severity of the labor. A traditional 0 to 10 Likert scale can be used by the patient to quantify the pain (a range of 7 to 10 is typical of strong contractions). Next, the Paramedic should ask about the length of the contractions (duration) and the time between contractions. The timing of a contraction starts at the beginning of one contraction and ends with the start of the next contraction.

While asking about the medical conditions, the Paramedic should perform a risk assessment. Certain pregnancy-related conditions may make a mother more likely to have a complicated birth, so the Paramedic should ask about pregnancy-induced hypertension and/or pre-eclampsia. These conditions can lead to convulsions and eclampsia during labor or childbirth.

The Paramedic should also ask the patient about medications, being particularly alert for any potential teratogenic drugs and category D or category X drugs, such as valium, lithium, phenytoin, warfarin, and even birth control pills.[8–10] Delivery of an infant exposed to these drugs may be complicated by congenital anomaly.

The Paramedic should also inquire about diabetes, and particularly gestational diabetes. Risk factors for gestational diabetes include a history of prior stillbirth, polyhydramnios, a history of prior gestational diabetes (65% of patients with gestational diabetes have the disorder again in a subsequent pregnancy), and obesity. Complications of gestational diabetes include larger than average babies (creating difficulties with delivery) and increased risk of birth trauma and fetal hypoglycemia.

Next, the Paramedic should ask about previous deliveries, typically using the TPAL or GPA system of notation. If the woman is multipara, the Paramedic may anticipate a shorter labor and/or imminent childbirth. Asking about complications of previous deliveries, such as placenta previa or placental abruption, can help the Paramedic anticipate potential problems with this delivery.

The Paramedic should also inquire if the births were either vaginal or cesarean section. A previous cesarean section carries the attendant (but fortunately rare) risk of uterine rupture. What may be of greater importance is the reason for the cesarean section; for example, whether the infant was delivered by cesarean section because it was breech or a footling presentation is relevant to the present pregnancy.

Although asking about the last meal (an element of the AMPLE mnemonic) is important, the Paramedic should also consider asking the patient about her last prenatal visit. This question opens the door for further conversation about prenatal care and who is the nurse–midwife or obstetrician attending the patient.

The events preceding the labor typically include the **bloody show**, a discharge of blood-tinged mucus, and the rupture of the bag of waters. This rupture is sometimes described as a trickle, whereas others describe it as a gush of water. If the woman's bag of waters has ruptured, the Paramedic should ask about the quantity (was it copious or scant) as well as the quality. A port wine-colored fluid may lead the Paramedic to suspect placental abruption whereas a green-tinged fluid is suggestive of meconium staining (**meconium** is the infant's first bowel movement). Of particular concern is foul-smelling fluid, as this may indicate uterine infection. These events may be used to document the start of the labor.

Special Case of Premature Rupture of Membranes

A premature rupture of membranes occurs in about 3% of pregnancies.[11] The Paramedic's primary concern with premature rupture of membranes is infection. If the bag of waters ruptures prematurely (i.e., two or more hours before labor), there is a greater risk of uterine infection. A **premature rupture of membranes (PROM)** (a rupture of the bag of waters before the expected date of delivery) can signal a premature birth. In fact, upwards of 40% of premature births begin with premature rupture of membranes.

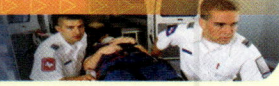

STREET SMART

Some women have difficulty distinguishing the amniotic fluid from urine. Urine is generally acidotic whereas amniotic fluid is alkaline. Using litmus paper, the Paramedic can distinguish urine from amniotic fluid because the litmus paper will turn blue.

CASE STUDY (CONTINUED)

The patient says, "I think it's coming!" At this point, the Paramedic asks if she could please examine the patient. The patient, now squatting at the end of the bed, agrees and hops onto the edge of the bed and lays back. At the vaginal orifice, the Paramedic sees a round scalp with a tuft of hair and prepares for an imminent delivery.

CRITICAL THINKING QUESTIONS
1. What are the elements of the predelivery physical examination of a patient?
2. Why is a vaginal assessment for crowning a critical element in this examination?

Examination

The primary assessment proceeds similar to all other examinations. Although childbirth should not be viewed as a medical emergency, the Paramedic should nevertheless focus on supporting the mother's airway, breathing, and circulation. There is some debate whether the Paramedic needs to provide high-flow, high-concentration oxygen or establish intravenous access in this situation. However, the Paramedic should be prepared to do so if needed.

Although a comprehensive review of systems and physical examination would be ideal, obtaining one will depend upon the situation. The Paramedic should use judgment to ascertain what is most pertinent given the situation at hand, and focus the examination accordingly.

It is essential that the Paramedic, before anything else, protect the patient's modesty, maintain a degree of privacy, and be empathetic. Childbirth, especially for a first-time mother, is a time of great anticipation and excitement. A misspoken word can be devastating to the patient–Paramedic relationship.

With proper draping in place, the Paramedic should start by examining the abdomen, looking for cesarean scars and inspecting for fetal movements. Next, the Paramedic should attempt to listen for fetal heart tones, if possible. The infant's heart rate should be almost too fast to count (usually greater than 140 beats per minute). A fetal heart rate of <120 beats per minute (bpm) may indicate an infant in distress. The Paramedic should immediately consider the possibility of a prolapsed cord or placental insufficiency secondary to either abruption of the placenta or placenta previa. Fetal bradycardia (<120 bpm) is a medical emergency. The mother should be placed in the left lateral recumbent, or side-lying, position; given high-flow, high-concentration oxygen; and transported immediately. Almost every emergency department is capable of performing an emergency cesarean section, if needed.[12]

As part of the abdominal examination, the Paramedic should palpate the abdomen. The Paramedic proceeds first to Leopold's maneuvers to determine the lie of the infant (whether the infant is side-lying or breech).[13] Estimating fundal height, for purposes of determining fetal age and development, is inaccurate at this stage. While one hand is on the abdomen, the Paramedic assesses the strength of contractions and determines the duration of contraction. A strong contraction should not allow the Paramedic to indent the abdomen.

On occasion, the Paramedic may also appreciate fetal movement. Although the absence of fetal movement during the third trimester may have ominous implications, fetal movement usually decreases during labor. Therefore, the presence—or absence—of fetal movements is a spurious finding.

With proper draping in place and the patient's privacy foremost in the Paramedic's mind, the Paramedic should

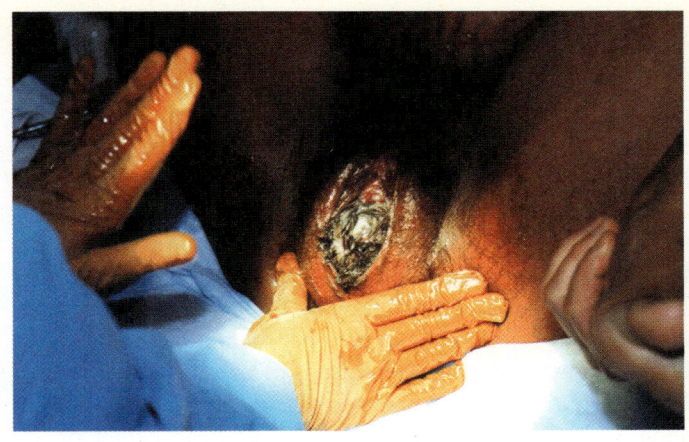

Figure 37-4 Crowning.

examine the patient's vagina. First, the external genitalia should be examined for evidence of vaginal bleeding, suggestive of placenta previa. If the patient experienced PROM, the Paramedic should immediately assess for a prolapsed cord. Next, the Paramedic should examine the vagina for bulging of the perineum and/or rectum. This may indicate the infant has started the descent into the birth canal. A widening of the vaginal opening during contractions, and the appearance of the top (crown) of the infant's head (called crowning), implies imminent delivery (Figure 37-4).

In some rare cases, the Paramedic may see a yellowish balloon-like protrusion during contractions. This is the amniotic sac (bag of waters). The fact that the mother has not ruptured the bag of waters is not a cause for concern as it may either rupture naturally or may need to be ruptured by the Paramedic during delivery.

Although nurse–midwives and physicians often perform an internal bimanual examination to determine cervical dilation, Paramedics typically do not perform this examination in the field. This is, in part, to reduce the risk of infection—especially if the bag of waters has ruptured—by minimizing the number of internal examinations.

CASE STUDY (CONTINUED)

The Paramedic is convinced that the child's birth is going to occur before they can get to the hospital and thus she prepares for a home delivery. While asking the mother what position she would prefer to deliver in, she prepares the birthing kit.

CRITICAL THINKING QUESTIONS

1. What is the significance of the crowning?
2. Why did the Paramedic ask the mother what position she would prefer to be in for the delivery?

Assessment

A pregnant patient's urge to push, or to move her bowels, coupled with crowning, is indicative of imminent delivery. As noted previously, first-time mothers may take up to three hours of pushing to give birth in what is considered a normal labor. Therefore, determining whether birth is imminent so as to prepare for birth or to make the decision to transport to the hospital or birth center depends on a number of factors.

If the patient is a primigravida; has not had strong, regular contractions; has not ruptured her membranes; has had no bloody show; and denies sensations of pressure or an urge to bear down, the decision is rather straightforward. The patient should be transported to the hospital or birth center of her choice.

If, on the other hand, the woman is a multipara, has a history of previous rapid labors, and is telling the Paramedic that the baby is coming, the Paramedic should prepare for a delivery. Most decisions are not as clear-cut as the scenarios just described. However, best judgment must be used, keeping the safety and welfare of the mother and child foremost in the Paramedic's mind. Delivery in the back of a moving ambulance is not an ideal situation and should be avoided whenever possible.

An irresistible urge to bear down or push signals the second stage of labor and eventually birth. Imminent birth is suspected when rectal bulging, perineal bulging, defecation, and/or progressive visibility of the fetal head are observed.

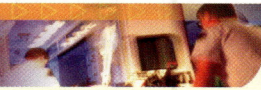

PROFESSIONAL PARAMEDIC

Many women attend childbirth classes and learn breathing techniques to help them cope with the discomfort and pain of labor. The Paramedic may elect to permit the patient's birthing companion to accompany the patient so that the patient may utilize the breathing techniques. The birthing companion should use proper restraints to avoid injury during transport.

CASE STUDY (CONTINUED)

After advising communications of a field delivery, the Paramedic prepares for the childbirth. Her EMT partner retrieves the shower curtain for the floor, gets several gowns from the ambulance, and retrieves every towel he can get his hands on and then starts to take the mother's vital signs.

CRITICAL THINKING QUESTIONS

1. What is the standard of care for childbirth?
2. What are some of the patient-specific concerns that the Paramedic should consider when preparing to deliver in the field?

Treatment

The woman should be given as much privacy as possible. She will likely be apprehensive, frightened, and in great discomfort, and her family will be very anxious. The Paramedic must reassure, comfort, and support the patient.

The Paramedic should protect the woman from exposure as much as possible. A sheet, blankets, or even a shower curtain may be placed underneath her, with towels rolled up to support her, and pillows or blankets placed where she finds them most comfortable. She may be on a bed, on the floor, or wherever she feels safe. She should be encouraged to assume a position that she finds most acceptable, while avoiding being flat on her back. Although lying supine in the lithotomy position may be convenient to the Paramedic, it is not—physiologically speaking—the best position for the patient. A good position for the mother to be in is the lateral recumbent position (Sim's position). Alternatively, the patient may prefer to squat, or sit on the edge of a chair. This position takes advantage of gravity and helps the pelvis widen.

During normal uterine contractions, there is a rise in central venous pressure, arterial pressure, and stroke volume and a reflexive decrease in pulse rate. These changes are magnified in the supine position, and minimized in the lateral recumbent position. In the lateral recumbent position, the woman herself (or a support person) may hold up her anterior leg behind the knee.

Another option is a semi-seated or semi-Fowler's position. As long as the supine position is avoided (due to risk of maternal supine hypotension), any position that the woman finds comfortable is encouraged.

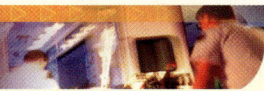
The expectant mother should be spoken to calmly, with respect, and allowed to birth in the way that works for her. She needs little direction; for example, she does not need to be coached to "push" or to "breathe," as often is seen in depictions of childbirth. Her body will do what it needs to do.

Preparations

The Paramedic should make routine preparations; for example, providing suction and an emesis basin. Many women in labor experience nausea, especially if lying flat. High-flow, high-concentration oxygen should be available on standby. In addition, equipment for neonatal resuscitation (discussed in Chapter 39) should be available.

As previously mentioned, there is some controversy about intravenous access. Under emergency conditions, such as a precipitous delivery, it may be prudent for the Paramedic to establish an intravenous access with a liter of normal saline solution available in case the patient becomes hypotensive and/or requires medication.

Equipment should be set up (on a sterile field, if possible), including clamps (at least two are ideal), scissors for cutting the umbilical cord, a bulb syringe, oxygen and suction (if available), equipment for neonatal resuscitation, extra towels or pads, and personal protective equipment (Table 37-1). Adequate lighting should be provided as well since illumination is important.

As the Paramedic prepares to assist with the delivery, she should take full body substance isolation precautions, including eye protection (either goggles or face shield), a fluid repellent gown, and examination gloves. The Paramedic can anticipate encountering blood, amniotic fluid, stool, and urine during the delivery process.

Table 37-1 Childbirth Preparation

- Privacy drapes (sheets)
- Gauze pads
- Cord clamps
- Scalpel or umbilical scissors (preferred)
- Sanitary pads
- Plastic bag with tie wrap (for placenta)
- Towels (drying)
- Bulb syringe
- Meconium aspirator
- Oxygen with tubing (blow-by oxygen)

The area immediately surrounding the patient's area should be covered with absorbent material such as towels, trauma dressings, and even newspaper if nothing else is available. Then, a clean sheet should be placed under the patient's buttocks.

Vaginal Birth

First, the patient should be assured that the process of childbirth is natural. The Paramedic should position herself to be able to completely visualize the birth canal and therefore be most able to help with delivery. The patient should be encouraged to use breathing techniques such as panting and blowing to control the delivery. Normally, the mother will bear down with contractions.

As the head starts to emerge (crowning), the Paramedic should place a gauze pad against the perineum and apply gentle counterpressure with the pads of the fingers. This will allow for a slower distention of the perineum, reducing the risk of perineal lacerations. Some Paramedics may place the index finger just inside the birth canal and gently rub back and forth to help thin the perineum and to help prevent tears; this is referred to as *ironing* the perineum.

If the amniotic sac is still intact and bulging through the vaginal opening, it may be necessary for the Paramedic to grasp the sac with a pair of forceps (or, if necessary, even the thumb and forefinger) and gently twist the sac to tear it. If the sac will not tear, the Paramedic can use a scalpel. However, great caution must be exercised to avoid cutting the newborn.

As the newborn begins to crown in a normal head first, or **vertex delivery**, the Paramedic should provide gentle pressure on the occiput or top of the baby's head to slow flexion. However, she should avoid applying any pressure to the fontanels. With a towel draped over the dominant hand, the Paramedic should allow the head to gradually extend, by exerting gentle control on the newborn's chin, while being careful not to impede the progress of the head with overly aggressive counterpressure (called the **Ritgen maneuver**).

Once the head is born, the Paramedic supports the newborn's head in one hand by sliding it below the baby's neck, and uses the other hand to feel below the neck, sweeping in both directions to feel for the umbilical cord and determine whether the umbilical cord is around the baby's neck. If an umbilical cord is present around the neck, called a **nuchal cord**, the Paramedic has to judge whether the cord is tightly or loosely wrapped around the neck. If the cord is loose, it should be slipped over the baby's head. If the cord is too tight to slip over the baby's head, but loose enough to move (not tight around the neck), the umbilical cord should be slipped over the shoulders as the baby's body is born. Alternately, if this cannot be done but the cord has some slack or looseness to it, the Paramedic can keep the baby's head close to the perineum as the body is born and, literally, somersault the baby as it is delivered. This will allow the Paramedic to untangle the cord after the body is born.

If the cord is too tight and not reducible (i.e., it is not possible to deliver the baby "through" the cord by guiding it past the shoulders or somersaulting the baby), the only option available is double clamping and cutting the cord before the baby is born.[14,15] The mother is directed to pant or blow during this maneuver, so that the cord may be double clamped, cut, and unwound from the neck prior to the birth of the body. Once the newborn's head is out of the birth canal, a bulb syringe may be used to suction the baby's mouth and then the nose.

At this point the baby will change position to permit delivery of the shoulder and will externally rotate. The Paramedic supports the baby's head by placing a hand underneath it, without directing the head in any direction. Unless the umbilical cord has been cut, there is no reason to interfere with the progression of the delivery. If the umbilical cord has been cut, the Paramedic should direct the mother to push to evoke a more rapid birth of the body.

Once the baby rotates, the Paramedic cradles the head on either side, providing very gentle downward and outward pressure to allow for the delivery of the anterior shoulder. Then she directs the body upward to allow delivery of the posterior shoulder.

The Paramedic will slide the posterior hand down the baby's body as the body delivers, keeping the head supported by the other hand or the forearm. She then places the baby immediately on the mother's abdomen, skin-to-skin, and dries the baby with a clean towel. The Paramedic then sets the towel aside and places another dry towel or blanket over the baby. Assessment of the newborn takes place immediately, as described in Chapter 38 (**Skill 37-1**).

For a step-by-step demonstration of Emergency Childbirth, please refer to Skill 37-1 on pages 732–734.

Special Case of Meconium

During gestation, the fetus forms a plug to prevent passage of stool while in the uterus. This first stool is called meconium. When a fetus is distressed, the meconium plug may pass into the amniotic fluid, staining it yellow, green, and even black-green. Upon delivery, the Paramedic may note the presence of meconium staining.

The decision to routinely suction an infant's airway upon delivery is often a matter of local protocols. Suctioning may unnecessarily stimulate a vagally induced bradycardia. However, in the presence of meconium staining the Paramedic should clear the airway.[16]

In extreme cases, the meconium may be so viscous, like pea soup, that it causes an obstruction, in which case the Paramedic may be required to intubate the newborn using a meconium aspirator (discussed in Chapter 39 on neonatal resuscitation). Meconium aspiration can result in significant neonatal hypoxia, brain injury, and meconium aspiration syndrome. **Meconium aspiration syndrome** consists of airway obstruction, disruption of the surfactant fluid coating that helps keep the alveoli open, a chemically induced inflammation of the lungs, and pulmonary hypertension.

Shoulder Dystocia

On rare occasions, the newborn's shoulders will fail to deliver through the pelvic outlet, known as **shoulder dystocia**. This problem is more common in large newborns (e.g., those born to diabetic mothers). The difficulty occurs when the umbilical cord becomes compressed during each fruitless contraction, leading to neonatal hypoxia.

One sign of shoulder dystocia is the "turtle sign." As the newborn is delivered, the head suddenly retracts after a contraction. If this happens, it is important that the Paramedic not apply forceful downward pressure in an effort to free the shoulder. Excessive traction can injure the brachial plexus and cause permanent injury such as wrist drop.

There are two maneuvers which the Paramedic may perform to free the shoulder.[17,18] In the first maneuver, called the **McRoberts maneuver**, the mother pulls her knees to her chest, along each side of the abdomen, to maximize the pelvic opening. This maneuver can increase the diameter of the pelvic opening by 30%. With the mother in this position, the Paramedic applies suprapubic pressure while another Paramedic applies gentle downward pressure to free the shoulder.

If this is unsuccessful, then the Paramedic may consider placing two fingers into the vagina, along the fetal scapula, and slowly rotating the posterior shoulder one half turn, in a corkscrew fashion, as the mother bears down. This maneuver, referred to as "Wood's corkscrew maneuver," should only be performed if a McRoberts maneuver fails as there is a risk of neck injury for the newborn.

When assisting a newborn in delivery, the Paramedic should avoid the temptation to try and "hook" the newborn under the arms and provide traction. Pressure to the newborn's nerve plexus in the upper extremity can lead to paralysis.

Breech Delivery

Whenever the presenting part of the newborn is not the head, then the delivery is considered breech. **Breech delivery** is, at best, a mechanical problem and, at worst, a potential cause of infant hypoxia. Fortunately, only about 3% to 4% of deliveries are breech.

Breech deliveries are placed in three categories. **Frank breech**, which makes up about 65% of all breech deliveries, starts with the buttocks presenting first, with the newborn's hips flexed and the knees extended. In a **complete breech**, which makes up about 10% of all breech deliveries, both hips and knees are flexed (Figure 37-5). The last category is the **incomplete breech**, which makes up about 25% of all breech deliveries. In an incomplete breech, either one leg (i.e., single footling) or both legs (double footling) presents.

One of the dangers of the breech delivery is a prolapse of umbilical cord, leading to cord compression and subsequent fetal hypoxia. Incomplete footling breeches have the highest incidence of prolapsed cords.

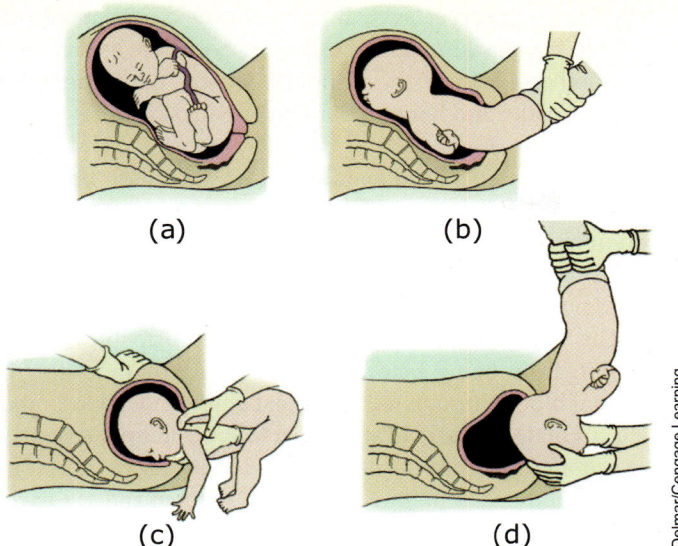

(a)   (b)

(c)   (d)

Figure 37-5 Birth of fetus in complete breech presentation. (a) Descent and internal rotation. (b) Extension of fetal back under symphysis (towel on legs used for traction). (c) Paramedic maintains head flexion by putting pressure on lower face with fingers of left hand (suprapubic pressure is applied by assistant to keep fetal head flexed). (d) Assistant holds fetal legs with towel while Paramedic assists the face and head over the perineum.

The Paramedic should suspect a breech delivery if the fetal heart sounds can be heard above the level of the umbilicus. Upon inspection of the vagina for crowning, the Paramedic may note either the fetus's feet or buttocks presenting.

Breech delivery can be performed in the field, especially if the newborn is small (less than 3,600 grams) and there is complete dilation of the cervix. However, unless conditions absolutely prevent transport to a childbirth center, the Paramedic should not deliver a breech infant in the field. Tocolysis should be considered instead.

If delivery is unavoidable, and the buttocks have entered the birth canal, then the Paramedic should encourage the mother to bear down and allow the buttocks to deliver. When the buttocks and lower back are visible, the Paramedic can hold the buttocks in one hand while gently delivering the legs with the other by grasping the legs with the forefinger in a hook-like fashion. With the legs delivered, the Paramedic should hold the newborn's hips for support (Figure 37-6).

If the newborn's arms are felt along the chest, the Paramedic should allow the arms to deliver spontaneously and only assist when necessary. After the first arm delivers, the newborn's buttocks should be raised to allow the other arm to deliver. If the arm(s) do not deliver, then the Paramedic may need to assist, using the forefinger as a hook and grasping the arm at the elbow.

If both arms are above the newborn's head, then the Paramedic will need to perform **Lovset's maneuver** (Figure 37-7).

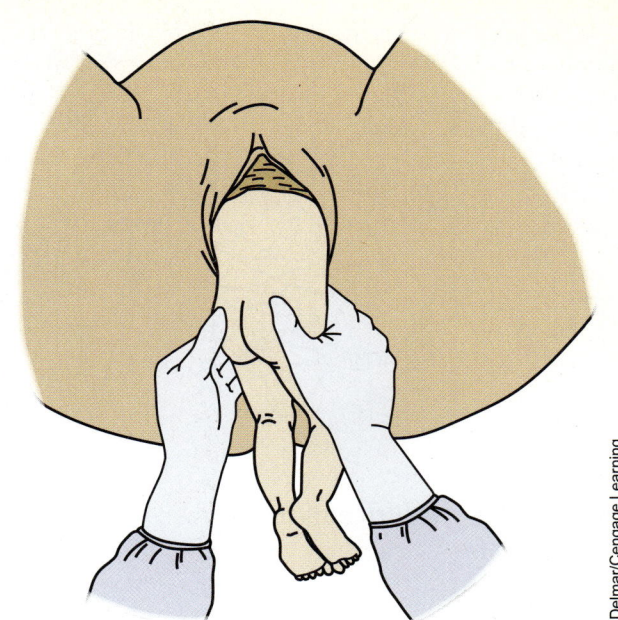

Figure 37-6 Supporting the hips.

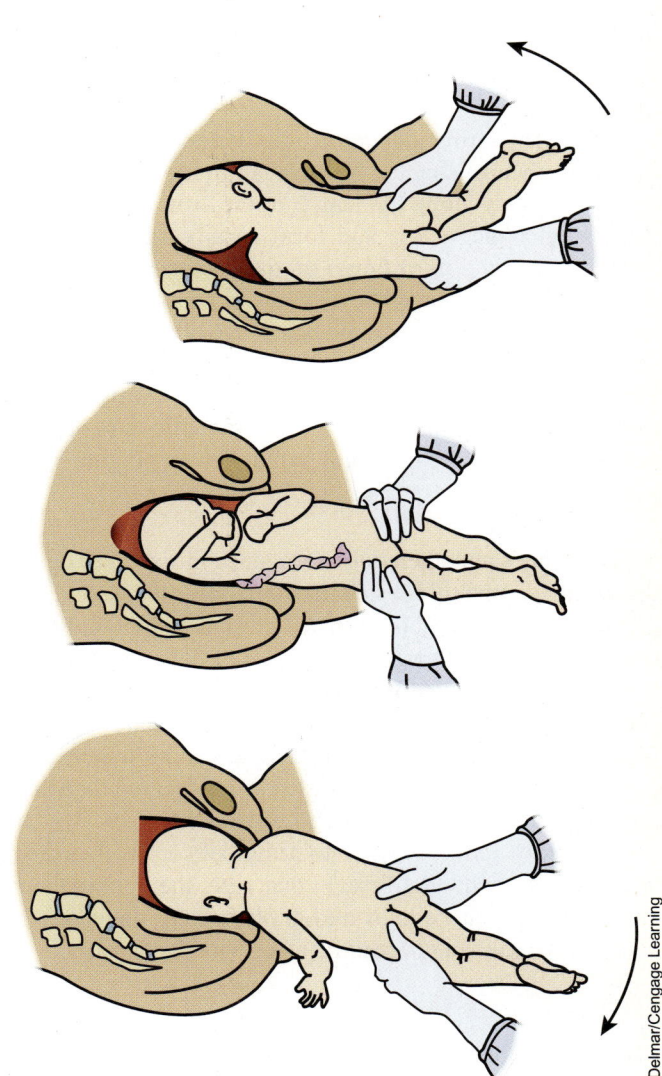

Figure 37-7 Lovset's maneuver.

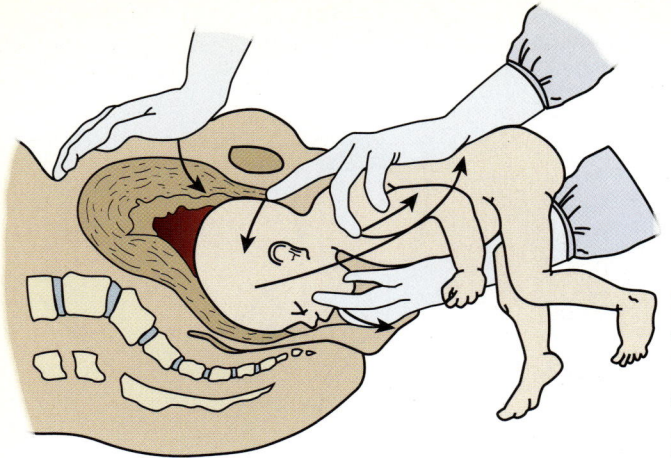

Figure 37-8 Mauriceau maneuver.

Holding the newborn by the hips, the Paramedic turns the newborn in a one-half circle, like a corkscrew, while applying downward pressure. This allows the formerly posterior arm to deliver anteriorly and to pass under the pubis. The Paramedic then reverses the corkscrew maneuver and delivers the other arm.

With the arms delivered, the Paramedic prepares to deliver the head, using the **Mauriceau maneuver**. Laying the newborn's body along the length of the arm, the Paramedic's fingers enter the vagina and form an airway for the infant. With the first and third finger on the newborn's cheekbones, and the second finger in the newborn's mouth and pulling the jaw downward, the Paramedic places the other hand on top of the newborn, grasping the shoulders in a pincer-like maneuver. Another assistant then places downward pressure above the mother's pubic bone, while the Paramedic raises the newborn's body until the nose and mouth deliver (Figure 37-8).

Multiple Gestation

If the mother's abdomen does not reduce in size after delivery, the Paramedic should consider the possibility of a second infant. Although the delivery of twins is unusual and the delivery of triplets in the field is rare, the process of delivery remains the same. The Paramedic must be prepared to provide supportive care to a number of newborns as well as neonatal resuscitation (discussed in Chapter 39), as multiple gestations tend to deliver prematurely. The Paramedic must also be prepared for a breech delivery as at least one infant will be breech.

The only addition of the footling delivery is the obvious need to deliver the feet first. In that case, the Paramedic first ensures both feet are delivered, pulling them down gently if necessary, and then proceeding as previously described.

Immediate Postdelivery Care

Once the newborn's body is clear of the birth canal, the Paramedic should firmly grasp the newborn's ankles and shoulders to lift the newborn and then place it on the mother's abdomen.

This maneuver serves several purposes. One, it removes the newborn from accumulated fluids (newborns are at great risk for hypothermia from drying fluid). Second, the skin-to-skin contact on the mother's abdomen provides warmth to the newborn.

The newborn's head should be lower than the body and the baby placed on its side, to permit passive drainage of secretions. At no time should traction be pulled on the umbilical cord. If the umbilical cord is too short, then the infant should not be placed on the mother's abdomen.

The Paramedic should exercise caution to prevent the newborn from being below the mother. Retrograde flow of maternal blood through the umbilical cord can lead to immediate circulatory overload and **hyperbilirubinemia**, an excessive amount of bilirubin in the blood that makes the infant appear jaundiced. The time of delivery is noted and sex of the infant is often announced as the Paramedic prepares to enter the last (third) stage of labor.

▷▷▷▷▷▷▷▷▷▷▷▷▷
CULTURAL/REGIONAL DIFFERENCES

If delivery takes place during transport to the hospital, the Paramedic should note the location as well as the time. Some states register births by the parish or county in which the child was born.

Newborn Care

With the newborn on the mother's abdomen, the Paramedic should vigorously dry the newborn with a towel. This serves the two-fold purpose of drying the infant (and thereby preventing hypothermia) as well as stimulating the newborn. If the newborn needs more stimulation to encourage it to breathe, then the Paramedic may elect to rub the newborn's back or smartly flick the soles of the newborn's feet. It is not appropriate for a Paramedic to grasp a newborn by the heels, invert it, and slap it on the buttocks, as use of force in this fashion can cause spinal cord damage.

Hypothermia

Hypothermia is a potential life-threat to a newborn. Newborns cannot shiver; therefore, the Paramedic must take affirmative steps to prevent hypothermia and to increase the newborn's temperature.

Signs of hypothermia in a newborn include irritability, then lethargy, pallor, bradycardia, and respiratory distress. Most newborns will have **acrocyanosis** (cyanosis of the extremities). This is the result of a combination of hypothermia and inadequate circulation and is generally not a cause for concern unless it progresses to central cyanosis. The effects of cold stress on the newborn include hypoglycemia, hypoxia, and acidosis.

To prevent cold stress, the newborn should be towel dried completely. A large portion of the infant's heat is lost from the head and neck. Therefore, placing a stockinet cap and draping a dry blanket over the newborn's head and shoulders can greatly improve the situation.

Clamping and Cutting the Umbilical Cord

Normally there is no need for the Paramedic to clamp and cut the umbilical cord immediately. However, the umbilical cord is clamped and cut immediately if the baby requires neonatal resuscitation (discussed in Chapter 39).[19] Otherwise, there may be benefits to delayed cord clamping, as long as the newborn is not held high above the mother's abdomen, resulting in blood loss from the newborn, or well below the maternal abdomen.

When ready to clamp and cut the cord, the Paramedic should palpate the cord. When pulsations cease, the Paramedic clamps the cord by placing two instrument clamps, commonly called Kelly clamps, in place. Some Paramedics prefer the use of silk tape over Kelly clamps as an umbilical tie. The clamps should be placed approximately 4 to 6 inches from the infant's abdomen, this length permits surgical revision of the umbilical cord later. The Paramedic may also need to access the umbilical vein during neonatal resuscitation. Finally, the neonatologist may need a sample of blood from the umbilical cord for analysis. With enough room between the clamps to allow for cutting of the cord, with either umbilical scissors (preferred) or a scalpel, the cord should be cut. In some instances, the mother's birth attendant or significant other may wish to cut the cord.

The umbilical cord should not be "milked" (stripped of blood). Milking the cord, and destroying red blood cells in the process, may contribute to hyperbilirubinemia later. Once an umbilical clamp, or tie, is in place, it should not be removed unless the Paramedic is attempting to access the umbilical vein with an umbilical catheter during a neonatal resuscitation.

APGAR Scoring

In the 1920s, Dr. Virginia Apgar developed a simple scoring method for purposes of trending a newborn's progress. This scale, called the APGAR score, takes into account the newborn's **A**ppearance, the newborn's **P**ulse, reactivity via facial **G**rimace, **A**ctivity as a function of muscle tone, and **R**espirations. These elements are rated on a 0 to 2 scale at one minute following birth and at five minutes of life (Table 37-2). There is more discussion of the APGAR score in Chapter 38 on newborn care.

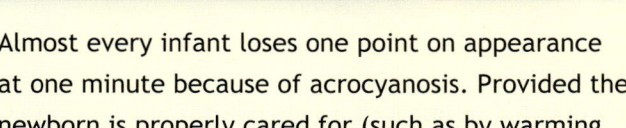

STREET SMART

Almost every infant loses one point on appearance at one minute because of acrocyanosis. Provided the newborn is properly cared for (such as by warming and drying), the score should be 10 at five minutes.

Delivery of the Placenta

The last stage of labor is the delivery of the placenta. The placenta usually separates from the uterine wall within 5 to 10 minutes after the baby is born; however, up to 30 minutes is considered to be within normal limits. Signs of placental separation include a small trickle or sudden gush of blood and/or lengthening of the umbilical cord as it extrudes from the vagina. The Paramedic may note a change in the shape or contour of the fundus, and the woman may report a sense of fullness or urge to bear down again as well.

Aggressive traction on the umbilical cord must be avoided, as it may result in pulling the cord off the placenta, leaving the placenta behind. As a result, hemorrhage (and in rare cases, inversion of the uterus) could occur.

The Paramedic should "guard" the uterus by placing a hand above the symphysis pubis on the mother's abdomen. The Paramedic should not massage the uterus at this time. Instead, the Paramedic should encourage the woman to push. If the placenta does not deliver after several pushes, and the woman is not bleeding excessively, the Paramedic should stop, allow the mother to rest, and try again in a few minutes. As long as vital signs are stable and there is no evidence of excessive bleeding, a normal third stage may last up to 30 minutes. If the delivery of the placenta

Table 37-2 APGAR Score

Item Assessed	Score		
	0	1	2
Appearance	Blue, pale	Body pink, extremities blue	Completely pink (light skinned); absence of cyanosis (dark skinned)
Pulse	Absent	Slow (<100)	Over 100
Grimace	No response	Grimace	Cry, cough, or sneeze
Muscle activity	Flaccid	Some flexion of extremities	Well flexed
Respiratory rate	Absent	Slow, weak cry	Good cry

is progressing slower than expected (greater than 30 minutes), the Paramedic may ask the mother to squat in an upright position to allow gravity to assist in the delivery of the placenta.

Once the placenta is delivered, the Paramedic should examine the margins of the placenta. The margins should be relatively smooth and make a complete oval or circular shape.

An incomplete placental detachment leaves partial products of conception in the uterus. Placental fragments can bleed, resulting in life-threatening hemorrhage.[20] The Paramedic should note the time of the delivery of the placenta and then place the placenta in a rip-proof plastic bag to be delivered with the mother and child to the hospital for inspection by the physician.

CASE STUDY (CONTINUED)

The first Paramedics to arrive call for a second unit and police to assist. A quick evaluation shows that the mother has already delivered the infant on the floor of the bathroom onto towels and a blanket. The infant is crying and remains attached to the placenta by an intact umbilical cord. The placenta appears torn and the mother is bleeding profusely from the vagina. She asks weakly about her baby.

One Paramedic takes care of clamping and cutting the cord, then wrapping and warming a baby girl. The other medic assesses the fundus of the mother. It is very soft and does not firm up with massage. The Paramedic notes that as the mother asked about her baby, she seemed to have difficulty breathing. After the delivery of a healthy female infant and the placenta, the Paramedic goes about preparing to transport the patient to the hospital. She notices that the mother continues to bleed despite fundal massage. She suggests to the mother that she put the baby to breast and encourage suckling. After a few minutes, the bleeding still has not stopped.

CRITICAL THINKING QUESTIONS

1. What are some of the predictable complications associated with childbirth?
2. What are some of the treatments for postpartum hemorrhage?

Evaluation

A major cause of concern for the Paramedic in the immediate postpartum period is maternal hemorrhage. To prevent hemorrhage, the muscular uterus must contract and constrict blood vessels. If the uterus does not contract (**uterine atony**), then the mother is at risk for severe maternal hemorrhage and hemorrhagic shock.[21]

Although some bleeding (about 250 to 500 mL) is a natural outcome of childbirth, blood loss in excess of 500 mL is cause for concern. Possible causes of maternal blood loss include retained products of conception (such as incomplete placental detachment), lacerations to the vagina and/or cervix, and maternal clotting disorders, such as von Willebrand disease. Risk factors for maternal hemorrhage include placenta previa, placental abruption, grand multipara (greater than six childbirths), and multiple deliveries (twins, for example).

Following delivery, the Paramedic typically places a sanitary pad in front of, but not inside, the patient's vagina to absorb blood. It is not unusual to use three to four pads, with approximately 100 mL absorbed per pad. However, when the pad count (the number of pads bled through) exceeds five, the Paramedic should be concerned about maternal hemorrhage.

The first step in controlling maternal hemorrhage is to perform uterine massage. After the placenta is delivered, the Paramedic should massage the fundus to decrease the risk of obstetric hemorrhage from uterine atony. Initially, the uterus will be soft or "boggy" and the Paramedic will have to massage the uterus until it is firm. To massage the uterus, the Paramedic "traps" the uterus by placing one hand at the top of the symphysis pubis horizontally and another at the top of the fundus of the uterus. The upper hand should massage the fundus of the uterus until it starts to contract, ultimately contracting to about the size of a softball and the consistency of a grapefruit. The fundus of the uterus should be at about the level of the mother's umbilicus when the uterus is firm. If the uterus is above the bladder, it may be because the bladder is full. In that case, the mother should be encouraged to void, after which the uterus is reevaluated.

If the uterus is not responding to uterine massage, or the hemorrhage is severe, then the Paramedic should encourage the mother to nurse the newborn. Nursing stimulates the release of oxytocin, which stimulates uterine contraction. If the newborn is unable to suckle, then the mother should be encouraged to perform self-stimulation of the nipples.

There is some evidence that 10 units of oxytocin (Pitocin), administered intramuscularly after the birth of the baby, may decrease the risk of postpartum hemorrhage. The Paramedic may consider using prophylactic oxytocin if the mother is in one of the high risk groups listed previously.[22]

If the mother is actively hemorrhaging, an infusion of oxytocin, 10 to 20 units in 1 liter of normal saline—infused at keep vein open (KVO), or 30 cc/hr—can be initiated and then titrated to produce uterine contractions and thereby control hemorrhage.

Amniotic Fluid Embolism

Although very rare, **amniotic fluid embolism** has a mortality rate as high as 80%.[23,24] Although there are other causes of amniotic fluid embolism, including uterine trauma, the most common cause is labor. During delivery, amniotic fluid and fetal debris can enter the central circulation via tears in the uterine walls or endocervical veins.

Originally it was thought that the amniotic fluid then traveled to the pulmonary tree, obstructing the pulmonary veins and causing a pulmonary embolism. Consequently, there would be a sudden drop in venous return to the left ventricle (preload), and acute left ventricular failure would occur. Alternatively, some physicians suggest that amniotic fluid and fetal debris enter the central circulation and cause an "anaphylactoid" reaction. Regardless of the etiology, the onset is sudden and unpredictable. Within the first minute, acute respiratory distress presents, often with associated cyanosis. This is quickly followed by hypotension, pulmonary edema, seizures, and even cardiac arrest. In fact, upwards of 80% of patients with this condition suffer cardiac arrest.

Treatment of the patient with suspected amniotic fluid embolism is focused on supportive care (if the patient survives) and rapid transport or standard resuscitation. In many cases, the mother dies while the infant survives, making the childbirth a bittersweet event. If the mother is still with child, then an immediate perimortem cesarean section is required. A perimortem cesarean section is outside of the scope of practice of Paramedics; therefore, the patient must be rapidly transported to an emergency department or a physician must be brought to the scene.

CASE STUDY CONCLUSION

A second unit sets up IV access; high-flow, high-concentration oxygen; and some warm, dry blankets to treat the mother for hypoperfusion. The Paramedic's uterine massage is ineffective in firming up the uterus and decreasing blood flow, so the infant is given to the mother to nurse, which she does quite well. Nursing leads to firming of the uterus. Mother and infant are transported together to the hospital while the police unit assists in obtaining temporary care of the other children until family members can arrive.

CRITICAL THINKING QUESTIONS

1. What is the most appropriate transport decision that will get the patient to definitive care?
2. What are the advantages of transporting a patient for postpartum follow-up?

Disposition

The woman and baby are transported to the receiving hospital or birth center together, ideally with the mother holding the baby skin-to-skin and breastfeeding, if she desires. Upon arrival, and after turning the mother and child over to the hospital or birthing center personnel, the Paramedic should, minimally, document the EDD, the time of delivery, the initial APGAR score, the appearance of the amniotic fluid, and the presence or absence of a nuchal cord.

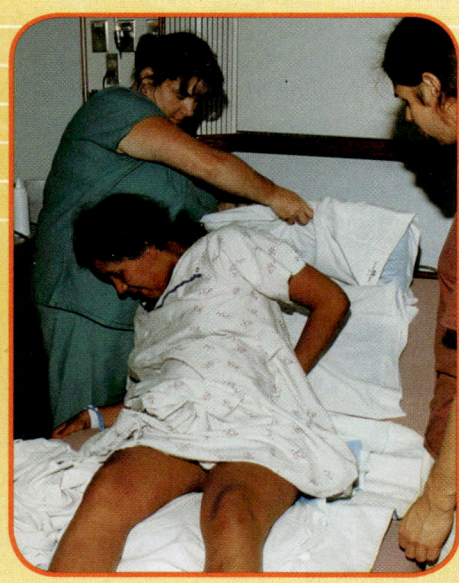

1 The Paramedic should position the mother supine with knees drawn up and spread apart and can assist the mother by helping her to elevate her buttocks on a pillow or blankets.

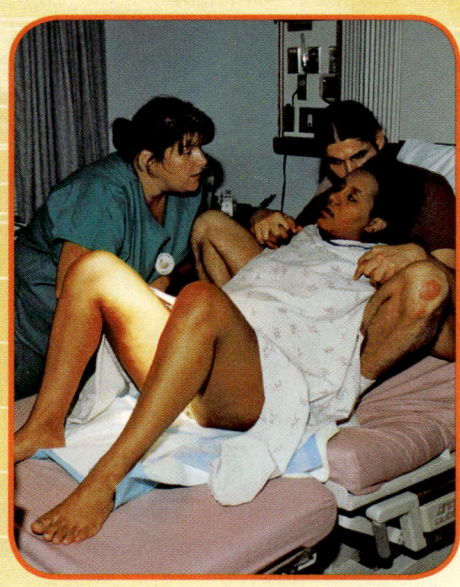

2 The Paramedic should create a clean area around the vaginal opening with clean towels or paper barriers.

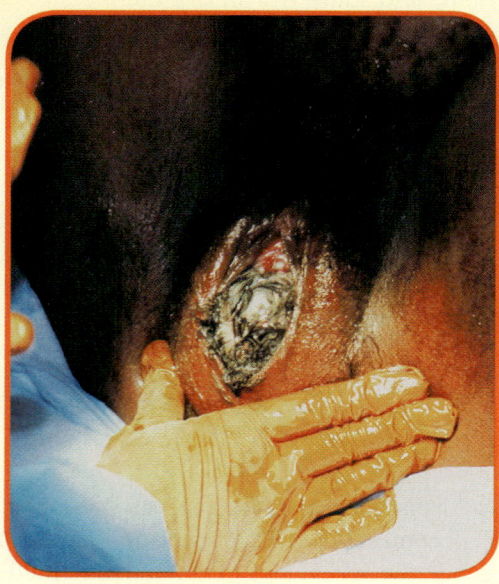

3 As the infant's head appears during crowning, the Paramedic should place her fingers gently on the skull and exert very gentle pressure to prevent explosive delivery.

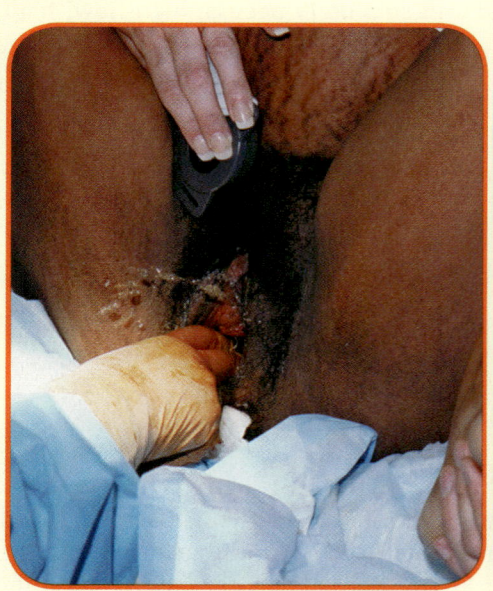

4 If the amniotic sac has not broken, the Paramedic should use her thumb and forefinger—or a clamp—to puncture the sac and push it away from the infant's head and face.

Delmar/Cengage Learning

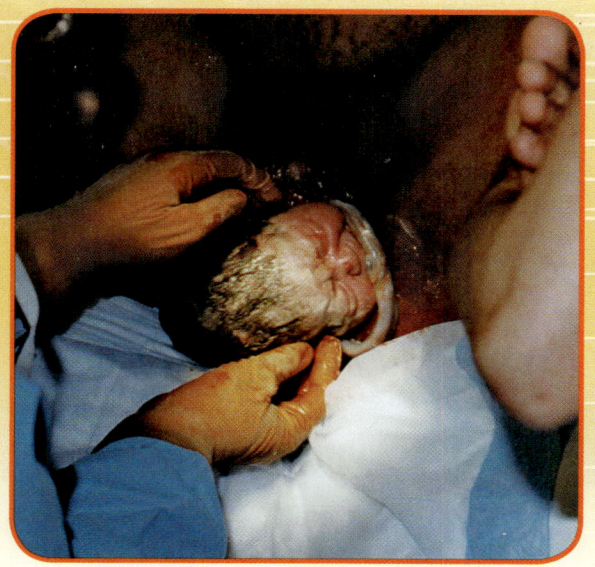

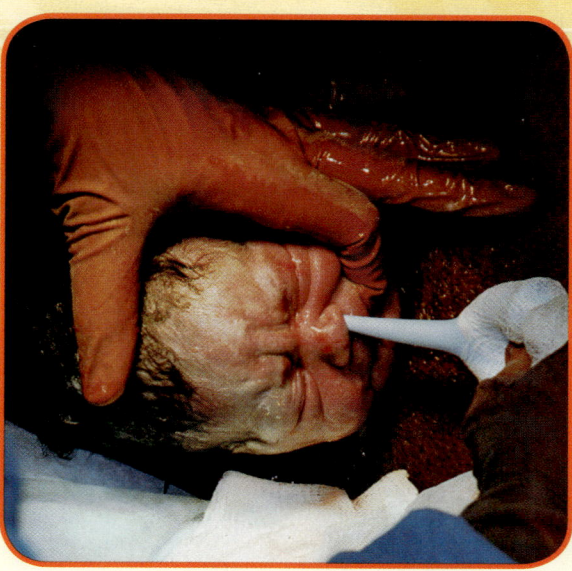

5 As the infant's head is delivered, the Paramedic should determine whether the umbilical cord is around the newborn's neck. If it is, the Paramedic should slip it over the infant's head or shoulder. If it is not possible to slip the cord, the Paramedic should clamp the cord in two places, cut the cord between the clamps, and unwrap the cord from the infant's neck.

6 After the infant's head is born, the Paramedic supports the head while suctioning the newborn's mouth and then the nose several times with the bulb suction device.

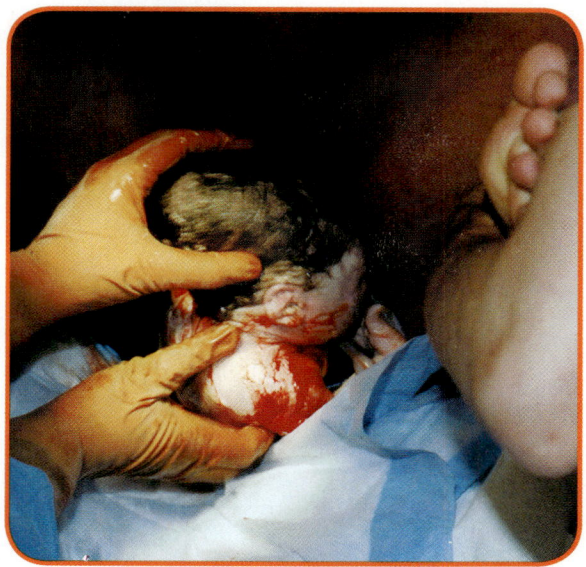

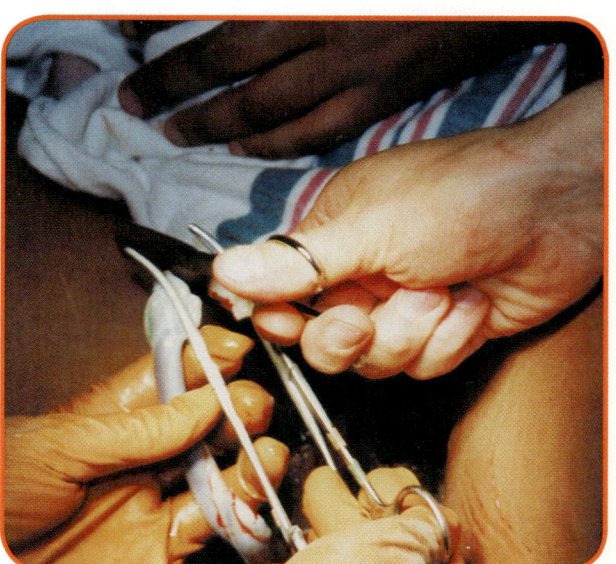

7 As the torso and full body are born, the Paramedic supports the infant with both hands. As the feet are born, the Paramedic should grasp them firmly.

8 After pulsations cease in the umbilical cord, the Paramedic should clamp the cord in two places, with the closest clamp about four fingers' width away from the infant, and then cut the cord between the clamps.

Delmar/Cengage Learning

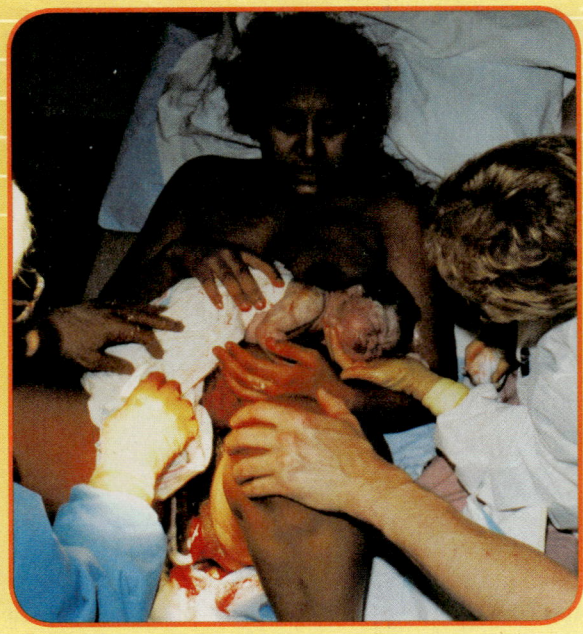

9 The Paramedic should gently dry the infant with towels and wrap the infant in a warm blanket. The infant should be placed on his side, preferably with the head slightly lower than the trunk.

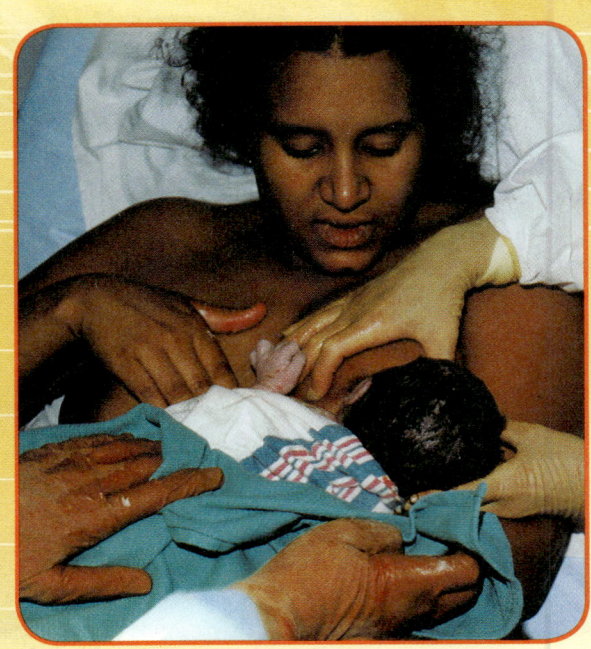

10 Another Paramedic or EMT should monitor the infant and complete initial care of the newborn.

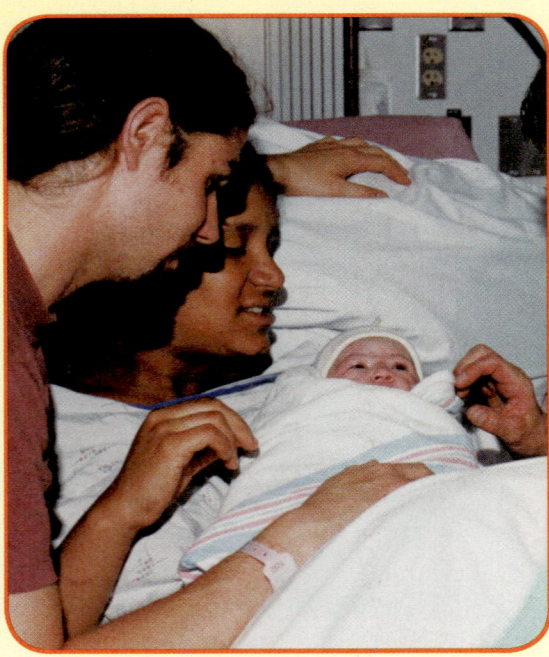

11 The Paramedic should place a sterile sanitary napkin between the mother's legs and have her close them around it. The Paramedic should also comfort the mother and monitor vital signs.

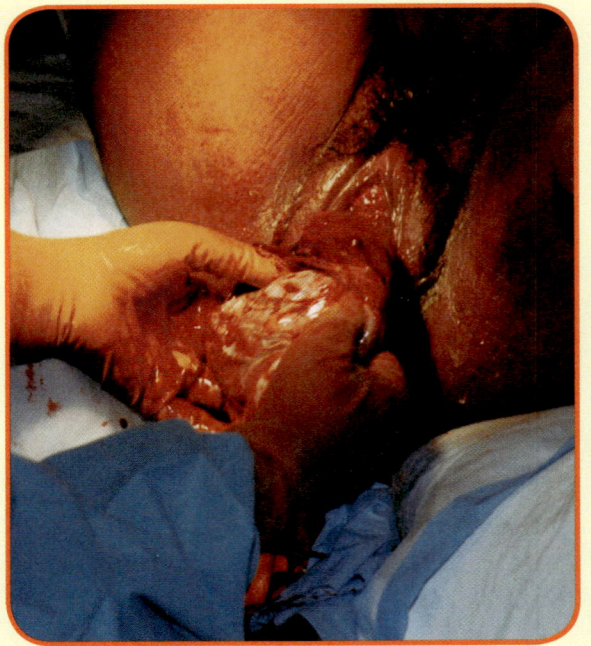

12 While preparing the mother and infant for transport, the Paramedic should watch for delivery of the placenta. When the placenta is delivered, the Paramedic wraps the placenta in a towel, places it in a plastic bag or container, and transports it to the hospital with the mother.

Delmar/Cengage Learning

CONCLUSION

Normal childbirth is a wonderful event that some Paramedics are called upon to share with the expectant parents. Even though most prehospital deliveries tend to be uncomplicated, the Paramedic is well equipped to handle and assist in the process of normal childbirth as well as any complications that may arise during the delivery.

KEY POINTS:

- During pregnancy, the uterus expands. Immediately after birth, it begins a process of shrinking, called involution.

- The placenta provides nutrition to the fetus, secretes hormones, and acts as a barrier to some potentially harmful substances.

- The umbilical cord serves to connect the fetus to the placenta.

- The fetus, umbilical cord, and placenta are contained within the amniotic sac.

- Normal childbirth proceeds through the three stages of labor:
  - The first stage extends to full dilation of the cervix.
  - The second stage extends from complete dilation to birth of the infant.
  - The third stage extends from birth of the infant to the birth of the placenta.
  - The puerperium, sometimes called the fourth stage, extends from the birth of the infant to six weeks postpartum.

- The infant moves the pelvis in a predetermined sequence of movements called the cardinal movements of labor.

- Assessment of the laboring mother begins with obtaining the estimated date of delivery.

- The Paramedic should ask when the contractions began:
  - Frequency (beginning of one contraction to beginning of the next)
  - Duration (from beginning of one contraction to the end of the same one)
  - Severity (intensity using pain scale)

- The Paramedic should determine the presence of bloody show and rupture of membranes.

- The Paramedic should complete a routine history using SAMPLE.

- Fetal heart tones should be equal to, or faster than, 140 per minute.

- The external genitalia is examined for bleeding, crowning, or evidence of a prolapsed cord.

- If the amniotic sac has not ruptured, it can be ruptured by the provider during delivery.

- An urge to push coupled with crowning is usually indicative of imminent delivery.

- The Paramedic should ensure as much privacy as possible during exam and delivery:
  - Allow the patient to be in a position of comfort for delivery
  - Prepare equipment, lighting, and comfort items
  - Use full body substance isolation
  - Provide counterpressure to the infant's head during delivery to reduce the likelihood of lacerations

- After the newborn's head is born, the Paramedic should assess for a cord around the neck, called a nuchal cord:
  - If loose, slip it over the head.
  - If tight, clamp it in two places and cut between the clamps.

- The Paramedic should use a bulb syringe to clear the mouth and then the nose.

- Meconium staining is an indicator of fetal distress.

- Thick meconium should be cleared from the airway.

- In shoulder dystocia, the shoulders are too large to deliver through the pelvic outlet.
  - Assessment reveals the "turtle" sign.

- Breech presentations include the newborn's buttocks, one foot, or both feet.

- If the mother's abdomen does not reduce in size after delivery, the Paramedic should consider the possibility of a second infant.

- Postdelivery care includes
  - Placing the newborn onto the mother's abdomen for warmth
  - Drying the infant
  - Stimulating the infant
  - Covering the infant's head with a cap

- In addition to initial assessment, the mnemonic APGAR is used to assess the infant at one minute and five minutes postdelivery.

- The placenta usually delivers within 30 minutes after delivery of the infant. The Paramedic should
  - Assess the margins
  - Bring it to the hospital

- Oxytocin may be required to control postpartum uterine hemorrhage if massage and nursing the infant are ineffective.

- Amniotic fluid embolus is a rare but often deadly complication from the entry of amniotic fluid into central circulation.
  - Signs and symptoms include respiratory distress and cardiovascular collapse with arrest.

REVIEW QUESTIONS:

1. Define the EDD.
2. How does the bloody show differ from the rupture of membranes?
3. What signs/symptoms are usually indicative of imminent delivery?
4. How should a loose nuchal cord be handled? A tight nuchal cord?
5. Name an indicator of fetal distress.
6. Describe shoulder dystocia. Name a common sign associated with shoulder dystocia.
7. Describe postdelivery care of the newborn.

CASE STUDY QUESTIONS:

Please refer to the Case Study in this chapter, and answer the questions below:

1. Based on normal physiology, what concerns are there for an infant born onto the floor of the bathroom?
2. What differential diagnoses exist for the mother in the Case Study?
3. Name the drugs available to assist in firming a boggy uterus. How are they dosed?

REFERENCES:

1. Caine D. Homebirth and maternal death. *Pract Midwife.* 2008;11(3):30–31.
2. Anthony S, Buitendijk SE, et al. Maternal factors and the probability of a planned home birth. *BJOG.* 2005;112(6):748–753.
3. Murphy PA, Fullerton J. Outcomes of intended home births in nurse–midwifery practice: a prospective descriptive study. *Obstet Gynecol.* 1998;92(3):461–470.
4. Dodd JM, Flenady V, et al. Prenatal administration of progesterone for preventing preterm birth. *Cochrane Database Syst Rev.* 2006;1:CD004947.
5. Harman CR. Amniotic fluid abnormalities. *Semin Perinatol.* 2008;32(4):288–294.
6. Friedman EA. An objective approach to the diagnosis and management of abnormal labor. *Bull N Y Acad Med.* 1972;48(6):842–858.
7. Hofmeyr GJ, Abdel-Aleem H, et al. Uterine massage for preventing postpartum haemorrhage. *Cochrane Database Syst Rev.* 2008;3:CD006431.

8. Nahum GG, Uhl K, et al. Antibiotic use in pregnancy and lactation: what is and is not known about teratogenic and toxic risks. *Obstet Gynecol*. 2006;107(5):1120–1138.

9. Gentile S. The safety of newer antidepressants in pregnancy and breastfeeding. *Drug Saf*. 2005;28(2):137–152.

10. Regesta G, Tanganelli P. Old and new anti-epileptic drugs in pregnancy. *Saudi Med J*. 2000;21(1):18–23.

11. Goldenberg RL, Culhane JF, et al. Epidemiology and causes of preterm birth. *Lancet*. 2008;371(9606):75–84.

12. Stallard TC, Burns B. Emergency delivery and perimortem C-section. *Emerg Med Clin North Am*. 2003;21(3):679–693.

13. McFarlin BL, Engstrom JL, et al. Concurrent validity of Leopold's maneuvers in determining fetal presentation and position. *J Nurse Midwifery*. 1985;30(5):280–284.

14. Crowther S. Nuchal cord at birth: to cut or not to cut? *Pract Midwife*. 2007;10(10):43–44.

15. Mercer JS, Skovgaard RL, et al. Nuchal cord management and nurse–midwifery practice. *J Midwifery Womens Health*. 2005;50(5):373–379.

16. Wiswell TE, Fuloria M. Management of meconium-stained amniotic fluid. *Clin Perinatol*. 1999;26(3):659–668.

17. Allen RH. On the mechanical aspects of shoulder dystocia and birth injury. *Clin Obstet Gynecol*. 2007;50(3):607–623.

18. Gottlieb AG, Galan HL. Shoulder dystocia: an update. *Obstet Gynecol Clin North Am*. 2007;34(3):501–531, xii.

19. Rahm SJ. Newborn resuscitation. *Emerg Med Serv*. 2002;31(7):61–65.

20. Chandraharan E, Arulkumaran S. Surgical aspects of postpartum haemorrhage. *Best Pract Res Clin Obstet Gynaecol*. 2008;22(6):1089–1102.

21. Ramanathan G, Arulkumaran S. Postpartum hemorrhage. *J Obstet Gynaecol Can*. 2006;28(11):967–973.

22. Gulmezoglu AM, Forna F, et al. Prostaglandins for prevention of postpartum haemorrhage. *Cochrane Database Syst Rev*. 2004;1:CD000494.

23. Stafford I, Sheffield J. Amniotic fluid embolism. *Obstet Gynecol Clin North Am*. 2007;34(3):545–553, xii.

24. Moore J, Baldisseri MR. Amniotic fluid embolism. *Crit Care Med*. 2005;33(10 Suppl):S279–S285

CHAPTER 38

CARE OF THE NORMAL NEWBORN

KEY CONCEPTS:

Upon completion of this chapter, it is expected that the reader will understand these following concepts:

- The transition the newborn undergoes from relying upon the mother to relying upon self for physical survival
- The cardiovascular and pulmonary systems as the key factors to transitioning
- The risk of hypothermia and hypoglycemia faced by the newborn
- Pre- or post-maturity and congenital anomalies that may increase the difficulties of transitioning

ANATOMY CONCEPTS:

Prior to reading this chapter the Paramedic student should be familiar with the following anatomy and physiology concepts:

- Neonatal anatomy
- Neonatal physiology
- Placental circulation

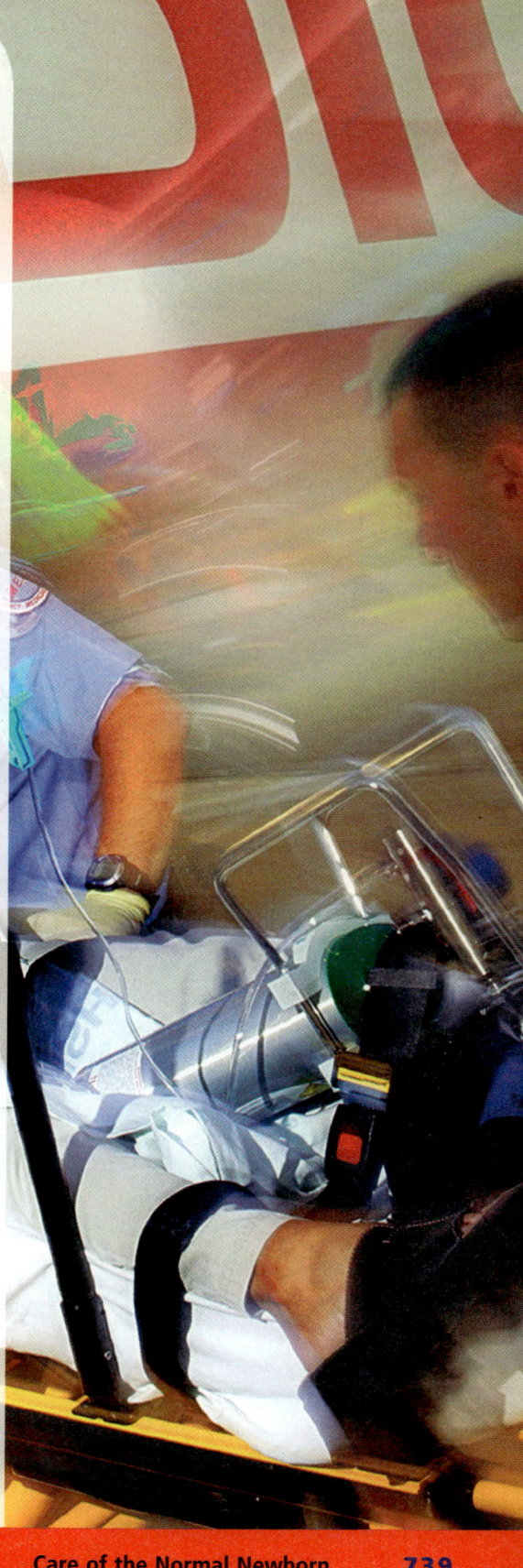

The dispatch indicates that a man called 9-1-1, saying that his girlfriend is in labor, her contractions are one right after the next, and the couple have no transportation to the nearest hospital-based birth center. The only information the Paramedics have is that this is her third newborn, and her due date is next week.

As the Paramedics make their way to the address given, the first Paramedic starts to think out loud to his partner. "The caller said the newborn's due date is next week, so they may have had prenatal care of some kind, and the newborn is likely to be a term newborn, not premature. That reduces the risk significantly that the newborn will need special care or that there will be a malpresentation, such as a breech newborn."

CRITICAL THINKING QUESTIONS

1. Are the Paramedic's statements accurate?
2. What emergencies should the Paramedic prepare for?

OVERVIEW

This chapter will deal with care of the normal newborn immediately following birth. Like in the childbirth process, the Paramedic functions in the role of caregiver, supporting mother and child during these important first moments of life.

Chief Concern

The pivotal issue the newborn must overcome to survive is the transition from dependence on the mother to physiologic independence. The newborn must also achieve thermoregulation, in order to maintain an ideal body temperature. Finally, the newborn must obtain glucose as a source of energy.[1,2]

Fetal Circulation

Fetal circulation is unique, owed to the fact that the mother provides the fetus with all necessary nutrients and substrates, including oxygen. The **fetal circulation** starts at the point where the umbilical vein emanating from the placenta, carrying oxygenated blood, enters the newborn's body and almost immediately divides. One-half of the blood from the mother passes through the fetus's liver and one-half of the blood enters the newborn's central circulation via a shunt known as the **ductus venosus**, where it joins with the vena cava. Eventually, blood leaving the liver combines with the blood in the ductus venosus in the inferior vena cava. Once in the vena cava, the blood travels to the right atrium, bypassing the lungs, and travels directly into the left atrium via the **foramen ovale**, the opening between the right and left ventricle. This shunting of blood past the lungs occurs because the lungs are largely nonfunctional in the fetus.[3]

The next fetal circulatory adaptation involves how the fetus discharges deoxygenated blood returning from the body. A large portion of the deoxygenated blood returning to the heart, from the fetal body via the superior vena cava, is shunted past the heart via the ductus arteriosus. The **ductus arteriosus**, a blood vessel that connects the pulmonary trunk to the aorta below the aortic arch, prevents deoxygenated blood from flowing to the brain. As the mixed venous and arterial blood is carried down the descending aorta, it passes out of the fetus's body via the umbilical arteries which branch from the iliac arteries (Figure 38-1).

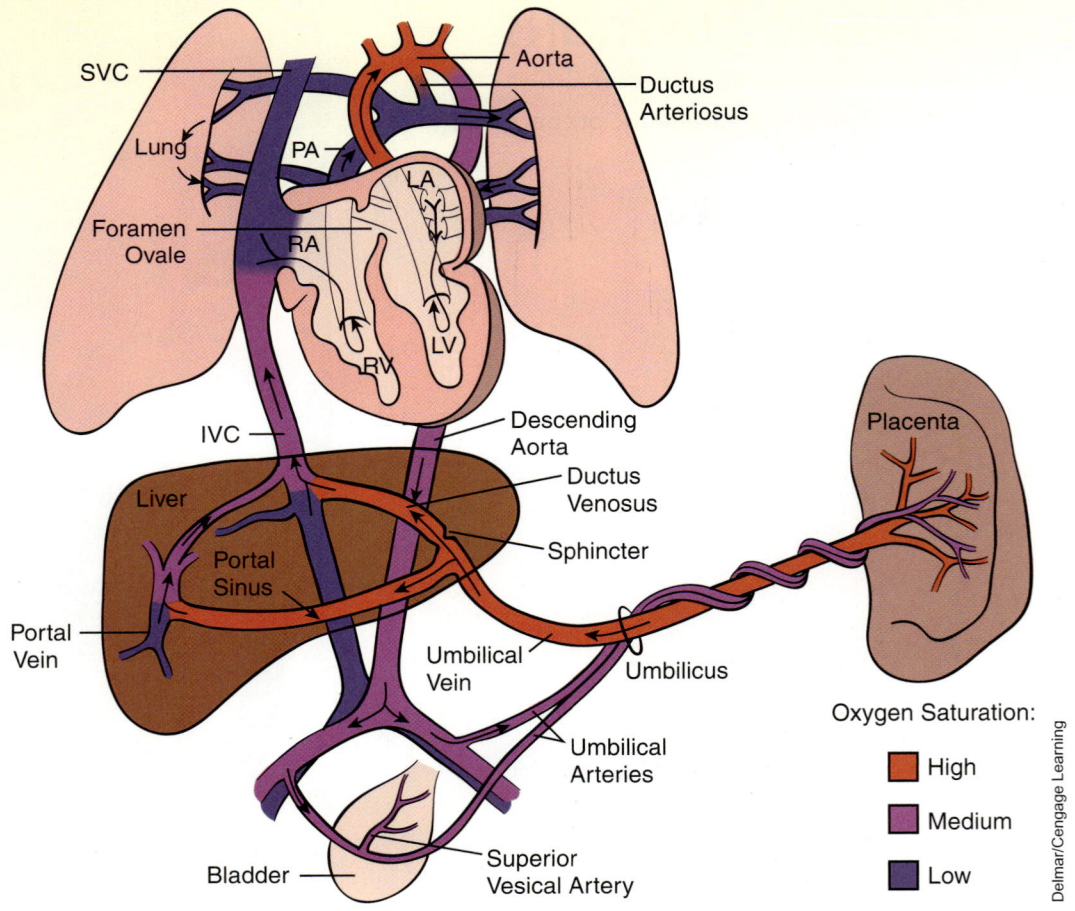

Figure 38-1 Fetal circulation.

Newborn Respiratory Adaptations

The newborn's first breath initiates a number of changes in the newborn's cardiopulmonary system. Although not clearly understood, the mechanism by which the newborn takes its first breath is believed to depend upon a variety of factors. These factors include chemoreceptors in the brain which sense hypoxia, the newborn's ability to produce **surfactant** (a phospholipid that reduces surface tension in the alveoli of the lungs), and mechanical pressure on the newborn's thorax as it descends in the birth canal. This pressure compresses the newborn's thoracic cavity, whereby the chest expands with the first breath, creating a negative intrathoracic pressure.

With the negative pressure of that first breath, air fills the newborn's trachea and bronchi, expanding the surface and pushing fluid into the periphery of the lungs where it is absorbed.[4] These first breaths cause the pulmonary vasculature to expand and open.

Prior to birth, fetal circulation is a "low pressure" system, with fluid-filled lungs that do not do the work of oxygenating the fetus. Rather, most fetal blood bypasses the lungs, flowing through the foramen ovale, an opening between the right and left atria. Once the newborn is born and the umbilical cord is clamped, this low-pressure system is shut off. The newborn's own circulation increases blood flow and blood pressure on the left side of the heart, from the pulmonary arteries, forcing closure of the foramen ovale.

The increased blood volume, returning from the now-functional lungs via the pulmonary veins and entering the left ventricle, is ejected under higher pressure from the left ventricle and rushes past the now largely dysfunctional ductus arteriosus. The ductus arteriosus eventually becomes a strip of connective tissue, called the **ligamentum arteriosum**, which tethers the heart to the aorta.

Thermoregulation in the Newborn

Heat loss is a major concern for the newborn, who was previously accustomed to a relatively stable 98.6°F (37.5°C) intrauterine environment. All that changes when the infant is born, as the extra-uterine environment starts to immediately drain heat from the newborn. Heat loss begins to take place due to evaporation of moisture from the skin, via conduction from contact with cold surfaces, and as a result of radiant heat loss to the ambient environment. The resulting cold stresses the newborn, prompting the newborn's immature thermoregulatory system to try to adjust. Significant heat loss, and the resulting cold stress, can cause hypoglycemia, hypoxia, and, if left unchecked, acidosis in the newborn.[5] This acidosis, in turn, leads to respiratory distress.

CASE STUDY (CONTINUED)

The Paramedic's partner, following up on this train of thought, says, "There was no mention of bleeding or trauma. They also didn't say whether the woman had ruptured membranes, and they didn't say how long she's been having contractions, how long her last labors have been, whether her previous births were vaginal or by caesarian section, or whether she is feeling any sense of pressure or bearing down." The Paramedic prepares herself mentally for transport to the birth center, or to assist with the birth and care of the newborn if birth is imminent. As the Paramedic enters the apartment, she hears a groan and, a second later, a crying newborn, along with exclamations from the family members present. The Paramedic observes the maternal-newborn dyad, and starts to assess the situation.

CRITICAL THINKING QUESTIONS

1. What are the important elements of the history that a Paramedic should obtain?
2. What is the importance of obtaining the mother's medical history as well?

History

As is the case with any patient, the care of the newborn begins with a history, in this case the prenatal and **intrapartum history** (i.e., the history of labor and delivery including contractions). If at all possible, the history should be obtained prior to birth, as it may have implications for the immediate care of the newborn. The Paramedic's focus when compiling a **perinatal history** (i.e., prenatal and intrapartum history) is to predict the newborn's risk of problems of transition and to determine the probability of the need for neonatal resuscitation.

Prenatal Care

One of the first questions that a Paramedic should ask the new mother is if she had prenatal care or if she is under the care of a physician or nurse–midwife. A physician or nurse–midwife can predict the presence of potential problems, such as **congenital anomalies** (physical abnormalities of a structure or function of the body).

The presence of congenital anomalies in the fetus is one of the positive predictors of problems of transition. These congenital anomalies may have been detected by amniocentesis or ultrasound during a prenatal visit. Without prenatal care, the diagnosis of underlying maternal conditions may not have occurred. Maternal conditions such as cardiac disease, renal disease, gestational diabetes, or pregnancy-induced hypertension each place the fetus at risk for problems of transition.

Furthermore, the risk of prematurity may be higher without prenatal care as the mother may not be aware of fetal development and progression.[6,7] A Paramedic may even be dealing with an undiagnosed multiple gestation. For these reasons, the first question that a Paramedic often asks is whether the patient has received prenatal care.

Estimated Date of Delivery

The estimated date of delivery (EDD) establishes if the baby will be term, premature, or post-date. Premature babies are more likely to require resuscitation at birth. They are also more likely to be in a **noncephalic** (i.e., breech) position and therefore be a difficult delivery with risks of cord compression, fetal hypoxia, and other complications during childbirth. Premature newborns, when delivered, have difficulty transitioning to extra-uterine life.

Prematurity

Up to one in eight babies are born before their due date.[8] Prematurity may be due to advanced maternal age or the youth of the mother (<18), maternal diabetes, pregnancy-induced hypertension, or pre-eclampsia.

A significant risk factor for prematurity is multiple gestations (54% of twins are delivered preterm). The risk of multiple gestations is an increasing reality in an era of technology-assisted reproductivity. Other risks for prematurity include use of alcohol during the pregnancy and cigarette smoking, as both have been shown to increase prematurity.

The complications of prematurity are numerous, including **retinopathy of prematurity (ROP)** leading to blindness, **patent ductus arteriosus (PDA)** leading to heart failure and hypoglycemia, thrombocytopenia, and sepsis.[3] Of greatest immediate concern to the Paramedic is the respiratory distress syndrome associated with premature birth.

A newborn who is at less than 34 weeks' gestation has an increased risk of respiratory distress syndrome (i.e., **hyaline membrane disease**). The premature infant's lungs have not developed sufficient surfactant, a complex lipid–protein compound that reduces the surface tension of the fluid that covers the intra-alveolar space, so as to inflate the lungs at birth.[9–11] The resulting atelectasis causes hypoxia. The incidence of respiratory distress syndrome increases with prematurity and is the single most common cause of death during the neonatal period.

Post-Date Pregnancy

Conversely, the Paramedic may be dealing with a post-date pregnancy. By definition, a post-date pregnancy is a pregnancy that goes to 42 weeks or more. The newborn who is born post-date often has classic signs of postmaturity including wrinkled and peeling skin, somewhat resembling a superficial burn.

Perinatal morbidity is high for the postmature newborn. Risks for the postmature newborn include **oligohydramnios** (scant amniotic fluid) and **macrosomia** (excessive birth weight, greater than 4,000 grams). Oligohydramnios may be the result of leaking membranes. The loss of amniotic fluid from premature rupture of membranes (PROM) increases the risk of intrauterine infection. Intrauterine infection, in turn, has been associated with a greater risk of meconium aspiration syndrome (discussed shortly).

Of greater concern, oligohydramnios may be an indication of placental problems, including placental abruption or placenta previa. This declining placental function can cause fetal distress.

The mother of a postmature newborn who is macrosomic (i.e., has excessive birth weight) is at greater risk for perineal lacerations, leading to hemorrhage. In some cases, the woman may even require blood transfusions. However, the risks of macrosomia to the postmature newborn may be even greater. During birth, the macrosomic newborn is at greater risk for shoulder dystocia and other birth trauma. The risk is 20 times greater if the newborn is larger than 4,500 grams.

Maternal Medical History

A maternal medical history should be routinely obtained during the case of caring for the mother and newborn. Although the importance of obtaining a comprehensive maternal medical history was discussed in Chapter 37, the following specific points in the maternal medical history have specific impact upon the infant.

Poorly controlled diabetes—either gestational diabetes or diabetes existing prior to pregnancy—can delay fetal lung maturity, cause macrosomia in a newborn, and cause hypoglycemia after birth in the newborn.[12] Uncontrolled diabetes also places the newborn at higher risk for congenital malformations and stillbirth.

Drug use, especially narcotic use within four hours of birth, may cause respiratory suppression in the newborn, and many drugs are associated with newborn withdrawal symptoms. Some medications are associated with birth defects, while others, such as certain antidepressants, may cause persistent pulmonary hypertension of the newborn.

Finally, the Paramedic should inquire about the risk of intrapartum infection. For example, the Paramedic should determine whether there was a premature rupture of membranes greater than 18 hours, a history of foul-smelling amniotic fluid, a recent history of sexually transmitted infections, presence of fever in labor, or fetal tachycardia (fetal heart tones greater than 160 beats per minute). All of these findings are suggestive of intrapartum infection and may impact the newborn's transition to extra-uterine life.

CASE STUDY (CONTINUED)

There are gasps of relief from the mother and father. Two other children are wide-eyed and smiling at the new baby. The Paramedic's partner has noted that while the baby doesn't evidence any respiratory difficulties, she seems lethargic with cyanotic limbs. The Paramedic's partner begins the newborn exam.

CRITICAL THINKING QUESTIONS

1. What are the elements of the physical examination of a newborn?
2. Why is a head-to-toe examination a critical element in this examination?

Examination

As most childbirths are uneventful, the Paramedic—keeping in mind the need for thermoregulation—can proceed to a physical examination. After airway, breathing, and circulation are established to be within normal limits (the ABCs), a brief general survey of the newborn is appropriate.

Starting at the head and working to the feet, the Paramedic should perform a systematic examination of the newborn. The newborn's head should be evaluated for signs of birth trauma. **Birth trauma** occurs because of the mechanical forces that occur during birth—including compression, torque, and traction—that injure the infant. Infants at risk for birth trauma are macrosomic newborns, breech deliveries, and those newborns born to small mothers with small hips and narrow pelvic outlets (i.e., **cephalopelvic disproportion**).

Signs of minor, and typically self-resolving, birth trauma on the skull include abrasions, ecchymosis, erythema, and **petechiae** (small red spots under the skin). More significant signs of birth trauma to the head are **caput succedaneum** (a diffuse swelling under the scalp), **cephalohematoma** (bleeding under the skull from interruption of blood vessels in the periosteum), and linear skull fractures (discernable by palpation of the cranium). A cephalhematoma, seen most commonly over the parietal bone, can only be appreciated indirectly by noting displaced suture lines.[13] Conversely, caput succedaneum is extraperiosteal accumulation of blood and fluids that can be felt as a softness of the skull. Caput succedaneum crosses over suture lines.[14] Any displaced bone not along a suture line can be assumed to be a linear skull fracture.

Examination of the newborn's face may reveal dysmorphic features (e.g., an enlarged ear, obvious congenital malformation such as cleft lip, or facial asymmetry). A cleft lip or palate may create problems with nursing and risks of aspiration due to difficulty with swallowing.

The Paramedic may also notice subconjunctival hemorrhage, a collection of blood in the conjunctiva. This is usually self-resolving without further intervention.

A hoarse cry or respiratory stridor may suggest a laryngeal nerve injury. **Laryngeal nerve injury** sometimes occurs when the head is flexed laterally and rotated during delivery. There is unilateral laryngeal nerve paralysis and subsequent difficulties with swallowing. If this is observed, the Paramedic should continuously monitor the airway and discourage the mother from breastfeeding.

Spinal cord injury may occur if excessive traction or rotation occurs during childbirth. As a result of these forces, epidural and intraspinal hemorrhage occurs. Typically, the newborn with a spinal cord injury is either stillborn or in respiratory arrest. The cause of the death or arrest is usually determined at autopsy.

Next, the Paramedic should inspect and palpate the abdomen, which should be soft and nondistended. A scaphoid abdomen, one that is concave instead of proturbant or potbelly, along with associated respiratory distress could indicate a **diaphragmatic hernia**.[15,16] Positive pressure ventilation often temporarily resolves the diaphragmatic hernia.

Obvious abdominal wall defects such as an omphalocele and gastroschisis require special care until they may be surgically treated. An **omphalocele** is a mid-abdominal wall defect characterized by an abdominal organ, such as bowel and liver, which protrudes through a defect in the abdominal wall, and is covered by a membrane. In **gastroschisis**, known as "split abdomen," a loop of bowel protrudes from the belly. The defect is typically lateral to the umbilicus, on the right side of the abdominal wall, and the bowel is external to the body without the covering membrane. In either case, special care must be taken to protect the organs while minimizing the risk of infection. The newborn should be transported as quickly as possible to a hospital. In both omphalocele and gastroschisis, the Paramedic must be aware that the greatest concerns are hypothermia, dehydration, and infection. The newborn should be kept as warm as possible. A sterile, warmed, saline-soaked gauze pad is applied to the abdomen, after which the abdomen is wrapped in sterile gauze to keep the sterile saline-soaked gauze in place.

The most common internal abdominal injury is a hepatic injury. Owing to its large size and its relationship to the umbilical cord, the liver can be injured, resulting in a subcapsular hematoma. The hepatic hematoma then expands until it ruptures. Hepatic rupture should be suspected in any newborn with signs of shock, including tachycardia (>160 bpm) and pallor, and abdominal distention.

Extremities are evaluated for signs of trauma such as bruising, nerve palsies, or fractures. The Paramedic should examine the extremities for injury, starting at the clavicles. Clavicle fractures, the most common newborn fractures, are often the unavoidable consequence of childbirth. Although macrosomic newborns and shoulder dystocia are often associated with clavicular fractures, clavicular fracture can occur spontaneously during delivery through the birth canal. Bony crepitus and sternocleidomastoid muscle spasm are suggestive of a clavicular fracture. The Paramedic need only limit motion by immobilizing the affected limb to the newborn's side.

One of the more common extremity injuries is a **brachial plexus injury**. Three patient populations are at risk for a brachial plexus injury: newborns with shoulder dystocia, breech delivery, and macrosomic newborns. Injuries associated with brachial plexus injury include clavicular fractures, fractures of the humerus, and Erb's palsy.[17,18] Erb's palsy is the result of C5 to C6 injuries, such as subluxation. As a result of brachial plexus injury, the arm lies adducted and internally rotated and therefore lacks motion. However, a grasp reflex is generally still intact. The Paramedic does not need to reset the injury, but only needs to protect the affected limb and notify the receiving hospital of the finding.

Polydactyly (extranumerary fingers or toes) and **syndactyly** (fused digits or webbed fingers) are common birth defects that are not a cause for concern in the prehospital setting, although they can be very disconcerting to the parents. It should be noted that approximately 25% of newborns with polydactyly have other congenital anomalies as well.

Finally, the Paramedic should inspect the newborn's back for indications of **spina bifida** or "split spine." Inspection of the back and spine may reveal sacral dimpling, a finding that is suggestive of spina bifida occulta, or more obvious neural tube defects. The most common open neural tube defects are meningocele or a myelomeningocele.

Meningocele, or meningeal cyst, involves a bony defect of the spinal cord where the meninges protrude through an opening in the spinal column, typically proximal to the sacrum.

In **myelomeningocele**, the spinal cord is encased in an external sac, most often in the area of the lumbar spine or sacrum. The greatest risk to these newborns is a meningeal infection (meningitis). To help prevent meningitis, and to protect the cyst, a sterile, warm saline dressing is applied to the area, which is then wrapped in additional sterile gauze. The newborn is then transported in the prone position (or any position that will keep pressure off the defect). Thermoregulation, hydration, and minimization of infection risk are paramount while the newborn is transported to a tertiary care facility.

CASE STUDY (CONTINUED)

"From all appearances, this seems like a normal newborn," states the Paramedic. After opting to leave the mother and child alone for a few moments, so that they may start to bond, the Paramedic steps out to report the delivery and to contact medical control for advice and consultation.

CRITICAL THINKING QUESTIONS

1. What is the significance of "bonding"?
2. What diagnosis did the Paramedic announce to the patient?

Assessment

Barring any finding from the previous list, the newborn is classified as a "normal newborn." Fortunately, most newborns are normal; as such, keeping the mother–newborn dyad together, warm, and supported emotionally and physically is the standard of care. Typically, the Paramedic continues on to obtain an APGAR score.

APGAR Score

At one minute and again at five minutes after birth, a Paramedic should obtain an APGAR score to establish a baseline and to trend the newborn's physiological status. In 1952, Dr. Virginia Apgar developed the system that bears her name in an effort to quantify the cardiorespiratory and basic neurologic condition of any given newborn.[19] The scale is still in general use today.

Assignment of a "score" is based on five elements: appearance (color), pulse (heart rate), grimace (reflex irritability), activity (muscle tone), and respiratory effort. All five elements are evaluated at one minute of age and again every five minutes until a score of greater than or equal to seven is reached, or neonatal death has been declared. It bears reinforcement that the APGAR score is not used to determine the need for neonatal resuscitation. Evaluation and assessment of the newborn begins immediately at birth, and intervention takes place within the first 30 seconds of life, if needed. The Paramedic cannot wait for a full minute before deciding to intervene for a newborn that is experiencing a difficult transition to extra-uterine life.

In assigning the APGAR score (Table 38-1), for each element a score of zero, one, or two is given. The five-minute APGAR score is more predictive of long-term morbidity and mortality than the score at one minute. Factors that influence the APGAR score are many and varied, and include obstetric issues, prematurity, trauma, maternal medication or drug use, and congenital issues such as heart defects in the newborn, to name just a few.

Table 38-1 APGAR Score Chart

Item Assessed	Score		
	0	1	2
Heart rate	Absent	Slow (<100)	Over 100
Respiratory rate	Absent	Slow, weak cry	Good cry
Muscle tone	Flaccid	Some flexion of extremities	Well flexed
Reflex irritability	No response	Grimace	Cry, cough, or sneeze
Color	Blue, pale	Body pink, extremities blue	Completely pink (light skinned); absence of cyanosis (dark skinned)

CASE STUDY (CONTINUED)

After completing the APGAR score, the Paramedic thoroughly dries the infant, swaddles the infant in a dry towel to help preserve body heat, and then returns the infant to the mother's arms.

CRITICAL THINKING QUESTIONS

1. What is the APGAR score?
2. What are some of the patient-specific concerns when caring for the newly born?

Treatment

The period of transition from intrauterine life to extra-uterine life is one that requires straightforward, supportive care in over 90% of cases. There are instances, however, when more than supportive care is needed and prompt action is imperative. Therefore, the Paramedic must evaluate the newborn immediately following birth to determine whether advanced respiratory or circulatory support is needed. The Paramedic must be able to recognize when intervention beyond basic care is indicated, and act immediately to perform neonatal resuscitation (this topic will be covered in Chapter 39; additional resources are also available through the American Heart Association).

For the large majority of newborns, supportive care, thermoregulation, and observation are the only interventions needed as the healthy newborn makes the transition from intra- to extra-uterine life.

As noted in Chapter 37, the vigorous newborn is placed on the maternal abdomen, skin-to-skin with the mother, to increase heat gain from the mother's abdomen, and to avoid heat loss due to contact with cold surfaces. After the newborn has been placed on the mother's abdomen, the newborn is dried with a towel or blanket (preferably prewarmed), after which this wet cloth is set aside. A clean, dry cloth is then placed over the newborn. Paramedics use this swaddling technique to keep the newborn warm (Figure 38-2).

The newborn is positioned so that the Paramedic can monitor the newborn's breathing, color, and tone and the newborn can be assessed in general. If the newborn has good tone (may be crying), good color, and good heart rate, there is research evidence to support delaying umbilical cord clamping until after the cord stops pulsing (this procedure was covered in Chapter 37).

A bulb syringe may be used to suction the newborn's mouth first, then the nares of the newborn to clear secretions, whenever obvious secretions are seen at the newborn's mouth or coming from its nose (Figure 38-3). Overvigorous suctioning is not recommended, however. Healthy newborns who are crying or sneezing are doing the work of clearing these secretions quite well on their own.

If a newborn has depressed respiratory effort at birth in the presence of meconium, the Paramedic should suction the oropharynx and nares, utilizing a catheter connected to mechanical suction, if available, before stimulating the newborn. Meconium can be aspirated, blocking the airway, and thus prevent adequate ventilation. However, use of a suction catheter can cause bradycardia, trauma, and edema to the respiratory tract and mucous membranes. An active, vigorous, crying newborn with good tone does not require intubation.

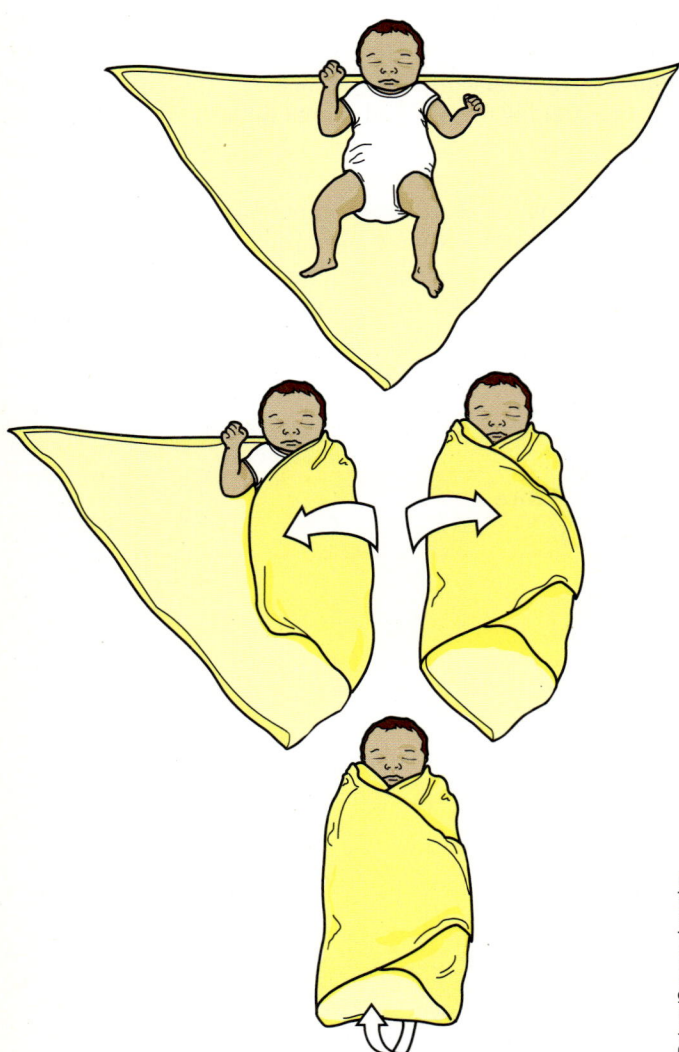

Figure 38-2 Swaddling.

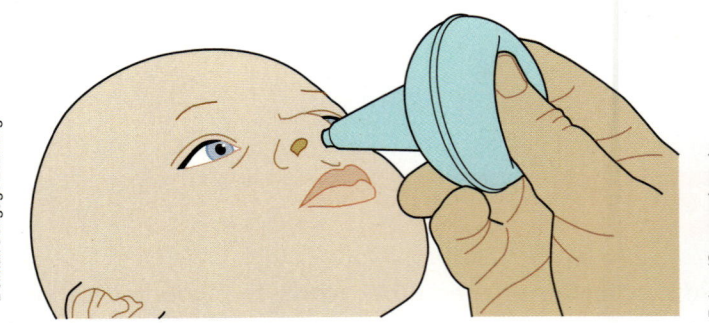

Figure 38-3 Bulb suctioning.

CASE STUDY (CONTINUED)

The Paramedic notes that the newborn is starting to become less active, which triggers her memory to check a blood glucose by heel stick. Fortunately, the blood glucose comes back within the normal range.

CRITICAL THINKING QUESTIONS

1. Why is a blood glucose reading important for a newborn?
2. What is the treatment for hypoglycemia in a newborn?

Evaluation

Hypoglycemia is a common problem for the neonate, one the Paramedic must immediately address. Up to 90% of the newborn's blood glucose is consumed by the brain. However, the newborn's glucose regulatory mechanisms are immature, which in some cases causes the newborn's brain to be starving for glucose. For these reasons, the newborn is very susceptible to hypoglycemia.[20] If left untreated, newborn hypoglycemia can lead to development delays or even permanent neurological damage.

Conditions that can make a newborn more prone to hypoglycemia include low birth weight (limited glucose stores), macrosomic newborns (diabetic mothers), perinatal asphyxia (breech delivery), and especially cold stress and increased work of breathing. Although the first conditions may be beyond the Paramedic's control, the Paramedic can prevent and/or treat the last two conditions.

The signs of neonatal hypoglycemia can be variable, from jitteriness to lethargy, and the typical signs (such as sweating) are not dependable. Therefore, a blood glucose level should be obtained for any newborn who may be at risk for hypoglycemia.

Typically, a newborn's blood glucose is obtained by performing a heel stick using a standard glucometer. The newborn can tolerate a blood glucose that is much lower than expected. However, a blood glucose of less than 40 mg/dL should be treated with a gentle infusion of either 2 to 3 mL/kg of $D_{10}W$ or, preferably, 5 mL/kg of D_5W. The Paramedic should perform repeat blood glucose measurements to monitor for rebound hypoglycemia.

CASE STUDY CONCLUSION

The mother and infant are transported together to the birth center for further assessment. The Paramedic understands that their examination in the field is very limited and that the newborn needs to be assessed by a neonatologist or pediatrician. As this was an unscheduled home delivery, the parents agree to the decision.

CRITICAL THINKING QUESTIONS

1. What other medical conditions may be present that the Paramedic cannot assess?
2. What post-childbirth procedures would a hospital perform?

Disposition

In general, a mother and newborn should be transported to the nearest facility that provides obstetrical care. In many rural areas, small community hospitals no longer provide obstetrical services. If the mother and newborn are stable, it is ideal to take them to a facility that is equipped to deal with the special concerns of mothers and babies. In the case of an unstable mother or newborn, the closest receiving facility is the ideal choice as emergency care may be initiated and patients may be stabilized prior to transport to a tertiary care center or neonatal intensive care unit, as the situation demands.

CONCLUSION

During the birth process, the newly born child's physiology rapidly transforms from one that was dependent on the mother for survival to independence in a matter of a few breaths. During this process, the child may become distressed. With an understanding of the birthing process and the physiologic changes that occur immediately after birth, the Paramedic will be able to accurately and rapidly assess the newborn and manage any complications.

KEY POINTS:

- At birth, the infant must transition from complete dependence upon the mother to physical independence.

- The infant's circulatory system shifts from receiving oxygen from the mother and bypassing the lungs to sending blood to the lungs for oxygenation.

- Arteries and veins necessary for fetal circulation close secondary to pressure changes and become connective tissue anchoring various structures within the thoracic and abdominal cavities.

- At the infant's first breath, the pulmonary system opens, alveoli fill with air, and fluid is pushed back toward the vasculature.

- Heat loss is a stressful event for the newborn.

- History of the pregnancy and birth includes prenatal care, estimated date of delivery, and the maternal medical history.

- Births occurring outside of term (pre- or postmature) place the infant at risk for complications.

- A stressed fetus may release meconium, placing the infant at risk for respiratory difficulties postdelivery.

- Postdelivery exam of the newborn begins with the ABCs, and then proceeds in a head-to-toe fashion.

- At one and five minutes, the Paramedic performs an APGAR assessment to establish a baseline and trend of physiologic status.

- The five minute APGAR score is more predictive of long-term progress than the one minute score.

- The APGAR score is not used to determine resuscitation needs.

- Most newborns require warmth and support only.

- Additional interventions may include drying, positioning, and suctioning.

- Newborns are at risk for hypoglycemia.

- For heel stick results below 40 mg/dL, the Paramedic should administer a dilute glucose infusion (2 to 3 mL/kg of $D_{10}W$ or 5 mL/kg of D_5W).

- The mother and infant should be transported for further evaluation.

1. What changes occur in the newborn's cardiovascular system at birth?
2. Name three components of the history of the pregnancy.
3. How can meconium lead to respiratory distress in the newborn?
4. For each body location, name a congenital anomaly and describe how it may impair transitioning to extra-uterine life.
   - Head, face, neck
   - Back
   - Abdomen
   - Limbs
5. What are the components of the APGAR score? Why is the APGAR useful?
6. List the interventions commonly required by newborns.
7. Describe the administration of glucose to the hypoglycemic newborn.

CASE STUDY QUESTIONS:

Please refer to the Case Study in this chapter, and answer the questions below:

1. Name at least two risks to transitioning present for the newborn in the Case Study.
2. What are the likely causes of lethargy with good respiratory effort and peripheral cyanosis in a newborn?
3. What interventions would be most effective for the infant in the Case Study?

REFERENCES:

1. Asakura H. Fetal and neonatal thermoregulation. *J Nippon Med Sch*. 2004;71(6):360–370.
2. Gunn TR, Gluckman PD. Perinatal thermogenesis. *Early Hum Dev*. 1995;42(3):169–183.
3. Myron J, Judith M, et al. *Current Pediatric Diagnosis & Treatment*. New York: McGraw-Hill; 2004.
4. Greer JJ, Funk GD, et al. Preparing for the first breath: prenatal maturation of respiratory neural control. *J Physiol*. 2006;570 (Pt 3):437–444.
5. Zayeri F, Kazemnejad A, et al. Hypothermia in Iranian newborns. Incidence, risk factors and related complications. *Saudi Med J*. 2005;26(9):1367–1371.
6. Iams JD, Romero R, et al. Primary, secondary, and tertiary interventions to reduce the morbidity and mortality of preterm birth. *Lancet*. 2008;371(9607):164–175.
7. Khan KS, Honest H. Risk screening for spontaneous preterm labour. *Best Pract Res Clin Obstet Gynaecol*. 2007;21(5): 821–830.
8. Furdon SA, Clark DA. Prematurity. 2006. Available from: **http://emedicine.medscape.com/article/975909-overview**. Accessed September 22, 2008.
9. Parmigiani S. The 5 W's of surfactant for respiratory distress syndrome of the premature infant. *J Matern Fetal Neonatal Med*. 2004;16 Suppl 2:25–27.
10. Morley C, Davis P. Surfactant treatment for premature lung disorders: a review of best practices in 2002. *Paediatr Respir Rev*. 2004;5 Suppl A:S299–S304.
11. Corbet A. Clinical trials of synthetic surfactant in the respiratory distress syndrome of premature infants. *Clin Perinatol*. 1993;20(4):737–760.
12. Satpathy HK, Fleming A, et al. Maternal obesity and pregnancy. *Postgrad Med*. 2008;120(3):E01–E09.
13. Feinberg AN, Greydanus D, et al. *Pediatric Diagnostic Examination*. New York: McGraw-Hill Professional; 2007.

14. Durward H. *Examination of the Newborn*. Washington, DC: Taylor & Francis; 2007.

15. Downard CD. Congenital diaphragmatic hernia: an ongoing clinical challenge. *Curr Opin Pediatr*. 2008; 20(3):300–304.

16. Hartnett KS. Congenital diaphragmatic hernia: advanced physiology and care concepts. *Adv Neonatal Care*. 2008;8(2): 107–115.

17. Backe B, Magnussen EB, et al. Obstetric brachial plexus palsy: a birth injury not explained by the known risk factors. *Acta Obstet Gynecol Scand*. 2008;87(10):1027–1032.

18. Sandmire H, Morrison J, et al. Newborn brachial plexus injuries: the twisting and extension of the fetal head as contributing causes. *J Obstet Gynaecol*. 2008;28(2):170–172.

19. Carlo WA, Schelonka R. The outcome of infants with an APGAR score of zero at 10 minutes: past and future. *Am J Obstet Gynecol*. 2007;196(5):422–423.

20. Jain A, Aggarwal R, et al. Hypoglycemia in the newborn. *Indian J Pediatr*. 2008;75(1):63–67.

CHAPTER 39

SPECIAL CONSIDERATIONS IN NEONATOLOGY

KEY CONCEPTS:

Upon completion of this chapter, it is expected that the reader will understand these following concepts:

- The risks preterm infants face due to their immature systems
- Hypothermia, decreased fluid volume, and respiratory distress represent the primary complications for preemies
- The need for premature infants to receive specialized care in a neonatal intensive care unit (NICU)

ANATOMY CONCEPTS:

Prior to reading this chapter the Paramedic student should be familiar with the following anatomy and physiology concepts:

- Neonatal cardiovascular physiology

The dispatch call is for a 23-year-old pregnant female who, although only about six months pregnant, felt her water break and feels as though she now has to "push." The Paramedic realizes that, instead of one patient, she now will have two that need treatment. She assesses the need in dispatching a second ambulance, one for each patient.

CRITICAL THINKING QUESTIONS

1. What are some of the possible problems of prematurity?
2. What is the implication of the patient's statement that she has the feeling like she wants to push?

Care of a premature newborn may be one of the most challenging tasks a Paramedic is confronted with in the field. Many times women go into preterm labor without the cause ever being determined. Some women have a history of preterm labor which may or may not be due to an incompetent cervix. Sometimes labor can be brought on by dehydration, such as occurs from nausea, vomiting, and diarrhea from the flu. Other times, a simple urinary tract infection may be the culprit. Whatever the cause, the woman delivers a premature infant that will require the Paramedic's care.

Chief Concern

A preterm newborn is a unique and complex patient that has many immature organ systems that complicate the patient's care. The most critical organ system affected by prematurity may be the respiratory system.

Neonatal Respiratory Insufficiency

Newborns who are born before 34 weeks' gestation do not have sufficient quantities of surfactant. This substance, composed of lipoproteins that are secreted by the alveolar cells of the lungs, help to keep the alveoli pliable and open, as well as aid in gas exchange at the alveolar level.[1] Neonates with a surfactant deficiency will have chest wall rigidity and may be more difficult to ventilate and oxygenate. This is due to diffuse alveolar atelectasis, pulmonary edema, and cell injury.

Preterm neonates should be brought to the closest appropriate facility capable of stabilizing a preterm newborn. These facilities can intratracheally administer **exogenous surfactants**, alveolar lipoproteins obtained from an outside source that rapidly improve the neonate's oxygenation and lung compliance. Injected surfactant also allows the Paramedic to use less pressure during ventilation, thereby reducing the possibility of barotrauma to the alveoli and any subsequent pneumothorax of the lungs.

Neonatal Hypothermia

The preterm newborn is also at greater risk for hypothermia than the full-term newborn. **Thermoregulation**, the body's ability to control its warmth, is difficult for the newborn to maintain directly after birth, even for the term newborn. However, hypothermia can be potentially life-threatening for the preterm newborn.

Neonatal survivability is based, in part, on the Paramedic's ability to help the neonate to maintain the body's temperatures between 36°C to 37°C (96°F to 98.6°F). The Paramedic's maintenance and ongoing assessment of the neonate's temperature is paramount. Poor outcomes including increased rates of sepsis and death have been reported due to hypothermia. A neutral thermal environment is the Paramedic's goal. The **neutral thermal environment** is the ideal state where body temperature is maintained within the normal range, thereby reducing oxygen demand, glucose consumption, and metabolic rate to a minimum. The neutral thermal environment is determined by the environment, the neonate's health status, and the neonate's activity level.

Unlike adults, newborns do not shiver to produce heat. Instead, they rely on metabolism of brown adipose tissue for heat production.[2,3] Premature newborns have decreased amounts of brown adipose tissue for **thermogenesis**, the ability to make heat, due to their prematurity. Because a neonate has decreased subcutaneous fat, as well as a large body surface area to weight ratio, the heat transfer from organs to skin is increased and subsequently heat is lost to the environment.

The Four Means of Heat Loss

There are four means of heat loss for the preterm newborn: conduction, convection, evaporation, and radiation. The Paramedic must address each of these means of heat loss in order to prevent neonatal hypothermia (Figure 39-1).

The first means of heat loss is **conduction**, the heat transfer from direct contact. For example, placing a neonate on a cold bed will cause a heat transfer from the neonate to the bed. The Paramedic's solution to preventing heat loss by conduction is to create a warm dry surface for the patient. The ideal surface for a newborn is the mother's abdomen. However, since a preterm newborn may need resuscitation away from the mother, a warm dry surface should be used.

The next means of heat loss is **convection**, the heat transfer due to air currents. For example, having a neonate exposed to drafts will cause a heat transfer. To prevent heat loss from convection, the Paramedic should wrap the full-term newborn

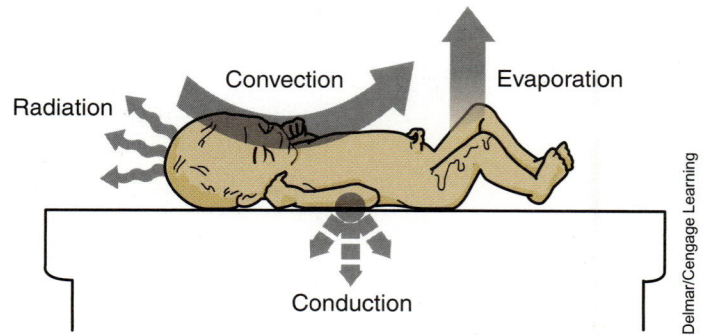

Figure 39-1 Neonatal heat loss.

in warm blankets and keep the child away from drafts. Again, the preterm newborn may need resuscitation that requires exposure of the body. In this case, the Paramedic should take efforts to minimize the time of exposure to a minimum and only expose the child as long as is medically necessary.

Evaporation is the transfer of heat by conversion of liquid to a vapor. For example, due to the fragile gelatinous state of a premature neonate's skin, the average preterm neonate can lose up to 150 mL of water in the first few days of life. This cannot only lead to heat loss, but when the skin dries and cracks it is a portal of entry for infection. To help prevent evaporation, as well as protect the neonate's fragile skin, the Paramedic can wrap the newly born neonate in clear plastic wrap prior to wrapping in warm blankets.

Radiation is the last means of heat loss for the neonate. **Radiation** is the heat transfer of radiant energy without direct contact through absorption and emission of infrared rays. The rate at which heat is transferred is dependent upon several factors including the surface area of the neonate, the temperature gradient between the neonate and the object, and the object's surface absorptive properties.

To reduce heat loss secondary to radiation, the Paramedic should wrap the newborn in clear plastic wrap prior to wrapping in warm blankets, and keep the neonate away from cold surfaces or other objects. Again, the best surface for a newborn is on the mother's abdomen. If possible, have the mother "kangaroo" the neonate, meaning the neonate placed skin-to-skin on her chest with a blanket covering both of them.

CASE STUDY (CONTINUED)

Just after the first ambulance arrives on scene, dispatch notifies both crews that the mother has delivered a tiny infant onto the edge of her bed. She is currently trying to dry off the infant and keep a hold on the child.

CRITICAL THINKING QUESTIONS

1. What are the important elements of the history of the delivery that a Paramedic should obtain?
2. What are the important elements of the maternal history that a Paramedic should obtain?

History

If a preterm delivery is anticipated, the Paramedic should try to obtain a maternal history. The maternal history for a preterm delivery is the same as the maternal history for a term delivery (Chapter 37), with a few additional questions.

Maternal History

Central to the question of prematurity is the estimated date of delivery (EDD). Any childbirth that occurs before week 37 in the pregnancy is considered premature, thus leading to a preterm newborn. The Paramedic should try to ascertain the EDD as close as practical.

Additionally, the Paramedic may want to inquire about multiple gestations. Twins, triplets, and so on, tend to deliver earlier than the EDD. While on the topic of gestations, the Paramedic should ask the patient about other pregnancies, particularly if she has a history of preterm delivery. There is a greater risk of preterm delivery in mothers who have had previous preterm deliveries.

If the patient has had preterm labor before, or is under care for preterm labor presently, the Paramedic should ask if she was given the medication betamethasone. Betamethasone is a glucocorticosteroid that crosses the placenta barrier and accelerates fetal lung development in anticipation of preterm delivery.[4]

CASE STUDY (CONTINUED)

The newborn's breathing is somewhat erratic. As this is a cause for concern for the Paramedic, she starts to assemble her respiratory equipment. In the interim, she asks an EMT to go to the kitchen and get some clear plastic wrap, the kind that is used to protect sandwiches. The EMT looks at the Paramedic quizzically and asks, "Plastic wrap?"

CRITICAL THINKING QUESTIONS

1. What are the initial problems of transition that a newborn must overcome?
2. Why is wrapping the preterm newborn in plastic wrap important?

Examination

The case presentation, history, and examination suggest that the Paramedic should prepare for the delivery of a preterm newborn. As the risks of prematurity include peripartum asphyxia, the Paramedic should be prepared for the eventuality of a neonatal resuscitation.

Newborns normally respond to hypoxia experienced initially during childbirth by increasing their respirations. However, preterm newborns who are hypoxic have an altered respiratory pattern. Preterm newborns may initially start with tachypnea but the continued hypoxia, secondary to their immature lungs, eventually leads to bradypnea, termed **primary apnea**.

During primary apnea, the preterm newborn can be encouraged to breath with stimulation; however, if the hypoxia continues the newborn will begin to have gasping breaths that become agonal, after which breathing ceases altogether. This condition is termed **secondary apnea**. The disciplined and algorithmic approach to neonatal resuscitation under these conditions gives the preterm newborn the best chance for survival.[5]

As these events are predictable for preterm newborns, the Paramedic should gather the appropriate respiratory equipment (Table 39-1), including oxygen tubing for blow-by oxygen, a bag–mask assembly with a variety of face masks from 0 to 1, as well as a laryngoscope and blades sizes 0 and 1.

The preterm newborn is also at great risk for hypothermia. Therefore, the Paramedic should prewarm the ambulance to greater than 80°F (between 80°F and 88°F cabin temperature

Table 39-1 Neonatal Resuscitation Equipment

Neonatal resuscitation supplies
- Bulb syringe
- Portable suction
- Suction catheters (5F, 6F, 8F, 10F, and 12F)
- Feeding tube (8R)
- Syringe (20 mL)
- Oropharyngeal airways (0, 00, and 000 size)
- Bag–mask assembly
- Face mask (neonate and infant)
- Portable oxygen
- Laryngoscope
- Straight (Miller) blades (0 and 1)
- Endotracheal tubes (2.5, 3.0, 3.5, and 4.0 ID)
- Meconium aspirator
- Endotracheal securing device
- Stethoscope with a neonatal diaphragm
- ECG monitor
- End-tidal CO_2 monitor
- Pulse oximeter
- Stockinet cap
- Swaddling blanket
- Aluminum foil wrap
- Plastic bag (1 gallon food grade and resealable)

Additional preterm supplies
- Clear plastic wrap
- Chemical hot pack or warming pad

STREET SMART

Preterm newborns have extremely fragile skin that is prone to tears. To protect the preterm newborn's skin, the Paramedic should cover the oxygen saturation probe with a bio-occlusive covering, such as Tagderm®, so that adhesive will not touch the neonate's skin.

is recommended) and prepare warmed blankets to swaddle the newborn.

Finally, the Paramedic should cut three pieces of clear plastic wrap to cover the neonate: one for the head, one for the upper body, and one for the lower part of the body. The umbilicus should be left exposed for umbilical catheterization, if necessary.

CASE STUDY (CONTINUED)

The mother is crying and saying that no baby that small could possibly live. The Paramedic tries to reassure the mother and tells her that most preterm newborns respond well to some very basic treatment. The mother senses the confidence in the Paramedic and becomes visibly relaxed.

CRITICAL THINKING QUESTIONS

1. What is the most common "pathway" for newborn care?
2. What is the current thinking about meconium?

Assessment

Neonatal resuscitation should be considered whenever the newborn appears limp and lifeless (i.e., without muscle tone), has absent or depressed respirations, or has a heart rate less than 100 beats per minute.

The steps of the neonatal resuscitation are algorithmic and are analogous to the primary assessment, beginning with basic techniques and then moving to advanced techniques. Neonatal resuscitation, like adult resuscitation, starts with stimulation (i.e., level of consciousness). The Paramedic then proceeds through airway, breathing, and circulation, with minor variations in technique attributed to the newborn's unique physiology.

Routine Care and Assessment

The Paramedic starts routine newborn care (discussed in Chapter 38) by drying and warming the newborn. While the Paramedic is drying the newborn, the Paramedic is also assessing the newborn's responsiveness (i.e., level of consciousness). The newborn should have a vigorous cry. Most newborns do not need more resuscitation than these simple maneuvers.

The Paramedic then proceeds to position and open the newborn's airway. The optimal position to place the newborn is in the sniffing position, with padding under the shoulders in order to keep the trachea in-line. Both overextension backward and hyperflexion forward can compromise the airway.[6]

With the airway opened, the Paramedic suctions the infant's nose and mouth with a basic bulb syringe. Suctioning with a catheter should be avoided unless there is concern for meconium aspiration. In addition, deep orotracheal suctioning may illicit a vagal response including bradycardia and apnea. Use of sterile saline to loosen secretions has also been shown to produce a vagal response and should be avoided at this stage of resuscitation.

Next, the Paramedic assesses the newborn. A healthy newborn will be breathing, preferably crying. The Paramedic should be concerned if the newborn is not crying, has a weak cry, or appears to be gasping—either a single deep noisy inspiration or a series of inspirations that might be misperceived as breathing. For the newborn, gasping is synonymous with apnea.

Finally, the newborn should also have good color (i.e., pink) and be vigorously moving (with arms and legs in the flexion and extension). It should take the Paramedic no more than 30 seconds to perform the procedures and assessments listed.

To this point, all of the newborn care has been routine. If this is the case, then the Paramedic should continue routine care of the newborn (i.e., provide warmth) and prepare for delivery of the placenta.

Meconium Aspiration Syndrome

Term and post-date deliveries are often associated with meconium-stained amniotic fluid. Newborn aspiration of the meconium can lead to meconium aspiration syndrome, a condition which does not usually occur in preterm infants.

Meconium aspiration syndrome is thought to occur in post-date pregnancy because of increased peristalsis in the postmature infant. Meconium aspiration syndrome is one of the most common causes of respiratory distress in the newborn and carries a mortality rate as high as 20%.[7,8]

Meconium aspiration syndrome causes respiratory distress in the neonate by creating an airway obstruction, causing surfactant dysfunction, and eventually leading to chemical pneumonitis.

Meconium aspiration can create either a complete lower airway obstruction, and subsequent atelectasis, or a partial airway obstruction. The partial airway obstruction of meconium creates a ball–valve effect, which allows air to enter the lungs but not to escape. Over time, alveolar hyperextension leads to hyperinflation and pneumothorax.

Meconium aspiration can also cause surfactant dysfunction. Surfactant, which is necessary for lung inflation, is stripped from the alveolar surfaces by free fatty acids in the meconium, resulting in atelectasis and subsequent hypoxia.

In the past, using a meconium aspirator to intubate and suction the airway of the neonate delivered through meconium-stained amniotic fluid was a routine practice. Some evidence suggests that meconium exists in the trachea and (in 10% of cases) below the cords, even if there is an absence of meconium in the pharynx during routine bulb syringe aspiration during childbirth. Therefore, all newborns delivered through meconium-stained amniotic fluid should be emergently intubated and suctioned with a meconium aspirator.

Although meconium-stained amniotic fluid is present in up to 15% of all childbirths, and up to one-third of these newborns may have meconium below the vocal cords, some 95% of these newborns spontaneously clear the inhaled meconium and suffer no harm. At risk are the remaining 5%, or 2 of 1,000 childbirths.[9] These newborns may have suffered in utero asphyxia secondary to pulmonary vasospasm and hyperreactivity secondary to the aspiration of meconium, resulting in respiratory distress.

For this subset of the newborn population, emergent intubation and meconium aspiration may be indicated (**Skill 39-1**). Current practice suggests that the newborn's condition—not the presence of meconium—should be the indication for emergent intubation and use of a meconium aspirator (Figure 39-2).

For a step-by-step demonstration of Meconium Aspiration, please refer to Skill 39-1 on page 769.

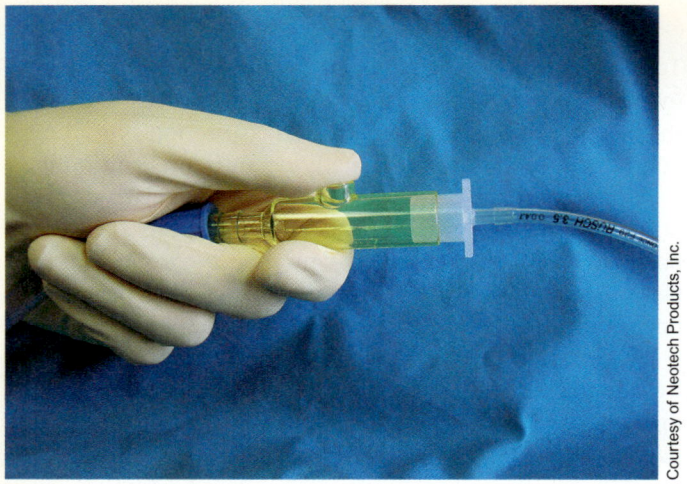

Figure 39-2 Meconium aspirator.

CASE STUDY (CONTINUED)

One Paramedic switches the wet bed linen for dry towels, completes the drying of the infant, and swaddles the infant in plastic and warm baby blankets. The newborn's respirations are gasping, so the Paramedic begins positive pressure ventilation with a bag-valve mask. Heart rate is monitored and remains above 100 bpm but is less than ideal.

CRITICAL THINKING QUESTIONS

1. What is the national standard of care for neonatal resuscitation?
2. What are some of the patient-specific concerns of a Paramedic during a neonatal resuscitation?

Treatment

The start of the delivery of the preterm newborn is the same as occurs with the term newborn. The Paramedic should dry and stimulate the neonate, making sure to pull used cold wet towels or blankets away from the neonate and then replace them with dry blankets. The goal is to dry the preterm newborn completely and then wrap him in clear plastic wrap, followed by warm blankets. This will decrease heat loss and minimize water loss of the preterm neonate's skin.

A systematic approach to assessment of the neonate will prevent the omission of critical information. Due to the instability of the preterm neonate (any newborn born less than 37 weeks' gestation), assessment must be thorough yet done in a timely manner to prevent hypoxia and hypothermia. Life-threatening emergencies must be dealt with prior to a more comprehensive exam.

Resuscitation

After drying and rubbing the newborn's back for 30 seconds, the Paramedic should reassess the newborn's vital signs (i.e., respirations and heart rate). Good chest rise and/or a strong cry are signs of good respiration, whereas gasping is not. In addition, the newborn's pulse should be above 100 bpm. To take the newborn's pulse, the Paramedic may either palpate the base of the umbilical cord, or auscultate for apical heart sounds (both methods are effective). The easiest means of calculating the newborn's pulse is to count the pulse for six seconds, then multiply by 10 to estimate the beats per minute.

If the newborn is breathing, pink, and has a heart rate greater than 100 bpm, then the Paramedic should provide supportive care. If the newborn is apneic or gasping, or the newborn's heart rate is less than 100 beats per minute, then the Paramedic should proceed to the ABCs. It can

Efforts should be made to provide the newborn with a warm environment. Cold stress further complicates the newborn's care. One source of cold stress is unheated, nonhumidified oxygen, which results in hypothermia and dehydration. Where available, warm humidified oxygen should be used during the resuscitation

be assumed at this point that the newborn is experiencing secondary apnea (**Skill 39-2**).

For a step-by-step demonstration of Initial Care of the Newborn, please refer to Skill 39-2 on page 770.

Breathing

If the newborn is apneic or has a heart rate less than 100 bpm, then the Paramedic should provide positive pressure ventilation using a bag–mask assembly. The Paramedic's first step in using a bag–mask assembly is to choose the correct mask. The mask should either be round (preferred) or anatomically shaped. The mask should have a soft inflatable face cushion to minimize trauma and maximize mask seal, and should cover the patient's mouth, nose, and chin without covering the eyes. Pressure applied to the eyes by the mask can produce a vagal response and subsequent bradycardia, further complicating the clinical picture.

Standing at the head of the newborn, where the Paramedic can visualize adequate chest rise, the Paramedic should very gently seat the mask on the newborn's face. It is not necessary or desirable to apply pressure to the face, as it may leave bruises.

With the airway in position, the mask applied to the face, and a good mask seal obtained, the Paramedic should gently start to ventilate the newborn at a rate of 40 to 60 breaths a minute. Whereas a volume of 5 to 7 mL per kg is optimal, the Paramedic should focus on watching the chest rise and fall.[6] After a trial of 30 seconds of positive pressure ventilation, the Paramedic should stop to reassess the newborn. If the newborn's heart rate is greater than 100 bpm, then the Paramedic can continue with supportive care (**Skill 39-3**).

For a step-by-step demonstration of Ventilation with Bag–Mask Assembly, please refer to Skill 39-3 on page 771.

Special Case of Choanal Atresia

Newborns are obligate nose breathers, meaning that they prefer to breathe through their nose. However, some newborns have a congenital narrowing of the nasal airway, called

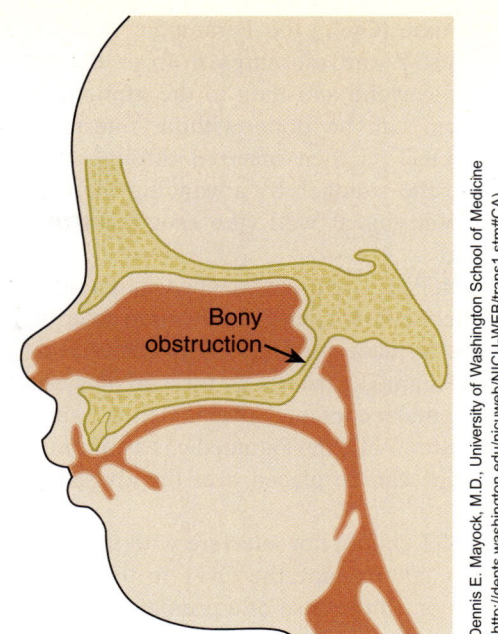

Dennis E. Mayock, M.D., University of Washington School of Medicine (http://depts.washington.edu/nicuweb/NICU-WEB/trans1.stm#CA).

Figure 39-3   Choanal atresia.

choanal atresia, that prevents them from breathing through their nose. These newborns will manifest with difficulty breathing (Figure 39-3).

Although a French catheter can be passed into each nostril to verify patency of the nasal airway, it may be more prudent for the Paramedic to simply place an oropharyngeal airway, or electively intubate the newborn in order to ensure a patent airway.

Special Case of Pierre Robin Syndrome

Some newborns have a congenitally small mandible that causes a narrowing of the airway (i.e., **Pierre Robin syndrome**, a form of dysmorphism). Subsequently, these newborns will have difficulty with breathing, especially when supine. This difficulty with breathing is owed, in part, to the tongue falling posteriorly into the pharynx, obstructing the airway.

The easiest technique to treat this condition is to place the newborn prone on her stomach. If this does not resolve the difficulty, it may be necessary for the Paramedic to intubate the neonate. Oral intubation is made very difficult by the short axis created by the pharyngeal airway malformation; therefore, a nasopharyngeal intubation may be needed.

Orogastric Tube Placement

Because of the immature glottis, the newborn is prone to gastric insufflations and abdominal distention that interferes with ventilation. To remove the air from the stomach, the Paramedic may elect to insert an orogastric tube. To place an orogastric tube (OGT) the Paramedic typically selects an 8 French OGT and measures it from the bridge of the nose to the earlobe and then to the xiphoid process. This measurement can be done without interrupting ventilation. The OGT is then inserted through the mouth and placed into the stomach by advancing the OGT along the posterior pharyngeal wall (the esophagus is posterior to the trachea).

The first Paramedic can resume ventilation with the OGT in place. Ventilation should not be interrupted for more than 15 seconds to place the OGT. With the OGT at the proper depth, the Paramedic takes a 20 mL slip tip syringe and aspirates for stomach contents, after which the abdomen should visibly deflate. While the Paramedic is aspirating stomach air, a stethoscope can be placed over the epigastrium to verify placement.

The OGT should not interfere with the mask seal. Most Paramedics simply tape the OGT to the side of the newborn's face or, in the case of a premature newborn, leave it open to air in order to passively decompress the stomach (**Skill 39-4**).

> **For a step-by-step demonstration of Insertion of an Orogastric Tube, please refer to Skill 39-4 on page 772.**

Special Case of Congenital Diaphragmatic Hernia

In some newborns, the diaphragm does not form completely and abdominal contents enter the thoracic cavity, resulting in a congenital diaphragmatic hernia. As a result, one lung is underdeveloped. When this occurs, it can be difficult to ventilate the newborn.

The Paramedic should suspect a congenital diaphragmatic hernia if it is difficult to ventilate the newborn, smaller than usual volumes are needed to cause chest rise, breath sounds are diminished on one side, and the newborn's abdomen is scaphoid in appearance. In these cases, intubation and careful titration of ventilation volumes is important as well as immediate placement of an orogastric tube to help decompress the stomach.

Intubation of the Neonate

There are several points along the neonatal resuscitation algorithm where intubation may be considered. Some advocate endotracheal intubation immediately following a trial of bag–mask assembly ventilation. However, there is some evidence that suggests that intubation of the neonate is unnecessary, provided adequate ventilation is being provided by bag–mask assembly. In the case of the preterm newborn, obtaining an adequate mask seal is very difficult and early intubation should be considered.

The traditional indications for intubation of the newborn include prolonged bag and mask ventilation (secondary to long transport times), ineffective bag–mask ventilation (secondary to prematurity), and tracheal suctioning for meconium.

Although preoxygenation would be optimal prior to intubation in some cases, the reason the newborn is being intubated is poor mask seal. In those cases, the newborn should be given blow-by oxygen via the bag–mask assembly.

Using clean technique, the Paramedic places the appropriate straight (Miller) blade and visualizes the vocal cords (Table 39-2). Grasping the correct cuffless endotracheal tube, the Paramedic advances the endotracheal tube into the trachea until the vocal cord guide (the black line at the end of the endotracheal tube) passes through the glottic opening. (**Skill 39-5**).

> **For a step-by-step demonstration of Intubation of the Neonate, please refer to Skill 39-5 on pages 773–774.**

STREET SMART

Although some Paramedics prefer the stiffness that a stylet provides to an endotracheal tube, it is often unnecessary as the distance from the opening of the mouth to the glottis opening is short. Furthermore, a stylet can be difficult to remove from the endotracheal tube and takes time to remove during the intubation.

Table 39-2 Neonatal Intubation Equipment

Gestational Age	Weight of Newborn		Endotracheal Tube	Miller Blade Size
(weeks)	(grams)	(pounds)	(mm)	
<28	<1,000	<2	2.5	0
28 to 34	1,000 to 2,000	2.0 to 4.5	3.0	0
34 to 38	2,000 to 3,000	4.5 to 7.0	3.5	0 to 1
>38	>3,000	>7.0	4.0	1

The importance of resuming ventilation cannot be over-emphasized. Many Paramedics place the finger into the newborn's mouth and press the endotracheal tube against the hard palate to stabilize it while the bag–mask assembly is reattached and the newborn ventilated.

With the endotracheal tube in place, it is important for the Paramedic to verify its placement using end-tidal carbon dioxide detectors and/or capnography. However, the Paramedic should be cautious when using the end-tidal carbon dioxide detector reading. Premature, low birth weight, and hypovolemic newborns may produce little carbon dioxide for the detector.

While the newborn is being ventilated, the Paramedic should place the stethoscope over the newborn's epigastrium and under each arm. Auscultation of the anterior chest may produce false findings as the newborn's chest is so small that sound transmits easily across the entire chest wall. Therefore, it is important that the Paramedic auscultate in the axilla. Finally, the Paramedic should observe for chest rise and fall as well as improvement in the newborn's heart rate.

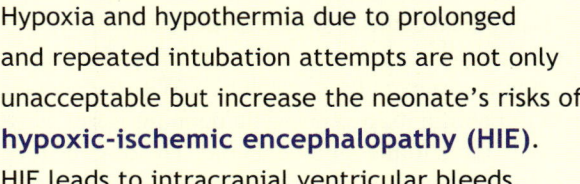

STREET SMART

Hypoxia and hypothermia due to prolonged and repeated intubation attempts are not only unacceptable but increase the neonate's risks of **hypoxic-ischemic encephalopathy (HIE)**. HIE leads to intracranial ventricular bleeds.

Causes of Difficulty with Positive Pressure Ventilation

Whenever positive pressure ventilation via the endotracheal tube seems ineffective, the Paramedic must assess the problem and try to resolve the issue. The mnemonic DOPE is helpful in divining the problem.

The D in DOPE stands for a **D**isplaced endotracheal tube. It is not difficult to accidentally pull the endotracheal tube into the hypopharynx. This delivers air to the stomach which, in turn, impairs ventilation. If this is the case, the patient should be extubated and the stomach decompressed with an orogastric tube.

Alternatively, it is possible to push the endotracheal tube into the right main stem. This effectively reduces the lung capacity in half, making delivery of a standard volume more difficult. If this is the case, then the endotracheal tube should be withdrawn until even chest rise is observed and compliance with positive pressure ventilation improves.

In some cases, the endotracheal tube becomes **O**bstructed (e.g., by meconium). This is the O in DOPE. In those cases, the Paramedic should consider the use of a meconium aspirator and then re-intubate the newborn.

In a fast-paced neonatal resuscitation, it is easy to forget that the newborn has to be ventilated carefully. On occasion, increased intrathoracic pressure leads to barotrauma and a **P**neumothorax (the P in DOPE).

If the Paramedic suspects a pneumothorax, then it may be necessary to perform a needle thoracostomy. Using a small 21 gauge or 23 gauge needle, the Paramedic inserts the needle into the chest at the fourth intercostal space at the midaxillary line, approximately in the nipple line. This site is preferentially chosen in order to avoid the heart and great vessels on the anterior wall.[6] With a syringe attached to a three-way stopcock, the air is aspirated, and the pneumothorax reduced. Compliance should improve with positive pressure ventilation via the bag–mask assembly.

Finally, it is possible that the **E**quipment (the E in DOPE) has failed. Starting at the patient, the Paramedic should work backwards over the respiratory circuit, from endotracheal tube to oxygen tank, to see if there is any equipment failure.

STREET SMART

Even with proper intubation and use of the bag-mask assembly, it may be difficult for the Paramedic to ventilate the premature infant. These newborns require higher than usual pressures in order to ventilate. The Paramedic must pay close attention to chest rise and other signs in these cases.

Chest Compressions

After 30 seconds of positive pressure ventilation, the Paramedic should reassess the newborn's heart rate. If the newborn's heart rate is less than 100 bpm, then the newborn's heart is too depressed (despite the presence of adequate oxygen) to pump blood. In this case, the Paramedic should proceed with external chest compressions.

The goal of cardiac compressions is to squeeze the heart between the sternum and the spine. This increase and release of intrathoracic pressure, as well as the direct pumping action, helps to circulate blood. There are two techniques Paramedics use to perform cardiac compressions.

The first technique, which may be more useful for full-term and post-term newborns, is the two finger technique.[10] The Paramedic identifies the lower third of the sternum and places two fingers (usually the index and middle finger) straight down on that point. With the other hand under the newborn's back, to act as a support, the Paramedic starts compressions.

For low birth weight and preterm newborns, the Paramedic should consider using the thumb technique of chest compressions. The Paramedic would encircle the chest wall with two hands and place each thumb on the midline of the

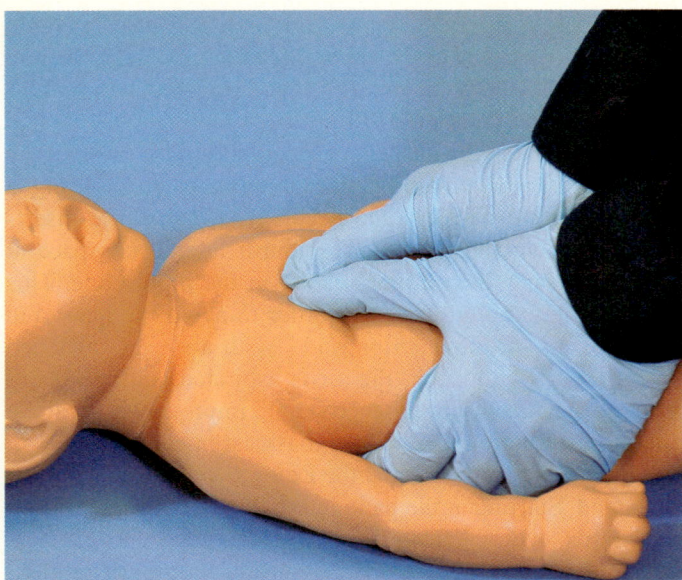

Figure 39-4 Neonatal chest compressions.

sternum. With the fingers acting as a support, and sometimes interlocked, the thumbs (one overlying the other if the newborn is small) would be used for compression. It is important that the tips of the thumbs, and not the pads of the thumbs, be used in order to compress the heart.

Although the thumb technique is less tiring, the two finger technique also allows the Paramedic access to the abdomen for umbilical catheterization. In both techniques, chest compression and ventilation must be coordinated in order to deliver 30 ventilations and 100 to 120 compressions a minute (Figure 39-4). An average cycle of three compressions and one ventilation should take about two seconds.

Drug Administration

After 30 seconds of combined ventilations and compressions, the Paramedic should stop and assess the newborn. If the newborn's heart rate has greatly improved (i.e., greater than 100 bpm), then the Paramedic should resume ventilation only

for another 30 seconds and then reassess to see if the newborn has further improved. If the newborn's heart rate is greater than 60 bpm but still less than 100 bpm, the Paramedic may continue ventilation and compressions.

If the newborn's heart rate remains below 60 beats per minute despite adequate ventilation and chest compressions, then the Paramedic should consider administering epinephrine.[11] Epinephrine increases the rate and strength of cardiac contractions and causes peripheral vasoconstriction.

Venous Access

Administration of epinephrine to a newborn can be a challenge, as the traditional routes of drug administration (intravenous and intraosseous) are not available. Instead, the Paramedic must use alternative routes of drug administration.

The first route is umbilical catheterization (Table 39-3). With practice, the Paramedic can become very proficient at umbilical catheterization. First, the Paramedic should loosely tie off the base of the umbilical cord with umbilical tape. A slight amount of bleedback is desirable, as it permits the Paramedic to identify the various structures more easily. If the bleeding is profuse, the tie can be tightened.

Next, the Paramedic should clean the cord with an antiseptic solution (often povidone–iodine solution) and then prepare the 3.5F or 5F umbilical catheter while the antiseptic solution dries.[6] The umbilical catheter should be filled with 0.9% saline solution by use of a three-way stopcock, with syringe and extension tubing to a bag of saline solution. With the necessary equipment out and in place, and while donning sterile gloves, the Paramedic turns to the umbilical cord. The umbilical cord should be cut, perpendicularly, approximately 1 to 2 cm from the clamp closest to the newborn.

Looking at the end of the umbilical cord, the Paramedic should identify the umbilical vein, which is usually found at the 1 o'clock position. The two smaller umbilical arteries are identifiable by their thicker walls and are typically at the 4 and 8 o'clock positions, respectively.

Next, the Paramedic carefully inserts the umbilical catheter into the umbilical vein, carefully threading the catheter approximately 2 to 4 cm or until a flash of fresh blood is observed (whichever occurs first).

With the umbilical catheter in place, as observed by the flash, the Paramedic flushes the catheter by opening

Table 39-3 Umbilical Catheterization Supplies

- Sterile gloves
- Antiseptic solutions (e.g., Betadine® wash)
- Umbilical scissors (preferred) or scalpel
- Syringes (sizes 1 mL, 3 mL, 5 mL, 10 mL, and 20 mL)
- Umbilical catheters (3.5F and 5F)
- Normal saline solution
- Three-way stopcock

the stopcock in the direction of the catheter and irrigating the catheter with approximately 5 mL of 0.9% saline solution.

With the umbilical catheter in place, the umbilical tape can be tightened to prevent bleedback and to ensure the passage for drug administration. At this time, the premeasured epinephrine is injected, followed by a saline flush (Skill 39-6).

For a step-by-step demonstration of Umbilical Catheterization, please refer to Skill 39-6 on page 775.

The alternative method of drug administration in a newborn is via the endotracheal tube. In this case, epinephrine can be absorbed through the lung and into the pulmonary veins, where it will travel directly to the heart.

One obstacle to endotracheal administration of epinephrine is the small volume. Often the volume of epinephrine has to be supplemented with a small 0.9% saline flush of 0.5 to 1 mL in order to provide a sufficient volume to reach the lungs. Without this additional flush, the epinephrine will only coat the walls of the endotracheal tube and never reach the lungs.

Alternatively, some Paramedics use a 5F feeding tube as a conduit for the epinephrine and follow the epinephrine with a 0.5 mL flush of 0.9% saline solution. The feeding tube is then removed from the endotracheal tube and ventilation resumes to help distribute the drug across the lung fields for absorption. Recent research suggests that more epinephrine is administered when placed directly down the endotracheal tube as opposed to down a feeding tube within the endotracheal tube.

Although this may be the easiest means of drug administration in a neonatal resuscitation, drug absorption via the lungs is slower than if the epinephrine is injected directly into the umbilical vein. Therefore, if the endotracheal route is chosen the larger dose of 0.3 mL/kg, followed by a 1 mL flush, should be considered.[12]

STREET SMART

Some Paramedics use a small 1 mL syringe to draw the drug from a standard 1 mg ampule of epinephrine and then draw an additional 0.5 mL 0.9% saline solution into another syringe for flush.

Additional Considerations

When the newborn has not responded adequately to ventilation, compressions, and epinephrine administration, the Paramedic should consider some other possible etiologies. Early consideration and intervention in these cases may lead to a better outcome for the newborn.

Narcotic-Induced Respiratory Depression

If the newborn has failed to respond to positive pressure ventilation, as demonstrated by poor muscle tone and/or apnea, and respiratory depression secondary to narcotics is suspected, the Paramedic might consider the administration of naloxone. However, naloxone should only be given in the field if the Paramedic administered morphine, or a similar opiate-based medication, to the mother within the last four hours. As this is a rare event, naloxone is seldom given in a prehospital neonatal resuscitation.[13–15]

The dose of naloxone is 0.1 mg/kg intravenously or endotracheally. As naloxone has a shorter half-life than some opiate-based medications, the Paramedic should be prepared to repeat the naloxone, as needed.

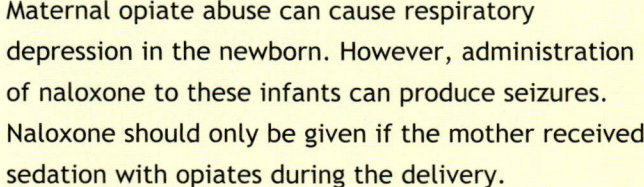

STREET SMART

Maternal opiate abuse can cause respiratory depression in the newborn. However, administration of naloxone to these infants can produce seizures. Naloxone should only be given if the mother received sedation with opiates during the delivery.

Hypovolemia

Some preexisting conditions—such as placental abruption, placenta previa, and hemorrhage from the umbilical cord—can make a newborn hypovolemic. If hypovolemia is suspected, as evidenced by pallor despite oxygenation, weak pulses with a good heart rate, and poor response to resuscitative efforts, the use of normal saline or lactated Ringer's as a volume expander can be considered. The initial volume of administration is 10 mL/kg, with a repeat of the same dose if indicated. The use of a stopcock and syringe attached to the extension tubing that is attached to the umbilical catheter can help to ensure administration of accurate volume.

Because of the fragile nature of the newborn's brain, the administration of a fluid challenge should be slow, over 5 to 10 minutes, and not in a bolus. Rapid intravenous bolus of solution puts the newborn at risk for intracranial hemorrhage.

Acidosis

Sodium bicarbonate solution, sometimes thought of as the drug of last resort, is administered when metabolic acidosis is suspected. Metabolic acidosis can dampen the strength of myocardial contraction as well as pulmonary vasoconstriction, leading to hypoxia and worsening acidosis. If metabolic acidosis is suspected, from lactic acid production secondary to anaerobic respiration, then the Paramedic can consider sodium bicarbonate administration.

The dose of sodium bicarbonate is 2 mEq/kg, or 4 mL/kg of 4.2% solution, administered intravenously very slowly, at 1 mEq/kg/min or 2 mL/kg/min. Sodium bicarbonate should only be used if adequate ventilation is provided. Because it is a hyperosmotic solution, it should be given slowly, at least over 30 minutes, in order to minimize the risk of intraventricular hemorrhage of the brain.[16]

For sodium bicarbonate to be effective, there must be adequate ventilation. Since sodium bicarbonate joins with acid to form carbon dioxide, ventilation is needed to rid the body of the excess carbon dioxide. Otherwise, it will remain in the blood as carbonic acid. Sodium bicarbonate should never be administered via the endotracheal tube, as sodium bicarbonate is caustic and can cause a chemical burn to the newborn's lungs. The Paramedic must be sure to use the proper drug dosages during a neonatal resuscitation (Table 39-4).

Table 39-4 Pediatric Resuscitation Drug Chart

Drug Name	Dose	Concentration
Epinephrine	0.1 to 0.3 mL/kg	1:10,000
Sodium bicarbonate	2 mEq/kg	4.2% solution (5 mEq/mL)
Naloxone	0.1 mg/kg	1.0 mg/mL
Dextrose	0.25 to 0.5 gm/kg	2.5 to 5 mL/kg of D_{10} 1 to 2 mL/kg of D_{25}

CASE STUDY (CONTINUED)

During transport, the preterm newborn is stabilized, and is receiving warmed, humidified oxygen by blow-by. The Paramedic is able to complete a neonatal examination while attending to the newborn's warmth and skin protection. The mother, who is being transported in a different ambulance, is given a quick update on her baby's condition by radio.

CRITICAL THINKING QUESTIONS

1. What are some of the predictable complications associated with neonatal resuscitation?
2. What are the elements of a neonatal examination?

Evaluation

When the preterm newborn is stabilized, the Paramedic may have the opportunity to do a head-to-toe examination of the child, reviewing critical organ systems in what is called a systems review. The first system to be examined, and perhaps the most important system, is the neurological system.

Neurological

The premature neonate's neurological system is not fully intact at birth as evidenced by the preterm neonate's inability to handle the stresses of light, touch, and sound stimulation. The Paramedic should strive to not startle the infant as sudden stimulation can lead to a change in vital signs. Containment of the neonate, by either wrapping the child in blankets or laying of hands on the neonate to restrict movement, will help the neonate remain calm and will help vital signs return to baseline.

During the examination, the Paramedic should attempt to keep the preterm newborn's head in a neutral alignment to prevent uneven buildup of pressure within the brain. This uneven intracranial pressure can lead to cerebral injury as manifest by abnormal movements or alteration in reflexes in the days or weeks that follow.

Typically, the Paramedic checks the newborn's papillary response as the first step in the neurological exam. The Paramedic should not be alarmed if the newborn's eyes are fused shut. It is not uncommon to find the premature neonate, especially who is under 27 weeks' gestation, with the eyes still fused and unable to open. The eyes will open on their own in a few days to a few weeks.

Next, the Paramedic should examine the newborn's cranium. The cranial suture lines of premature newborns are usually overriding and the head moldable secondary to prolonged positioning on one side. Well-approximated suture lines are seen more commonly in the term neonate. The Paramedic should be assessing for separation of the suture lines, which is seen in **hydrocephalus** (increased spinal fluid surrounding the brain) (Figure 39-5).

The Paramedic may then proceed to examine the fontanels. **Fontanels** (i.e., soft spots) are the openings between the skull's bones in the suture line. Fontanels that are tense, full, or bulging indicate different degrees of increased intracranial pressure. Flat fontanels indicate an appropriate fluid balance whereas sunken fontanels can indicate dehydration or conditions where cerebral spinal fluid production is not adequate. The condition of the fontanels should be noted in the Paramedic's report and documentation.

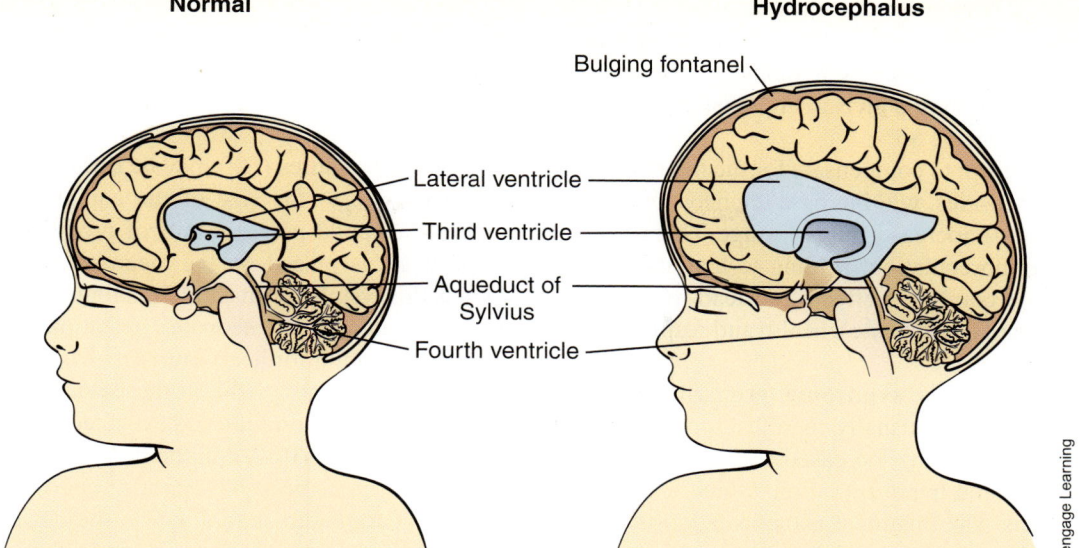

Normal   **Hydrocephalus**

Bulging fontanel

Lateral ventricle

Third ventricle

Aqueduct of
Sylvius

Fourth ventricle

Delmar/Cengage Learning

Figure 39-5 Hydrocephalus.

Intraventricular Hemorrhage

Periventricular hemorrhage (PVH) and **intraventricular hemorrhage (IVH)** are two life-threatening complications of prematurity. Complications of PVH and IVH, if the newborn survives, are cerebral palsy, developmental delays, and seizure disorders.

PVH and IVH occur when fragile capillaries within the germinal layer matrix rupture and bleed, secondary to sudden increases in blood pressure. Events that can cause PVH and IVH include asynchronous ventilation, hypoxia or hypercarbia, endotracheal suctioning, pneumothorax from overventilation, rapid intravenous bolus, infusion of dextrose 25% (D_{25}), and even rough handling.[17]

As a result of PVH and IVH, neurological damage can occur. Although this neurological damage can lead to abnormal movements and reflexes, these abnormal movements are not usually seen within the first few days of life. Bleeds are categorized according to severity on a scale of I to IV, with IV being the most severe. These intraventricular bleeds can have devastating, if not fatal, consequences.

Thoracic

After examination of the central nervous system, the Paramedic should assess the thoracic area for signs of respiratory difficulty. A hypoxic neonate (one in extremis) will exhibit nasal flaring, grunting, retractions, and low oxygen saturations.

The normal respiratory rate of a neonate is 40 to 60 breaths per minute. Since respiratory rates less than 40 breaths per minute are cause for concern, the Paramedic should continue the assessment in this situation.

The Paramedic should look for signs of increased work of breathing by checking for nasal flaring, grunting noises, and retractions. Audible expiratory grunting is caused by forcing air past a partially closed glottis. This mechanism creates a back pressure, called auto-PEEP (positive end expiratory pressure), that helps keep the lower airways and alveoli open.[10] Nasal flaring will also accompany grunting noises and is a sign of increased work of breathing.

The Paramedic may also note, especially during positive pressure ventilation using a bag–mask assembly, that the preterm neonate's rib cage is much more compliant than that of a toddler or adult. This is because the ribs are primarily cartilage.

When there is parenchymal disease, such as hyaline membrane disease or surfactant deficiency, the increased resistance to ventilation requires the newborn to work harder to breathe and therefore produces greater negative pressure, resulting in retractions. It is not uncommon to see a dip in excess of a few centimeters in the chest wall when the neonate is breathing normally. Therefore, when the neonate has an increased work of breathing, retractions will be more notable. These retractions are rated as slight (i.e., normal), mild, moderate, or severe, depending on the depth of the retractions.

The Paramedic may also want to check the newborn's oxygen saturation, often by placing a soft adhesive probe, covered in a transparent membrane, around the great toe (most of the newborn's skin is too fragile for an adhesive). There are commercially available, soft non-adhesive wraparound pulse oximeter probes for newborns.

Oxygen saturation for neonates differs from that of children and adults because of fetal hemoglobin. Oxygen saturations at or above 85% are acceptable for a newborn. However, because of the changing internal physiology, it may take a newborn 15 minutes to one hour to achieve an oxygen saturation of 95%. If oxygen is needed, it should not be withheld. Rather, the Paramedic should give an FiO_2 that keeps the oxygen saturation at or above 85%.

The body's attempt to compensate for the hypoxia, by the use of accessory muscles, will increase the neonate's oxygen demand, and will also increase glucose usage. This will affect the neonate's thermoregulation, leading to hypothermia and more stress. These combined effects can lead to a spiraling downward decline of the neonate's health and respiratory distress syndrome.

Respiratory distress syndrome primarily occurs in the preterm neonates and usually manifests in the first few hours. It is characterized by increased respiratory difficulty, leading to hypoxia and hypoventilation, which leads to progressive atelectasis. The treatment is the installation of intratracheal exogenous surfactant and respiratory support, either in the form of continuous positive airway pressure (CPAP), mechanical ventilation, or high frequency oscillator ventilations. These tools are all available in a neonatal intensive care unit (NICU).

Cardiovascular System

A number of remarkable changes occur in the newborn's cardiovascular system during the peripartum period. In most cases, the newborn's cardiovascular system will adjust to a more adult-like configuration within hours of birth. However, some newborns have cardiac defects, or anomalies. If a neonate has a cardiac defect, usually it will not affect the vital signs for the first few hours because the patent ductus arteriosus (PDA) will remain open.

Therefore, the newborn's cardiovascular status, as represented by heart rate, is more of reflection of the health of the respiratory system than a sign of cardiovascular disease. For this reason, it is the heart rate—not the respiratory rate—which drives the clinical decisions during resuscitation. If the heart rate falls below 60 bpm while the newborn is ventilated, the Paramedic should reposition and attempt ventilations again. If the heart rate does not increase, the Paramedic should start compressions as discussed previously.

The newborn's heart rate and rhythm is assessed by auscultation of the chest with a stethoscope rather than by the use of ECG leads. The Paramedic can obtain the heart rate at the umbilical stump. If no pulse is appreciated by palpation, then the apical heart rate should be obtained by auscultation. The normal heart rate of a premature neonate ranges from 140 to 180 beats per minute and will rise and fall due to oxygen saturations, temperature, and external stimuli.

If the Paramedic can appreciate a pulse at the umbilical stump, the quality of the pulse should be obtained. Bounding pulses signal to the Paramedic that the PDA is open, a common occurrence in the preterm neonate. If coupled with poor capillary refill (discussed shortly), diminished pulses may be a sign of hypotension.

Capillary refill, a dependable sign of perfusion in newborns, may be best obtained on the newborn's forehead. The normal capillary refill of the central body is between two and three seconds, and is even more important than the blood pressure.

Blood pressures (BP) may be difficult for the Paramedic to obtain due to the size of the equipment required. If an automated blood pressure cuff of proper size is used, more importance is placed on the mean arterial pressure (MAP) versus the systolic or diastolic readings. The MAP should be relatively equal to the neonate's gestational age in weeks.

Auscultation for heart murmurs in a newborn is not productive for the Paramedic in the field. Murmurs in the preterm neonate are common and expected, secondary to a patent ductus arteriosus (PDA). In the first few hours of life, almost every preterm neonate has a murmur and is asymptomatic.

The Paramedic should assess the newborn for signs of total body edema. Excessive edema to the entire body of the neonate may identify a condition known as **fetal hydrops** (i.e., hydrops fetalis). This condition is the generalized subcutaneous edema accompanied by ascites, pleural effusions, and or pericardial effusions.[18] Hydrops fetalis was more common before the creation of RhoGAM. RhoGAM was created to treat an isoimmune hemolytic disease that lead to erythroblastosis fatalis. Non-immune-related forms of hydrops fetalis, resulting in an imbalance of interstitial fluid production and lymphatic return, still exist today. Hydrops fetalis, a serious life-threatening condition, requires immediate neonatal intensive care as the treatment of the individual signs and symptoms of the various body systems is different.

Gastrointestinal

The abdomen of the neonate should be slightly rounded, soft, and nontender when the neonate is relaxed. Bowel sounds in the preterm neonate will be absent or hypoactive. It will take time for GI motility to start and bowel sounds to be audible; therefore, auscultation of bowel sounds may not be indicated. However, if the abdomen is firm or rigid, the Paramedic should investigate further. A rigid abdomen may be due to excess air in the gastric body from resuscitation efforts. Decompression of the stomach with an orogastric tube is essential at this time, since failure to decompress the stomach may lead to increased respiratory difficulty.

Genitourinary

In the preterm neonate, the appearance of genitalia varies according to gestation age. In rare occasions, the genitalia may be ambiguous. Urination may occur at birth or may take several hours. Normal urinary output in a neonate is between 2 and 4 mL per kg per hour.

Skin

The skin of preterm neonates, especially the **extremely low birth weight (ELBW)** neonate (a neonate weighing less than 1 kg or 2.2 pounds), is fragile and can be damaged easily.

The preterm newborn's skin is so thin that it will appear translucent, with blood vessels being visible directly under the skin. For this reason, warm packs are not to be used to warm a neonate. Instead, dry warm blankets should be used.

The integumentary system functions to protect the neonate against pathogens, topical teratogens, infection, and insensible water losses. The stratum corneum, the uppermost layer of the skin, may only be a few cells thick. Skin tears and skin shears easily happen during even routine care. For this reason, no adhesives should be placed directly on the skin of an extremely low birth weight neonate. Instead, adhesives should be covered with a bio-occlusive dressing prior to application to the skin. For example, the Paramedic, after applying the oxygen saturation probe that is covered with a bio-occlusive dressing, may now defer ECG leads and obtain a heart rate from the oxygen saturation probe. Many NICUs defer ECG leads during the first week of life in the extremely low birth weight neonate.

Because the newborn's skin is largely dysfunctional, the Paramedic must take steps to protect the newborn. Directly after birth and resuscitation, the neonate should be swaddled in a clear plastic wrap, followed by warm dry blankets, to decrease insensible water loss through the skin and to help with thermoregulation.

A premature rupture of membranes can be problematic for the newborn. If the amniotic sac protecting the neonate has been ruptured for an extended period of time, creating a potential portal of entry for infection, it can also create skin problems. Amniotic fluid in the womb acts as a cushion and exists for the neonate's protection. If there has been a lack of fluid prior to delivery, the neonate may be born with pressure ulcers of the skin that may even penetrate the muscle.

Extremities/Hips/Spine

At delivery, all neonates should be placed on their side directly after birth and the back inspected for possible undiagnosed myelomeningocele (protrusion of the spinal cord and nerves through an opening in the skin along the spine).

Table 39-5 Ballard Scoring

Gestational Age/Score	24 to 26 wk Score = 0	35 to 40 wk Score = 4
Skin	Gelatinous, red, translucent	Parchment, deep cracks, no visible vessels
Lanugo	Sparse	Mostly bald
Plantar surface	No crease	Creases over entire sole
Breast	Barely perceptible	Full areolae: 5 to 10 mm bud
Eye and ear	Lids open, pinna flat and stays folded	Thick cartilage, ear stiff
Genitalia (male)	Scrotum empty, faint rugae	Testes pendulous, deep rugae
Genitalia (female)	Prominent clitoris, small labia minora	Majora covers clitoris and minora

If a myelomeningocele is found, the area should be covered with sterile gauze, moistened with normal saline, then the trunk of the neonate should be wrapped with clear plastic wrap and blankets to decrease heat and water loss. This newborn should be left in a side-lying position and transported immediately to a tertiary care center containing a neonatal intensive care unit.

Ballard Scale and Prematurity

If time permits and the neonate remains stable, the **Ballard scoring system** can be used to approximate gestational age using a neuromuscular maturity score combined with a physical maturity score (Table 39-5). This can be particularly helpful if the mother is a poor historian. Although gestational age is important to report if known, it should be deferred in favor of stabilization and transport of the unstable neonate.

CASE STUDY CONCLUSION

The infant and mother are each transported to the Regional Medical Center, which has a level one NICU. The initial bonding activities are continued with the kangaroo care method. When the Paramedics run into the father one month later, he says his son is growing well but has had some setbacks as he continues to adjust to life outside of his mom. He thanks the team for their professional care of his family.

CRITICAL THINKING QUESTIONS

1. What is the most appropriate transport decision that will get the patient to definitive care?
2. What are the advantages of transporting a preterm neonate to these hospitals, even if that means bypassing other hospitals in the process?

Disposition

When transporting a preterm neonate and the mother by separate ambulances, the preterm neonate should be taken to the closest appropriate facility. However, both mother and neonate should be transported to the same facility if possible. Although this makes sense for ease of obtaining consents from the mother to treat her neonate, the even bigger reason is to help ensure mother–child bonding. Studies have shown that premature neonates have a higher risk for abuse, including shaken baby syndrome, due to lack of diminished bonding related to the mother and newborn being separated.[19]

The importance of the mother–child dyad cannot be overemphasized. While en route to the hospital, the mother should be encouraged to have contact with the infant.

One means is kangaroo care (i.e., placing the newborn to the mother's chest and swaddling mother and child). Kangaroo care encourages skin-to-skin contact between mother and child and fosters maternal bonding. Kangaroo care has also been shown to help stabilize the newborn's temperature, breathing, and heart rate. In the absence of an incubator, kangaroo care can provide the necessary warmth for newborn survival. Kangaroo care also provides ready access to nourishment through breastfeeding.

It is important for the Paramedic to identify the most appropriate facility for the preterm neonate. A preterm neonate will require stabilization and treatment in a neonatal intensive care unit (NICU). A NICU has specialized mechanical ventilators, infant incubators (open warmers), and a team of specialists to care for the newborn.

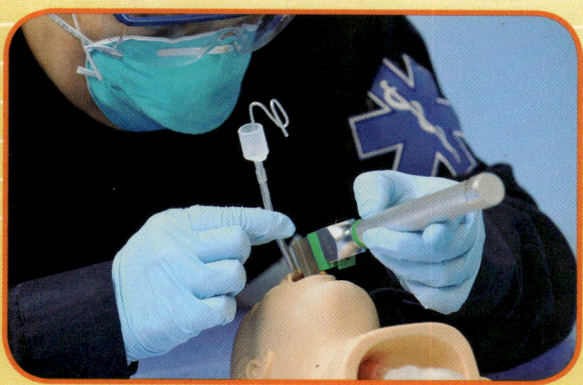

1 Intubation with straight blade.

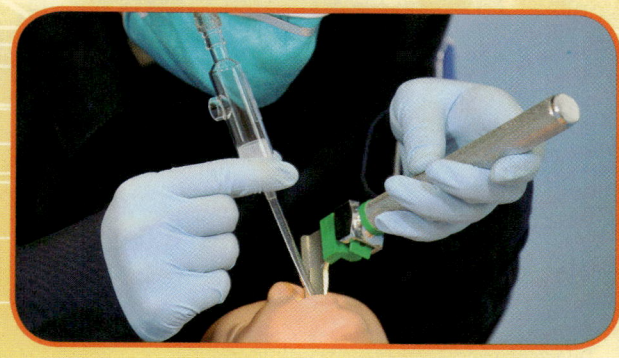

2 Use of endotracheal tube with meconium aspirator attached.

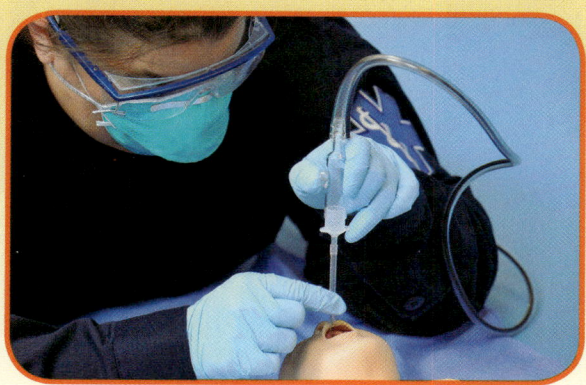

3 Withdrawal of endotracheal tube/meconium aspirator assembly.

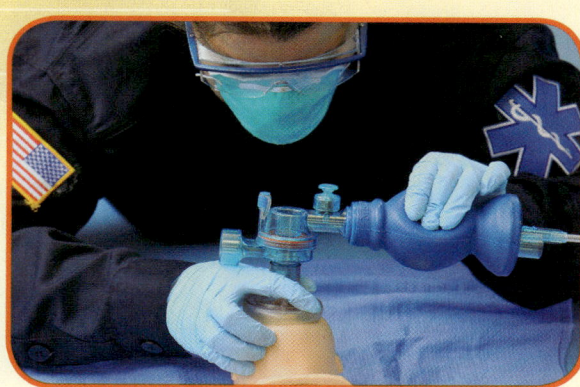

4 Ventilation and reassessment.

Delmar/Cengage Learning

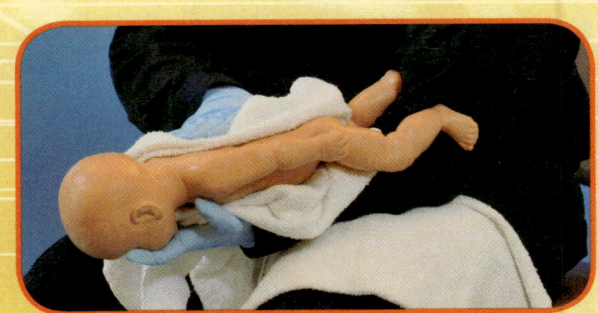

1 Drying newborn—changing towels frequently.

Rubbing infant's back to stimulate.

2

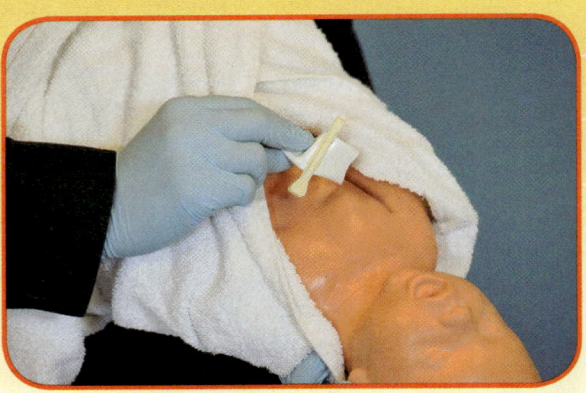

3 Assessing heart rate at umbilical stump.

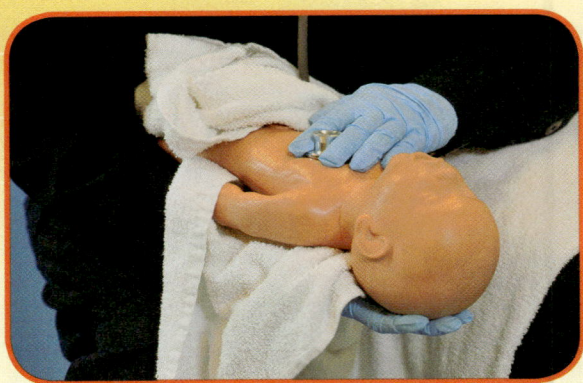

4 Assessing heart rate at apical point with neonatal stethoscope.

Delmar/Cengage Learning

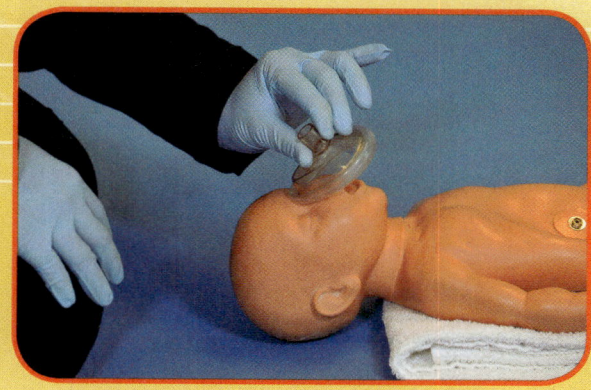

1 Selection of correct mask—attention to eyes and chin.

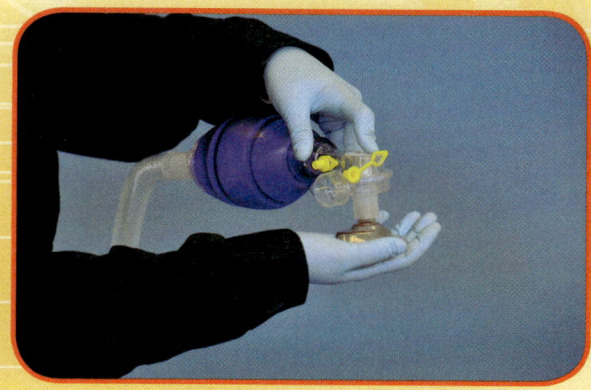

2 Application of BVM to mask.

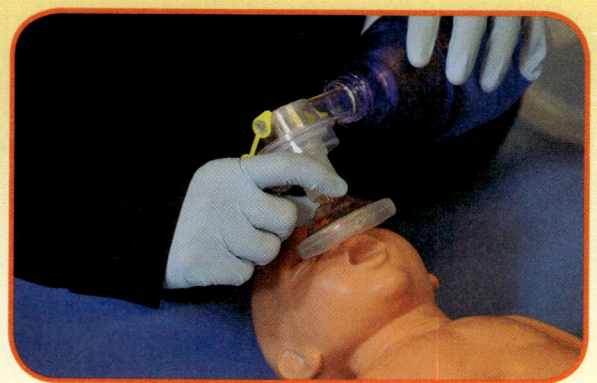

3 Seating mask on face.

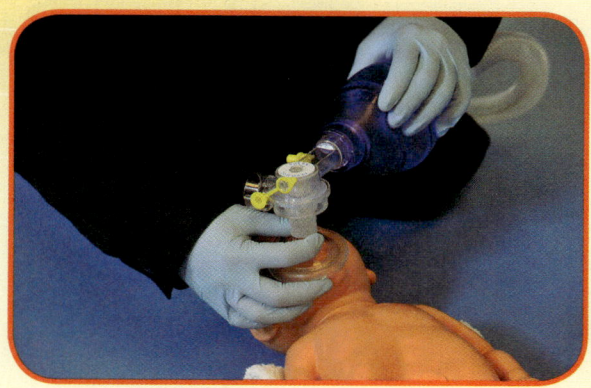

4 Gentle ventilation.

Delmar/Cengage Learning

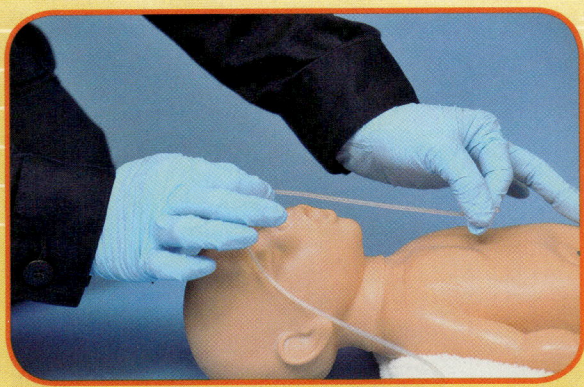

1 Measurement of 8F OGT from bridge of nose to earlobe to xiphoid process.

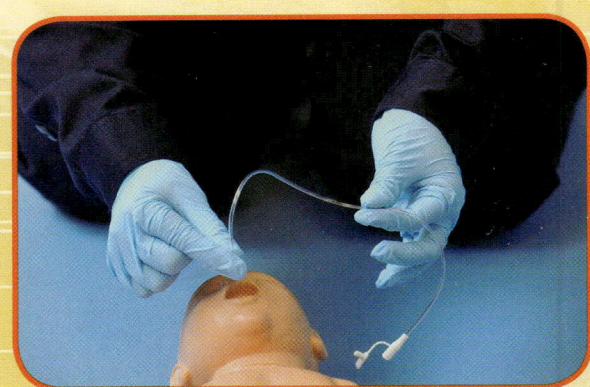

2 Insertion of OGT posteriorly.

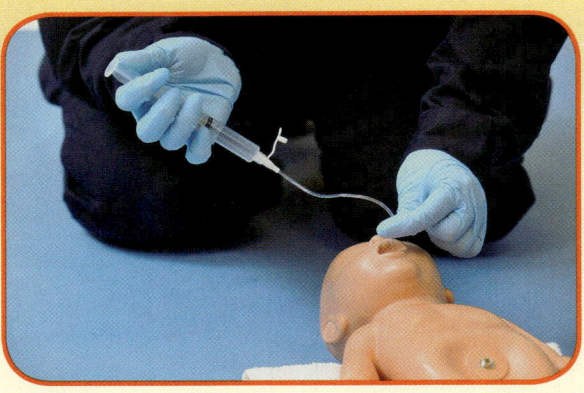

3 Aspiration of OGT.

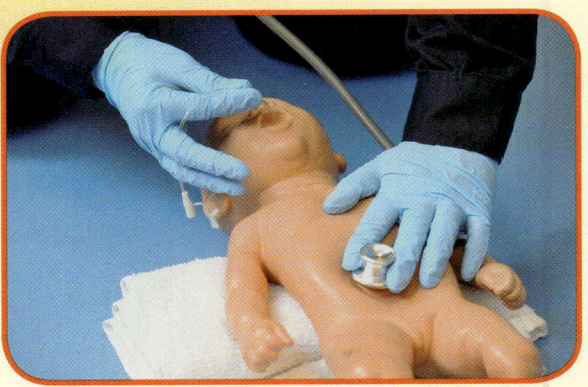

4 Confirmation with neonatal stethoscope.

Delmar/Cengage Learning

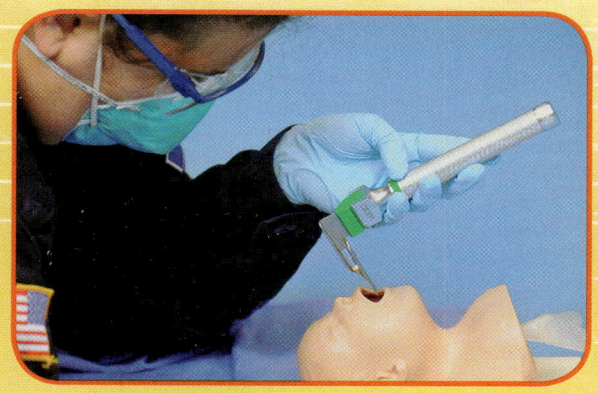

1 Left hand position—choked down on handle.

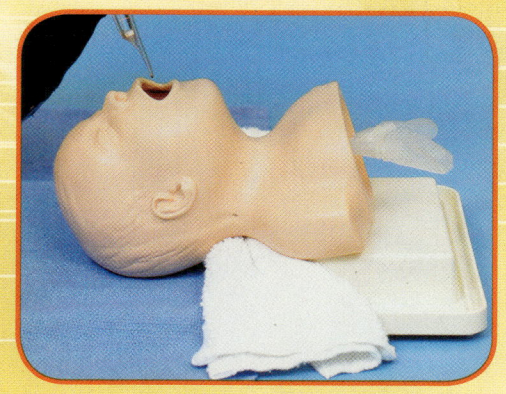

2 Newborn's head in neutral position—towel under shoulders.

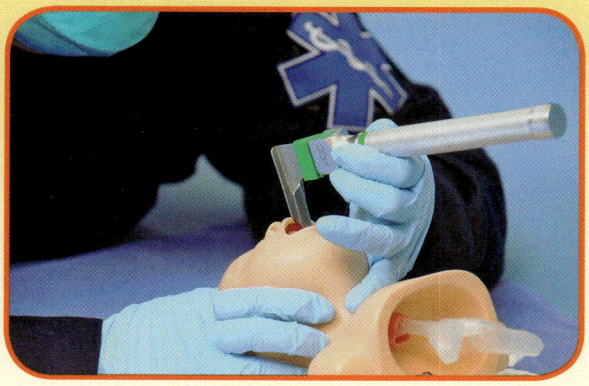

3 Insertion of blade midline with gentle forward traction—not pivoting—small finger applying pressure on larynx.

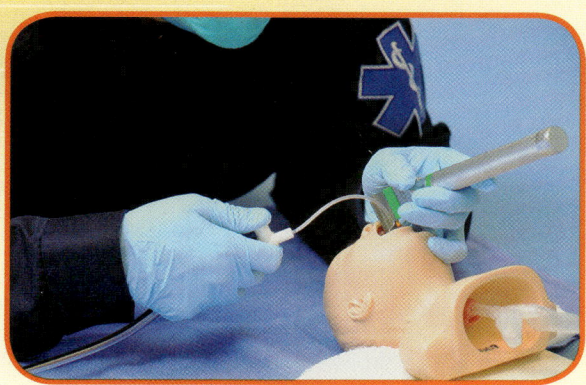

4 Suctioning with French catheter to clear secretions.

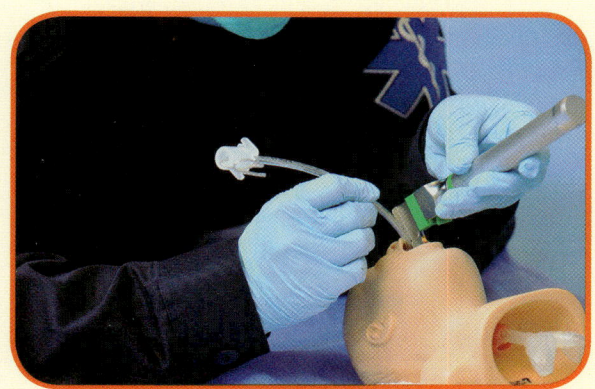

5 Insertion of endotracheal tube from right side—not midline.

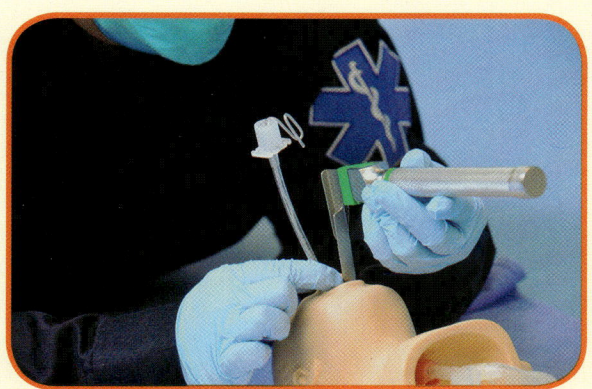

6 Stabilizing endotracheal tube with right forefinger while withdrawing blade.

Delmar/Cengage Learning

Special Considerations in Neonatology **773**

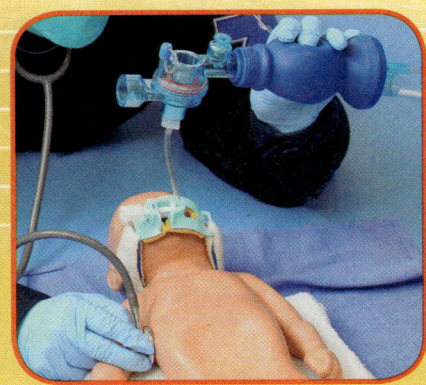

7 Ventilation while ascultating axilla.

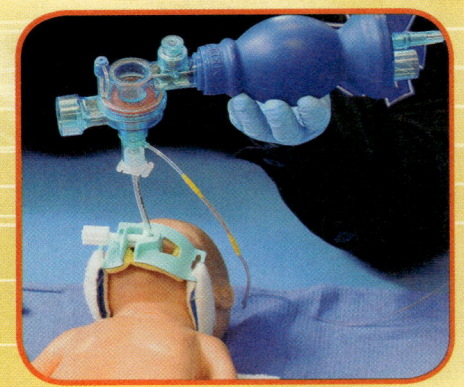

8 Use of end-tidal CO_2 and commercial securing device.

Delmar/Cengage Learning

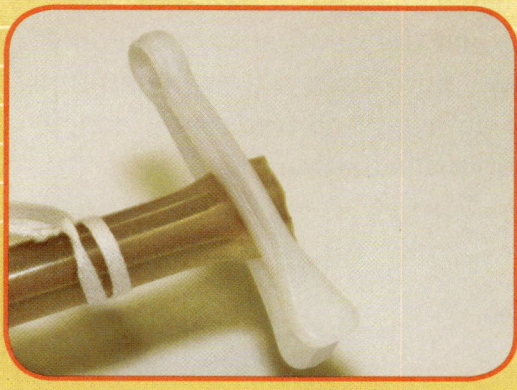

1 Apply umbilical tie and clamp.

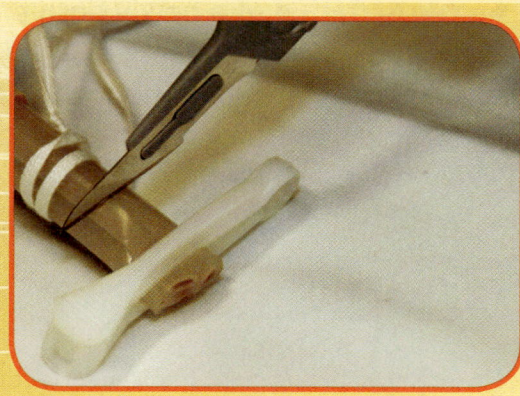

2 Prepare and cut the umbilical cord using sterile technique.

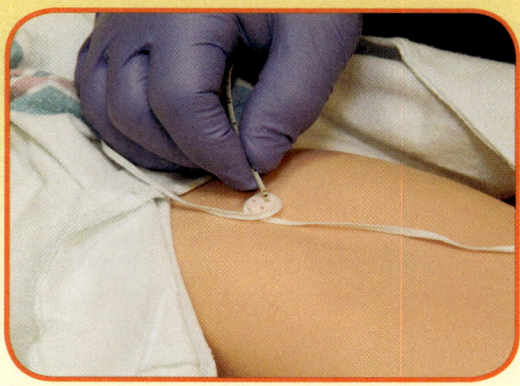

3 Insert the umbilical catheter approximately 1 to 2 cm into the umbilical vein.

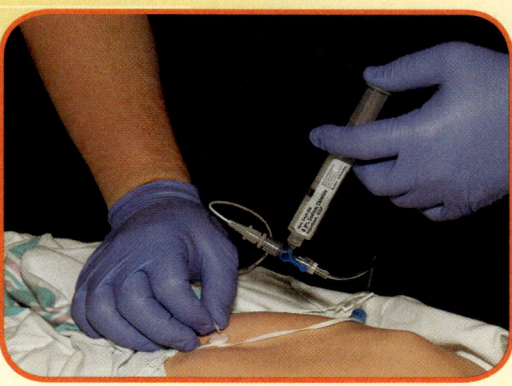

4 Open the stopcock and flush the vein in preparation of epinephrine administration.

Delmar/Cengage Learning

CONCLUSION

The resuscitation of a newly born child can be a highly charged situation for the Paramedic. Although most deliveries go smoothly and the newly born often only requires drying and stimulation, occasionally the newly born child will be in extremis. Thorough understanding of a treatment algorithm or pathway and frequent practice will allow the Paramedic to expertly handle this emotional situation.

▶ KEY POINTS:

- Preterm infants often have insufficient surfactant.

- Hypothermia is potentially life-threatening to preterm infants.

- A neutral thermal environment is the environmental goal for preterm infants.

- The four means of heat loss are conduction, convection, evaporation, and radiation.

- Paramedics can reduce the newborn's heat loss by wrapping the infant in plastic or using skin-to-skin contact called the kangaroo method.

- Primary apnea occurs in preterm infants when continued hypoxia leads to bradypnea. They can be stimulated to breathe.

- Secondary apnea occurs when prolonged hypoxia leads to gasping agonal respirations prior to apnea.

- In both cases, the Paramedic should apply the same early interventions of drying and warming the infant.

- Neonatal resuscitation is algorithmic in approach.

- Choanal atresia, or narrowed nasal airway, will prevent the infant from breathing through the nose.

- Robin's syndrome, a congenitally small mandible, will impair breathing when the infant is supine.

- To reduce abdominal distention that interferes with ventilation, the Paramedic may place an orogastric tube.

- Congenital diaphragmatic hernia occurs when the diaphragm is incompletely formed, allowing abdominal organs into the thoracic cavity.

- The mnemonic DOPE is used to find the cause of ventilation difficulty.

- The Paramedic should start chest compressions if the newborn's heart rate is below 100 and not improving with oxygen and ventilation.

- Failure to respond to chest compressions and ventilations should lead the Paramedic to employ epinephrine.

- Naloxone is indicated only if the mother has received an opiate four hours or less before delivery.

- Initial volume replacement for a preterm infant is 10 mL/kg of normal saline or lactated Ringer's.

- Sodium bicarbonate is indicated for metabolic acidosis in the face of good ventilation.

- A head-to-toe exam includes:
  - Eyes—may be fused shut at less than 27 weeks' gestational age
  - Suture line—separated in hydrocephalus
  - Fontanels—tense in increased intracranial pressure or depressed in dehydration
  - Chest—look at work of breathing
  - Abdomen—may be rigid due to air in stomach, bowel, or anal abnormalities
  - Genitalia—gender may be ambiguous in the preterm infant
  - Skin—fragile and thin
  - Extremities/hip/spine—look for myelomeningocele

- Vital signs
  - Heart rate and rhythm are checked by stethoscope or at the umbilical stump.
  - Capillary refill of two to three seconds is normal and best obtained at the forehead.

- The Ballard scoring system is one method of estimating gestational age.

REVIEW QUESTIONS:

1. Describe the consequences of hypothermia on the preterm infant.
2. Name two methods of preventing heat loss in the preterm infant.
3. Describe the algorithmic approach to neonatal resuscitation.
4. Explain each letter in the mnemonic DOPE as related to ventilation difficulties.
5. When should the Paramedic consider the use of the following medications in the treatment of the preterm infant?
   a. Epinephrine
   b. Naloxone
   c. Sodium bicarbonate
6. What is the usual fluid replacement calculation for a preterm infant? Which fluids are usually chosen for volume replacement?

CASE STUDY QUESTIONS:

Please refer to the Case Study in this chapter, and answer the questions below:

1. What methods exist for estimating gestational age?
2. Based on a gestational age of approximately 28 weeks, what exam results do the Paramedics expect in the following exams?
   a. Eyes
   b. Suture lines
   c. Fontanels
   d. Chest
   e. Abdomen
   f. Genitalia
   g. Skin
3. Explain why preterm infants are at risk of shaken baby syndrome or other forms of child abuse. How can initial Paramedic care influence that risk?

REFERENCES:

1. Hay W, Hayward A, et al. *Current Pediatric Diagnosis & Treatment*. New York: McGraw-Hill/Appleton & Lange; 2002.
2. Asakura H. Fetal and neonatal thermoregulation. *J Nippon Med Sch*. 2004;71(6):360–370.
3. Gunn TR, Gluckman PD. Perinatal thermogenesis. *Early Hum Dev*. 1995;42(3):169–183.
4. Brownfoot FC, Crowther CA, et al. Different corticosteroids and regimens for accelerating fetal lung maturation for women at risk of preterm birth. *Cochrane Database Syst Rev*. 2008;4:CD006764.
5. Hermansen CL, Lorah KN. Respiratory distress in the newborn. *Am Fam Physician*. 2007;76(7):987–994.
6. Association A. *PALS Provider Manual*. Dallas: American Heart Association; 2002.
7. Gonzalez de Dios J, Moya Benavent M, et al. Neonatal morbidity associated with meconial amniotic fluid. *An Esp Pediatr*. 1998;48(1):54–59.
8. Katz VL, Bowes WA, Jr. Meconium aspiration syndrome: reflections on a murky subject. *Am J Obstet Gynecol*. 1992;166(1 Pt 1):171–183.
9. Carbine DN. Meconium aspiration. *Pediatr Rev*. 2008;29(6):212–213; discussion 213.
10. Drew D, Jevon P, et al. *Resuscitation of the Newborn: A Practical Approach*. England: Books for Midwives; 2000.
11. Ziino AJ, Davies MW, et al. Epinephrine for the resuscitation of apparently stillborn or extremely bradycardic newborn infants. *Cochrane Database Syst Rev*. 2003;2:CD003849.
12. Lindemann R. Resuscitation of the newborn. Endotracheal administration of epinephrine. *Acta Paediatr Scand*. 1984;73(2):210–212.
13. McGuire W, Fowlie PW, et al. Naloxone for preventing morbidity and mortality in newborn infants of greater than 34 weeks' gestation with suspected perinatal asphyxia. *Cochrane Database Syst Rev*. 2004;1:CD003955.
14. McGuire W, Fowlie PW. Naloxone for narcotic exposed newborn infants: systematic review. *Arch Dis Child Fetal Neonatal Ed*. 2003;88(4):F308–F311.
15. Herschel M, Khoshnood B, et al. Role of naloxone in newborn resuscitation. *Pediatrics*. 2000;106(4):831–834.
16. Reichert EM, Fuller PW. Relationship of sodium bicarbonate to intraventricular hemorrhage in premature infants with respiratory distress syndrome. *Nurs Res*. 1980;29(6):357–361.
17. Altman DI, Volpe JJ. Cerebral blood flow in the newborn infant: measurement and role in the pathogenesis of periventricular and intraventricular hemorrhage. *Adv Pediatr*. 1987;34:111–138.
18. Jauniaux E. Diagnosis and management of early non-immune hydrops fetalis. *Prenat Diagn*. 1997;17(13):1261–1268.
19. De Sevo MR. Learning from tragedy: comments on "Reason to connect". *Nurs Womens Health*. 2007;11(1):11–12; author reply 12.

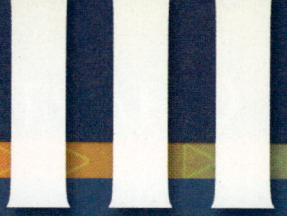

SECTION III

PEDIATRICS

Children are more than just small adults. However, Paramedics should not be fearful of treating these pediatric patients! This section presents the assessment, physiology, and pathophysiology of children. This allows the Paramedic student to become more confident in assessing and treating pediatric patients.

- **Chapter 40:** Assessment of the Stable Child
- **Chapter 41:** The Critically Ill Child
- **Chapter 42:** Pediatric Medical Emergencies
- **Chapter 43:** Child Abuse and Neglect

ASSESSMENT OF THE STABLE CHILD

KEY CONCEPTS:

Upon completion of this chapter, it is expected that the reader will understand these following concepts:

- The essential need for a quick initial assessment to differentiate whether there is a need for immediate hands-on care or if time allows for an opportunity to develop rapport with the child
- Ways to determine chronological age and developmental milestone achievement when planning history gathering and interventions for the stable child
- Methods to determine and use the correct size equipment for pediatric interventions

ANATOMY CONCEPTS:

Prior to reading this chapter the Paramedic student should be familiar with the following anatomy and physiology concepts:

- Child developmental stages

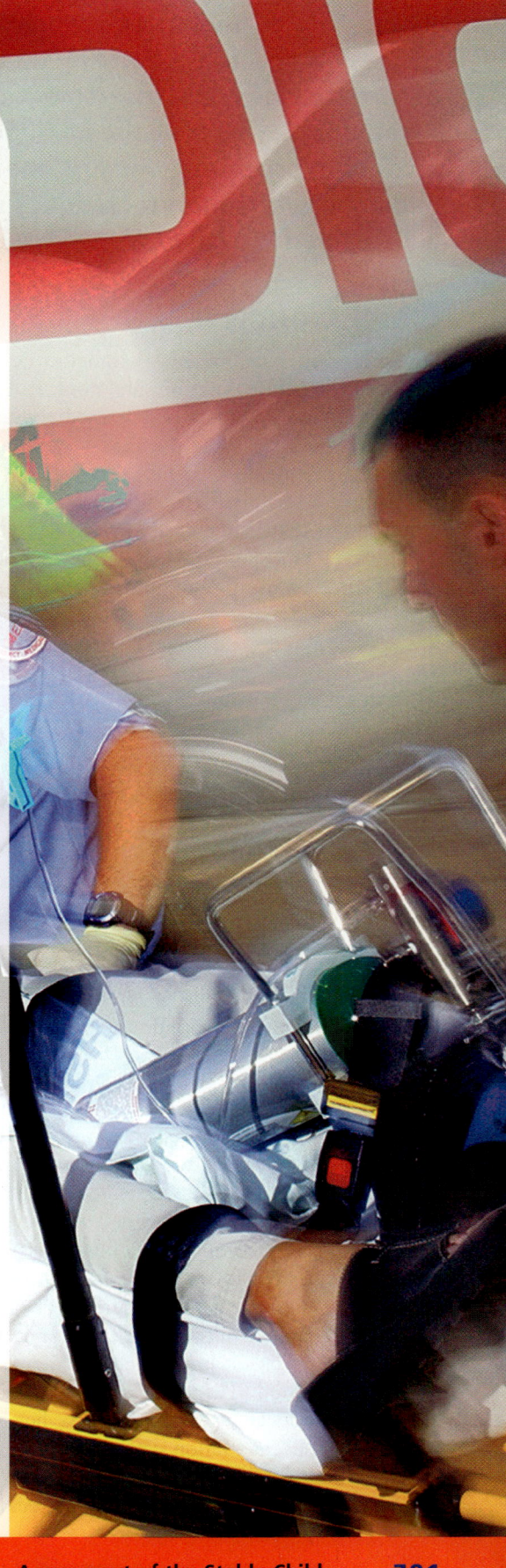

CASE STUDY:

The Springville Ambulance Squad with two Paramedics on board is dispatched to 127 Hollow Grove Drive for a child who has fallen from a bicycle. The child was initially unconscious but now is awake. The driver navigates the intersections in emergency response mode while his partner is considering the possible injuries. Both recently took a pediatric refresher class and attended several continuing education sessions at the local pediatric emergency department, so there is minimal anxiety from the crew about the call while en route.

On arrival, they step out of the ambulance and pause for a split second to notice Bobby Smith, lying flat on the ground next to a damaged bicycle with his mother kneeling beside him. Bobby appears to be about 6 years old, is talking with his mother, is moving all his extremities, appears to be breathing normally, and has normal appearing skin color. With their initial impression completed, the Paramedics each grab gear and move toward Bobby and his mother.

CRITICAL THINKING QUESTIONS

1. What are some of the possible causes of pediatric syncope?
2. What is the significance of the unconsciousness and then regained consciousness?

OVERVIEW

The field of pediatrics encompasses a significant age and developmental range of patients, often extending up to the age of 21. With variations of development at different stages, the assessment of pediatric patients can pose unique challenges to the Paramedic called to assist an ill or injured child. This challenge sometimes produces anxiety in providers who are uneasy in working with children. A solid understanding of pediatric assessment techniques will help Paramedics ease their anxiety when working with pediatric patients.

Chief Concern

As with adult patients, the Paramedic develops an initial impression when making his first contact with a child. This first impression provides the Paramedic with an initial indication of the severity of the illness or injury sustained by the pediatric patient. One tool that was developed to assist the Paramedic in rapidly identifying pediatric patients who require immediate intervention is the **Pediatric Assessment Triangle (PAT)** (Figure 40-1).[1] The Pediatric Assessment Triangle is most useful for younger pediatric patients and will allow the Paramedic to differentiate between those patients that require an immediate hands-on assessment and intervention and those that are stable enough so that more time can be taken in gaining the child's trust.

PROFESSIONAL PARAMEDIC

The Pediatric Assessment Triangle is an objective tool developed by the American Academy of Pediatrics that can be used to determine the severity of illness or injury in a child. The assessment criteria are determined during the general impression portion of the assessment.

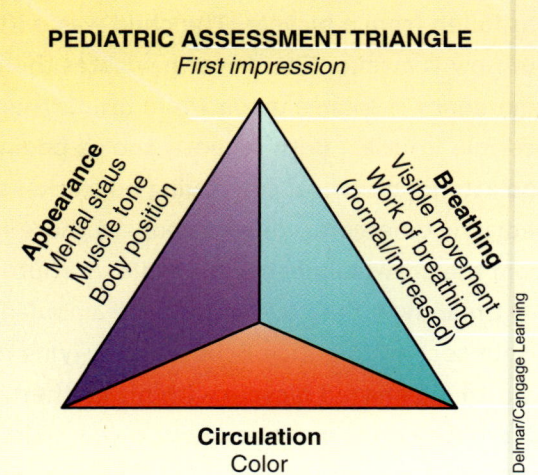

Figure 40-1 The Pediatric Assessment Triangle.

Table 40-1 The TICLS Mnemonic Used to Guide the Paramedic's Initial Assessment of a Child's Appearance

Category	Examples
Tone	Vigorous movement, limp, flaccid
Interactivity	Alert, attentive to surroundings, makes eye contact, reach for objects
Consolability	Crying alleviated by comforting
Look/Gaze	Eyes follow Paramedic's movement vs. blank stare
Speech/Cry	Strong, weak, hoarse

The three sides of the PAT consist of appearance, breathing, and circulation. Although these are three different aspects of the initial assessment, they are highly interrelated and can be thought of more as a three-legged stool than a triangle. If one of the legs of the three-legged stool is broken, the stool will fall over. In the same way, a child who, on initial assessment, has an issue with one of the three arms of the triangle is a sick patient and needs to be aggressively treated.

The appearance of the child, the first part of the PAT, can be assessed by observing the child's mental status, muscle tone, and position. The child's mental status is judged by assessing her level of consciousness, her interaction with parents, and her interaction with others. Some providers find the mnemonic **TICLS (Tone, Interactivity, Consolability, Look/Gaze, Speech/Cry)** helps them recall the important factors in assessing the child's appearance (Table 40-1).[2] Most children without severe distress should be alert and interact continuously with their environment and people around them at an age and developmentally appropriate level. The child should be interactive and make eye contact with the Paramedic as he enters the room. Children down to 6 months old should recognize their parents' voice and look toward their parent if the parent calls the child's name. A child who displays irritability, decreased responsiveness, poor interaction with parents, and does not acknowledge the Paramedic's presence as he moves closer to the patient should be rapidly assessed for a life-threatening condition.

Muscle tone and body position are assessed at the same time. Younger children and infants normally maintain slightly flexed extremities when their tone is normal. After the age of 6 months, most infants are able to sit up and look around without assistance. All children should spontaneously move their arms and legs. An infant or small child that lays with arms and legs extended and does not make eye contact with the Paramedic is likely sick and requires an immediate hands-on assessment and management.

The next side of the triangle is an assessment of the child's work of breathing. A child who is breathing normally should have a free, rhythmic excursion of the chest with inspiration and expiration without using any of the accessory muscles of respiration. In younger children and infants, abdominal movement with breathing is normal, whereas in older children this movement is abnormal. Any signs of an increased work of breathing during the initial assessment require immediate intervention by the Paramedic. As children are highly dependent on breathing, increased work of breathing can be an early sign of decompensation.[2]

The third side of the PAT is circulation. The Paramedic assesses the child's circulation during the initial assessment by observing the child's skin color. The skin color can be

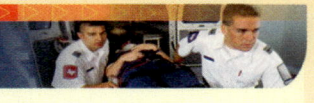
assessed on any exposed skin or mucous membrane surface (e.g., the lips, tongue, palms of the hands, or the soles of the feet). Normally, these surfaces should have a pink hue or normal coloration for the child's race. Cyanosis, pallor, mottled skin, or a gray tone indicates a significant circulatory problem that requires aggressive management.

If the child passes the initial assessment with all three sides of the PAT intact, then the Paramedic can continue obtaining a history and performing a more detailed physical examination, using the parents to assist him in gaining the child's trust. However, if any one of the three sides of the PAT has an issue, then the Paramedic must move quickly to provide supportive care while the more detailed assessment is performed.

CASE STUDY (CONTINUED)

The Paramedics introduce themselves to the child and then to the mother. "What happened?" one asks. She finds out that Bobby was riding his bicycle near the edge of the driveway when he lost his balance on a crack in the sidewalk. Bobby is crying and upset and tells her that he hurts all over. Bobby's mother denies that Bobby lost consciousness but also states she did not see him fall. Throughout the interview, the Paramedic speaks calmly and reassures Bobby and his mother.

CRITICAL THINKING QUESTIONS

1. What are the important elements of the history that a Paramedic should obtain?
2. Is obtaining a history from a child different than obtaining a history from an adult?

History

If the child is assessed as noncritical after the initial assessment, the Paramedic often has time to obtain a detailed history. Although many of the same questions are asked of pediatric patients as are asked of adult patients, the Paramedic may have to alter his method of questioning to be more effective at gathering an appropriate history. Much of this depends on the physical and emotional age of the child, with the understanding that most children, even teens, will emotionally regress when placed in a situation of stress, pain, or anxiety. If that is the case, the Paramedic may have to use the same techniques

to gain the trust of—and a history from—an older child who has emotionally regressed.

Regardless of age, the Paramedic can use some general principles in obtaining a history from a pediatric patient. The Paramedic can introduce himself and other crew members to both the patient and the family, making eye contact during the introduction.

The Paramedic should kneel down to the child's level to allow better eye contact and gain the child's trust. He should speak softly, calmly, and clearly while looking at the child, and use age-appropriate language, providing examples the child may understand. The Paramedic should be

In some cultures, it is considered disrespectful or challenging to make direct eye contact. The Paramedic should use the caregiver's actions as an example. Additionally, it may also be disrespectful for a child to make eye contact with an adult or to answer before his elders answer.

honest with the child and answer her questions to the best of his ability.

For infants, the history is going to come from the caregivers or bystanders. The Paramedic should assess stable children while they are in a caregiver's arms or sitting on the caregiver's lap. This will help the Paramedic gain the child's trust. The Paramedic should speak softly and calmly, since infants are disturbed or startled by loud sounds. By exhibiting a calm demeanor, the Paramedic will help instill confidence in the parents, trust in the child, and provide overall reassurance. Calming the parents or caregivers will help calm the infant and allow the Paramedic to gather a more accurate history and complete physical examination.

Toddlers (ages 1 to 3 years old) are often a bit more interactive than infants. However, this will vary as toddlers go through the natural periods of separation anxiety. It is often best to allow the child to sit in his caregiver's arms if it is medically possible until the Paramedic develops a rapport with the child. Again, loud speech may frighten the child, whereas a soft and clear voice will be comforting. The Paramedic should kneel down to talk with the child and the parent, looking the child in the eyes during the introduction. Speaking to the child before making physical contact will allow the toddler time to get comfortable with the Paramedic's presence and allow a more reliable physical examination. Small bits of praise (e.g., commenting on their appearance, clothing, or toys) can also build a sense of trust with the toddler and calm fears about the Paramedic's presence. Finally, toddlers and young children are very literal. Therefore, the Paramedic should use concrete terms with toddlers to avoid confusion and issues later.

Past medical history that the Paramedic should obtain on children in the infant and toddler age groups include information about the pregnancy, delivery, development, and immunizations. Complications that occurred during the pregnancy may include trauma, gestational diabetes, poor growth, and bleeding. Delivery complications may include presence of Group B strep or active herpes, the need for an emergent cesarean section, poor APGAR scores, or other complications during the delivery process.[3] Learning about the child's achievement of **developmental milestones** (physical or behavioral signs of development) will help the Paramedic

adjust his interview and assessment technique based upon the child's developmental age and provide an indication as to what may be normal for the child. Immunizations are designed to significantly decrease the risk of certain diseases that have historically been responsible for the death and disability of many children and young adults. Some parents choose not to have their children immunized due to religious beliefs or due to fears the vaccines are linked with autism and neurological diseases. The paramedical differential may be broadened in patients who have not been properly immunized. In many situations, it is also helpful to briefly ask about the child's feeding and elimination habits as part of the history of present illness. Inadequate feeding may indicate a primary respiratory problem and increases the likelihood that the patient is dehydrated. Dehydration and poor feeding may be confirmed by a history of a recent decreased urine output. One helpful way to ask this question for the pre-potty trained child is to ask the caregiver when the child's diaper was last changed and how soaked it was. If the diaper was changed recently, the Paramedic should ask about the timing and sogginess for the diaper change before the most recent one.

Preschoolers (ages 3 to 6 years old) are also very literal in their thinking and will take what the Paramedic says very literally. The Paramedic should approach the child at eye level and introduce himself to the child first to ease her anxiety and provide the child with some control. The preschooler is generally a little more curious than the toddler and may want to play with the Paramedic's equipment, which will provide a distraction and defuse the situation. As with toddlers, praise goes a long way toward winning trust and providing common ground. The Paramedic should use simple, concrete language and terms when asking questions and discussing care. Although most preschoolers begin the encounter shyly, most will open up and begin to play with the Paramedic during their contact.

School-age children (ages 6 to 12 years old) begin to develop more logical thinking and better communication skills. As a result, they may be able to answer a lot of questions themselves. Again, the Paramedic should introduce himself to the child at eye level and begin the interview with the child by obtaining her version of the events. At the appropriate time, the Paramedic should tell the child that he will now ask some questions of the caregiver, allowing the Paramedic an opportunity to obtain information that the child may not be able or willing to give. Depending on the situation, the child may be afraid to provide information when her caregiver is present for fear of disapproval or getting into trouble. If the Paramedic senses that may be the case, he should turn to the caregiver and ask that individual to provide some history to a Paramedic partner, affording the child some privacy to talk about the events. The Paramedic should reassure the child that his intention is only to help her, not to get her into trouble. Praise will also help the Paramedic gain trust and alleviate anxiety in this age group as it does in younger age groups. The Paramedic should ask questions using simple terms the child can understand.

Adolescents and teenagers can be very challenging as they tend to develop risk-taking behaviors at that age, along with a sense of immortality. Paramedics may be looked upon as authority figures, which will cause some teens to develop a rebellious attitude toward them. Their caregivers may feed into this situation, causing the conflict to escalate. As with other age groups, the Paramedic should introduce himself to the patient first and then her caregivers. At this point, the Paramedic should be able to obtain most of the history directly from the patient. Teenagers and young adults are capable of, and frequently interested in, being sure their side of the story is heard. It may be appropriate for the Paramedic to try to interview the patient in private while the caregivers are either in another room or involved in a conversation with a Paramedic partner. The Paramedic should be straightforward, honest, and nonjudgmental with the patient and address any questions or concerns that surface during the interview. The maturity level in this age group will vary, with some patients acting more like an adult and some more like a school-ager. The Paramedic should attempt to defuse uncooperative teens by addressing their issues rather than by becoming angry at the uncooperative patient. Friends may be able to provide collateral information in the event that the patient is not able to provide a history.

As discussed in the prior section, in times of stress and anxiety, children may regress to an earlier developmental stage regardless of their physical age. If the Paramedic senses this is happening, he will need to change his approach to fit the child's developmental age.

CASE STUDY (CONTINUED)

After rapidly determining that Bobby's airway, breathing, and circulation are intact, the Paramedic explains to Bobby that she wants to make sure he is OK. To do so, she will listen to Bobby with her stethoscope and will touch his bones, his belly, and his chest. Through his tears, Bobby says it is OK for her to do those things. She then performs a quick head-to-toe assessment. In the meantime, her partner has retrieved the pediatric immobilization equipment from the ambulance and is now checking Bobby's vital signs.

CRITICAL THINKING QUESTIONS

1. What are the elements of the physical examination of a pediatric patient?
2. Why is the Pediatric Assessment Triangle a critical element in this examination?

Examination

Using the PAT during the initial assessment will allow the Paramedic to rapidly identify the patient's need for immediate intervention. If the initial assessment indicates to the Paramedic that a potentially life-threatening situation exists, the Paramedic should quickly move to a hands-on assessment and intervention as appropriate. In this situation, the Paramedic will most likely have only been able to get the essentials of the patient's history of present illness from the caregivers while simultaneously rapidly assessing the child's airway, breathing, and circulation. Once the airway, breathing, and circulation are stabilized, the Paramedic can move toward a focused physical examination.

If the PAT does not immediately reveal a life-threatening condition, the Paramedic can approach the child while observing the airway, breathing, and circulation in more detail than during the initial examination. As with adult patients, the Paramedic should ensure the airway is patent, the patient is oxygenating and ventilating appropriately, and circulation is adequate. In contrast to adult patients, children have an amazing ability to compensate for stressors and maintain a somewhat normal blood pressure in early shock. Shock, which can be classified as compensated or uncompensated, is defined as inadequate tissue perfusion with oxygen.[4] Compensated shock is indicated by signs of poor perfusion (e.g., pallor, cool skin, and delayed capillary refill), combined with a normal or near normal blood pressure. In uncompensated shock, perfusion has worsened and the patient's blood pressure has dropped below what is considered normal for the child's age (Table 40-2). In adults, the transition from normal perfusion to compensated shock and then to decompensated shock occurs fairly smoothly and rapidly. In contrast, the pediatric patient will compensate for a longer period of time and then suddenly decompensate, sometimes progressing rapidly to cardiopulmonary arrest in a matter of minutes.[5] Aggressive treatment by the Paramedic while the critically ill child is in compensated shock will prevent the child from progressing to decompensated shock.

Vital signs and weight for pediatric patients varies based upon the child's age. Once the child reaches late school age (early adolescence), vital signs approach those of

Table 40-2 Normal Vital Signs and Weight by Age

Age	Weight	Respirations	Heart Rate	Systolic Blood Pressure
Newborn	4 to 5 kg	30 to 50/min	120 to 160 bpm	60 to 90
Infant	4 to 11 kg	20 to 30/min	80 to 140 bpm	87 to 105
1 to 3 years	11 to 14 kg	20 to 30/min	80 to 130 bpm	95 to 105
3 to 6 years	14 to 25 kg	20 to 30/min	80 to 120 bpm	95 to 105
6 to 13 years	25 to 63 kg	(12 to 20) to 30/min	(60 to 80) to 100 bpm	97 to 112
13 to 16 years	62 to 80 kg	12 to 20/min	60 to 100 bpm	112 to 128

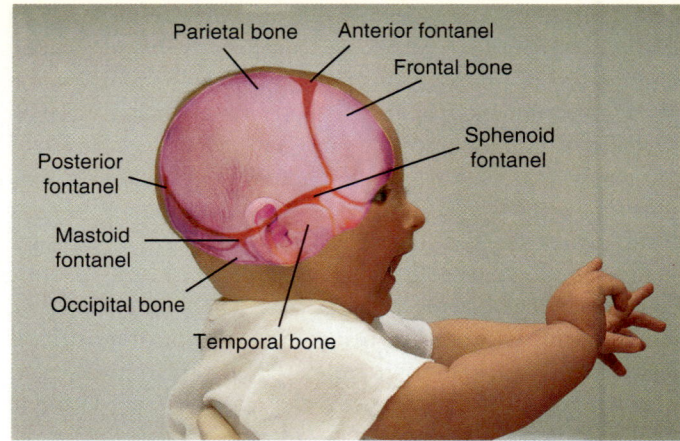

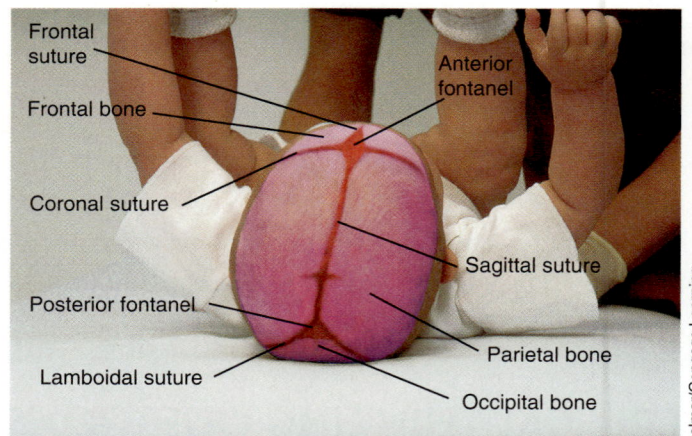

Delmar/Cengage Learning

Figure 40-2 The bones that form the skull do not fuse until the child is approximately 18 months old, with the anterior fontanel disappearing last.

adult patients as their physiology becomes more like adults (Table 40-2). However, these vital signs are approximate and may differ slightly based upon the child's size. Similar charts are often available in EMS reference guides as well as on commercially available length-based tapes.

As with history taking, there are several modifications to the usual examination process that the Paramedic should consider based on different age groups. For some age groups, there are physical features that are not present in adults that can provide useful information to the Paramedic during the physical examination. Especially with the infant and younger children, temperature control is an issue. Children who become relatively hypothermic do not breathe as effectively and easily become bradycardic. Older children from preschooler to adolescent are also very modest. For these reasons, the Paramedic should maintain the patient's modesty while exposing the stable pediatric patients during the physical exam. For critical pediatric patients, the Paramedic should expose the patient as necessary to perform interventions and then cover the child immediately after to help preserve heat.

Infants are often more comfortable when assessed in a caregiver's arms or seated on the caregiver's lap. First, the Paramedic will assess the infant with observation as the infant becomes accustomed to the Paramedic's presence. It is much easier to obtain a respiratory rate while the infant is calm and not crying. The Paramedic starts the physical assessment at the feet, moving toward the head last. In this manner, the Paramedic is not as threatening to the infant. Older infants may want to grab hold of the Paramedic's stethoscope or penlight, which makes them the perfect objects to distract the infant during the examination. A toy or pacifier can also soothe the infant. The Paramedic should make sure the stethoscope head is warmed before performing auscultation. As auscultation is

affected by crying, it is usually best to perform that examination early on before the infant tires of the encounter and starts crying.

Infants' skulls are not fully fused until approximately 18 months of age and can provide the Paramedic with valuable information. A depressed anterior fontanel (Figure 40-2) indicates to the Paramedic that the infant is likely dehydrated.[6] A protruding fontanel indicates the presence of increased pressure, which may occur for several reasons including trauma, cerebral bleeding, and infection.

Toddlers are often a bit more interactive than infants; however, they do become shy very quickly and often remain in the caregiver's lap during the physical examination. Using a toe-to-head strategy when examining toddlers may allow the toddler time to become accustomed to the Paramedic. At this age, the Paramedic may be able to provide the toddler with small choices that allow her to participate in her care (e.g., asking the toddler if she wants her leg or her tummy looked at first). Choices such as the ones displayed in this example do not allow for a "no" answer, but do allow the toddler to have some control over the situation. The Paramedic should also avoid showing needles or other sharp objects to the child before using them to avoid escalating the child's anxiety. Most toddlers do not want to see wounds, and anything that is wet that comes from their body is often thought to be blood. The Paramedic should keep the wounds covered and only uncover them enough for *the Paramedic* to visualize the wound. Paramedics should be mindful that parents may unintentionally gasp or react when they see their child's wound, which potentially sets off a seemingly endless loop of panic between the child and the parent.

Preschoolers are generally more curious than toddlers and not as afraid. Therefore, they may be interested in playing with the Paramedic's medical equipment. Since preschoolers are also interested in helping the Paramedic, he should take advantage of this quality and ask the preschooler to help in age-appropriate ways (e.g., breaking an ice pack or holding the package of roller gauze). It may be helpful for the Paramedic to demonstrate assessments or procedures on a doll before performing them on the apprehensive preschooler.

School-age children have a better capacity to understand explanations regarding the Paramedic's examination and treatment; however, the Paramedic should still use clear and simple language when explaining what he is doing to the school-age child. At this age, the Paramedic will likely be able to perform a physical examination in the usual head-to-toe fashion as the school-age child has likely had enough experience visiting the doctor's office for annual checkups to be used to this examination sequence. The Paramedic should verbalize what he is doing before he does it, whether it is an examination or procedure.

Adolescents also tend to be accustomed to the usual head-to-toe examination. As with younger children, the Paramedic should preserve the patient's modesty, especially in the younger adolescent who is often uncertain and embarrassed about the normal developmental changes occurring with her body.

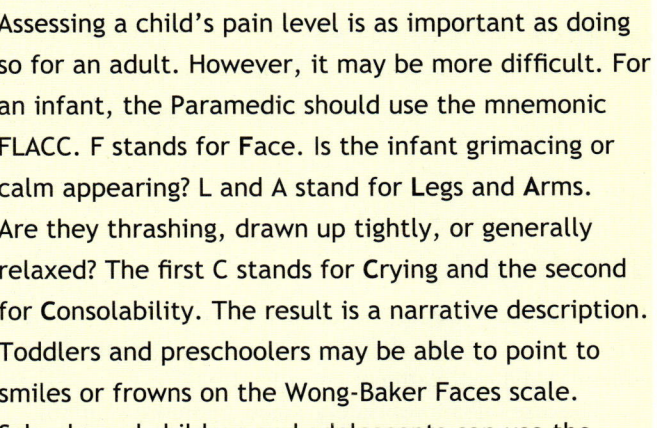

STREET SMART

Assessing a child's pain level is as important as doing so for an adult. However, it may be more difficult. For an infant, the Paramedic should use the mnemonic FLACC. F stands for **F**ace. Is the infant grimacing or calm appearing? L and A stand for **L**egs and **A**rms. Are they thrashing, drawn up tightly, or generally relaxed? The first C stands for **C**rying and the second for **C**onsolability. The result is a narrative description. Toddlers and preschoolers may be able to point to smiles or frowns on the Wong-Baker Faces scale. School-aged children and adolescents can use the numerical pain scale.

CASE STUDY (CONTINUED)

After performing a history and physical examination on Bobby, the Paramedic finds that Bobby has tenderness along his posterior midline cervical spine and the posterior portion of his left thorax. He is not having any trouble breathing but did grimace when he took a deep breath during lung auscultation. The Paramedic is concerned Bobby may have fractured his rib and injured his neck in the fall.

CRITICAL THINKING QUESTIONS

1. What is the significance of the neck injury to breathing?
2. What diagnosis did the Paramedic explain to the mother and child?

Assessment

The Pediatric Assessment Triangle assists the Paramedic in rapidly differentiating between pediatric patients who are critically ill and those who are not critically ill. A small number of patients pass the initial assessment using the PAT and are later found to be critically ill on closer examination. However, the Paramedic can be assured that those patients who do not pass the PAT during the initial assessment will indeed be critically ill and require aggressive intervention to prevent decompensation.

The Paramedics place Bobby on oxygen and carefully immobilize him to an appropriate-size immobilization device with the help of the police officer and an off-duty EMT who also responded to the call. Bobby screams in pain during the immobilization.

Bobby is moved to the ambulance and kept warm. The Paramedic explains that she wants to make Bobby feel better and to do that she needs to give him a shot of medicine in his arm to ease his pain. She asks Bobby in which arm he would like to receive the shot.

CRITICAL THINKING QUESTIONS

1. What is the standard of care of pediatric patients with suspected spinal injury?
2. What are some of the patient-specific concerns and considerations that the Paramedic should consider when applying this plan of care to a pediatric patient?

Treatment

The Paramedic's treatment for specific conditions will be discussed in subsequent chapters. This section simply discusses general pediatric treatment considerations.

The use of appropriately sized pediatric equipment is also essential to caring for pediatric patients.[7-9] The physical proportions of pediatric patients are different than those of adult patients (Figure 40-3). For the infant, a significantly greater proportion of the body is made up from the head. As the infant grows, the proportions change until the child reaches the normal adult proportions. This not only affects the equipment used to immobilize the pediatric patient but also the methods used to accomplish immobilization. Intravenous equipment also must be smaller to allow access into the child's smaller veins.

Drug dosing and fluid dosing for pediatric patients is based on the child's weight in kilograms, which makes the approximate weight or weight at the last pediatrician's visit important. To help reduce error by minimizing calculations, the use of a **length-based tape** (Figure 40-4) is recommended. These tapes are used by laying the tape out next to the supine patient as directed on the tape (Figure 40-5). The tape is divided into sections based on the patient's length, placing the patient into a weight range. The length-based tapes typically

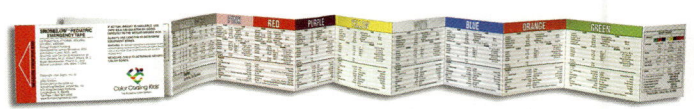

Figure 40-4 An example of a commercially available length-based tape.

Photo courtesy of Armstrong Medical, Inc. Copyright Vial

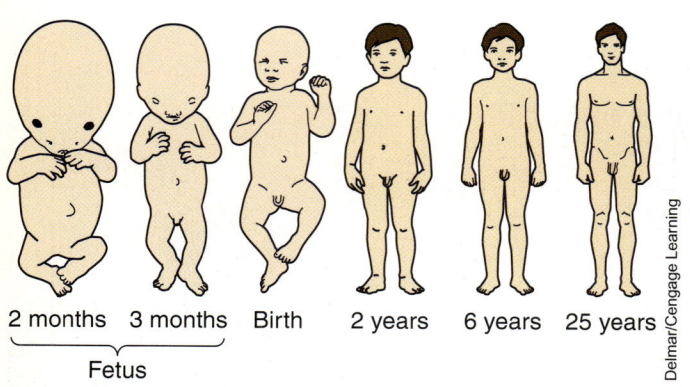

2 months   3 months   Birth   2 years   6 years   25 years

Fetus

Delmar/Cengage Learning

Figure 40-3 The physical proportions change as the infant grows into an adult.

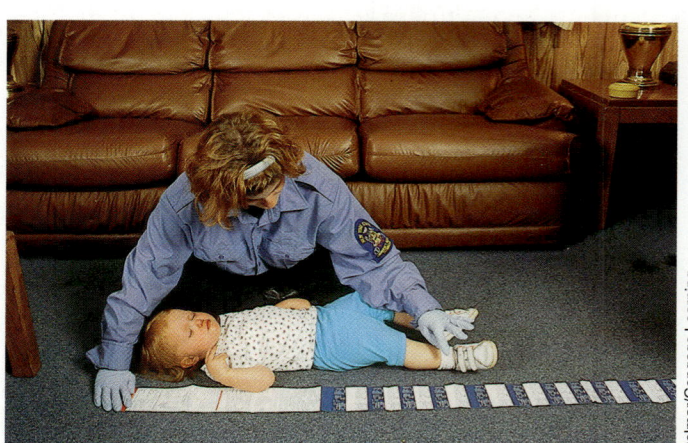

Delmar/Cengage Learning

Figure 40-5 Use of a length-based tape to determine proper medication dosing for a pediatric patient.

include information regarding dosing for common resuscitation medications as well as airway equipment. Other helpful information may also be present on the tape. These guides provide a rapid reference for information and provide the Paramedic with an opportunity to decrease error and improve patient safety.

Fluid administration can also produce error, especially in the younger patients. A seemingly small volume of fluid can be enough to produce volume overload in the infant or younger toddler. Two methods allow the Paramedic to deliver intravenous fluids more accurately. For infants, a simple solution is to attach a three-way stopcock to the extension tubing from the catheter. The second port is attached to the intravenous fluid line while the third is attached to a large syringe, between 20 and 60 mL. The Paramedic calculates the volume of the fluid bolus and then turns the stopcock so that the syringe is able to draw up the appropriate volume from the intravenous fluid bag. The stopcock is then rotated and the syringe slowly instills the fluid bolus into the intravenous catheter. This process may be repeated if the fluid bolus needed is larger than the volume of the syringe. A second method is to use a burette that is placed in line between the intravenous fluid bag and the intravenous line. The burette is filled with the appropriate volume from the intravenous bag and then allowed to infuse from the burette to the intravenous line.

The pediatric patient is not the only individual who requires treatment on scene. The Paramedic must also take care of the caregivers, who may display a wide range of emotions and actions based on the severity of the situation and their own coping mechanisms. Caregivers may fear that the child will have a permanent disability, disfigurement, or pain. There is often a sense of helplessness in that the caregiver is not able to help alleviate the child's suffering or intervene to help make things better. There may also be guilt associated with the events that led up to the call for assistance, even if there was nothing the caregiver could have done to prevent the situation.

The Paramedic can use several strategies to help provide reassurance to the caregivers. With the initial encounter, the Paramedic should make sure to introduce himself and his team to the caregivers and reassure them that his focus is on providing comfort for the child. The Paramedic should then explain what he is doing and why he is doing it to the child using clear, nonmedical terms so the caregivers can understand. The Paramedic should encourage the caregivers to ask questions and provide honest answers. By involving the caregivers in the child's care, it allows them to feel less helpless regarding the situation. If appropriate, the Paramedic should reassure them that the events could not have been prevented. Through these strategies, the Paramedic will calm the caregivers, which in turn will calm the child.

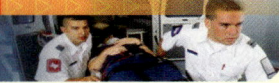

STREET SMART

Caregivers may experience a grief response when notified of their child's illness or injury. The stages of grief, which are not necessarily sequential and which may overlap or jump back and forth, are

- Denial
- Anger
- Bargaining
- Depression
- Acceptance

CASE STUDY (CONTINUED)

The Paramedic reassesses Bobby a few minutes down the road. She notices that Bobby's heart rate has increased slightly; however, his blood pressure remains the same and he is not in as much pain as he was earlier. When she reassesses Bobby's capillary refill in his lower extremities, which were covered and warm, she discovers that his capillary refill is now three seconds whereas during her on-scene examination it was less than two seconds, indicating worsening perfusion. Bobby is given a 20 mL/kg bolus of fluid over five minutes.

CRITICAL THINKING QUESTIONS

1. What are some of the predictable complications associated with pediatric trauma?
2. What are some of the predictable complications associated with the treatments for pediatric trauma?

Evaluation

As with adults, pediatric patients require constant reevaluation. As discussed earlier, although the pediatric patient may be able to maintain a normal blood pressure for an extended period of time, once the patient decompensates, she does so rapidly. The Paramedic must continuously monitor and reassess for changes in perfusion that may indicate deterioration.

CASE STUDY CONCLUSION

Given Bobby's change in condition, the Paramedic tells Bobby's mom of the concern of internal bleeding and changes the destination from the community pediatric emergency department to the pediatric level one trauma center 15 minutes down the road.

The single intravenous fluid bolus improves Bobby's perfusion and his capillary refill stays at approximately two seconds for the remainder of the transport. The Paramedic's report to the assembled trauma team includes concerns of internal hemorrhage given the change in status.

Bobby's evaluation in the emergency department reveals that he sustained two lower left-sided rib fractures in the fall along with a low grade laceration of the spleen. Bobby is admitted to the intensive care unit and observed for several days. His spleen laceration does not develop into a rupture, and he is released from the hospital two weeks later.

CRITICAL THINKING QUESTIONS

1. What is the most appropriate transport decision that will get the patient to definitive care?
2. What are the advantages of transporting a patient with suspected trauma-induced hemorrhage to these hospitals, even if that means bypassing other hospitals in the process?

Disposition

The disposition of pediatric patients often varies from community to community. Some communities have a dedicated pediatric emergency department, either as part of a small number of freestanding pediatric hospitals or as part of a larger general hospital. However, some communities do not have a separate pediatric emergency department. Special care needs of the patient (e.g., multisystem trauma or conditions requiring subspecialty care) may dictate transport directly to a tertiary care center. In some areas, emergency departments may be categorized by pediatric capability where not all emergency departments are credentialed for pediatric patients.[10] The Paramedic must learn the resources available in his region. The Paramedic may also need to rely on caregivers of those pediatric patients with chronic diseases who may indicate the patient should be transported to a specific emergency department. Unless the patient is critically unstable and not responding to the Paramedic's interventions, it is usually wise for the Paramedic to honor the caregivers' destination request.

CONCLUSION

The assessment of a pediatric patient should not be scary or anxiety provoking for the Paramedic. During training, the Paramedic student should seek out opportunities to interact with pediatric patients, both those who are sick and those who are stable. Through experience, the Paramedic student will reduce any anxiety present in dealing with pediatric patients.

KEY POINTS:

- The Pediatric Assessment Triangle is useful in differentiating the unstable child from the stable child.

- The three sides of the Pediatric Assessment Triangle are appearance, breathing, and circulation.

- Appearance involves assessment by level of consciousness, interaction with caregivers and others, and body posture and movement.

- Work of breathing is assessed through rate, rhythm, and accessory muscle use.

- Circulation is best assessed by skin color.

- Children and teens may regress to a previous emotional level when faced with a stressful situation.

- In stable infants and toddlers, the Paramedic should assess the child
  - In the caregiver's lap
  - From toe to head
  - Using simple, concrete terms
  - By offering simple choices that do not involve a yes or no answer
  - Without showing needles, sharp instruments, or the injury

- The Paramedic should obtain the history about the pregnancy, delivery, developmental milestones, and immunizations.

- In stable preschoolers, the Paramedic should assess the child
  - After developing rapport
  - While praising the child and answering questions
  - Using simple, concrete terms

- After allowing the child the opportunity to manipulate clean equipment
- After a demonstration of some interventions on a doll or toy

- In the stable school-age child, the Paramedic should assess the child
  - By speaking with the child first
  - Providing privacy as appropriate
  - Using a head-to-toe approach

- In the adolescent, the Paramedic should assess by
  - Speaking with the adolescent privately
  - Being honest and straightforward
  - Avoiding judgment
  - Protecting modesty

- Vital signs vary by age. Generally, the younger the child, the lower the blood pressure and the faster the pulse and respiratory rate.

- The Paramedic should use appropriately sized equipment.

- The Paramedic should use a length-based tape for drug and fluid dosing.

- The Paramedic should use a three-way stopcock or a burette to reduce fluid administration errors.

- The Paramedic should consider the emotional needs of caregivers.

- Pediatric patients decompensate very quickly.

- The Paramedic should know the availability of local pediatric services and try to honor specific caregiver transport requests.

1. What is the value of the Pediatric Assessment Triangle? Name its components.
2. How is mental status assessed in a child?
3. What is the common body position of a stable infant or young child?
4. When is abdominal breathing normal?
5. Describe normal skin color.
6. What changes are expected in maturation when a pediatric patient is stressed, in pain, or anxious?
7. Describe the physical assessment of a stable infant or toddler.
8. How does the Paramedic use developmental milestones when obtaining a history?
9. What are the normal ranges of vital signs for a/an
   a. Infant
   b. Toddler
   c. Preschooler
   d. School-age child
   e. Adolescent
10. Describe the assessment of the anterior fontanel and the implications of each result.
11. Drug and fluid administration is based on what particular aspect of the child? How will you obtain information on that aspect?
12. Name two techniques used to decrease fluid dosing errors.

Please refer to the Case Study in this chapter, and answer the questions below:

1. What are Bobby's possible injuries based on the initial dispatch information? What other information will be necessary to narrow the list?
2. What differences are noted between the initial dispatch information and the answers that Bobby's mother gives? How can the Paramedics obtain a clearer picture of what happened?
3. Based on the physical exam, what injuries might Bobby have sustained?

REFERENCES:

1. Diekmann RA, ed. *Pediatric Education for Prehospital Professionals,* second edition. Boston: Jones and Bartlet; 2006.

2. Pediatrics AA. *Basic Life Support Provider: Pediatric Education for Prehospital Professionals.* Boston: Jones & Bartlett Publishers; 2008.

3. Deterding RR, Hay WW, et al. *Current Pediatric Diagnosis and Treatment.* New York: McGraw-Hill Professional; 2008.

4. Dellinger RP, Levy MM, et al. Surviving Sepsis Campaign: international guidelines for management of severe sepsis and septic shock: 2008. *Crit Care Med.* 2008;36(1):296–327.

5. American Heart Association. *PALS Course Guide and PALS Provider Manual.* American Heart Association: Dallas; 2007.

6. Manz F. Hydration in children. *J Am Coll Nutr.* 2007;26 (5 Suppl):562S–569S.

7. Luten RC, Zaritsky A, et al. The use of the Broselow tape in pediatric resuscitation. *Acad Emerg Med.* 2007;14(5):500–501; author reply 501–502.

8. Nieman CT, Manacci CF, et al. Use of the Broselow tape may result in the underresuscitation of children. *Acad Emerg Med.* 2006;13(10):1011–1019.

9. Deboer S, Seaver M, et al. Color coding to reduce errors. *Am J Nurs.* 2005;105(8):68–71.

10. Wertz EM. *Emergency Care for Children.* Clifton Park, NY: Delmar Cengage Learning; 2002.

CHAPTER 41

THE CRITICALLY ILL CHILD

KEY CONCEPTS:

Upon completion of this chapter, it is expected that the reader will understand these following concepts:

- The categorization of critical pediatric illnesses as respiratory failure, circulatory collapse, cardiopulmonary arrest, bradycardia, or tachycardia
- The emphasis placed on airway, breathing, circulation, disability, and exposing the critically ill patient during examination
- The need, regardless of etiology, for frequent reevaluations of children who may rapidly decompensate

ANATOMY CONCEPTS:

Prior to reading this chapter the Paramedic student should be familiar with the following anatomy and physiology concepts:

- Child developmental stages

"Squad 22, Engine 7, respond to 4755 Broadway, upper floor, for a 6-month-old male, acting fussy with trouble breathing," squawks the Central Rapids Fire Department Dispatch.

The Paramedics assigned to Squad 22 jump into the quick response truck and head to the scene. Their battalion had completed their pediatric life support review two months prior. En route, they discuss some of the possible causes for the patient's concern. Five minutes later, they pull up on-scene to find the crew of Engine 7 already there. Dispatch notifies Squad 22 that their transport ambulance has an ETA of seven minutes.

CRITICAL THINKING QUESTIONS

1. What are some of the possible causes of pediatric shortness of breath?

2. How is the child acting fussy related to the child's trouble breathing?

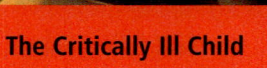

OVERVIEW

Caring for a critically ill or injured neonate, toddler, or child may prove to be the most stressful part of a Paramedic's practice. Fears of not doing the right thing, missing a critical action in the Pediatric Advanced Life Support (PALS) algorithm, or unfamiliarity with pediatric patients may prevail when caring for an ill child. Medico-legal, social, and ethical issues may also be of greater concern in this patient population versus the adult population. Because of these issues, it is imperative for the Paramedic to learn a systematic approach to evaluating these patients so that evaluation, early treatment, and stabilization will be more intuitive.

Children are not just little adults. Instead, they have distinct anatomical and physiological differences as compared to their adult counterparts. These differences require Paramedics to have a specialized subset of skills to appropriately manage pediatric patients. This chapter explores the evaluation and treatment of the critically ill pediatric patient.

Chief Concern

No single chief concern indicates to the Paramedic that a child is critically ill. In fact, not all critically ill children will even have a clear chief concern (e.g., difficulty breathing). In some cases, the chief concern is irritability, fever, or poor feeding. These situations without a clear chief concern challenge the Paramedic's history taking and examination skills.

The many different critical pediatric illnesses can be broadly categorized as respiratory failure, circulatory collapse, cardiopulmonary arrest, bradycardia, and tachycardia. In this section we will discuss the underlying pathophysiology of the conditions that fall into these broad categories.

Respiratory Failure

The primary cause of cardiac arrest in the pediatric patient is respiratory failure.[1] Pediatric patients do not have the years of atherosclerosis buildup commonly seen in adults and which generally causes cardiovascular disease. Pediatric patients are also more sensitive to changes in oxygenation and ventilation than adults. Hypoxia commonly causes altered mental status, bradycardia, and hypotension in the pediatric patient.

Respiratory failure can occur due to a variety of causes, including infection, asthma, dehydration, trauma, and metabolic causes.[2] Respiratory infections are a common cause of respiratory failure and include pneumonia, bronchiolitis, and other viral causes of respiratory infection. Asthma can be severe in younger children who have proportionately smaller airways than adult patients. Dehydration can cause metabolic problems that manifest as tachypnea, respiratory distress, and respiratory failure, if left untreated. Trauma can cause direct pulmonary injury and respiratory failure from the injury.

Circulatory Failure

Hypoperfusion is inadequate perfusion of nutrients, fluids, and removal of waste products from the tissues. The key difference between a child and an adult in shock is how their bodies address this hypoperfused state. Since children typically have strong healthy vessels and organs, they are able to compensate very well initially. When their compensatory mechanism fails, children physiologically deteriorate rapidly. Children compensate for hypoperfusion by constricting their blood vessels and increasing their heart rate, but are not able to increase their force of contraction as well as adults. Although children can generally tolerate hypoperfusion better than adults, they generally cannot tolerate hypoperfusion for extended periods of time.

Although there are numerous types of shock children succumb to, they are similar to those seen in adults. Vomiting and diarrhea are two of the more common causes of shock in children.[3] The child's inability to rehydrate after significant volume losses causes electrolyte imbalance, which can worsen dehydration and in turn produce dysrhythmias.

Bacterial infection is another common cause of shock. As the body fights the infection, the bacteria release toxins that cause inflammation, vasodilatation, and shifting of fluids from the vessels into the interstitial spaces. The body's metabolic needs steadily increase, in part as a response to the infection itself, but also in response to the increased energy needs to maintain normal bodily functions. Once the process overwhelms the various organ systems, the patient decompensates. Other types and causes of shock are similar to those of the adult and are cared for in similar manners.

Cardiopulmonary Arrest

Cardiac arrest is the absence of heart activity characterized by unconsciousness, apnea, and pulselessness. As previously discussed, in the pediatric population the most common cause of cardiac arrest is respiratory arrest. Children who suffer a respiratory insult will develop hypoxemia, followed by cardiac dysrhythmias, followed by a cessation of cardiac activity.[4] Pediatric causes of cardiac arrest are varied but are closely linked with trauma, sudden infant death syndrome (SIDS), drowning, poisoning, choking, asthma or other lung diseases, foreign body aspiration, and pneumonia.

As in adults, pulseless electrical activity (PEA) is the absence of a pulse with organized activity on cardiac monitoring. The mnemonic of the 5 H's and T's (Table 41-1) can assist the Paramedic in remembering the etiology of PEA.

Asystole is a terminal rhythm indicating that the electrical system has been completely exhausted. In adults, asystole is usually preceded by an agonal rhythm, pulseless ventricular tachycardia, or ventricular fibrillation. Pediatric patients, especially infants and younger children, more often present with asystole as the initial rhythm in cardiac arrest.[5] This may be due to increased vagal tone in younger pediatric patients or may be indicative of a more rapid decline in condition. The 5 H's and T's that provide a helpful reminder of the causes of PEA also provide a reminder of the causes of asystole.

Symptomatic Bradycardia

Hypoxemia is the most frequent cause of bradydysrhythmias in children. Bradycardia may resolve with initiation of oxygen therapy. Nonpathological sinus bradycardia is rare in the pediatric population. However, heart blocks often occur from increased vagal tone or are a congenital condition. A heart rate of less than 60 bpm is often not tolerated in the younger pediatric patient and will cause severe hypoperfusion.

Tachycardia with a Pulse

Sinus tachycardia often occurs in response to a systemic process or increased body energy demand. Causes of sinus tachycardia include pain, respiratory distress, hypoxemia, hypovolemia, fever, stimulants, or low blood sugar. Although sinus tachycardia is usually not suggestive of significant pathology, the rhythm may precede an unstable tachydysrhythmia or nonperfusing rhythm and should not be taken lightly. It may be difficult at times, when dealing with faster heart rates, to differentiate between sinus tachycardia and supraventricular tachycardia. Sinus tachycardia may reach up to 180 beats per minute in children and up to 220 beats per minute in infants

while supraventricular tachycardia often presents with a rate above 180 for children and 220 for infants.

Supraventricular tachycardia (SVT) is a narrow complex tachycardia of atrial origin that occurs due to an accelerated rate of firing from the SA node or rogue atrial cell. The majority of pediatric patients who develop SVT have an accessory pathway or a re-entry circuit which allows bypass of electrical impulses around the AV node (Figure 41-1).[6]

Older children will frequently present around 150 beats per minute, which is the maximum rate allowed by the AV node, whereas others with a more complex re-entry pattern will have a higher heart rate. Up to 90% of infants in SVT will present with a heart rate greater than 230 bpm due to a re-entry circuit.[7] Re-entry SVT is a prominent cause of syncope in the pediatric age group and may be responsible for syncopal episodes in the pediatric patient.

Ventricular tachycardia (VT) and fibrillation (VF) are life-threatening rhythms that occur in 5% to 15% of all pediatric out-of-hospital cardiac arrests.[8] When a single cell in the ventricle begins to overpace the AV node, VT ensues. Cardiac output plummets when the rate is too fast to allow the heart to fill. This process further decompensates as ventricular cells become further starved of oxygen and nutrients. Ultimately, it will degrade into fibrillation when the heart's electrical energy is nearly exhausted and organized cardiac contraction comes to a near standstill.

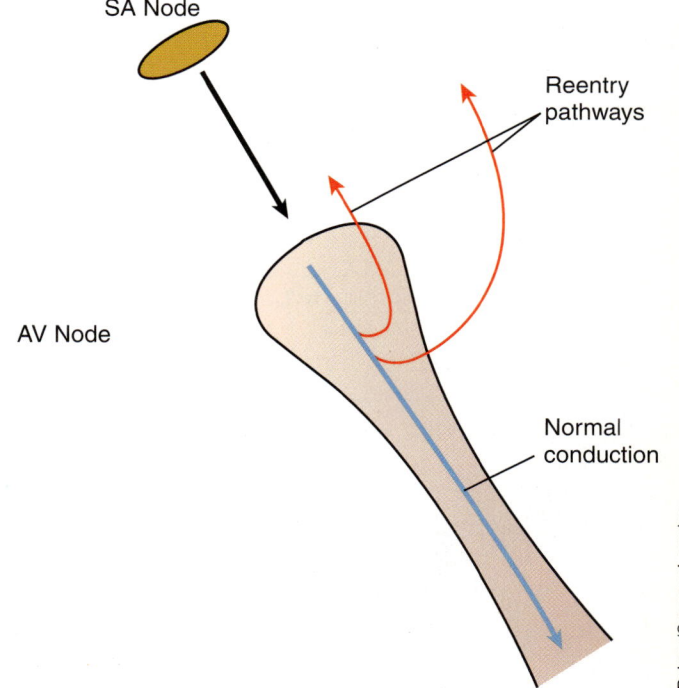

Figure 41-1 A re-entry pathway allows the electrical impulse to reverse and re-discharge the atrium, bypassing the AV node. When active, this re-entry pathway can produce atrial rates exceeding 230 beats per minute in the pediatric patient.

Table 41-1 The Common Causes of PEA and Asystole

The H's	The T's
• Hypoxemia	• Tamponade
• Hypovolemia	• Tension pneumothorax
• Hypothermia	• Toxins/poisons
• Hyper/Hypokalemia and metabolic acidosis	• Thromboembolism
• Hypoglycemia	• Trauma

Ventricular tachycardia and fibrillation are uncommon rhythms in pediatric patients. These rhythms are usually seen in patients with preexisting heart disease or failure, severe hypoxemia, drug overdose or poisoning, electrolyte imbalances, or metabolic acidosis. Prehospital providers may encounter this rhythm in pediatric patients who have received bystander CPR which has prevented asystole.

Torsades de pointes is a subset of ventricular tachycardia with alternating amplitudes above and below the isoelectric line (Figure 41-2) resulting from multiple irritable foci in the ventricles, essentially producing a multiform ventricular tachycardia. The usual rate for torsades is between 150 and 250 bpm. The definition of torsades includes a markedly prolonged QT interval (sometimes over 600 ms) and is confirmed by the prolonged QT interval once the rhythm is terminated (Figure 41-3).[9] It is now known that Long QT syndrome can be both congenital and acquired. Congenital **Long QT syndrome** (an infrequent, hereditary disorder of the heart's electrical rhythm that can occur in otherwise healthy people)

is one of several genetic conditions that can affect the cardiac conduction system.[10] The more common of these genetic conditions are dominant, in that if one of the parents passes the gene to the child, the child will have Long QT syndrome. Specific ion channel dysfunctions have been implicated as the cause of Long QT syndrome. It is believed that this syndrome may be a significant contributor to undiagnosed pediatric cardiac syncope and death, and perhaps SIDS.[11]

CULTURAL/REGIONAL DIFFERENCES

Abnormal heart rhythms or arrest caused by blunt trauma to the chest is called **cordis commotio**. Many states now require school districts to have AEDs available during sporting events if a child may be at risk for cordis commotio.

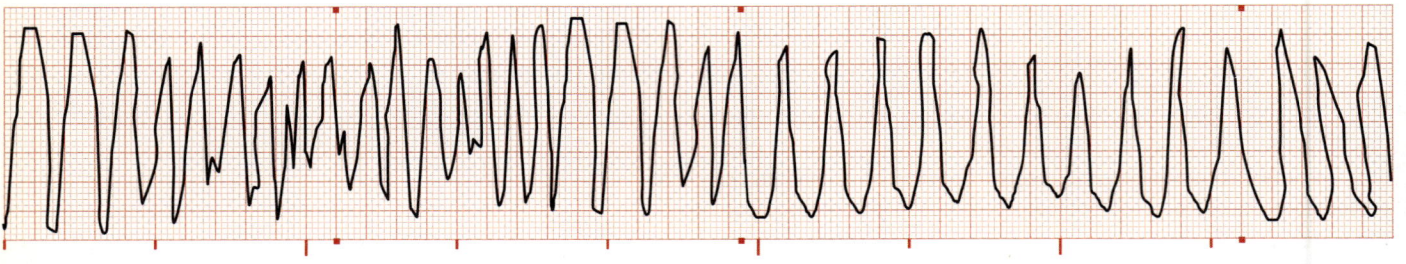

Figure 41-2 Torsades de pointes.

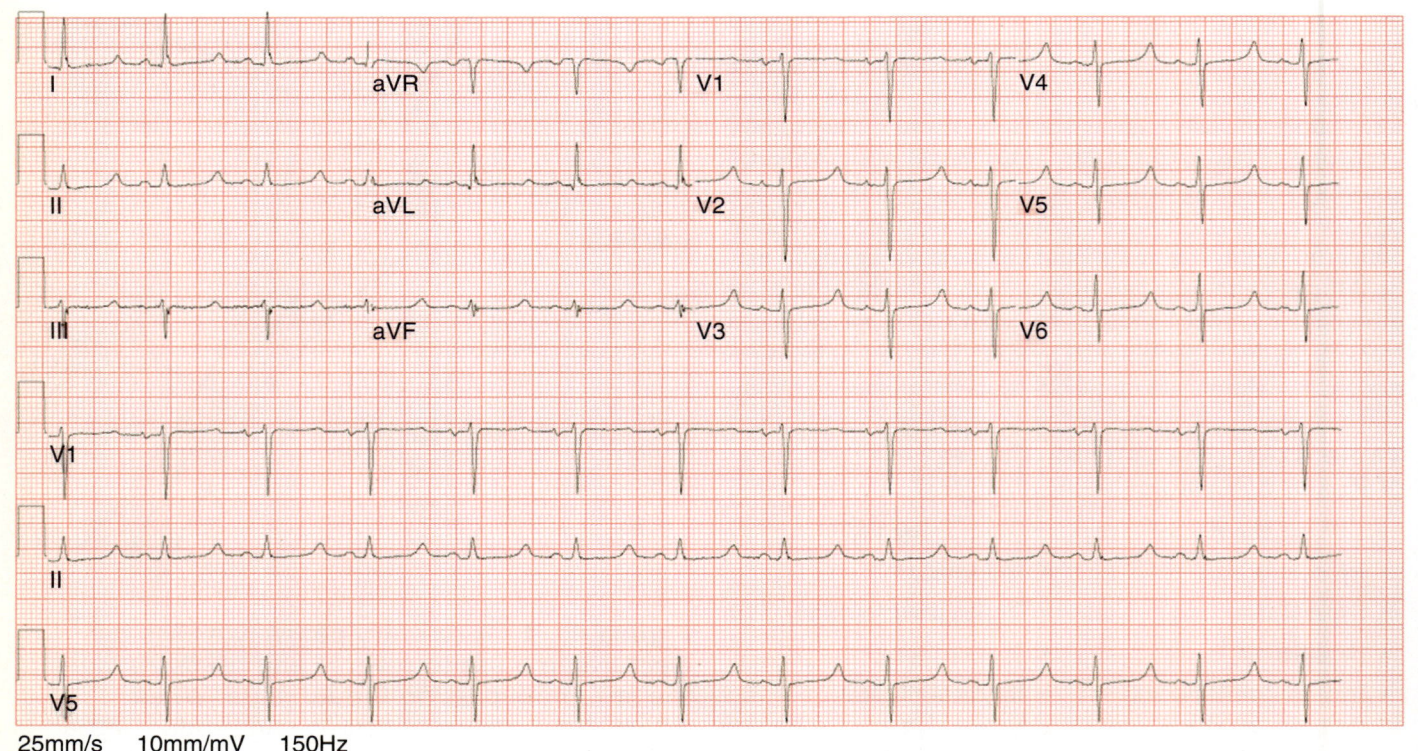

25mm/s   10mm/mV   150Hz

Figure 41-3 This 12-lead electrocardiogram demonstrates a prolonged QT interval.

Although overall a rare rhythm, torsades is more common in pediatric patients than in adults. In adults, a prolonged QT interval is frequently caused by medications or chest wall trauma. Medications such as procainamide, quinidine, amiodarone, digitalis, erythromycin, fluconazole, and the class of tricyclic antidepressants have all been indicated in prolonging the QT segment and the development of torsades.[12] Chest wall trauma which occurs at the peak of the R wave or at some susceptible point during ventricular repolarization may cause torsades or VT in children and may be the cause of sudden death in patients who have sustained localized blunt chest trauma without a vascular injury.

CASE STUDY (CONTINUED)

During their introduction to the child's caregiver, both Paramedics rapidly assess Tonele, the 6-month-old child, using the Pediatric Assessment Triangle. Both notice that the child does not make eye contact when they approach and appears to be in respiratory distress.

While one proceeds to do a rapid hands-on assessment, the other obtains a history from the child's mother. She reports the child had an uneventful birth and normal development. The mother noticed that while Tonele was feeding well two days ago, he drank less and less formula. She had not noticed a fever. There was no diarrhea or vomiting, and his last wet diaper was eight hours before. She noticed that Tonele was "breathing hard," so she called 9-1-1.

CRITICAL THINKING QUESTIONS

1. What are the important elements of the history that a Paramedic should obtain?
2. What may be the significance of the heavy breathing?

History

Many of the historical features discussed in Chapter 40 on assessment of the stable pediatric patient apply to critically ill children as well. For children that appear to be unstable after the initial assessment using the Pediatric Assessment Triangle, much of the initial history of present illness will focus on rapid identification of the cause of the patient's condition. A detailed history of the present illness will provide the Paramedic with the clues necessary to direct the treatment. The Paramedic will often have to rely on caregivers to provide a history as most critically ill children will not be able to provide sufficient history themselves.

Factors the Paramedic must consider are the patient's specific symptoms and duration of those symptoms. Feeding and urination history are important in all younger children and infants. Poor feeding and decreased urine output are obvious signs of dehydration; however, they can also be subtle signs of an underlying cardiac or respiratory condition. In addition, abnormal mental activity can also be a subtle sign of an underlying cardiac, respiratory, toxic, metabolic, or infectious condition. In this case, the abruptness of onset of the abnormal mental activity can help the Paramedic identify the underlying cause.

A patient's history of fever is also important. Any fever, defined as a body temperature above 38°C or 100.4°F in an infant younger than 30 to 60 days old, is a significant concern. The child with such a fever needs to be fully evaluated at the emergency department and admitted to the hospital.[13,14] A fever above 39.4°C or 102.9°F in the child between 2 and 36 months old also carries the same concern, although this child may not require hospital admission.

When obtaining a past medical history, the Paramedic should think about three additional items pertaining to pediatric patients over and above the usual past history. In younger children, especially younger infants, a birth history including complications during pregnancy, labor, or delivery can point toward issues relating to these early events in the child's life. Developmental history is also important as it can help the Paramedic gauge the younger child's abilities and put them into the correct context with the current illness. The third important item in the pediatric past medical history is immunizations. The patient's lack of immunizations or delayed immunizations brings about the possibility of certain infectious diseases that may not otherwise cause an issue in a child who has been immunized.[15]

CULTURAL/REGIONAL DIFFERENCES

In some cultures and religions, immunizations are viewed with distrust. The Paramedic should act in a nonjudgmental fashion when gathering the patient's history if the patient has not been immunized.

During his exam, Tonele is breathing at approximately 56 breaths per minute, has a capillary refill of approximately six seconds with cool skin, and does not have a peripheral pulse. Tonele's apical pulse is over 200 beats per minute, which is really too fast to count. The team applies a cardiac monitor which reveals a wide complex tachycardia at 260 beats per minute that appears to be a ventricular tachycardia.

CRITICAL THINKING QUESTIONS

1. What are the elements of the physical examination of a patient with suspected tachydysrhythmia?
2. Why is a blood pressure a critical element in this examination?

Examination

In the critically ill child, much of the Paramedic's focus of the examination will be on airway, breathing, circulation, disability, and exposing the patient. The Paramedic should examine the patient's airway for patency and address immediate concerns. Gurgling, stridor, or snoring sounds indicate an upper airway obstruction that may be due to secretions, foreign material, or upper airway edema.

The signs of respiratory distress in a pediatric patient include sternal and intercostal retractions, accessory muscle use, and pursed lip breathing. These signs of respiratory distress are often more dramatic in children than in adults because of the flexibility and pliability of the child's thoracic cage. Another sign of increased work of breathing in the pediatric patient is nasal flaring, in which the nares dilate during inspiration (Figure 41-4). The young child may also demonstrate increased abdominal excursion when in respiratory distress. Until their thoracic cage stiffens, younger children use their abdominal muscles during normal breathing. The abdominal excursion will increase when these young children have difficulty breathing. A rapid assessment of breath sounds will help the Paramedic determine if the cause of the child's illness is primarily respiratory in nature or from another cause. Wheezing or stridor on auscultation indicates airway obstruction whereas an absence of breath sounds may indicate a pneumothorax.

Skin color is another important indicator of the child's oxygenation. **Acrocyanosis** is the development of cyanosis in the peripheral parts of the body such as the nail beds, palms of the hands, and soles of the feet. As hypoxemia worsens, cyanosis will move centrally. Blue discoloration of the lips and oropharynx indicates to the Paramedic that the body's circulatory needs are not being met.

Inadequate perfusion is an early sign of shock in children. Cool, mottled, pale, or dusky skin and delayed capillary refill are ominous signs of hypoperfusion and need to be addressed immediately, even if the blood pressure is normal for the child's age.[16] In younger children, the Paramedic should assess the patient's pulse rate and quality at the brachial and femoral arteries as radial pulses may be difficult to obtain. Delayed capillary refill is an early indicator of hypoperfusion and will occur in children before the blood pressure falls.

Table 40-2 in the previous chapter displayed normal blood pressures for children. However, the Paramedic can use a quick method to determine the low normal systolic blood pressure for children. To use this method, the Paramedic doubles the patient's age in years and adds that to 70. For example, a 6-year-old child should have a systolic blood pressure of 82 mmHg (Figure 41-5). This threshold marks the change in status from compensated shock to decompensated shock for the critically ill child. Once the child decompensates, respiratory and cardiac arrest will rapidly develop.

Flared nostrils

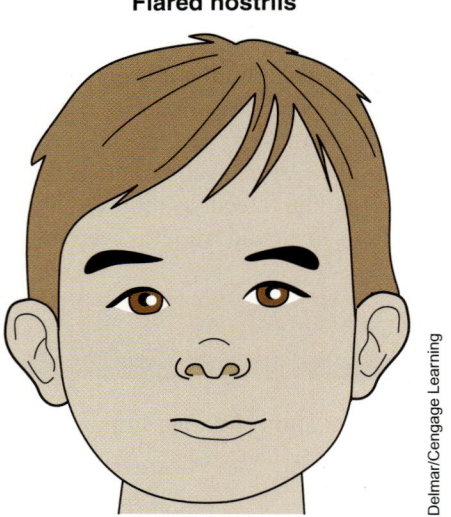

Delmar/Cengage Learning

Figure 41-4 This child has nasal flaring during inspiration, a sign of increased work of breathing.

Child's Age × 2 + 70 = Low Normal Blood Pressure

Example:

Question: What is the low normal blood pressure for a 6-year-old child?

Answer: 6 × 2 = 12; 12 + 70 = 82 mmHg

Delmar/Cengage Learning

Figure 41-5 Rapid method to calculate the low normal blood pressure in children.

As discussed previously, the fontanels (soft spots) in children from birth until approximately 18 months old are still open and allow the Paramedic to assess the child for dehydration. In the infant and young toddler, assessing the fontanels is a rapid means of determining the child's fluid status. For example, if the fontanel is depressed (i.e., the skin sinks below the level of the surrounding bone at the fontanel), the child is hypovolemic.[17] In contrast, a bulging fontanel in an infant or early toddler may indicate increased intracranial pressure.

Disability assessment in the older child is similar to that of an adult. The Paramedic rapidly assesses the patient's pupil reaction and obtains an overall indication of peripheral motor ability and mental status by asking the conscious child to wiggle the toes or hold up a finger. In younger children, assessing the pupils remains an important step in assessing disability. All children, regardless of age, should look toward or make eye contact with the Paramedic as she approaches and makes physical contact. The Paramedic may assume a child without a history of cognitive and developmental delay who does not make eye contact or acknowledge the Paramedic has altered mental status until proven otherwise. In some children, especially those with cognitive disabilities, it may be difficult to determine whether the child is acting normally or not. In those cases, the Paramedic should ask the parent whether the manner in which the child is acting is normal or abnormal and, if abnormal, what makes it seem that way. Increased intracranial pressure, infection, or hemorrhage in an infant, evidenced by a bulging fontanel, may be a cause for the patient's altered mental status.

CASE STUDY (CONTINUED)

The Paramedics realize that Tonele has an unstable wide complex tachycardia. They explain to Tonele's mother that he is very ill due to a heart rhythm that is too fast. Visibly upset, the mother starts to ask a barrage of questions.

CRITICAL THINKING QUESTIONS

1. What is the significance of the wide complex tachycardia segment?
2. What diagnosis did the Paramedic announce to the patient's mother?

Assessment

Critically ill children will clearly have an airway, breathing, or circulatory problem that requires immediate attention in order to intervene and prevent death. However, the Paramedic's treatment priority may not necessarily follow the A-B-C order. The Paramedic must determine the most likely primary problem—airway, breathing, or circulation—and address that problem first.

Airway issues are usually obvious and indeed take priority over breathing and circulatory issues. On closer assessment, however, if noisy airway noises are due to fluid, blood, or other secretions in the airway, that takes priority and should be addressed first. True stridor in children indicates an upper airway partial obstruction that may progress to a complete airway obstruction if untreated.

The cause of the patient's increased work of breathing may be more difficult to determine. If the cause of increased work of breathing is primarily a respiratory problem, then the Paramedic should address the respiratory problem first.

Hypoxia and adventitious lung sounds suggest a respiratory origin for respiratory distress. Signs of poor perfusion, in the absence of adventitious lung sounds, suggest a circulatory origin.

Dysrhythmias also may have a respiratory or cardiac origin. Bradycardia is more commonly caused by hypoxia in children than cardiac disease. The Paramedic's initial treatment priority should focus on optimizing oxygenation and ventilation and keeping the patient warm.[3] If bradycardia is secondary to inadequate oxygenation, ventilation, or warmth, these interventions should improve the bradycardia. If they do not, the child likely requires pharmacologic intervention to improve bradycardia and a search for other potential causes, including primary cardiac and toxicologic causes.

Tachycardia in critically ill children is often related to hypoperfusion or primary rhythm disturbances. The patient's history will often help the Paramedic determine which cause is the more likely. Fever, vomiting, diarrhea, and dehydration produce sinus tachycardia, and the patient will develop hypoperfusion from a decreased fluid volume. Primary rhythm disturbances often cause a significant tachycardia, above 180 in children and above 220 in infants. These patients will develop hypoperfusion because the rate does not allow the heart to fill adequately and thus the patient cannot produce sufficient forward flow of blood into the arterial system. In some cases, there will be a mixed picture, such as when tachycardia initially was secondary to dehydration and a supraventricular tachycardia then developed as a result of an electrolyte disturbance that occurred along with dehydration. The opposite can happen as well. When the SVT began, the child may have had poor oral intake and became dehydrated. In these mixed presentations, it can be challenging to determine which condition is the primary issue.

CASE STUDY (CONTINUED)

The firefighters from the BLS engine company place Tonele on high-flow, high-concentration oxygen. The Paramedics decide to obtain venous access via the intraosseous route and administer a mild sedative. Tonele then receives a synchronized shock to convert his rhythm.

CRITICAL THINKING QUESTIONS

1. What is the national standard of care for tachydysrhythmia in pediatric patients?
2. What are some of the patient-specific concerns and considerations that the Paramedic should consider when applying this plan of care?

Treatment

The critically ill pediatric patient requires aggressive management to correct the underlying cause of the critical illness. High-flow, high-concentration oxygen should be administered quickly to the critically ill child. Younger children who are awake may be scared of the nonrebreather mask when it is placed over their mouth and nose. In this situation, blow-by oxygen is an appropriate alternative. The caregiver can assist by holding the oxygen mask near the child's face.

Respiratory failure is best addressed by early assisted ventilations using a bag–valve mask. Early use of assisted ventilations may reverse respiratory failure and stimulate more appropriate spontaneous breathing. Bag–valve–mask ventilation is often easier to accomplish in children due to the lack of extra tissue in and around the airway. When compared with more invasive airway management techniques in one study, outcomes in pediatric patients who were treated with adequate bag–valve–mask ventilation compared with intubation were not different. In fact, in two of the study's subgroups, children had improved outcomes when using bag–valve mask alone.[18] Based on this study, the focus of pediatric airway management has shifted from immediately moving to invasive airway management to that of delayed invasive airway management as long as bag–valve–mask ventilations are adequate. Invasive airway techniques involve endotracheal intubation, supraglottic devices, and cricothyrotomy. Indications for endotracheal intubation include a pediatric patient in respiratory failure who cannot be adequately oxygenated and ventilated using a bag–valve mask and basic airway adjuncts. If the gag reflex is absent, the patient may be intubated without pharmacological assistance; otherwise, the Paramedic may need to use rapid sequence intubation in order to successfully place the endotracheal tube.

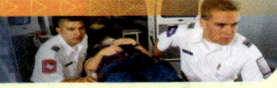

STREET SMART

Intubation may place the child at risk for infection secondary to the tube placement. Among 6,290 pediatric ICU patients surveyed between 1992 and 1997, the incidence of nosocomial invasive bacterial and fungal infections were as follows:[19]

- Ventilator-associated pneumonia: 21%
- Lower respiratory infection: 12%
- Ear, nose, and throat infections: 7%

Supraglottic devices provide a reasonable alternative to endotracheal intubation in patients who are obtunded and without a gag reflex. Multiple sizes of the laryngeal mask airway are available down to infants weighing 5 kg. Pediatric sizes of the King LT airway® are available for children 35 inches tall and taller who weigh at least 12 kg. The Combitube® is available for patients who are four feet tall and taller. The needle cricothyrotomy technique is used in children under the age of 12 in the rare situations in which both bag–valve–mask ventilations are inadequate and an endotracheal tube or supraglottic airway device cannot be placed. Surgical and percutaneous cricothyrotomy techniques are contraindicated in children under the age of 12 due to significant tracheal stenosis that can occur from the other surgical techniques.[20] These situations are rare and are likely related to maxillofacial trauma, neck trauma, or foreign body aspiration. Although rare and invasive, cricothyrotomy can be a life-saving procedure. When indicated, it will allow for oxygenation until a more definitive airway can be placed.

Circulatory Failure

As discussed earlier in this chapter, circulatory failure most often occurs secondary to hypoxia from respiratory failure. Therefore, it is important for the Paramedic to maximize oxygen delivery with supplemental oxygen or bag–valve–mask ventilation. Absence of a palpable central pulse or a heart rate less than 60 in a pediatric patient warrants initiation of CPR to temporarily improve circulation until the cause can be found and corrected.[20]

Intravenous or intraosseous vascular access should be obtained rapidly. Peripheral vascular access in the antecubital fossa may be the easiest to achieve in pediatric patients. Scalp veins are frequently prominent and may be accessed with a 24 gauge or higher venous catheter in the neonatal and younger infant patient populations. If the Paramedic cannot obtain intravenous access within 90 seconds or it takes more than three attempts to cannulate a vein, the Paramedic should obtain intraosseous access. In obtunded, critically ill children with circulatory collapse and poor perfusion, the Paramedic should obtain intraosseous access without attempting intravenous access. For the newly born, umbilical line placement may be utilized to obtain intravenous access.

Normal saline (0.9% NaCl solution) is the first-line fluid used in fluid resuscitation for the critically ill child. Boluses are administered with a volume of 20 mL/kg IV/IO push. The 20 mL/kg dose can be repeated up to three times (60 mL/kg) with vital signs and assessments repeated between each bolus. In non-trauma causes of shock, the total volume provided over a 24-hour period may exceed many times the 20 mL/kg dose. The Paramedic should reassess the child between boluses to look for improvement as well as prevent fluid overload. For the newly born child, the fluid dose is reduced to 10 mL/kg with reassessment between each bolus.

The pediatric patient with poor perfusion in the prehospital setting would rarely require a pharmacological agent to treat shock. Most often, the patient will respond to repeated intravenous or intraosseous fluid boluses. If a vasopressor medication is required, however, epinephrine is the initial drug of choice.[21,22] It is fast acting, highly effective, its actions and reactions are well known to most Paramedics, and it has a short half-life. The beta/adrenergic stimulation also aids in cardiac output and bronchial dilation. The recommended dose for continuous infusion of epinephrine is 0.1 to 1 mcg/kg/min, starting with a rapid infusion of 2 mcg/kg/min to initiate the effect and then titrating the infusion downward as needed.

A rapid way to mix the appropriate dose for an epinephrine drip was presented in McLeroy's paper in 1994.[23] First, the Paramedic should take the child's weight in kg and multiply it by 0.6. The Paramedic then takes that amount of epinephrine in mg and mixes it with normal saline in a burette up to a total volume of 100 mL. The Paramedic initially infuses the epinephrine drip at a rate of 20 mL/hour, which is equivalent to a rate of 2 mcg/kg/min. As the child responds to the epinephrine infusion, the Paramedic should titrate the drip down to a rate of 1 to 10 mL/hour to provide the dose of 0.1 to 1 mcg/kg/min (Figure 41-6).

Cardiopulmonary Arrest

Pediatric patients have specific CPR ratios, rates, and measures (Table 41-2). Compressions should be initiated if the patient's central pulse is not palpable or the child with hypoperfusion and hypotension has a heart rate below 60 beats

Example: Your patient is a 7-year-old boy who weighs 20 kgs.
1. Add 0.6 × 20 mg or 12 mg of epinephrine in a burette.
2. Add normal saline to a total volume of 100 mL. This provides a concentration of 120 mcg/mL of epinephrine.
3. Begin infusion at 20 mL/hr or 20 drops per minute using a 60 drops/mL infusion set.
4. Once the child responds with an adequate blood pressure, drop the rate to 10 mL/hr.
5. Titrate to between 1 mL/hr and 10 mL/hr in order to maintain adequate perfusion.

Figure 41-6 Calculation of appropriate epinephrine drip dosing.

Table 41-2 Pediatric Basic Life Support

Age	Breaths	Compression Rate	Compression Depth	Compression Method	Ratio of Compression: Ventilation
Infant (birth to 1 year)	15 to 20/minute (8 to 10/minute with advanced airway)	100/min	1/3 to 1/2 of the chest	Two thumbs encircling the body just below nipples	30:2 single rescuer 15:2 if two rescuers
Child (1 year to adolescent)	15 to 20/minute (8 to 10/minute with advanced airway)	100/min	1/3 to 1/2 of the chest	Heel of one hand at center of chest between nipples	30:2 single rescuer 15:2 if two rescuers

per minute, regardless of age. Priority should be given to compressions followed by ventilation, with a return to compressions in a regular and orderly fashion in children.[24] The pediatric literature has favored continuous compressions with as little interruption as possible during the resuscitation. Maintaining compressions improves the blood flow into the coronary arteries as well as out to the brain and organs. The best outcomes in patients who are in a poorly perfusing cardiac dysrhythmia, respiratory distress, or cardiac distress are achieved with early and aggressive CPR. The quality of compressions delivered by one person deteriorates in as little as two minutes, even if the provider performing compressions denies fatigue. If sufficient resources are available, the provider assigned to chest compressions should be rotated frequently.[25]

Paramedics can use the standard treatment algorithm for pediatric pulseless cardiopulmonary arrest (Figure 41-7). At the top, the opening reminds the Paramedic to perform basic cardiac life support treatments, including adequate ventilations with a bag–valve mask attached to high-flow, high-concentration oxygen and to provide adequate chest compressions based on the child's age and weight. As cardiac arrest in children is usually preceded by respiratory arrest, the focus initially is on beginning excellent basic cardiopulmonary resuscitation.

Once the cardiac monitor is attached to the child, the Paramedic interprets the rhythm and decides whether the rhythm is either shockable (i.e., ventricular tachycardia or ventricular fibrillation) or nonshockable (i.e., pulseless electrical activity or asystole). This decision point divides the algorithm in half and directs further treatment.

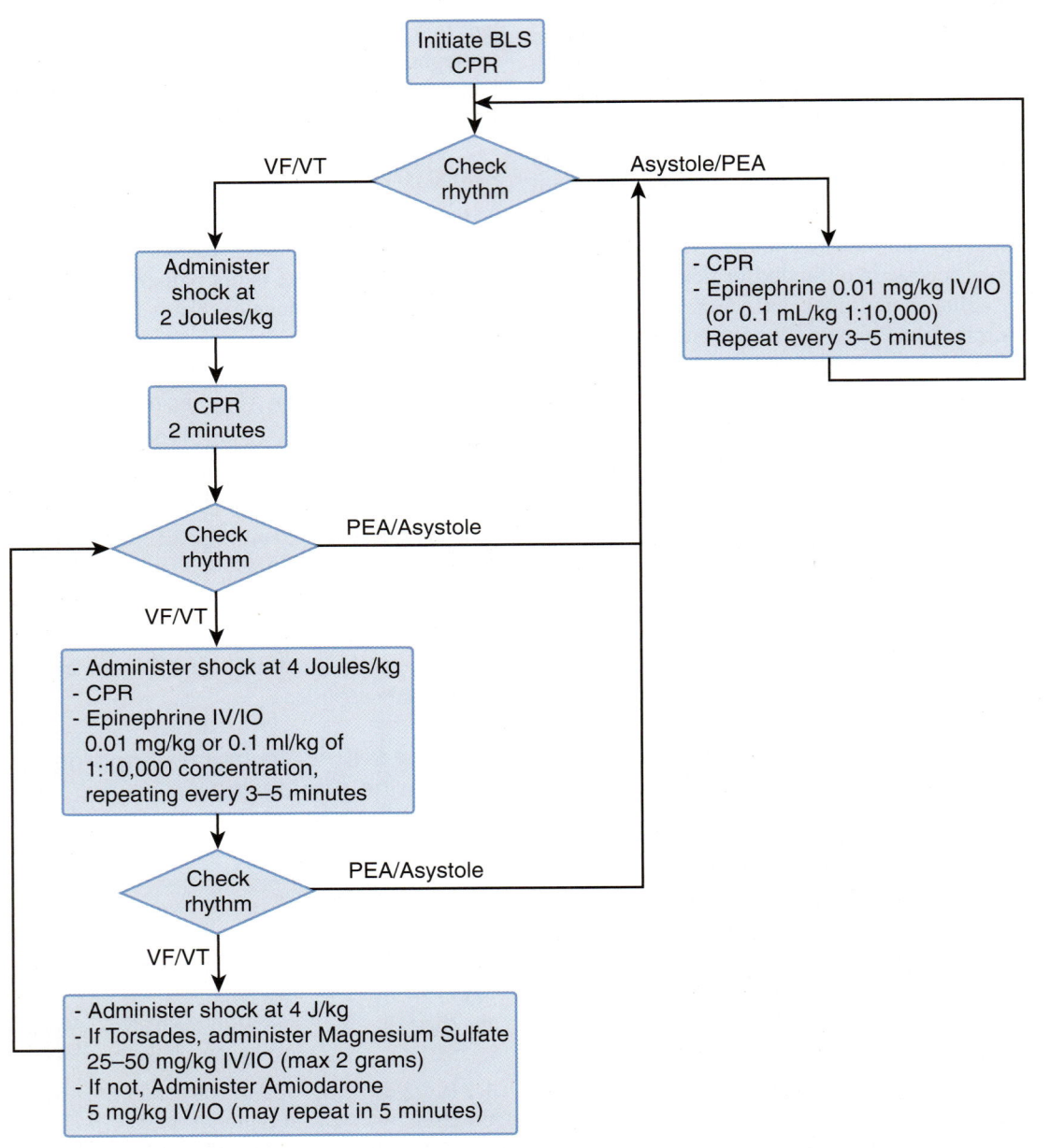

Figure 41-7 The pediatric pulseless arrest algorithm.

Delmar/Cengage Learning

If the patient has a shockable rhythm, the Paramedic's first step is to administer a single shock at an energy level of 2 joules/kg. Small paddles or gel pads which measure approximately 4.5 cm should be used for patients up to 1 year old or 10 kg. Adult paddles may be used on children 1 year of age or older, or those children larger than 10 kg or longer than 30 inches. If there is a clear indication for defibrillation and only adult paddles are available, the Paramedic may use an anterior–posterior approach. The Paramedic should place one electrode posterior on the patient's back and the second anterior, just left of the sternum. Firm application must be ensured with approximately 10 lbs of pressure applied over each paddle to ensure skin contact. The Paramedic should liberally apply conducting gel. If paddles or pads are not in sufficient contact with the skin, the electrical pulse may arc over the skin. This may result in skin burns, shock the rescuers, and deliver a subtherapeutic energy dose to the patient.[26]

After the shock, the Paramedic should immediately resume CPR without a pulse check and before rhythm analysis. The focus should be on minimal interruption of compressions during CPR, so the Paramedic should complete five cycles of CPR and then perform a simultaneous rhythm and pulse check. If the patient remains in a shockable rhythm, the Paramedic will administer one shock at an energy level of 4 joules/kg. From this point forward in the resuscitation, all electrical countershocks should be administered at an energy level of 4 joules/kg. After the electrical countershock, the Paramedic should immediately resume compressions and obtain intraosseous or intravenous access. Once intraosseous or intravenous access is obtained, the Paramedic administers epinephrine in a dose of 0.01 mg/kg (0.1 mL/kg of the 1:10,000 concentration). Epinephrine should be repeated every three to five minutes during the resuscitation.

After the next five cycles of CPR, the Paramedic should pause for another rhythm and pulse check. If the patient remains in ventricular fibrillation or pulseless ventricular tachycardia, the Paramedic administers a third electrical countershock at 4 joules/kg and immediately resumes compressions. At this point, the Paramedic has three options for antiarrhythmics. The first option is amiodarone administered as a 5 mg/kg bolus intraosseously or intravenously. The second option is to administer lidocaine at a dose of 1 mg/kg bolus intraosseously or intravenously. Both the first and second options attempt to treat the ventricular tachycardia or fibrillation rhythm. If, however, the rhythm on the monitor is torsades de pointes, then the Paramedic should administer magnesium sulfate at a dose of between 25 and 50 mg/kg intraosseously or intravenously, with a maximum dose of 2 grams. CPR is continued for another 5 cycles before the next pulse and rhythm check. This process continues as long as the patient remains in ventricular tachycardia or ventricular fibrillation (Figure 41-7). If the Paramedic places an invasive airway at any time, compressions should be continuous and not timed with ventilations and the pulse and rhythm check should occur every two minutes rather than after every five cycles of CPR.

The right half of the algorithm (Figure 41-7) handles the situation in which the rhythm is either asystole or pulseless electrical activity (PEA). Once the rhythm and pulse check confirm a nonshockable rhythm of asystole or PEA, the Paramedic resumes compressions and obtains intraosseous or intravenous access. Once vascular access is obtained, the Paramedic administers epinephrine every three to five minutes and provides five cycles of CPR. After the five cycles of CPR, the Paramedic checks the pulse and rhythm. If the rhythm at this point is ventricular tachycardia or ventricular fibrillation, then the Paramedic should jump to the top of the left side of the algorithm and proceed to administer an electrical countershock. If the rhythm remains PEA or asystole, the Paramedic repeats the five cycles of CPR, pulse and rhythm check, and administration of epinephrine every three to five minutes.

During the resuscitation, the Paramedic should address the causes of cardiopulmonary arrest in children that were presented earlier (Table 41-1). These five H's and five T's help to remind the Paramedic of several causes of cardiopulmonary arrest that can be addressed during the resuscitation. Hypoxemia can be addressed by providing excellent bag–valve–mask ventilations or ventilation through an advanced airway in order to provide sufficient oxygen to the lungs. Effective compressions also assist in the delivery of oxygen by providing forward circulation of oxygenated blood to the brain, heart, and other organs. Hypovolemia is addressed by either running an appropriate amount of fluid during the resuscitation or administering fluid boluses during resuscitation. Hypothermia, as previously mentioned, is a common cause for bradycardia. Although the Paramedic should keep the child covered and warm, exposing only what needs to be exposed in order to provide care, accidental hypothermia is the concern here. Hypothermia protocols should be followed (i.e., active external rewarming or internal rewarming at the hospital). Hyperkalemia is uncommon in the pediatric patient, although it is a possibility for children who are on dialysis. Acidosis can occur from prolonged hypoxia or from a metabolic cause (e.g., diabetic ketoacidosis). In these cases, the use of sodium bicarbonate may be indicated. Finally, hypoglycemia can be corrected by administering D_{10} or D_{25} in infants and children and D_{50} in adolescents.

The T's cover several traumatic causes of cardiac arrest, and more likely PEA, including pericardial tamponade, tension pneumothorax, and hypovolemia secondary to trauma. If a tension pneumothorax is suspected, needle decompression with an appropriate-sized needle is indicated. If a specific toxin is suspected and an antidote is available, the Paramedic should consider administering the antidote. Examples include administering naloxone for opioid toxicity, atropine for organophosphate ingestion, and high-flow, high-concentration oxygen for carbon monoxide exposure. A significant thromboembolism in the pulmonary arteries can cause sudden death due to circulatory collapse. In the prehospital setting, the focus is on providing excellent compressions, oxygenation, and ventilation.

In the setting of successful return of spontaneous circulation at any time during the resuscitation, the Paramedic should reassess the child's airway, breathing, and circulatory status. If the airway is not patent, the Paramedic should place an advanced airway to maintain patency. If the patient has inadequate spontaneous respirations, the Paramedic should continue to ventilate the patient to ensure appropriate oxygenation and ventilation.

If signs of poor perfusion are present, the Paramedic administers a fluid bolus and reassesses the response. The Paramedic will use smaller fluid boluses (5 to 10 mL/kg) with caution in patients who may have poor cardiac function. This will reduce the chance of fluid overload after resuscitation. It is not uncommon for the myocardium to be stunned for a period of time after cardiac arrest and have poor function which then improves. If the patient still has poor perfusion after appropriate fluid boluses have been given, then a vasopressor is indicated. If the patient is hypotensive, the Paramedic should consider using either epinephrine at 0.1 to 1 mcg/kg/min or dopamine at 10 to 20 mcg/kg/min. If the patient is normotensive and has poor perfusion, the Paramedic should consider using dobutamine at 2 to 20 mcg/kg/min or dopamine at 2 to 20 mcg/kg/min. The Paramedic will titrate the dose of the vasopressor to the minimum dose required to improve perfusion. At the present time, there is no data to suggest a benefit to initiating therapeutic hypothermia in children who have sustained a cardiac arrest. However, studies are underway to explore therapeutic hypothermia as a treatment option.[27]

Symptomatic Bradycardia

When encountering a patient who is bradycardic, the Paramedic must first determine if the bradycardia is causing poor perfusion. If the bradycardia does not produce signs of poor perfusion, then close monitoring and observation is indicated. For the patient who is bradycardic with a pulse but has poor perfusion, the Paramedic's initial treatment is to administer oxygen; ensure the patient is warm; support the airway, breathing, and circulation; and attach an ECG monitor (Figure 41-8). At this point, the Paramedic will reassess the patient's perfusion. If the patient is perfusing poorly and has a heart rate below 60 beats per minute, then the Paramedic starts chest compressions to augment the child's circulation. If CPR still does not improve the patient's perfusion, then the Paramedic should obtain intraosseous or intravenous access and administer epinephrine 0.01 mg/kg (0.1 mL/kg of a 1:10,000 concentration). The Paramedic should then reassess and repeat the epinephrine every three to five minutes. If the child's rhythm demonstrates an atrioventricular block or if the history suggests an increase in vagal tone as the cause for the child's bradycardia, then the Paramedic should administer atropine at 0.02 mg/kg, with a minimum dose of 0.1 mg and a maximum dose of 1 mg. Except for these circumstances, routine use of atropine in bradycardic children is not indicated as it is in the adult population.

For patients who experience hemodynamic instability with bradycardia, transcutaneous pacing is an option although

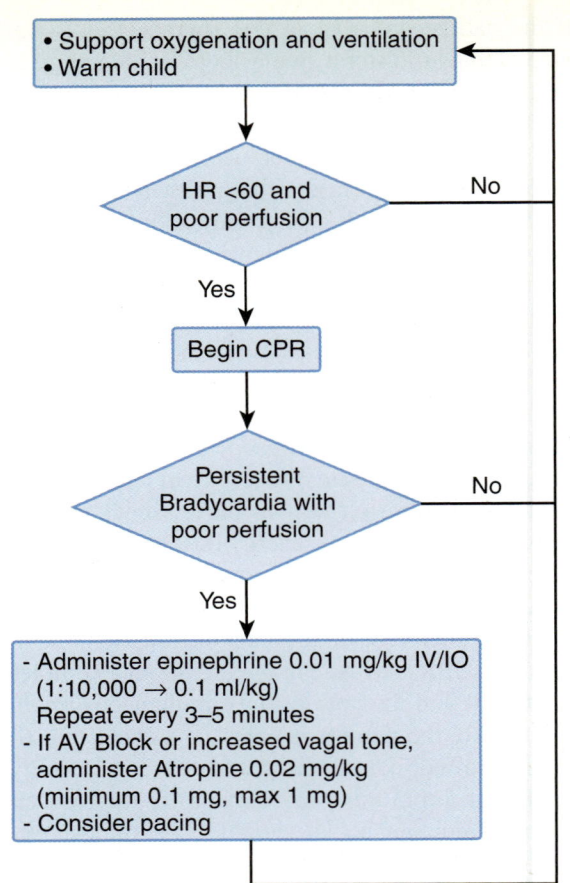

Figure 41-8 The treatment algorithm for pediatric patients who present with bradycardia and a pulse.

the benefit is questionable in pediatric patients.[28] One pad is placed on the anterior chest wall and the other on the back. The left midaxillary line is acceptable if the region of the midback is not accessible. Initial pacing is begun by setting the rate to 100 bpm with maximum energy output, which may be decreased until continuous capture of ventricular contraction (a pacing spike followed by a QRS complex) is obtained on the monitor. Pacing is a painful procedure and should be reserved for patients who are bradycardic and hemodynamically unstable. The Paramedic should strongly consider the use of sedation when pacing a patient.

Tachycardia with a Pulse

Pediatric patients who present with a tachycardia and are hemodynamically stable will likely be uncomfortable but will not appear **toxic**. A toxic child is one that appears very ill. For pediatric patients who present with a tachycardia and poor perfusion, the Paramedic should manage the patient's airway and breathing, and obtain vascular access to support the circulation. At this point, the Paramedic should assess the cardiac rhythm to help decide the most appropriate treatment for the patient (Figure 41-9).

A QRS duration which is greater than 0.08 seconds wide is more likely ventricular tachycardia and should be treated with synchronized cardioversion as a first-line treatment. The dose for

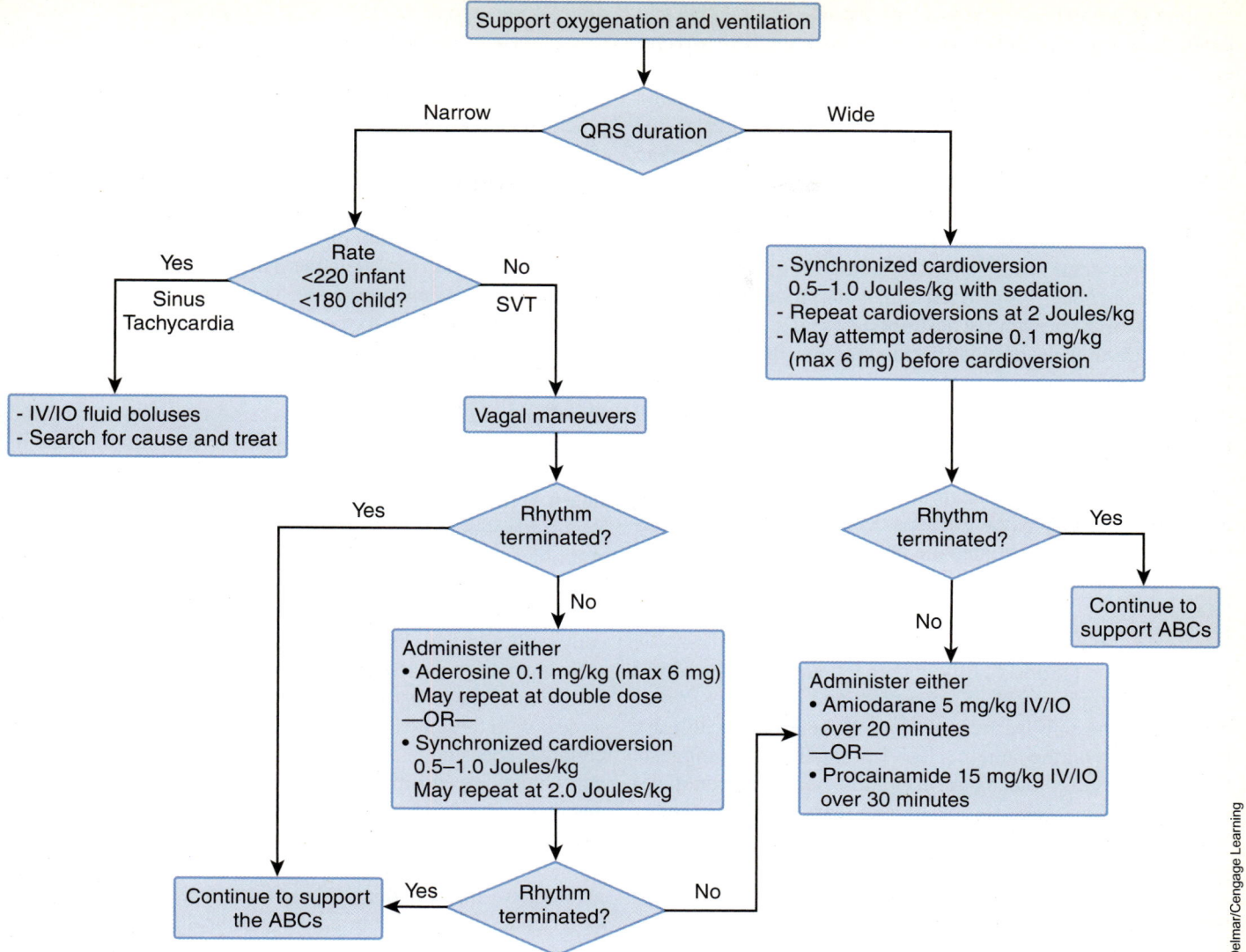

Figure 41-9 Treatment algorithm for a pediatric patient who presents with tachycardia with a pulse and poor perfusion.

initial cardioversion is 0.5 to 1 J/kg. The energy level for subsequent synchronized cardioversion attempts should be increased to 2 J/kg. Although cardioversion should not be delayed, it is acceptable to attempt a dose of adenosine at 0.1 mg/kg (maximum 6 mg) prior to cardioversion if there is a delay in administering the synchronized shock. If cardioversion is not effective, the Paramedic should consider administering amiodarone at 5 mg/kg intravenously or intraosseously over the next 20 minutes or procainamide 15 mg/kg over the next 30 minutes.

On the other hand, a QRS duration less than or equal to 0.08 seconds is normal and consistent with a narrow complex tachycardia. This narrow complex tachycardia may be a sinus tachycardia or a supraventricular tachycardia (SVT). The differentiation between these two rhythms was discussed earlier in this chapter.

Treatment of sinus tachycardia with poor perfusion consists of fluid boluses and addressing the underlying cause of the tachycardia. For SVT, vagal maneuvers may be attempted

initially to break the tachycardia by slowing conduction through the AV node. Asking the patient to bear down as if having a bowel movement, preferably against a closed glottis, will increase the patient's vagal tone on the heart. This slows electrical conduction through the AV node, offering the opportunity to terminate the tachycardia. The Paramedic may ask the older child to blow through a straw as another means of bearing down. Doing so may break the rhythm.[29] Carotid massage is a valuable option for patients who are unable to follow instructions. This technique, which is performed by massaging the carotid artery at the carotid bifurcation at the point of maximum impulse in the neck, stimulates baroreceptors and chemoreceptors, which signal the brain to decrease the heart rate. The maneuver is safer to perform in pediatric patients than in adults as children's carotid atherosclerotic plaque burden is much less. Ice water or ice packs placed directly on the face for 10 to 15 seconds will induce a vagal response as well. Finally, anal stimulation with a rectal thermometer is another vagal maneuver. Some patients will respond well to these maneuvers, although others will break the SVT rhythm only to return to SVT within seconds or minutes.

SVT refractory to the previous situations may respond to adenosine. Adenosine offers the chemical equivalent of defibrillation, and asystole may actually be noted on cardiac monitoring. The pediatric dose is 0.1 mg/kg up to an initial dose of 6 mg. If SVT continues, it should be treated with a second dose of adenosine at 0.2 mg/kg or a maximum of 12 mg. If vascular access is not immediately available or the patient is unstable, it is also reasonable to proceed directly to cardioversion as previously described.

One rhythm deserving special mention due to the difference in management is torsades de pointes. For pediatric patients who are hemodynamically stable, the Paramedic should consider administering magnesium sulfate at a dose of between 25 and 50 mg/kg intravenously or intraosseously over 20 minutes. Magnesium stabilizes the myocardial cell membrane and helps treat torsades. Hemodynamically unstable patients should be treated the same as those with pulseless ventricular tachycardia and receive defibrillation.

Family Presence during Resuscitation

During resuscitation, family members are often escorted out of the room for fear of immediate and long-term consequences to the family, the patient, and the entire healthcare team working on the patient. However, the literature suggests a family presence during resuscitation could be beneficial to both the family and the healthcare team. The Emergency Nurses Association and the American Heart Association both endorse family-witnessed resuscitation.[30]

Healthcare professionals report two primary reasons for their reluctance to invite patients' families to be present at a resuscitation attempt: the unpleasantness of what the families will see and anxiety that family members will become disruptive. Less frequently mentioned concerns include patient confidentiality, possible increase in litigation if patients' families are present, and more aggressive and prolonged treatment if patients' families are present.[31]

Several studies have shown that having a family member presence during the resuscitation is beneficial for both the parents and family members involved. Some programs have gone so far as to have a dedicated person stay with the family to explain actions during the code process and answer specific questions the family may have regarding the resuscitation, patient death, and organ donation. Although this may not be practical in the prehospital setting due to lack of personnel, if an individual is available to explain to the caregivers what is going on, it will not only help provide some reassurance to the caregivers but will also help prevent them from interfering with the resuscitation efforts. Witnessing the team effort of the resuscitation may help them understand everything that could have been done was done. This also offers the family a chance to say goodbye to their loved one.

Pediatric Death

Few things in life are more distressing than the unexpected death of a child. Trauma remains the most common cause of death in children 6 months and older whereas **sudden infant death syndrome (SIDS)** predominates in children younger than 6 months of age.[32] Death in neonates, infants, toddlers, and older children evokes strong emotional responses among healthcare workers at all levels.

After the death of a child, the patient's caregivers are typically confused and distraught. The members of the healthcare team involved in the resuscitation may also be upset at the unsuccessful attempts at resuscitation. However, there's often not time to deal with these feelings. Healthcare workers are expected to continue, focusing on the family and the patient, in these emergent situations and maintain professionalism. The Paramedic and her crew involved in the pediatric resuscitation should debrief each other at an appropriate time after the incident.

Most hospital systems have counselors or faith directors available to speak with and share in the healthcare provider's experience. The literature addressing healthcare professionals' experiences caring for dying children indicates telling stories about deceased patients to supportive peers is frequently used for finding meaning. There are mechanisms in place to help healthcare providers cope with loss regardless of how they choose to deal with it. Taking the approach of keeping the incident to oneself has been found to be unhealthy. In contrast, talking with peers, friends, or family can help alleviate the discomfort of the situation and assist the Paramedic in coping with the experience.

► CASE STUDY (CONTINUED)

After the synchronized cardioversion, Tonele's rhythm changes to a sinus tachycardia at 140 beats per minute, his respiratory rate slows, and his capillary refill falls to four seconds. He receives a 20 mL/kg saline bolus via syringe and three-way stopcock to help stabilize his hemodynamics.

CRITICAL THINKING QUESTIONS

1. What are some of the predictable complications associated with synchronized cardioversion?
2. Why would the cardiovascular system be unstable?

Evaluation

The treatment algorithms for critically ill children discussed in the previous section include reminders to reevaluate the patient. It is essential for the Paramedic to perform continuous monitoring and reassessment during the resuscitation of critically ill children, as changes in patient status can occur rapidly. If the child is stabilized during the initial resuscitation, the Paramedic should periodically reassess the airway, breathing, and circulatory status during transport. Any change in cardiac rhythm, end-tidal carbon dioxide, pulse oximetry, or blood pressure warrants a reassessment of the patient's airway, breathing, and circulation.

CASE STUDY CONCLUSION

The ambulance arrives to transport Tonele to Rapids General emergency department, which is across town, because they have a pediatric emergency department and a pediatric intensive care unit. The remainder of the transport is uneventful and Tonele's condition improves during transport.

CRITICAL THINKING QUESTIONS

1. What is the most appropriate transport decision that will get the patient to definitive care?
2. What are the advantages of transporting an unstable pediatric patient to these hospitals, even if that means bypassing other hospitals in the process?

Disposition

Critically ill children should be taken to the closest appropriate pediatric-equipped emergency department. If a specialized pediatric emergency department is within a reasonable transport distance, it may be appropriate to transport the patient directly to the pediatric emergency department rather than the closest facility. As with trauma, spending the time up front transporting a patient to a specialty center saves a significant amount of time for the patient to reach definitive specialty care. Significant delays can occur when the patient is taken to an emergency department which must then transfer the patient. In the event of a cardiac arrest or an unstable airway, the Paramedic must travel to the closest emergency department.

CONCLUSION

When caring for the critically ill child, the majority of the EMS contact time will be spent obtaining a rapid history and examination, intervening appropriately given the potential underlying condition, and performing constant reassessments of the child. Focusing on these critical aspects and continual reassessment will allow the Paramedic to expertly care for critically ill children.

KEY POINTS:

- No single chief concern indicates that a child is critically ill.

- Critical pediatric conditions fall into one or more of the following categories:
  - Respiratory failure
  - Circulatory collapse
  - Cardiopulmonary arrest
  - Bradycardia
  - Tachycardia

- The primary cause of pediatric cardiac arrest is respiratory failure.

- Hypoxia in the pediatric patient causes altered mental status, bradycardia, and hypotension.

- Children are able to compensate well for a hypoperfused state but will deteriorate rapidly.

- Asystole is a more common initial arrest rhythm for children than for adults.

- Bradydysrhythmias commonly result from hypoxemia.

- Increased vagal stimulation may also cause a significant bradycardia in children.

- Tachycardia results from a stressor such as pain, fever, anxiety, or metabolic alterations.

- Ventricular tachycardia and ventricular fibrillation are uncommon in the child.

- A specific form of VT, torsades de pointes, is more common in children than adults.

- Fever, feeding, and urination history are important factors to consider in younger children and infants.

- Additional history for infants and young children includes:
  - Birth history
  - Developmental progress
  - Immunizations

- The assessment focus in the critically ill child is on the initial assessment of airway, breathing, circulation, disability, and exposure.

- Decompensated shock leads rapidly to respiratory and cardiac arrest.

- Assessment of the fontanels yields information regarding hydration status and intracranial pressure.

- The Paramedic should address the primary problem found in the A-B-C assessment first.

- High-flow, high-concentration oxygen is an essential treatment for the critically ill child.

- Assisted ventilation may reverse respiratory failure and stimulate more normal breathing.

- Advanced airways include endotracheal intubation, King tubes, LMA mask, and needle cricothyrotomy.

- Surgical and percutaneous cricothyrotomy are contraindicated in children under age 12 due to scarring and stenosis of the airway.

- Circulatory failure most often results from respiratory failure.

- CPR is indicated for pediatric patients with heart rates less than 60.

- Vascular access may be obtained via the IV or IO route.

- Scalp veins may provide access in the infant.

- Normal saline is the fluid of choice and is administered at 20 mL/kg.

- If vasopressor medication is indicated, epinephrine is the drug of choice.

- Pediatric CPR should maximize compressions while keeping any interruptions to a minimum.

- Further treatment of the child in cardiac arrest is based on whether a shockable rhythm exists.
  - Shock at 2 J/kg and resume two minutes of CPR. Any additional shocks are at 4 J/kg, then follow guidelines for antiarrhythmic therapy.
  - Perform CPR for asystole or pulseless electrical activity, administer epinephrine, and consider the causes:
    - Hypoxemia, hypothermia, hypovolemia, hypoglycemia, hyperkalemia
    - Tamponade, tension pneumothorax, trauma, toxins, thromboembolism

- With any return of pulses, the Paramedic should immediately reassess the patient's airway, breathing, and circulation.

- For bradycardia, the Paramedic should determine if the rate is causing poor perfusion:
  - Treat poor perfusion and bradycardia initially with oxygen and support of body systems
  - Initiate CPR for rates below 60 per minute
  - Use epinephrine as the drug of choice unless the rate has been caused by increased vagal tone, then administer atropine
  - Consider a pacemaker

- For bradycardia that is not causing poor perfusion, the Paramedic should monitor closely for changes.

- For hemodynamically stable tachycardia, the Paramedic should determine the rhythm and treat per algorithm.

- For hemodynamically unstable tachycardia, the Paramedic should administer oxygen, obtain venous access, and determine the rhythm:
  - Ventricular tachycardia should be cardioverted.
  - SVT may be converted by vagal maneuvers, pharmacologic methods, or electricity.

- Torsades de pointes should be treated with magnesium sulfate administered over 20 minutes.

- The literature suggests that a family presence during a resuscitation has benefits to the family and team members.

- Pediatric death causes strong emotions in the healthcare team.

- During pediatric care, the Paramedic should frequently reevaluate patients.

REVIEW QUESTIONS:

1. What is the likely cause of pediatric cardiac arrest?
2. Name two common causes of bradydysrhythmias and four common causes of tachycardia in the child.
3. Why is torsades de pointes more common in children than in adults?
4. Name six categories of medical history that are more important to obtain in young children than adults.
5. What vasopressor is the drug of choice if needed in the pediatric population?
6. What drug is indicated for a child with a bradycardia caused by increased vagal tone?
7. What is the treatment for the child with SVT? The child with torsades de pointes?

CASE STUDY QUESTIONS:

Please refer to the Case Study in this chapter, and answer the questions below:

1. Which aspects of the Pediatric Assessment Triangle were abnormal upon initial assessment? Explain the relationship of Tonele's problem to the exam results that were ultimately found.

2. Explain why the Paramedics chose to treat Tonele's heart rhythm rather than first treating his respiratory rate and effort.

3. Should family members be permitted to view interventions or a resuscitation? Why or why not?

REFERENCES:

1. Levin M, Sondheimer M, et al. *Current Pediatric Diagnosis & Treatment*. New York: McGraw-Hill; 2004.

2. Baren JM, Brennan J, et al. *Pediatric Emergency Medicine*. St. Louis: Saunders; 2007.

3. Kochanek, P. (ed) *Pediatric Critical Care Medicine (Pediatric Critical Care Medicine (Slonim))*. Philadelphia: Lippincott Williams & Wilkins; 2006.

4. Wheeler, W. et al. *Science and Practice of Pediatric Critical Care Medicine*. New York: Springer; 2009.

5. Association AH. *PALS Provider Manual*. Dallas: American Heart Association; 2002.

6. Allen HD, Driscoll DJ, et al. *Moss and Adams' Heart Disease in Infants, Children and Adolescents: Including the Fetus and Young Adult, 2 Volume Set*. Philadelphia: Lippincott Williams & Wilkins; 2007.

7. Kugler JD, Danford DA. Management of infants, children, and adolescents with paroxysmal supraventricular tachycardia. *J Pediatr*. 1996;129(3):324–338.

8. Mogayzel C, Quan L, et al. Out-of-hospital ventricular fibrillation in children and adolescents: causes and outcomes. *Ann Emerg Med*. 1995;25(4):484–491.

9. Bessette M. Torsades de pointes. Available at: **http://emedicine.medscape.com/article/760667-overview**. Accessed May 16th 2009.

10. Sovari A. Long QT syndrome. Available at: **http://emedicine.medscape.com/article/157826-overview**. Accessed May 16th 2009.

11. Wedekind H, Smits JP, et al. De novo mutation in the SCN5A gene associated with early onset of sudden infant death. *Circulation*. 2001;104(10):1158–1164.

12. Gongadze N, Kezeli T, et al. Prolong QT interval and "torsades de pointes" associated with different group of drugs. *Georgian Med News*. 2007;153:45–49.

13. Chiu CH, Lin TY. Application of the Rochester Criteria in febrile neonates. *Pediatr Infect Dis J*. 1998;17(3):267–269.

14. Ferrera PC, Bartfield JM, et al. Neonatal fever: utility of the Rochester criteria in determining low risk for serious bacterial infections. *Am J Emerg Med*. 1997;15(3):299–302.

15. Wooten KG, Janssen A, et al. Associations between childhood vaccination status and medical practice characteristics among white, black, and Hispanic children. *J Natl Med Assoc*. 2009;101(3):229–235.

16. Brierley J, Carcillo JA, et al. Clinical practice parameters for hemodynamic support of pediatric and neonatal septic shock: 2007 update from the American College of Critical Care Medicine. *Crit Care Med*. 2009;37(2):666–688.

17. Ivan LP, Badejo A. Clinical and experimental observations with fontanel pressure measurements. *Childs Brain*. 1983;10(6):361–368.

18. Gausche-Hill M, Lewis RJ, et al. Design and implementation of a controlled trial of pediatric endotracheal intubation in the out-of-hospital setting. *Ann Emerg Med*. 2000;36(4):356–365.

19. Nguyen QV. Hospital acquired infections. E-medicine. Available at: **http://emedicine.medscape.com/article/967022-overview**. Accessed May 16, 2009.

20. Sofferman RA, Johnson DL, et al. Lost airway during anesthesia induction: alternatives for management. *Laryngoscope*. 1997;107(11 Pt 1):1476–1482.

21. Irazuzta J, Sullivan KJ, et al. Pharmacologic support of infants and children in septic shock. *J Pediatr (Rio J)*. 2007;83(2 Suppl):S36–S45.

22. Sharman M, Meert KL. What is the right dose of epinephrine? *Pediatr Crit Care Med*. 2005;6(5):592–594.

23. McLeroy PA. The rule of six: Calculating intravenous infusions in a pediatric crisis situation. *Hospital Pharmacy*. 1994;29(10):939–940, 943.

24. Greingor JL. Quality of cardiac massage with ratio compression-ventilation 5/1 and 15/2. *Resuscitation*. 2002;55(3):263–267.

25. Larsen MP, Eisenberg MS, et al. Predicting survival from out-of-hospital cardiac arrest: a graphic model. *Ann Emerg Med*. 1993;22(11):1652–1658.

26. Caterine MR, Yoerger DM, et al. Effect of electrode position and gel-application technique on predicted transcardiac current during transthoracic defibrillation. *Ann Emerg Med*. 1997;29(5):588–595.

27. Hutchison JS, Doherty DR, et al. Hypothermia therapy for cardiac arrest in pediatric patients. *Pediatr Clin North Am*. 2008;55(3):529–544, ix.

28. Quan L, Graves JR, et al. Transcutaneous cardiac pacing in the treatment of out-of-hospital pediatric cardiac arrests. *Ann Emerg Med*. 1992;21(8):905–909.

29. Manole MD, Saladino RA. Emergency department management of the pediatric patient with supraventricular tachycardia. *Pediatr Emerg Care*. 2007;23(3):176–185; quiz 186–189.

30. Eppich WJ, Arnold LD. Family member presence in the pediatric emergency department. *Curr Opin Pediatr*. 2003;15(3):294–298.

31. Twibell RS, Siela D, et al. Nurses' perceptions of their self-confidence and the benefits and risks of family presence during resuscitation. *Am J Crit Care*. 2008;17(2):101–111; quiz 112.

32. Hunt CE. Sudden infant death syndrome and other causes of infant mortality: diagnosis, mechanisms, and risk for recurrence in siblings. *Am J Respir Crit Care Med*. 2001;164(3):346–357.

CHAPTER 42

PEDIATRIC MEDICAL EMERGENCIES

KEY CONCEPTS:

Upon completion of this chapter, it is expected that the reader will understand these following concepts:

- The organization of pediatric concerns necessitating prehospital care into a subset of conditions among the cardiovascular, respiratory, neurological, and gastrointestinal systems
- The focus of general pediatric treatments on airway, breathing, and circulation

ANATOMY CONCEPTS:

Prior to reading this chapter the Paramedic student should be familiar with the following anatomy and physiology concepts:

- Child developmental stages

"Centerport Rescue, respond to 312 Hudson Street apartment 7, for an 18-month-old child with a cough and respiratory distress." The address is one of the tenement houses located along the city's manufacturing strip. After the Paramedics knock on the apartment door, it is opened by a young woman holding a crying toddler who has a barking cough and clear nasal discharge.

CRITICAL THINKING QUESTIONS

1. What are some of the possible causes of a barking cough?
2. How is trouble breathing related to the nasal discharge?

OVERVIEW

Children are relatively healthy and do not have to contend with many of the chronic diseases and conditions that plague adults. Because of their relative good health, the Paramedic will only encounter a relatively small number of critically ill children during a typical career. However, even if a child passes the initial assessment with the Pediatric Assessment Triangle, the child may still have an underlying severe illness. A child who does not pass the initial assessment may have one of the conditions discussed in this chapter that has worsened, leading the child to decompensate and become critically ill. This chapter discusses the wide range of medical emergencies which can affect children.

Chief Concern

The diversity of medical conditions that occur in pediatric patients spans the entire breadth of medicine. In Paramedic practice, the Paramedic will encounter a subset of these conditions among the cardiovascular, respiratory, neurological, and gastrointestinal systems. In this population, there are also several infectious diseases that occur more commonly in pediatric patients than in adults.

Cardiac

Cardiovascular disease is uncommon in the pediatric patient population. Many of the significant cardiac issues that occur in children are either secondary to respiratory disease, related to dysrhythmias, or related to congenital conditions. Chapter 41 covered many of the life-threatening cardiovascular-related conditions facing children. These are often acute onset conditions in which the child appears critically ill on the initial examination.

However, some congenital cardiovascular conditions may go undetected in the first several months to years of life. Although these are not commonly encountered in prehospital practice, there is a good chance that at some point in a Paramedic's career the Paramedic will encounter a patient who has a congenital cardiac condition.

Before discussing the common congenital cardiac abnormalities that may occur, a discussion of normal fetal circulation is appropriate (Figure 42-1). Oxygenated blood starts at the placenta, travels along the umbilical vein, and follows the ductus venosus around the liver and into the inferior vena cava. This oxygenated blood flows through the foramen ovale into the left side of the heart and is pumped out the aorta into the fetal circulation. Deoxygenated blood returns to the right atrium and flows into the right ventricle. Rather than circulating through the lungs, the majority of the deoxygenated blood flows from the pulmonary artery through the ductus arteriosus and into the aorta. This deoxygenated blood flows back to the placenta via the two umbilical arteries. Much of the blood flowing through the fetal circulation is mixed oxygenated/deoxygenated blood that flows in the appropriate direction preferentially in order to maintain gas exchange.

Fetal hemoglobin is different from adult hemoglobin in that it has a greater affinity, or binding potential, for oxygen.[1] This allows the fetus to survive and grow in a relatively hypoxemic environment. It also means the fetus is sensitive to maternal hypoxia or maternal distress. After delivery, the infant's first several breaths cause these bypass vessels to clamp down and circulation shifts to the normal direction of blood flow. These ducts are closed within the first 10 hours of life and are permanently closed within three weeks of delivery.

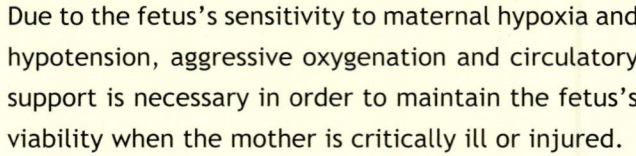

STREET SMART

Due to the fetus's sensitivity to maternal hypoxia and hypotension, aggressive oxygenation and circulatory support is necessary in order to maintain the fetus's viability when the mother is critically ill or injured.

Congenital cardiac conditions can be broken down into three major categories; conditions that cause a right-to-left shunt, conditions that cause a left-to-right shunt, and conditions that cause obstruction of either the left ventricle or right ventricle outflow.[2] In all three classifications of congenital cardiac conditions, there is an abnormality of circulation that occurs either due to inadequate closure of one of the bypass pathways of fetal circulation or a structural abnormality that does not allow normal circulation. In some conditions, the bypass pathways will temporarily stay open as a means of allowing somewhat normal circulation to occur.

In conditions that cause a right-to-left shunt, instead of deoxygenated blood flowing from the right side of the heart to the lungs, deoxygenated blood bypasses the lungs and ends up in the neonatal circulation. Conditions that cause a right-to-left shunt are also called **cyanotic heart disease** due to the cyanosis that occurs from the mixing of oxygenated and deoxygenated blood in the systemic circulation. The most common congenital condition that causes a right-to-left shunt, and is present in 10% of all neonates with congenital

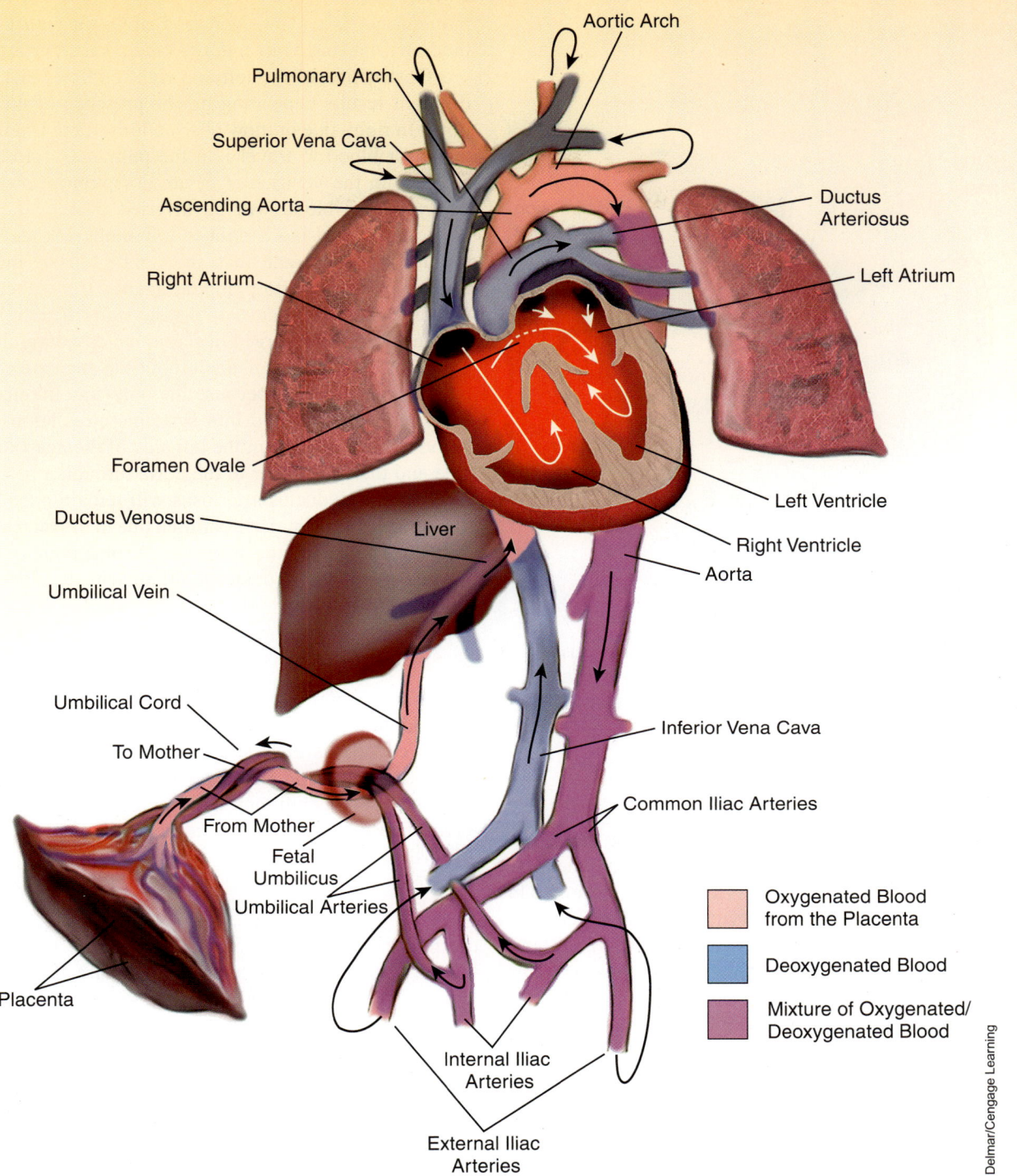

Labels on figure:
- Pulmonary Arch
- Aortic Arch
- Superior Vena Cava
- Ascending Aorta
- Ductus Arteriosus
- Right Atrium
- Left Atrium
- Foramen Ovale
- Left Ventricle
- Ductus Venosus
- Liver
- Right Ventricle
- Umbilical Vein
- Aorta
- Umbilical Cord
- To Mother
- Inferior Vena Cava
- From Mother
- Fetal Umbilicus
- Common Iliac Arteries
- Umbilical Arteries
- Placenta
- Oxygenated Blood from the Placenta
- Deoxygenated Blood
- Mixture of Oxygenated/Deoxygenated Blood
- Internal Iliac Arteries
- External Iliac Arteries

Delmar/Cengage Learning

Figure 42-1   Normal fetal circulatory anatomy. The umbilical arteries, umbilical vein, ductus venosus, and ductus arteriosus close within the infant's first several breaths, converting fetal circulation to the more familiar circulatory system.

cardiac disease, is the Tetralogy of Fallot.[3] **Tetralogy of Fallot** was first described in the late 1800s and consists of four congenital abnormalities (Figure 42-2). Pulmonary artery stenosis restricts blood flow to the lungs. With the increased resistance of blood flow to the lungs, deoxygenated blood preferentially flows through the ventricular septal defect into the left ventricle. It then flows out into systemic circulation through an aorta that overrides and has a direct pathway to the right ventricle rather than accepting all of its blood from the left ventricle. Due to the increased pressure the right ventricle must pump against, the right ventricular myocardium enlarges in order to overcome the higher pressure.

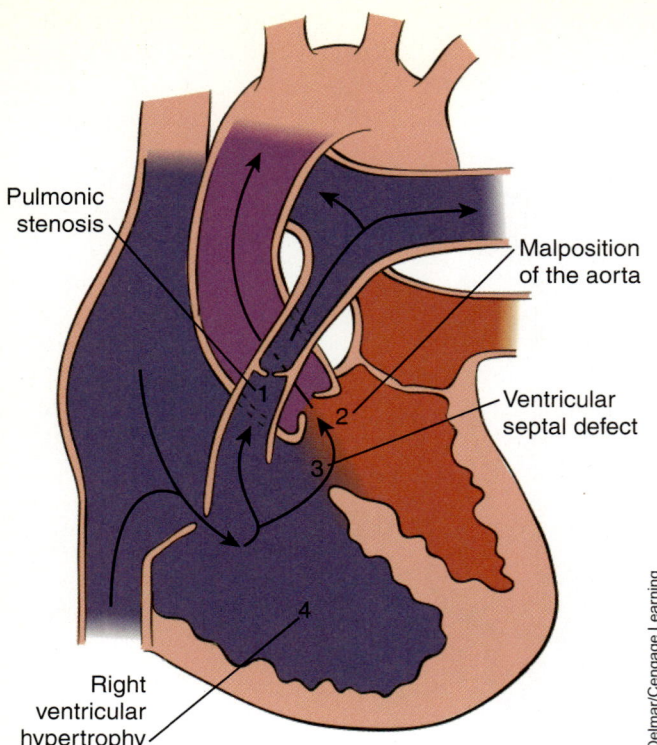

Pulmonic
stenosis

Malposition
of the aorta

Ventricular
septal defect

Right
ventricular
hypertrophy

Delmar/Cengage Learning

Figure 42-2 Diagram of the classic congenital abnormalities associated with Tetralogy of Fallot. (1) Pulmonary stenosis. (2) Overriding aorta. (3) Ventricular septal defect. (4) Right ventricular hypertrophy.

Infants who have Tetralogy of Fallot can have **TET spells** (short for Tetralogy of Fallot spells) in which the infant becomes suddenly cyanotic and has a syncopal episode. This is typically due to feeding and crying, although older children will have TET spells during physical exertion. During a TET spell, the pressures in the neonate's pulmonary circulation increase while the resistance of the system circulation decreases, resulting in a significant increase in blood flow which bypasses the lungs. With more deoxygenated blood bypassing the lungs, the neonate's oxygen saturation rapidly falls. Surgical repair of the congenital defects is possible and typically occurs later in the first year of life. Adults who had surgical repair of Tetralogy of Fallot are at risk for sudden cardiac death and heart failure and often have ECG abnormalities due to the surgical incisions made to the myocardium during the surgery.[4] Until surgical repair is made, the Paramedic may be called for an infant who has a TET spell.

In conditions with a left-to-right shunt, flow of oxygenated blood from the left side of the heart preferentially travels into the pulmonary circulation due to the lower resistance of the pulmonary circulation as compared with systemic circulation. Conditions that cause a left-to-right shunting of blood are often termed **acyanotic heart disease** because these conditions do not produce cyanosis. The additional blood in the pulmonary vascular system can cause congestion in the pulmonary vessels and increased stress on the right side of the heart, causing heart failure in the neonate or infant.

Obstruction of the left and right outflow tract produces different results depending on the presence of other conditions. In right-side outflow obstructions, there is a high resistance for blood to travel into the pulmonary circulation. If a defect in the ventricular or atrial septum is present, then deoxygenated blood will be diverted over to the left side of the heart, causing a right-to-left shunt. If a defect in the septum is not present, then the right ventricle muscle will thicken in response to pumping against the higher pressure and the neonate will develop classic signs of right heart failure, including an enlarged liver and increased jugular venous pressure. Obstructions in the left outflow tract are called ductal dependent lesions because the only way the neonate can have any flow of blood into systemic circulation is for the blood to cross over from the left side of the heart to the right side and then back over to the aorta through a patent ductus arteriosus. The ductus arteriosus will remain open for a longer period of time in these children due to the increased blood flow through the ductus. However, at some point it will close. At that point, the neonate or infant will develop profound shock and likely die.

Respiratory

There are several common respiratory conditions that occur in children, often with a chief concern of dyspnea or cough. These conditions include asthma, bronchiolitis, croup, bacterial tracheitis, and pneumonia. In addition, two congenital respiratory conditions the Paramedic may encounter in children are cystic fibrosis and neonatal respiratory distress syndrome.

Asthma

Asthma is prevalent in 5% to 10% of the pediatric population, most commonly presenting before the age of 4 or 5 years.[5] Boys are more likely than girls to be affected until adolescence, when the prevalence is equal in both genders. The pathophysiology of the disease is the same in adults as it is in children. Two differences between adult and pediatric patients are the greater effect edema has on the diameter of the airways and the impact the increased work of breathing has on the child's transition from compensation to decompensation. The child's bronchial tree is much smaller in diameter than those of adults. Even a small amount of lower airway edema can decrease the airflow through the respiratory system and lead to significant air trapping. Children in severe respiratory distress will use up a large amount of energy when the work of breathing is increased. Fatigue and progressive airway edema cause the child to decompensate more rapidly than an adult.

The two types of asthma are intermittent asthma and chronic asthma. The child with intermittent asthma is symptom free for extended periods of time without medication intervention. In contrast, a child with chronic asthma has more frequent symptoms that require frequent or continuous medication.[6] Both types of asthma can vary in intensity with the patient developing an acute asthma exacerbation.

Status asthmaticus is a severe prolonged asthma attack with significant air trapping and respiratory distress that does not respond to usual treatment aimed at bronchodilation and decreasing inflammation. Without aggressive treatment, the child in status asthmaticus may rapidly progress to respiratory failure and cardiac arrest.

Wheezing is the classic sign that develops with asthma due to swelling in the mucous lining of the respiratory tree. Coughing is also commonly associated with asthma and may be an early sign that a child either has asthma or is about to develop an asthma exacerbation. As in adults, a child's asthma exacerbation may be initiated by an upper or lower respiratory infection, secondhand smoke, or other irritants. Viral upper respiratory infections tend to cause a significant amount of clear nasal discharge, with much of the discharge flowing backward from the sinuses down the pharynx and into the airways, producing bronchospasm. Secondhand smoke is a leading cause of asthma and other upper respiratory infections in children, even in homes where the caregivers smoke outside. The irritants remain on the caregiver's clothing and are transferred to the child during physical contact.[7,8]

Bronchiolitis

Bronchiolitis is a viral infection of the bronchioles caused by the respiratory syncytial virus (RSV), the parainfluenza virus, or the influenza A virus. The infection produces a bronchospasm that decreases the size of the bronchioles and increases the production of mucus. This combination causes a decrease in ventilation and an increase in respiratory effort. Frequently confused with asthma, bronchiolitis characteristically presents with a fever, dry cough, runny nose, and nasal congestion. Upon examination, the child may have wheezing (both inspiratory and expiratory) and rhonchi. Dehydration is always of concern due to the patient's fever and increased work of breathing. In some patients, there may be a significant bronchospastic component to the illness that responds to asthma medications. In younger children, bronchiolitis can cause life-threatening respiratory failure.[9]

Croup

Croup is a common viral upper respiratory illness that causes edema in the larynx, upper trachea, and larger bronchi. The medical name for croup is laryngotracheobronchitis, indicating the three sites of inflammation associated with the condition. The edema leads to the variety of symptoms associated with croup including a hoarse voice, a barking cough that sounds similar to a seal barking, stridor on inhalation, and varying degrees of respiratory distress. Croup is most commonly seen in children 3 months to 3 years of age, although it can be seen in older children as well. The caregivers often report that the child appears perfectly well during the day with the symptoms worsening at night time. Typically, the symptoms will be at their worst on the second or third night of the illness and then begin to improve. The patient may have a copious amount of clear nasal discharge associated with the illness. Fevers are not common, but may be present.

Croup improves in cool dry air, which helps alleviate some of the upper respiratory edema. As croup is common in the fall and winter months, it is not unusual for the Paramedic to arrive on-scene in the middle of the night to find the child has improved simply by moving out into the cold air. Croup also improves with warm moist air, which is why some pediatricians recommend that parents bring their child into a bathroom with a warm shower running to humidify the air. The humidity helps thin the secretions, making it easier for the child to expel them. However, humidity does not help in reducing the upper airway inflammation that occurs in croup.

Bacterial Tracheitis

Bacterial tracheitis is an uncommon bacterial infection of the trachea that produces significant tracheal and upper bronchial edema and mucus.[10] Bacterial tracheitis has symptoms similar to croup as the airway narrowing that occurs in both conditions reduces the diameter of the trachea. The main clinical difference between the two conditions is that croup typically will get worse and then improve whereas bacterial tracheitis will progress and the child will appear very ill. Bacterial tracheitis also typically occurs in the fall and winter months, the same time croup occurs. Bacterial tracheitis was found to occur in approximately 2% of patients who were admitted to one hospital for croup.[8] The mortality from bacterial tracheitis is higher than croup and is related to airway obstruction from edema.

Pneumonia

Pneumonia can develop in the child just as in the adult and can be responsible for high or persistently elevated fever. As in the adult, pneumonia can be caused by a virus or by bacteria affecting the lungs. When assessing children, it may be difficult for the Paramedic to appreciate the typical changes in lung sounds that occur in pneumonia. The signs and symptoms in younger children may only include fever and increased respiratory rate. Older children and teens will develop the more typical cough that produces green sputum, difficulty breathing, fever, and tachypnea. Some children, as in adults, will also develop bronchospasm associated with their pneumonia and may benefit from the same treatment as patients with an asthma exacerbation.

Congenital Respiratory Conditions

As with the cardiovascular system, patients may be affected by congenital conditions that affect the respiratory system. Two congenital respiratory conditions which the Paramedic may commonly encounter that affect not only the pediatric patient but also the adult patient are cystic fibrosis and neonatal respiratory distress syndrome.

Cystic Fibrosis

Cystic fibrosis is the most common of the serious genetic pulmonary diseases. However, with the advancements made in care, many children with this major disease will live well into adulthood. Cystic fibrosis is a genetic condition in which the patient has increased viscosity of mucosal secretions among other enzymatic and autonomic nervous system dysfunctions. It is a recessive condition, meaning the child needs to have genes from both his parents in order to develop the disease.[11] Specific respiratory system issues of patients who have cystic fibrosis include chronic respiratory infections due to the inability to clear the secretions as effectively as a person without cystic fibrosis. Children with cystic fibrosis frequently may have a **failure to thrive** in which there is decreased feeding and weight gain along with a gradual deterioration of the respiratory system. The symptoms can present at birth or be delayed for a number of years. Although cystic fibrosis affects several body systems, the majority of the fatalities occur due to the respiratory complications of the disease.

Neonatal Respiratory Distress Syndrome

Neonatal respiratory distress syndrome, also referred to as **hyaline membrane disease** or infant respiratory distress syndrome, is the most common complication of premature newly born infants who have not had the opportunity to fully develop their lungs before birth. The disease is caused by the lack of surfactant production. Surfactant aids the alveoli in remaining partially open during exhalation and in decreasing the effort required to open the alveoli during inspiration. Surfactant production does not start until approximately 24 to 28 weeks of gestation and increases over the next several weeks.[12] By approximately 36 weeks' gestation, the amount of surfactant should be sufficient to prevent neonatal respiratory distress syndrome. If there is concern about a premature delivery, the obstetrician may administer betamethasone, a type of steroid, to the mother who is less than 36 weeks' gestation in order to help speed up the maturity of the lungs in case of a premature delivery.[13] In the situation in which the premature birth is unexpected, synthetic surfactant can be administered in the neonatal intensive care unit if the infant develops respiratory distress syndrome.

Neonatal respiratory distress syndrome will develop within the first eight hours of life, most frequently within the first minutes of life. Depending on how long it takes for the newly born child to develop signs of neonatal respiratory distress syndrome, the neonate will either retain or develop a cyanotic appearance, including that of the mucous membranes. Signs include a rapid and/or shallow respiratory rate accompanied by grunting, nasal flaring, and apnea. Respiratory distress and failure will ensue shortly and the child often requires assisted ventilations and intubation. If caught early, appropriately sized nasal continuous positive airway pressure may support the neonate's respiratory status until he can be treated with surfactant.

Neurological Emergencies

Seizure disorders are the most common neurological emergencies the Paramedic will encounter. There are many conditions that cause seizures, including toxicologic issues, head injury, infections (e.g., meningitis and encephalitis), brain tumors, hypoglycemia, congenital conditions, and epilepsy. Some of these causes are discussed in other sections. In the vast majority of cases, the seizure is brief and will have terminated by the time the Paramedic arrives on-scene.

In children who have frequent seizures, caregivers are often instructed to call EMS only if the seizure lasts greater than 10 minutes, is different from the usual seizure, or the child has more frequent seizures. Some caregivers administer rectal diazepam to the patient if the seizure lasts longer than 10 minutes and only call EMS if the seizure lasts an additional five minutes longer. These are children with chronic and frequent seizures with close linkage to the healthcare system and not those with new onset seizures or a history of infrequent seizures. In children with a seizure history who suddenly develop more frequent seizures, the Paramedic should look for an infectious source as the most likely cause. Especially in those children with disabilities and developmental delays, urinary infections are common triggers for increased seizures. Another common cause for frequent seizures occurs after a period of rapid growth when the medication dose may then be inadequate to control the seizures and may therefore need to be increased by the physician.

Status epilepticus traditionally has been defined as seizure activity which lasts for 30 minutes with or without treatment or two seizure episodes without a return to normal mental status in-between seizures. Some experts in the field recommend that the definition of status epilepticus be changed to a seizure that lasts more than five minutes.[14] The epilepsy foundation echoes that recommendation and suggests parents call EMS for any seizure lasting more than five minutes, noting that approximately 42,000 deaths occur from episodes of status epilepticus.[15]

Patients with status epilepticus typically develop prolonged tonic–clonic seizures with massive oxygen, glucose, and energy requirements of the neurons involved. Metabolic acidosis develops from the drop in glucose and increased muscle contraction as the seizure continues. As hypoxia worsens, cerebral function is affected and the risk of an anoxic brain injury is increased. The risk of aspiration and respiratory distress also increases with the length of seizure. Other injuries may develop from seizure, whether from a fall or from the patient striking objects during the seizure. Some of these injuries include soft tissue injuries, extremity injury, head injury, drowning, or multiple trauma if the seizure occurs while riding a bicycle or other physical activity.

Altered Mental Status

Altered mental status may present in many ways, including agitation, confusion, or complete unresponsiveness. There is a wide Paramedical differential of acute causes of altered

Table 42-1 Common Conditions That Cause Altered Mental Status

T	Trauma
I	Infection
P	Psychogenic
S	Seizure, suicide attempt, subarachnoid hemorrhage
A	Alcohol
E	Electrolyte imbalance, encephalopathy
I	Insulin (blood sugar too high or low)
O	Opiates, oxygen (hypoxemia), overdose (drugs)
U	Uremia (renal failure)

mental status including respiratory insufficiency, respiratory failure, hypoxemia, shock, hypoglycemia, traumatic brain injury (including shaken baby syndrome), seizures, poisoning, drug overdose, sepsis, meningitis, hyperthermia, and hypothermia. The mnemonic TIPS AEIOU (Table 42-1) may help remind the Paramedic of the more common causes of altered mental status.

Altered mental status lies along a continuum and can sometimes be subtle. What is an altered mental status? The 2-year-old who clings to the mother like an octopus with a death grip? The 6-year-old who doesn't flinch when the Paramedic attempts to start the IV? The 15-year-old who, when standing next to a parent, does not acknowledge the parent's existence? All three of these children might have an altered mental status, However, they also might be acting normally for the individual, for their age, or for the situation. Mental status is only altered if it is different from baseline for that specific patient. Special consideration must be afforded for the various developmental phases of childhood and their impact on normal mental status.

Hyper- and Hypoglycemia

Diabetes mellitus, an endocrine disorder which is one of the most common chronic diseases among children in the United States, is related to either an absent or significantly decreased production of insulin (type 1) or a resistance to insulin produced by the body (type 2). Insulin is required to transport glucose from the blood into the cell for use in energy production.

As of 2007, approximately 180,000 people under the age of 20 have the disease and its prevalence is increasing at alarming rates.[16] The typical diabetic child is of American Indian, African, Asian, or Hispanic/Latino descent; is overweight; and has a family history of the disease. The data suggests that as many as 43% of the new cases of pediatric diabetes are type 2. Signs and symptoms of diabetes in children are the same as those in the adult population. Altered mental status can occur due to either hyperglycemia or hypoglycemia.

Toxicologic

Accidental ingestion is another common cause of altered mental status in the younger child, especially older infants and toddlers who are still in the oral stage of development.

At this developmental stage, anything the child can grasp is placed in the mouth. Improperly stored chemicals and medications can be accidently ingested by the curious child. In older preschoolers and school-age children, the child may intentionally take a medication because he thinks it will help him feel better if ill or because the pill is mistaken for candy. Younger children may also mistake alcohol or recreational drugs as other edible items and ingest them with significant consequences. Toxic exposures can also occur from accidental exposure to household chemicals (e.g., cleaning fluids and fertilizers) and carbon monoxide. An older child might be involved in a hobby or play that might cause an inadvertent exposure to these toxins.

Adolescents and teenagers may become involved in ingesting alcohol and other recreational drugs. Overdoses of these substances may be recreational, in which the adolescent or teen has intentionally taken too much of the substance in an effort to get high. Overdoses may also be intentional as a means for the adolescent or teen to cause self-harm. In some cases, it may be difficult for the Paramedic to differentiate between the recreational and non-recreational overdose. It is prudent for the Paramedic to assume the patient was trying to harm himself and transport the patient to the emergency department for a more complete evaluation.

Apparent Life-Threatening Event and Sudden Infant Death Syndrome

An **apparent life-threatening event (ALTE)** typically affects children under 1 year of age and is characterized by any combination of apnea, change in skin color, change in muscle tone, coughing, or gagging.[17] Any of these events may require physical stimuli to rouse the infant; however, in some cases, the event resolves on its own. Nearly half of the children seen in the medical system for these nondescript events are ultimately diagnosed with an underlying condition which explains the event itself. The Academy of Family Practice states that only half the cases of ATLE have a source found, with up to 50% of cases of ATLE diagnosed as digestive problems, approximately 30% neurological, approximately 20% respiratory, and 5% cardiac, with endocrine and metabolic causes making up less than 5%. Unfortunately, the other 50% of these events are idiopathic and no cause is found.[18] ALTE is most prevalent among infants 10 weeks old or less. It is believed that ALTE may occur in up to 6% of infants and is believed to be a major cause of sudden infant death syndrome (SIDS).

The most frequent cause of ALTE presentations is believed to be GI related in up to 50% of the cases. The child chokes, gags, and possibly foams at the mouth and may become temporarily cyanotic during the process. This is thought to be related to the still developing nerve pathways between the newborn brain and intricate network of nerves which control the swallowing process. Approximately 30% of ALTE events are due to neurologic complications such as CNS bleeding, infection, or congenital abnormalities. Respiratory and cardiac causes comprise the remaining 20% of diagnosed causes and occur from infection, congenital abnormalities, and arrhythmias. Several factors—the first event occurring after two months of age, abnormal vital signs on physical examination, and a history of a previous ALTE—are associated with a higher risk of death, making these questions an essential part of the history. Unfortunately, most causes of ALTE are never discovered.

Some patients are sent home on an apnea monitor after hospital evaluation of an ALTE. The apnea monitor may alert the parents to another apneic episode, prompting the request for EMS. On arrival, the infant may appear well, after having been stimulated by the parents and due to the resumption of breathing. Regardless of history, all infants with a questionable ALTE should be transported to the hospital for further evaluation.

Sudden infant death syndrome (SIDS) affects approximately 0.5 out of every 1,000 live births.[19] SIDS typically affects infants under the age of 12 months, but has also been deemed the cause of death in some older children. The common scenario is the parent checking on the sleeping child only to find the child apneic and pulseless. The caretaker sometimes reports the child had a recent viral upper respiratory infection and nasal congestion. Some of the risk factors for SIDS include teenage pregnancy; lack of prenatal care; previous SIDS children; drug, alcohol, or tobacco use during pregnancy; and exposure to secondhand smoke and smoking by-products.[15] Although most of the time it is not clear what caused the infant's death, congenital dysrhythmias (e.g., Long-QT syndrome) and gastric reflux may cause a significant percentage of SIDS deaths.

There is no doubt that the Paramedic's response to this emotionally charged event will make a difference in the caregivers' ability to mourn the child's death. Knowing everything was done that could have been and having the Paramedics' kind and gentle presence there to help make the horrible situation a slight bit more tolerable will stay with the caregivers forever.

Abdominal Pain

Abdominal pain is a common and nonspecific chief concern in the pediatric patient. There are many causes of abdominal pain, from the less concerning (e.g., cramping) to the severe (e.g., appendicitis and intussusception). Food, illness, trauma, irregularity, monthly cycles, dehydration, overhydration, chemical ingestions, allergies, inflammation, and spasm are but a few of the causes of abdominal pain. Although some conditions may occur regardless of the child's age, most conditions have an age group in which the condition is more prevalent (Table 42-2).

Preschool-age children often complain of "belly or tummy pain" regardless of what is actually ailing them. This phenomenon is understandable since much of a parent's history taking during an illness relates to the abdomen. "Does your tummy hurt? Did you eat too much? When was the

Table 42-2 Causes of Abdominal Pain in Children Broken Down by Age Group

Age Group	Conditions
Infants	• Colic • Hernia • Intussusception
Children	• Appendicitis • Constipation • Gastroenteritis • Urinary tract infection
Adolescents and teenagers	**Both Genders** • Appendicitis • Constipation • Gastroenteritis • Renal colic **Female** • Urinary tract infection • Menstrual cycle • Pregnancy • Ectopic pregnancy • Pelvic inflammatory disease • Ovarian cyst • Ovarian torsion **Male** • Testicular torsion • Inguinal hernia

last time you went potty?" are all questions that caregivers routinely ask children. As the child gets older, the nondescript tummy pain is used to explain maladies of unknown description including ones the caregiver can't quite put her finger on. In the adolescent and teenage age groups, the causes of abdominal pain are identical to those of their adult counterparts.

Common causes of abdominal pain in infants include colic, congenital hernias, and intussusception. **Colic** is a very common condition that is caused by spasm of the stomach and intestines, typically in response to gas. Some infants consume special formulas or end up trying many different formulas before finding one that does not cause gas. The infant typically pulls his knees up to the abdomen and cries during the period of pain and then relaxes as the wave of pain concludes. Sometimes the infant has relief after passing gas. A hernia is a protrusion of an organ through an opening in the abdominal wall. In male infants, **congenital inguinal hernias** are the most common type of hernia.[20] These hernias can be severe enough that bowel loops pass into the scrotal sac or twist and strangulate, producing significant pain. In most cases, however, the hernia does not produce significant pain. An **intussusception** occurs when one section of the small bowel or large bowel telescopes into another section of bowel (Figure 42-3). As this happens, the blood supply to the overlapping segment of bowel is reduced or blocked completely. If not recognized

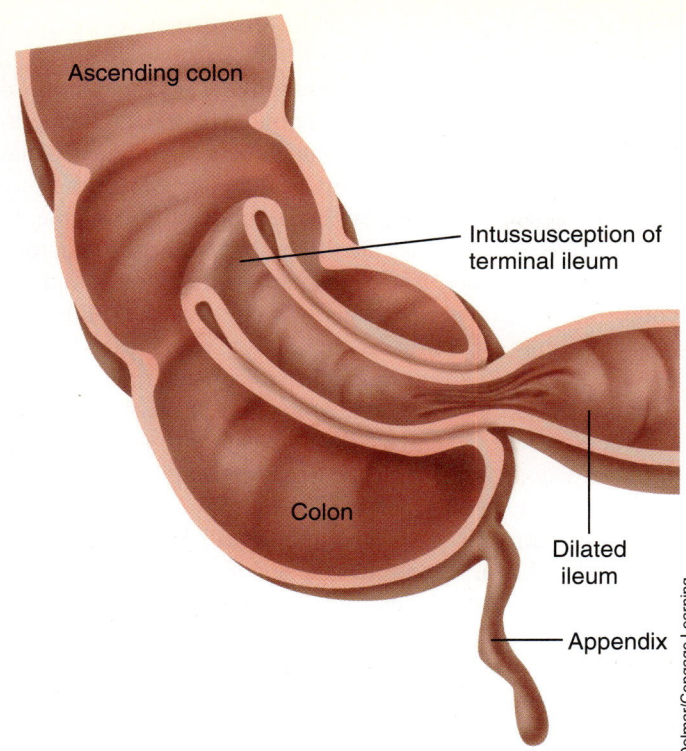

Delmar/Cengage Learning

Figure 42-3 An intussusception most commonly occurs at the terminal ileum, which is the junction between the small bowel and the large bowel.

Labels on figure: Ascending colon, Intussusception of terminal ileum, Colon, Dilated ileum, Appendix

and treated within 24 hours, that segment of bowel can die and cause sepsis.[20] Inflammation of that segment of bowel may cause bleeding and increased mucous production, resulting in stool that is described as currant jelly red. The pain occurs in waves in intervals between 5 and 30 minutes apart. Vomiting is usually associated with intussusception.

In toddlers, preschoolers, and school-age children, the common causes of abdominal pain include constipation, gastroenteritis, urinary tract infection, and appendicitis. Constipation is very common at various stages of a child's development. In early school-age children, there may be a fear of having a bowel movement outside the home. Caregivers typically do not monitor urination and bowel movements as much as when the child was potty training and may not be aware of the volume of stool a child expels daily. Children who are constipated often still have bowel movements that are smaller in volume than usual. When constipation worsens, the caregivers will often report that the child has diarrhea because the only material that can get around the concreted stool in the child's rectum and colon is liquid. In the extreme, the child's bowel can dilate, thus increasing the risk of perforation, sepsis, or chronic issues with bowel motility.

Gastroenteritis is a viral illness that causes abdominal cramping, nausea, vomiting, and diarrhea. Rotavirus is a common pathogen in the fall, winter, and early spring, although many viruses will cause diarrhea and vomiting at various points in the infection. It is not common to have a high fever with gastroenteritis unless the child has become moderately dehydrated. Gastroenteritis commonly sweeps through a family because the virus is excreted in the stool. Most children and many caregivers do not follow appropriate hand washing techniques after wiping; therefore, the virus spreads rapidly among close family members.

A urinary tract infection affects the portion of the lower urinary tract from the urinary bladder through the urethra. When the infection affects the urinary bladder, the irritation and inflammation will often cause suprapubic pain located just above the pubic symphysis, pelvic pain, or lower abdominal pain. Urinary tract infections are more common in females due to their shorter urethra. This is especially true in toddlers who are potty training and preschoolers who wish to be independent but may not clean themselves adequately. Urinary tract infections often cause dysuria, frequent urination, crampy spasm-quality pain in the lower abdomen, and sometimes a fever.

Appendicitis can be more challenging to detect in children, especially younger children, because they don't always have the classic symptoms of fever, right lower quadrant abdominal pain, anorexia (lack of appetite), and nausea. Early in the disease, the pain may be more diffuse and located around the umbilicus rather than in the right lower quadrant. Diarrhea may also be present and the clinical picture may mimic gastroenteritis. The younger child may not be able to describe the classic symptoms associated with appendicitis. As with adults, the appendix can rupture and spread the infection throughout the abdomen. Typically, the pain worsens at the time of rupture and then improves as the stretching of the appendix stops. The pain will again worsen as the infection spreads. The body can respond to the inflamed appendix and create a wall surrounding the appendix so that the rupture is contained, which is referred to as a walled off rupture of the appendix.

Adolescents and teenagers have the same common causes of abdominal pain as younger children. Although not common, renal colic may also occur in the teenage group in a small number of patients who complain of unilateral flank pain. In addition, there are conditions which the Paramedic must consider as the reproductive systems of this age group mature.

In the female, pelvic pain may be related to pregnancy and menstrual cycle changes, ovarian cyst, urinary tract infection or (more serious) an ovarian torsion, pelvic inflammatory disease, or ectopic pregnancy. The pathophysiology of these conditions in the adolescent and teenager is similar to those of the adult and were discussed in detail in prior chapters.

In the adolescent and teenage male, two common causes of testicular and lower abdominal pain are testicular torsion and inguinal hernias. This age group tends to be the most physically active, with many children actively engaged in contact sports. Both conditions are related to congenital changes in the lower abdominal wall. The pathophysiology for these conditions was discussed in detail in earlier chapters.

Children who present with red flag abdominal signs and symptoms (Table 42-3) should be considered to have a

Table 42-3 Red Flag Signs and Symptoms in the Pediatric Patient Complaining of Abdominal Pain

- Sudden or acute onset
- Any signs or symptoms of shock
- Radiating pain
- Increase in pain upon exertion
- Changes in mental status due to the abdominal complaint
- Respiratory distress or changes in ventilation
- Changes in vital signs without cause (running around will increase the heart rate)
- Abdominal distention, especially acute distention
- Dark and tarry or bloody stools

serious underlying condition until proven otherwise after full evaluation in the emergency department.

Infectious Disease

Chief concerns related to infectious disease also are common among pediatric patients. Most of these conditions produce a fever and can range from the benign to the more serious.

Fever and Febrile Seizures

Fever is not only one of the common medical conditions seen in the pediatric population; it is probably the only aspect of hyperthermia that is different in children than in adults. Fever is defined as a child's body temperature that rises above 100.4°F (38°C). Fever is a normal physiological reaction which occurs in response to infection, dehydration, exposure to high environmental temperatures, reaction to medications or vaccinations, and other bodily stresses. Children with a fever may be flushed, warm to the touch, and diaphoretic. The child may complain of chills and sweats. More concerning signs include an increased respiratory and pulse rate, an increased work of breathing, and altered mental status. Dehydration is more common in children compared with adults due to the relative difference in respiratory rates.

Although most of the time a fever is helpful to the body in fighting an invading organism, any fever in children between birth and 30 to 60 days old is most concerning due to the immature immune system, even in the well-appearing child.[21] There is enough of a concern for a serious bacterial infection in this age group that all of these children are admitted to the hospital, given intravenous antibiotics, and observed closely. In infants 60 days old and older up to children 3 years old, the cutoff for concern of a serious cause of the fever is 102.4°F or 39°C. This does not mean that a fever over 102.4°F (39°C) is caused by a serious or life-threatening infection. It simply means the chance of bacteremia, or bacteria from the source of infection gaining access to the bloodstream, is significantly increased. In the emergency department, the practitioner attempts to locate a source for the child's fever. The child may or may not be admitted to the hospital for observation depending on the results of the emergency department evaluation.

Febrile seizures occur in children ages 3 months to 6 years old and are triggered by a rapid rise in body temperature. Although the exact cause is not known, it is believed that some of the factors that are part of the body's fever production pathway make the neurons in the brain more excitable. In some children, this causes the full brain discharge of neurons that causes a seizure. Although scary to the parents and the child, febrile seizures are usually benign and self-limiting. The child may awaken after the seizure without the typical post-ictal state usually seen in other seizure disorders. Febrile seizures can occur in any child, not only those with seizure disorders. A fever in children with a history of seizure disorders may trigger a seizure, even in children well controlled on anti-seizure medication.

Febrile seizures can be classified as either simple or complex (Table 42-4). Simple febrile seizures occur more often than complex seizures and are generally benign. Complex febrile seizures usually indicate a more serious underlying condition, such as meningitis, encephalitis, a brain mass, or cerebral bleed. Children who have a febrile seizure are more prone to have future febrile seizures.[22]

Meningitis and Encephalitis

Meningitis and encephalitis are severe infections that affect the meninges (thin covering surrounding the spinal cord and brain) or the brain itself (encephalitis) and are a serious cause of altered mental status and seizures in children. Meningitis may be of viral or bacterial origin, with viral origins as a more common cause. Several viruses—such as the enterovirus, paramyxoviruses, adenoviruses, herpes, and influenza virus—have been implicated. The typical child who has viral meningitis will appear ill, tired, confused, lethargic, or sedate with some degree of mental status change. Transmission is environmental; it involves droplet (nasal or oral secretion) spread and is communicable with persons in close contact. The bacterial variant of meningitis has a much more moribund prognosis. Bacterial meningitis produces a toxic appearing, lethargic, possibly septic and hypotensive ill child. Bacterial meningitis often worsens rapidly. It progresses from the child showing only vague symptoms to developing altered mental status to death within several hours. Some patients who have bacterial meningitis will develop a classic **petechial rash** (purplish discolorations) caused by one specific bacterium, neisseria meningitidis (Figure 42-4). Infection

Table 42-4 Comparing and Contrasting Simple and Complex Febrile Seizures

Simple	Complex
• Generalized seizure	• Focal seizure
• Less than 15 minute duration	• Prolonged seizure
• Does not recur in under 24 hours	• More than one seizure in 24 hours

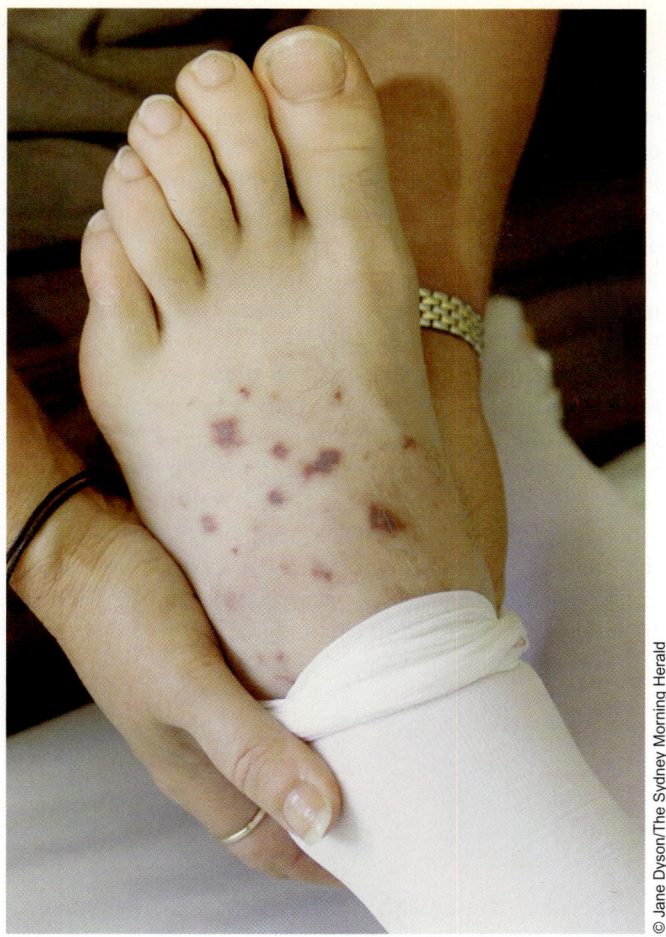

Figure 42-4 Petechial rash, which is typical in a patient who has meningitis from the bacterium neisseria meningitidis.

© Jane Dyson/The Sydney Morning Herald

with other bacteria may not cause this rash. Infection with neisseria meningitidis has a high mortality.[23] As the bacteria are transmitted in respiratory and oral secretions, if neisseria meningitidis is suspected, those Paramedics who performed airway management should receive antibiotic prophylaxis to prevent infection. Others in the household should also be given prophylactic antibiotics to prevent infection. The patient's age may help in determining which pathogen is most likely involved (Table 42-5).

Table 42-5 Typical Pathogens Responsible for Bacterial Meningitis by Age

Age	Most Common Pathogen
Birth to 30 days	Group B streptococci present in the mother's vagina
Infants over 2 months old to school-age children	Streptococcus pneumoniae
Adolescents and teenagers	Neisseria meningitidis

Encephalitis is an inflammation of the brain parenchyma or tissue itself by either a viral or bacterial pathogen. Viral encephalitis occurs when pathogens gain access to the brain via hematogenous spread through the blood or retrograde travel along neurons. The most common pathogens that cause viral encephalitis involve the togavirus, flavivirus, and bunyavirus families, along with West Nile virus, which is spread by mosquito bites. Mosquitoes and migrating birds pass the virus between each other and spread the virus to humans via bites. Any mosquito vector virus is not contagious between humans and can only be spread directly from the mosquito to humans.

Bacterial encephalitis most often occurs from hematogenous spread. Rarely, bacterial encephalitis will be caused by direct spread of bacteria from a sinus or middle ear infection or through direct inoculation in penetrating trauma. Children who have encephalitis will appear ill and develop altered mental status with rapid progression to unresponsiveness. The caregivers may report a history of a headache, photophobia, nausea, or vomiting before the child became unresponsive.

Epiglottitis

Epiglottitis, a bacterial infection involving the epiglottis, is now an uncommon condition in the pediatric population as most children are immunized against haemophilus influenzae bacteria, which has historically been responsible for the majority of cases. Epiglottitis historically has been a disease of major concern because of its affinity to completely close the patient's upper airway and cause death. Since the development of the H. flu type B vaccine in the mid-1980s, the incidence of epiglottitis in children has diminished dramatically. In children who have received all appropriate immunizations, other bacteria cause the few remaining cases of epiglottitis. Although epiglottitis was most commonly seen in children at 3 to 5 years of age, now more adults than children are diagnosed with the disease.[24] The signs and symptoms include a reduced ability or inability to speak due to vocal cord edema, sudden onset of high fever (102°F to 105°F), painful swallowing, drooling, and stridor. The patient who has epiglottitis also sits in a characteristic tripod or leaning forward position to allow oral secretions to drain from the mouth. Epiglottitis can easily advance to respiratory failure as the swollen epiglottis occludes the airway (Figure 42-5).

Pertussis

Pertussis, a bacterial respiratory tract disease caused by the bordetella pertussis bacteria, acquired its common name—whooping cough—from the persistent cough associated with the infection. Although pertussis was nearly eradicated through childhood vaccination, a resurgence of the disease in the late 1990s led to the identification of the need for a booster which is administered to the adolescent. There has also been a resurgence of adults who develop pertussis, although the signs and symptoms in adults are consistent with a persistent bronchitis without the whoop.

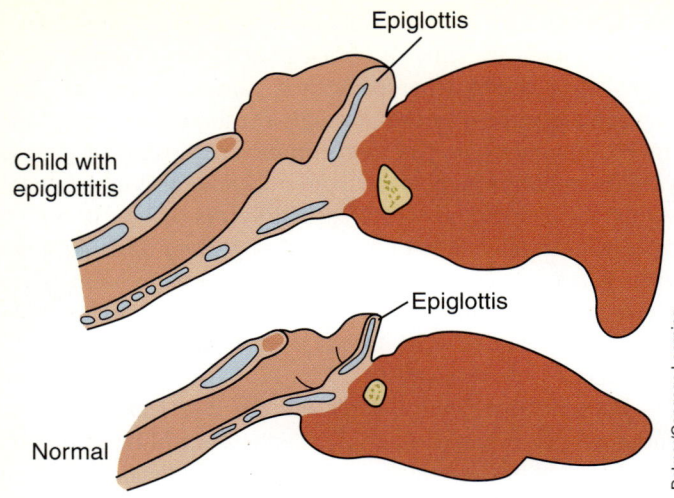

Figure 42-5 Comparison of a normal pediatric airway (lower) to that of a child who died of epiglottitis (upper).

Pertussis infects the lining of the upper airways, producing a thick mucus that can plug the smaller airways. The whoop component of the cough, which is actually stridor heard during the inspiratory phase of the cough, occurs secondary to laryngeal and tracheal buildup of the mucous excretions. In the infant, plugging of the smaller airways can cause significant problems with oxygenation and ventilation. Pertussis typically occurs in children between the ages of 3 months and 5 years of age, although most of the deaths occur in children who are less than 6 months old.

Coughing in younger children often occurs in response to feeding or physical exertion. During the initial stage of the infection, the child has clear nasal discharge, a mild cough, and decreased appetite. The coughing episodes become more severe and prolonged with time, and finally the classic whooping sound develops. Vomiting may occur with or after the coughing episode. In rare cases, a child can develop a cerebral hemorrhage which occurs as a result of the increased intracranial pressure from coughing.

CASE STUDY (CONTINUED)

The Paramedic introduces himself and his partner. "This is Marcus," the child's mother replies. "He has not been feeling well the last couple of days."

"Marcus has had a runny nose for about a week and started coughing two days ago. He keeps getting worse. He has only been coughing at night and he doesn't have a fever," the child's mother states while trying to calm her child.

The Paramedic continues taking the history and learns that Marcus is her only child, there have been no other sick contacts, past medical and surgical history are unremarkable, and no one smokes in the household.

CRITICAL THINKING QUESTIONS

1. What are the important elements of the history that a Paramedic should obtain?
2. What is the symptom pattern for upper airway infections?

History

In obtaining a history, the Paramedic should ensure the child is involved in the process and addressed at the appropriate developmental level. In gathering histories on neonates, infants, and toddlers, the Paramedic should ask the caregiver about pregnancy and birth history, as this information is quite important. Immunization history is also important as some caregivers choose not to immunize their children. Specific historical questions related to the conditions previously discussed should be covered by the Paramedic as appropriate. If the Paramedic allows the caregiver and child to tell their stories, the most likely paramedical diagnosis will often be readily apparent. Smoking is a key social history point to obtain as the risk of asthma and other respiratory conditions increases significantly in households where someone smokes.

At the doorway, both Paramedics independently assess Marcus using the Pediatric Assessment Triangle and determine the child is not critical. On further examination, they find he is breathing at 36 respirations a minute, has a pulse rate of 120 beats per minute, has a blood pressure of 82/42, and has warm and dry skin. Auscultation reveals clear lung sounds with a slight upper airway stridor. A large amount of clear nasal discharge is found. The remainder of the examination is unremarkable.

CRITICAL THINKING QUESTIONS

1. What are the elements of the physical examination of pediatric patients with suspected upper respiratory infection?
2. Why is auscultation of the chest a critical element in this examination?

Examination

Enlisting the assistance of the caregiver will not only help the Paramedic ease any anxiety the child has, but can also calm the caregivers. Often the chief concern and history will direct the Paramedic toward the key portions of the physical examination where she should focus.

The Paramedic runs through the list of common paramedical differential diagnoses in his mind. Given Marcus's classic barky cough and the timing at which his cough worsened, it appears Marcus has croup.

CRITICAL THINKING QUESTIONS

1. What is the list of potential diagnoses?
2. What diagnosis did the Paramedic announce to the patient's mother?

Assessment

The Paramedic's process of differentiating between the several paramedical diagnoses is the same in the pediatric patient as in the adult patient. Narrowing down the differential requires the Paramedic looking at the entire picture, identifying which system is affected, and then narrowing it down to the common pediatric conditions.

The EMT starts humidified oxygen, asking Marcus's mother to hold the mask a few inches from the child's face so Marcus can breathe the cool mist. After bundling the child up to keep him warm in the cool winter night, she assists his mother in carrying Marcus to the ambulance.

CRITICAL THINKING QUESTIONS

1. What is the standard of care of patients with suspected upper respiratory assessment?
2. What are some of the patient-specific concerns and considerations that the Paramedic should consider when applying this plan of care?

Treatment

General treatment of the pediatric patient, regardless of age and condition, starts with ensuring the airway is patent, the child is oxygenating and ventilating adequately, the circulatory system is supported, and the child is kept warm. Regardless of the specific pathophysiology involved, these four basic tenets of pediatric care should be assessed and addressed on every encounter with a pediatric patient. The following sections will cover specific treatment issues for the various conditions.

Cardiovascular Conditions

Caring for a child who has a TET spell can be anxiety provoking due to the severe cyanosis that accompanies the spell. For a known TET spell, the child's knees should be brought up to his chest, or the older child can be asked to squat. These maneuvers increase the pressure in the left side of the heart and may help stop the diversion of circulation away from the lungs.[25] Pharmacologic treatment may include administering morphine (which is thought to decrease pressure in the pulmonary system) and epinephrine (which increases system pressure), thus encouraging blood to resume a normal flow through the pulmonary system. The child with a right-to-left shunt may not improve on high-flow, high-concentration oxygen because the problem is not with oxygen transport, but with a lack of blood flow through the lungs.

Pediatric patients with suspected or known congenital cardiovascular disease who are hypotensive may or may not respond to fluid. Administration of the standard 20 mL/kg intravenous or intraosseous fluid bolus may worsen CHF, especially if the patient has a left-to-right shunt or left-sided outflow obstruction. In these patients, it would be appropriate to administer smaller volume boluses (10 mL/kg) over a longer period of time with constant reassessment. Consultation with an on-line physician may assist the Paramedic in sorting out these complex patients.

Respiratory Conditions

Airway and respiratory support are of the utmost importance in respiratory conditions. Asthma and status asthmaticus in the pediatric patient are treated in a fashion similar to the adult patient: with nebulized albuterol and atrovent, oral or intravenous steroids, epinephrine or terbutaline (in children over 6 years old), and magnesium in the extreme cases. If the child in status asthmaticus requires rapid sequence intubation, the use of ketamine to induce sedation may have the added benefit of bronchodilation.

The Paramedic's treatment of the pediatric patient with bronchiolitis includes supporting the airway, breathing, and circulation as previously noted. The Paramedic should administer humidified oxygen if the child has signs of respiratory distress or hypoxemia. In general, bronchiolitis does not produce bronchospasm that responds to nebulized albuterol treatments. Therefore, nebulized albuterol is only indicated if wheezing is auscultated on examination.

As previously discussed, many pediatric patients who have croup will appear improved on arrival or after bringing the patient out to the ambulance. Humidified oxygen will help improve the child's breathing. The definitive treatment is administering either intramuscular or oral dexamethasone or nebulized budesonide.[26] These steroids help reduce the swelling present in the larynx and upper trachea, alleviating the patient's stridor. In severe cases, nebulized epinephrine or racemic epinephrine may be administered to help vasoconstrict the arterioles in the upper airway and reduce the airway edema by that mechanism. Bacterial tracheitis may be difficult to discern from croup in the prehospital environment. With viral croup significantly more common, it would be reasonable for the Paramedic to treat bacterial tracheitis in a fashion similar to croup. Children with bacterial tracheitis will ultimately require antibiotics in the hospital.

Children who present with pneumonia are often mildly dehydrated both from the fever and from the extra fluid loss due to increased respiratory rate. Ultimately in the emergency department the child will require antibiotics if a bacterial cause is found. Some children may have a component of bronchospasm from the pneumonia and will respond well to nebulized albuterol. Similarly, patients with a history of cystic fibrosis are prone to pneumonia and bronchospasm and may benefit from rehydration and nebulized albuterol.

Neonatal respiratory distress syndrome may not manifest itself immediately after delivery.

Neurological Emergencies

The Paramedic's treatment for the child in status epilepticus, or seizing on the Paramedic's arrival, includes managing the airway, breathing, and circulation. Diazepam is the first-line medication in the treatment of seizures and can be administered intravenously, intramuscularly, rectally, or intranasally.[27,28] Lorazepam and midazolam are also acceptable for first-line use to treat an active seizure.

In many cases, the seizure will have resolved before the Paramedic's arrival on-scene. In these situations, the patient may be post-ictal or the mental status may be improving. If this happens, it is acceptable for the Paramedic not to administer a benzodiazepine and instead simply observe the patient. However, the Paramedic should administer the benzodiazepine if the patient has a second seizure while in her care. The patient should be placed in a position of comfort and the Paramedic should monitor the airway, breathing, and circulation.

Altered Mental Status

The Paramedic care for pediatric patients with altered mental status is focused on supportive care. The Paramedic should exclude immediately treatable causes (e.g., hypoglycemia and opiate overdose). If the blood glucose level is decreased, the Paramedic should administer the appropriate weight-based dose of D_{25} or D_{10} intravenously or glucagon intramuscularly and reassess the patient. If signs of an opiate toxidrome are present, the Paramedic should administer naloxone. The use of a coma cocktail (i.e., thiamine, intravenous glucose, and naloxone) without evidence to support the presence of hypoglycemia or opiate overdose is not appropriate and is potentially harmful.[29]

Hyperglycemia can be another cause of altered mental status, especially if the patient has developed diabetic ketoacidosis. As with adults, the Paramedic should support the patient's airway, breathing, and circulation. Children in diabetic ketoacidosis will have relatively large body fluid deficits and may require several 20 mL/kg boluses of normal saline, especially if perfusion is poor. The Paramedic should reassess the respiratory status after each bolus to ensure the child does not develop fluid overload from overaggressive rehydration. Although the intravenous fluids will help lower the blood glucose through dilution, the child will ultimately require insulin in order to transport the glucose from the blood into the cells where it can be used for energy, halting the production of acids.

Apparent Life-Threatening Event and Sudden Infant Death Syndrome

Many infants who have suffered an ALTE may have completely recovered and appear well to the Paramedic. If this is the first time the child has had an ALTE, the history may help identify that the child had an ALTE. The Paramedic can inform the caregivers of his suspicion and concern and strongly recommend transport to the emergency department for a full evaluation into the cause of the event.

In a small number of cases, the infant will remain in distress or be in cardiopulmonary arrest when the Paramedic arrives on-scene. The focus at this point will be ensuring the infant has an adequate airway, is adequately oxygenating and ventilating, and has adequate circulation.

Abdominal Pain

The treatment of the child who has a chief concern of abdominal pain is primarily supportive care, ensuring the child is well-oxygenated and well-perfused. The Paramedic should consider analgesia; however, the use of analgesia in patients who complain of abdominal pain is controversial with some physicians concerned that administering morphine will decrease their ability to accurately diagnose surgical abdominal conditions. Most literature suggests that administering analgesia does not affect the ability of physicians to diagnose life-threatening causes of abdominal pain, does not cause complications, and improves patient comfort.[30] The Paramedic may need to consult with the destination emergency department.

Infectious Disease

Excellent infection control precautions are important with every single patient encounter and even more important in obtunded children who are febrile. Meningitis is a highly contagious disease. Respiratory protection during airway management is critical to protecting the crew from transmission. Ensuring a patent airway, adequate oxygenation and ventilation, and adequate circulation are the Paramedic's treatment goals. Children with meningitis can become septic very quickly and show signs of poor perfusion, which should be treated with intravenous or intraosseous fluid boluses.

Paramedic care for children with a suspected febrile seizure includes supportive measures, rehydration, and antipyretics (e.g., acetaminophen if the child is post-ictal). Benzodiazepines should not be administered unless the child is seizing on arrival or seizes again during EMS contact. Pediatric patients who have had a suspected febrile seizure should be transported to the emergency department for further evaluation.

Epiglottitis can cause a true airway emergency. Supportive care includes humidified blow-by oxygen and calm transport in a position of comfort for the child. Stimulation of the airway may result in total occlusion. Therefore, airway management should be avoided unless the child cannot be adequately ventilated by bag–valve mask. If airway management is attempted, the Paramedic will likely have to use an endotracheal tube size smaller than typical for the child's age. If unable to adequately ventilate or intubate the child, the Paramedic will need to perform a needle cricothyrotomy to obtain an airway in this critically ill child.[31]

Paramedic care of the child with pertussis is intended to ensure adequate respiratory status. The Paramedic should transport the patient in the position of comfort with humidified oxygen.

CASE STUDY (CONTINUED)

After securing Marcus into the car seat attached to the stretcher, the Paramedic continues administering the humidified oxygen. Marcus's cough appears to have improved in the last few minutes, supporting the Paramedic's suspicion of viral croup. He keeps the heat off in the back of the ambulance to prevent warming and drying out the air too much during transport.

CRITICAL THINKING QUESTIONS

1. What are some of the predictable complications associated with croup versus epiglottitis?
2. What are some of the predictable complications associated with the treatments for reactive upper airway disease?

Evaluation

As discussed in the previous pediatric chapters, continuous reassessment during prehospital contact is essential, allowing the Paramedic to detect the subtle changes that can occur if the child's condition worsens. Pediatric patients have the ability to compensate for a longer period of time than adults but will decompensate faster once their reserves are exhausted. Through constant monitoring and reevaluation, the Paramedic will detect these changes and intervene early.

CASE STUDY CONCLUSION

Marcus's mother requests that he be taken to Crawford Memorial Hospital two blocks away because of transportation issues. The Paramedic reassesses Marcus and determines he is stable enough to be evaluated at the community hospital.

The remainder of the EMS contact time is uneventful. After finishing the run report, the Paramedic talks with Dr. Imbruglia, the emergency physician on that night. Dr. Imbruglia confirms that the Paramedic was correct in his evaluation and administers oral steroids to Marcus. After being observed for about two hours, Marcus is discharged from the emergency department and has an appointment with his pediatrician the following afternoon.

CRITICAL THINKING QUESTIONS

1. What is the most appropriate transport decision that will get the patient to definitive care?
2. What are the advantages of transporting a patient with suspected croup to the hospital?

Disposition

Disposition of the pediatric patient often depends on the child's chief concern, history of chronic illnesses, physiologic condition, and resources available in the community. Pediatric patients with airway issues that cannot be addressed by the Paramedic should be taken to the nearest qualified emergency department. Critically ill children are best cared for in a facility with a pediatric intensive care unit. A neonate in distress after a field delivery is best cared for in a hospital with a neonatal intensive care unit. If these resources are available in the community within a reasonable travel distance, the pediatric patient will receive definitive care significantly faster than if the patient is brought to a community emergency department, who will then transfer the patient later. In some communities, those tertiary care services are not available within a reasonable travel distance, and the Paramedic will have to transport the pediatric patient to the closest appropriate emergency department. The Paramedic must know what services are available within the community in order to make appropriate destination decisions.

In some situations, the patient may appear reasonably well upon the Paramedic's initial assessment and during a more detailed assessment. In these situations, the caregivers may want to decline treatment or transport to a facility. Several of the medical conditions discussed previously may initially present in a child who does not appear to be in distress. In most situations, it is better to recommend transport to an appropriate emergency department than to allow the caregivers to decline transport. If the caregivers would like to decline transport, the Paramedic should inform them of her concerns and stress the importance of the more thorough work-up at the emergency department. In some cases, discussing the concerns and allowing the caregivers to talk to the child's pediatrician or with an on-line medical control consultant in the emergency department may convince the caregivers to allow transport of the child to the emergency department.

CONCLUSION

The breadth of pediatric medical emergencies can be both challenging and rewarding for the Paramedic. Through continued education, the Paramedic will become comfortable identifying and managing these conditions.

KEY POINTS:

- Cardiovascular disease is uncommon in the pediatric population. Cardiac events stem from respiratory issues, dysrhythmias, or congenital issues.

- Congenital cardiac problems stem from right-to-left shunt, left-to-right shunt, or obstruction to either the right or left ventricle.

- Asthma may be intermittent or chronic.

- Bronchiolitis causes bronchospasm and increased mucus, limiting ventilation and increasing the patient's work of breathing.

- Croup causes edema in the larynx, trachea, and large bronchi.

- Bacterial tracheitis leads to edema in the trachea along with an increase in mucus.

- Pneumonia can stem from
  - Bacteria
  - Viruses

- Young children with pneumonia may present with fever and an increased respiratory rate. In older children, the pattern of sputum production, difficulty breathing, fever, and tachypnea is likely.

- Cystic fibrosis, a genetic condition, causes multiple organ changes; however, mortality is usually related to respiratory failure.

- Neonatal or infant respiratory distress syndrome results from inadequate surfactant production, causing increased work of breathing and respiratory failure.

- In a child with a seizure history, any change in pattern or frequency should be investigated as a possible infectious process.

- Status epilepticus causes an increased use of oxygen and glucose.

- Altered mental status is based on the usual or baseline status for the specific patient.

- Accidental ingestion is a common cause of altered mental status in the younger child.

- Many pediatric patients are discharged on apnea monitors after an apparent life-threatening event.

- Paramedic actions during a possible sudden infant death call help set the stage for family and caregiver mourning.

- Abdominal pain is a common complaint for children.
  - Abdominal pain in infants is often related to colic, hernia, or intussusception.
  - In toddlers, preschoolers, and school-age children, abdominal pain is usually related to constipation, gastroenteritis, urinary tract infections, or appendicitis.
  - In adolescents and teens, the Paramedic should consider all adult reasons for abdominal pain.

- Appendicitis presents differently from the adult presentation. The pain is more diffuse and closer to the umbilicus. Diarrhea may occur in the patient.

- In the febrile state, dehydration is more common in children due to the difference in respiratory rates.

- Fever in an infant up to 60 days old is of concern due to the immaturity of the immune system.

- Febrile seizures occur in children between 3 months and 6 years and are related to the rapid rise in temperature.

- Children are at risk for meningitis with viral meningitis occurring more often.

- Epiglottitis, an infection involving swelling of the epiglottis, is uncommon due to the haemophilus influenza B (HiB) immunization.

- Pertussis or whooping cough causes a profuse thick mucus that obstructs the smaller airways.

- The presence of cigarette smoking in the home is an important risk factor for respiratory conditions in the pediatric population.

- General pediatric treatments focus on airway, breathing, and circulation.

- The Paramedic should treat TET spells by drawing the child's knees up or having the child squat.

- For altered mental status, the Paramedic should seek reversible causes and provide supportive care.

- Children with a suspected febrile seizure should be transported to the emergency department for evaluation.

- Epiglottitis is an airway emergency.

REVIEW QUESTIONS:

1. How does right-to-left shunting affect the child's presentation?
2. What is the most common condition of right-to-left shunting in a child?
3. How do right-sided outflow tract obstructions differ in presentation from left-sided outflow tract obstructions?
4. What are the signs and symptoms of bronchiolitis? With what other condition is it often confused?
5. What locations of the airway are affected by croup? What is the usual symptom pattern of croup? What is the best treatment?
6. Name two causes of an increase in the frequency of seizures in a child with a diagnosed seizure history.
7. Why is dehydration more common in children with fevers than in adults during the febrile state?
8. What triggers a febrile seizure?

CASE STUDY QUESTIONS:

Please refer to the Case Study in this chapter, and answer the questions below:

1. What are the treatment options for a "barking cough"? How does each option affect the pathophysiology associated with the condition?

2. Describe the components of history that should be gathered when the complaint is difficulty breathing in an infant or toddler.

REFERENCES:

1. Bank A. Regulation of human fetal hemoglobin: new players, new complexities. *Blood*. 2006;107(2):435–443.

2. Baren JM, Brennan J, et al. *Pediatric Emergency Medicine*. St. Louis: Saunders; 2007.

3. Kirklin JW. *The Tetralogy of Fallot from a Surgical Viewpoint*. St. Louis: Saunders; 1970.

4. Gatzoulis M, Murphy D. (eds). *The Adult with Tetralogy of Fallot: The ISACCD Monograph Series*. Malden, MA: Wiley-Blackwell; 2001.

5. Sharma GD. Asthma. E-medicine. Available at: **http://emedicine.medscape.com/article/1000997-overview**. Accessed May 16, 2009.

6. Main C, Shepherd J, et al. Systematic review and economic analysis of the comparative effectiveness of different inhaled corticosteroids and their usage with long-acting beta2 agonists for the treatment of chronic asthma in children under the age of 12 years. *Health Technol Assess*. 2008;12(20):1–174, iii–iv.

7. Carlsen KH, Carlsen KC. Respiratory effects of tobacco smoking on infants and young children. *Paediatric Respiratory Reviews*. 2008;9(1):11–19.

8. Tager IB. The effects of second-hand and direct exposure to tobacco smoke on asthma and lung function in adolescence. *Paedistric Respiratory Reviews*. 2008;9(1):29–37.

9. Bont L. Current concepts of the pathogenesis of RSV bronchiolitis. *Adv Exp Med Biol*. 2009;634:31–40.

10. Rajan S. Bacterial tracheitis. E-medicine. Available at: **http://emedicine.medscape.com/article/961647-overview**. Accessed May 16, 2009.

11. Rosaler M. *Cystic Fibrosis (Genetic Diseases)*. New York: Rosen Publishing Group; 2006.

12. Escande B, Kuhn P, et al. [Secondary surfactant deficiencies.]. *Arch Pediatr*. 2004;11(11):1351–1359.

13. Grier DG, Halliday HL. Effects of glucocorticoids on fetal and neonatal lung development. *Treat Respir Med*. 2004;3(5):295–306.

14. Lowenstein DH, Bleck T, et al. It's time to revise the definition of status epilepticus. *Epilepsia*. 1999;40(1):120–122.

15. Epilepsy Foundation. Seizures and syndromes: prolonged or serial seizures (status epilepticus). Available at: **http://www.epilepsyfoundation.org/about/types/types/statusepilepticus.cfm**. Accessed May 16, 2009.

16. American Diabetes Association. Total prevalence of diabetes and pre-diabetes. Available at: **http://www.diabetes.org/diabetes-statistics/prevalence.jsp**. Accessed May 16, 2009.

17. Hay WW, Hayward AR, et al. *Current Pediatric Diagnosis & Treatment*. New York: McGraw-Hill/Appleton & Lange; 2002.

18. Hall KL, Zalman B. Evaluation and management of apparent life-threatening events in children. *Am Fam Physician*. 2005;71(12):2301–2308.

19. Burnett LB, Adler J. Sudden infant death syndrome. E-medicine. Available at: **http://emedicine.medscape.com/article/804412-overview**. Accessed May 16, 2009.

20. Lawrence PF. *Essentials of General Surgery*. Philadelphia: Lippincott; 2000.

21. Baraff LJ. Management of fever without source in infants and children. *Ann Emerg Med*. 2000;36(6):602–614.

22. Gordon KE, Dooley JM, et al. Is temperature regulation different in children susceptible to febrile seizures? *Can J Neurol Sci*. 2009;36(2):192–195.

23. Prasad K, Karlupia N, et al. Treatment of bacterial meningitis: An overview of Cochrane systematic reviews. *Respir Med*. 2009 103(7):945–950.

24. Carey MJ. Epiglottitis in adults. *Am J Emerg Med*. 1996;14(4):421–424.

25. Evans-Berro EA. How to defeat a "tet spell." *Am J Nurs*. 1991;91(7):46–48.

26. Geelhoed GC. Budesonide offers no advantage when added to oral dexamethasone in the treatment of croup. *Pediatr Emerg Care*. 2005;21(6):359–362.

27. Sofou K, Kristjansdottir R, et al. Management of prolonged seizures and status epilepticus in childhood: a systematic review. *J Child Neurol*. 2009.

28. Sreenath TG, Gupta P, et al. Lorazepam versus diazepam-phenytoin combination in the treatment of convulsive status epilepticus in children: a randomized controlled trial. *Eur J Paediatr Neurol*. 2009. [ePub ahead of print]

29. Bledsoe BE. No more coma cocktails. Using science to dispel myths & improve patient care. *JEMS*. 2002;27(11):54–60.

30. Green R, Bulloch B, et al. Early analgesia for children with acute abdominal pain. *Pediatrics*. 2005;116(4):978–983.

31. Mace SE, Khan N. Needle cricothyrotomy. *Emerg Med Clin North Am*. 2008;26(4):1085–1101, xi.

CHAPTER 43

CHILD ABUSE AND NEGLECT

KEY CONCEPTS:

Upon completion of this chapter, it is expected that the reader will understand these following concepts:

- Awareness that child neglect or abuse can occur in any family, but is more likely to occur with families that have increased stressors and decreased resources for support
- The need for Paramedics to maintain a degree of suspicion regarding child neglect or abuse
- The items to include in documentation: assessments made regarding the child, the environment, and what was said regarding the situation, but not judgments
- The methods used to report the suspicion of child abuse in a Paramedic's area

ANATOMY CONCEPTS:

Prior to reading this chapter the Paramedic student should be familiar with the following anatomy and physiology concepts:

- Child developmental stages

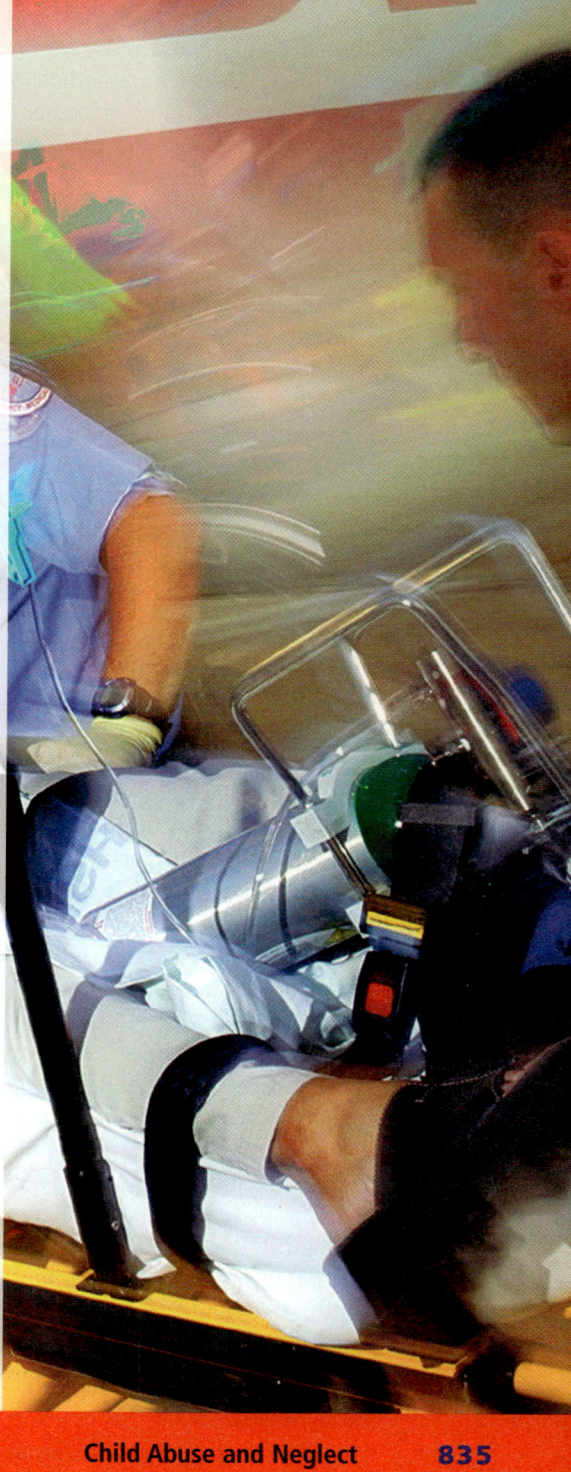

The call comes in for a 5-month-old infant who is "not acting right." The call location is a second story walk up in the center of the city. Both Paramedics express concern that the center of the city is economically depressed and many of the residents in the city's central area do not have health insurance.

CRITICAL THINKING QUESTIONS

1. What are some of the possible causes for a 5-month-old infant to "not act right"?
2. How is the fact that the area is economically depressed related to the infant's behavior?

OVERVIEW

Parents rarely report child abuse. Therefore, it is the Paramedic's responsibility to maintain a high index of suspicion that child abuse may have occurred.[1–4] Paramedics are in a unique position that affords them an unusual opportunity to detect and report child abuse. Paramedics can enter the patient's house and assess the home environment—including interactions of family members within that home—without the guise of law enforcement.

Chief Concern

To be effective, the Paramedic must first acknowledge that child abuse can occur. Most Paramedics, and most people, cannot imagine a parent harming his or her child. It is important for the Paramedic to suspend that disbelief in order to have any measure of suspicion.

It is also important for the Paramedic to maintain a nonjudgmental attitude. Although the Paramedic, based on the facts of the abuse, may not believe that the parent loves the child, studies indicate that parents who abuse their children generally do love them. In many cases, these parents are simply doing what their parents did and they have not been taught how to parent effectively. The cycle of the abused becoming the abuser is called the **cycle of abuse**. By maintaining a nonjudgmental attitude and using effective intervention, the Paramedic can help break the cycle. In the end, most children who are abused are returned to their parents to be loved and raised.

Child Abuse

Every child in the United States has a right to nourishing food, proper clothing, and a safe shelter to rest in at night as well as an education which helps in preparation for the future. Perhaps more importantly, a child should grow up in an environment without fear, especially fear of harm at the hands of loved ones and caregivers. A child should grow up without shame or fear of humiliation. Parents, adult family members, and caregivers directly involved in the care and upbringing of the child have the responsibility to ensure that all of these conditions are met. Whenever these rights are abridged, either through an act of omission or commission, then the possibility of child abuse or neglect has to be considered.

Broadly, the term "child abuse" encompasses acts of violence as well as willful acts of neglect. Using the term more narrowly, **abuse** involves non-accidental injury to a dependent person. This injury may lead to serious disfigurement or permanent disability. Abuse also occurs when the responsible person creates a substantial risk of death. Child abuse can also include the infliction—or allowance of the infliction—of excessive corporal punishment on a child.

Federal law defines child abuse as any act, or failure to act, on the part of responsible adults which results in death, serious physical or emotional harm, sexual abuse or exploitation, or an act or failure to act which presents an imminent risk of serious harm.[5]

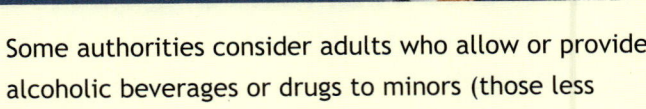

STREET SMART

Some authorities consider adults who allow or provide alcoholic beverages or drugs to minors (those less than 18 years of age) to be guilty of child abuse.

Sexual Abuse

Children should not have sexual relations until they are at the age of consent. Although the risks of sexually transmitted diseases and unintended pregnancy can be potentially life-threatening, the psychological ramifications for the child can have life-long implications.

It has been estimated that one out of every four girls and one out of every ten boys will be sexually assaulted in their childhood, and a number of these incidents will be the result of **sexual abuse** (sexual relations with a parent or caregiver before the age of consent).

Sexual abuse is a subset of child abuse that includes the traditional definitions of rape and sodomy. More specifically, sexual abuse includes the vaginal or rectal penetration of the child with any body part or object including the mouth, fingers, or penis.[6]

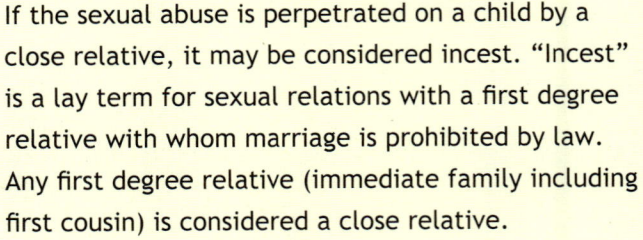

STREET SMART

If the sexual abuse is perpetrated on a child by a close relative, it may be considered incest. "Incest" is a lay term for sexual relations with a first degree relative with whom marriage is prohibited by law. Any first degree relative (immediate family including first cousin) is considered a close relative.

Sexual molestation is a lesser degree of sexual abuse that includes acts without penetration that are performed for

Table 43-1 Sexual Abuse

- Penetration
  - Oral—penile
  - Anal—either penile or digital
  - Genital—either penile or digital
- External manipulation (fondling)
  - Breast
  - Anus
  - Genitals
  - Buttock
- Indecent exposure
- Exploitation
  - Prostitution
  - Pornography
    - All media

the sexual gratification of the perpetrator, who may be the child's caregiver. Key to the description of sexual molestation is unwanted or improper sexual contact. Examples of sexual molestation include permitting a child to watch adults having intercourse, masturbating in front of a child, or having a child touch an adult's genitals (Table 43-1).

Some experts include sexual exploitation under sexual molestation. **Sexual exploitation** occurs when an adult uses a child in a sexual performance or in the production of pornography. Sexual exploitation also occurs when an adult uses a child for purposes of, or to obtain, sexual arousal. If the adult involved in the act is a parent or caregiver, then the act is sexual abuse. If the adult involved in the act is not a parent or caregiver, or does not have custodial responsibilities, then that adult is a **pedophile**. Pedophilia is considered a psychological pathology.

It has been suggested that the shame and guilt associated with these sexual acts experienced by the victim has led to underreporting.[7,8] Referred to as the "conspiracy of silence," adults convince impressionable children that reporting such acts to others would harm the family. By looking for subtle

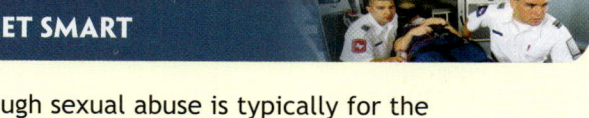

STREET SMART

Although sexual abuse is typically for the perpetrator's self-pleasure, sexual exploitation can have other motivations including commercial interests. An adult arrested for promoting child prostitution or sexual performance could be charged with sexual exploitation even though no sexual contact occurred between the child and the adult.

signs or behavioral indicators, alert Paramedics may be able to detect and reveal sexual abuse.

Psychological Maltreatment

Actions do not have to be physical to be considered child abuse. Psychological or emotional maltreatment is also considered child abuse and can lead to criminal charges. Psychological maltreatment includes any act(s)—however well-intentioned—leading to a state of substantially diminished psychological or intellectual functioning.

At one level, a parent who prevents a child under the legally mandated age from attending school could be perceived as being psychologically abusive and therefore constitute child abuse (i.e., impaired intellectual functioning). However, the more typical cases involve reports of bizarre punishments, such as forced imprisonment, or verbally abusive parents.

Psychological child abuse, the third most reported form of child abuse, is often difficult to detect, as there may be no physical signs. These facts lead authorities to suspect that there is more psychological abuse occurring than is being reported.[9]

Neglect

Typically child abuse is thought of as an act of violence against a child. However, the most common form of child abuse is not the result of an action but the result of inaction. Child **neglect** occurs when an adult with custodial responsibilities fails to provide legally mandated care for the child (Table 43-2). Parent(s) and custodial caregivers are obligated to provide a child with food, clothing, shelter, and medical, surgical, and dental care as well as compulsory education. Caregivers who fail to meet these responsibilities risk charges of child neglect. To be actionable (permit the intervention of the courts in the child's care), the neglect must result in physical and/or psychological impairment of the child.

Although physical neglect, such as the lack of clean clothes or provision of medical care, may seem more obvious, many cases of neglect stem from the lack of supervision of minor children. Supervisory neglect can lead to juvenile delinquency. For example, a Paramedic responding to care for an underage driver at the scene of a motor vehicle collision might suspect supervisory neglect.

Parents make decisions as to whether a child is responsible enough to be left alone every day. That decision should be made after careful consideration of the quality of the child's previously demonstrated independent judgments and the child's physical, cognitive, and emotional capabilities. In addition,

Table 43-2 Physical Neglect

- Inadequate supervision
- Expulsion
- Abandonment
- Delay of health care
- Refusal of health care

that decision should be tempered with contemplation of potential dangers the child could face. Parental decisions which put a child at risk for physical, emotional, or psychological harm make up supervisory neglect, another form of child abuse.

Historical Perspective

In the past, corporal punishment was a parental expectation, as illustrated by the saying, "Spare the rod, spoil the child," which was first found in a poem by Samuel Butler. In fact, acts of infanticide (for religious purposes) and abandonment (for illegitimacy) were not unheard of in the 1800s. However, at the end of the century it was recognized that severe corporal punishment might be doing more harm than good.

In 1874, the case of Mary Ellen Wilson of New York City brought the issue of child abuse to the public's attention.[10,11] Mary Ellen Wilson was a child who was being brutally beaten by her stepmother, Mary Connolly. Henry Bergh, founder of the American Society for the Prevention of Cruelty to Animals (ASPCA), had Mary Connolly successfully prosecuted for child abuse and subsequently formed the Society for the Prevention of Cruelty to Children. This early effort has helped lead to a national child abuse reporting system.

Epidemiology

Child abuse, in its various forms, is thought to occur relatively frequently (16.1 cases per 10,000 people) according to the National Child Abuse and Neglect Data System.[12] The clear majority of cases are reports of neglect (60%), while the rest of the cases are physical abuse (18%), sexual abuse (10%), or emotional abuse.[13]

Although the popular press may make it seem like child abusers are male paramours (unmarried partners of women), the reality is that 79% of accused abusers are parents of the child and the majority of abusers are women (as high as 58%). Combining the number of unmarried partners accused of child abuse with other relatives, the total of this group accounts for only about 10% of reported cases.

Certain patient populations are more at risk for child abuse. When interviewing children, the Paramedic should

Table 43-3 Situational Indicators of Child Abuse

- History of intimate partner violence
- Alcohol abuse and illicit drug use
- Medically fragile children

keep these patient populations in mind. However, the Paramedic should also keep an open mind, as child abuse knows no economic, social, racial, or ethnic boundaries (Table 43-3).

Children living in single-parent households are statistically more at risk for child abuse. These single parents struggle with maintaining a family without the benefit of extended family support. This problem has become more pronounced in the last 25 years, with a 200% increase in the number of single-parent households.

By race, the children at highest risk for child abuse appear to be African Americans, Pacific Islanders, and First Americans. Euro–Americans and Hispanic children have about the same rates of child abuse.

Children with chronic medical conditions, which put extraordinary demands on the family and family resources, are at higher risk of child abuse.[14] Examples of these medically fragile children include premature infants, colicky babies, children born with cerebral palsy or spina bifida, or others with developmental disabilities.

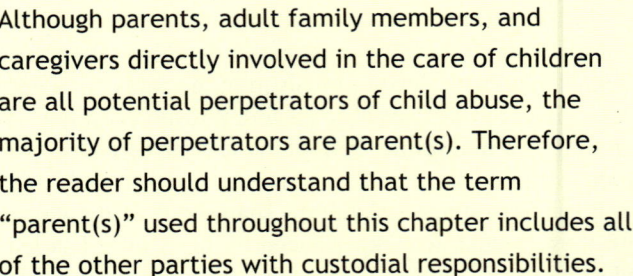

STREET SMART

Although parents, adult family members, and caregivers directly involved in the care of children are all potential perpetrators of child abuse, the majority of perpetrators are parent(s). Therefore, the reader should understand that the term "parent(s)" used throughout this chapter includes all of the other parties with custodial responsibilities.

CASE STUDY (CONTINUED)

Upon their arrival, the Paramedics find a 15-year-old girl holding a small infant. She tells the Paramedics that she had put her son down for a nap and when he awoke, he wasn't acting right. The child had been born at the County Hospital. He was full term and reported as healthy even though his mother had not received any prenatal care. While one of the Paramedics takes the child to begin an examination, the other Paramedic begins eliciting a history.

CRITICAL THINKING QUESTIONS

1. What are the important elements of the history that a Paramedic should obtain?
2. Why is the psychosocial evaluation also part of the history?

History

While addressing the patient's chief concern, the Paramedic should start to obtain a psychosocial history of the child under the guise of obtaining a thorough medical history. If the child is less than 8 years of age but over 2 years of age, the Paramedic should ask if the child sleeps alone, as a fear of sleeping alone may be a sign of regression. Another sign of regression is enuresis. **Enuresis**, or bedwetting, can occur at night or be an "accident" during the daytime. **Encopresis**, or self-soiling, can be associated with enuresis and is another sign of regression. Some children have even been observed to regress to thumb sucking. All of these psychosocial indicators should be documented.

While on the topic of sleep and sleep habits, the Paramedic should ask if the child is sleeping well, or whether the child experiences nightmares or night terrors. Poor sleep may be an indicator of anxiety, and fatigue can impact on other associated activities, such as school.

School is a central focus for this age group. The Paramedic should ask about school attendance and changes in behavior (such as a drop in grades or fear of school). A drop in grades may indicate delinquency and a fear of school may indicate sexual or physical abuse at school.

The Paramedic's first priority is to treat the presenting medical emergency. However, in the course of that care the Paramedic may suspect that child abuse is occurring and/or has occurred in the past. The following psychosocial evaluation (Table 43-4) may help the Paramedic to put the issue into focus and provide a foundation for the Paramedic's diagnosis of suspected child abuse.

The Paramedic should first observe the parent(s). Adults who have mistreated children often have a shaky self-esteem. These adults may be easily threatened by the presence of authority figures, such as Paramedics, and may react angrily

Table 43-4 Psychosocial Evaluation

- Parental behavior
- Familial situation
- Child behavior

to questions about the care of the child. Alternatively, they may offer only scant information about the child's medical history and other facts. Instead of focusing on the child, the parent may focus on "intruders"—such as Paramedics, law enforcement officers, or firefighters—in their home. Abusive parents often withdraw assistance when questioned and may even retaliate against the Paramedic by demanding that all emergency services personnel leave the house. It is important for the Paramedic to not respond to the parent's behavior but to simply document the parent's response.

Child abuse can occur, or reoccur, when extraordinary circumstances occur in the family. The Paramedic should investigate whether there has been a recent death in the family, loss of custodial support from other adults, loss of employment, or any acute life stressor that would contribute to the risk of child abuse. Any potentially contributing situational crisis should be noted on the patient care report.

Finally, the Paramedic should observe the child. Children with chronic medical conditions (such as cerebral palsy or spina bifida) or who have frequently reoccurring exacerbations of chronic conditions (such as a seizure disorder) may be at greater risk of child abuse. These medically fragile children demand more exhaustive care.

In the same way, there are periods of a child's life when the child's care puts more demands on the child, such as teething and toilet training. The Paramedic should observe if the parent(s) have inappropriate expectations of children during these times.

CASE STUDY (CONTINUED)

The physical exam shows an irritable infant with a high-pitched cry. There is bilateral periorbital bruising and his anterior fontanel is tense to the touch. The child's mother states that he hasn't received any shots since she hasn't gotten to a clinic and he last saw a pediatrician at birth. Since his birth, she has moved three times.

CRITICAL THINKING QUESTIONS

1. What are the elements of the physical examination of a patient with suspected child abuse?
2. Why is a behavioral assessment a critical element in this examination?

Examination

Behavioral signs, not physical signs, are central to the examination of an abused child. These behavioral signs are apparent in both the child and the parent. Behavioral signs of possible child abuse include visible apprehension when other children are crying and inappropriate fear of the Paramedic. The child may display a mood which is inappropriate in light of the situation, or demonstrate extreme mood swings (e.g., from tearfulness to elation).

Table 43-5 Parental Indicators of Child Abuse
• Delay in seeking medical care • Parental indifference • Alcohol abuse and illicit drug use • Conflicting histories

Table 43-6 Children's Behavioral Indicators of Child Abuse
• Inappropriate affection • Extremes of behavior • Wary of adult contact

Similarly, the parent may display either agitation over the Paramedic's questioning or a complete indifference to the child's plight. These observations are important to note.

Child Abuse

Specific behavioral indicators are suggestive of child abuse. Both the parent(s) and the child will manifest these behaviors. Careful observation of these indicators during the course of the Paramedic–parent–patient interaction should alert the Paramedic to the potential of child abuse.

Parental Behavior

Certain parental behaviors should alert the Paramedic to possible child abuse. For example, it is natural for a parent to be concerned about his or her child. Therefore, it is abnormal for a parent to appear indifferent or unconcerned about the child's welfare. This indifference may be demonstrated by a delay in seeking medical attention (Table 43-5).

Inconsistency is another red flag. The Paramedic should be concerned if the parent gives an inadequate explanation of the child's injury or the parent's explanation conflicts with the child's story.

All too often, alcohol abuse and illicit drug use play into child abuse. Parental intoxication or signs of intoxication—such as empty bottles of alcohol or visible drug paraphernalia—are causes for concern.

Acts of anger toward the child while in the presence of a Paramedic may require immediate action and police intervention. Whether these acts are statements of shame in which the parent describes the child as evil or bad, or attempts at physical discipline in the presence of the Paramedic, these acts can demonstrate poor impulse control.

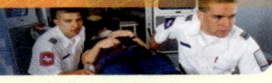

STREET SMART

In order to avoid suspicion, some parent(s) will ask to have the child taken to different hospitals for each injury. So called "doc shopping" is another indicator of potential child abuse.

Child Behavior

Fear is probably the greatest single source of an abused child's behavior. Abused children may be wary—or even fearful—of adults, including their parents. As such, they will cower and may even physically tremble around adults. The child may express dread about going home, fearing a beating upon arrival.

The behavior of an abused child may demonstrate extremes of behavior, from aggressiveness to withdrawal, that will often be inappropriate to the situation (Table 43-6). Of particular concern is when the child appears apprehensive when other children cry.

Alternatively, the child may attempt to endear herself to adults—any adults—by seeking the adult's sympathy and protection. However, attempts at affection should be viewed cautiously. Any sexual talk from the child is a red flag to the Paramedic. Even more alarming is sexual acting out, which can be subtle (such as inappropriate touching) or brazen (such as exposure and even public masturbation). If the Paramedic observes any of these behaviors, firm boundaries should be immediately established and another provider asked to accompany the Paramedic and the patient.

Special Case of Adolescents

Generally, child abuse is limited to young children. However, adolescents can be the victims of child abuse as well, especially sexual abuse. As friends are the focus of attention for most adolescents, the Paramedic should ask the patient about social interactions. Fear of being alone, peer problems, and even substance abuse may be signs of child abuse. Reports of special concern are self-mutilation, sexual promiscuity, suicidal ideation, and violent fantasies.

Sexual Abuse

The pattern of violence surrounding sexual abuse of a child makes it difficult for the Paramedic to obtain the history. Pedophiles often begin a conditioning process when the child is as young as 5 or 6 years old. The child, not knowing better, is taught that questionable sexual activity, such as observation of masturbation, is acceptable. The abuser then progresses to the fondling stage and then to the oral stage. Studies indicate that oral sexual abuse occurs for years (3 or 4 years) before penile–vaginal or penile–anal penetration in many cases. Genital warts have been found in the back of the throat of some abused children.

At each stage, the child is made to believe that the child and the abuser share a secret that must not be shared with others. This conspiracy of silence makes it difficult for the Paramedic to obtain a history of the event because the child does not believe that anything has gone wrong and may actually become defensive if it is suggested. Therefore, the Paramedic should focus on the patient's concerns. For example, painful discharge of urine or repeated urinary tract infections may indicate early sexual promiscuity and sexual abuse. Other psychological indicators of sexual abuse may be precocious behavior, inappropriate sexual behavior, and dropping grades in school.

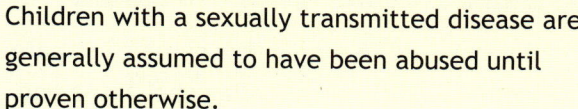

STREET SMART

Children with a sexually transmitted disease are generally assumed to have been abused until proven otherwise.

Child Behavior

A child's unwillingness to disrobe for examination or excessive fear of being touched may be indicators of sexual abuse. In addition, a child's hypersexuality and premature sexual knowledge may also be signs of sexual abuse.

Child Neglect

Although at its surface charges of child neglect could appear to be indictments of the poor, child neglect knows no economic boundaries. In the United States, there are sufficient social resources (e.g., Women, Infants and Children's (WIC) food and nutrition service) to ensure that no child need be neglected. Child neglect is a conscious decision on the part of the parent.

CULTURAL/REGIONAL DIFFERENCES

The Paramedic must take care not to compare the care of the child with the care provided or received in her own home. An example is in bathing. Although it is common in the United States to take frequent (even daily) baths or showers, many cultures do not bath as frequently. However, an obviously dirty child with ripped or inappropriate clothing for weather is cause for concern. The Paramedic should take care not to mix cultural bias with an assumption of neglect.

Parental Behavior

Two key attitudes can be used to sum up the behavior of parents who neglect their children: hopelessness and helplessness. Parents who neglect their children often have disorganized home lives and may express feelings of apathy

Table 43-7 Parental Behavioral Indicators of Child Neglect

- Alcohol abuse
- Chronic illness
- Unsafe living conditions

Table 43-8 Children's Behavioral Indicators of Child Neglect

- Truancy and tardiness
- Listlessness and fatigue
- Alcohol abuse or drug use

(Table 43-7). Often the parent is isolated, without the support of an extended family or friends. In some cases, the parent may have chronic health concerns that may detract from the child's care. In other instances, the parent has limited intellectual capacity and is unable to access social services without assistance.

Child Behavior

Behaviors which demonstrate a child's survival instinct are indicators of child neglect (Table 43-8). For example, because of constant hunger the child may resort to begging for food or stealing food. Similarly, problems at home, or lack of shelter, may cause the child to arrive early or stay late at school. These problems at home can cause sleeplessness. The child may also have failing grades or be observed falling asleep in class.

Infanticide and Abandoned Infants Acts

Some mothers do not realize that they are pregnant until they deliver. Overwhelmed by the sudden appearance of the infant and all of the life-changing events that surround parenting, these mothers may choose to abandon—or even kill—their babies.[15,16]

To protect the lives of these infants, some states have enacted an abandoned infant act. These acts permit the mother, or legal guardian, to relinquish care of the newborn to a "safe haven" such as a public safety agency. Typically, the individual is not asked for a name or any other identifying information. The person is simply asked, in a nonjudgmental manner, if there is medical information that would help in the care of the infant.

Psychological Maltreatment

Psychological maltreatment can have far more devastating, and long-lasting, effects on a child's psyche than the harm caused by physical abuse. By its definition, psychological maltreatment leads to substantial psychological and intellectual impairment that has a ripple effect throughout the child's life.

Parental Behavior

The key to psychological maltreatment is the lack of love. Like Cinderella, the child is made to feel unwanted and the parent is cold and rejecting. Characteristically, the child is treated differently than other members of the family. Even in times of personal turmoil, the parent withholds love from the child. These behaviors (Table 43-9) are so ingrained in the family life that they are evident even when the Paramedic is involved.

Child Behavior

A number of behavioral disorders occur in this patient population, each a manifestation of the psychological maltreatment. In order of severity, these disorders include habit disorders, conduct disorders, neurotic disorders, and psychiatric disorders (Table 43-10).

Habit disorders may be the most easily identified. In an effort to self-soothe, the child will be observed to be sucking fingers or rocking to and fro, mimicking maternal behaviors.

Paramedics are made aware of conduct disorders when the child becomes injured in an antisocial act or from some destructive behavior. The latter (destructive behaviors) are attention-seeking behaviors, including suicide attempts, which are intended to cause parental concern.

As the child matures, he may start to develop maladaptive coping mechanisms in response to the psychological maltreatment. These can be of the level of neurosis, and include sleep and speech disorders, or can rise to the level of psychosis. Examples of induced psychotic behaviors include obsessions, compulsions, and phobias.

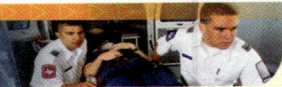

STREET SMART

The child's exposure to extreme or chronic intimate partner violence (IPV), as well as alcohol abuse and drug use, may constitute emotional neglect.

Physical Examination

While trying to appear unobtrusive, so as not to alert the patient, the Paramedic should assess the child, in a head-to-toe fashion, for signs of physical abuse (Table 43-11). After proper introductions and age-appropriate explanations of the examination, the Paramedic should form a general impression of the child at the start of the examination.

The Paramedic should carefully examine the patient's head and face, as approximately 50% of child abuse victims have injuries to these areas.[17] The Paramedic should examine the head for the absence of patches of hair or bleeding beneath the scalp. These findings are suggestive of hair pulling and traumatic hair loss.

If the child is an infant, then the Paramedic should observe for bulging of the posterior and the anterior fontanel. A bulging fontanel may be indicative of increased intracranial pressure, possibly secondary to intracerebral hemorrhage.

The Paramedic should examine both of the patient's eyes for evidence of bilateral periorbital ecchymosis (raccoon's eyes). Bruising around the eyes is suggestive of a basilar skull fracture, which may occur when a child is thrown to the floor.

Table 43-9 Parental Behavioral Indicators of Psychological Maltreatment

- Terrorizing
  - Threatened violence
  - Placing child in danger
- Isolating
  - Confinement
  - Social isolation
    - Truancy
- Corrupting
  - Criminality
    - Prostitution
    - Shoplifting
  - Permitted substance abuse
- Rejecting
  - Belittling
  - Ridicule

Table 43-10 Children's Behavioral Indicators of Psychological Maltreatment

- Habit disorders
- Conduct disorders
- Neurotic disorders
- Psychiatric disorders

Table 43-11 Physical Indicators of Child Abuse

- Bruising
  - Unexplained bruising
  - Atypical bruising
  - Multiple stages of healing
- Human bites
- Burns
  - Cigarette
  - Hot water immersion
  - Stoves
- Fractures
  - Multiple fractures
  - Spiral fractures

Next, the Paramedic should observe the patient for lacerations or abrasions to the lips and gums. Lip tears may occur because of a direct blow to the mouth or forced feeding. While looking into the mouth, the Paramedic should observe the frenulum, the short flap of tissue that attaches the lips to the gums and the tongue to the floor of the mouth. Although it is normally difficult to tear the frenulum, forced bottle feeding can cause a laceration to the tissues.

After finishing the assessment of the child's head, the Paramedic should perform a complete examination of the body, with the exception of the genitals, observing for bruises and other signs of child abuse.

Bruising

The single most significant indicator of physical child abuse may be bruises in unusual places, unexplained bruises, or bruises in various stages of healing.[18] A bruise (contusion or ecchymosis) is a collection of blood under the skin that occurs as a result of trauma. Bruises typically heal in approximately one week or so. During the healing process, the bruise changes colors. Initially, and for the first few days, the bruise is a deep purple, referred to as black and blue. By week's end, the bruise will lighten to become brown and then greenish. After the first week, the bruise becomes yellow or tan. The presence of multiple bruises in various stages of healing suggest repeated trauma and should be viewed suspiciously.

Similarly, bruises in unusual places should be cause for concern. Usual locations for bruises are the knees and the elbows, such as might result from a fall. Unusual places for bruises include the inside of the upper arm, the ribs, or the thighs. These bruises may be the result of forceful grabbing of the child. This "non-accidental distribution" of bruises is suggestive of child abuse.

Bruises are the result of trauma; therefore, an event can be linked to each bruise. In the case of child abuse, the mechanism of injury that supposedly caused the bruise often does not match the location of the bruise, or the healing of the bruises by stages does not match the timing of the incident.

The Paramedic should also make note of the time of the incident and which parent was responsible for the child. Bruises that appear after the parent has had visitation, such as weekends or vacations, may be cause for concern.

Bruises to the face are of particular concern. Loss of vision, loss of teeth, and traumatic brain injury, which can all result from facial trauma, can have life-long implications. Bruises of the face, lips, and mouth can be the result of a fall, but also can result from a slap or a punch.[19] Slap or punch injuries may reflect a parent's problem with anger control and inappropriate coping mechanisms.

Of special concern are bruises that are clustered and that form regular recurrent patterns (Figure 43-1). These regular recurrent patterns can reflect the shape of articles that were used to inflict trauma. Objects used as a whip or switch will leave a distinctive mark. For example, electrical cords will leave loops of bruises on the skin or the buckle of a belt may leave a squared bruise on the skin.

STREET SMART

A deficiency of vitamin C, which is necessary for blood vessels, can make capillaries friable (easily ruptured) by weakening the collagen in the blood vessels. Any slight trauma to these vulnerable blood vessels can lead to bruising.[20] In addition, infants fed bottled milk may develop scurvy, as vitamin C is destroyed in pasteurization.

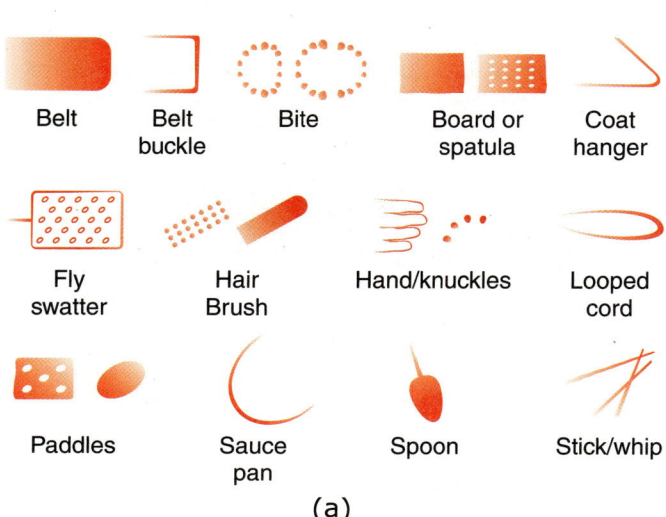

Belt — Belt buckle — Bite — Board or spatula — Coat hanger

Fly swatter — Hair Brush — Hand/knuckles — Looped cord

Paddles — Sauce pan — Spoon — Stick/whip

(a)

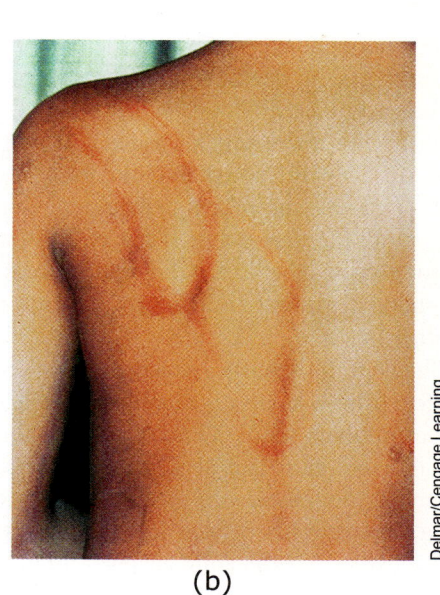

Delmar/Cengage Learning

(b)

Figure 43-1 Pattern bruises suggestive of child abuse.

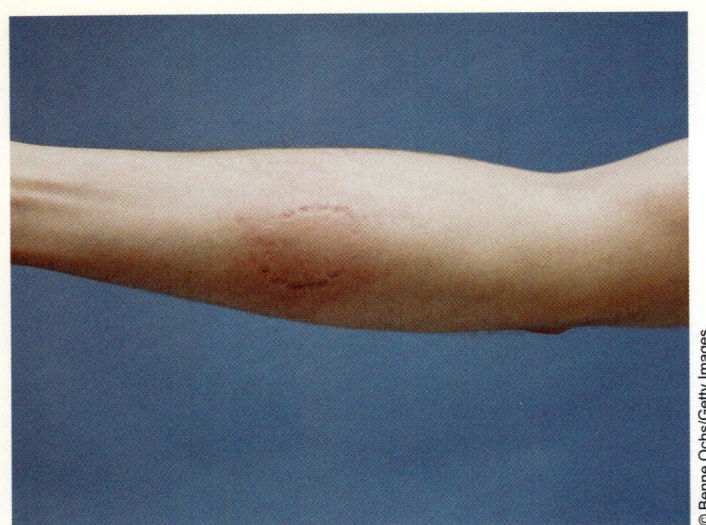

Figure 43-2 Adult bite mark indicators.

© Benne Ochs/Getty Images

Bites and Burns

Many parents have experienced the dismay of finding out their child has bitten someone else's child. Although this behavior is natural, it is not acceptable and the child is quickly corrected. However, an adult biting a child is never acceptable.

Adult bite marks are, logically, a larger semicircle of puncture marks than a child's (Figure 43-2). The shape of the punctures also helps to differentiate adult human bite marks from other puncture wounds. Incisors leave a narrow rectangular puncture mark whereas the canines leave a triangular puncture mark. Again, the location of the bite mark may help distinguish accidental from intentional injury as well. Children typically bite each other on the hand or forearm. Bites on a child's shoulders, back, or thighs would be suspicious.

By accident, a child may pull a saucepan from the stove and receive a burn or run water that is too hot into the bathtub and get burned. These unfortunate burns are an experience of youth. Burns of concern (non-accidental burns) are cigarette burns, immersion burns, and pattern burns. These should never be part of a childhood.

Parents, in a moment of rage, will use any convenient object to inflict pain upon their child. In some cases, the object is the lit cigarette the parent is smoking. Using the cigarette like a brand, the parent burns the child's palms, back, buttocks, or soles of the feet. A cigarette leaves a characteristic small round burn that is distinctive and cannot be confused with other burns.

When a toddler pulls a saucepan from the stove, or a cup of coffee from a table, it usually leaves a superficial burn called a toddler's scald. The typical distribution of burn is across the shoulders and neck (the toddler reflexively averts the face). A non-accidental immersion scald, which occurs when a parent holds a limb underwater, is the result of a forceful restraint of the child, as even infants will reflexively withdraw their legs. Burns from immersion in scalding hot water will leave a characteristic dunking pattern. If just the

child's hands or feet are immersed, then the burn will have a glove-like or sock-like appearance. Since the child cannot pull away, or kick, there are not burns from side splash and there is a clear line of demarcation.

If the child's entire torso is immersed in the scalding hot water in the bathtub, a characteristic "donut" burn may occur.[21] As the child's buttocks rest on the bottom of the bathtub, and away from the scalding hot water, the genitalia are spared. This action leaves a characteristic bull's eye appearance to the burn.

Another burn of concern is a patterned burn (Figure 43-3). These burns are the result of forced contact with an object, such as an iron, the burner of a stove, or a hot water radiator. The result is a characteristic striped or circular burn.

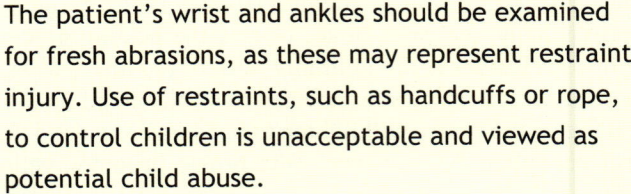

STREET SMART

The patient's wrist and ankles should be examined for fresh abrasions, as these may represent restraint injury. Use of restraints, such as handcuffs or rope, to control children is unacceptable and viewed as potential child abuse.

Fractures

Fractured bones are the result of trauma. More specifically, certain fractures are indicative of certain traumas. For example, a spiral fracture (a fracture that runs up the shaft of the bone like the ribbon on a barber's pole) is the result of a twisting action (Figure 43-4). Other injuries, such as dislocations, are the result of distracting forces that pull joints apart.

Not all spiral fractures or dislocations are the result of child abuse. For example, "nursemaid's elbow" is a dislocation of the radius from the humerus. It can be the result of pulling on a child's arm to coax the child to move along and may be seen as a natural consequence of parenting. Fractures of concern are skull fractures, nasal fractures, and multiple fractures. The Paramedic should view the latter (multiple fractures in various stages of healing) like bruises in multiple stages of healing—with suspicion.

STREET SMART

Osteogenesis imperfecta is a congenital medical condition that results in easily fractured bones, often from no apparent trauma. Interestingly, the sclera of children with osteogenesis imperfecta may have a blue-gray tint and the face of the child may be triangular.

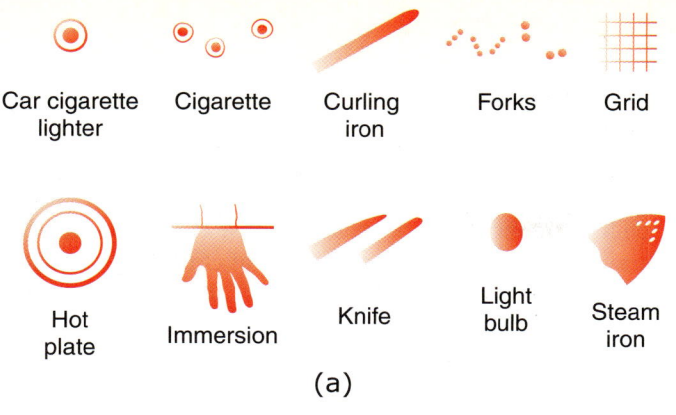

Car cigarette lighter   Cigarette   Curling iron   Forks   Grid

Hot plate   Immersion   Knife   Light bulb   Steam iron

(a)

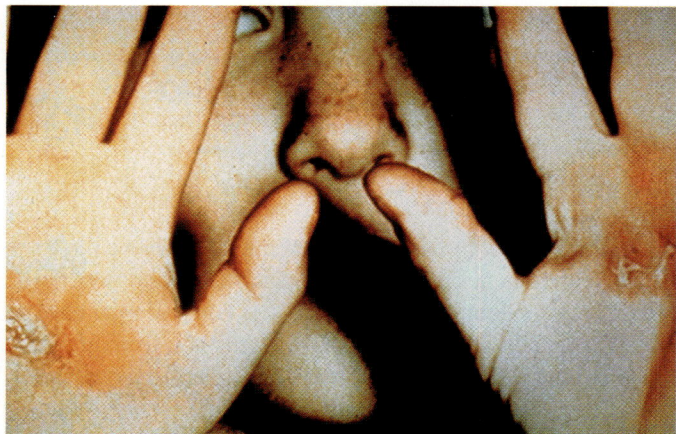

(b)

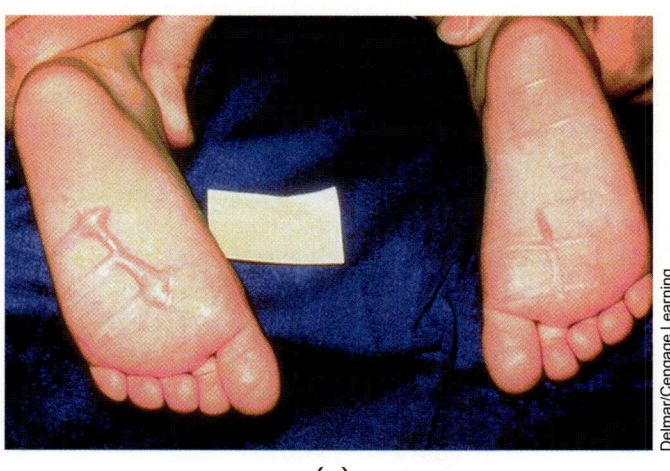

(c)

Figure 43-3 Patterned burns suggestive of child abuse.

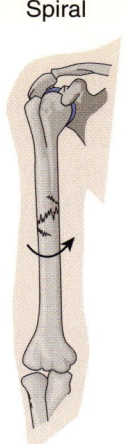

Spiral

Delmar/Cengage Learning

Figure 43-4 Fracture suggestive of child abuse.

Table 43-12 Munchausen Syndrome by Proxy
• Maternal menstrual blood
○ Mixed with child's stool
○ Smeared on child's genitals
○ Mixes with urine sample
• Stirred with tampon
• Child's feces mixed with child's vomit
○ Vomiting induced with syrup of ipecac
• Feigned seizure disorder
○ Strangulation
• Enforced invalidism
○ Hazards of bedrest

Munchausen refers to Baron Von Munchausen, a soldier and teller of outrageous war stories.

A bogus illness can be created by rubbing a thermometer until the temperature suggests a fever, or creating a friction burn that appears like a rash. In some cases, the parent will be an active inducer, meaning that the parent will poison the child in order to make the child ill (Table 43-12). The mortality rate of MSP is thought to be as high as 10%.[22]

Paramedics have a unique role in identifying MSP. These parents often seek medical care at multiple facilities (doctor shopping) in order to avoid suspicion. The common denominator in these situations is EMS. A Paramedic who repeatedly cares for the same dependent child should be concerned about MSP.

Special Case of Munchausen Syndrome by Proxy

In order to gain attention for themselves, a parent may either fabricate or induce an illness in the child so that medical professionals will have to treat it. This behavior is known as **Munchausen Syndrome by Proxy (MSP)**. The name

Cultural Practices

Every culture has common folk remedies which originated in earlier times before Western medicine was widely practiced. These traditional forms of healing include some practices that a Paramedic might perceive as child abuse.

For example, some Southeast Asians practice cao gio, or coin rubbing, to relieve pain, fever, abdominal pain, and even the cough from a common cold. Usually an oil (such as tiger balm, containing camphor), oil of wintergreen or peppermint, or similar aromatic solution is applied liberally over the person's back and then a coin is rubbed repeatedly in a linear pattern until blood raises to the surface. This dermal abrasive technique leaves distinctive patterns on the patient's back.

It should be emphasized that cao gio is not child abuse. The purpose of the use of cao gio is well-intentioned and is not intended to cause injury or harm to the child. The Paramedic must keep this in mind. False claims of child abuse can lead to alienation of this patient population and seed distrust among people.

Sexual Abuse

The suspicion of sexual abuse, in the field, is largely based on history (Table 43-13). However, there are some physical signs that the Paramedic may observe. For example, the child may have difficulty in walking or sitting after a rape or assault. The patient may also complain of pain or itching in the genitals.

Children also have a right to privacy for their bodies and can refuse examinations. A child should never be forced to have an examination, even by the parent, if the child refuses. This is especially important if sexual abuse is suspected. Generally, an examination should only be performed if it is medically necessary. Even if the child consents to an examination, it is inappropriate for a Paramedic to perform an external examination of the genitalia for contusions, lacerations, bleeding, and so on. If the Paramedic is given torn, stained, or bloody underclothing from a child, it should be placed in a paper bag and given to a law enforcement officer.

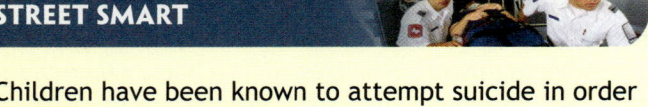

STREET SMART

Children have been known to attempt suicide in order to draw attention away from another sibling. This attention-seeking behavior is intended to distract the parent's attention in order to prevent further abuse of the sibling.

Table 43-13 Physical Indicators of Sexual Abuse

- Nonspecific abdominal pain
- Dysuria
- Pain in the vagina or rectum
- Bleeding from the vagina or rectum
- Discharge from the urethra, vagina, or rectum

Child Neglect and Psychological Maltreatment

Although child neglect and psychological maltreatment do not have the more obvious signs of trauma that are seen with child abuse, they nevertheless have clear markers. In some respects, child neglect (the failure to provide legally mandated care for a child) may be more devastating for a child than physical abuse. Although the physical injuries of child abuse heal, the psychosocial harm of child neglect has life-long implications.

An environmental assessment can help establish if neglect has occurred. For example, an empty refrigerator or the lack of running water may indicate a lack of proper food or shelter. Structural hazards or unsanitary conditions also indicate a lack of proper shelter.

Evidence of drug abuse or alcohol use is another key indicator of neglect, as these represent a clear danger to the child. Anytime a child has been poisoned, then neglect must be suspected.

Failure to Thrive

An infant with poor physical development may leave the Paramedic with a general impression that the infant is not well cared for, as may be the case. However, the child may have an inborn error of metabolism which prevents him from growing, or the child may have been a premature infant. In some cases, where the mother suffers from postpartum depression, the child may not be receiving nurturance. In this case, the mother's psychological state is responsible for the child's health.

Some infants are identified by the label **failure to thrive (FTT)**. FTT is not a diagnosis, but rather a description of the child's subaverage growth for age. FTT may be the result of maternal smoking or alcohol consumption during pregnancy or problems with diet (such as inborn errors of metabolism or food allergies).

Children with FTT may have signs of muscle wasting or skin changes, such as poor turgor, suggestive of malnutrition. These children may also have signs of dehydration, such as sunken anterior fontanels and/or dry mucous membranes.

In the past, the assumption was made that FTT occurred as a result of maternal rejection or maternal neglect. However, a number of medical conditions can lead to FTT. Therefore, although the Paramedic must have a suspicion of child neglect, it is important to recognize that the child may have other legitimate medical conditions.

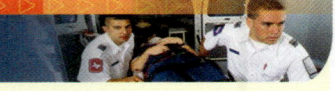

STREET SMART

The newborn child can naturally lose as much as 10% of the birth weight in the first week. These newborns would not be characterized as failure to thrive, as these newborns should regain that weight within two weeks to a month.

Special Case: Sudden Infant Death Syndrome

When an infant dies unexpectedly and without apparent cause, the patient's death may be labeled as sudden infant death syndrome (SIDS). SIDS is not due to child abuse.

However, child abuse can result in the death of an infant. Regardless of the cause of death, the Paramedic should proceed with routine care, focusing on the emergency at hand, and the parent(s) should be given care and compassion during these trying times.

CASE STUDY (CONTINUED)

The mother explains that the "raccoon's eyes" occurred after the baby rolled off the bed while she was changing him. However, as she explains the source of the injury she looks away from the Paramedic.

Based on the physical findings (bilateral periorbital ecchymosis and a tense fontanel) and the incongruity of the mother's story to the developmental age of the child, the Paramedic suspects child abuse.

CRITICAL THINKING QUESTIONS

1. What is the significance of the infant's developmental age to the injury?
2. What diagnosis did the Paramedic announce to the patient's mother?

Assessment

To make a proper assessment, the Paramedic must first suspend disbelief and embrace the possibility that child abuse may exist. Then the Paramedic must maintain a nonjudgmental attitude toward the parents, always keeping the child's best interests in mind. All this is done while assessing the child for the chief concern.

The Paramedic's diagnosis of suspected child abuse is based on focused observation and critical thinking. The Paramedic should support the diagnosis by, for example, illustrating that the mechanism of injury does not match the developmental age of the child or that the behaviors demonstrated by the parent and child are inconsistent with expected behaviors of this dyad.

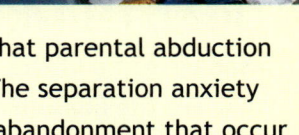

STREET SMART

Many authorities believe that parental abduction of a child is child abuse. The separation anxiety and the fears of parental abandonment that occur during a parental abduction result in psychological maltreatment of the child.

CASE STUDY (CONTINUED)

The mother starts to tell the Paramedic that she has changed her mind and that she will take the infant to the clinic down the street instead. The Paramedic explains to the mother that the child is ill and needs immediate medical attention, while his partner steps out, on the pretense of getting equipment, to call law enforcement to the scene.

CRITICAL THINKING QUESTIONS

1. Does the mother have the right to refuse care for the infant?
2. What are some of the patient-specific concerns that relate to the patient's injuries?

Treatment

Treatment in the case of suspected child abuse should proceed as normal, focusing on the chief concern and transporting the patient to the hospital for further treatment. It is not the Paramedic's place—nor does a Paramedic have the education and preparation—to therapeutically intervene when child abuse is suspected.

Refusal of Care

Although under ordinary circumstances a parent may refuse care for a child, preferring to transport the child to a family physician or pediatrician instead, when child abuse or neglect is suspected the Paramedic must take steps to ensure the safety of the child and to prevent further child abuse.

In some cases, certain religious or ethnic practices may appear to be child abuse. Some laws (e.g., the Child Abuse and Prevention Treatment Act, or CAPTA), make specific exemptions for religious beliefs, allowing a parent to decide about medical treatment for their child. However, most of these laws do not provide this exemption in cases of suspected child abuse.

Ideally, Paramedics would canvas their communities and meet with local ethnic and religious leaders to improve understanding of these practices and to establish guidelines for treatment. Often, however, these decisions are made on-scene.

In many jurisdictions, Paramedics enlist the assistance of law enforcement officers or child protective services to convince the parent(s) that medical care is necessary. However, for the refusal of health care to rise to the level of physical neglect, the parent(s) must fail to provide (or allow) needed medical care in accordance with physician recommendations. Therefore, Paramedics should enlist the assistance of their local medical control physician in these cases.

▷ ▷ ▷ ▷ ▷ ▷ ▷ ▷ ▷ ▷ ▷ ▷ ▷ ▷
CULTURAL/REGIONAL DIFFERENCES

Many regional EMS systems or law enforcement jurisdictions automatically dispatch law enforcement officers for EMS calls concerning children and trauma.

CASE STUDY (CONTINUED)

During the exchange between the mother and the Paramedic, the infant becomes unresponsive and begins to seize. The mother screams as both Paramedics protect the child from injury and seek to protect the airway. Blow-by oxygen is started and the child's blood glucose is checked, which is normal at 88.

CRITICAL THINKING QUESTIONS

1. What are some of the predictable complications associated with abusive head trauma?
2. What are the anatomical factors that contribute to shaken baby syndrome?

Evaluation

A number of possible causes exist for convulsions in infants without a fever, including hypoxia, hypoglycemia, and head injury. The latter is seen with abusive head trauma, such as **shaken baby syndrome (SBS)**.[23]

During SBS, the infant is violently shaken to and fro, resulting in shearing forces during acceleration and deceleration. These forces tear fragile bridging veins in the skull and cause subsequent subdural bleeding, as well as cause metaphyseal fractures and retinal hemorrhage. These anatomical factors contribute to shaken baby syndrome (Table 43-14).

Reports of a short fall from a bed or from a changing table might increase the Paramedic's suspicion of shaken baby syndrome. Death from head injuries from falls of less than 4 feet is unlikely (less than one in a million) and rarely result in subdural or epidural hematoma.

Up to 50% of deaths attributed to child abuse are from shaken baby syndrome and up to 25% of babies who are victims of shaken baby syndrome die. Other complications associated with SBS include blindness, cerebral palsy, and long-term cognitive impairment.

The shaking, often done by the father or boyfriend of the mother, is the result of frustration with the infant's crying. Although there are a number of techniques to soothe a baby, when all else fails, the infant should be left to cry. This approach, "It's OK to walk away," could save many infants.

Table 43-14 Anatomical Factors Contributing to Shaken Baby Syndrome

- Newborn's head is 10% to 15% of total body weight (adult is 2% to 3%)
- Shallow subarachnoid space
- Weak neck muscles
- Demyelinated brain gelatin-like
- Higher water content

Infants who have been shaken may present as irritable, inconsolable, or lethargic.[24] Many of these infants may have difficulty breathing, as manifest by irregular breathing patterns, or may even convulse.

After completing the primary assessment, the Paramedic should perform a thorough head-to-toe examination. Close inspection of the scalp may reveal contusions or lacerations from impact on hard surfaces. The cranium should be palpated for an uneven surface, especially along the sutures, that would suggest a step-off from a displaced fracture or split suture. The ears and nose should be examined for signs of otorrhea and rhinorrhea.

Although over 80% of SBS have associated retinal hemorrhage, Paramedics do not have the tools to examine for this condition.[25] Therefore, the Paramedic should examine the patient's pupils, using a bright light source, to check for equality and reactivity.

Proceeding to the torso, the Paramedic should palpate the patient's ribs for fractures and observe for bruises, which are signs of a forceful grab. Similarly, the long bones of the upper arm should also be examined for fractures and bruises. On occasion, "grab bruises," the finger bruises created when the child was shaken, may be visible on the upper arm.

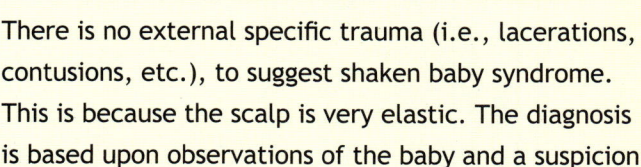
SBS can cause a rapid neurological dysfunction, culminating in seizures and death. It is imperative that the infant be expeditiously transported to a medical facility capable of caring for pediatric patients.

CASE STUDY CONCLUSION

The Paramedics transfer care of the infant to the physician and nurse in the ED. They then follow their state's regulations for reporting a suspicion of child abuse.

Several days later, they are contacted by their medical director, who reports that the infant had suffered a subdural hemorrhage likely caused by shaking. The mother had told the emergency department nurse that she didn't know how to get the baby to stop crying and she hadn't had any sleep in several nights. The baby's father provided some financial support but she was alone in taking care of the infant.

CRITICAL THINKING QUESTIONS

1. What is the most appropriate transport decision that will get the patient to definitive care?
2. What is the responsibility of the Paramedic to report suspected child abuse?

Disposition

After proper delivery of the patient to the hospital and the turnover of care to other healthcare professionals, the Paramedic should report the suspicion of child abuse. Every state in the United States has a mandated reporter law. Certain classes of individuals—such as educators, law enforcement, and day care workers—who are in a position to observe a child are mandated reporters.

As mandated reporters, Paramedics must document, usually on state approved forms (Figure 43-5), and report, usually on a selected telephone line, their suspicions. Generally, that report must include the basis for the suspicion, actions taken to protect the child, the identity of the child, and often the location of other children at risk.

In many states, the failure to report suspected child abuse can expose the Paramedic to both criminal and civil penalties including imprisonment and fines. However, to encourage reporting, Paramedics who report suspected child abuse in good faith are granted immunity from liability.

The importance of proper reporting is revealed by child abuse statistics. The National Child Abuse and Neglect Data

SUSPECTED CHILD ABUSE REPORT

To Be Completed by **Mandated Child Abuse Reporters**
Pursuant to Penal Code Section 11166
PLEASE PRINT OR TYPE

CASE NAME: _____

CASE NUMBER: _____

A. REPORTING PARTY

NAME OF MANDATED REPORTER	TITLE			MANDATED REPORTER CATEGORY

| REPORTER'S BUSINESS/AGENCY NAME AND ADDRESS | Street | City | Zip | DID MANDATED REPORTER WITNESS THE INCIDENT? ☐ YES ☐ NO |

| REPORTER'S TELEPHONE (DAYTIME) ( ) | SIGNATURE | TODAY'S DATE |

B. REPORT NOTIFICATION

☐ LAW ENFORCEMENT ☐ COUNTY PROBATION
☐ COUNTY WELFARE / CPS (Child Protective Services)   AGENCY

| ADDRESS | Street | City | Zip | DATE/TIME OF PHONE CALL |

| OFFICIAL CONTACTED - TITLE | TELEPHONE ( ) |

C. VICTIM *One report per victim*

| NAME (LAST, FIRST, MIDDLE) | BIRTHDATE OR APPROX. AGE | SEX | ETHNICITY |

| ADDRESS | Street | City | Zip | TELEPHONE ( ) |

| PRESENT LOCATION OF VICTIM | SCHOOL | CLASS | GRADE |

| PHYSICALLY DISABLED? ☐ YES ☐ NO | DEVELOPMENTALLY DISABLED? ☐ YES ☐ NO | OTHER DISABILITY (SPECIFY) | PRIMARY LANGUAGE SPOKEN IN HOME |

IN FOSTER CARE? IF VICTIM WAS IN OUT-OF-HOME CARE AT TIME OF INCIDENT, CHECK TYPE OF CARE: TYPE OF ABUSE *(CHECK ONE OR MORE)*
☐ YES   ☐ DAY CARE ☐ CHILD CARE CENTER ☐ FOSTER FAMILY HOME ☐ FAMILY FRIEND   ☐ PHYSICAL ☐ MENTAL ☐ SEXUAL ☐ NEGLECT
☐ NO   ☐ GROUP HOME OR INSTITUTION ☐ RELATIVE'S HOME   ☐ OTHER (SPECIFY)

| RELATIONSHIP TO SUSPECT | PHOTOS TAKEN? ☐ YES ☐ NO | DID THE INCIDENT RESULT IN THIS VICTIM'S DEATH? ☐ YES ☐ NO ☐ UNK |

D. INVOLVED PARTIES

VICTIM'S SIBLINGS

NAME	BIRTHDATE	SEX	ETHNICITY		NAME	BIRTHDATE	SEX	ETHNICITY
1.				3.				
2.				4.				

VICTIM'S PARENTS/GUARDIANS

| NAME (LAST, FIRST, MIDDLE) | BIRTHDATE OR APPROX. AGE | SEX | ETHNICITY |

| ADDRESS | Street | City | Zip | HOME PHONE ( ) | BUSINESS PHONE ( ) |

| NAME (LAST, FIRST, MIDDLE) | BIRTHDATE OR APPROX. AGE | SEX | ETHNICITY |

| ADDRESS | Street | City | Zip | HOME PHONE ( ) | BUSINESS PHONE ( ) |

SUSPECT

| SUSPECT'S NAME (LAST, FIRST, MIDDLE) | BIRTHDATE OR APPROX. AGE | SEX | ETHNICITY |

| ADDRESS | Street | City | Zip | TELEPHONE ( ) |

OTHER RELEVANT INFORMATION

E. INCIDENT INFORMATION

IF NECESSARY, ATTACH EXTRA SHEET(S) OR OTHER FORM(S) AND CHECK THIS BOX ☐   IF MULTIPLE VICTIMS, INDICATE NUMBER: _____

| DATE / TIME OF INCIDENT | PLACE OF INCIDENT |

NARRATIVE DESCRIPTION (What victim(s) said/what the mandated reporter observed/what person accompanying the victim(s) said/similar or past incidents involving the victim(s) or suspect)

SS 8572 (Rev. 12/02)   ***DEFINITIONS AND INSTRUCTIONS ON REVERSE***

DO NOT submit a copy of this form to the Department of Justice (DOJ). The investigating agency is required under Penal Code Section 11169 to submit to DOJ a Child Abuse Investigation Report Form SS 8583 if (1) an active investigation was conducted and (2) the incident was determined not to be unfounded.

WHITE COPY-Police or Sheriff's Department; BLUE COPY-County Welfare or Probation Department;   GREEN COPY- District Attorney's Office; YELLOW COPY-Reporting Party

Figure 43-5 Example of a mandated child abuse reporting form.

System (NCANDS) reports that two-thirds of cases of child abuse reported are investigated and the majority (56%) of those reports are made by healthcare professionals. These investigations have substantiated approximately 30% of reported cases of child abuse. The majority of child abuse cases (80%) involve children less than 4 years old.

Documentation

Proper reporting of suspected child abuse is important, in part, because the Paramedic is in a unique position to observe evidence of child neglect or maltreatment in the home setting. Paramedics are also the first "reporters" of child abuse, reporting the explanations offered to them. An abusive parent may collaborate with others or with the child to fabricate a story to explain the injuries. This deceit is often discovered when the physician compares the Paramedic's report to the parent's report.

When documenting child abuse, the Paramedic should avoid judgmental terms, such as "the mother was drunk," in favor of descriptive terms, such as "half empty beer bottles were strewn around the floor." These descriptions should be as specific and objective as possible.

The Paramedic should first start by describing the scene, then documenting the history, using the parent's and patient's own words as much as possible (the Paramedic should be sure to identify each quote). Next, the Paramedic should state what aroused the suspicion of child abuse. Finally, the Paramedic should note all protective actions taken, including calling for law enforcement (if needed), transporting the patient safely, reporting the suspicion to other mandated reporters, and fulfilling responsibilities as a mandated reporter.

Hearsay Exceptions

Under rules of law, hearsay testimony is generally not admissible in court as evidence of the truth of a matter. However, there is an exception made in certain situations.

When a person makes a statement while in the excitement of an event, called an excited utterance, this statement may be allowed into evidence. Not only is the verbal utterance considered a statement but the child's demeanor also has meaning. For example, a child's emotional response to a question, such as "Did Daddy hit you?" or a finger pointed at the genitals would be considered a statement. It is understood that a child may not be able to express himself in words but that he does have other means to express himself. Therefore, a Paramedic should note the child's response—such as trembling, crying, or pressured speech—when asked specific questions.

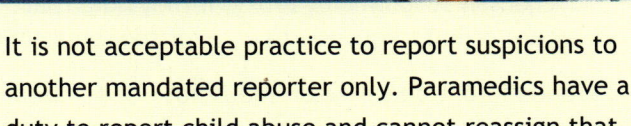

STREET SMART

It is not acceptable practice to report suspicions to another mandated reporter only. Paramedics have a duty to report child abuse and cannot reassign that responsibility to others.

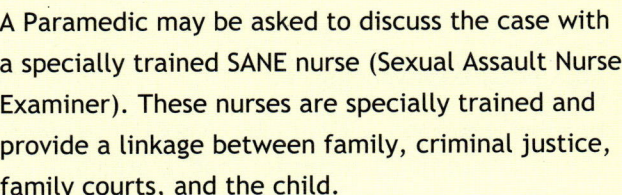

STREET SMART

A Paramedic may be asked to discuss the case with a specially trained SANE nurse (Sexual Assault Nurse Examiner). These nurses are specially trained and provide a linkage between family, criminal justice, family courts, and the child.

CONCLUSION

Although EMS scenes are often chaotic, especially when children are involved and comparatively little time is actually spent with the patient, the Paramedic's timely observation and reporting of child abuse can prevent the reoccurrence of child abuse and even save the child's life.

KEY POINTS:

- Child abuse includes both actions and inactions that predispose a child to risk of death or serious injury.

- Sexual abuse may include rape or sodomy, lesser degrees of fondling or exposure, or exploitation such as prostitution or pornography.

- Abuse may be psychological.

- Neglect occurs when adult caregivers fail to meet the child's responsibilities for food, clothing, shelter, medical care, or education.

- The Paramedic should obtain a complete psychosocial history from (about) the child and document answers plus behaviors.

- Some states have enacted "safe haven" acts enabling parents to leave infants in safe care as opposed to abandoning or killing them. The Paramedic should be aware of such an act in your state.

- After completing an initial exam, the Paramedic should perform a head-to-toe exam for bruising, human bites, burns, or fractures.

- Paramedics may be the key to recognizing Munchausen Syndrome by Proxy, if they note that they are called frequently to care for the same child.

- Sudden infant death syndrome is not due to child abuse.

- Parents may refuse care for their minor children. The Paramedic should contact medical control for assistance in convincing parents of the need for care.

- In addition to medical reasons for seizures, the Paramedic should consider the possibility of head trauma due to shaken baby syndrome.

- The Paramedic should know the procedure for reporting suspicion of child abuse in her state.

REVIEW QUESTIONS:

1. What is the definition of
   a. Child abuse
   b. Sexual abuse
   c. Sexual molestation
   d. Sexual exploitation
2. How does neglect differ from abuse?
3. What situational indicators predispose children to abuse?
4. What is the cycle of abuse? How does it affect families?

5. Describe each of the following physical patterns suggestive of child abuse.
   a. Bruising
   b. Bites
   c. Burns
   d. Fractures
6. What is Munchausen by Proxy Syndrome?
7. Name four possible causes of failure to thrive other than child neglect.

Please refer to the Case Study in this chapter, and answer the questions below:

1. What concerns should the Paramedics have based on their first interactions with the child and his mother?

2. What other assessments should the Paramedics perform when the child begins seizing?

3. Discuss the rationale for requesting a police unit for the mother's transport to the hospital.

4. What is the procedure for reporting suspicions of child abuse in your region?

> ◢ REFERENCES:

1. Markenson D, Tunik M, et al. A national assessment of knowledge, attitudes, and confidence of prehospital providers in the assessment and management of child maltreatment. *Pediatrics.* 2007;119(1):e103–e108.

2. Kinnane JM, Garrison HG, et al. Injury prevention: is there a role for out-of-hospital emergency medical services? *Acad Emerg Med.* 1997;4(4):306–312.

3. Vasquez E., Pitts K. Red flags during home visitation: infants and toddlers. *J Community Health Nurs.* 2006;23(2):123–131.

4. Markenson D, Foltin G, et al. Knowledge and attitude assessment and education of prehospital personnel in child abuse and neglect: report of a National Blue Ribbon Panel. *Prehosp Emerg Care.* 2002;6(3):261–272.

5. Child Abuse Prevention and Treatment Act, 42.U.S.C.A. §5106g.

6. Makoroff KL, Brauley JL, et al. Genital examinations for alleged sexual abuse of prepubertal girls: findings by pediatric emergency medicine physicians compared with child abuse trained physicians. *Child Abuse Negl.* 2002;26(12):1235–1242.

7. Besharov DJ. Responding to child sexual abuse: the need for a balanced approach. *Future Child.* 1994;4(2):135–155.

8. Lawson C. Mother-son sexual abuse: rare or underreported? A critique of the research. *Child Abuse Negl.* 1993;17(2):261–269.

9. Leonard BJ, Hellerstedt WL, et al. Association of maternal psychological functioning to pathology in child sexual abuse victims. *Issues Ment Health Nurs.* 1997;18(6):587–601.

10. Available at: **http://en.wikipedia.org/wiki/Mary_Ellen_Wilson**. Accessed February 10, 2009.

11. Available at: **http://www.americanhumane.org/about-us/who-we-are/history/mary-ellen.html**. Accessed February 10, 2009.

12. Fluke JD, Yuan YY, et al. Recurrence of maltreatment: an application of the National Child Abuse and Neglect Data System (NCANDS). *Child Abuse Negl.* 1999;23(7):633–650.

13. Kaplan SJ, Pelcovitz D, et al. Child and adolescent abuse and neglect research: a review of the past 10 years. Part I: Physical and emotional abuse and neglect. *J Am Acad Child Adolesc Psychiatry.* 1999;38(10):1214–1222.

14. Geist R, Grdisa V, et al. Psychosocial issues in the child with chronic conditions. *Best Pract Res Clin Gastroenterol.* 2003;17(2):141–152.

15. Denny C, Isaac R. The relation between child death and child maltreatment. *Arch Dis Child.* 2006;91(3):265–269.

16. Spinelli MG. Infanticide: contrasting views. *Arch Womens Ment Health.* 2005;8(1):15–24.

17. Oral R, Yagmur F, et al. Fatal abusive head trauma cases: consequence of medical staff missing milder forms of physical abuse. *Pediatr Emerg Care.* 2008: 24(12):816–821.

18. Kos L, Shwayder T. Cutaneous manifestations of child abuse. *Pediatr Dermatol.* 2006;23(4):311–320.

19. Thompson S. Accidental or inflicted? *Pediatr Ann.* 2005;34(5):372–381.

20. Mudd SS, Findlay JS. The cutaneous manifestations and common mimickers of physical child abuse. *J Pediatr Health Care.* 2004;18(3):123–129.

21. Ayoub C, Pfeifer D. Burns as a manifestation of child abuse and neglect. *Am J Dis Child.* 1979;133(9):910–914.

22. Galvin HK, Newton AW, et al. Update on Munchausen syndrome by proxy. *Curr Opin Pediatr.* 2005;17(2):252–257.

23. Altimier L. Shaken baby syndrome. *J Perinat Neonatal Nurs.* 2008;22(1):68–76; quiz 77–78.

24. Wyszynski ME. Shaken baby syndrome: identification, intervention, and prevention. *Clin Excell Nurse Pract.* 1999;3(5):262–267.

25. Tang J, Buzney SM, et al. Shaken baby syndrome: a review and update on ophthalmologic manifestations. *Int Ophthalmol Clin.* 2008;48(2):237–246.

SPECIAL PATIENTS

The final section of this volume covers the unique needs of several different types of patients. These special patient populations include geriatric patients, who have special considerations due to changes in physiology that come with aging as well as other potential impairments. Patients who are technology dependent, who are chronically ill, or who have different cultural backgrounds from our own are all patient populations that may have special needs. Finally, the subject of domestic violence and sexual assault is covered, providing the Paramedic with the tools to sensitively handle these situations.

44

GERIATRICS

KEY CONCEPTS:

Upon completion of this chapter, it is expected that the reader will understand these following concepts:

- How the increasing geriatric population affects emergency medical services
- That aging may contribute to disease, although not all diseases are the result of aging
- The change in communication style, assessment, treatment modalities, lifting, moving, and packaging required because of the older patient's bodily changes of aging

ANATOMY CONCEPTS:

Prior to reading this chapter the Paramedic student should be familiar with the following anatomy and physiology concepts:

- Baseline functions of all organ systems

Medic 32 is dispatched to the home of a 77-year-old female who has, according to her husband's 9-1-1 call, fainted several times and is experiencing dizziness and difficulty breathing. En route, the Paramedics discuss the possible reasons for the patient's problems and what their approach to the patient will be when they arrive.

CRITICAL THINKING QUESTIONS

1. What are some of the possible causes of syncope?
2. How is the patient's age related to the syncope?

OVERVIEW

Geriatric patients present with ailments that are unlike other patient populations due to changes in physiology that are a result of aging. It is also true that the human population as a whole is aging. For this reason, it is important that the Paramedic be familiar with the physical, cognitive, and psychosocial differences in the geriatric patient. But it is just as important for the Paramedic to realize that this population can also be active and vital contributors to society. The Paramedic must recognize that aging in itself is not a disease—but simply a development event beginning before birth. This chapter covers the last stage of life and how to respond to and treat this special patient population.

Geriatrics

"The aging of the U.S. population is one of the major public health challenges we face in the 21st century."

—Julie Louise Gerberdine, MD, MPH
*Director, Centers for Disease Control and Prevention,
U.S. Department of Health and Human Services 2007*

People are living longer than ever. In fact, the number of Americans ages 65 or older will double during the next 25 years.[1] Life expectancy in the United States has increased from 47 years for those born in 1900 to 77 years for those born in 1971. Because of this and the number of aging baby boomers, by 2030 the number of older Americans will reach 71 million, or roughly 20% of the U.S. population. [2,3]

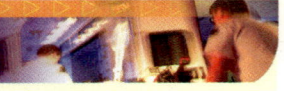

PROFESSIONAL PARAMEDIC

The U.S. Census Bureau reports that elderly persons 85 years old and over are projected to be the fastest growing part of the elderly population into the next century.

These factors have a major effect upon emergency medical services. Obesity, hip fractures, deteriorating mental health, and poor oral hygiene (including loss of all teeth) contribute to conditions that emergency care providers deal with every day in the elderly population. Although most think of the elderly as being thin (44% of elderly patients lose weight as they age), 19% gain weight and one in five is obese. Obesity in the elderly leads to cardiovascular disease, diabetes, and falls. [4] In addition, mental deterioration leads to malnutrition, falls, and noncompliance with medication schedules, as well as environmental problems. Oral problems also lead to malnutrition. Among the elderly population, falls accounted for 14,900 (43%) of all unintentional injury deaths in 2004. Hip fracture, the most serious

fall-related fracture, is a major contributor to death, disability, and diminished quality of life among older adults, and accounts for a significant number of EMS responses. [5,6]

Geriatrics is the study of all aspects of aging, including the psychological, pathological, economic, and sociological problems connected with aging. Aging can be defined as a progressive functional decline with age,[7] or the intrinsic, inevitable, and irreversible age-related process of loss of viability and increase in vulnerability.[8] Aging and senescence are often used interchangeably; however, senescence also refers to the ultimate disability of cells to reproduce themselves, leading to death of the organism.[9] Disease, on the other hand, is a disruption of bodily function, systems, or organs. Aging may contribute to disease, but not all diseases are the result of aging.

Chief Concern

In aging, there is a decline in every organ system, beginning at the cellular level. The total number of body cells decreases. There is a decline in total body water from around 60% of body weight to perhaps 40% to 50%. Body fat decreases 15% to 30% in the majority of people, but may increase in others. Metabolic rates remain fairly constant. The Paramedic must be aware of the changes due to aging in order to adequately assess the aging patient.

Cardiovascular System

Changes in the cardiovascular system begin with puberty and involve changes that occur in the arteries throughout life. Deposition of plaque and thickening of the arterial walls leads to atherosclerosis, arteriosclerosis, and hypertension due to decreased elasticity of the vessels. Atherosclerosis forms in all vessels, not preferentially to one location within the circulatory system. The presence of coronary artery disease increases the risk of stroke, ischemic heart disease, dysrhythmia, myocardial infarction (MI), and sudden cardiac death. By age 70, approximately 70% of individuals will have significant atherosclerosis, including asymptomatic disease.

Uncontrolled hypertension causes cardiomyopathy, left ventricular hypertrophy (LVH), and congestive heart failure due to the constant increased pressure the ventricle needs to overcome in order to maintain forward blood flow. Hypertension increases atherosclerosis, increases the likelihood of plaque rupture, and increases the likelihood of both hemorrhagic and ischemic stroke. Exercise tolerance decreases as the arterial system loses its elasticity. The patient's cardiac output decreases with normal aging, but is accelerated in patients with uncontrolled hypertension.

On the right side of the heart, cor pulmonale, or right heart failure, results from increased pressures in pulmonary circulation that can arise from any of a number of causes including emphysema, fibrotic tissue changes in the lungs, tumors, and other changes in lung tissue.

Blood vessels lose elasticity with age, leading to varicose veins. These are most commonly seen in the legs because of the increased venous pressures in the legs from standing. Coupled with a general slowdown in circulation, the risks of deep vein thrombosis (DVT) and pulmonary embolism (PE) are increased.

Respiratory System

Significant changes in lung tissue and pulmonary function result in loss of elasticity of lung tissue and loss of lung compliance. Normal lungs experience some regional atelectasis, or lower airway collapse, from time to time, often as a result of position. The amount of atelectasis increases with age due to the loss of elasticity in the airways. This increases the risk of developing pneumonia after surgery or with immobility.

Although the maximum size of the lungs (total lung capacity) does not change with age, functional residual capacity (FRC) and residual volume (RV) both increase so that inspiratory capacity (IC) and vital capacity (VC) both decline. This leads to decreased exercise tolerance, reduced ability to adjust to stress, and a decline in the activities of daily living. The differences of lung capacities from an average 25-year-old to an average 75-year-old can be striking (Figure 44-1).

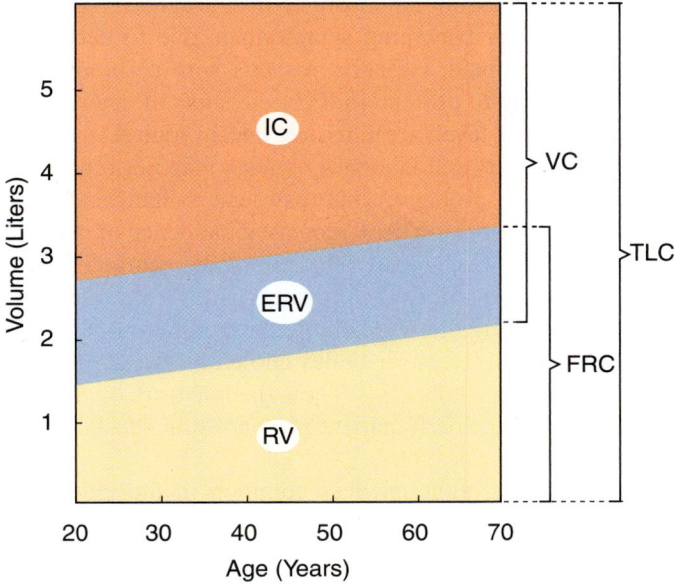

Figure 44-1 Differences in lung capacities.

Elderly patients are susceptible to many chronic lung diseases, including emphysema, chronic bronchitis, bronchiolitis, lung cancer, and interstitial fibrosis. Many of these conditions develop after chronic bombardment with toxic substances (e.g., cigarette smoke or asbestos). As the immune system declines, patients with underlying chronic lung diseases become more susceptible to pulmonary infections. Those patients who continue to smoke compound their risks.

Respiratory system problems also often coexist with other chronic diseases such as diabetes, coronary heart disease, arthritis, kidney disease, and immune system decline.

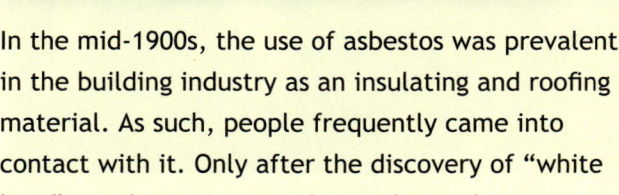

STREET SMART

In the mid-1900s, the use of asbestos was prevalent in the building industry as an insulating and roofing material. As such, people frequently came into contact with it. Only after the discovery of "white lung" or asbestosis was asbestos banned as an insulating material.

Nervous System

The nervous system declines in many different ways with age. In disease-free individuals, intellectual performance may remain quite normal until the eighth and ninth decades of life, although processing of thoughts and tasks may take longer.[10] There are also changes in the size of the brain. Brain weight decreases an average of 10% between early adulthood and age 90, and the area of the brain occupied by the ventricles increases with age-related brain atrophy. However, these changes do not appear to correlate with changes in intelligence.

Several neurological changes and conditions may impair activities of daily living.[11] Brain atrophy and decreased brain size increase the risk of subdural hematomas due to stretching of the bridging veins that span the space from the dura to the brain tissue. Decreased cerebral blood flow, especially in diabetics, also contributes to atrophy and microvascular disease and ischemia. For example, synapse time and decreased nerve conduction velocity slows reflexes as people age. Decreased dopamine synthesis and Parkinson's disease both produce movement disorders that can cause falls. As people age, many people develop insomnia and an impaired ability to adjust to temperature changes. As a result, elderly patients typically find that they are more prone to forgetfulness, fatigue, and trouble with balance, which can increase the risk of fall injuries.

Some patients experience various types of dementia, including Alzheimer's disease (Figure 44-2), depression, increased susceptibility to drug effects, and tumors. An abrupt decline in any system or function is always due to disease,

Delmar/Cengage Learning

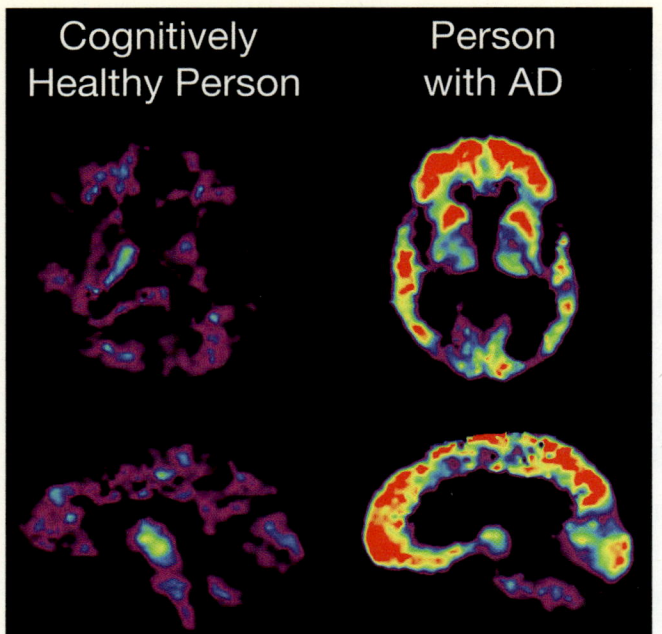

Figure 44-2 Brain scan comparison of normal brain and brain of patient with Alzheimer's disease.

not aging. Patients react differently to aging; however, some aspects of aging can be attenuated by limiting risk factors such as smoking, hypertension, and sedentary lifestyle.[11]

One of the challenges in evaluating elderly patients is differentiating between delirium and dementia. EMS are often requested when a family member, close friend, or nursing home staff member identifies a change in mental status from the patient's usual baseline. An elderly patient with an altered mental state should not automatically be assumed to be senile or suffering from dementia. As discussed previously, many patients suffer from one of the many forms of **dementia**, causing a gradual cognitive decline as the condition progresses. In contrast, **delirium** occurs as an acute and typically reversible change in mental status from the patient's baseline mental status. Any of a large number of disease processes can produce temporary delirium, causing changes that may present along a spectrum from an alert patient who is confused to a completely unresponsive patient. The most common cause of delirium is an infection, with urinary tract and respiratory infections as the most common infections in the elderly.

▷▷▷▷▷▷▷▷▷▷▷▷▷▷▷

STREET SMART

If a patient experiences any abrupt decline in any system or function, its cause should be considered to be due to disease and not aging.

Endocrine System

All organs decline in function as people age. However, a decline in thyroid function, ovarian function, and testicular function can result in decreased energy, decreased heat or cold tolerance, and weight gain. Weight gain may lead to type 2 diabetes with insulin resistance. In some cases, insulin production may decrease.

Diabetes has serious implications for the elderly. Effects on the vascular system lead to heart disease and increased risk for heart attack. Peripheral circulatory problems can result in impaired circulation in the extremities, particular in the lower extremities. These circulatory issues cause neuropathy and poorly healing ulcers and infections in the lower extremities, which may worsen over time to the point where amputation is required. Circulatory changes from diabetes can also cause failure of the kidneys and other organs. Neurological effects of diabetes result in decreased pain sensation, which is responsible for "silent myocardial infarction," or a myocardial infarction that presents without the usual chest pain. Elderly females are particularly prone to "silent MI."

Gastrointestinal System

Many gastrointestinal system changes occur with aging For example, saliva production decreases, leading to dry mouth, tongue soreness, and difficulty chewing and swallowing. Hydrochloric acid production decreases, leading to increased digestion time. Bowel motility decreases, leading to slower movement of food through the intestines. Taste buds fail so that food tastes bland, leading to overuse of salt and other seasonings, as well as a diminished desire to eat. Gums atrophy and become sore, leading to difficult and inefficient chewing. Tooth loss makes chewing difficult and inefficient.

Abdominal disorders also constitute a significant problem for the elderly. Abdominal disorders may progress to dangerous levels before becoming symptomatic due to decreased ability to sense pain. Geriatric patients with peritonitis are much less likely to present with classic signs of acute abdomen, as their pain levels are much less than in younger patients, many are afebrile, and laboratory values may not reflect the seriousness of a problem. This may lead to increased time intervals before seeking help, increased incidence of delay in treatment, and misdiagnosis. The Paramedic can be of great value in ensuring proper treatment by taking careful patient histories and doing thorough physical examinations.[12]

Biliary tract disease includes cholelithiasis, cholecystitis, and ascending cholangitis. These disorders are often more serious, with the elderly patient presenting in sepsis due to diminished pain sensation.

Appendicitis, although less common in the elderly, is much more serious. Whereas only about 10% of acute appendicitis cases occur in patients over 60 years of age, half of all deaths from appendicitis occur in this group. The rate of perforation in elderly patients is approximately 50% higher than in younger adults, largely because elderly patients tend to wait more than 24 hours before seeking help.[12]

Although mesenteric ischemia is rare, the condition is 70% to 90% fatal, and delay in treatment increases the risk greatly. The pathophysiology of mesenteric ischemia is similar to that of embolic stroke or myocardial infarction where a clot lodges in the arterial supply to the gut, causing ischemia and necrosis. Risk factors for mesenteric ischemia include untreated atrial fibrillation, vascular disease, and low cardiac output.[12] Mesenteric ischemia produces pain that is diffuse and out of proportion to the findings on the abdominal examination.

Bowel obstruction accounts for about 12% of abdominal pain in the elderly, exacerbated by decreased physical activity and overuse of laxatives to treat perceived constipation.[12] Chronic constipation increases the risk of a volvulus, or a twisting of the large intestine at the sigmoid colon. Malignancy is another leading cause of bowel obstruction in the elderly, whether from primary colon cancer or from metastatic cancer. Malignancy accounts for approximately 10% of abdominal problems in the elderly.

Abdominal aortic aneurysm is more common in the elderly than other populations, and men are seven times more likely to develop an abdominal aortic aneurysm than women. Abdominal aortic aneurysms can mimic renal colic (kidney stones) and musculoskeletal back pain. Among patients with abdominal aneurisms, 80% who present in shock will not survive.[12]

Peptic ulcer disease (PUD) is increasing in the elderly, possibly because of increased use of nonsteroidal anti-inflammatory drugs. Mortality in elderly patients with peptic ulcer disease is about 100 times higher than in younger patients. The most common sign of PUD is melena, but even perforation may be painless.[12] The Paramedic should rule out gastroenteritis in elderly patients who present with vomiting and diarrhea. Half of elderly patients with appendicitis are initially diagnosed as having gastroenteritis.[12]

Diverticulosis and diverticulitis are 85% likely to present with pain in the left colon. Elderly patients with left lower quadrant pain should be assumed to have diverticulitis until proven otherwise. Hematochezia may or may not be present in these cases. Even though infection is present, many patients will be afebrile and misdiagnosed as simply being constipated.[12]

Other conditions in the paramedical list of differential diagnoses of abdominal pain in elderly patients include hernias, herpes zoster, myocardial infarction, pancreatitis, pneumonia, urinary tract obstruction, and pneumonia.

Urinary System

The patient's kidney structure and function deteriorate with aging and senescence. As one ages, the number of nephrons is decreased, arterial blood flow to the kidneys is reduced, and there is less clearance of waste products from the blood. Arterial changes result in decreased renal blood flow, decreased renal clearance of drugs and toxins, decreased glomerular

function, and chronic kidney failure. These changes may be accelerated by comorbid conditions such as hypertension, atherosclerosis, and heart failure.

Most Paramedics will encounter patients in end-stage renal failure at some time. Many of these patients, who may be encountered either in the patient's home or a dialysis center, will be dialysis dependent. It is important for the Paramedic to understand the problems caused by kidney failure.

The Paramedic should be familiar with the terminology used in describing patients with kidney disease. **Chronic kidney disease (CKD)** is the preferred term for patients who have impaired kidney function but are not in end-stage disease. **End-stage renal disease (ESRD)** describes those who will progress to the stage where they will need continuous dialysis or kidney transplant. Other terms, such as pre-ESRD, chronic renal insufficiency, chronic renal failure, acute kidney injury (AKI), and chronic renal disease, may be seen in patient records and in articles on the subject.

The Paramedic should understand the five stages of CKD, since patients with kidney disease will often relate what stage of disease they are in during their interactions with the Paramedic. The basic laboratory tests that identify CKD are an increase in serum urea nitrogen (BUN) and serum creatinine, along with a decrease in glomerular filtration rate (GFR). The stages of CKD are based upon GFR (Table 44-1), the rate at which the kidneys filter toxins from the blood.

Patients in Stages 4 or 5 may present with significant electrolyte imbalances, cardiac dysrhythmias, and even cardiac arrest. Calls for cardiac arrests at dialysis centers require that the Paramedic be familiar with the special demands of resuscitation of dialysis patients.

Table 44-1 The Five Stages of Chronic Kidney Disease

Stage 1:	Normal or increased GFR ($>= 90$ mL/min/1.73m²) with some evidence of kidney damage. The emphasis is on diagnosis, treatment, and prevention of disease progression.
Stage 2:	Mildly decreased GFR (60 to 89 mL/min/1.73m²) with some evidence of kidney damage. There is still interest in diagnosis and treatment of the underlying cause but the emphasis is shifting toward prevention of disease progression.
Stage 3:	Moderately decreased GFR (30 to 59 mL/min/1.73m²). The emphasis is still on preventing disease progression but the evaluation and treatment of complications are becoming more of an issue.
Stage 4:	Severely decreased GFR (15 to 29 mL/min/1.73m²). The emphasis is generally on treating complications and preparing for dialysis or kidney transplantation.
Stage 5:	Very little GFR left (< 15 mL/min/1.73m²). Treating complications becomes increasingly difficult and dialysis is usually started at this point.

Besides renal problems, elderly patients commonly experience bladder problems. Women experience bladder incontinence, which may be caused by decreased bladder sphincter tone or damage to the nerves that control bladder function. Incontinence can range from minor leakage to involuntary bladder emptying at inappropriate times. Women are also more prone to urinary tract infections. Men typically experience problems with urination resulting from enlargement of the prostate gland. The term **benign prostatic hyperplasia or hypertrophy (BPH)** applies to most men over the age of 50. The cardinal signs of BPH are **urinary hesitancy** (difficulty beginning to urinate), **urinary urgency** (a sudden, compelling urge to urinate), and **urinary frequency** (the need to urinate often). Because of the inability to empty the bladder completely, many patients with BPH experience **nocturia**, or frequent waking during sleep to urinate, that interrupts the sleep cycle. Patients may also have to strain to urinate, and often there is a weak urinary stream with stopping and starting. Acute urinary retention, or inability to urinate at all, may lead to extreme lower abdominal distress and distention requiring catheterization. BPH also increases the elderly male's risk of developing a urinary tract infection.

Many older men with BPH will be taking alpha 1 adrenergic receptor blockers such as terazosin (Hytrin®), prazosin (Minipres®), and dutasteride (Avodart®), a testosterone-converting enzyme inhibitor, which is used to shrink the prostate and reverse the effects of BPH. The Paramedic should be familiar with the drugs commonly prescribed for BPH patients. Some EMS services allow Paramedics to insert Foley catheters in patients with acute urinary retention where transport times to a hospital are prolonged.

Musculoskeletal System

Muscle mass decreases with aging, leading to loss of strength and loss of height. Height loss, a common occurrence with aging, reflects osteoporosis as well as loss of muscle tone and connective tissue. Women experience greater height loss than men; however, significant height loss (>3 cm) correlates to increased mortality from cardiovascular and respiratory conditions.[13]

Arthritis can affect any joint and result in stiffness, loss of flexibility, and pain. Calcium loss leads to osteoporosis, which can lead to loss of bone strength and size, and increase the risk of falls and fractures.

Kyphosis, or an increase of the normal forward curve of the thoracic spine (Figure 44-3), can result from a number of processes, including normal loss of muscle tone, osteoporosis, arthritis, ankylosing spondylitis, and tumors, among other things. Kyphosis in the elderly patient presents a problem for EMS providers when a patient must be placed on a spineboard. Padding must be used in all spaces when transporting these patients to minimize the possibility of pressure injury. Kyphosis in itself may cause reduced ventilatory function and volumes because rib excursion and lung expansion are affected by the thoracic curvature. Studies show that elderly patients with kyphosis are at greater risk for respiratory and cardiovascular diseases and higher mortality rates.[14,15] Patients with ankylosing spondylitis present challenges in intubation, since vertebrae are fused together and hyperextension of the neck can result in spinal fracture or limited neck mobility.

Sensory Organs Changes

Several changes occur in the sensory organs as people age, which may impair some activities of daily living. Balance and ambulation may also become an issue with some patients due to these changes.

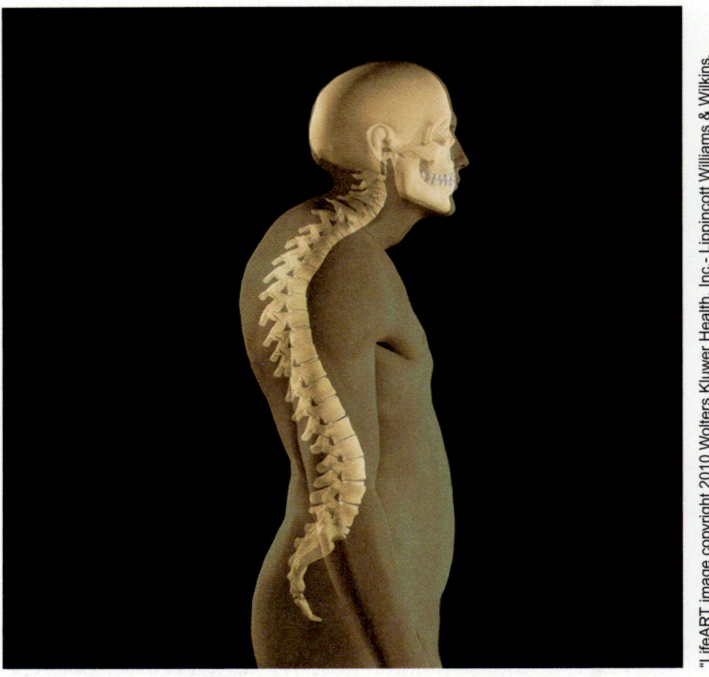

Figure 44-3 This patient has kyphosis, an increase in the normal forward curvature of the thoracic spine.

Eyes and Vision

Beginning with middle age, many patients develop **hyperopia** or **presbyopia**, also known as farsightedness. This is a steadily progressive occurrence and often requires patients to have prescription lenses that must be changed at regular intervals.

Pupil size decreases with age, resulting in a lessened ability to compensate for changes in light. The patient's ability to focus is decreased, and the amount of light reaching the retina is greatly diminished, leading to poor night vision and increased time to accommodate to low light. Color vision and contrast discrimination also diminish, and green–blue vision may decline. Peripheral vision narrows, leading to patients bumping into things and failing to see obstacles in their path. Glare is more apparent. All these changes can lead to traumatic injuries and lifestyle changes, such as preventing driving.

The lenses of the eye thicken, causing cataracts which result in blurred vision. Decreased lacrimation, or tear production, leads to dry eye. Eyelid drooping, or ptosis, may be noticeable, along with changes in pigment deposition that produce a bluish circle around the outer edge of the iris, called **arcus senilis**. Diabetic patients may experience diabetic retinopathy, which can result in blindness.

Hearing

Hearing loss due to aging is known as **presbycusis**. The aging patient often experiences loss of the high frequency range of hearing due to atrophy of the structures of the ear. Further, loss of cochlear hair cells may lead to impaired balance, increasing the risk of falls. Hearing problems are generally described as conductive or sensorineural. Conductive hearing problems may be caused by obstructions in the external ear canal such as buildup of cerumen, tumors, a collection of blood or fluid in the inner ear, and tympanic membrane injury. Sensorineural hearing problems may be caused by prolonged exposure to loud noise, head trauma, and some medications (e.g., aspirin).[16]

Immune System

As one ages, there is a decreased number and function of some of the specific immune system cells that affect the individual's ability to fight infection and other conditions (e.g., cancer). The thymus gland, located in the upper chest, is at its largest and most active during childhood and decreases in size with age starting in puberty. The thymus gland is responsible for producing T-cells, which fight certain invasive conditions (e.g., cancer). As the thymus gland decreases in size, the T-cells produced do not function as well as T-cells manufactured during childhood.

B-cells, another type of immune cell, also do not function as well as one ages even though the number of cells remains somewhat constant throughout life. The B-cells primarily fight infections. With the decline in B-cell function that accompanies aging, the elderly are more susceptible to illness.

Antibody production and function also decline with age. As one ages, fewer antibodies are produced, which also decreases the body's ability to fight infections. As antibody function declines, the elderly individual may start to lose immunity against conditions he was immunized against. Finally, as one ages it becomes more likely that one's immune system will turn against the body's own tissues and develop one of the many autoimmune diseases.

The Skin and Connective Tissue

The body's appearance changes because of changes in the skin and connective tissue. Collagen and connective tissue loss lead to loss of thickness and elasticity of skin, wrinkling, and increased risk of injury. Minor falls and contusions can lead to skin tears and bleeding into the tissues. In addition, the number of sweat glands declines, leading to dry skin and poor cooling in hot environments.

Damage from exposure to the sun increases the incidence of **melanoma** (a form of skin cancer) and causes **senile keratosis**, a small rough spot on skin. **Lentigines**, also called liver spots, age spots, or sun spots, are so-called because of their liver-like color. They are not related to liver problems. True lentigines are harmless and do not require treatment.

One risk for elderly patients who are immobilized or bedridden are decubitus ulcers (Figure 44-4a–d). **Decubitus ulcers** form from pressure on the skin, typically over bony prominences, secondary to immobility. Decubitus ulcers are graded from 1 through 4 based on the depth of the ulcer (Table 44-2).[17] Necrotic tissue often forms around or within the ulcer and must be removed, or debrided, periodically. The tissue inside the ulcer, at the ulcer edges, or the surrounding intact tissue can become infected, causing fever and delirium in the bedridden patient.

Another common occurrence is skin and muscle breakdown when an elderly person falls and is unable to get up, either secondary to injury or lack of strength. These patients are at risk for developing hypothermia from lying uncovered on a floor that is typically a lower temperature than room temperature. These patients are also at risk for developing rhabdomyolysis, the rapid breakdown of muscle from trauma, secondary to lying immobile on the hard surface for a significant amount of time. Rhabdomyolysis in seen in patients who are immobile for prolonged periods of time. Patients with normally decreased kidney function, secondary to aging, can develop acute renal failure faster than a younger person with healthier kidneys. Patients immobilized on the floor for long periods of time often urinate or defecate on themselves, setting the stage for cellulitis and other infections.

Table 44-2 Staging System for Decubitus Ulcers

Stage 1	Intact skin with erythema that does not blanch with palpation
Stage 2	Partial thickness skin loss that does not extend deeper than the dermis
Stage 3	Full thickness skin loss that does not extend below the fascia
Stage 4	Full thickness skin loss involving the muscle and bone

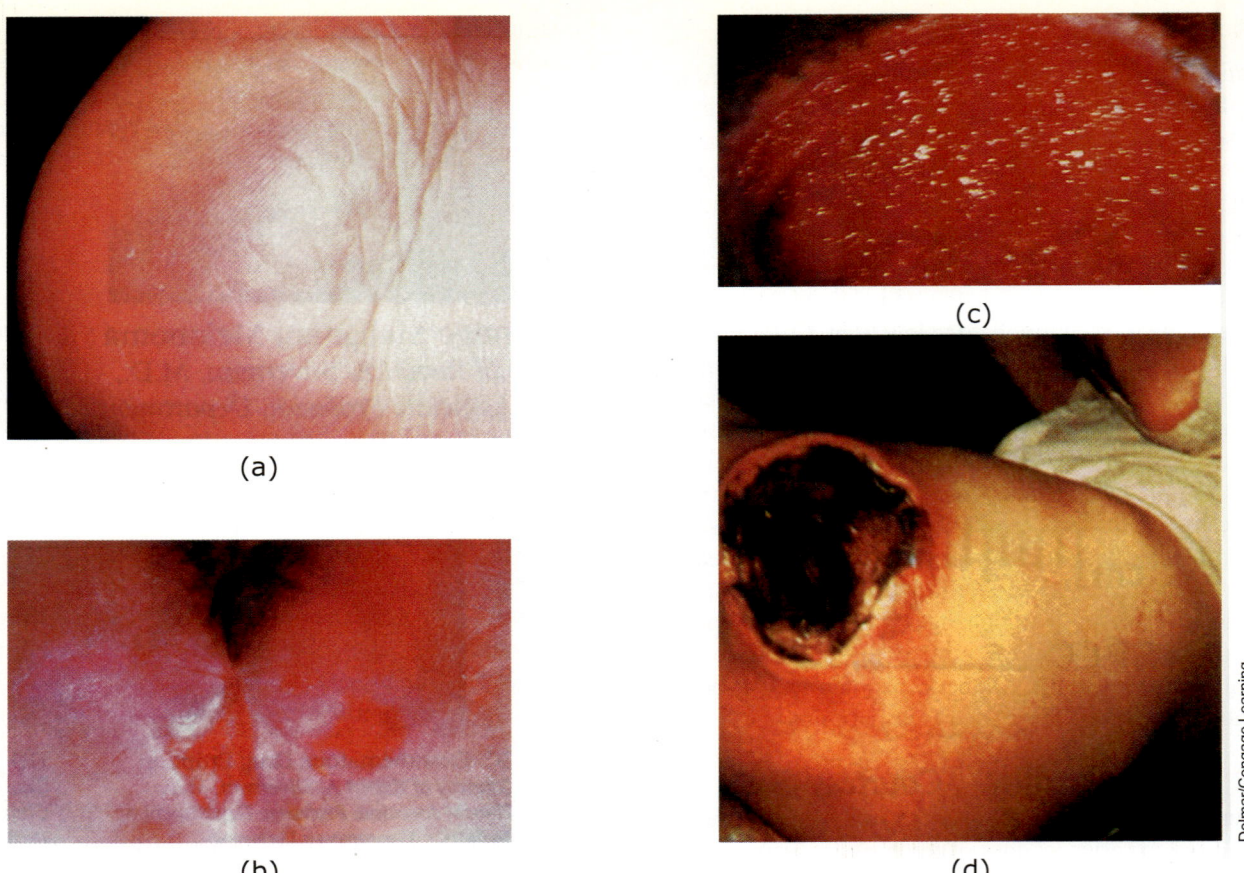

Figure 44-4 Decubitus ulcer by stage: (a) Stage 1, (b) Stage 2, (c) Stage 3, (d) Stage 4.

CASE STUDY (CONTINUED)

The Paramedics arrive at a residence in an upscale subdivision and are met at the door by Herb Jones, the patient's husband. He appears to be agitated and concerned. He leads them into the den where they find Barbara, his wife, seated in a recliner.

The Paramedics' first impression is of a woman who looks to be her stated age of 77, about 5'6" in height, and approximately 200 pounds. Her skin is pale and diaphoretic. She appears to be frightened. Mrs. Jones tells them that she has fainted several times and that now she is dizzy and short of breath. She was incontinent during one of her syncopal episodes. She denies any chest pain, but says that she has vomited once and feels nauseated. She states that she has difficulty walking because she has had a recent knee replacement, and that her feet and ankles are swollen. She further advises that she has type 2 diabetes which was diagnosed approximately 10 years ago.

Herb presents her medication bottles and the Paramedics note that Barbara takes lisinopril, metoprolol, aspirin, Metformin, and Glipizide. She has been taking her medications as prescribed.

CRITICAL THINKING QUESTIONS

1. What are the important elements of the history that a Paramedic should obtain?
2. What is the symptom pattern for cardiac-related syncope?

History

Although the history taking process is similar in elderly patients to non-elderly patients, the Paramedic may need to modify some of his questions in order to obtain an accurate history. In some cases, the elderly patient's chief concern is generic or vague; for example, "I am weak and dizzy" or "I don't feel well." The Paramedic may need to ask specific clarifying questions in order to get at the root of the concern. It is also important for the Paramedic to ask about episodes of chest pain or pressure and difficulty breathing. These may not be the patient's chief concern but are pertinent positives or negatives when the chief concern is vague.

In elderly patients who suffer from chronic disease processes, it is important to identify acute changes in function and condition, especially when the chief concern is vague. Symptoms that may be easily brushed off by the Paramedic since they have been present for a long period of time may indeed have a pertinent acute change the Paramedic will miss if the patient is not questioned. When encountering symptoms or a chief concern that on the surface appears to have been present for a long time, it is important for the Paramedic to ask what is different about the chief concern or the symptom today in relation to the normal symptom. In other words, what has changed about the concern or symptom that made the patient call for an ambulance? These questions may help the patient reflect on her symptoms and help the Paramedic better focus his history.

The decline in the patient's sensory organs may also provide challenges to obtaining an accurate history. Loss of hearing may affect the accuracy of information obtained by the Paramedic. Rather than speaking louder, the Paramedic should position herself in front of the patient so she can be seen by the patient and speak clearly, annunciating her words. The Paramedic should allow sufficient time for the patient to answer the questions without interrupting. For patients with visual impairment, the Paramedic should verbalize any assessments or procedures before performing them on the patient. Positioning oneself in front of the patient will help for patients who have difficulties with their peripheral vision.

Patients with difficulty breathing may have any number of medical problems including bacterial, viral, and fungal infections in the lungs; congestive heart failure and acute pulmonary edema; tumors; pneumothorax; pulmonary embolism; and chronic lung conditions such as interstitial fibrosis, emphysema, bronchiolitis, and chronic bronchitis.

A patient with dizziness and syncope may have any number of possible problems. Heart failure is a common cause of dizziness and syncope in the elderly patient. Cardiac dysrhythmias can produce syncope and dizziness if cardiac output is not sufficient to maintain adequate perfusion of the brain. Low blood pressure can result in dizziness, and may be the result of medical problems or overmedication. Dehydration and bleeding must also be ruled out in the patient with syncope.

Any elderly patient complaining of dizziness and syncope should be suspected of having a myocardial infarction or congestive heart failure. The diabetic patient is at increased risk for both. The risks of "silent MI" in diabetics, particularly diabetic women, are magnified. Alterations in blood glucose level may also produce somewhat vague symptoms.

When the Paramedic is obtaining a past medical and surgical history, the mnemonic SAMPLED is useful for obtaining a thorough history. **Polypharmacy**, or the use of a large number of prescribed medications, increases the risk of side effects and errors that may account for vague or unrelated symptoms. Ascertaining the presence of advanced directives is important for any patient with potentially critical pathology so that her wishes can be honored. Prior medical problems, surgeries, and current medications all may provide clues to the Paramedic in determining the cause of a patient's symptoms. After obtaining the patient's current medications, the Paramedic should ask if any doses have changed, medications have stopped, or new medications have been added. The timing of these changes may also provide important clues to the origin of the patient's chief concern.

The Paramedic assesses Mrs. Jones's vital signs and determines that her pulse rate is normal. She is placed on the pulse oximetry, and the monitor on her finger reveals that her oxygen saturation is 94% on room air. The Paramedic places her on oxygen by nasal cannula at 4 liters per minute and continues assessing her vital signs The Paramedic reports that her pulse rate is 64, her blood pressure is 106/66, her respirations are 24, her blood glucose level is 276, her temperature is 98.4°F, and her oxygen saturation is now 100% on oxygen.

The other Paramedic recognizes the potential that Mrs. Jones may be having a "silent MI" because of her diabetic history and therefore acquires a 12-lead ECG, which shows ST-elevation in Leads II, III, and aVF, with ST-depression in aVL and in Leads V2, V3, and V4. The Paramedic then obtains a right-sided ECG which demonstrates a 2 mm ST-elevation in the V4R lead. The rest of the Paramedic's physical examination reveals that Mrs. Jones has elevated jugular venous pressure while sitting upright, clear lungs, normal heart tones, and no peripheral edema.

CRITICAL THINKING QUESTIONS

1. What is the significance of the elevated ST-segment?
2. Why is a 12-lead ECG a critical element in this examination?

Examination

As with all encounters, the Paramedic first assesses the patient for life-threatening conditions that require immediate attention during the primary survey. If no immediate life-saving interventions are necessary, the Paramedic should perform a focused physical assessment in a conscious and responsive patient based upon the patient's chief concern. Assessment of the elderly patient presents unique challenges to the Paramedic. Not only must the Paramedic understand the physical changes that occur with age, but he must also understand how those changes alter vital signs and presentation of medical conditions.

The first task in assessing any patient is to do a visual head-to-toe assessment. Does the patient look sick or not sick? If the patient looks sick, does she look "a little sick" or "really sick"? If the patient looks "really sick," is there something that must be done immediately to save her life?

The patient's airway must be assessed for patency. However, elderly patients may have false teeth or bridgework that may obstruct the airway. Elderly patients also choke on food more easily than younger patients, and the possibility of upper airway obstruction must always be considered. Noisy respirations always trigger further investigation and immediate intervention in the case of upper airway obstructions. Since noisy respirations may be the result of fluid in the upper airway, suction should always be quickly available. Stroke patients often lose the ability to swallow their saliva and other upper airway secretions. If your patient cannot speak clearly, she may not be able to swallow.

On respiratory examination, it is normal for some elderly patients to have mild fine rales (crackles) in the bases of their lungs on auscultation. However, rales in the setting of acute dyspnea or diffuse among all lung fields often requires immediate intervention. The Paramedic should note other adventitious sounds during auscultation, as consolidation of lung tissue produces a loud sound compared to normal breath sounds. Tumors, blood, or fluid collection will produce no sounds at all. The Paramedic should be aware that some patients may have had a lung surgically removed, which will also demonstrate absent or decreased lung sounds. Tactile fremitus, or vibrations caused by speech, may also be present in the setting of pneumonia or bronchitis.

Vital signs may signal significant changes from normal. For example, a resting sinus tachycardia is unusual and should be investigated. Causes of sinus tachycardia can be hypovolemia, hypoxemia, and altered cardiac function. Sinus tachycardia may also be a response to stress such as exertion, emotional distress, responses to temperature changes, and other stressful conditions.

Elderly patients generally have higher blood pressures than younger patients when not controlled by medications. A rule of thumb for normal systolic blood pressure is to take the patient's age plus 100, up to 140 systolic. Target blood pressures for patients on antihypertensive medications are around 120/80; therefore, a blood pressure below the target range may signal shock. Any patient with a blood pressure lower than normal for the patient's age—showing other signs of shock such as cool, pale, and diaphoretic skin; nausea; and vomiting—should immediately be evaluated for shock and treated accordingly.

Assessment of an elderly patient with dizziness and syncope involves obtaining vital signs, assessment of the cardiorespiratory system, and acquisition of a 12-lead electrocardiogram. Assessment of heart sounds are limited in the field as it is difficult to hear heart sounds in a noisy environment; however, the Paramedic should be able to identify the S1 and S2 sounds easily. Some patients with heart failure will have an S3 sound, which may be audible. When assessing a patient with dizziness and syncope, the Paramedic should consider the possibility of stroke or medication interaction.

An elderly patient with signs of shock and no obvious reason for hypovolemia must be evaluated for occult bleeding, dehydration, vasogenic (septic) shock, hypoxia, and cardiogenic shock. A patient's heart rate may not respond as expected due to beta blockers or other medications; thus, subtle signs of shock may be absent. Patients may not be able to adjust for shock as easily as younger individuals and, as such, advance more rapidly through the stages of shock.

The Paramedic should also consider the possibility of a cardiovascular or neurologic event preceding a fall. Often, the events leading up to a fall may not be clear to the patient. Some patients may blame the fall on tripping on a rug or other object or being unsteady. The Paramedic should examine the patient thoroughly not only for injuries but for signs that may indicate an alternative cause for the fall.

CASE STUDY (CONTINUED)

Despite the absence of a complaint of chest pain, the Paramedic treats the patient as if she has acute coronary syndrome. This treatment includes starting an intravenous access. However, the nitroglycerine is withheld at this time because of the possibility of an inferior wall ischemia with right ventricular extension.

CRITICAL THINKING QUESTIONS

1. What are the elements of the physical examination of an elderly patient with suspected acute coronary syndrome?
2. What diagnosis did the Paramedic announce to the patient?

Assessment

As discussed previously, the Paramedic must always consider underlying cardiovascular, neurological, and diabetic conditions that affect the patient's symptoms. This is especially true when the history is vague or difficult to obtain because of the patient's mental status. This uncertainty broadens the paramedical differential diagnosis and in some cases makes the Paramedic's decision making more complex. A thorough history and physical will often lead the Paramedic to the most likely conditions responsible for the patient's symptoms.

CASE STUDY (CONTINUED)

The Paramedic administers aspirin 325 mg and starts two intravenous lines in each of Barbara's antecubital veins. The Paramedic advises her partner that rapid transport is indicated and starts giving a fluid bolus of 500 mL normal saline while her partner prepares the stretcher for Barbara. Barbara says that she can walk to the stretcher, but they tell her not to try to get up. They place Barbara on the stretcher and move her to the ambulance. They also place her in the high Fowler's position to minimize breathing difficulty.

CRITICAL THINKING QUESTIONS

1. What is the national standard of care of patients with suspected acute coronary syndrome?
2. What are some of the patient-specific concerns and considerations that the Paramedic should consider when applying this plan of care that is intended to treat a broad patient population presenting with acute coronary syndrome?

Treatment

Some treatments may require modification in the elderly population. For example, medication dosages often need to be decreased in the elderly due to decreased medication clearance through the liver and kidneys. This is especially true with medications that may cause sedation or respiratory depression as a side effect. Baseline dementia or delirium caused by the acute condition decreases the patient's mental status to compensate for certain medications. In cases where the mental status issues are combined with a decreased respiratory functional capacity, the elderly patient is more at risk for apnea with sedating medications. It is better for the Paramedic to use shorter acting medications that are titrated to effect and avoid overadministration of medications.

Spinal motion restriction and splinting are other treatments that may require modification. Additional padding is often required during spinal immobilization due to the loss of muscle mass, thinner skin, and spinal deformity, such as occurs with kyphosis. Spinal motion restriction on a long spine board causes increased tissue pressures in healthy volunteers.[18] This places the elderly patient at risk for tissue ischemia. Padding not only provides a more comfortable immobilization surface, but also allows sturdier immobilization and decreases the risk of tissue breakdown.

Similarly, suspected or obvious fractures should be immobilized with additional padding in order to protect the skin. This is especially important when the bone is tenting the skin. This increased pressure, combined with less physiological padding, puts the elderly patient at risk for turning a closed fracture into an open fracture. Additional padding also prevents additional pressure from affecting the fragile skin, which may lead to the beginning of pressure sores.

The Paramedic should calmly and clearly explain any assessments or procedures performed on the elderly patient. Changes in the senses accompanying age combined with rough handling can produce significant anxiety in the elderly patient. This anxiety can exacerbate the patient's current condition.

Maintaining normal body temperature is also important when treating the elderly patient. Between the loss of skin thickness, fat layer, and muscle thickness and the decreased ability to regulate body temperature, the elderly patient is more susceptible to hypothermia, even in mild temperatures. Conversely, if the patient is bundled too much, his body temperature can rise dangerously due to the inability to regulate temperature.

CASE STUDY (CONTINUED)

During the course of the transport to the hospital, the patient's blood pressure starts to drop precipitously. Fortunately, the Paramedic had already established two intravenous lines and is able to counteract the hypotension with a fluid bolus.

CRITICAL THINKING QUESTIONS

1. What are some of the predictable complications associated with acute inferior wall myocardial ischemia?
2. What are some of the predictable complications associated with acute inferior wall myocardial ischemia with right ventricular extension?

Evaluation

Reassessing the patient is a key factor to evaluating the response of the therapies administered by the Paramedic and detecting changes in physiological status. Continually monitoring vital signs in the elderly is especially important when the Paramedic has administered medications that can affect the patient's vital signs. Nitrates, rate control medications, analgesics, sedatives, and vasopressors are all medications that can significantly affect the elderly patient's vital signs, even in small doses. Maintaining a normal body temperature and providing comfortable transport with reassurance will also decrease the stressors on the elderly patient.

One Paramedic calls the hospital by radio while they are still on-scene and advises that they are bringing Mrs. Jones in with a possible inferior wall STEMI as confirmed by 12-lead ECG.

At the end of the conversation, the Paramedics are told to take Barbara directly to the cath lab on arrival where she undergoes successful primary angioplasty. Barbara returns home three days later.

CRITICAL THINKING QUESTIONS

1. What is the most appropriate transport decision that will get the patient to definitive care?
2. What are the advantages of transporting a patient with suspected acute coronary syndrome to these hospitals, even if that means bypassing other hospitals in the process?

Disposition

As with younger patients, if the elderly patient requires specialty care, and a specialty care center is within a reasonable transport distance from the scene, the patient should be taken to the specialty care center. If specialty care is not required, then the patient should be transported to the hospital her physician is affiliated with to ensure continuity of care, especially when the patient has a complex medical history and conditions. A patient who has critical airway, breathing, or circulation issues must be taken to the closest appropriate facility unless the patient can be stabilized and taken to her usual facility.

CONCLUSION

Caring for geriatric patients can often be challenging for the Paramedic, especially in cases where the history is vague or not reliable due to altered mental status, chronic conditions, or unclear causes. Some treatments require modification in order to accommodate the patient's needs or provide safer treatment for the patient. As the geriatric population increases, Paramedics must be more aware of the issues presented in this chapter to care for this growing sector of society.

KEY POINTS:

- Aging is a progressive functional decline, not a pathologic occurrence.

- Changes in the cardiovascular system include
  - Plaque formation and atherosclerosis
  - Increase in blood pressure
  - Left ventricular hypertrophy
  - Loss of vessel elasticity
  - A typical decrease in cardiac output
  - Increased pulmonary venous pressures
  - Decreased speed of circulation systemically

- Changes in the respiratory system include
  - Loss of lung elasticity
  - Loss of lung compliance
  - Increased atelectasis
  - Decreased inspiratory capacity and vital capacity
  - Increased risk for pulmonary infections

- Changes in the nervous and endocrine systems include
  - Increased time for processing thoughts though intelligence may remain unchanged
  - Decreased brain weight
  - Decreased cerebral blood flow
  - Decreased nerve conduction velocity
  - Decreased thyroid function

- Changes in the gastrointestinal and genitourinary systems include
  - Decreased production of digestive juices
  - Altered blood flow in the GI tract
  - Decreased renal blood flow
  - Decreased sphincter tone at the urethra and prostate enlargement

- Changes in the musculoskeletal system include
  - Decreased muscle mass
  - Demineralization of bone

- Changes in sense organs include
  - Changes in lens, resulting in farsightedness
  - Changes in pupils, resulting in difficulty in responding to light or distance
  - Thickening of the lens, causing cataracts
  - Loss of hearing, especially in the high frequency range

- Changes in the immune system include
  - Decrease in antibody production
  - Decrease in the size of the thymus gland

- Changes affecting the skin include
  - Decreased number of sweat glands, causing inability to respond to changes in temperature

- The Paramedic must differentiate life-threats from chronic conditions or age-related changes.

- The Paramedic should consider cardiovascular, neurological, or endocrine explanations for acute changes in condition, especially if the patient's complaint is vague.

- The elderly patient's treatment may need adjustment, such as lower medication dosages or increased padding for immobilization.

- Reassessment remains important.

REVIEW QUESTIONS:

1. Is an acute change in functioning in an elderly patient likely due to age or disease/injury? Explain your answer.
2. What disease or injury pattern is likely to result from each of the following changes?
   a. Cardiovascular system
      i. Plaque formation and atherosclerosis
      ii. Increase in blood pressure
      iii. Left ventricular hypertrophy
      iv. Loss of vessel elasticity
      v. Usually a decrease in cardiac output
      vi. Increased pulmonary venous pressures
      vii. Decreased speed of circulation systemically
3. What disease or injury pattern is likely to result from each of the following changes?
   a. Respiratory system
      i. Loss of lung elasticity
      ii. Loss of lung compliance
      iii. Increased atelectasis
      iv. Decreased inspiratory capacity and vital capacity
      v. Increased risk for pulmonary infections
4. What disease or injury pattern is likely to result from each of the following changes?
   a. Nervous and endocrine systems

i. Increased time for processing thoughts, although intelligence may remain unchanged
      ii. Decreased brain weight
      iii. Decreased cerebral blood flow
      iv. Decreased nerve conduction velocity
      v. Decreased thyroid function
5. What disease or injury pattern is likely to result from each of the following changes?
   a. Gastrointestinal and genitourinary systems
      i. Decreased production of digestive juices
      ii. Altered blood flow in the GI tract
      iii. Decreased renal blood flow
      iv. Decreased sphincter tone at the urethra and prostate enlargement
6. What disease or injury pattern is likely to result from each of the following changes?
   a. Musculoskeletal system
      i. Decreased muscle mass
      ii. Demineralization of bone
   b. Immune system
      i. Decrease in antibody production
      ii. Decrease in the size of the thymus gland
7. What system changes are likely explanations for vague complaints?

CASE STUDY QUESTIONS:

Please refer to the Case Study in this chapter, and answer the questions below:
1. What is the value of the observation that Mrs. Jones appears to be her stated age?
2. Give at least two explanations for Mrs. Jones's heart rate of 64.

3. What is the likely explanation for Mrs. Jones's complaint of syncope and weakness rather than chest pain?

REFERENCES:

1. Centers for Disease Control and Prevention and The Merck Company Foundation. *The State of Aging and Health in America 2007*. Whitehouse Station, NJ: The Merck Company Foundation; 2007. Available at: **http://www.cdc.gov/aging and www.merck .com/cr**.

2. Centers for Disease Control and Prevention. Public health and aging: trends in aging—United States and worldwide. *Morbidity and Mortality Weekly Report.* 2003;52(06):101–106.

3. Wan H, Sengupta M, et al. U.S. Census Bureau. *65+ in the United States: 2005* (Current Population Reports). Washington DC: U.S. Government Printing Office. Available at **http:// www.census.gov/prod/2006pubs/p23–209.pdf.** Accessed August 20, 2008.

4. Villareal DT, Apovian CM, et al. A joint position statement reviews the clinical issues and weight-management guidelines related to obesity in older persons: obesity in older adults: technical review and position statement of the American Society for Nutrition and NAASO, The Obesity Society. *Obes Res.* 2005;13:1849–1863.

5. Wolinsky FD, Fitzgerald JF, et al. The effect of hip fracture on mortality, hospitalization, and functional status: a prospective study. *Am J Pub Health.* 1997;87(3):498–503.

6. Hall SE, Williams JA, et al. Hip fracture outcomes: quality of life and functional status in older adults living in the community. *Aus N Z J Med.* 2009; 30(3):327–332.

7. Partridge L, Mangel, M. Messages from mortality: the evolution of death rates in the old. *Trends Ecol Evol.* 1999;14(11): 438–442.

8. Comfort A. *Ageing: The Biology of Senescence*. Routledge & Kegan Paul, London; 1964.

9. Hayflick L, Moorhead PS. The serial cultivation of human diploid cell strains. *Exp Cell Res.* 1961;25:585–562.

10. *The Merck Manual of Geriatrics*, Ch. 42, Aging and the nervous system. Available at: **http://www.merck.com/mkgr/mmg/sec6/ ch42/ch42a.jsp.** Accessed August 23, 2008.

11. Resnick NM, Dosa D. Geriatric Medicine. In: Kasper, D. et al, eds. *Harrison's Principles of Internal Medicine*, 16th ed., New York: McGraw-Hill; 2005.

12. Bryan ED. Abdominal pain in elderly persons. eMedicine Online. Available at: **http://www.emedicine.com/EMERG/ topic931.htm.** Accessed August 25, 2008.

13. Wannamethee G, Shaper A, et al. Height loss in older men: associations with total mortality and incidence of cardiovascular disease. *Arch Intern Med.* 2006;166:2546–2552. Available at: **http://archinte.ama-assn.org/cgi/content/full/166/22/2546.** Accessed August 25, 2008.

14. Kado DM, Huang MH, et al. Hyperkyphotic posture predicts mortality in older community-dwelling men and women: a prospective study. *J Am Geriatr Soc.* 2004 Oct;52(10):1662–1667.

15. Ryan SD, Fried LP. The impact of kyphosis on daily functioning. *J Am Geriatr Soc.* 1997 Dec;45(12):1479–1486.

16. Campen AS. Hearing loss. eMedicine Online. Available at: **http:// www.emedicinehealth.com/hearing_loss/page2_em.htm.** Accessed August 23, 2008.

17. Barbul A. Chapter 8: wound healing. In: Brunicardi CF, ed. *Schwartz's Principles of Surgery*, eighth edition. New York: McGraw-Hill; 2005:223–248.

18. Cordell WH, Hollingsworth JC, et al. Pain and tissue-interface pressures during spine board immobilization. *Ann Emerg Med.* 1995;26(1):31–36.

CHAPTER 45

PATIENTS WITH SPECIAL CHALLENGES

KEY CONCEPTS:

Upon completion of this chapter, it is expected that the reader will understand these following concepts:

- How the increasing cultural diversity of the United States can pose challenges for prehospital providers
- The advances in technology which allow more patients to live at home
- How EMS calls tend to occur after patients and families have tried everything to solve their own problem

ANATOMY CONCEPTS:

Prior to reading this chapter the Paramedic student should be familiar with the following anatomy and physiology concepts:

- Respiratory physiology
- Upper airway anatomy

Medic 4 is called to the home of a 36-year-old male complaining of difficulty breathing. Dispatch advises that the patient weighs approximately 600 pounds.

The Paramedic requests that the bariatric unit be dispatched, as well as a ladder company from the fire department, to assist with lifting and moving the patient.

CRITICAL THINKING QUESTIONS

1. What are some of the possible causes of shortness of breath?
2. How is trouble breathing related to the patient's weight?

OVERVIEW

A Paramedic will encounter many patients with special needs during an EMS career. This chapter will review some of the challenges the Paramedic might face while providing care to patients who have special challenges. Since much of the clinical information regarding specific conditions has been discussed in previous chapters, this chapter will focus on the operational aspects of caring for these patients.

Chief Concern

Patients with sensory impairments—whether due to disease, trauma, or aging—sometimes present a challenge to the Paramedic as he attempts to obtain a history and perform a physical examination. Three specific impairments that may affect the Paramedic's assessment and treatment of the patient are hearing impairments, visual impairments, and speech impairments.

Hearing Impairment

Hearing impaired patients may be completely deaf or suffer from differing degrees of hearing loss, either unilaterally or bilaterally. Paramedics can recognize patients with hearing impairments by the fact that they are wearing a hearing aid, speaking with poor diction, or having an inability to respond to verbal communication in the presence of direct eye contact.

CULTURAL/REGIONAL DIFFERENCES

Persons with hearing loss may have grown up in the Deaf Culture and generally identify themselves as Deaf. Those who have acculturated to a hearing society usually use the term "deaf" or "deafened." Those in the Deaf Culture do not acknowledge deafness as a loss of something but rather as the presence of something different from hearing.

Patients who had intact hearing up until age 12 or 13 will usually have intelligible speech, whereas those who never had hearing or who developed hearing loss before age 12 or 13 will often have distorted or unintelligible speech. Although patients will often appear to understand the speaker, they may actually have no idea what is being said. Sometimes the Paramedic may encounter a patient who displays frustration with his communication difficulties.

Patients with impaired hearing may use speech reading (also known as lip reading), hearing aids, or a combination of the two to help them understand speech. By asking the patient what method of communication he prefers, the Paramedic

can avoid difficulties. Speech reading ability varies widely among patients with hearing impairments, and only about 30% of speech sounds are communicable by lip movement. The patient relies upon her general knowledge to fill in the rest of the speech.[1] Since the Paramedic's use of medical terminology presents a significant challenge to the patient with hearing impairment, it should be avoided.

Communication with the hearing impaired may require a combination of speech, writing, speech reading, interpreters, visual aids, and visual language systems (sign language). However, before resorting to writing, it is wise for the Paramedic to determine whether or not the patient understands her speech, since if she does writing may not be necessary. In addition, Paramedics with facial hair or masks may pose some difficulty for the patient who wants to speech read. If the patient is not wearing an obvious hearing aid, the Paramedic should ask whether he has one and retrieve it, if possible. The Paramedic should speak in a normal tone of voice, stay about three to six feet away from the patient, and remain in good light. Using loud speech may distort what little hearing the patient has or cause his hearing aid to produce a painful noise.

Writing is naturally a slower process than speech. Many patients with hearing impairment use **American Sign Language (ASL)** (speaking with their hands) in addition to their writing. The language context of ASL is quite different from standard English, so the Paramedic may have difficulty interpreting the patient's writing since the sentence structure will be different. The Paramedic should keep her writing as simple as possible and avoid long sentences. The Paramedic must keep in mind that if the patient who is communicating through writing or ASL is restrained, he had lost all means of communicating.

Visual language takes a variety of forms. Some persons use finger spelling, whereas others use a combination of finger spelling and body movements, including facial expressions and mime. Still others use ASL. Visual aids such as charts and graphs may be helpful when communicating with the patient and are widely available. The Paramedic should note that many patients with impaired hearing communicate using a seamless combination of all of these methods.

When the Paramedic uses an interpreter, the rules are the same as for other language interpreters. The Paramedic should speak directly to the patient as she normally would. The interpreter then interprets the Paramedic's speech just as she says it. The Paramedic should refrain from saying things like, "Ask him whether he has any pain," which address the interpreter. Instead, she should say, "Do you have any pain?" The Paramedic should maintain constant eye contact with the patient, as glancing around may give the impression that the Paramedic is impatient with the patient or that someone else is occupying her attention. The Paramedic should keep the interpreter close by so that the patient does not have to constantly focus his eyes in different directions.

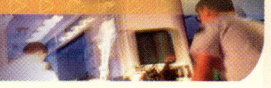

PROFESSIONAL PARAMEDIC

Ideally, the Paramedic should try to use an interpreter who is not a member of the patient's family. Some medical questions may be embarrassing for either the interpreter to ask or the patient to answer.

Paramedic problems in communication with patients who are deaf or hearing impaired—such as failure to properly assess, failure to discover medication allergies, inadequate history taking, and missing critical findings—can have legal implications. Although the Paramedic may become frustrated with the patient and become distracted, she must try to communicate as well as possible.[2]

Visual Impairment

Vision difficulties may not be immediately apparent to the Paramedic during the initial patient contact. If in doubt about the patient's visual abilities, the Paramedic should ask about them. As patients may have some residual vision, it is helpful for the Paramedic to know what they can see and what they cannot. The Paramedic should look for specialized visual aids such as prismatic glasses. Other clues hinting at visual impairment may be canes and service animals. If the patient has a service animal, the service animal should be transported with the patient, in as safe and secure a manner as possible. Service animals are an accommodation recognized by the **Americans with Disabilities Act** and have legal protection. Additionally, many states and services have rules and regulations that deal with accommodation of service animals.[3,4]

When encountering a patient who is blind or visually impaired, the Paramedic should introduce herself and let the patient know what is going to be done before touching him. The Paramedic should then provide continuing information about her actions. If the patient is ambulatory, he should be allowed to take the Paramedic's arm as a guide when moving. The Paramedic should not pull or push him. If the Paramedic is in the patient's home, she should ask about the location of medications and retrieve them. After asking permission, the Paramedic should look for purses or wallets, hospital discharge papers, home health medical records, and other items that may assist caregivers in managing the patient's care and permit the patient's family and friends to be contacted; it may

be wise to enlist the help of a law enforcement officer when looking for this information.

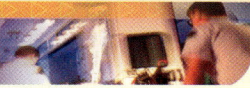

PROFESSIONAL PARAMEDIC

A service animal is considered a working animal and should be treated with the same respect as any other "employee." The Paramedic should not touch the animal without the patient's permission.

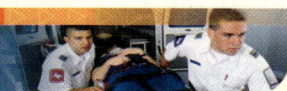

STREET SMART

Roughly 21.2 million Americans report experiencing vision loss. Although there has been a reduction in the number of people who are blind or visually impaired from the effects of infectious diseases, there has been an increase in the number of people who are blind from conditions related to longer life spans.

Speech Impairment

Speech impairment may have many causes including language disorders, articulation disorders, voice production disorders, and fluency disorders.[5]

Language disorders involve a sluggish ability to understand speech and slow growth in vocabulary and sentence structure. They can be caused by stroke, head injury, brain tumor, delayed development, hearing loss, lack of stimulation, emotional disturbance, shock, and other conditions.

Articulation disorders involve the cranial nerves that control speech. They are characterized by differences in the way words are pronounced, such as substituting the "w" sound for the "r" sound (e.g., "wabbit" instead of "rabbit") and may arise from damage to nerve pathways passing from the brain to the muscles in the larynx, mouth, or lips. Delayed development from hearing problems and slow maturation of the nervous system can also affect articulation.

Voice production disorders may be exhibited by inappropriate pitch, tone, volume, or quality resulting from conditions affecting the vocal cords, hormonal or psychiatric disturbances, and severe hearing loss. **Fluency disorders** are stuttering and inappropriate lapses and pauses in speech.

When caring for a patient with a speech disorder, the Paramedic should allow the patient time to respond to questions and not "pressure" him to respond. Displaying frustration with the patient will cause the Paramedic to miss key elements of the history and physical exam (which provide clues as to the patient's condition).

Technology-Dependent Patients

With the move toward expanded home care capabilities, the Paramedic will encounter patients classified as **technology dependent**. These patients rely on advancing medical technologies to allow them to undergo long-term treatment at home. In some cases, the devices allow the patient who would otherwise be institutionalized to live at home with family. The Paramedic will often encounter technology-dependent patients when an issue develops that is beyond the patient's or the patient's family's ability to manage.

Airway and Ventilation Devices

Two airway devices the Paramedic may see in the home are tracheostomy tubes and home ventilators. Patients who are on home ventilators all have tracheostomy tubes in place. However, a patient can be at home with a tracheostomy but not necessarily require home ventilation. In some cases, the patient places himself on the home ventilator only at nighttime or only if he develops difficulty breathing.

There are two general types of tracheostomy tubes: cuffed and uncuffed. The cuffed tubes are necessary for ventilation as the cuff closes the space between the tracheostomy tube and the trachea, allowing positive pressure ventilation. Tracheostomy tubes all have three parts to them: an outer cannula, an inner cannula, and an obturator (Figure 45-1). The outer cannula has a flange attached to the more proximal aspect of the tube which allows the tube to be secured to the patient by either sutures or, more commonly, by a fabric tie that goes around the patient's neck. At the proximal end of the tracheostomy tube is the standard adapter used to attach a BVM or ventilator circuit to the tracheostomy tube. The inner cannula is removable so it can be cleaned regularly by the patient or a caregiver; this should be done several times a day depending on the amount of sputum production.[6] The inner cannula locks in place with a twisting motion when fully inserted in order to prevent dislodgement by coughing. The obturator is inserted through the inner cannula and has a blunt end that protrudes slightly past the end of the tracheostomy tube. The obturator is used during insertion of a new tracheostomy tube to prevent airway injury during insertion. Some tracheostomy tubes are **fenestrated tubes**, or tubes that have a hole in the cannula. This hole allows air to flow outside the tracheostomy tube proximally up to the larynx, allowing the patient to speak with the tube in place and improve swallowing in patients requiring long-term tracheostomy.[7]

Paramedics may encounter two specific complications when working with patients who are tracheostomy dependent: dislodgement or obstruction of the tracheostomy tube. Dislodgement of the tracheostomy tube can be an anxiety provoking event for the patient and family. Depending on the length of time that the patient has had the tracheostomy, the tracheostomy itself will begin to narrow and close. A recently placed tracheostomy will close rather quickly, whereas one in place more than several months will close more slowly. Patients should have a spare tracheostomy tube available that is the same size. Occasionally, the patient may have a second spare tracheostomy tube that is a size smaller than the one currently in place, in case the tracheostomy closes a bit. If a tracheostomy tube is dislodged, the patient may require suctioning with a flexible catheter to clear sputum prior to placement of a new tracheostomy tube. Supplemental oxygen administered via blow-by from a nonrebreather mask may be appropriate while the new tracheostomy tube is prepared. The Paramedic lubricates the end of the new tracheostomy tube with water-soluble lubricant and places the tube with gentle constant pressure in the direction of the airway (Figure 45-2). Once the tube is in place, the Paramedic should remove the obturator, insert and lock the inner cannula, and secure the tracheostomy tube with the fabric tie supplied with the tube. The patient will likely cough during tube replacement and may require suctioning. Positive pressure ventilation assistance is generally not needed during tube replacement; however, the Paramedic must assess the patient's oxygenation and ventilation for underlying respiratory problems.

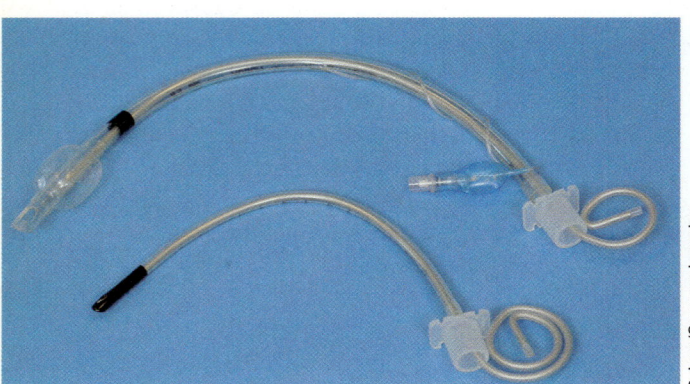

Figure 45-1 Anatomy of cuffed and uncuffed tracheostomy tubes.

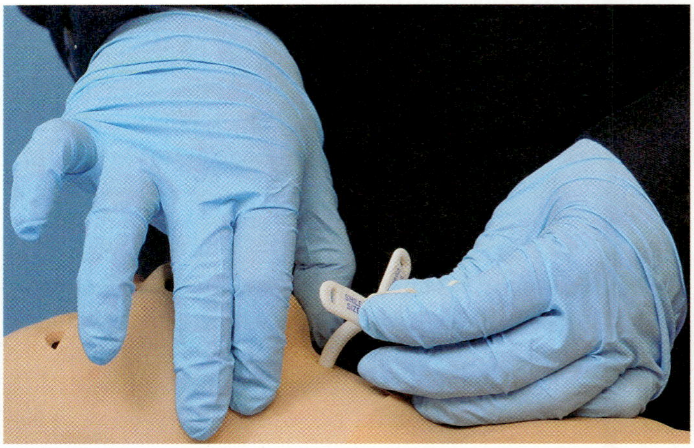

Figure 45-2 Placement of a new tracheostomy tube.

Some patients utilize home ventilators to assist their breathing, allowing a patient who otherwise would be institutionalized to live at home. Some patients require continuous ventilatory support, whereas others use their ventilation support only at night or if tired. If a patient who does not normally need to continuously use a home ventilator begins using it more often, it is often a signal that the patient has a respiratory infection or a change in the underlying chronic disease that necessitates home ventilation.

Patients who are on home ventilators should have a bag–valve–mask device available in the event the ventilator suffers a mechanical failure or the patient's home loses power. In the event of a home ventilator failure, the patient or his family often calls EMS for assistance until the issue with the ventilator can be resolved. The patient may have a backup ventilator available in the event of a mechanical failure or a battery-powered ventilator in the event of a power failure. The ventilator manufacturer or distributor often has a 24-hour access number if replacement is necessary. In some cases, the ventilator-dependent patient may require transport to the hospital until the issue can be resolved. This is especially the case for patients who use the home ventilator around the clock.

STREET SMART

The Paramedic may apply the mnemonic DOPE— where the D is for displacement, the O is for obstruction, the P is for pneumothorax, and the E is for equipment failure—as a method of determining the problem with ventilation. The Paramedic need not try to fix a ventilator, since BVM ventilation can sustain the patient until an expert is able to fix the ventilator.

The Paramedic should review the home ventilator settings and note any changes made by the patient. Many home ventilators have the ability to adjust to the same parameters as the Paramedic's transport ventilator or hospital ventilators. This may include FiO_2, the tidal volume (Vt), respiratory rate, and positive end expiratory pressure (PEEP). Different ventilator modes may also be available including continuous modes as well as intermittent or pressure support modes.

Parenteral and GI Feeding Devices

At times, patients in the home environment will require either supplemental nutrition or be completely dependent on feeding tubes to supply nutrition. Nutrition can be supplied either through feeding tubes placed into the gastrointestinal tract or parenterally through a vascular access device. Overall, feeding the patient through the gastrointestinal tract is the preferred method of supplying nutrition, although that is not always a feasible method in all patients.

Feeding tubes can either be inserted through the patient's nose and into the gastrointestinal tract or surgically placed through the abdominal wall directly into the gastrointestinal tract (Figure 45-3). Tubes that are placed through the nose or mouth are temporary feeding tubes meant for short duration of supplemental nutrition. This method is sometimes used initially when it is not clear how long a patient will require supplemental nutrition. If the patient responds slowly to the supplemental nutrition, or it is felt that the patient will be

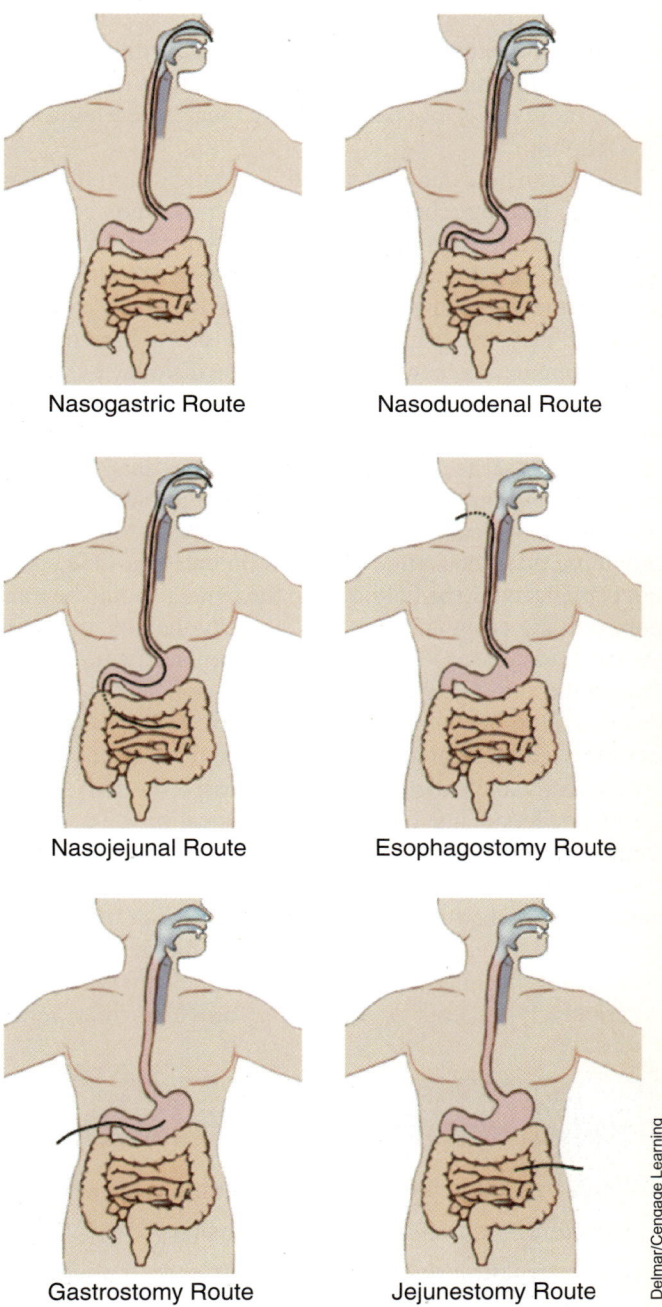

Nasogastric Route   Nasoduodenal Route

Nasojejunal Route   Esophagostomy Route

Gastrostomy Route   Jejunestomy Route

Delmar/Cengage Learning

Figure 45-3 Feeding tubes may be placed nonsurgically through the mouth or nose or surgically through the abdomen into the stomach or small intestine.

better served by longer duration supplemental nutrition, then a feeding tube is surgically placed across the abdominal wall. Regardless of the method used, caretakers are able to administer nutrition, hydration, and oral medications through the feeding tube. However, oral medications often need to be crushed before administration.

The distal tip of the feeding tube is placed either in the stomach or in the jejunum, the second section of the small bowel. **Jejunostomy tubes**, also known as J tubes, are often used in patients who have problems with either poor stomach emptying or who are at risk of aspiration.[8] Allowing the feeding tube to enter the gastrointestinal tract further downstream will decrease the patient's risk of aspirating feeding contents. **Gastrostomy tubes**, also known as G tubes, are placed more easily, but patients using them have a higher risk of aspiration.

A Paramedic may be called for patient complications related to feeding tubes. One of the most common complications is feeding tube dislodgement. Although feeding tubes are often secured by sutures, tape, or through an internal balloon, if the external portion of the feeding tube is caught, the tube may be dislodged. Although not a life- or limb-threatening emergency, replacement of a dislodged G tube or J tube should occur as soon as possible as the tract through the abdominal wall will start to narrow and close rapidly if the tube has been placed recently. Tubes that have been placed more than a few weeks prior tend to have developed more permanence to the tract through the abdominal wall, providing additional time for replacement. The tube should not be replaced in the field; rather, the patient should be transported to the designated hospital (usually the hospital where the tube was placed) for insertion of a replacement tube. The Paramedic should assess patients for complications that may develop from not receiving medications, as the patient may have missed medication doses while the tube was dislodged. Additionally, the patient should be assessed for dehydration.

The second most common complication of a feeding tube is an obstructed tube. Over time, material builds up on the inside wall of the feeding tube that can obstruct flow and cause an obstruction. In addition, the tip of the tube can become obstructed by other material in the gastrointestinal tract. Often flushing the tube can help alleviate obstruction. Alternatively, parents or other care providers may relieve the obstruction by pouring several milliliters of cola into the feeding tube, waiting approximately 20 minutes, and then attempting to flush the tube. The acids in the cola often dissolve any material that may be obstructing the tube. If these measures are unsuccessful, the feeding tube requires replacement and EMS may be summoned for patient transportation to a medical facility.

Vascular Access Devices

Central lines are placed into the larger caliber subclavian vein, internal jugular vein, or femoral vein. These lines are larger caliber and often have several lumens, allowing simultaneous infusion of multiple medications. Central lines are placed under sterile conditions and can be left in place for prolonged periods of time. These lines need to be flushed after each medication infusion and three times a day to prevent clotting from developing. Often 1 to 3 mL of heparin is instilled into the line after it is flushed to help minimize the chance of clotting. However, the line can still clot off, even with these preventative measures. Clots may also form at the tip of the catheter, occluding the catheter or causing a deep vein thrombosis and swelling in the patient's upper extremity. Implanted vascular devices are similar to central lines in that the line is placed in the subclavian vein; however, it is different in that there is only one lumen. The proximal end of the catheter is tunneled under the skin and attached to a port that is implanted just beneath the skin inferior to the clavicle. This implanted port can be accessed by a **Huber needle**, a noncoring needle with a 90-degree angle midshaft to permit easier entry. Often these ports are placed for extended periods of time and are only removed when clotted. They need to be accessed on a regular basis—often at least once a month—and flushed to keep the line patent.

Dialysis catheters are large bore double-lumen catheters that are placed in the internal jugular vein. They are used to provide temporary dialysis in a patient requiring short-term dialysis or in a patient who requires long-term dialysis but is awaiting a surgical procedure to form a fistula in an extremity for long-term dialysis. One style of catheter is tunneled under the skin with the line emerging from the skin inferior to the clavicle, whereas the other type of line exits at the site of the initial venipuncture. The tunneling provides a greater distance for bacteria to travel and theoretically reduces infection. Several mL of heparin are always instilled into these types of central venous access after dialysis. Should the Paramedic be required to access this type of central line, 5 to 10 mL of blood should be withdrawn and discarded before infusing intravenous fluids and medications.

Peripherally inserted central catheters, or **PICC lines**, are inserted into either the basilic or cephalic vein in the antecubital fossa and advanced until the catheter tip is either in the subclavian vein or near the right atrium. PICC lines are often used for prolonged intravenous antibiotic administration in the outpatient setting. These lines have a narrow lumen. If the Paramedic should be required to use a PICC line, she should withdraw and discard 10 mL of blood before

STREET SMART

When treating a patient with a feeding tube who experiences difficulty breathing or signs of a pulmonary infection, the Paramedic should always ask for the time of the last feeding, position of the patient after the feeding, and the color and consistency of the patient's sputum.

infusing medications or intravenous fluids. When administering a medication, the Paramedic should take care not to administer the medication too rapidly as the narrow lumen of the PICC may not withstand the pressure produced by the intravenous push and rupture.

Urinary Devices

Urinary devices include two different types of catheters that are inserted into the bladder to allow drainage of urine from the bladder. They are used in patients who cannot ambulate due to critical illness, mental status, or neurologic impairment.

Foley catheters are easily placed in a nonsurgical fashion through the urethra and advanced into the urinary bladder. Patients with a chronic indwelling urinary catheter are prone to urinary tract infections. Those patients with chronic neurologic disorders that affect the process of urination may perform self-catheterization four to six times a day to drain the urinary bladder. Although requiring more work on the part of the patient, self-catheterization significantly reduces the risk of urinary tract infection.

Suprapubic catheters are surgically placed through the lower abdominal wall just superior to the pubic symphysis. Their purpose is also to drain the urinary bladder. Although a more invasive procedure, suprapubic catheters have a lower incidence of urinary tract infection. These catheters are most often used in patients requiring a long duration catheter who are not capable of self-catheterization due to other disabilities.

Neurologic Devices

The Paramedic may encounter patients who have one of several types of implanted neurologic devices. The most common of these is a ventriculoperitoneal shunt that is often placed in children but which may also be present in adults. Other devices include pumps and nerve stimulators that provide a variety of functions.

Ventriculoperitoneal Shunt

A **ventriculoperitoneal (VP) shunt** is an implanted tube that is placed inside the ventricle in the brain, exits the skull, and runs under the skin to the abdomen. The purpose of the VP shunt is to divert cerebrospinal fluid (CSF) from the brain to the peritoneum in patients who produce CSF at a faster than normal rate. Due to the skull's relative inability to expand, a marked increase in CSF production can produce an elevated intracranial pressure. VP shunts are most commonly placed for patients who have congenital or acquired **hydrocephalus**, or increased production of cerebrospinal fluid, and are sometimes placed close to birth in children born with the condition. Older adults can develop hydrocephalus as well and may require placement of a VP shunt as treatment. Although a less common use for VP shunts, they are sometimes placed in patients who have suffered a traumatic brain injury. Although most shunts drain excess CSF into the peritoneal cavity where it is absorbed by the body, some shunts are directed into the thorax. Often a port is placed under the skin on the top of the skull that allows for sampling of the CSF without performing a lumbar puncture. Other types of shunts are placed in the spinal column and drain CSF from the spinal column into the peritoneum, although these are not as common as VP shunts. The Paramedic may encounter complications of VP shunts such as infection, dislodgement, and obstruction.

It is estimated that approximately 3% to 12% of patients with VP shunts will develop infections related to the shunt. Although these infections most often occur shortly after the shunt has been placed, they can occur up to a year out and are often due to contamination during the surgical procedure.[9] Signs of a shunt infection include fever, lethargy, irritability, redness along the shunt, and abdominal discomfort. Occasionally, peritoneal infections may occur.[10]

Shunt malfunctions often involve obstruction of the shunt. A patient with a blocked shunt needs emergency intervention that may involve surgery to clear the device. In some cases, the shunt will become disconnected as the child grows or kinked due to movement. Signs of shunt malfunction include those of increasing intracranial pressure (ICP): headache, nausea, vomiting, decreased level of consciousness, and development of Cushing's triad (increased systolic blood pressure with widened pulse pressure, bradycardia, and irregular respiratory patterns). Children with bradycardia should always be assessed not only for adequate ventilation but for increased ICP as well.[11]

Analgesia Pumps

Analgesia pumps provide continuous low level analgesia directly to the epidural space around the spinal cord. The pump, which may be implanted under the skin in the abdomen or may be external to the patient, is connected to a flexible catheter that is placed into the epidural space surrounding the spinal cord (Figure 45-4). It typically delivers analgesia to between two and four spinal segments depending on the pump's flow rate.[12] The analgesia used may be an opioid medication (e.g., morphine or hydromorphone), a local anesthetic (e.g., lidocaine or marcaine), or a mixture of both.

Complications with analgesia pumps that the Paramedic may encounter can be broken down into situations involving infection, situations where too much analgesia is delivered, and situations where too little analgesia is delivered. Although these devices are placed under sterile conditions, there is still a small risk of infection. As the distal end of the catheter is placed within the epidural space, infection that occurs within the line may progress to meningitis, diskitis, vertebral osteomyelitis, or epidural abscess. More commonly, the skin surrounding the catheter will become infected and may progress to a more serious condition.

Two issues may occur if the patient receives too much analgesia. In general, the analgesia does not produce systemic effects. However, if the pump is delivering too high of a dose (either a higher concentration medication or at a higher flow rate), then the patient may develop signs and symptoms consistent with an opioid overdose, including altered mental status, pinpoint pupils, and respiratory depression. Although

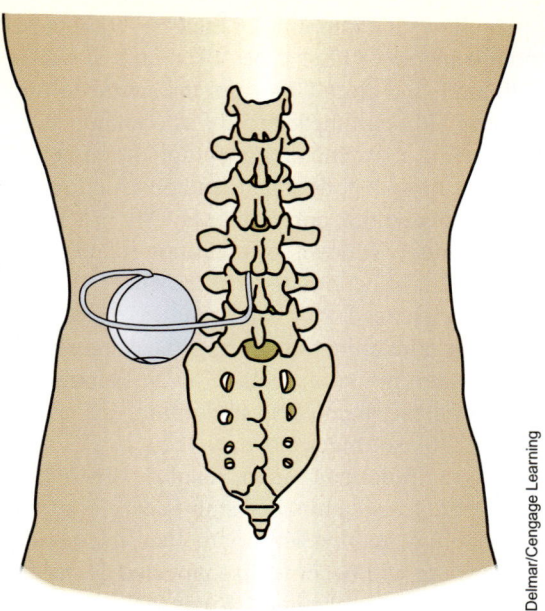

Figure 45-4 Analgesia pump with the catheter tip in the epidural space in the thoracic spine.

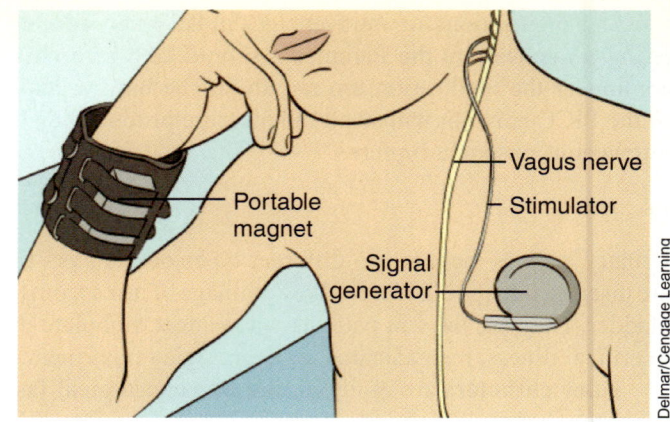

Figure 45-5 Vagal nerve stimulator.

this may be more likely to occur with an external pump, it can also occur after an implanted pump's flow rate has been changed or medication reservoir has been refilled. Although pump malfunctions that cause an underdelivery of medication may not be life-threatening, they can be devastating to a patient who depends on the analgesia pump for reasonable pain control. In these cases, the Paramedic may encounter a patient who has activated the EMS system for analgesia.

Nerve Stimulators

Nerve stimulators are implanted devices that provide electrical pulsations to certain nerves in an effort to control epilepsy and other seizure disorders as well as treat chronic pain.[13–15] Nerve stimulators have also been used to treat depression, urinary incontinence, Alzheimer's disease, and Parkinson's disease. Finally, nerve stimulators have also been used to treat hemiplegia from stroke.[16] In all of these applications, the effectiveness is not clear. However, the Paramedic may encounter patients who have implanted or transcutaneous nerve stimulators.

Implanted nerve stimulators consist of a generator box that is placed just under the skin in either the patient's upper chest or in the abdomen. An electrode is run from the generator box to the nerve to be stimulated. In the case of seizure disorders, the electrode is wrapped around the right vagus nerve (Figure 45-5) and helps inhibit the electrical impulses in the brain that cause seizures. Some vagal nerve stimulators are activated by a magnet that the patient wears around her wrist. The magnet is held over the stimulator either when a pre-seizure aura is sensed or when a seizure starts. When used to decrease pain, the electrical impulses interrupt the impulses that transmit pain sensation to the brain.

Complications may include infection, electrode dislodgement, and low battery. Infection most commonly occurs soon after implantation. If the electrodes are placed directly into the brain or spinal cord, an infection can travel into the CSF and cause meningitis. Most often, however, infections are limited to the surface of the skin.

In situations where the electrode is dislodged or the battery is low, the stimulator will not fire and the patient may develop seizures or increased pain, depending on the application of the nerve stimulator. The Paramedic will often be called to assess and treat a patient who develops additional pain or recurrent seizures.

Insulin Pumps

Insulin pumps are used by some patients who have diabetes to more closely regulate the blood glucose level throughout the entire 24-hour period, operating on the idea that the amount of insulin secreted by the pancreas changes over a 24-hour time period based on intake and activity. **Insulin pumps** are small programmable pumps approximately the size of a cell phone which hold a cartridge of insulin. A catheter exits the pump and is placed in the subcutaneous tissues of the abdomen, typically at one of the flanks near the anterior axillary line. Insulin pumps deliver a constant amount of insulin 24 hours a day, which is called the basal rate, while allowing the user to administer additional boluses of insulin based on food intake.[17] Newer pumps also allow the patient to program different basal rates and automatic boluses, depending on the time of day and an individual's own pattern of blood glucose readings. Insulin pump catheters typically have a port that allows the pump to be disconnected for up to one to two hours to allow water-based activities, including showering and bathing, without the pump. Although it can take a while to become accustomed to the insulin pump, some patients find using the pump fits their lifestyle better than periodic insulin injections. The results of one study indicated that both the incidence of diabetic ketoacidosis and the rate of severe hypoglycemia were lower, the glucose control was better, and less insulin was used overall by patients who used insulin pumps as compared with those administering insulin multiple times a day.[18]

Complications of insulin pump therapy include both underadministration and overadministration of insulin.[19] Underadministration of insulin can be caused by running out of insulin, being disconnected from the pump for more than two hours, having an obstructed administration line, or using inadequate bolus dosing. Underadministration of insulin often leads to hyperglycemia and may lead to diabetic ketoacidosis. Overadministration of insulin does not occur as often, but can occur from overbolus administration, an elevated basal rate, or inadequate oral intake. Overadministration of insulin can cause altered mental status from hypoglycemia.

Mental and Emotional Challenges

Any patient encountered by Paramedics may have an underlying mental or emotional disorder. The causes of mental and emotional challenges are many and varied. The line between physical and mental disorders is vague, as many emotional disorders may, in fact, be organic in origin. Behavioral disorders may be caused by physiological imbalances, drug ingestion, psychotic disorders, or a combination of these actions. It is often difficult to determine the origin of a disorder that is manifested by a behavioral problem.

A part of the Paramedic's patient assessment involves asking about a history of mental illness if there is any indication of the presence of one. Asking about medications being taken will often reveal a neuroleptic or psychotherapeutic medication, such as an antipsychotic or antidepressive. Since patients may be noncompliant with medication regimes, the Paramedic should always ask whether the patient is taking medications as prescribed. Also, the Paramedic should try to find out whether or not the patient has ingested alcohol or other drugs.

Mentally impaired patients experience the same acute trauma and medical conditions as other patients. Therefore, the Paramedic should treat their complaints just as she would those of any other patient, keeping in mind possible interactions between drugs the patient may be taking and those the Paramedic may administer.

Developmental Disabilities

Developmental disabilities are a diverse group of severe chronic conditions that occur due to mental and/or physical impairments. People with developmental disabilities have problems with major life activities such as language, mobility, learning, self-help, and independent living. Developmental disabilities begin anytime during early development up to 22 years of age and usually last throughout a person's lifetime.[20] There are many developmental disabilities.

Autism spectrum disorders are characterized by significant impairments in social interaction and communication and the presence of unusual behaviors and interests. Patients with autism, including Asperger syndrome, may present challenges in management including difficulty cooperating and communicating, displaying repeated behaviors and routines, and have accompanying disorders such as mental retardation and intellectual impairment.[21] The Paramedic should always maintain a patient and respectful attitude. The patient's normal caregivers and mentors can be helpful in managing emergencies in patients with autism.

Cerebral palsy (CP) refers to a group of disorders that affect one's ability to move and maintain balance and posture. People with CP have nonprogressive damage to the part of the brain that controls muscle tone. There are four main types of CP: spastic, athetoid (dyskinetic), ataxic, and mixed (Table 45-1). Patients who have CP have varying degrees of disability. The Paramedic must take into consideration the types of dysfunctions displayed when lifting, moving, and securing the patient with CP.[22]

Down syndrome is a genetic disorder that results from having an extra copy of one of the chromosomes, usually chromosome 21 (thus, the nomenclature trisomy 21 because there are three copies of chromosome 21 instead of two), and causing a set of mental and physical symptoms. Instead of the normal 46 chromosomes, the Down syndrome patient will have 47 chromosomes.

Down syndrome is characterized by a small, flat face with an upward slant at the corners of the eyes, and skin folds on either side of the nose extending to the inner corners of the eye (Figure 45-6). Other physical features include a short neck, a large and protruding tongue, abnormally shaped ears, white spots on the iris of the eye, a deep crease in the palm of the hand, a flattened posterior portion of the head, poor muscle tone and loose ligaments, and small, short hands.

Patients with Down syndrome may also have other accompanying conditions such as congenital heart disease, subglottic stenosis, hearing problems, eye problems (e.g., cataracts), intestinal problems, thyroid dysfunction, and dementia.[23] Approximately 50% of patients with Down syndrome have a structural cardiac defect.

Life expectancy for people with Down syndrome is much longer than it once was due to improved medical care and support systems. Average life expectancy is now 55 years, with many living into their sixties and seventies.[24] Life expectancy

Table 45-1 The Four Main Types of Cerebral Palsy

1. *Spastic:* Characterized by increased muscle tone, stiff movements, and awkward movements. Between 70% to 80% of CP patients have spasticity.

2. *Athetoid or dyskinetic:* Characterized by slow, writhing movements which are unable to be controlled, involving hands, arms, feet, legs, and sometimes the face and tongue. Patients may have difficulty talking. Between 10% to 20% of CP patients have this form.

3. *Ataxic:* Characterized by problems with balance and depth perception, causing patients to walk with unsteady gait. Between 5% to 10% of CP patients have this form.

4. *Mixed:* Characterized by a combination of the other types.

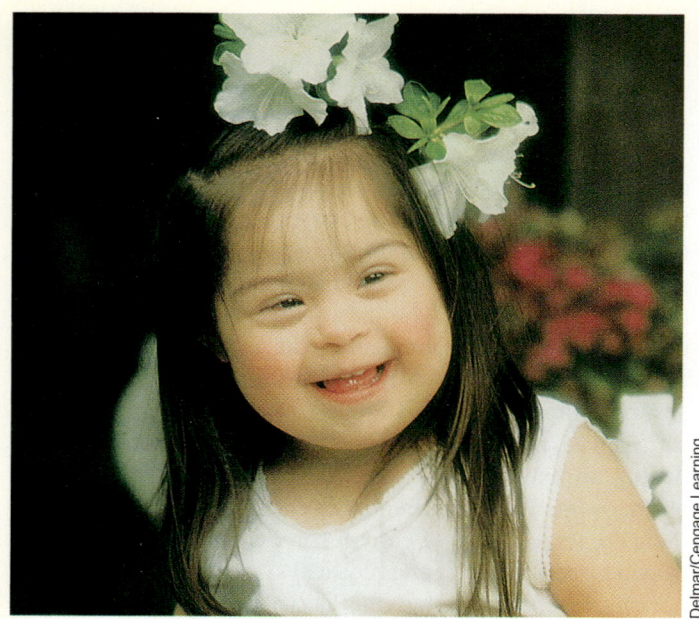

Figure 45-6 Facial features commonly seen in patients with Down syndrome.

may, however, be shorter for those with congenital heart defects. Many people with Down syndrome attend regular schools, hold jobs, and lead productive lives. However, they may present some special challenges to the EMS provider; for example, facial features may make ventilation with the BVM difficult, and intubation may be difficult as well. A small mouth opening, short neck, and subglottic stenosis may be present, causing endotracheal intubation to be a real challenge. The Paramedic should consider using a smaller-than-normal ET tube, and always have an alternative supraglottic airway available.[25]

Fragile X syndrome, the most common form of inherited mental retardation, is caused by a mutation in a single gene called the *fragile X mental retardation 1 (FMR1) gene*. This gene normally causes production of a protein the body needs for brain development. People who have a mutation of this gene do not produce enough of this protein, causing issues during brain development. The patient with this disorder may experience mild or unrecognizable disabilities as well as severe intellectual disabilities.

Fetal alcohol spectrum disorders include fetal alcohol syndrome (FAS), fetal alcohol effects (FAE), alcohol-related neurodevelopmental disorder (ARND), and alcohol-related birth defects (ARBD). FAE has been used to describe behavioral and cognitive problems in children who were exposed to alcohol prenatally but who do not have all the features of FAS. ARND refers to functional or mental disorders linked to FAS, and ARBD refers to those with heart, kidney, bone, or hearing problems. FAS is the most commonly used term to describe all these conditions.

Patients with fetal alcohol spectrum disorders are usually small for their gestational age, or of small stature in relation to their peers. Many have facial abnormalities such as small eye openings; a wide, flat nose; small jaw; and lack of a groove between the nose and lip. These patients may present a challenge for intubation. Poor coordination, hyperactive behavior, learning and developmental disabilities, and sleep disorders round out the characteristics displayed by the fetal alcohol spectrum patient.[26] All these conditions have a negative effect on the activities of daily living. These patients are sometimes confused with patients with Down syndrome due to the similarities in their features. The same airway difficulties may be found in patients with FAS as those with Down syndrome.

Cultural Diversity

Patients who are from cultures that are different from one's own may present challenges involving language differences, religious beliefs that prohibit certain kinds of health care, and other products of ethnic and cultural diversity. The Paramedic may encounter patients who challenge her patience due to their lifestyles, personal hygiene, and living situation.

Language Barriers

The Paramedic must be aware of provisions for language translation used by the service (e.g., Language Line®) or the availability of family members or other translators. Most dispatch centers have the ability to patch into language translation services. In addition, many field language translation pocket guides are available that the Paramedic can use in emergency language communication. Computer-based translation programs are also available. The Paramedic should have tools available to help in communication with non-English speakers who are commonly encountered. The Paramedic should also recognize that family members may not be the ideal translators, especially those who do not understand the context of the history questions asked by the Paramedic. Family members who serve as translators may begin answering questions for the patient and affect the accuracy of the history obtained. Difficulty may also exist when the Paramedic needs to ask questions of a sensitive nature (e.g., dealing with sexual orientation or alcohol and drug abuse) when using a family member to translate. Ideally, the Paramedic should use professional translation services.

Religious Beliefs

A patient's religious beliefs may affect his willingness to receive treatment. For example, many members of the Jehovah's Witnesses do not accept blood products in treatment. Christian Scientists often do not allow administration of medications, although this is a personal choice by each individual and can vary. The Paramedic should not make any assumptions about the beliefs of any individual regardless of his religious persuasion. It is important for the Paramedic to understand that these patients, if they are adults with the present mental capacity to refuse care, have the right to do so. However, the Paramedic should discuss the reason for the individual treatments and the consequences of declining those treatments. The Paramedic should also carefully assess and document the patient's level of mental capacity and the refusal of the declined treatments. Although adults have the ability to refuse to accept treatments if they have the mental capacity to understand the consequences of refusing treatment, courts have uniformly held that parents with such religious beliefs cannot withhold medical care from their minor children. This may present difficulties that can only be remedied through the aid of law enforcement and child protective services.

Cultural Beliefs

Some cultural groups now in the United States employ practices that may appear strange to the Paramedic. For example, acupuncture is a Chinese method of treatment that has become widely accepted by Western medicine. However, other practices may be new to the Paramedic. One example of these practices comes from the Hmong people from Southeast Asia. Some of the Hmong medical practices employed for sick children include the use of herbs, diet, religious symbols and ceremonies, cupping, coining, spooning, and poking with needles (Table 45-2 and Figure 45-7).[27–29] These

Table 45-2 Hmong Medical Practices

- *Cupping*, also known as *fire cupping*, employs a vacuum created on the patient's skin by applying heated glass cups. It leaves purplish circles on the skin that may take several days to go away.

- *Coining* involves rubbing oil on the skin and firmly abrading it with a coin, leaving red streaks.

- *Spooning*, or *gua sha*, is a variation on coining using a spoon-shaped object, typically a Chinese soup spoon.

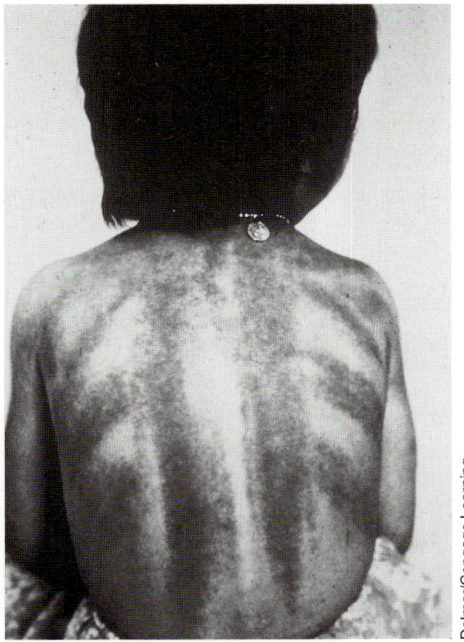

Delmar/Cengage Learning

Figure 45-7 Coining is a practice where hot coins are rubbed over a child's back or chest to cure a fever.

practices leave marks that have been incorrectly identified with child abuse. However, these practices do not actually constitute child abuse.[30] Hmong people and some other ethnic groups believe that talking about an illness is an invitation for it to appear; thus, they may be reluctant to discuss signs and symptoms with the Paramedic. Although many Hmong may still practice traditional medicine, most are quite open to modern medicine once good communication is established and interventions are explained.

Cultural Response to Death

The Paramedic will inevitably be present when a patient has died or is close to death. The Paramedic's own reaction to the situation will vary according to her experience and the situation. For example, the traumatic death of a child is especially hard for most caregivers of any experience level. Paramedics on the scene of such a tragedy must not only deal with their own emotions but also those of other caregivers, and ultimately those of the family and loved ones of the deceased. As society becomes more culturally diverse, the Paramedic will encounter differing cultural practices involving death. It is important for the Paramedic to become familiar with traditions in the local community.

Race, ethnicity, and religion all influence the actions and expectations of both patients and their families and friends. Notions about end-of-life care vary among the different cultures and religions. In fact, a number of books have been written on the death and dying rituals, as cultural differences vary widely. Many cultural beliefs deal with disposition of the body after death. Traditionally, African Americans and Hispanics have been less prone to organ donation, although that may be changing. African Americans also have more negative attitudes toward hospice.[31] Some traditional Chinese patients may choose to avoid death at home because of traditional beliefs about ghosts inhabiting dwellings where someone has died.[32]

Moreover, family members and friends present while resuscitation is taking place may have differing reactions and need special understanding. Although it is possible to list some of the basic practices and beliefs of different cultures (Table 45-3), the caregiver must guard against stereotyping patients by racial, ethnic, or cultural background, because there are so many variations in practices among groups. Good communication between the caregiver and family members and friends can go a long way toward understanding any of the family's special needs and considerations. In an ideal situation, one member of the EMS team would be available to act as an intermediary between the team and the family, explaining what is happening to their loved one. Although some services may be able to provide that extra person, perhaps in the form of a shift supervisor, oftentimes the lack of manpower prohibits assigning one person dedicated just to care for the family. It is important for the lead Paramedic to both direct the resuscitation and communicate effectively and clearly with the family, being realistic about the situation and condition of their loved one.

Table 45-3 Cultural Responses to Dying

- *Asian*
  - Chinese view the whole family as a part of the patient's care team.
  - Decisions about care are made by the whole family, often without the patient's knowledge. They believe that if you tell a patient what's wrong, he may get worse.
  - Chinese often favor traditional medicine but are usually willing to combine it with modern Western medical treatments.[32]
- *Latin Americans*
  - Latin Americans tend to be quite religious, and many are Catholic. The Catholic Church's last rites, commonly referred to as the Anointing of the Sick, will be important for them.
  - Latin Americans also have a strong history with traditional medicine and a native practitioner may be involved with their care.
  - Language barriers may get in the way of good communication and result in inadequate pain management simply because the patient is unable to express his discomfort to the caregiver.
- *Jewish*
  - Jews believe that a dying man is considered the same as a living man in every respect, and a dying person must be treated as he always was treated: as a complete person capable of decision making and managing his affairs.
  - The dying patient is never left alone, and friends and relatives are always at the bedside, 24 hours a day. Thus, the Paramedic must be prepared for relatives to insist upon staying in the room during resuscitation.[33]
- *Muslim*
  - Islam holds life as sacred and belonging to God.
  - Muslims believe that death is only a transition between two different lives.
  - Islamic families may desire to perform certain rituals at the time of death.
  - Do not resuscitate orders are acceptable.
  - The family may ask that the Paramedic place the body facing east after death.[34]
- *Buddhist*
  - The dying Buddhist or his family may wish to have an ordained Buddhist minister perform blessings or chant over the dying person.
  - Most of the time, the family will want to remain with the patient.
  - In some Buddhist cultures (Vietnamese), the family may desire that the patient die at home; however, they will not resist transport by Paramedics if appropriate.
  - Buddhists believe that death is merely the separation of the body and mind, and the mind is believed to continue on and take rebirth in a new body.
  - The family may want the body disturbed as little as possible in the moments before death and immediately thereafter.
  - Some Buddhists are reluctant to take any kind of medication that may cloud the mind; thus, pain management may be resisted. A careful explanation of the effects of the analgesic may allow them to accept some level of analgesia.
  - Some believe that it takes a period of time after death for the spirit to leave the body, and they will not allow the body to be moved until prayers to assist the departure of the spirit are finished.[35]
- *Native American*
  - There are hundreds of different groups of Native Americans and their customs vary widely.
  - Native American medicine, which is thousands of years old, is holistic medicine that addresses imbalance on every level of life including mind, body, spirit, emotions, social group, and lifestyle.
  - In the colonization process, many Native Americans became Christians, and with that came Western ways, including the acceptance of medical practice.
  - Native American medicine is practiced by elders who learned the techniques through word of mouth; traditions are still transferred that way.
  - Combining native therapy with Western approaches is generally accepted.
  - The Paramedic must be aware that some herbal substances taken in native medicine may react with medications and seek advice when appropriate.
  - There may be many different customs that patients and their families desire to carry out, such as burning certain plants and so forth. The Paramedic should seek to accommodate these wishes to the greatest extent possible.[36]

During history taking, the Paramedic should ask about traditional medicines and treatments. Some cultural groups easily blend traditional folk medicine with modern medicine. By asking about traditional therapies the Paramedic may learn about their practices and rituals connected with death and dying. Herbal compounds may interact with the Paramedic's medications just as other prescribed medications may interact.

Sometimes when Paramedics arrive on-scene, it will be apparent that the patient is dead. This may be true in traumatic deaths where injury is incompatible with life, or in so-called "natural deaths" where death is apparent. The presence of rigor mortis, dependent lividity, and decomposition are undeniable signs of death. The patient who is pulseless and apneic with fixed and dilated pupils may or may not be a candidate for attempted resuscitation, depending upon the circumstances. At one time, once resuscitative efforts were begun, the patient was almost always transported to the hospital where CPR and other resuscitative efforts were continued. However, recently, the American Heart Association has recommended that resuscitative efforts that are clearly not effective be stopped in the field and the resuscitation terminated.[37] In either case, the Paramedic will generally be the person who will have to notify family and friends of the patient's death.

Whether or not family members should be allowed to be present during resuscitation efforts depends upon several factors: the physical location of the patient, the circumstances of the death, the availability of areas away from the patient's location, and the reactions of family and friends to the situation.

Many experts now advocate that family members be given the option to observe resuscitation efforts. This may be particularly true when attempting to resuscitate the pediatric patient. Sometimes, however, it is not physically appropriate for all family members to stay in the room due to space limitations. Also, family members and bystanders cannot be allowed to interfere with the Paramedic's efforts.

If family and friends are removed from the immediate work area, one member of the resuscitation team should regularly communicate with them and let them know what is happening. If resuscitation efforts are not effective, the Paramedic should prepare the family for the inevitable by using an approach something like this: "When we got here your mother was not breathing and her heart had stopped. We immediately started CPR and attached the cardiac monitor to her. The monitor showed that her heart had completely stopped, and we were not able to shock her heart back into beating. We have started IVs and given her drugs, and we have put a breathing tube in. So far she has not responded in any way to any of our efforts, but we're still working with her. I have to tell you that it doesn't look good, but we'll keep trying for the time being. We're going to keep on working with her here because we're doing everything that could

be done in the hospital at this time. I'll keep you posted. Do you have any questions?" A few minutes later, the Paramedic should approach the family again and let them know that, "We have now been working with your mother for about 30 minutes without any response to our efforts. We'll keep working for a few minutes more, but it is time to think about stopping." Often, at that time the family will tell the Paramedic not to continue. However, this is widely dependent on cultural differences.

When the Paramedic decides to cease resuscitative efforts, she should remember to follow the procedures set forth in her department's policies and protocols and make the proper notifications to medical control, the police, and the medical examiner, as appropriate. At this time, the Paramedic should approach the family and tell them that she has stopped all efforts to resuscitate the patient and that the patient is dead. The best way to do this is to be direct. The Paramedic should not use expressions such as "she's gone," "passed away," "passed on," "is in a better place," "has expired," or "is deceased." The Paramedic should have the family sit down, sit down with them, and then state, "As you know, we have been working with your mother for 45 minutes now, and she has not regained a heart beat or breathing. I am sorry, but your mother has died." At that point, the Paramedic should stop talking and let the message sink in. Silence is acceptable here. If appropriate, the Paramedic should reach out and take the hand of a surviving spouse or child. Hugs may be appropriate, depending upon the situation. The Paramedic should let her instincts be a guide. Because the Paramedic has given appropriate updates, the family has had time to process the fact of death and is now more able to accept it. After a few minutes, the Paramedic might ask if there is anything she can do, someone to call, and so forth. Sometimes a simple act of kindness such as, "Can I make you some coffee?" is the best thing to say. That starts a transition from shock to reality and coping.

End-of-life issues confront Paramedics regularly. After the patient has died, the Paramedic has new patients—the family and friends who are present. By showing professionalism and compassion, the Paramedic can help the survivors with their grief and acceptance of what has happened.

Financial and Social Challenges

Paramedics often see patients without health insurance, personal physicians, or the means to pay for care. Many patients today use the emergency departments of hospitals as their personal medical clinics. Some patients face other challenges relative to their financial and economic status as well, including lack of transportation, restricted mobility, and inability to get prescriptions filled. This can affect their health. For example, the insulin-dependent diabetic may run out of insulin and either lack the money to purchase more, or have no means of transportation to the pharmacy to buy it. Some of these patients will call 9-1-1 when they need non-emergency medical services and tie up the system. Some services are experimenting with alternative responses and destinations for patients whose needs do not involve emergency medical care or transportation. However, the Paramedic should always remember that a patient with high system utilization can always have a legitimate complaint that requires emergency treatment. The Paramedic should never make assumptions about the legitimacy of a patient's call, as such assumptions can lead to serious medical consequences for the patient and legal consequences for the Paramedic.

Other social considerations involve homelessness, drug and alcohol addiction, malnutrition, lack of routine health and dental care, poor nutrition, and other situations that affect the patient's state of health. The Paramedic must not only be aware of these considerations but must also understand how they affect the patient's general health and well-being.

▶ CASE STUDY (CONTINUED)

Medic 4 reaches the patient at the same time as Engine 6. They find Roy, a morbidly obese man, sitting in a reclining chair in his living room. His chest is heaving as he tries to breathe. His lips and face are blue, and he appears to be tugging at his tracheostomy tube. Relatives and friends who are present advise that his tracheostomy tube is clogged up and the suction machine they have is not working. The Paramedic asks whether the patient has had a total laryngectomy, and learns that he had one almost five years ago.

CRITICAL THINKING QUESTIONS

1. What are the important elements of the history that a Paramedic should obtain?
2. What is the importance of understanding whether the patient has a tracheostomy or a laryngectomy?

History

The same principles of history taking apply to patients with special challenges as they do to patients who do not have those challenges. The Paramedic may need to obtain some collateral information for some patients to either confirm what is being said or to gain additional information that the patient is unable to provide. Sensitivity to cultures different than the Paramedic's own is also important to consider. As previously discussed, some cultures have practices that may differ from one's own. Taking a non-judgmental and caring approach will allow the Paramedic to build a rapport quickly and obtain as much history as possible.

The Paramedic may need to be more patient with people who have sensory issues or language barriers. To do this, the Paramedic should utilize available translators as necessary in obtaining the history, but understand that using the patient's family or friends as a translator may not provide an accurate history. The Paramedic should speak clearly and slowly, using common terminology instead of medical terminology in an effort to be understandable.

For patients who are technology dependent, the Paramedic should inquire as to the operation of the devices as part of the history. History related to the devices may assist the Paramedic is determining if a device failure has occurred and the likelihood of device malfunction causing the patient's chief concern. For implanted devices, the Paramedic should inquire about the date of insertion or revision, especially in the case of a patient with a fever or altered mental status.

The Paramedic should always ask about the patient's compliance with prescribed medications, both in dose and in frequency. Patients from a different culture may not view prescribed medications as beneficial or may see them as being in conflict with traditional therapies from their culture. Patients from different cultures may also use different terminology than the Paramedic. For example, the term "fever" in some cultures equates to a flushing or warm feeling as opposed to an elevated body temperature. Finally, those with socioeconomic issues may have problems in obtaining chronic medications, or not be compliant with chronic medications either due to mental capacity or substance abuse. These historical factors should be taken into account by the Paramedic as she develops her list of paramedical differential diagnoses.

The Paramedic performs a quick review of Roy's ABCs and knows he needs to intervene immediately to clear Roy's airway. Although Roy's skin color is cyanotic, his skin temperature is very warm to touch and Roy is observed to attempt to cough and clear his tracheostomy tube.

CRITICAL THINKING QUESTIONS

1. What are the elements of the physical examination of a patient with a plugged tracheostomy?
2. Why is a pulmonary assessment a critical element in this examination?

Examination

As with all patients, the Paramedic will rapidly assess the airway, breathing, and circulation during the initial assessment and immediately handle any issues discovered to restore these critical functions. Technology-assisted patients who have a tracheostomy and may or may not be on home ventilation may develop critical airway issues if the tracheostomy tube becomes plugged with mucus, sputum, or blood. Although most families and patients are trained to handle these situations, at times they have difficulty in effectively or completely clearing the airway and may call for Paramedic assistance.

Once the airway, breathing, and circulation are stabilized, the Paramedic should continue on with the physical examination. Ideally, the Paramedic would perform a focused examination pertinent to the chief concern. In some instances, however, whether due to cultural or language barriers or the patient's mental capacity, when the chief concern is vague and the history is difficult to clearly obtain, the Paramedic may be required to perform a more comprehensive physical examination than usual.

Cultural issues may also dictate the extent of the physical examination. In many male-centered cultures, a female patient can only be examined by a female healthcare provider or may be examined by a male healthcare provider only with the permission of a male family member (e.g., a husband or father). Extra care for modesty should be taken in these situations as the patient's culture may have a different viewpoint on the amount of bare skin allowed to be seen in public.

Based on the limited history and rapid physical, the Paramedic determines that Roy's tracheostomy tube is plugged. The family also provides information suggestive of pneumonia, including a fever over the past few days and abnormal lung sounds on rapid auscultation of the right lower lobe.

CRITICAL THINKING QUESTIONS

1. What is the significance of the abnormal breath sounds over the right lung?
2. What diagnosis did the Paramedic announce to the patient?

Assessment

The development of a paramedical differential diagnosis and impression is the same for patients with special challenges as for patients without those challenges. The only difference with technology-dependent patients is the Paramedic must always take into account the operation of those assist devices, considering malfunction and infection as possibilities.

Patients who have a tracheostomy in place often have issues with plugging of their tracheostomy when mucus and other secretions increase, which is often the first sign of a respiratory infection. When historical or physical examination is limited by language, cultural, or communication barriers, the Paramedic must keep a higher index of suspicion for a wider range of possible paramedical diagnoses.

The EMT already has the airway kit open as the Paramedic hooks up a catheter to the portable suction. Suspecting a mucous plug, the Paramedic puts on sterile gloves and, using sterile technique, attempts to thread the suction catheter into the tracheostomy tube. It is blocked. The Paramedic removes the inner cannula of the tube and tries again, without success.

Recognizing that the problem is now very serious, the Paramedic deflates the cuff on the tracheostomy tube and removes it. Once again inserting the suction catheter, it advances a little way and he suctions thick mucus from the airway. The EMT places the BVM over the stoma and ventilates with high-concentration oxygen using a pediatric mask. He notes some compliance and gives several breaths. The Paramedic rinses the suction catheter and suctions more mucus. After several cycles of ventilations and suction, the airway is clear and the patient's normal color returns.

CRITICAL THINKING QUESTIONS

1. What is the standard of care of patients with a plugged tracheostomy tube?
2. What are some of the patient-specific concerns that the Paramedic should consider when applying this plan of care?

Treatment

In general, the treatments that a Paramedic has to offer a patient will not change in the population of patients with special needs. However, some patients may decline treatments based upon their religious or personal beliefs. It is important for the Paramedic to gain the patient's verbal acceptance prior to initiating treatment if the patient is alert enough to interact with the Paramedic. This can be as simple as stating, "I'm going to start an IV line and give you some medication for pain." This provides the patient with an opportunity to disagree with the treatment and provide an avenue for the Paramedic to discuss the patient's concerns.

Technology-dependent patients should also be treated as per usual routines. Patients with indwelling catheters or intravenous access that become dislodged should be transported in a position of comfort while the Paramedic treats any acute issues that may have arisen. The Paramedic's access to central venous access devices will depend on local protocol and procedures. If the line is accessed by the Paramedic, she should always follow sterile procedures such as cleaning off the claves or ports before attaching tubing or syringes to minimize infection. Prior to administering any intravenous fluids or bolus medications, the Paramedic should withdraw at least 10 mL of blood from the line and discard it to prevent over-anticoagulation in the event the line was flushed with heparin during the last access. Once the Paramedic is certain the line draws with ease, she should flush the line with 10 mL of normal saline to ensure the line flushes appropriately. Once the Paramedic is sure the line draws and flushes appropriately, the line should be acceptable to use. Again, the Paramedic's ability to use indwelling vascular access devices will depend on local protocols and procedures.

Three other technology-dependent issues that may require different interventions by the Paramedic are tracheostomy tubes, insulin pumps, and vagal nerve stimulators. Patients who have a plugged tracheostomy tube often require aggressive suctioning in order to clear the tracheostomy. This is accomplished by inserting a flexible catheter into the tracheostomy, applying suction, and twisting the suction catheter while withdrawing from the tracheostomy. Instilling 1 to 2 mL of normal saline into the tracheostomy tube prior to suctioning will often help break up secretions and facilitate suctioning. If the tracheostomy cannot be cleared quickly in the setting of severe hypoxia, then the tracheostomy tube needs to be removed, the stoma aggressively suctioned and cleared, and either a new tracheostomy tube or endotracheal tube inserted in the stoma. Patients who have been breathing against a plugged tracheostomy often tire and may benefit from positive pressure ventilation to allow the patient time to rest.

In treating patients who have an insulin pump and have become hypoglycemic, the Paramedic should turn off the pump to prevent continued insulin administration until the patient is stabilized. The Paramedic should then make a note of the basal rate before turning off or disconnecting the pump. If disconnecting the pump, the Paramedic should maintain the sterility of the tubing ends to prevent infection; administer oral glucose, glucagon, or 50% dextrose as appropriate for the situation; and monitor the patient for response to treatment.

Patients who have an implanted vagal nerve stimulator for seizures often wear a magnet that can activate the stimulator and treat the seizure. The patient's caregivers also typically have their own magnet. While managing the airway, the Paramedic should place the magnet over the implanted stimulator. If the seizure does not terminate, then it would be appropriate to treat the seizure with benzodiazepines.

CASE STUDY (CONTINUED)

The Paramedic asks if there is a new tracheostomy tube available, and Roy advises that he does not have a spare. Noting that the old tube is a 6.5 mm tube, the Paramedic places a 6.5 mm ET tube into the stoma. Although the patient now wishes to refuse transport to the hospital, the Paramedic explains that a new tracheostomy set will be required and that he does not have one on his ambulance. He also completes a thorough assessment and determines that Roy has a tympanic membrane temperature of 100.4°F and some sounds of consolidation in his right lower lobe. The Paramedic explains to Roy that he may have pneumonia, and Roy agrees to transport.

CRITICAL THINKING QUESTIONS

1. What are some of the predictable complications associated with replacing a tracheostomy tube with an endotracheal tube?
2. Why was transport important in this case?

Evaluation

The Paramedic should continually reevaluate the patient during transport, assessing the airway, breathing, and circulation for continued patency and addressing new issues that arise.

This is especially true with technology-dependent patients. For patients who have persistently altered mental status, the Paramedic should constantly monitor the airway to ensure patency and monitor oxygenation and ventilation with pulse oximetry and capnography.

CASE STUDY CONCLUSION

The members of Engine Company 6 have, in the meantime, put in a call for the department's specialized bariatric ambulance which is now on location. Using the oversized stretcher, the four firefighters lift Roy onto it and transport him outside where he is winched into the ambulance.

The Paramedic climbs in with the crew of B1 and transport begins. The Paramedic acquires a 12-lead ECG en route and monitors Roy's oxygen saturation and carbon dioxide levels. The ECG shows sinus rhythm with some signs of ischemia, SaO_2 is 92%, and capnography shows a carbon dioxide level of 52 torr. The Paramedic places Roy on the unit's transport ventilator at 15 breaths per minute at 800 mL, and 40% oxygen. Within five minutes, Roy's carbon dioxide level is at 40, his SaO_2 is 98%, and his next ECG shows normal sinus rhythm. Roy is transferred to the ED where he is admitted to the ICU for pneumonia.

CRITICAL THINKING QUESTIONS

1. What is the most appropriate transport decision that will get the patient to definitive care?
2. What are the advantages of transporting a bariatric patient in a bariatric ambulance?

Disposition

Ideally, the Paramedic will transport the patient with special challenges to the facility in which the patient receives most of his chronic care. However, in the situations of critical illness, the Paramedic may decide it is more appropriate to transport the patient to the closest facility for stabilization, especially if the patient's usual hospital is some distance away.

CONCLUSION

Paramedics often encounter patients with special needs. Caring for such patients is as much a part of health care as is the prompt delivery of oxygen, CPR, or defibrillation. Meeting the challenges of everyday emergency medical care and transportation is stressful and difficult. The Paramedic has special needs and must take care of himself as well as his patients. Both actions are necessary for a full and rewarding career as an emergency medical provider.

KEY POINTS:

- The sensory impairments of hearing loss, vision loss, and speech difficulties can affect the Paramedic's ability to obtain a good history and physical.

- The sensory impairments may be present in combination or in varying degrees.

- Service animals are an accommodation recognized by the Americans with Disabilities Act.

- Technology advances allow more patients who require assistance to remain in the home.

- Tracheostomy tubes vary by size, presence of a cuff, or accommodation for speech.

- During replacement of a tracheostomy tube, the Paramedic should be prepared with suction, a BVM, and an alternative type of airway device.

- Home ventilators support various therapy modes such as continuous or intermittent ventilation or pressure support.

- Home ventilators allow for adjustments in FiO_2, tidal volume, rate, and positive end expiratory pressure. The Paramedic should document the home settings.

- Nutrition can be provided through a feeding tube placed into the GI tract or by a vascular access device.

- G and J tubes should not be replaced in the field.

- Obstructed tubes may be flushed. If flushing is unsuccessful, the tube needs to be replaced.

- Vascular access devices may be peripherally or centrally inserted.
  - Peripheral lines include a PICC line.
  - Central lines include access ports, dialysis lines, and other devices that are implanted or tunneled.

- Urinary devices include Foley catheters (which are placed in the urethra) or suprapubic catheters (which are placed through the abdominal wall). Suprapubic catheters have a lower incidence of infection.

- Ventriculoperitoneal shunts divert cerebrospinal fluid to the abdomen to prevent or alleviate hydrocephalus.

- Analgesia pumps deliver a set dose of medication into the epidural space surrounding the spinal cord.

- Nerve stimulators deliver an electrical pulse to specific nerves to control a variety of neurological abnormalities such as pain, epilepsy, or Parkinson's disease.

- Insulin pumps deliver a basal dose of insulin plus bolus doses related to carbohydrate intake.

- Mental and emotional disorders can affect the Paramedic's care. It is important to remember that physical disorders can cause mental or emotional problems.

- Developmental disabilities include
  - Autism spectrum disorders, which are characterized by social and communication disorders

- Cerebral palsy, which affects movement, balance, and posture
- Down syndrome, which causes both physical and mental symptoms
- Fetal alcohol spectrum disorders, which include physical, mental, and emotional problems

- Differing cultures with varying languages, customs, and beliefs often challenge Paramedic providers.

- Cultures have different responses to illness and end-of-life rituals.

- Paramedics will need to make decisions regarding the presence of family members at resuscitations.

- After a death, the Paramedic has new patients: members of the family.

- Health insurance, homelessness, addiction, and poor nutrition affect the patient's state of health. Many patients with such challenges will use EMS and the ED as a means of primary care.

- The Paramedic should keep cultural issues in mind when questioning a patient or performing a patient exam.

- Paramedics need to care for each other in this stressful and demanding profession.

REVIEW QUESTIONS:

1. Describe the varying degrees of hearing impairments, visual impairments, and speech impairments displayed by patients.
2. Name at least three methods of communication for a patient with a hearing impairment.
3. Describe an appropriate method of working with a patient with a visual impairment.
4. How should a displaced G or J tube be managed in the field? An obstructed G tube?
5. How does a peripheral vascular access device differ from a central device?
6. How does a ventriculoperitoneal shunt work?
7. What complications can occur with analgesia pumps? Insulin pumps?

CASE STUDY QUESTIONS:

Please refer to the Case Study in this chapter, and answer the questions below:

1. Explain why the Paramedics continued to engage Roy in the conversation even though he had a hard time communicating as opposed to using only the family to obtain a history.
2. Would you have complied with Roy's request to decline transport and stay at home? Why or why not?

REFERENCES:

1. Brown WS. Communicating with hearing-impaired patients. *West J Med.* 1977 (August);127(2):164–168.
2. Iezzoni LI, O'Day BL, et al. Communicating about health care: observations from persons who are deaf or hard of hearing. *Ann Intern Med.* 2004 Mar 2;140(5):356–362.
3. Americans with Disabilities Act of 1990, 42 U.S.C. §§ 12101, *et seq.*
4. For example, State of New York SEMAC Advisory. Service animals. Available at: **http://www.health.state.ny.us/nysdoh/ems/pdf/07-01.pdf**. Accessed August 30, 2008.
5. Speech-language disorders and the speech pathologist. American Speech-Language Hearing Association. Available at: **http://www.asha.org/students/professions/overview/sld.htm**. Accessed August 30, 2008.

6. American Head and Neck Society. Tracheostomy care. Available at: **http://www.headandneckcancer.org/ patienteducation/docs/tracheostomy.php**. Accessed January 6, 2009.

7. St. Joseph's Hospital Ireland. Care of fenestrated tracheostomy tube. Available at: **http://www.stjames.ie/PatientsVisitors/ Departments/Otolaryngology/TracheostomyCareGuidelines/ CareofFenestratedTube/**. Accessed January 6, 2009.

8. Duszak R. Percutaneous gastrostomy and jejunostomy. E-medicine/Medscape. Available at: **http://emedicine.medscape .com/article/421427-overview**. Accessed January 10, 2009.

9. Simkins CJ. Ventriculoperitoneal shunt infections in patients with hydrocephalus. *Pediatric Nursing.* November/December 2005;31(6):457–462.

10. Medscape Today. Patient care after shunt insertion. Available at: **http://www.medscape.com/viewarticle/541771_4**. Accessed September 5, 2008.

11. National Institutes of Health. MedlinePlus. Hydrocephalus. Available at: **http://www.nlm.nih.gov/medlineplus/ency/ article/001571.htm**. Accessed September 5, 2008.

12. Ropper AH, Brown RH, eds. Pain. In: Adams and Victors, *Principles of Neurology,* eighth edition, New York: McGraw-Hill; 2005.

13. Balabanov A, Rossi MA. Epilepsy surgery and vagal nerve stimulation: what all neurologists should know. *Seminars in Neurology.* 2008; 28:355–363.

14. Jasper J, Hayek S. Occipital nerve stimulators. *Pain Physician.* 2008;11:187–200.

15. Mailis-Gagnon A, Furlan MD, Sandoval JA, Taylor RS. Spinal cord stimulation for chronic pain. *Cochrane Database of Systematic Reviews.* 2004, issue 3. Art. No.: CD003783. DOI: 10.1002/14651858.CD003783.pub2.

16. Chae J, Sheffler L, et al. Neuromuscular electrical stimulation for motor restoration in hemiplegia. *Topics in Stroke Rehabilitation.* 2008;15(5):412–427.

17. American Diabetes Association. Insulin pumps. Available at: **http://www.diabetes.org/type-1-diabetes/insulin-pumps.jsp**. Accessed January 2, 2009.

18. Bode BW, Steed RD, et al. Reduction in severe hypoglycemia with long-term continuous subcutaneous insulin infusion in type I diabetes. *Diabetes Care.* 1996;19(4):324–327.

19. Guerci B. Acute complications of insulin pump therapy. *Diabetes Research and Clinical Practice.* 2006;74(Supplement 2): S104–S107.

20. United States Centers for Disease Control. Development disabilities. Available at: **http://www.cdc.gov/ncbddd/dd/dd1 .htm**. Accessed September 3, 2008.

21. United States Centers for Disease Control. Autism. Available at: **http://www.cdc.gov/ncbddd/autism/symptoms.htm**. Accessed September 3, 2008.

22. United States Centers for Disease Control. Cerebral palsy. Available at: **http://www.cdc.gov/ncbddd/dd/cp2.htm**. Accessed September 3, 2008.

23. National Institutes of Health, National Institute of Child Health and Development. Down syndrome. Available at: **http://www .nichd.nih.gov/health/topics/down_syndrome.cfm**. Accessed September 3, 2008.

24. National Association for Down Syndrome. Facts about down syndrome. Available at: **http://www.nichd.nih.gov/health/ topics/down_syndrome.cfm**. Accessed September 3, 2008.

25. Kahairi A, Ahmad R, et al. Down's syndrome child with subglottic stenosis: a case report. *The Internet Journal of Otorhinolaryngology.* 2006;402. Available at: **http://www .ispub.com/ostia/index.php?xmlFilePath=journals/ijorl/ vol4n2/downs.xml**. Accessed September 3, 2008.

26. U.S. Department of Health and Human Services, Centers for Disease Control and Prevention. Fetal alcohol spectrum disorders. Available at: **http://www.cdc.gov/ncbddd/fas/fasask .htm**. Accessed September 3, 2008.

27. Dinulos JG, Graham EA, Skin manifestations of cultural practices. University of Washington Harborview Medical Center. Image available at: **http://ethnomed.org/ethnomed/clin_topics/ dermatology/pigment40.html**. Accessed September 5, 2008.

28. Dinulos JG, Graham EA, Skin manifestations of cultural practices. University of Washington Harborview Medical Center. Image available at: **http://ethnomed.org/ethnomed/ clin_topics/dermatology/pigment35.html**. Accessed September 5, 2008.

29. Huard P, Wong M. (Smith DN trans.) *Oriental Methods of Mental and Physical Fitness: The Complete Book of Meditation, Kinesitherapy, and Martial Arts in China, India, and Japan.* New York: Funk & Wagnalls; 1977.

30. United States Department of Health and Human Services, Centers for Disease Control. Ethnographic Guides/Hmong. Available at: **http://www.cdc.gov/tb/EthnographicGuides/ Hmong/chapters/chapter2.pdf**. Accessed September 5, 2008.

31. Neubauer BJ, Hamilton CL. Racial differences in attitudes towards hospice care. *Hospice J.* 1990; 6(1):37–48.

32. Koenig B, Gates-Williams J. Understanding cultural difference in caring for dying patients. *WJM.* September 1995;163:245.

33. Gordon A. The Psychological Wisdom of the Law. In: Jack Riemer, ed. *Jewish Reflections on Death.* NY: NY Knopf Publishing Group; 1997.

34. Koenig B, Gates-Williams J. Understanding cultural difference in caring for dying patients. *WJM.* September 1995;163:248.

35. Death, dying and religion: Buddhism. Karuna Hospice Services. Available at: **http://www.karuna.org.au/2007/02/death-dying-and-religion-buddhism**. Accessed January 14, 2009.

36. Avery C. Native American Medicine: traditional healing. *JAMA.* 1991;265(17):2271–2273; Native American History/Philosophy. Available at: **http://www.healthandhealingny.org/tradition_ healing/native.html**. Accessed January 14, 2009.

37. American Heart Association. *Handbook of Emergency Cardiovascular Care for Healthcare Providers.* Dallas, Tx: American Heart Association; 2008.

CHAPTER 46

CARE OF THE CHRONICALLY ILL PATIENT

KEY CONCEPTS:

Upon completion of this chapter, it is expected that the reader will understand these following concepts:

- How simple complaints may be (or may become) complicated in the face of chronic conditions
- How the presence of chronic conditions may alter the Paramedic's treatment and stabilization options
- The recognition that patients with chronic conditions may have advanced directives in place
- How the presence of chronic conditions does not automatically exclude patients from donating organs and tissues

ANATOMY CONCEPTS:

Prior to reading this chapter the Paramedic student should be familiar with the following anatomy and physiology concepts:

- Neuromuscular junction
- Nervous control

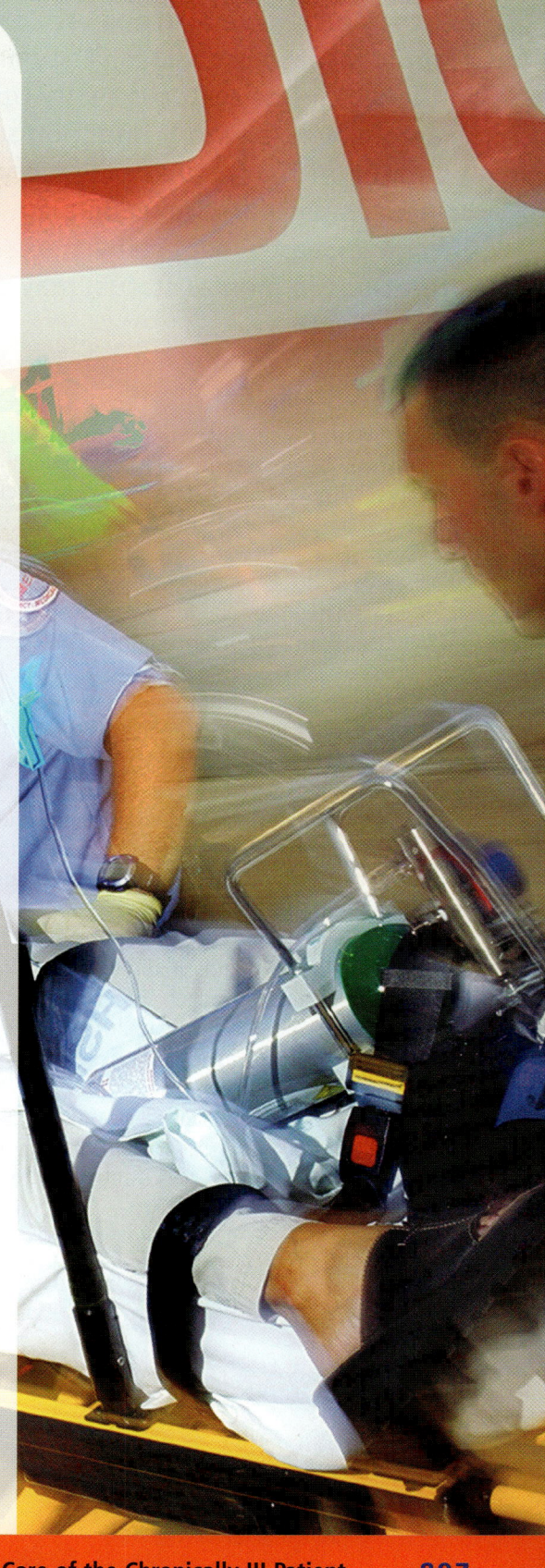

CASE STUDY:

"Medic 14, respond to Grove Heights Assisted Living, Apartment 219, for a 92-year-old woman who has fallen. Medic 14, your time is 14:12. Grove Heights Fire Department Ambulance 7 is en route BLS."

About 15 minutes later, the Paramedic arrives at Grove Heights Assisted Living, which is an enriched living senior citizen apartment complex. She grabs her gear and proceeds to Apartment 219. The patient, Mabel Gray, is an elderly woman lying supine on the kitchen floor who appears to be responsive. There is a small amount of blood on the floor from a small laceration on the side of her head, but the bleeding has stopped. She is being attended to by the two EMTs from Grove Heights Fire Department.

CRITICAL THINKING QUESTIONS

1. What are some of the possible causes of falls in the elderly?
2. How is the fall related to the patient's advanced age?

OVERVIEW

Patients with chronic illnesses face many challenges not faced by the average patient. Not only can they suffer exacerbations of their underlying disease process, but they also have a strong tendency to develop complications as a result of these chronic disease processes. They are **medically fragile** because the balance that exists in their baseline status is easily tipped by relatively minor illnesses and trauma. For example, a respiratory infection such as influenza often progresses to pneumonia in a patient with a fragile respiratory status due to chronic lung disease, heart disease, or neuromuscular disease like amyotrophic lateral sclerosis. Patients with many chronic diseases, especially those affecting the neuromuscular system or those causing alterations in mental status, may also be more prone to trauma, especially from falls.

Chief Concern

It is important to note that not all chronic illnesses have the same effects. Some chronic diseases, including certain types of cancer or end-stage AIDS, may have a relatively short course over a period of months to a few years, and have a high incidence of complications, especially related to infection. Other chronic diseases, such as chronic lung and heart diseases, most often produce a slow decline over several years, but may cause a rapid deterioration when the patient is faced with stressors such as infection or trauma. Chronic diseases such as diabetes and autoimmune diseases like lupus may allow the patient to have a relatively normal life span with frequent exacerbations, producing changes in body functions over time. Other chronic diseases, particularly those affecting neuromuscular function (such as muscular dystrophies or multiple sclerosis), may lead to a higher tendency toward trauma, particularly from falls.[1] Elderly patients not only have to contend with the normal decline in body functions relating to aging, but often have (or develop) several chronic diseases, especially lung, heart, and renal diseases.[2] Almost all chronic diseases can influence both the chief concerns of the patient, as well as how the patient responds to the current stressor, whether it is medical or traumatic.

A relatively minor head injury, secondary to a fall, can be complicated by the patient's chronic health status. There may be issues related to the patient's health status that led to the fall, as well as issues that might lead to a more serious underlying problem than would be expected from the mechanism of injury. A possible slight alteration in mental status manifesting itself as confusion expands the differential diagnosis beyond a simple head laceration. Possibilities for the Paramedic to consider include a more severe head injury, such as a concussion or subdural, epidural, or intracranial bleeding. However, the differential diagnosis should also include the possibility of a syncopal event leading to the fall. Therefore, causes of syncope—including cardiac dysrhythmias, electrolyte or fluid imbalances, acute gastrointestinal bleeding, and seizures—may also need to be considered for treatment. Other factors that affect elderly patients include problems with balance and the ability to care for themselves. Often the first indication of a change in health status is a series of falls.

PROFESSIONAL PARAMEDIC

Some EMS organizations have instituted fall prevention programs designed to reduce the number of patient falls and the severity of falls in their geriatric population. A starting point for such programs is the CDC website, http://www.cdc.gov/ncipc/duip/preventadultfalls.htm.

The Paramedic interviews Mrs. Gray, who knows that she fell, but is not able to say why she fell or the circumstances of the fall. The Paramedic asks Mrs. Gray several direct questions about symptoms preceding her fall, how long she has been on the floor, and why she tripped, but Mrs. Gray just shrugs her shoulders and states that she is not sure. Mrs. Gray can give her name and can tell you she is in her house but can't recall her address or telephone number. The aide that works in the apartment building states she had just been in to visit Mrs. Gray and was walking out the door when she heard Mrs. Gray fall, but she did not witness the fall. The aide states that while Mrs. Gray does have short-term memory problems, she usually does not have problems with orientation.

The EMT obtains a past medical history from a card on the refrigerator which indicates Mrs. Gray has insulin-dependent diabetes mellitus, "heart trouble," hypertension, and chronic renal failure necessitating dialysis three times a week. The aide tells the Paramedic that the patient's last dialysis treatment was two days ago and she is scheduled for transport for another treatment tomorrow. Dialysis is done through a double-lumen venous catheter, which is prominent under a dressing in the patient's right upper chest wall. The patient is on multiple medications including digoxin, potassium, captopril, erythropoietin, and Coumadin. Her allergies include penicillin, codeine, and latex. The patient has a medical order for life-sustaining treatments and a medication list on the refrigerator.

CRITICAL THINKING QUESTIONS

1. What are the important elements of the history that a Paramedic should obtain?
2. What are MOLST?

History

Although many of the questions asked of chronically ill patients may be similar to those asked of other patients when eliciting past history and history of present illness, there may be a difference in emphasis or a deeper probing of past events. In addition to asking what symptoms the patient is having, it may be useful for the Paramedic to ask how the symptoms are different from similar episodes in the past, how many times the patient has needed hospitalization, when the last episode was, and what the treatment was at that time. In particular, it is important to know whether intensive care or advanced procedures such as intubation were needed.[3] If the symptoms include pain, the Paramedic needs to ask questions related to the onset, quality, and severity of the pain, as well as what provokes or improves the pain, whether it radiates anywhere, and how long the pain has lasted. These are questions asked of all patients with pain. However, in chronically ill patients, it may also be helpful to know if they have had the pain previously, and if there are any differences in the pain during the current episode as compared to previous episodes.

As with other patients, the Paramedic should ask questions about allergies and medications. It is important to specifically ask chronically ill patients about latex allergies, particularly if they have needed frequent procedures requiring the use of gloves. For example, patients whose bladder function is impeded by spinal trauma or neuromuscular disease may require frequent urinary catheterizations, potentially exposing them to latex at a much higher frequency than most patients and increasing the potential for developing an allergy. Patients with renal failure requiring dialysis also have an increased potential for exposure to latex during their frequent procedures. Patients with chronic illness often take multiple medications, making medication reactions more likely. Additionally, certain medications—such as steroids, insulin, or blood thinners like Coumadin—increase the likelihood of complications or may decrease the patient's ability to respond to trauma or illness.

A detailed past history assessment may be very important in determining the potential severity of the patient's problem and the possibility of complications. Small stressors such as an infection or a traumatic event can throw off the balance in the chronically ill patient's cardiac, respiratory, or metabolic status. Renal patients have the possibility of electrolyte imbalances, especially hyperkalemia, acid–base imbalances, encephalopathy, or neuropathy, any of which can increase the potential for dizziness or loss of balance, leading to falls.[4] These factors can also complicate a patient's response to trauma or illness. For example, renal patients often have cardiac function changes including dysrhythmias as a result of their kidney problems. Additionally, medications such as digoxin may be difficult to maintain within normal therapeutic levels because of diminished kidney function and alterations in levels due to dialysis with a resultant higher possibility of toxicity.

Poor nutrition and dehydration also may play a role in many patients with chronic diseases, including patients with gastrointestinal disease or cancer, especially if chemotherapy is involved. Renal patients have similar problems because of a tendency toward frequent nausea, vomiting, or unpleasant tastes in their mouths, but they are also often restricted on their fluid and dietary intake, especially protein foods. In addition to asking about the patient's last meal, it may be helpful for the Paramedic to elicit information about any dietary issues related to the patient's chronic health problem, and if there have been any problems in the past several days with oral intake. For example, even a small increase in sodium intake from a ham dinner may be enough to increase sodium and fluid retention, potentially resulting in an exacerbation of congestive heart failure in a cardiac or renal patient.

While eliciting information about the events leading up to the need for emergency services, additional questions may be useful in assessing a patient with chronic health problems. In some cases, symptoms may have been occurring over hours or even days. Asking the patient what finally caused the decision to call for assistance may provide the Paramedic with additional information about increased symptoms or decreased ability to cope with the situation. Other useful questions may include when the last chemotherapy or dialysis treatment occurred.

Information about the patient's current stage of disease may be very important in making treatment and transport decisions. Patients with end-stage cancer, cardiac disease, neuromuscular or renal dysfunction, or severe lung disease may have already made decisions about their care. They may have some form of advanced directive which can assist with making care decisions, at least in events that may be terminal.[5] The Paramedic should elicit this information while gathering other past medical history information. If the patient's current condition is relatively serious or has the potential for deterioration, it may be prudent to bring any advanced directives to the hospital with the patient.

Additional insight into the patient's current health status may also be surmised from the patient's place of residence and the living conditions at that location. A patient with chronic health problems may have little or no support, which could cause issues of safety or increase the potential for worsening of the patient's condition. Some patients may need little additional support between exacerbations of their disease process, whereas others may need ongoing support either in their private residence or in a group setting. Some may be able to live independently with outside services such as dialysis or chemotherapy. Other patients may need periodic nursing, physical therapy, or occupational therapy services in their home, or may even have daily nursing aide service. It is often useful for EMS providers to relay information to the hospital or others about the patient's living conditions, especially if there are concerns about the adequacy of care or patient safety.

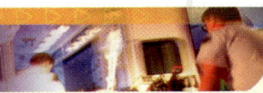

PROFESSIONAL PARAMEDIC

Although aging is not a disease, the normal changes of aging may predispose the patient to illnesses or injuries that are less likely to be found in the younger population. The Paramedic should consider the patient's current concern within a framework of the developmental and physiological changes of aging. Paramedics should not view aging as the problem.

An increasing number of patients with chronic diseases, especially if they are elderly, now live in group living situations ranging from **skilled nursing facilities**, which provide medical care for the residents, to **independent living apartments**, which have added resources but no direct oversight of residents' medical needs. Categories, definitions, and requirements for group living or care facilities vary considerably from state to state, but in general they all provide additional support to individuals based on their needs. However, although there are more supportive services for a patient in these settings, there may also be some additional issues. Patients living in a group setting are at a higher risk of exposure to infectious diseases, which may complicate their status.[6–8] There is also a greater potential for the patient to be in a group setting when EMS arrives, which may add to the confusion of trying to assess and treat the patient quickly. Information about a patient's condition and history may be easier to obtain in some group settings than in others, depending on staff availability and their direct involvement with the patient. For example, a patient's medical history will in many cases be easier to obtain in a skilled nursing facility with multiple staff members than in an assisted living center with records kept in a central office or where medical information is limited to information posted in the patient's apartment.

Patients who live in an assisted living center usually need more physical or medical support for the effects of their chronic illness or of aging than patients living at home or in an independent senior living center, but not as much as a patient living in a nursing home. There is usually meal support, medication administration, housekeeping, transportation, and recreational services. However, patients in facilitated living centers usually maintain their own activities of daily living and are mobile. There are no individual ongoing nursing services; instead, there is usually just a nurse for medication administration and general oversight, along with aides who may occasionally assist with daily living activities as needed. Patients in these facilities usually have call devices, most often on their wrists or around their necks, to summon assistance if they feel ill or fall. Historical information other than allergies, medications, and some past medical history would probably be limited.

Medical group homes have considerable variation in the services they provide, but they often have patients with similar problems living within a relatively small group center. For example, psychiatric-related group homes may be similar to enriched living centers with primarily supportive and oversight features. Although the patients are usually responsible for their own physical care, there may be more oversight of patient status by staff members. Group homes for medical patients such as those with cerebral palsy or other neuromuscular deficits, however, might have much more physical assistance.

Staff members in these assisted living centers would be more aware of ongoing changes in the patient's status. Patients with senility or Alzheimer's disease may also live in a group setting with the primary focus on providing safety and consistency to deal with the loss of memory. Additional care may also be provided to a patient that needs more physical or emotional support. Patients in group homes tend to be relatively stable, but as with all chronically ill patients they may have complications related to their disease such as behavioral issues in the psychiatric-related homes, or a higher tendency toward seizures or trauma in the neuromuscular-related homes.

Nursing homes or skilled living facilities usually have a considerable amount of ongoing physical care and status oversight. Patients are assigned to staff members each shift who provide physical care as well as medical oversight. There is often a wide range in the types of patients in nursing homes or skilled nursing facilities. Patients may range from those who just need assistance with daily living needs to patients with significant chronic disease. Some patients may be technologically dependent on ventilators or have other adjuncts such as colostomies, ileostomies, pacemakers, or indwelling venous catheters, any of which may have related complications requiring transport to a hospital.

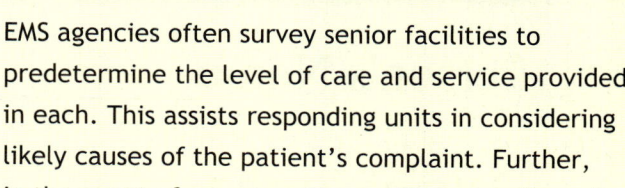

Patients with end-stage disease may be involved with hospice services either at home or in a **palliative care facility**, an organization whose purpose is to provide comfort to a dying patient. The goal of **hospice services** is to provide patients with quality comfort care rather than increasing the patient's lifespan.[9,10] Emphasis is placed on relief of pain and other symptoms and on supportive services. Patients in hospice care have DNRs (Figure 46-1), DNARs, "comfort care only," or "allow natural death" orders. Families or other caretakers are usually advised not to call EMS if the patient goes into cardiac or respiratory arrest. However, a family member may call EMS for verification of a patient's death, or may find that he or she cannot handle the emotional stress of watching the loved one's final stages of dying. Paramedics need to be sensitive to the family's needs in these cases even though they may be doing little or no actual patient care. Of course, there may be instances even in a palliative care facility in which EMS is called to transport a hospice patient for a non-life-ending event, such as an injury.

State of New York
Department of Health

Nonhospital Order Not to Resuscitate
(DNR Order)

Person's Name ______________________________

Date of Birth __ / __ / __

Do not resuscitate the person named above.

Physician's Signature ________________

Print Name ________________________

License Number ________________

Date __ / __ / __

It is the responsibility of the physician to determine, at least every 90 days, whether this order continues to be appropriate, and to indicate this by a note in the person's medical chart. The issuance of a new form is NOT required, and under the law this order should be considered valid unless it is known that it has been revoked. This order remains valid and must be followed, even if it has not been reviewed within the 90-day period.

DOH-3474 (04/09)

Courtesy of New York State Dept of Health

Figure 46-1 Prehospital DNR form.

The Paramedic looks under the bandage applied by the EMT and notes a small laceration on the side of Mrs. Gray's head. However, the bleeding has stopped. There is a small amount of blood on the floor from the laceration. During the head-to-toe examination, the Paramedic notes that Mrs. Gray appears to have tenderness along her upper cervical spine; however, her distal motor and neuro function is intact. The Paramedic does not note any abnormalities in Mrs. Gray's cardiac or respiratory examination. However, her skin color appears a little pale and her temperature is a little cool, but dry.

One EMT obtains a set of vital signs including a respiratory rate of 24, an irregular heart rate of 92, and a blood pressure of 156/90. The EMT reports Mrs. Gray's Glasgow Coma Score to be 14 because she seemed slightly confused when asked questions.

CRITICAL THINKING QUESTIONS

1. What are the elements of the physical examination of a patient with suspected head injury?
2. Why is a 12-lead ECG a critical element in this examination?

Examination

The primary physical assessment of a chronically ill patient is essentially the same as for any other patient: checking for life-threatening problems and treating them as needed. It is important that an EMS provider question whether any abnormalities are consistent with the patient's baseline mental status. The same questioning may be pertinent for airway, breathing, and circulation findings as well, since chronically ill patients often have changes in their **baseline status**, their usual level or condition. For example, a patient who has ongoing problems with chronic hypoxia or anemia may always have some degree of dyspnea or always appear pale. Asking about the patient's usual status and how things are different currently can be very helpful to the Paramedic in determining the severity of the problem at the present time. Another helpful question to ask a patient who has chronic symptoms is why the decision was made to call EMS, since there is almost always some change in the symptoms that prompted the emergency call. Baseline vital signs may be higher or lower than the normal range in many chronic disease processes such as thyroid dysfunction or cardiac disease. The medications taken by chronically ill patients can also have an impact on the patient's usual vital signs. For example, beta blockers may cause a relative brady-cardia and prevent a patient from increasing her heart rate even in response to a stressor such as hypovolemia.[12] It is important for the Paramedic to elicit information when available about the patient's baseline status in order to determine the severity of the patient's present condition. Although potentially life-threatening symptoms are usually treated as they are found, there could be a difference for patients with advanced directives, since life-saving treatments such as intubation, CPR, or defibrillation may be withheld when findings in the primary assessment would normally call for action.

Secondary assessment focuses particularly on the parts of the body or body systems suggested by the patient's chief concern or symptoms. However, chronically ill patients may have changes in their baseline from the typical patient. For example, chronic lung disease patients may have diminished lung sounds, wheezes, or basilar rales, even when they are relatively stable. Decreased oxygen saturation levels may be a chronic issue for patients with ongoing lung or heart disease or patients with anemia, including sickle cell disease. Ongoing problems with mobility are found in many patients, including those with arthritis and neuromuscular disease, whereas sensation changes may be due to diabetes or nerve impairment.

CASE STUDY (CONTINUED)

The Paramedic is concerned that, with this fall, Mrs. Gray may have developed a head injury that is causing her disorientation. Mrs. Gray is also on dialysis and has other chronic medical issues, all of which could cause disorientation, that may have preceded her fall.

CRITICAL THINKING QUESTIONS

1. What is the significance of the dialysis to the fall?
2. What diagnosis did the Paramedic announce to the patient?

Assessment

The Paramedic will often have multiple potential conditions to consider in the chronically ill patient. In the Case Study presented, the Paramedic could consider concussion and head trauma on first impression, but it would also be prudent to consider a rule-out for intracranial bleeding based on the patient's chronic illness and current medications. As the case progresses, and the patient deteriorates, the likelihood of increasing intracranial pressure due to bleeding correspondingly increases. However, there are other conditions that should be considered related to the cause of the fall. Syncope is a strong consideration as the cause of the patient's fall. With this patient's history of diabetes and chronic renal failure, the syncope could be a result of cardiac dysrhythmias, abnormal blood glucose levels, electrolyte imbalances (especially related to potassium), or fluid imbalances. A seizure related to the patient's renal status is also a potential cause of the fall, especially since she is probably due for another dialysis treatment and her electrolytes may be abnormal. All of these potential problems should be evaluated during the assessment process and treated appropriately if found or if the problem recurs during transport.

CASE STUDY (CONTINUED)

While the EMTs secure Mrs. Gray to a long spine board, the Paramedic takes the sheet with the list of her medications and the medical orders for life-sustaining treatments form so she can bring that to the hospital. The Paramedic asks the EMTs to apply supplemental oxygen by nasal cannula and bring Mrs. Gray out to the ambulance while she sets up to start an intravenous line and acquire a 12-lead ECG. The Paramedic also pulls out the glucometer so she can check Mrs. Gray's blood glucose level when she starts the intravenous line.

CRITICAL THINKING QUESTIONS

1. What is the national standard of care of extreme elderly patients with suspected spine trauma?
2. What are some of the patient-specific concerns and considerations that the Paramedic should consider when applying this plan of care that is intended to treat a broad patient population?

Treatment

Patient treatment can also become more complicated in a chronically ill patient. Spinal immobilization may be difficult in a patient with bony deformities such as kyphosis, or in a patient with a congestive heart disease history who becomes more dyspneic when supine. Oxygen should be administered to all patients with altered mental status.[13] When and if a patient becomes unresponsive and the breathing begins to be irregular, use of a bag–valve mask and simple airway adjunct become important to maintain ventilation and oxygenation. Advanced airway devices may also be a consideration, especially with a longer transport time or difficult-to-maintain airway. It is essential for the Paramedic to maintain an even oxygen flow and ventilation rate to minimize damage to the brain from the increasing intracranial pressure. The need for ventilation in this patient is related to the increasing pressure on the brain's respiratory centers. Other chronically ill patients may have other needs for early ventilatory control. For example, patients already dependent on ventilators (either fully or partially) may need immediate support with a bag–valve device either through their tracheotomies or by mask. This is often the case for patients with neuromuscular disease or previous brain damage.

Fluid administration needs to be monitored very closely in patients with ongoing cardiac, pulmonary, or renal problems because of the possibility of the patient developing pulmonary edema. Although the patient in the Case Study does not immediately need fluid resuscitation, intravenous access should be considered because of the potential for deterioration. It can be difficult to obtain intravenous access on patients with chronic illnesses because of the disease process itself, or because they have needed frequent blood draws or intravenous treatments. Some patients, such as the current patient in the Case Study, have some type of indwelling intravenous device. However, because the device can easily be infected, most EMS systems do not allow access by Paramedics. In some cases, the devices may be used under direct medical control authorization in cases of extremis when no other access is available. However, with the advent of intraosseous devices, this should be a rare occurrence, at least in the unconscious patient.

Although the patient in the presented Case Study is primarily a head injury concern, medications may need to be considered if cardiac dysrhythmia, seizures, or cardiac arrest occurs. Medication doses may need to be modified for some patients with chronic illnesses, or in some cases the choice of medication administered or frequency may need to be altered. For example, with the current patient, mannitol (if permitted by local protocols for increased intracranial pressure) should be avoided because of the patient's chronic renal failure. A patient on high doses of furosemide may not respond to the typical starting dose for congestive heart failure, whereas low doses (if any at all) would be more suitable for patients with renal failure. A patient with atrial fibrillation and Wolff-Parkinson-White syndrome probably would not be given adenosine or a calcium channel blocker for symptomatic tachycardia. Atropine and ipratropium bromide would be a problem for patients with acute angle glaucoma. Haloperidol should be avoided in patients with Parkinson's disease or epilepsy and should be used with great caution in patients with liver or cardiac disease. Morphine can be problematic in patients with diseases causing a decreased respiratory drive or in patients taking MAO inhibitors. It is very important for the Paramedic to do frequent reassessments for the effects of drugs that are administered to patients with chronic illness.

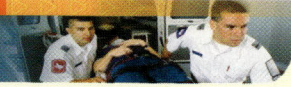

STREET SMART

Drugs are not tested in all combinations before being made available for prescription. The Paramedic should consider a potential drug reaction anytime a new drug is added to a previous regimen. This includes the emergency drugs carried in the field.

CASE STUDY (CONTINUED)

Mrs. Gray is concerned that if she should die that no extraordinary means of resuscitation be taken and again refers to her POLST form.

CRITICAL THINKING QUESTIONS

1. What are some of the predictable complications associated with a traumatic head injury in the elderly?
2. What are some of the implications of the POLST form?

Evaluation

It is important for the Paramedic to recognize that patients with chronic problems can deteriorate very quickly, as they may not have any reserve stores of strength to draw on when they are under stress. It is therefore essential for the Paramedic to continually reassess the patient's status and response to treatment and make adaptations in care as needed based on the changes.

In some cases, there may also be deterioration in the patient's health over time to the point where end-of-life issues begin to surface. Patients may be involved with hospice care in their own home or in other settings. **Living wills**, DNR orders, **Medical Orders for Life-Sustaining Treatment (MOLST)** or **Physician Orders for Life-Sustaining Treatment (POLST)** forms, or other advanced directives may be in place, expressing the patient's desires about resuscitation issues.[14] These factors may play a big role in the Paramedic's treatment and transport decisions. It is essential for Paramedics to know how the presented information can impact their care and what documents can be honored in their region. In many cases, state laws may permit direct acknowledgement of a patient's wishes if documented on a specific legal form, whereas in other cases, advanced directives may only be used to consult with medical control for direction on performing or withholding medical care.

Do Not Resuscitate (DNR), or the more currently adopted term **Do Not Attempt Resuscitation (DNAR)**, forms are probably the earliest and most widely recognized versions of advanced directive. Studies detailing the use of DNR forms in hospitals date back to the early 1980s, primarily for terminally ill patients. In 1984, the Supreme Court in *Bartling v. Superior Court* decided that a competent adult patient had the constitutional right to refuse medical treatment. The passage of the Patient Self-Determination Act of 1990 expanded the right to have advanced directives to nonterminal patients. It required hospitals, nursing homes, home health services, and others receiving Medicare funding to provide written information to all patients about state-specific advanced directives, and to document whether the patient did or did not sign a DNR/DNAR.

Although there were some local initiatives in the mid-1980s, state legislation allowing recognition of DNR/DNAR forms by EMS began to be passed in the early 1990s. There is considerable variation between state laws—and even within a state, based on local interpretation. It is therefore very important that EMS providers know what the prehospital DNR/DNAR statutes or regulations are in the state in which they practice. For example, although most states allow DNR/DNAR for any competent adult, a few states only allow recognition of the forms when the patient has a terminal condition. Most states require a physician's signature, but there are a few states that only require the signature of two competent adult witnesses. Some states allow the forms to be signed by a parent, guardian, or surrogate, especially if a durable power of attorney for health care (DPAHC) exists. A few states only allow prehospital DNR/DNAR recognition for patients 18 years of age or older. Although some states require the presence of a valid DNR form, in most states a DNAR bracelet, medallion, or wallet card is sufficient to withhold resuscitative measures. A few states require the presence of a bracelet as the only recognized DNR/DNAR authorization in the prehospital setting.

Immunity for the EMS provider also varies from state to state. Almost all of the states have either an explicit recognition of immunity from civil and criminal liability for withholding resuscitative measures when a valid DNR/DNAR is available, or immunity is implicit in other portions of state health codes. However, in some cases, there is a modification to the immunity stating that the decision to withhold care be "reasonable" and/or done in "good faith." On the other hand, there is considerable variation in immunity from liability if resuscitative measures are started in spite of the presence of a DNR/DNAR.

In some states, honoring a DNR or DNAR is optional. In other states, there are specific indications for not honoring a DNR or DNAR listed in the legislation. These may include objection by family members, questionable validity, or possible revocation of the DNR/DNAR. In a few states, there may be a modification based on the moral beliefs/conscience of the EMS provider. In such cases, the EMS provider is required to turn the patient's care over to another provider willing to carry out the patient's wishes. Other conditions such as lack of knowledge of the existence of a DNR/DNAR, or the safety of the EMS provider, usually have immunity implicit or based on other general statutes regulating EMS providers.

The common features of most state-specific DNR/DNAR legislation include a limitation to cardiac and/or respiratory arrest events only.[15,16] The care withheld usually includes CPR, intubation, defibrillation, and resuscitation medications. DNRs/DNARs in most states have little validity in pre-arrest conditions or in conditions potentially reversible by airway measures or medications. Such is the case with foreign body aspiration, in which removal of the foreign body may prevent progress to a full arrest situation. Comfort care measures are permitted in all states with legislation, and in some cases comfort care measures are outlined within the state's legislation. Permitted treatments in non-arrest situations usually include oxygen, suction, and pain relief measures. In recent years, some areas of the country have begun to utilize "allow natural death" or "comfort care only" orders, but few of these initiatives are currently in state EMS legislation. Beyond their applicability to resuscitation issues, most of the issues addressed by these initiatives relate primarily to ongoing patient care rather than to situations involving EMS providers, since they usually involve ongoing feeding or use of antibiotics and other medications.

POLST or MOLST forms (Figure 46-2) are more expansive than DNR/DNAR forms.[17] In 1996, the state of Oregon modified its EMS scope of practice to allow its providers to honor a patient's wishes related to medical treatment beyond resuscitation measures. Unlike a DNR/DNAR form, the two-page pink POLST form allows positive decisions about care as well as refusals. POLST forms provide options for care which can be chosen by the patient for possible future care, and are not limited to situations when a patient is unresponsive. For example, patients can check off boxes indicating that they wish comfort care only, limited treatments, or full treatment in non-arrest situations as well as deciding on whether CPR should be attempted in an arrest situation. In 2005, New York State adopted MOLST, a four-page modified version of the POLST form, as an alternative to its DNR form with variations in its use in some regions of the state. EMS can accept the DNR or DNI (Do Not Intubate) portions of the document by regional authorization, or use the document as an expression of the patient's wishes in consultation with medical control. Other portions of the MOLST form include information about the patient's wishes related to artificial hydration and nutrition, antibiotics, and ventilator use. In the prehospital setting, the portions of the form related to CPR and intubation are the most pertinent in direct care decisions. However, relaying information from other parts of the form may assist the medical control physician in directing the Paramedic about intravenous and medication use or about BLS airway and ventilation measures. New York State's MOLST process also has additional forms available for minor children or for adults who lack the capacity to make decisions for themselves that can be signed by parents, guardians, and court-appointed advocates. Several other states have adopted or are considering adoption of POLST paradigms.

Early in an EMS call, the information on the MOLST form may not seem particularly pertinent because the patient may have a relatively minor injury or illness. However, because patients with chronic medical problems—especially those with significant cardiac, chronic lung, and renal problems—can deteriorate so quickly, it is prudent to transport the document to the hospital with the patient.

If the patient's status worsened en route to the hospital, significant information about the patient's desire for resuscitation could provide direction to the Paramedic about whether to provide CPR if the patient did proceed to cardiac or respiratory arrest. Even if arrest did not occur, information about the patient's desires related to fluid administration or medications for nonlethal cardiac dysrhythmias could be relayed to the medical control physician for appropriate orders.

There are other forms of advanced directives that might be in the possession of patients, especially those with chronic diseases, including living wills, healthcare proxies, and durable power of attorneys for health care (DPAHC). EMS recognition of these documents varies from state to state, but in most cases they have little impact on emergency care in the prehospital setting. Although EMS usually cannot honor the requests in these documents directly, they may be useful when contacting medical control about orders for treatment or for not instituting treatment.

Living wills may contain information about medical care preferences, but do not constitute medical orders. This differs from POLST or MOLST forms, which document agreement between a physician and patient over the medical treatments

Physician Orders
for Life-Sustaining Treatment (POLST)

First follow these orders, then contact physician, NP, or PA. These medical orders are based on the person's current medical condition and preferences. Any section not completed does not invalidate the form and implies full treatment for that section.

Last Name/ First/ Middle Initial

Address

City / State / Zip

Date of Birth (mm/dd/yyyy)   Last 4 SSN   Gender

☐ M   ☐ F

A *Check One*

CARDIOPULMONARY RESUSCITATION (CPR): **Person has no pulse and is not breathing.**
☐ Attempt Resuscitation/CPR   ☐ Do Not Attempt Resuscitation/DNR (Allow Natural Death)
When not in cardiopulmonary arrest, follow orders in **B**, **C** and **D**.

B *Check One*

MEDICAL INTERVENTIONS: **Person has pulse and/or is breathing.**

☐ **Comfort Measures Only** Use medication by any route, positioning, wound care and other measures to relieve pain and suffering. Use oxygen, suction and manual treatment of airway obstruction as needed for comfort. *Do not transfer to hospital for life-sustaining treatment. Transfer if comfort needs cannot be met in current location.*

☐ **Limited Additional Interventions** Includes care described above. Use medical treatment, IV fluids and cardiac monitor as indicated. Do not use intubation, advanced airway interventions, or mechanical ventilation. May consider less invasive airway support (e.g. CPAP, BiPAP). *Transfer to hospital if indicated. Avoid intensive care.*

☐ **Full Treatment** Includes care described above. Use intubation, advanced airway interventions, mechanical ventilation, and cardioversion as indicated. *Transfer to hospital if indicated. Includes intensive care.*

Additional Orders: _____

C *Check One*

ANTIBIOTICS
☐ No antibiotics. Use other measures to relieve symptoms.
☐ Determine use or limitation of antibiotics when infection occurs.
☐ Use antibiotics if medically indicated.

Additional Orders: _____

D *Check One*

ARTIFICIALLY ADMINISTERED NUTRITION: **Always offer food by mouth if feasible.**
☐ No artificial nutrition by tube.
☐ Defined trial period of artificial nutrition by tube.
☐ Long-term artificial nutrition by tube.

Additional Orders: _____

E

REASON FOR ORDERS AND SIGNATURES

My signature below indicates to the best of my knowledge that these orders are consistent with the person's current medical condition and preferences as indicated by the **discussion with:**

☐ Patient   ☐ Health Care Representative   ☐ Parent of Minor

☐ Court-Appointed Guardian   ☐ Other _____

Print Primary Care Professional Name

Print Signing Physician / NP / PA Name and Phone Number
(   )

Physician / NP / PA Signature (mandatory)   Date

Office Use Only

SEND FORM WITH PERSON WHENEVER TRANSFERRED OR DISCHARGED

© CENTER FOR ETHICS IN HEALTH CARE, Oregon Health & Science University, 3181 Sam Jackson Park Rd, UHN-86, Portland, OR 97239-3098 (503) 494-3965

Courtesy of Center for Ethics in Healthcare, Oregon Health & Science University

Figure 46-2 Physician Orders for Life-Sustaining Treatment (POLST) form used in Oregon. (*continues*)

that would or would not be ordered in a particular situation. Living wills must be signed or authorized by competent adult patients themselves, not by surrogates as is sometimes the case with DNRs, DNARs, and POLST or MOLST forms. Living wills only take effect in cases where the patient has been determined by a physician or other authorized healthcare provider to be terminally ill or injured, or in cases when the patient is permanently unconscious or in a permanent

vegetative state. They do not take the place of a DNR/DNAR form, which is usually a separate document. However, in some states signing a living will may generate the issuance of a DNR/DNAR if so desired by the patient.

Most states do not recognize provisions of a living will that refuse life-sustaining care in the case of a pregnant woman until the child is delivered or is no longer viable. This restriction usually also applies to the authority of healthcare

Information for Person Named on this Form

This form records your preferences for life-sustaining treatment in your **current** state of health. It can be reviewed and updated by your health care professional at any time if your preferences change. If you are unable to make your own health care decisions, the orders should reflect your preferences as best understood by your surrogate.

Signature of Person or Surrogate

Signature	Name (print)	Relationship (write "self" if patient)

Contact Information

Surrogate (optional)	Relationship	Phone Number	Address	
Health Care Professional Preparing Form (optional)	Preparer Title		Phone Number	Date Prepared
PA's Supervising Physician			Phone Number	

Directions for Health Care Professionals

Completing POLST

- Should reflect person's current preferences. Encourage completion of an advance directive.
- POLST must be signed by a physician/NP/PA to be valid. Verbal orders are acceptable with follow-up signature by physician/NP/PA in accordance with facility/community policy.
- Use of original form is encouraged. Photocopies and FAXes are legal and valid.

Using POLST

Section A:
- No defibrillator (including AEDs) should be used on a person who has chosen "Do Not Attempt Resuscitation."

Section B:
- When comfort cannot be achieved in the current setting, the person, including someone with "Comfort Measures Only," should be transferred to a setting able to provide comfort (e.g., treatment of a hip fracture).
- IV medication to enhance comfort may be appropriate for a person who has chosen "Comfort Measures Only."
- Treatment of dehydration is a measure which prolongs life. A person who desires IV fluids should indicate "Limited Additional Interventions" or "Full Treatment."

Section D:
- Oral fluids and nutrition must always be offered if medically feasible.
- A person with capacity, or the surrogate of a person without capacity, can void the form and request alternative treatment.

Reviewing POLST

This POLST should be reviewed periodically and if:
- The person is transferred from one care setting or care level to another, or
- There is a substantial change in the person's health status, or
- The person's treatment preferences change.

Draw line through sections A through E and write "VOID" in large letters if POLST is replaced or becomes invalid.

The POLST program was developed by the Oregon POLST Task Force and is housed at OHSU's Center for Ethics in Health Care. For permission to use the copyrighted form contact the Center. Information on the POLST program is available online at **www.polst.org** or at **polst@ohsu.edu**.

SEND FORM WITH PERSON WHENEVER TRANSFERRED OR DISCHARGED

© CENTER FOR ETHICS IN HEALTH CARE, OHSU   Form developed in conformance with Oregon Revised Statute 127.505 et seq   August 2008

Courtesy of Center for Ethics in Healthcare, Oregon Health & Science University

Figure 46-2 (*continued*)

proxies and those with durable powers of attorney in making decisions that may potentially end the life of a pregnant woman while her child is still viable.

In most states, patients may designate a **healthcare proxy** to make decisions for them if they become unconscious or mentally incapacitated.[18–20] This designation is written either as a separate document or as part of a living will. EMS providers usually cannot directly comply with the request of a healthcare proxy. However, in some states, EMS can recognize the requests of individuals who hold **durable power of attorney for health care (DPAHC)** for a patient, especially in connection with resuscitation, if the DPAHC is present at the scene with proof of identification and DPAHC status. DPAHC only takes effect if the patient is unable to express his own wishes. In some states, the decisions of a patient's DPAHC overrule the conditions expressed in the patient's living will because the DPAHC is responding to conditions in the actual situation rather than following an expression that was written in advance for a possible scenario. It is the highest level of healthcare proxy and takes precedence in decision making over family members or other healthcare proxies. All advanced directives have provisions for revocation by a patient at any time, even at the time of treatment by EMS.

At times DNR/DNARs or other advanced directives may not be discovered or verified until after resuscitative measures have begun. In most states, discovery of a valid DNR/DNAR allows immediate termination of resuscitation attempts. In other states, medical control must be contacted to terminate resuscitative measures once they have begun. In the absence of a DNR/DNAR, many states have provisions for termination of resuscitation in particular circumstances. In addition to injuries incompatible with life and EMS provider fatigue or exposure to danger, there may be a time element after which resuscitative efforts can be stopped. In some cases, medical control contact is required before stopping. Information provided in advanced directives may help a physician determine the appropriateness of terminating efforts. In the absence of advanced directives or a DPAHC's guidance about a patient's wishes, however, other information gathered by EMS during subjective and objective assessment may also be of value to the decision making of a medical control physician. This is particularly true in the case of a patient with chronic illness, especially if the patient has end-stage cancer or renal disease, versus the usually healthy patient with a sudden event.

If no DNR/DNAR or other advanced directive is in place, resuscitative efforts should be started on chronically ill patients just as on other patients, even though there is an even smaller likelihood of success because of the compromise to body systems caused by the chronic illness. Pre-arrest conditions such as those seen in the Case Study should also be appropriately treated, although the patient probably will not have a high likelihood of recovery.

CULTURAL/REGIONAL DIFFERENCES

Some Asian cultures and Native American cultures believe that it is unwise to speak of dying and therefore do not utilize advanced directives. The Paramedics should be nonjudgmental when faced with these situations.

CASE STUDY CONCLUSION

During the 30-minute transport to the hospital where she receives her dialysis, the patient becomes less responsive. She seems drowsy and can only hesitantly say her name. She thinks that she is on her bed at home. Mrs. Gray's blood glucose is 172 and oxygen saturation is 92. The monitor shows controlled atrial fibrillation in the 78 to 80 range and her 12-lead ECG does not show any acute changes. Repeat vital signs show a blood pressure of 178/94 and a respiratory rate of 18 which seems to be somewhat irregular in its rhythm. Mrs. Gray continues to deteriorate, becoming unresponsive with her heart rate continuing to decrease and her blood pressure continuing to increase. Respirations begin to follow a Cheyne-Stokes pattern.

Upon arrival at the emergency department, the Paramedic is assisting Mrs. Gray's ventilations with a bag-valve mask. Mrs. Gray's POLST form indicates that she does not wish intubation and prolonged mechanical ventilation and does not wish CPR. Mrs. Gray is rushed back into the resuscitation room where report is given to Dr. Jordan, the emergency physician. A stat CT scan of the brain shows a severe epidural hematoma that the consulting neurosurgeon evaluates and states is a non-survivable bleed. In the meantime, both Dr. Jordan and the neurosurgeon review the POLST form and discuss Mrs. Gray's condition with her son and two daughters. It is agreed among all parties that Mrs. Gray would not want surgery or to be kept alive in this situation and the physicians order comfort care measures to ease any discomfort Mrs. Gray may have. Mrs. Gray dies peacefully a few hours later with her close family beside her.

CRITICAL THINKING QUESTIONS

1. What is the most appropriate transport decision that will get the patient to definitive care?
2. What are the advantages of transporting a patient with a POLST form to these hospitals, even if that patient is going to die?

Disposition

Chronically ill patients are more likely to need hospitalization or transport to an emergency department by ambulance. It is usually best to take patients to the hospitals where they have been treated previously so that their medical records—and in some cases, medical personnel who are familiar with their histories—are more readily available. However, as with other patients, it may be necessary to transport the chronically ill patient to the closest hospital when there is a life-threatening condition. Transport to specialty centers, especially trauma centers, is often even more important than usual because the somewhat delicate balance for many chronically ill patients is so easily upset. Even if the patient looks relatively stable on first assessment, appropriate transport must be carefully considered. Despite the initial appearance, the patient's underlying disease process may not allow continued adequate response. For example, patients with cardiac deficits may be able to respond to trauma or infection with tachycardia in the short term, but even a small additional stress such as movement, body position changes such as supine immobilization, or coughing may be sufficient to overwhelm the heart's ability to compensate for the original insult. These patients are particularly prone to cardiac dysrhythmias as the myocardium fatigues or is deprived of sufficient oxygen, and prone to sudden pulmonary edema as the "pump" fails, causing back pressure of fluid into the lungs. Similarly, patients on anticoagulants may lose the ability to clot even small wounds, increasing the possibility of internal bleeding and shock. It is important for the Paramedic to recognize the potential for deterioration in a patient's status and decide on a transport destination accordingly.

It should be noted some chronically ill patients may be candidates for organ donation. For example, patients with some end-stage musculoskeletal diseases, spinal cord injury, or pulmonary disease may still have viable kidneys or corneas. On the other hand, chronic diseases such as diabetes, severe cardiac disease, or diseases involving infectious processes will most likely decrease the possibility of organ donation because of long-term changes in organ function. Organ donation, therefore, is not automatically precluded in many patients with chronic disease and may be a factor in transport and treatment decision making, especially in cases in which the patient is dying as the result of a brain injury.

Good documentation and communication of information related to a chronically ill patient is essential. Hospital admission, observation, and treatment may be more likely in many patients with chronic illnesses. The information that EMS provides may assist in decision making. This is particularly true when the patient's condition has improved by the time of arrival in the emergency department.

For example, a trauma patient with a cardiac or bleeding disorder may be observed for a longer period or have additional tests performed to detect potential complications. Additionally, patients with chronic mental status or memory changes might not be able to relay historical information. Thorough EMS documentation may be the only historical detail available not only to emergency staff but also to inpatient staff if the patient is admitted.

CONCLUSION

In summary, patients with chronic disease processes provide additional challenges to a Paramedic in all aspects of assessment and care. Such patients may have multiple potential morbidities beyond their original chief concerns or those which contributed to the cause of their current problem.

Complications from their disease process may be immediately evident or become apparent during treatment and transport. Treatment and transport decisions may be affected by the patient's ongoing health status, especially if the patient is terminally ill or other end-of-life issues are involved. Therefore, thorough history and assessment is essential to appropriate decision making and modification of care based on the patient's unique needs. Good communication to the receiving medical and nursing staff is also essential.

KEY POINTS:

- The chronic health status of a patient can have an impact on complications and recovery.

- A detailed history is essential in determining the likely severity of a patient's current condition.

- The patient's current living conditions affect the patient's treatment compliance and safety.

- Involvement with hospice services or palliative care may alter the patient's treatment options.

- Knowledge of the patient's physical and mental baseline status is important for making comparisons regarding the current condition or complaint.

- Multiple chronic conditions may lead to the patient's current condition.

- Alterations in treatment and stabilization are necessary due to chronic conditions and changes of aging.

- Patients with chronic conditions have few reserves for an acute condition.

- Advanced directives and EMS immunity vary from state to state.

- Patients with chronic diseases may be able to donate organs or tissues.

REVIEW QUESTIONS:

1. Describe at least three ways in which a chronic condition can alter treatment options by the Paramedic.
2. How does a patient's living arrangement affect treatment compliance, patient safety, and availability of past medical history?
3. How do hospice services offer palliative care?
4. How does a Paramedic use the patient's physical and mental baseline status in making treatment decisions?

5. How does the presence of skeletal deformities affect stabilization?
6. What are the differences between the advanced directives of DNR, DNAR, living wills, healthcare proxies, durable power of attorney for health care, and POLST and MOLST forms?

CASE STUDY QUESTIONS:

Please refer to the Case Study in this chapter, and answer the questions below:

1. Name at least three likely causes for a fall in the elderly patient.

2. Describe the professional communication that should take place between home health providers and the Paramedic.

3. Should the Paramedic bring the patient's medication bottles to the ED? Why or why not?

4. Did the Paramedic follow the intent of the POLST form by starting the IV, checking a blood sugar, and assisting ventilations with the BVM? Explain your answer.

REFERENCES:

1. Kennedy RL, Grant PT, et al. Low-impact falls: demands on a system of trauma management, prediction of outcome, and influence of comorbidities. *J Trauma*. 2001;51(4):717–724.

2. Aschkenasy MT, Rothenhaus TC. Trauma and falls in the elderly. *Emerg Med Clin North Am*. 2006;24(2):413–432, vii.

3. Arnold DH, Gebretsadik T, et al. Assessment of severity measures for acute asthma outcomes: a first step in developing an asthma clinical prediction rule. *Am J Emerg Med*. 2008;26(4):473–479.

4. Jorres AJ. Acute renal failure: pathogenesis, diagnosis and conservative treatment. *Minerva Med*. 2002;93(2):85–93.

5. Iserson KV. Prehospital advance directives—a better way. *J Emerg Med*. 2002;23(4):419–420.

6. Mathei C, Niclaes L, et al. Infections in residents of nursing homes. *Infect Dis Clin North Am*. 2007;21(3):761–772, ix.

7. Hughes CM, Smith MB, et al. Infection control strategies for preventing the transmission of meticillin-resistant Staphylococcus aureus (MRSA) in nursing homes for older people. *Cochrane Database Syst Rev*. 2008;1:CD006354.

8. Kenneley IL. Infection control and prevention in home healthcare: prevention activities are the key to desired patient outcomes. *Home Healthc Nurse*. 2007;25(7):459–467; quiz 468–469.

9. Younis T, Milch R, et al. Length of survival in hospice for cancer patients referred from a comprehensive cancer center. *Am J Hosp Palliat Care*. 2009; 5(23):205–211.

10. Claxton-Oldfield S, Gosselin N, et al. Imagine you are dying: would you be interested in having a hospice palliative care volunteer? *Am J Hosp Palliat Care*. 2009;26(1):47–51.

11. Purnell LD, Paulanka BJ. *Transcultural Health Care*. Philadelphia PA: FA Davis; 2003.

12. Kinsky MP, Vaid SU, et al. Effect of esmolol on fluid therapy in normovolemia and hypovolemia. *Shock*. 2008;30(1):55–63.

13. Association, American Heart. *Advanced Cardiovascular Life Support Provider Manual (American Heart Association, ACLS Provider Manual)*. Dallas: American Heart Association; 2007.

14. Physician Orders for Life Sustaining Treatment Paradigm. Available at: **http://www.ohsu.edu/ethics/polst/.** Accessed February 2, 2009.

15. Heffner JE, Barbieri C, et al. Procedure-specific do-not-resuscitate orders. Effect on communication of treatment limitations. *Arch Intern Med*. 1996;156(7):793–797.

16. Fleming C, Mallepalli J, et al. How—and when—to obtain consent for do-not-resuscitate orders. Clinical guidelines and strategies for resolving conflicts. *J Crit Illn*. 1995;10(10): 679–681, 686, 690–691.

17. Cantor MD. Improving advance care planning: lessons from POLST. Physician Orders for Life-Sustaining Treatment. *J Am Geriatr Soc*. 2000;48(10):1343–1344.

18. Crane MK, Wittink M, et al. Respecting end-of-life treatment preferences. *Am Fam Physician*. 2005;72(7):1263–1268.

19. Lo B. Advance care planning. *Am J Geriatr Cardiol*. 2004;13(6):316–320.

20. Nolde D. The New York State Health Care Proxy Law and the issue of artificial hydration and nutrition. *J N Y State Nurses Assoc*. 2003;34(2):22–27.

CHAPTER 47

VIOLENCE IN THE COMMUNITY

KEY CONCEPTS:

Upon completion of this chapter, it is expected that the reader will understand these following concepts:

- The important role of prehospital personnel in identifying the signs and symptoms of intimate partner abuse, sexual abuse, and elder abuse

- The importance to Paramedics of understanding the dynamics and impact of domestic violence, sexual assault, and elder abuse on the individual, the family, and the community

- The Paramedic's significant role as a member of the sexual assault response team

- The impact of appropriate treatment and referrals for victims of violence

ANATOMY CONCEPTS:

Prior to reading this chapter the Paramedic student should be familiar with the following anatomy and physiology concepts:

- Reproductive anatomy
- Head and face anatomy
- Abdominal anatomy

CASE STUDY:

Paramedics on board a Southeast Ambulance are dispatched to the home of a 72-year-female patient complaining of abdominal pain. Arriving on-scene approximately three to four minutes later, the Paramedics find a female sitting on the porch, crying. She is wearing a cotton summer dress with dried blood on the hem. As the Paramedics approach the patient, they notice multiple bruises on her arms bilaterally. The Paramedics introduce themselves and ask the female if she was the individual who summoned an ambulance.

CRITICAL THINKING QUESTIONS

1. What are some of the possible causes of abdominal pain?
2. How is dried blood on the dress related to the abdominal pain?

OVERVIEW

Victims of violence may suffer emotional, psychological, physical, and/or sexual abuse. Each of these types of violence can result in both acute and chronic signs and symptoms of physical illness and injury, as well as psychological, emotional, and financial injury. Frequently, the injuries sustained require abused victims to seek care from healthcare professionals immediately after their victimization.

Violence in the community is a serious health concern which affects people of all socioeconomic classes and backgrounds. Violence is also a worldwide problem affecting individuals of all ages, races, ethnicities, and religious affiliations. Violence encompasses a wide variety of topics and subjects, but the focus of this chapter will be on sexual assault (SA) and rape, intimate partner violence (IPV), domestic violence (DV), and elder abuse. These all represent forms of violence in the community aimed at an individual who may have a trusting relationship betrayed.

Chief Concern

The consequences or dynamics of domestic violence on society range from physical and emotional injuries to social and financial devastation. Examples of violence include gun violence, robbery or theft, sexual assault, intimate partner violence or domestic violence, elder abuse, and child abuse, to name a few.

Of particular concern is the rise in youth violence and youth dating violence. **Youth violence** has been defined as "the intentional use of physical force or power, threatened or actual, exerted by or against children, adolescents or young adults ages 10–19 which results in or has a high likelihood of resulting in injury, death, psychological harm, maldevelopment or deprivation."[1]

According to the Centers for Disease Control and Prevention (CDC), one out of four adolescents report some form of abuse each year. In addition, 20% of teenage girls and young women have experienced some form of dating violence (controlling, abusive, and aggressive behavior) in a romantic relationship.[2] Physical and sexual abuse are typically accompanied by social, psychological, and emotional abuse (Figure 47-1).

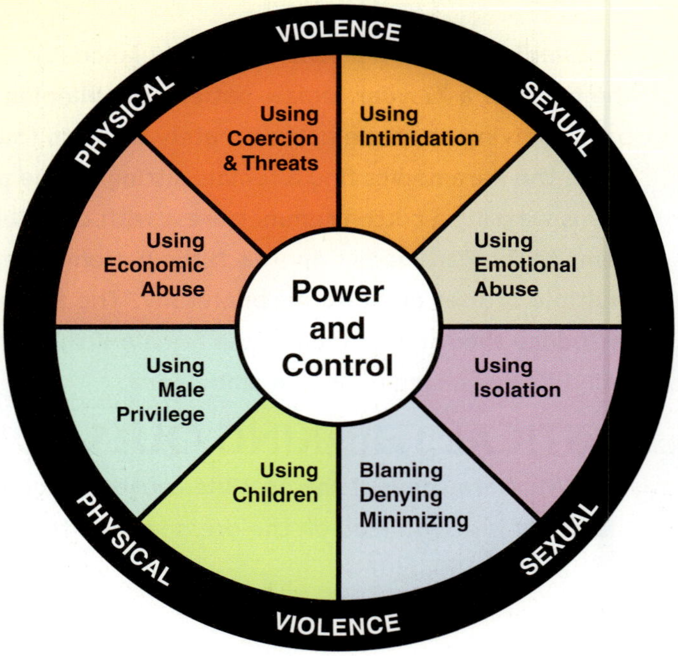

Intimate Partner Violence

Intimate partner violence (IPV), also referred to as **domestic violence (DV)**, can be described as violence between partners in an ongoing or past relationship regardless of marital status or sexual orientation. Domestic violence continues to be a prevailing problem in the United States and has, over the last several years, emerged as one of the most serious public health problems facing society, particularly women and youth.[3] According to the National Violence against Women Survey of 2002, approximately 25% to 50% of women who

Figure 47-1 Dynamics of abuse.

Courtesy of Domestic Abuse Intervention Programs

seek emergency services or care are victims of intimate partner violence (Table 47-1).[4]

The statistics related to intimate partner violence are not exact. This could be due to the manner in which the data is collected, how intimate partner violence is defined, and, more importantly, the underreporting of intimate partner violence. Most data that is collected is obtained from police departments, clinical settings, surveys, research, and other sources.[5]

Table 47-1 Domestic Violence Statistics

- 20% to 30% of American women are physically abused by partners.
- 1.3 million women and 834,732 men are physically assaulted by an intimate partner annually.
- 201,394 women are forcibly raped by an intimate partner annually.
- 11% of women involved in homosexual relationships and 23% of men in homosexual relationships report being raped or physically assaulted by an intimate partner.
- 1% to 25% of all pregnant women are battered during pregnancy.
- 30% to 40% of women's emergency room visits are from injuries related to DV.
- 30% of women killed in the United States are killed by husbands or boyfriends.
- 50% of men who assaulted their female partners also assaulted their children.
- 3.3 million children witness DV each year.

Source: http://www.ojp,usdoj.gov/bjs

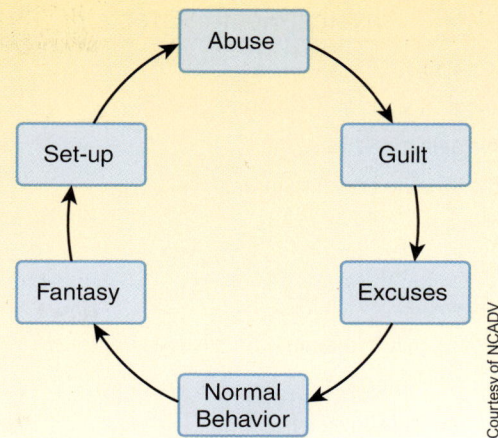

Figure 47-2 Cycle of abuse.

CULTURAL/REGIONAL DIFFERENCES

In some cultures and religious groups, physical violence toward women and children is perceived as discipline or "keeping one in line." Regardless of whether it is culturally or religiously sanctioned, physical violence is not permissible in the United States.

During the history and physical, the patient may admit to depression, anxiety, suicidal ideations, low self-esteem, fear, and distrust. In addition, the patient may disclose risky behaviors such as substance abuse, unprotected sex or multiple sex partners, unhealthy diet, and cigarette smoking. Therefore, it is important for the Paramedic to use a nonjudgmental therapeutic approach when providing care to patients who are victims of abuse.[6]

The phenomenon of intimate partner violence is frequently cyclical and the level of violence escalates over time (Figure 47-2).

The **cycle of abuse** is tension, crisis, and calm. The components of intimate partner violence may include financial, verbal, emotional or psychological, physical, and sexual abuse or the threat of violence and/or harm. Additional components include forced sex or sexual assault, sexual intimidation or degradation, unprotected sex, and nonnegotiable sex. According to the National Coalition against Domestic Violence, between one-third and one-half of battered women are raped by their partners at least once during their relationship.[7]

The physical and emotional effects of intimate partner violence have devastating long-term effects on victims and their families. Children may also become victims of intimate partner violence when the violence occurs between the parents of the children. Research has shown that an overlap exists between intimate partner violence and child maltreatment and abuse. One study demonstrated that children of abused mothers are 57 times more likely to be harmed because of violence between the parents.[8]

The significance for Paramedics is that the victim of intimate partner violence may present with either very specific complaints or vague nondescript complaints. Examples of the physical effects of intimate partner violence may include physical injuries and trauma, neurological symptoms, acute or chronic pain, hypertension, sexually transmitted infections, HIV/AIDS, and suicide attempts (Table 47-2).

The crimes of rape and **sexual assault (SA)** are defined in legal terms by legislation in every state. Specific laws vary by state, but sexual assault generally refers to any crime in which the offender subjects the victim to sexual contact that is unwanted and offensive. Sexual assault encompasses rape and thus includes nonconsensual sexual intercourse that is committed by physical force, or the threat of injury.[9] **Nonconsensual** (lack of permission) sexual intercourse includes situations in which the victim is unable to say "no" to intercourse or sexual contact. The inability may be due to mental capacity, developmental level, the effects of drugs or alcohol, or age of consent.

Drug-facilitated sexual assault (DFSA) is an assault facilitated by the offender's use of an "anesthesia-type" drug which, when administered to the victim, renders the victim physically incapacitated or helpless and thus incapable of giving or not giving consent (Table 47-3).[10,11] Signs and symptoms of this drug may include feeling very drunk (although the victim states only having one alcoholic drink), euphoria, not recalling events, cameo recall, awakening with articles of clothing missing, awakening with the sensation that he or

Table 47-2 Physical Health Effects of IPV/DV

- Physical injury
- Neurological signs and symptoms
- Chronic pain
- Chronic irritable bowel syndrome
- Hypertension
- Smoking
- STDs, HIV/AIDS
- Pelvic pain, pelvic inflammatory disease, infertility
- Urinary tract infections
- Risk of homicide, low self-esteem
  - Physical: ranges from minor injuries to life-threatening (even death)
  - Psychological: depression and anxiety, antisocial behavior, low self-esteem, loss of trust, and fear of intimacy
  - Social: risk-taking behaviors including promiscuity, substance abuse, social isolation, and restricted access to services
  - Economic: the cost of IPV exceeds billions of dollars in direct medical and mental health care costs and indirect costs in lost productivity

Table 47-3 Common Drugs Used in Sexual Assault

- Alcohol: Ethanol is the number one drug of choice
- GHB/GBL (Gamma Hydroxybutyrate): Colorless, thicker consistency than water, salty taste (i.e., easy lay, Liquid X)
- Benzodiazepines: Ativan, Valium, Xanax, Rohypnol
- Ketamine: Clear liquid, white powder, unstable
- Ecstasy: Decreases inhibitions, increases euphoria
- LSD: Powerful hallucinogenic, CNS depressant

Table 47-4 Sequela of Rape

- Isolation
- Depression
- Anxiety
- Suicide attempts

sodomy, fellatio, cunniligus, and analingus, just to name a few. The dynamics of sexual assault include power, control, and anger. Rape is a crime of violence that involves the use (or threat) of force that is motivated by power, control, aggression, anger, and rage. The sequela of rape may include isolation, depression, anxiety, and suicide attempts (Table 47-4).

The U.S. Department of Justice, Bureau of Justice Statistics reported that about 7 in 10 female rape or sexual assault victims stated the offender was an intimate partner, other relative, a friend, or an acquaintance.[12] Males were more likely to be violently victimized by a stranger than a non-stranger. The scope of the crime of rape cannot be truly appreciated because of underreporting. However, the U.S. Department of Justice statistical reports show that for persons age 12 and older, over 190,000 rapes and sexual assaults were reported to law enforcement, and over 112,000 attempted rapes and threats of sexual assault were reported. The interesting statistical data showed that 30% of the rapes and attempted rapes occurred between 6 p.m. and midnight and 4 out of 10 assaults occurred in the victims' homes.[9,13]

The sexual offender controls the victim and the experience. Gaining control of the victim, which can be done through the use of weapons or threats, is the first important component of the crime. What happens during the attack depends on the type and mind-set of the offender. Some offenders are sadistic and find sexual excitement in inflicting pain. The sex acts themselves also depend on the fantasy of the offender. What is very important to remember is that rape is about power and control and the sex or assault is the vehicle used to carry out the anger and aggression. Serial rapists repeat the pattern of sex acts and other behaviors involved in the crime. Law enforcement officials profile sexual offenders by examining behavior and the crime scene and by gathering information from or about the victim (Table 47-5).

Elder abuse and maltreatment is a public health problem which includes physical, sexual, emotional, and psychological

she had sex, or awakening in a location different from last remembered.

It is important to note that rape can occur when the offender and victim have a preexisting relationship (e.g., a "date rape") and even when the offender is the victim's spouse.

Sexual assault is an all-encompassing term that includes sexual activity with or without penetration. In some states, it is unlawful for an adult to engage in sexual intercourse with a person who has not reached the age of consent (usually 18 years of age); thus, that act is considered a sexual assault. Sexual assault is any form of nonconsenting sexual activity, which encompasses all unwanted sexual acts (vaginal, anal, oral, fondling, penetration).[9] The elements of sexual assault may involve lack of consent, age of consent, force, and the actual or attempted penetration of a victim's mouth, vagina, or rectum. The types of sexual offenses may include intercourse,

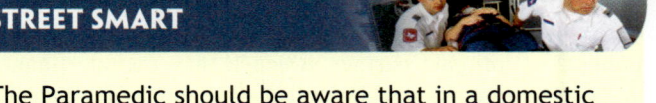

STREET SMART

The Paramedic should be aware that in a domestic violence situation both victim and perpetrator can turn on the Paramedic. Waiting for law enforcement officers prior to entering such a scene is a prudent course of action for the Paramedic.

Table 47-5 Types of Rapists

- The Power Re-Assurance "Peeping Tom" commits about 81% of reported rapes. This type strikes around midnight to 4 a.m.

- The Power Assertive rapist commits about 12% of reported rapes. This type "cruises for victims," chooses random victims, is charming, beats women, has a large ego, is antisocial, can be psychotic, and may use any force necessary.

- The Anger-Retaliatory rapist commits about 5% of reported rapes. This type is described as a "Tasmanian devil," who will beat women/victims, is very angry, and retaliates until anger is resolved.

- The Anger-Excitation rapist commits about 1% of reported rapes. This type is described as "Dr. Jekyll and Mr. Hyde" and is the most dangerous rapist. This type will kill the victim, is psychotic, has premeditated plans, will have tape, rope, and other accessories needed, will video or record attack/murder, is well-educated, has a white collar job, and takes victim to a second location.

abuse and neglect as well as control over the elderly person's finances. Neglect is the most prevalent form of elder abuse, accounting for 60% to 70% of elder abuse cases that are reported to Adult Protective Services each year. **Adult Protective Services (APS)** is a collection of governmental social service agencies that focus on the elderly.[5] Consisting of social workers and others, APS is typically responsible for investigating reports of domestic elder abuse. It is estimated that in the United States, 1.5 to 2.5 million older persons suffer from abuse each year, with the majority of the abuse cases being domestic abuse (occurring in the home, with abuse by close relatives and intimate partners) rather than in an institution such as a nursing home.[14] Family violence—including child physical and sexual abuse, child neglect and maltreatment, intimate partner violence, and elder abuse—takes place in homes across the country every day.

Elder sexual abuse has been defined as the coercing or the use of (or threat of) force against an elderly person to cause such person to engage in sexual acts against his or her will.[15] The exact prevalence of elder sexual abuse is not known and there is little research that has been conducted to investigate the breadth of the problem. Advanced age, female gender, poverty, depression, increased dependency, social isolation, and cognitive and functional impairment are factors that place the elderly at risk for abuse. The National Crime Victimization Survey in 2006 noted that, out of the 261,000 rapes and sexual assaults that occurred, 3,270 victims were age 65 or older.[12]

It is important to understand that the domestic violence/sexual abuse dynamic involves not only a victim but a perpetrator as well. Abused and neglected elders, who may be mistreated by their spouses, partners, children, and other relatives, are among the most isolated of all victims of violence. Many of the elderly live alone and may have little or no interaction with community organizations, which makes it difficult to detect elder abuse. For example, an adult son or daughter who lives with his or her parents may depend on the parents for financial support and may be in a position to inflict abuse.[15] Additional stressors that may precipitate the abuse by the offender include drug and alcohol use, legal problems, and a history of being abused themselves.

Medical personnel are not typically trained to identify sexual abuse of the elderly.[14] This may be due to lack of experience of the healthcare providers; unfamiliarity with the elderly patient's anatomy and physiology, physiological changes (normal aging process), mechanism of injury (cause of injury), or inability to communicate (cognitive ability); and/or the Paramedic's sociocultural beliefs (ageism).[16] Some of the first steps in providing care to elderly victims of abuse are to accurately assess, treat, and stabilize. The next important steps are to identify signs of abuse and accurately document and report physical findings. Lastly, the prehospital medical personnel must also be astute and preserve evidence. Some warning signs of elder abuse may include unexplained injuries and falls, bruises, malnourishment, inappropriate clothing, poor hygiene, significant dependence on caregiver, financial constraints, and delays in seeking medical care. If a Paramedic suspects elder abuse, he should contact the police or a law enforcement agency, or a welfare or social services agency, according to the state or employment agency law and policies. Most cities and counties will investigate and protect the elder adult from abuse. The website for the National Center on Elder Abuse maintains a list of phone numbers, by state, that can assist individuals who suspect elder abuse.

CASE STUDY (CONTINUED)

Through her tears, the patient relates that she was sexually assaulted by her nephew. Distraught, she keeps asking, "What did I do to deserve this?" She explains that her nephew often comes over to the house to help with odd jobs and often just hangs out with her. She is not sure that she can ever be safe in her house again.

CRITICAL THINKING QUESTIONS

1. What are the important elements of the history that a Paramedic should obtain?
2. What resources could the Paramedic request to help on-scene?

History

The Paramedic should ensure that the scene is safe for both the victim and himself prior to taking a history. The assessment should include the patient's feeling of danger and lethality, the patient's safety concerns, the patient's present health status, a review of the patient's medications, a physical assessment for trauma and other signs of illness, an evaluation of level of consciousness (LOC), and the ABC principles.

Paramedics are in a unique position to help recognize, intervene, and minimize the effects of sexual assault and IPV. Paramedics are usually the first healthcare providers that victims encounter and are in a critical position to identify victims of domestic violence and sexual abuse.

The Paramedic will be providing services and care to survivors, offenders, and family members of the parties. In addition, the uniqueness of IPV will require the Paramedic to work collaboratively with other healthcare professionals, crisis intervention advocates, law enforcement officials, and the judicial system. The healthcare provider's goals are to help reduce violence in the community; provide and offer support to victims, offenders, and family members; and to educate the public on the dynamics and effects of IPV on a community.[13] In addition to assessing for signs of domestic violence and sexual assault (i.e., choking, strangulation, ligature marks, bite marks, or burns), the Paramedic must use caution and maintain the integrity of evidence while treating the patient.

PROFESSIONAL PARAMEDIC

As sexual assault and other domestic violence incidents are often attempts at control, the professional Paramedic will give the patient as much control of the situation as is safely possible. This may mean backing away and allowing another provider of the same gender or age to work with the patient instead.

Paramedics should be aware of the **critical time frames** related to sexual assault evidence collection. The International Association of Forensic Nurses (IAFN) has well-established guidelines to aid healthcare professionals and a SANE nurse in providing care to victims of sexual assault. Briefly, a **sexual assault nurse examiner (SANE)** is a registered nurse who has undergone additional intensive training which consists of classroom and clinical education.[17,18] The post-education clinical requirements and skills include medical, legal, forensic, crisis intervention, and law enforcement competencies. Once completed, the SANE sits for the national certification examination. The IAFN guidelines for sexual assault investigations include steps in the collecting, processing, procuring, securing, and transferring of evidence (Table 47-6), as well as administering post-exposure medication, which must all be given in a very specific time frame.

The IAFN's purpose for developing standards is to fulfill the needs of registered nurses and/or healthcare providers and offer guidance in working with patients/clients who are victims/survivors of violence in all settings. The goal is to be able to provide the best possible medical, emotional, and psychological outcome for the victim as well as assist with the legal outcome.

Table 47-6 Role of EMS with Sexual Assault Victim: Critical Time Frames

- Identify any physical or psychological needs
- Stabilize patient and treat injuries
  - May supersede forensic exam
- Preserve evidence
- Critical time frames:
  - 96 hours for sexual assault forensic exam
  - 36 hours for post-exposure HIV medications
  - 72 hours for emergency contraception medication
  - 24 to 36 hours for DFSA evidence collection to be completed
- Documentation
- Judicial process

CASE STUDY (CONTINUED)

The woman, Mrs. Smythe, at first refuses any physical examination. However, after walking to the safety offered by the back of the ambulance and listening to the Paramedic's calm and reassuring voice, she agrees to let the Paramedic's partner take a set of vital signs. The Paramedic starts to talk to Mrs. Smythe about the bruises on her arms.

CRITICAL THINKING QUESTIONS

1. What are the elements of the physical examination of a patient who is a victim of sexual assault?
2. Why is a witness a critical element in this examination?

Examination

Accurate **wound identification** and location is essential when the Paramedic is documenting injuries for victims of sexual assault. A wound can be defined as a break or interruption in the continuity of tissue caused by physical or mechanical means (Tables 47-7 and 47-8). Depending on the length and severity of abuse, the physical findings may range from minor bruises, abrasions, and scratches to more life-threatening injuries such as gunshot or knife wounds, choking or respiratory difficulties, heart or circulatory problems, broken bones, or obstetric and gynecological emergencies.

Accurate recognition and assessment for signs of abuse and maltreatment will aid the Paramedic in determining the appropriate treatment options as well as help facilitate improving the patient's overall outcome.[19]

STREET SMART

In an effort to preserve evidence, the Paramedic should instruct the victim to avoid eating, drinking, gargling, brushing teeth, washing, or showering until evidence is collected. If possible, urination and defecation should also be avoided.

Clothing from the victim should be folded and placed in a paper bag. The Paramedic should not shake the clothing. The bag should be labeled and the patient care record should reflect to whom (by name and title) the bag was given. This is called the chain of evidence.

Table 47-7   Documentation Tool

Wound Documentation Tool: The BEARS mnemonic is often used to document injuries to victims of sexual assault.

B   Bruises, tears, lacerations, etc.

E   Ecchymosis/bruises

A   Abrasions

R   Redness

S   Swelling

Table 47-8   Mechanism of Wounds

- Mechanical (caused by some kind of trauma that damages the tissue)
  - Blunt trauma: created by items such as a hammer, a pipe, a fist, etc.; creates contusions, lacerations, and abrasions
  - Blunt-force trauma: sometimes creates a pattern in the design or shape of the injury that resembles the weapon
  - Bite mark: a form of patterned injury composed of contusions and lacerations that correspond to the offender's dental arch, tooth characteristics, and jaw
- Physical (may result from organisms, chemicals, thermal agents, or death of tissues or organs)
  - Bruise: usually results in swelling and pain
  - Ecchymosis: flat, blood underneath the skin, NOT PAINFUL
  - Laceration: jagged, caused by blunt force
  - Cut/incision: smooth edges, usually caused by a sharp object
  - Abrasion: removal of the top layer of skin (superficial)
  - Avulsion: tearing of a structure from its normal anatomical position, may be damage to vessels, nerves, etc.
- Stages of healing: acute, sub-acute, chronic, and old-chronic
  - Acute: immediately following incident, amount of bleeding determined by injury
  - Sub-acute: epithelialization, bleeding usually ceased, pain and swelling, less than three to four days after injury, this stage ends when scab is gone in a week or so
  - Chronic: skin's layer structure formed, smooth, firm, pink, "proud flesh"
  - Old-chronic: remodeling continues for years
- Most common sites of injury: nonconsensual penile–vaginal penetration
  - Mounting injuries are usually seen at 3-6-9 o'clock on posterior fourchette.
  - Injuries to these sites suggest that the human physiological response to sexual stimulation plays a significant role. For example, lack of pelvic tilt to assist with insertion of penis, lack of lubrication, lack of relaxation.
    - Posterior fourchette "BEARS"
    - Fossa navicularis "BEARS"
    - Labia minora "abrasions"
    - Hymen "ecchymosis"

Mrs. Smythe is clearly traumatized, both physically and psychologically, by the sexual assault. Trying to not be forceful or overbearing, the Paramedic recommends that Mrs. Smythe at least seek medical attention.

CRITICAL THINKING QUESTIONS

1. What is the common sequela of sexual assault and rape?
2. Why was the Paramedic concerned about not appearing to be overbearing?

Assessment

Each victim of sexual assault (rape) processes the psychological trauma associated with the assault differently. However, there are common patterns that emerge in these responses, commonly referred to as the rape trauma syndrome. The limbic system in the brain holds traumatic memory and is the body's alarm center as well as the center of arousal, sleep, rest, sexual response, and attachment. The psychological sequelae of sexual assault (rape) may include isolation, depression, anxiety, suicide attempts, and post-traumatic stress disorder (PTSD). There are four common signs and symptoms: (1) reliving the experience, (2) social withdrawal, (3) avoidance, and (4) increased physiological arousal (somatic complaints).[12]

Mrs. Smythe appears a little disoriented and becomes agitated by the presence of the Paramedics. The Paramedics elect to withdraw from Mrs. Smythe for a few minutes by stepping out of the ambulance and allowing her to be alone. She soon calls the Paramedics back into the ambulance, saying, "I am bleeding and I really need to go to the hospital."

CRITICAL THINKING QUESTIONS

1. What is the standard of care of patients when treating a sexual assault victim?
2. What are some of the patient-specific concerns that the Paramedic should focus on?

Treatment

Victims often report difficulties related to these processes. Many victims exhibit signs and symptoms of the rape trauma syndrome. **Rape trauma syndrome (RTS)** is defined as the temporary loss of ability to cope with life situations related to overwhelming stress. RTS is further defined as the behavioral, somatic, and psychological reactions that occur as a result of rape or attempted rape. This syndrome is an acute reaction to a life-threatening situation. Rape trauma syndrome has two stages: an acute (disorganization) stage and a long-term process (reorganization) stage (Table 47-9).[12] Treatment is focused on providing psychological "first aid" to the patient.

Table 47-9 Rape Trauma Syndrome: Acute and Long-Term Phase

- Rape trauma syndrome: acute phase
  - Expressed emotion: fear, anger, panic
  - Guarded and controlled emotions: guilt, abandonment
  - Physical reactions: G.I., G.U., musculoskeletal pain, and/or wounds
  - Change in sexual behaviors
  - Psychological: phobias, nightmares, depression, suicidal ideations, anxiety, and sleep disturbances
- Rape trauma syndrome: long-term phase
  - Physical changes: unkempt appearance
  - Psychological changes: phobias, personality, emotionally labile, and/or depression
  - Social changes: seek family and social network support
  - Changes in sexuality
  - Both acute and long-term phases can last days, months, and years post-sexual assault

During the quiet ride to the hospital, Mrs. Smythe relates how her nephew paid all of the bills, using her checkbook, and took care of all of her financial affairs. She was becoming concerned because she had received a telephone call from the power company telling her she was late in paying her bill and that they may be forced to turn off the power. She told them that was not possible as her nephew always paid the bills on time. The power company said they would send a representative to her house to discuss it. After hanging up the telephone, she started to become worried. However, the patient's nephew told her that the check was probably lost in the mail and he would send another one.

CRITICAL THINKING QUESTIONS

1. What is the definition of elder abuse?
2. Is diversion of financial resources for personal gain a crime?

Evaluation

Although sexual assault can be emotionally overwhelming to the Paramedic, he must keep in mind that sexual assault is, first, a trauma. Sexually assaulted individuals are often battered. In the case of an elderly patient, especially one on anticoagulant, a minor head wound could lead to a life-threatening subdural hematoma. The Paramedic must remain vigilant for signs of traumatic brain injury, internal bleeding (particularly intra-abdominal hemorrhage), and musculoskeletal injury. The patient may be distracted and fail to report other injuries.

The Paramedics escort Mrs. Smythe into the examining room and wait for the nurse to come to the bedside. They explain the situation and the fact that Mrs. Smythe did not want the police involved. The nurse thanks the Paramedics and asks them to speak to the attending physician on their way out.

CRITICAL THINKING QUESTIONS

1. What is the most appropriate transport decision that will get the patient to definitive care?
2. What are the advantages of transporting a sexual assault victim to a SAFE center, even if that means bypassing other hospitals in the process?

Disposition

Documentation is especially important. The medical record is a legal document and appropriate documentation that provides concrete evidence of violence and abuse may be critical to the outcome of any legal case. The Paramedic needs to be able to document accurately and objectively the physical injuries by means of a written record, body map, or diagram.[20] The prehospital professional may receive a subpoena ordering him to appear in court to testify in criminal cases involving alleged abuse. Courtroom preparation begins with the initial on-scene contact with the victim. It is important to note that the Paramedic may be the only individual who will hear the victim (or a perpetrator) issue a statement in the heat of the moment (called an excited utterance). The Paramedic must document these statements using the speaker's own words in quotation marks (Table 47-10).

Sexual assault forensic examination (SAFE) centers, as well as community response teams, provide victims of sexual assault with access to trained staff 24 hours per day 7 days per week to assist victims of sexual assault with forensic exams and other needed services (Table 47-11).

Community members typically consist of doctors, nurses, prehospital personnel, law enforcement, and social services agencies including Adult Protective Services. The APS is also responsible for providing families with guidance in seeking help with other services and needs.

Table 47-10 Documentation Tips

- Always write legibly. This can help keep you out of court and/or provide strong support if you are required to testify.
- Document the patient's complaints (use quotation marks if using patient's own words) and symptoms as well as the results of your assessment and observation.
- Document the patient's allergies, medical and trauma history, and *relevant* social history.
- Document a detailed description of the injuries, including type, number, size, location, and explanations given by the patient.
- When circumstances allow, elicit and document if there were any witnesses to the event, and where and when the event occurred.
- Document responding agencies: crisis intervention/advocacy, law enforcement agencies, prehospital personnel (EMS & fire department), and the time of arrival to facility.

Table 47-11 Community Resources: Sexual Assault Response Team (SART)

- Law enforcement
- Prehospital personnel
- Sexual assault nurse examiners (SANE)
- Crisis services/advocates
- Prosecutors/district attorneys
- Designated sexual assault forensic exam (SAFE) centers

Victims of sexual assault have encountered a frightening and traumatic experience. They often present to hospital EDs needing physical evaluation and emotional support. Each victim of sexual assault presenting at the ED deserves to have a medical and forensic screening exam by a healthcare provider who has access to consultative specialty services as indicated by the patient's medical and psychosocial needs. Victims of sexual assault should be immediately processed so that care can be provided following the *Protocol for the Acute Care of the Adult Patient Reporting Sexual Assault* and established SAFE procedures.[3]

Victims of sexual assault benefit from going to a SAFE center. They are offered prophylactic post-exposure treatment for sexually transmitted infections (STI), including the HIV post-exposure prophylaxis (HIV-PEP) kit and hepatitis B virus (HBV) immune globulin. All victims who are considered fertile are offered emergency contraception (EC). Each victim is given sexual assault literature including comprehensive sexual assault assessment forms, crime victims board claim forms, sexually transmitted diseases information, and counseling/advocacy program information. By deciding to transport the victim to a SAFE center, the Paramedic will help facilitate the goal of improving the medical, psychosocial, and legal outcomes for victims of sexual assault.

CONCLUSION

Violence in the community is a serious health concern that affects people of all socioeconomic classes and backgrounds. Violence is a worldwide problem affecting individuals of all ages, races, ethnicities, and religious affiliations. Violence encompasses a wide variety of topics and subjects including physical and sexual abuse, which is typically accompanied by social, psychological, and emotional abuse.

Accurate recognition and assessment for signs of abuse and maltreatment will aid the Paramedic in considering the appropriate treatment options as well as help facilitate improving the patient's overall outcome. Paramedics should be aware of the critical time frames related to sexual assault evidence collection. Victims of sexual assault have encountered a frightening and traumatic experience. They often present to hospital EDs needing a physical evaluation and emotional support. Paramedics play an integral role as a member of the SART team. The goal is to be able to obtain the best possible medical, emotional, psychological, and legal outcomes for the victim.

KEY POINTS:

- CDC records indicate that 25% of youth report experiencing personal violence, and 20% of teen girls report dating violence.

- Physical abuse is often accompanied by social, psychological, or emotional abuse.

- Intimate partner violence is cyclical and often escalates over time.

- The cycle of abuse is tension, crisis, and then calm.

- Sexual offenders control the victim and the experience.

- The history and exam must be conducted in a safe place for both the victim and the Paramedic.

- Taking a history, gathering evidence specimens, and administering medication must take place in a specific time frame.

- Documentation must include accurate wound identification and location.

- Common patterns of response to sexual assault are termed rape trauma syndrome.

- Elder maltreatment and abuse includes multiple types of actions as well as control over the elderly person's finances.

- Elders are often isolated, making abuse difficult to detect.

- Accurate documentation of incidents is crucial.

REVIEW QUESTIONS:

1. How prevalent is youth violence?
2. Name at least three other types of abuse that accompany physical abuse.
3. What are the three elements of the cycle of abuse?
4. Name the essential time frames for obtaining evidence and administering AIDS and contraceptive prophylaxis to victims of sexual assault.
5. List the individual meanings for the letters in the mnemonic BEARS as applied to wounds.
6. Define rape trauma syndrome.
7. Describe the forms of elder abuse.

CASE STUDY QUESTIONS:

Please refer to the Case Study in this chapter, and answer the questions below:

1. What concerns do you have regarding the initial presentation of the patient?

2. What forms of elder abuse do you suspect have occurred to Mrs. Smythe?

3. Using the tips on documentation, briefly write up the initial contact with Mrs. Smythe.

REFERENCES:

1. Valdez AM. Youth violence and injury prevention. *J Emerg Nurs.* 2007;33(4):379–381.

2. Catalano S. Intimate partner violence in the United States. 2005. Available at: **http://www.olp.usdoj.gov/bjs**. Accessed April 30, 2008.

3. International Association of Forensic Nurses. Sexual assault nurse examiner standards of practice. 2006. Available at: **http://www.iafn.org**. Accessed May 25, 2008.

4. Crane PA. Predictors of injury associated with rape. *J Forensic Nurs.* 2006;2(2):75–89. Available at: **http://www.iafn.org**. Accessed May 25, 2008.

5. Emergency Nurses Association. Emergency Nurses Association position statement: intimate partner and family violence, maltreatment and neglect. 2006. Available at: **http://www.ena.org**. Accessed May 25, 2008.

6. Berlinger J. Helping abuse victims part I: taking an intimate look at domestic. *Nursing2004.* 2004;34(10):42–46. Available at: **http://www.nursing2004.com**. Accessed May 25, 2008.

7. National Violence against Women Survey. (n.d.) Available at: **http://www.ncadv.org**. Accessed May 25, 2008.

8. Burgess AW, Roberts A. Violence and families. 2007. Available at: **http://www.nurse.com/ce/ptint.html?CCID=4113**. Accessed April 27, 2008.

9. Brown K. Sexual assault and rape: the nursing role. 2007. Available at: **http://www.nurse.com/ce/print.html?CCID=3225**. Accessed April 27, 2008.

10. Crawford E, Wright MO, et al. Drug-facilitated sexual assault: college women's risk perception and behavioral choices. *J Am Coll Health.* 2008;57(3):261–272.

11. Beynon CM, McVeigh C, et al. The involvement of drugs and alcohol in drug-facilitated sexual assault: a systematic review of the evidence. *Trauma Violence Abuse.* 2008;9(3):178–188.

12. Burgess A. Rape violence. 2007. Available at: **http://www.nurse.com/ce/print.html?CCID=4115**. Accessed April 27, 2008.

13. International Association of Forensic Nurses. *Standards of Intimate Partner Violence Nursing Practice.* 2006. Available at: **http://www.iafn.org**. Accessed May 25, 2008.

14. Burgess AW, Clements PT. Information processing of sexual abuse in elders. *J Forensic Nurs.* 2006;2(3):113–120.

15. Cooper GM, King MR. Interviewing the incarcerated offender convicted of sexually assaulting the elderly. *J Forensic Nurs.* 2006;2(3):130–146.

16. Schofield RB. Office of justice programs focuses on studying and preventing elder abuse. *J Forensic Nurs.* 2006;2(3):150–153. Available at: **http://www.iafn.org**. Accessed May 25, 2008.

17. Campbell R, Patterson D, et al. A participatory evaluation project to measure SANE nursing practice and adult sexual assault patients' psychological well-being. *J Forensic Nurs.* 2008;4(1):19–28.

18. Logan TK, Cole J, et al. Sexual assault nurse examiner program characteristics, barriers, and lessons learned. *J Forensic Nurs.* 2007;3(1):24–34.

19. Markson D, Tunik M, et al. A national assessment of knowledge, attitudes and confidence of pre-hospital providers in the assessment and management of child maltreatment. *Pediatrics.* 2007;119(1):103–108.

20. Brown K. Evidence collection and preservation in a healthcare setting. 2006. Available at: **http://www.nurse.com/ce/print.html?CCID=3311**. Accessed April 30, 2008.

ACRONYMS

AAA Abdominal aortic aneurysm
AAPCC American Association of Poison Control Centers
ABC Airway, breathing, circulation
ACE Angiotensin-converting enzyme
ACEP American College of Emergency Physicians
Ach Acetylcholine
ACLS Advanced cardiac life support
ACS Acute coronary syndrome
ACTH Adrenocorticotropic hormone
ADA American Diabetes Association
ADC AIDS dementia complex
ADH Antidiuretic hormone
ADL Activities of daily living
AED Automated external defibrillator
AFib Atrial fibrillation
AFE Amniotic fluid embolism
AF-RVR Atrial fibrillation with a rapid ventricular response
AHA American Heart Association
AIA Aspirin-induced asthma
AICD Automatic implanted cardiovertor—defibrillator
AIDS Acquired immunodeficiency syndrome
AIVR Accelerated idioventricular rhythms
AKA Alcoholic ketoacidosis
AKI Acute kidney injury
ALD Alcoholic liver disease
ALS Advanced life support
ALS Amyotrophic lateral sclerosis
ALTE Apparent life-threatening event
AMI Acute myocardial infarction
ANP Atrial natriuretic peptides
AODM Adult onset diabetes mellitus
APE Acute pulmonary edema
ARB Angiotensin II receptor blockers
ARBD Alcohol-related birth defects
ARDS Acute respiratory distress syndrome
ARF Acute renal failure
ARND Alcohol-related neurodevelopmental disorder
ASL American Sign Language
ASPCA American Society for the Prevention of Cruelty to Animals
ATP Adenosine-5'-triphosphate
ATV Automatic transport ventilator
AV Arteriovenous
AV Atrioventricular
AVNRT AV nodal re-entry tachycardia
AVPU Alert, voice, pain, unresponsiveness
AVRT AV re-entrant tachycardia

AWMI Anterior wall myocardial infarction
BAC Blood alcohol concentrations
BCG Bacillus Calmette—Guerin
Bi-PAP Bi-level positive airway pressure
BiVAD Biventricular assist device
BLS Basic life support
BMI Body mass index
BNP Brain natriuretic peptides
BP Blood pressure
BPH Benign prostatic hyperplasia/hypertrophy
BPPV Benign paroxysmal positional vertigo
BRBPR Bright red blood per rectum
BTE Biphasic truncated exponential waveform
BUN Blood urea nitrogen
BURP Backward, upward, rightward pressure
BVM Bag—valve mask
CABG Coronary artery bypass graft
CAD Coronary artery disease
CAP Community acquired pneumonia
CAPTA Child Abuse and Prevention Treatment Act
CBF Cerebral blood flow
CCPD Continuous cyclic peritoneal dialysis
CDC Centers for Disease Control
CFC Chlorofluorocarbons
CHB Complete heart block
CHF Congestive heart failure
CKD Chronic kidney disease
CO Cardiac output
CO Carbon monoxide
COHb Carboxyhemoglobin
COP Colloidal osmotic pressure
COPD Chronic obstructive pulmonary disease
CP Cerebral palsy
CPAP Continuous positive airway pressure
CPP Cerebral perfusion pressure
CPR Cardiopulmonary resuscitation
CSM Carotid sinus massage
CSP Carotid sinus pressure
CRPS Complex regional pain syndrome
CSF Cerebrospinal fluid
CSS Cincinnati stroke scale
CT Central terminal
CVA Cerebrovascular accident
D&C Dilation and curettage
DC Direct current
DCS Decompression sickness
DDS Dialysis disequilibrium syndrome
DFSA Drug-facilitated sexual assault

DGI Disseminated gonococcal infection
DIC Disseminated intravascular coagulation
DKA Diabetic ketoacidosis
DNAR Do not attempt resuscitation
DNI Do Not Intubate
DNR Do Not Resuscitate
DOE Dyspnea on exertion
DPAHC Durable power of attorneys for health care
DRSP Drug-resistant streptococcus pneumoniae
DSP Digital signal processing
DTaP Diphtheria, tetanus, and pertussis
DV Domestic violence
DVT Deep vein thrombosis
EC Emergency contraception
ECF Extracellular fluid
ECG Electrocardiographic
ED Emergency department
EDC Estimated date of confinement
EDD Estimated date of delivery
EDP Emotionally disturbed person
EEG Electroencephalogram
EGDT Early goal-directed therapy
ELBW Extremely low birth weight
ELM External laryngeal manipulation
EM Erythema migrans
EMC Emergency medical condition
EMD Electromechanical dissociation
EMG Electromyographic signal
EMI Electromagnetic interference
EMT Emergency medical technician
EMTALA Emergency Medical Treatment and Labor Act
EOM Extraocular eye movement
EPS Extrapyramidal syndrome
ESRD End-stage renal disease
FAE Fetal alcohol effects
FAS Fetal alcohol syndrome
FDA Food and Drug Administration
FRC Functional residual capacity
FTT Failure to thrive
FUO Fever of unknown origin
GABA Gamma aminobutyric acid
GAS Group A streptococcus
GCS Glascow Coma Scale
GDM Gestational diabetes
GERD Gastroesophageal reflux disease
GFR Glomerular filtration rate
GI Gastrointestinal
GIK Glucose, insulin, potassium
GN Glomerulonephritis
GPA Gravid, para, abortus
G6PD Glucose-6-phosphate dehydrogenase
GTD Gestational trophoblastic disease
HAART Highly active antiretroviral therapy

HAV Hepatitis A
HBV Hepatitis B
HCV Hepatitis C
HD Huntington's disease
HDV Hepatitis D
HEENT Head, eyes, ears, nose, throat
HEPA High-efficiency particulate air
HEV Hepatitis E
HFA Hydrofluoroalkanes
HHNS Hyperosmolar hyperglycemic nonketotic syndrome
HIE Hypoxic-ischemic encephalopathy
HIT Heparin-induced thrombocytopenia
HIV Human immunodeficiency virus
HIV-PEP HIV post-exposure prophylaxis
HJR Hepatic jugular reflex
HONKS Hyperosmolar nonketotic syndrome
HPV Human papilloma virus
HR Heart rate
HUS Hemolytic uremic syndrome
HVS Hyperventilation syndrome
IABP Intra-aortic balloon pump
IAFN International Association of Forensic Nurses
IBD Inflammatory bowel disease
IBS Irritable bowel syndrome
IC Inspiratory capacity
ICD Implantable cardioverter-defibrillator
ICP Intracranial pressure
ICS Inhaled corticosteroids
ICU Intensive care unit
I/O Intake/output
IO Intraosseous
IPV Intimate partner violence
ITP Idiopathic thrombocytopenic purpura
ITV Impedance threshold valve
IUD Intrauterine device
IWMI Inferior wall myocardial infarction
JET Junctional ectopic tachycardia
JVD Jugular venous distention
KSHV Kaposi's sarcoma-associated herpes virus
KVO Keep vein open
LAD Left anterior descending
LAE Left atrial enlargement
LASS Los Angeles Stroke Scale
LBBB Left bundle branch block
LBO Large bowel obstruction
LCA Left coronary artery
LED Light emitting diode
LGL Long-Ganong-Levine
LOC Level of consciousness
LPS Lipopolysaccharide
LTB Laryngotracheobronchitis
LVAD Left ventricular assist device

LVH Left ventricular hypertrophy
LMA Laryngeal mask airway
LMP Last menstrual period
MAHA Microangiopathic hemolytic anemia
MAO Monoamine oxidase
MAP Mean arterial pressure
MAT Multifocal atrial tachycardia
MCL Modified chest leads
MDI Metered dose inhaler
MDMA Methylenedioxymethamphetamine
MDR-TB Multi-drug resistant tuberculosis
MEND Miami emergency neurologic deficit
MetHb Methemoglobin
MI Myocardial infarction
MMAD Mass median aerodynamic diameter
MMR Mumps, measles, rubella
MMWR Morbidity and Mortality Weekly Report
MOLST Medical Orders for Life-Sustaining Treatment
MONA Morphine, oxygen, nitrates, aspirin
MRSA Multiple-resistant Staphylococcus aureus
MS Multiple sclerosis
MSDS Materials safety data sheet
MSE Mental status examination
MSE Medical screening examination
MSP Munchausen syndrome by proxy
NASH Nonalcoholic steatohepatitis
NCANDS National child abuse and neglect data system
NGT Nasogastric tube
NIBP Non-invasive blood pressure
NICU Neonatal intensive care unit
NIDDM Non-insulin dependent diabetes
NIHSS National Institutes of Health Stroke Scale
NINDS National Institute of Neurological Disorders
NIPD Nocturnal intermittent peritoneal dialysis
NIPPV Nasal intermittent positive pressure ventilation
NMS Neuroleptic malignant syndrome
NO Nitric oxide
NOI Nature of illness
NPA Nasopharyngeal airway
NPO Nothing by mouth
NSAID Non-steroidal anti-inflammatory drug
NSS Normal saline solution
NSTEMI Non-ST elevation myocardial infarction
OCD Obsessive-compulsive disorder
OGT Orogastric tube
OP Organophosphate pesticides
OPQRST AS/PN Onset, provocation, quality of pain, radiation, severity, timing, associated symptoms, pertinent negatives
OTC Over the counter
QTc Corrected QT interval
PAC Premature atrial complex
PALS Pediatric advanced life support

PAP Primary atypical pneumonia
PAT Paroxysmal atrial tachycardia
PAT Pediatric Assessment Triangle
PCP Pneumocystis carinii pneumonia
PDA Patent ductus arteriosus
PE Pulmonary embolism
PEA Pulseless electrical activity
PEEP Positive end expiratory pressure
PICC Peripherally inserted central catheter
PID Pelvic inflammatory disease
PIH Pregnancy-induced hypertension
PJC Premature junctional complex
PMI Point of maximal intensity
PND Paroxysmal nocturnal dyspnea
PNS Parasympathetic nervous system
POLST Physician Orders for Life-Sustaining Treatment
POPE Post-obstructive pulmonary edema
POTS Postural orthostatic tachycardia syndrome
PPD Purified protein derivative
PPE Personal protective equipment
PPI Proton pump inhibitors
PRI PR interval
PROM Premature rupture of membranes
PTCA Percutaneous transluminal coronary angioplasty
PTSD Post-traumatic stress disorder
PUD Peptic ulcer disease
PVC Premature ventricular complex
PVT Polymorphic ventricular tachycardia
RA Rheumatoid arthritis
RAAS Renin-angiotensin-aldosterone system
RAE Right atrial enlargement
RAP Repetitive complaints of abdominal pain
RAS Reticular activating system
RBBB Right bundle branch block
RBC Red blood cell
RCA Right coronary artery
ROP Retinopathy of prematurity
ROSC Return of spontaneous circulation
RP Refractory period
RRWP Reverse R wave progression
RSD Reflex sympathetic dystrophy
RSI Rapid sequence induction
RSV Respiratory syncytial virus
RTS Rape trauma syndrome
RUQ Right upper quadrant
RV Residual volume
RVAD Right ventricular assist device
RVH Right ventricular hypertrophy
RVR Rapid ventricular response
RWD Romano-Ward syndrome
SA Sexual abuse
SA Sinoatrial
SAFE Sexual assault forensic examination

SAH Subarachnoid hemorrhage
SANE Sexual assault nurse examiner
SARA Standing and raising aid
SARS Severe acute respiratory syndrome
SART Sexual assault response team
SBO Small bowel obstruction
SBS Shaken baby syndrome
SCA Sudden cardiac arrest
SCBA Self-contained breathing apparatus
SCFE Slipped capital femoral epiphysis
SIDS Sudden infant death syndrome
SITS Syndrome of inappropriate sinus tachycardia
SLE Systemic lupus erythematosus
SNS Sympathetic nervous system
SOB Shortness of breath
SP Septal perforators
SSCP Substernal chest pain
SSRI Selective serotonin reuptake inhibitors
STD Sexually transmitted disease
STEMI ST elevation myocardial infarction
STI Sexually transmitted infection
SV Stroke volume
SVN Small volume nebulizer
SVR Systemic vascular resistance
SVT Supraventricular tachycardia
TCA Tricyclic antidepressants
TCC Tunnel-cuffed catheter
TCP Transcutaneous pacing
TEP Transcutaneous external pacemaker
TESS Toxic exposure surveillance system
TEST Transmission, epidemiology, symptoms, and treatment

TdP Torsades de pointes
TIA Transient ischemic attack
TIPS Transjugular intrahepatic portosystemic shunt
TMJ Temporomandibular junction
TNF Tumor necrosis factor
TNM Tumors, nodes, metastasis
TOPV Trivalent oral polio vaccine
TPAL Term, preterm, abortions, living infants
TSH Thyroid-stimulating hormone
TTP Thrombotic thrombocytopenic purpura
UC Ulcerative colitis
UES Upper esophageal sphincter
URI Upper respiratory infection
UTI Urinary tract infection
VC Vital capacity
VCD Vocal cord dysfunction
VD Venereal disease
VF/VT Ventricular fibrillation/ventricular tachycardia
VP Ventriculoperitoneal
VPA Valproic acid
VPB Ventricular premature beat
VPC Ventricular premature complex
V/Q Ventilation/perfusion
VT Ventricular tachycardia
VTE Venous thromboembolism
VWF Von Willebrand factor
VZV Varicella zoster virus
WAP Wandering atrial pacemaker
WKS Wernicke—Korsakoff syndrome
WPW Wolff—Parkinson—White
XDR-TB Extensively drug-resistant tuberculosis

GLOSSARY

Abdominal crisis A medical emergency that occurs when there is infarction within abdominal organs during a sickle cell crisis.

Aberrant conduction Cell-to-cell conduction that circumvents the usual myocardial conductive pathway and results in an abnormal ECG tracing.

Abortus The patient's number of spontaneous abortions (miscarriages) and induced abortions.

Absence seizures Also called petit mal seizures, a condition that causes a short lapse of consciousness manifest by a staring gaze without loss of motor tone.

Absolute refractory period A period of time, during repolarization of the ventricles, seen in the first half of the T wave, in which the ventricles are unable to sustain a second depolarization.

Abuse Intentional physical injury to a dependent person that may lead to serious disfigurement or permanent disability.

Accelerated automaticity An increase in the spontaneous depolarization of the myocardium.

Accelerated idioventricular rhythms (AIVR) A rhythm that results from enhanced automaticity of the bundle of His-Purkinje fibers, which occur under certain conditions.

Accelerated junctional rhythm Any junctional rhythm faster than the inherent automaticity of the AV node (i.e., faster than 60 bpm).

Acetylcholinesterase An enzyme that breaks down acetylcholine (ACh).

Acidosis Excessive acid in the bloodstream that can have a profound effect upon the body's uptake, distribution, and the effectiveness of medications administered.

Acme The point during an illness at which the full force of the patient's immunological defenses are brought to bear on the infection.

Acquired immune deficiency syndrome (AIDS) A condition that occurs during the late phases of the HIV infection. In this condition, the patient's declining immune system response, specifically the C4 T cell count, leaves the patient vulnerable to a number of opportunistic infections (such as candidiasis) and cancers such as Kaposi's sarcoma.

Acrocyanosis A blue coloration to a newborn's extremities (nail beds, palms of the hands, and soles of the feet) that is common and self-limiting.

Acute abdomen Sometimes called a "hot belly," a sudden acute abdominal pain that may indicate a surgical emergency.

Acute alcohol poisoning Ingestion of excessive quantities of alcohol within a short period of time, leading to a peak alcohol level greater than 0.40 grams per deciliter.

Acute angle-closure glaucoma A condition in which the pressure within the anterior chamber of the eye increases rapidly and dramatically and can cause dysfunction of the optic nerve, leading to permanent loss of vision.

Acute arterial occlusion A situation caused by a thrombus or an embolus lodging in the blood vessel that occludes (or partially occludes) the arterial supply to an extremity.

Acute cardiac event (ACE) See Acute myocardial infarction.

Acute coronary syndrome (ACS) A complex of symptoms associated with the continuum of cardiovascular disease, emphasizing its morbidity (and more importantly, its mutability) and not simply its mortality.

Acute dystonic reactions Idiosyncratic reactions associated with the use of antipsychotic medications, characterized by involuntary spasmodic contractions of the face, neck, truck, and extremities.

Acute hypertensive episode Condition in which a patient presents with Stage II hypertension, but without signs or symptoms of end-organ damage.

Acute ischemic bowel syndrome An interruption of the blood supply to the intestines, often secondary to rupture of atherosclerotic plaque.

Acute liver failure Rapid deterioration of liver function, which is considered a medical emergency and has a high mortality rate.

Acute myocardial infarction (AMI) A blockage of a coronary artery that interrupts blood flow to part of the heart, resulting in the death of heart cells; commonly known as a heart attack.

Acute psychotic disorder A paramedical diagnosis it is owed to a longstanding mental illness or to a brief reactive psychosis with a symptom complex of hallucinations and delusions.

Acute respiratory distress syndrome (ARDS) A rapid inset of lung failure associated with increased permeability of the alveoli and the resultant interstitial edema.

Acute transplant rejection A situation in which the body's immune system attacks a transplanted organ in the weeks to years following transplant and causes symptoms that are related to the failure of that organ.

Acute vascular occlusion A situation which occurs in an extremity when a blood vessel is occluded (blocked).

Acyanotic heart disease Conditions that cause a left-to-right shunting of blood (flow of oxygenated blood from the left side of the heart preferentially travels into the pulmonary circulation) and do not produce cyanosis.

Adaptive immune system The body's specific system used to fight infection that features specialized cells, called antibodies.

Adrenocorticotropic hormone (ACTH) The hormone that controls the cortex of adrenal gland.

Adult Protective Services (APS) A collection of governmental social service agencies that focus on the elderly. Consisting of social workers and others, APS is typically responsible for investigating reports of domestic elder abuse.

Affect The outward expressions of feelings and emotions seen in a patient's body language and speech.

Affective disorders Those psychological disorders that affect a patient's mood, including depression, elation, panic, and anxiety.

Affective flattening A lack of emotional expressiveness.

Afferent nerves Nerves that carry impulses of stimulation from the senses to the central nervous system.

Affinity The tendency to chemically react with and/or bind to another substance.

Afterload The force against which the ventricle must contract, caused by systemic vascular resistance, that opposes outflow of blood from the heart to the lungs and systemic organs.

Agnosia Loss of the ability to recognize objects. Visual agnosia is the inability to recognize familiar faces or items. Agnosia is not blindness; the patient is able to see and describe objects, but cannot recognize them.

Akathisia A medication-induced movement disorder that is characterized by motor restlessness.

Alcoholic hallucinosis Auditory, tactile, and visual hallucinations a patient may experience during alcohol withdrawal. Characteristic hallucinations ascribed to alcohol withdrawal are a feeling of insects under the skin, the sound of ringing bells, or walls that seem to move.

Alcoholic hepatitis A complex inflammatory-immunological disease that results from the oxidation of alcohol.

Alcoholic ketoacidosis (AKA) A buildup of ketones in the blood, without hyperglycemia, caused by excessive alcohol consumption and not associated with diabetes specifically.

Alcoholic liver diseases Disorders caused by excessive alcohol use that ultimately damage the liver. Some common diseases are fatty liver disease, alcoholic hepatitis, and liver cirrhosis.

Alcoholism A chronic disease involving the persistent use of alcohol despite full knowledge of the physical, social, and/or psychological harm that will occur.

Algor mortis The natural cooling of the deceased body to the ambient temperature.

Allergen An antigenic substance that causes vasodilation and leaky blood vessels, producing the signs and symptoms associated with an allergic reaction: a pruritic (itchy), red, raised rash; throat swelling; limb and facial swelling; and wheezing.

Allodynia The presence of pain from a normally non-painful stimulus (e.g., light touch on the affected limb).

Alloimmune hemolytic anemia A condition that occurs when the person develops antibodies to red blood cells after an exposure to another individual's red blood cells.

Alogia A poverty of speech which is evident when the patient is unable to sustain a conversation.

Amenorrhea The absence of menstruation.

American Sign Language (ASL) A form of communication used by people with hearing impairments in which they "speak" with their hands.

Americans with Disabilities Act Legislation which recognized service animals as an accommodation and provided them legal protection.

Amniotic fluid embolism A condition that occurs during chilbirth in which amniotic fluid and remnants of fetal tissue can enter the maternal circulation via tears in the uterine walls or endocervical veins.

Amniotic sac A membranous bag that contains the fetus, placenta, and umbilical cord within about 1 liter of pressure-absorbing fluid.

Amoebic dysentery Also known as traveler's dysentery, a form of bloody diarrhea caused by ingestion of contaminated water which contains protozoa (unicellular life forms that consume bacteria).

Amyloidosis A group of infiltrative diseases that result from the abnormal deposition of a protein called amyloid into various body tissues, which damages the atrial muscle.

Amyotrophic lateral sclerosis (ALS) A degenerative disease, made famous by baseball player Lou Gehrig, that affects motor function and balance, creates cranial nerve dysfunction, and eventually causes dementia from destruction of frontal lobe neurons in the brain.

Anaphylactic reaction A situation in which a patient has been previously been sensitized to an antigen, and subsequent exposure can trigger a severe response.

Anaphylactoid Non—IgE mediated, allergic-like reaction.

Anasarca An excessive swelling or buildup of fluid in the body.

Anemia A condition of decreased red blood cells or hemoglobin in the body that can be either acute or chronic in nature. Nutrient deficiency, chronic gastrointestinal bleeding, and heavy menses are three common causes of anemia.

Anemia of pregnancy The imbalance of plasma volume to hematocrit that occurs as the percentage of red blood cells actually decreases secondary to hemodilation during pregnancy.

Aneurysm A bulge that forms in a weak area of a blood vessel wall.

Angina equivalents Atypical presentations (shortness of breath, diaphoresis, nausea) that may develop rather than pain in ACS events.

Angina pectoris Ischemic cardiac pain that occurs secondary to diminished blood flow as a result of the narrowing of the coronary arteries.

Angiodysplasia A vascular malformation whereby enlarged capillaries and veins in the bowel wall become fragile and bleed.

Angioedema A localized swelling of the deeper dermis of the lips, tongue, or upper airway in response to specific antigenic stimuli.

Angioplasty A surgical procedure used to widen vessels narrowed by stenosis or occlusions.

Anorexia A lack of desire to eat.

Anterograde Moving or extending forward.

Antibodies Lymphocyte B cells and T cells that are programmed to attack a specific pathogen with specific proteins, called antigens, which distinguish the pathogen from normal cells.

Antepartum hemorrhage Bleeding that occurs after 24 weeks of conception but before childbirth.

Anticholinergics Drugs that interfere with the body's parasympathetic neurotransmitter acetylcholine. These agents typically work in the neurons by blocking the binding of acetylcholine to the parasympathetic receptor.

Antidiuretic hormone (ADH) Also known as vasopressin, a substance released by the posterior pituitary that assists in increasing the body's intravascular volume by constricting blood vessels while also stimulating the reabsorption of water.

Antidote A substance used to counteract a toxic substance.

Antidromic Conducting impulses in the opposite of the normal direction as a result of one branch which conducts the impulse forward and the other which conducts the impulse backward.

Antigen Particles or organisms that stimulate an immune response. These can include dust, pollens, bacteria, fungi, viruses, antibiotics, or other medications.

Anuria A complete cessation of urine output.

Aortic outflow obstruction The narrowing of the artery due to hypertrophic cardiomyopathy, which can lead to the development of thromboembolism.

Aphasia The inability to comprehend or to utter speech, not the inability to utter sounds. It is another stereotypical sign of stroke.

Aplastic crisis A complication of sickle cell disease in which there is massive red blood cell hemolysis, often precipitated by a viral illness. The hemoglobin can drop rapidly and the patient may require blood transfusion.

Apoptosis A process of programmed cell death.

Apparent life-threatening event (ALTE) A condition that affects children under 1 year of age characterized by any combination of apnea, change in skin color, change in muscle tone, coughing, or gagging. Also called a "near-miss" sudden infant death syndrome.

Appendicitis Inflammation of the appendix. If left untreated, the appendix can rupture, causing peritonitis and sepsis.

Apraxia The patient's inability to carry out simple or learned purposeful movement, such as shaking one's hand.

Arcus senilis A benign white-gray ring that forms around the pupils of the eye as a result of deposits of cholesterol.

Arrhythmogenesis The origin of a dysrhythmia (abnormal rhythm).

Arteriovenous (AV) malformation A congenital anomaly that appears like a tangled bundle of blood vessels, called a nidus, which is prone to bleeding at the union where the higher pressure arterioles meet with the low pressure venuoles.

Arthralgia A general term indicating joint pain.

Arthritis A general term indicating inflammation of a joint.

Articulation disorders A set of abnormalities involving the cranial nerves that control speech. These disorders are characterized by differences in the way words are pronounced, such as substituting the "w" sound for the "r" sound (e.g., "wabbit" instead of "rabbit") and may arise from damage to nerve pathways passing from the brain to the muscles in the larynx, mouth, or lips.

Ascites Serous fluid that develops in the peritoneal cavity.

Ashman's phenomenon Short bursts of abnormally conducted supraventricular impulses seen in atrial fibrillation.

Asterixis A motor disturbance of sustained, uncontrolled contractions or tremors, sometimes called liver flap because of its occurrence during hepatic conditions.

Asthma A chronic respiratory disease whose history is punctuated with acute exacerbations manifested by airway hyperirritability, reversible bronchospasm, and inflammation.

Asynchronous mode A fixed mode of external cardiac pacing of the heart regardless of any underlying rhythm.

Ataxia An inability to coordinate muscular movement; a staggering gait similar to drunken staggers when walking.

Atelectasis The failure of the alveoli to expand naturally during inhalation.

Atonic seizure Formerly referred to as a drop attack, a condition characterized by a patient's sudden loss of muscle tone and a collapse to the ground.

Atopy A genetic, IgE antibody-induced hypersensitivity to allergens found in approximately 50% of the population.

Atrial fibrillation (AF) A common ECG dysrhythmia which can be divided into three classifications, according to presentation: uncontrolled atrial fibrillation, paroxysmal atrial fibrillation, and persistent atrial fibrillation.

Atrial flutter A re-entry phenomena that occurs in the atria; a slightly larger macrocircuit than in atrial fibrillation, it can break down and convert into an atrial fibrillation and then revert back into atrial flutter again.

Atrial pacemakers A heart regulator that returns the patient's atrial kick and improves cardiac output in patients with borderline heart function.

Attenuated The weakening of a virus's virulence.

Augmented leads A boosting of the signal between electrodes which makes the characteristics recorded easier to identify.

Aura The first indication of a tonic-clonic seizure, in which the patient reports feeling a sensation such as a bright light, characteristic smell or metallic taste, for example.

Autism spectrum disorders Abnormalities characterized by significant impairments in social interaction and communication and the presence of unusual behaviors and interests.

Autoimmune hemolytic anemia A condition in which the patient develops antibodies that work against the patient's own red blood cells.

Autoimmunity A situation in which people develop antibodies to their own body cells.

Automatic implanted cardiovertor-defibrillator (AICD) A device placed inside the body which is designed to defibrillate/cardiovert the patient if she has a tachyarrhythmia or ventricular fibrillation. Many AICD also have pacing functions.

Automatisms Repetitive unconscious movements such as lip smacking, eyelid fluttering, and finger tapping.

Autonomic hyperactivity The symptom pattern associated with alcohol withdrawal consisting of profuse sweating (particularly of the hands and face), tachycardia, and hypertension, as well as hand tremors and nausea.

A/V nodal re-entry tachycardia A fast rhythm initiated above the level of the ventricles.

Avolition The lack of desire to complete a task or assignment that the patient has the skills to do.

A/V re-entry tachycardia (AVRT) An accelerated rhythm that occurs when the early or premature activation of the ventricles, through the use of a congenital accessory tract that goes around the AV node, allows a movement to occur.

Axis The common direction, or vector, of the heart's energy of depolarization.

Axis deviation A deflection of the electrical axis as seen on an ECG. An axis deviation, also called an axis shift, that shows the heart's conduction is not normal.

Azotemia The accumulation of nitrogenous waste products, including urea, in the blood.

Bacterial tracheitis An uncommon bacterial infection of the trachea that produces significant tracheal and upper bronchial edema and mucus. While symptoms are similar to the viral infection laryngotracheobronchitis (croup), bacterial tracheitis does not respond to therapy for croup.

Bacterium A single unicellular, metabolically active life form, which is the source of many diseases.

Bacteriuria A bacterial urinary tract infection.

Ballard scoring system A tool used to approximate gestational age using a neuromuscular maturity score combined with a physical maturity score.

Balloon pump A device inserted by a cardiologist or cardiothoracic surgeon to mechanically augment blood flow from the heart.

Baseline status A patient's physical level or condition, against which later measurements are compared.

Behavioral emergency A situation in which a person exhibits aggressive behavior toward others or acts in a manner that may be cause himself harm. The person may engage in potentially self-destructive behaviors.

Bell's palsy An inflammation or paralysis of the seventh cranial nerve, which leads to an inability to control facial movements in the affected area.

Benign paroxysmal positional vertigo (BPPV) An abnormal sense of motion that occurs due to a change in head position. Although it usually resolves when the head is moved to a different position, it can persist after the motion ceases.

Benign prostatic hyperplasia or hypertrophy (BPH) A series of urinary issues (urinary hesitancy, urinary urgency, and urinary frequency) tied to enlargement of the prostate gland that applies to men over the age of 50.

Beta agonists A bronchodilator medicine that opens the patient's airways by relaxing the muscles surrounding the airways that may tighten during an asthma attack or in chronic obstructive pulmonary disease.

Beta receptors A site in the autonomic nervous system or terminal organ when adrenergic agents, such as norepinephrine and epinephrine, are released, are stimulated.

Bigeminy A sinus rhythm sequence in which every other complex is a premature beat; can be atrial or ventricular.

Bi-level positive airway pressure (Bi-PAP) A form of non-invasive pressure support ventilation that provides a lower pressure during expiration as compared to inspiration.

Biliary colic Right upper quadrant pain that occurs each time the gallbladder contracts.

Biphasic defibrillation Delivering part of the energy of defibrillation down the conduction system, then reversing the energy, to more naturally follow the heart's conductive pathway and allow for more complete depolarization of all of the myocardium.

Bipolar disease An affective disorder in which the patient rapidly moves from mania to depression to mania, cyclically, without spending an appreciable amount of time balanced in the middle.

Bipolar leads Standard limb leads that use two electrodes—one negative and one positive—to measure the electrical potential between these electrodes as it flows from negative to positive.

Birth trauma A situation that develops because of the mechanical forces that occur during birth—including compression, torque, and traction—that injure the neonate.

Bland aerosol administration A method to deliver humidification to the patient's upper airway and to help break up the mucous plugs by delivering either sterile water or sterile saline via a small volume nebulizer. The intent of a bland aerosol administration is to deliver moisture to the upper airways.

Blebs Also called bullae, these are bubble-like blisters on the pleural lining. When under increased intrathoracic pressure (such as might occur during positive pressure ventilation), blebs can rupture, leading to a spontaneous pneumothorax.

Bloody show A small amount of pinkish or brown-tinged mucous discharge that may be an indication of a child's imminent delivery.

Body habitus Physical characteristics that, when observed, would cause the Paramedic to suspect certain medical conditions may coexist. For example, a barrel chest suggests that the patient may have emphysema, a condition in which barrel chest is common.

Body mass index (BMI) A calculation of the patient's weight in kilograms divided by the patient's height, in meters, squared, which is often used as a determination of obesity.

Boerhaave syndrome A full thickness tear (perforation) of the esophagus that exposes the structures in the mediastinum—namely the heart, lungs, and great vessels—to stomach acids, food, and normal bacterial flora of the gastrointestinal tract.

Bohr effect An increase of carbon dioxide and a decrease in pH in the blood which results in a reduction of hemoglobin's affinity for oxygen.

Botulism A food-borne disease caused by the bacterium clostridium botulinum. The typical symptom pattern for botulism includes a dry mouth, slurred speech, and difficulty in speaking, mimicking the symptoms of a stroke.

Brachial plexus injury A common extremity injury seen in newborns with shoulder dystocia, during breech delivery, and with macrosomic newborns. Injuries associated with brachial plexus injury include clavicular fractures, fractures of the humerus, and Erb's palsy.

Bradydysrhythmia A cardiac rhythm with a slow rate.

Bradykinin A potent vasodilator that causes the capillaries to leak, allowing fluid to shift into the tissues in an action similar to—but more impressive than—the action of histamine.

Bradypnea Abnormally slow breathing, which may be a sign of respiratory failure and impending respiratory arrest.

Braxton-Hicks contractions Episodes of sporadic tightening of the abdomen or lower back that cause discomfort in pregnant women. These nonrhythmic, sporadic contractions are sometimes confused with labor.

Breakthrough pain A severe episode of pain that "breaks through" the regular analgesia prescribed for the patient. The pain can occur either spontaneously or from a number of causes, such as transferring the patient from a bed to a stretcher.

Breakthrough seizure An epileptic seizure that suddenly occurs in a patient who had typically managed seizures with medication.

Breech delivery A situation that occurs during childbirth whenever the presenting part of the newborn is not the head.

Broadcasting A patient's belief that the patient can insert their thoughts into the minds of others and can read others' thoughts (telepathy).

Bronchiolitis A viral infection of the bronchioles often caused by the respiratory syncytial virus (RSV), the parainfluenza virus, or the influenza A virus. The infection produces a bronchospasm that decreases the size of the bronchioles and increases the production of mucus.

Bronchospasm The sudden constriction, or spasm, of the bronchioles, which is a key clinical finding in obstructive respiratory disease.

Brudzinski's sign Flexion of the patient's hips and knees when the patient's neck is flexed due to meningeal irritation.

Bruit The sound of turbulent blood flow, which sounds like a low-pitched whooshing as blood passes through a narrowed blood vessel.

Bundle branch block A loss of conduction in either the right or left bundle branch; see Type II first degree AV block.

Bursitis An inflammation of a bursa sac, often from repetitive motion and stress on that joint. Bursitis can cause mild swelling around a joint and pain with movement of the affected joint.

Burst suppression An attempt to gain control of a tachydysrhythmia by increasing the rate of a transcutaneous pacer (TCP) until the TCP takes control and then gradually slowing the rate to a tolerable range. Also known as overdrive pacing.

Cachexia A wasting syndrome characterized by loss of weight and muscle mass generally caused by chronic disease.

Calculi A kidney stone commonly made of either calcium oxylate or calcium phosphate.

Cannon A waves Pulsations in the jugular neck vein as the atria contract against the closed tricuspid valves and pulsations flow backward; often seen in supraventricular tachycardia and ventricular tachycardia.

Capnography The monitoring of the concentration of carbon dioxide in the end expiratory phase of expiration or end–tidal carbon dioxide level (EtCO2).

Caput medusa Engorgement of the umbilical veins secondary to an enlarged liver and back up of portal blood seen in liver disease. These engorged veins are visible under the skin around the umbilicus and resemble the writing snakes of Medusa's hair.

Caput succedaneum An abnormal and diffuse swelling under a neonate's scalp following birth.

Carbuncles A painful, localized skin infection that forms an abscess deep in the skin.

Cardiac asthma Wheezing secondary fluid accumulation in the lungs, causing bronchoconstriction, from backwards heart failure.

Cardiac output The amount of blood pumped out of the heart over a minute. (CO = HR + SV).

Cardinal movements of labor The rotation a baby takes during the birth process to align with the birth canal: engagement, flexion, descent, internal rotation, and extension and external rotation.

Cardinal signs The typical symptoms from which a diagnosis of a disorder or disease is made. For example, in a patient with backwards heart failure, the cardinal signs are a jugular venous distention, ventricular gallop, pulmonary edema manifested by rales, hepatojugular reflex, dependent peripheral edema, and peripheral cyanosis.

Cardiogenic shock Loss of cardiac output resulting in systemic hypoperfusion, a.k.a. forward heart failure, it is the most extreme form of pump failure.

Cardiomegaly An abnormal enlargement of the heart.

Cardiomyopathy A general term that describes hypertrophy, dilation, rigidity of the myocardial walls, or constriction of the ventricles due to various disease processes. It may be caused by exposure to infectious disease or toxins, systemic connective tissue disease, or nutritional deficiencies.

Cardiotoxic medications Medications that negatively impact heart function and can be fatal, even in a dose as low as one pill.

Cardioversion A change in the heart's rhythm to a sinus rhythm. It can be accomplished by mechanical means such as vagal maneuvers, pharmacological methods after administration of dysrhythmia medication, or, electrically with a timed direct current countershock.

Carotid endarterectomy A surgical procedure in which a fatty buildup of plaque is removed from the wall of the carotid artery.

Carrier A person who has an infectious agent in his body, and is able to pass it to another, but does not have the symptoms of the disease itself.

Catabolism The digestion process in which complex carbohydrates such as starches and cellulose are broken down into their simple sugars (glucose, fructose, and galactose).

Catarrhal signs Classic signs of an infection, e.g., coughing and discharge the nose (rhinorrhea) that is often seen with upper respiratory infection.

Catatonic schizophrenia A mental disorder in which the patient typically presents with stupor, mutism, and waxy flexibility.

Cauda equina syndrome A loss of function of spinal nerve root at or below the lumbar plexus in the spine.

Cellulitis A bacterial infection on the superficial layers of the skin.

Central vertigo An abnormal sense of motion due to disorders of the central nervous system, particularly the cerebellum.

Cephalohematoma Bleeding under the skull of a neonate from interruption of blood vessels in the periosteum, secondary to birth trauma.

Cephalopelvic disproportion A problem of childbirth where the mother's pelvic outlet is narrow and is too small for the passage of the neonate.

Cerclage Surgical procedure wherein the cervix is sewn shut until the baby comes to term, which is roughly 36 to 38 weeks.

Cerebral palsy (CP) A group of disorders that affect one's ability to move and maintain balance and posture. People with CP have nonprogressive damage to the part of the brain that controls muscle tone. The four main types of CP are spastic, athetoid (dyskinetic), ataxic, and mixed.

Cerebral perfusion pressure (CPP) The net blood pressure to the brain, determined by subtracting the intracranial pressure from the mean arterial pressure (CPP = MAP − ICP).

Chain of infection A series of events that must occur between an agent and host before an infection occurs.

Chancres A small painless ulceration formed during the primary stage of syphilis.

Chemical pacing An alternative to electrical or percussion pacing that uses drugs like dopamine or epinephrine to regulate heart rate.

Chemotherapy The use of chemical agents to treat disease, primarily cancer.

Chest crisis A significant condition that can occur as part of a sickle cell crisis. A patient with chest crisis often complains of chest pain that is sharp and may change with inspiration and expiration, fever, a productive cough, and other signs of pneumonia.

Chest leads Electrodes placed so as to encircle the anterior ventricular wall from the septal wall on the right to the lateral wall on the left, which permits a complete view of the anterior myocardium.

Chickenpox A common childhood disease caused by the varicella zoster virus (VZV) that is characterized by small, itchy, irregularly shaped blisters and the classic catarrhal signs with or without conjunctivitis.

Chlamydia The most commonly transmitted STI in the United States. Although it has almost no associated mortality, it is a leading cause of pelvic inflammatory disease and infertility.

Choanal atresia A congenital narrowing of the nasal airway that prevents newborns from breathing through their nose.

Cholangitis An inflammation of the bile duct, which is one of the more serious complications of cholelithiasis and constitutes a medical emergency.

Cholecystitis An infection that may develop if a gallstone remains stuck in the gallbladder.

Choleliths Gallstones made of cholesterol that may be as small as a grain of sand or as large as a golf ball.

Chronic bronchitis Inflammation of the bronchi, leading to a productive cough, for three months during two consecutive years.

Chronic kidney disease (CKD) The preferred term for patients who have impaired kidney function but who are not in end-stage disease.

Chronic obstructive pulmonary diseases (COPD) A disease process that creates an obstacle to free airflow in the airway. The three primary obstructive pulmonary diseases are asthma, chronic bronchitis, and emphysema.

Chronic transplant rejection Repeated episodes of acute rejection due to a low level immune attack on the transplanted organ. The organ becomes permanently damaged and eventually is unable to function.

Chronotropy The timing of the heart's rhythm.

Chvostek's sign Twitching of the facial muscles when the facial nerve is tapped, seen in patients who have severe hypocalcemia.

Cincinnati Stroke Scale (CSS) A screening tool for stroke that uses three criteria to make a determination of stroke: facial symmetry, extremity weakness, and speech.

Circadian rhythm Cyclic phenomena of wakefulness and rest necessary for the body's rejuvenation.

Cirrhosis An chronic inflammation of the liver resulting in destruction of normal celss with fibrous tissue and functional failure of the liver.

Classic heart block See Type II second degree block.

Clinical depression Protracted and/or debilitating feelings of sadness and loss which interfere with the patient's activities of daily living.

Clonic phase Alternating contractions of muscles during a seizure. The clonic phase typically lasts one to two minutes and rapidly wanes as the patient becomes exhausted.

Clusters Events such as multiple cases of diarrhea or flu-like symptoms that are compared against the expected incidence of those symptoms within a given population in order to identify variation and identify potential disease outbreak.

Coagulation cascade A series of reactions that result in the formation, aggregation, and solidification of a blood clot in response to bleeding.

Coagulopathy Any bleeding disorder due to problems with the coagulation cascade.

Cogwheeling Hypertonia of muscle resulting in spasmodic movement of the extremities when performing an action like taking a blood pressure. This is often seen in patients with Parkinson's Disease.

Colic A very common condition that is caused by spasm of the stomach and intestines, typically in response to gas.

Collateral circulation A network of blood vessels that form a secondary and parallel circulation to a primary blood vessel that can keep blood flowing around an injury or occlusion in the primary blood vessel.

Command hallucinations An auditory hallucination in which the patient hears voices directing the patient to do something. These hallucinations can lead to self-destructive behaviors and violence.

Communicable period The time frame during which a patient is able to transfer an infection to an uninfected person.

Community acquired pneumonia (CAP) The spread of lung infection among a group of individuals, caused by bacteria, viruses, fungi, and parasites.

Compensatory pause A situation in which a premature depolarization does not reach the SA node, causing no change in the entire sinus node rhythm. The R-R-R rhythm—which includes a normal beat, a premature beat, and another normal beat—will be equal to a sinus node rhythm containing three normal beats.

Competitive inhibition The body's ability to prevent an infection from another microbe due to the presence of a benign microbe.

Complement system A process that helps the body continue its antimicrobial attack by marking invading microbes for easier identification by antibodies.

Complete abortion The body's expulsion of the products of conception.

Complete breech A situation during childbirth in which both the newborn's hips and knees are flexed and the buttocks present in the birth canal.

Complex regional pain syndrome (CRPS) Also known as reflex sympathetic dystrophy (RSD), a condition that produces severe and intense burning pain in an extremity.

Concordance In an ECG, the deflection of all R waves in the same direction across the precordial leads.

Conduction Heat transfer from direct contact. For example, placing a neonate on a cold bed will cause a heat transfer from the neonate to the bed.

Congenital anomalies Physical defects in the body's structure or function as a result of genetic abnormalities.

Congenital hemolytic anemia A decrease in red blood cells caused by a genetic condition that, when active, may result in an acute hemolytic anemia. An acute hemolytic anemia is an acute anemia that is caused by rapid red blood cell destruction (hemolysis) when the condition is active.

Congenital inguinal hernias The most common type of protrusion of an organ through an opening in the abdominal wall seen in male infants. These hernias can be severe enough that bowel loops pass into the scrotal sac or twist and strangulate, producing significant pain.

Congenital rubella syndrome A condition affecting unborn children whose mothers contract rubella. The newborn with congenital rubella syndrome is at risk for a number of congenital birth defects of the heart (including patent ductus arteriosus), hearing impairment, cataracts, and mental retardation.

Conjunctivitis An inflammation of the membranes that line the eyelids, leading to redness of the conjunctiva.

Consolidation A situation in which cellular debris, bacteria, and the like coalesce to form a pocket of pus within the lungs which does not permit the exchange of gasses and may lead to hypoxia.

Constitutional signs Symptoms that indicate general illness but are not specific to a certain disease, such as fever, muscle ache, headache, malaise, and fatigue.

Contact tracing An investigation conducted when an infectious disease breaks out to help determine who might have been exposed to the contagion (i.e., those who were in contact with the patient). This process can help prevent secondary cases of infection from occurring among these exposed individuals.

Contagious A disease's ability to be passed from one person to another person.

Contiguous leads Two or more leads that look at the same wall of the ventricle.

Continuous positive airway pressure (CPAP) A method of improving a patient's gas exchange by providing a constant pressure during both inspiration and expiration. In this way, it allows the alveoli to remain open during exhalation.

Contractility The capability of muscle fibers to shorten.

Convalescence The body's recovery period during which any needed repairs to heal the body are made.

Convection Heat transfer due to air currents. For example, having a neonate exposed to drafts will cause a heat transfer.

Cordis commotio Sudden cardiac arrest caused by blunt trauma to the chest.

Cor pulmonale A failure of the right side of the heart brought on by pulmonary hypertension, increased pulmonary vascular resistance, and myocardial infarction of the right ventricle of the heart.

Coryza Symptoms of a head cold including a runny nose.

Couplets Ectopic beats that appear two in a row.

Coupling interval The relationship of the premature complex to the preceding complex. A fixed coupling interval suggests a re-entry mechanism, whereas a variable coupling interval suggests an independent ectopic focus.

Crescendo angina An increasing frequency, duration, or intensity of chest pain that may indicate progressive coronary artery disease.

Crisis intervention A therapeutic technique using supportive communications to provide an immediate resolution of the patient's crisis.

Critical rate The rate at which aberrancy develops. If the rate decelerates, it must drop below the critical rate before normal conduction resumes.

Critical time frames A guideline for the period of time during which sexual assault evidence should be collected.

Crohn's disease A chronic autoimmune inflammatory disease of the upper and lower intestinal tract. The inflammation can cause abdominal pain, bloody diarrhea, and weight loss.

Croup A common viral upper respiratory illness that causes edema in the larynx, upper trachea, and larger bronchi. The condition presents with a characteristic raspy or brassy cough, often described as being like a seal bark, as well as an often audible inspiratory stridor that is aggravated by the cough.

Cushing's syndrome A disorder that occurs when there is an excess of adrenal hormones, particularly cortisol, causing hypertension, elevated blood glucose, insulin resistance, and hypokalemia (low potassium).

Cushing's triad The symptom pattern of rising blood pressure, decreasing heart rate, and abnormal respiratory pattern which serves as a sign of increased intracranial pressure.

Cyanosis A bluish discoloration of skin that can be observed peripherally, in the fingernails or toes, and centrally in the inside of the lips, the tongue, and the conjunctiva of the eyelids.

Cyanotic heart disease A congenital heart defect that leads to low blood oxygen levels, hypoexmia, visible as a bluish discoloration of the skin.

Cycle of abuse The stages that an incident of abuse typically goes through: tension, crisis, and calm. This also refers to the cycle of the abused victim becoming the abuser later in life.

Cyst An abnormal membranous sac, containing gaseous, liquid, or semisolid substances, that can sometimes form a protective covering.

Cystic fibrosis The most common of the serious genetic pulmonary diseases. In this genetic condition, the patient has increased viscosity of mucosal secretions among other enzymatic and autonomic nervous system dysfunctions.

Cystine stones Kidney stones formed as the result of an autosomal recessive disorder which leads to excessive cystine in the urine.

Cystitis An inflammation in the bladder often caused by a bacterial infection.

Cytokines Chemical mediators, i.e., signaling molecules, which are released by immune system to control the body's immune system.

Dalton's law A principle of physics that states the sum of partial pressures of nitrogen and oxygen in the ambient air equals the total pressure of the gas mixture.

Dead space The area in the upper and lower airway, to the level of the terminal bronchioles where gas exchange does not occur.

Debriefings A review of the care provided at the end of a medical procedure (e.g., resuscitation), special EMS call or mass casualty incident.

Decreased contractility Reduced force of ventricular muscular contraction resulting in diminished ejection of blood.

Decreased preload A reduction in the sum of venous return to the heart, specifically the right ventricle.

Decubitus ulcers Also called bedsores, a skin breakdown that forms as a result of prolonged pressure on the skin, typically over bony prominences, secondary to immobility.

Deep vein thrombosis (DVT) A blood clot that can form in deep veins of the legs, most commonly the popliteal, but also the fermoral or the pelvic veins.

Delirium An acute and potentially reversible decline in mental status often associated with illness.

Delirium tremens Mental and neurological changes that occur during alcohol withdrawal, featuring the triad of confusion, delirium, and seizures.

Delta wave A slurring of the upstroke of the R wave that broadens the QRS slightly, indicating an accessory pathway.

Delusions Beliefs that are contrary to the evidence. Thinking one is omnipotent despite being human would be an example of a delusion.

Delusions of grandeur A feeling that one is especially important and has been selected for a special mission or a quest. In some cases, the patient may take on the persona of an important person such as Jesus Christ.

Dementia A gradual and irreversible decline in mental function generally owed to an organic cause such as senility or Alzheimer's disease.

Dependent lividity A reddish-blue discoloration on the body's underside that results from blood pooling (i.e. livor mortis).

Developmental disabilities A diverse group of severe chronic conditions that occur due to mental and/or physical impairments. People with developmental disabilities have problems with major life activities such as language, mobility, learning, self-help, and independent living.

Developmental milestones Physical, cognitive, and behavioral achievements that children should reach within a certain age range.

Dextrocardia A condition in which a patient's heart is located in the right side of the chest.

Diabetes insipidus A condition characterized by excretion of large amounts of dilute urine secondary to decreased secretion of vasopressin (ADH).

Diabetes mellitus A condition in which the body does not produce, or properly utilize, insulin to transport glucose into the cells.

Diabetic ketoacidosis (DKA) A complication of diabetes in which the body, because it can't use sugar for fuel, uses lipids instead. The breakdown of lipids leads to an excess of free fatty acids, or ketones in the body.

Dialysis disequilibrium syndrome (DDS) A central nervous system disorder post-dialysis that is thought to be due to fluid shifts and transient cerebral edema.

Diaphragmatic hernia A birth defect in which the gastrointestinal organs protrude through the opening in the diaphragm, disrupting the mechanics of breathing.

Diaschisis A loss of function from a brain injury in a distant, but related, portion of the brain area. It is thought to be due to edema and inflammation from the ischemic tissue the symptoms may resolve spontaneously as the edema and inflammation subside.

Diastasis recti A separation of the rectus abdominis muscle along the midline, or linea alba, caused by the enlarged uterus. This abdominal muscle separation is usually benign and does not typically lead to an umbilical herniation.

Diastolic dysfunction A disorder in which there is less cardiac output due to elevated end-diastolic pressure and decreased ventricular filling during diastole.

Didelphys A uterine malformation in which the patient develops a double (paired) uterus, often accompanied by a double vagina.

Dilation Widening of the cervical os that occurs in labor.

Diplopia Double vision.

Disequilibrium A feeling of being off-balance or unsteady.

Diskitis Infections in the intervertebral disc.

Dissection A small tear or separation of body tissues.

Disseminated intravascular coagulation (DIC) A condition in which there is an overactivation of both the coagulation and fibrinolytic systems.

Diverticulosis A condition that occurs when berry-like pockets, or diverticula, develop in the colon's wall and become infected or inflamed, causing bleeding.

Doll's eyes The oculocephalic reflex, in which the patient's gaze is fixed when the patient's head is turned, which is suggestive of either intracranial hemorrhage or another space-occupying lesion such as a tumor.

Domestic violence (DV) See Intimate partner violence (IPV).

Dominance The concept that the heart's fastest pacemaker assumes control of the rate of depolarization of the atrium and ventricle.

Do Not Attempt Resuscitation (DNAR) A form completed by a competent adult patient, or healthcare proxy in the event the patient is incompetent, who requests that resuscitative efforts not be performed.

Dose The amount of medication administered at one time.

Down syndrome A genetic disorder that results from having an extra copy of one of the chromosomes, usually chromosome 21, and causing a set of characteristic mental and physical signs.

Drug-facilitated sexual assault (DFSA) An assault performed following the offender's use of an "anesthesia-type" drug which, when administered to the victim, renders the victim physically incapacitated or helpless and thus incapable of giving consent.

Dual chamber pacemakers Internal pacemakers that stimulate both the atria and ventricles to contract in a synchronous manner.

Ductus arteriosus A blood vessel in the fetus that connects the pulmonary trunk to the aorta below the aortic arch and prevents deoxygenated blood from flowing to the brain.

Ductus venosus A shunt through which blood from the mother joins with the inferior vena cava and enters the newborn's central circulation.

Durable power of attorney for health care (DPAHC) A legal document granting a person the right to make healthcare decisions for a patient who is unable to express their own wishes.

Duty cycle The time spent in compression and decompression during each set of external cardiac massage.

Dysautonomia A disorder of the autonomic nervous system which enhances sinus automaticity. It can cause a patient's heart rate to be abnormally high, even at rest, and cause the patient's heart rate to increase with the slightest provocation.

Dysentery Called bloody flux, often caused by an infection of the digestive tract, it leads to the frequent passage of diarrhea that may contain blood and mucus.

Dysfunction Impaired or abnormal operation (function).

Dysfunctional uterine bleeding Heavy menstrual flow that can occur at irregular times or with a prolonged duration and may be severe enough to cause severe anemia and hypotension.

Dysmenorrhea Painful menstruation.

Dyspnea Difficulty in breathing.

Dyspnea on exertion (DOE) Fatigue and shortness of breath felt by patients with heart failure which worsens when climbing stairs or with simple movement around the house.

Dysuria Painful urination.

Early goal-directed therapy (EGDT) A standardized treatment algorithm used to treat severe sepsis and septic shock.

Eclampsia A pregnancy-induced convulsion that complicates about 2% of pregnancies. It occurs in three phases: pregnancy induced hypertension, pre—eclampsia and eclampsia with convulsion after the 20th week of pregnancy.

Ectopic focus An area of irritability that causes an abnormal spontaneous depolarization; any pacemaker outside of the cardiac conduction system.

Ectopic pregnancy Situation in which an embryo implants anywhere outside the uterus. Although the most common site for ectopic implantation is in a fallopian tube, the embryo can implant in the abdomen.

Effacement Thinning of the cervix as labor begins.

Ejection fraction The percentage of blood of the end-diastolic volume expelled by the left ventricle with each contraction.

Elder abuse Physical, sexual, emotional, and/or psychological maltreatment of an older individual, which includes such actions as neglect.

Elder sexual abuse The coercion, or the use of (or threat of) force, against an elderly person to cause such person to engage in sexual acts against his or her will.

Electrical alternans A condition in which every other ECG complex has alternating amplitude (i.e., the one QRS complex is smaller compared to the next).

Electrical capture During electrical pacing when a QRS complex immediately follows the pacer spike.

Electromagnetic interference (EMI) A non-physiological source of ECG artifact (distortion) caused by electromagnetic fields.

Electromyographic signal (EMG) An electrical signal detected by an ECG as rapid spikes that occurs every time a muscle contracts.

Electroneurostimulators A system of probes placed on the brain's surface that are attached to a generator/computer assembly. The device takes continuous, real time, electroencephalograms (EEG) and detects spikes. When a spike is detected, an electrical stimulus is applied to the brain, via the electrodes, to neutralize the irritable focus. It is hoped this device might be used to control seizures.

Electrophysiologic mapping A method of electrophysiologic testing that identifies the temporal and spatial distributions of electrical potentials generated by the myocardium during normal and abnormal rhythms.

Embolic stroke A loss of blood flow to the brain caused by a blood clot that developed somewhere in the body other than the cerebral circulation.

Emotionally disturbed person (EDP) A person whose emotional behavior is dysfunctional or impairs activities of daily living.

Emphysema A respiratory disease with the essential characteristic of obstruction to airflow. That obstruction leads to hyperinflation of the alveolus and ultimately permanent destruction of the alveolar walls.

Empirically Treating someone based on the clinical presentation without diagnosis of a disease.

Empyema A space-occupying pulmonary abscess which prevents the exchange of gasses and causes hypoxia.

Encephalitis An inflammation of the brain parenchyma by either a viral or bacterial pathogen.

Encopresis Involuntary self-soiling; a condition in which a toilet-trained child loses the ability to control defecation.

Endocarditis An infection of the endocardial (inner) layer of the heart.

Endometriosis A painful pelvic condition related to the female reproductive system in which some endometrial tissue from the lining of the uterus migrates into the pelvis.

Endometrium The innermost layer of the uterus, which provides nutrients to the fetus via the placenta.

Endotoxin A destructive chemical compound that is released with the bacteria's destruction. These components not only act as pyrogens but also activate the inflammatory response system. They also release nitric oxide, a potent vasodilator.

End-stage renal disease (ESRD) A condition in which a person's kidney failure is complete or near-complete and is the fifth stage of chronic kidney disease.

Enterotoxin A toxin specific to the intestines which is responsible for the vomiting and diarrhea associated with food poisoning.

Enuresis Also called bedwetting, an inability for a toilet-trained child to control urination, especially at night while sleeping.

Epiglottitis An infection of the epiglottis, the flap-like cartilaginous tissue that protects the airway. When infected and inflamed, it swells and can cause an airway obstruction.

Epistaxis Nose bleed, which can occur for a variety of reasons and of concern when associated with profound hypertension.

Error in automaticity A cardiac disorder of impulse formation that produces enhanced spontaneous depolarizations of the myocardium, often due to hypoxia or chemical imbalance.

Error of automaticity An irritation that generally involves some biochemical derangement at the cellular level within the myocardium.

Error of conduction A cardiac disorder in impulse formation that takes an altered path within the cardiac conduction system of the heart.

Erythema An area of redness on the skin due to vasodilation or inflammation.

Escherichia coli (E. coli) A bacteria commonly found in the large intestine. Only certain strains of the bacteria are pathogenic.

Esophageal varices Distended veins in the esophagus, which are the result of portal hypertension.

Esophagitis An inflammation of the lining of the esophagus, which is often the result of acid backwash.

Estimated date of confinement (EDC) See Estimated date of delivery (EDD).

Estimated date of delivery (EDD) The best estimate of the date at which the fetus will be 40 weeks' gestation.

Evaporation The transfer of heat by conversion of liquid to a vapor.

Exacerbation The worsening of a pre-existing medical condition.

Exanthema A widespread rash seen with certain infectious diseases.

Excited delirium A condition characterized by an acute change in the patient's mental status which is followed by agitation, hostility, and a heightened physiologic state, often associated with use of sympathomimetics, that can lead to cardiac arrest and death.

Exercise-induced polymorphic ventricular tachycardia An increased heart rate thought to be caused by epinephrine, a catecholamine, following a patient's exertion.

Exogenous surfactants Alveolar lipoproteins obtained from an outside source that rapidly improve the neonate's oxygenation and lung compliance.

Exophthalmos The bilateral protrusion of the eyes and retraction of the eyelids from increased volume of tissue behind the eyes that is often seen in patients with hyperthyroid disease.

Exotoxin A poisonous chemical compound secreted by a bacteria.

Expressive aphasia Also called Broca's aphasia, a condition highlighted by the patient's inability to communicate. Although the patient may form words, the speech is grammatically incorrect and somewhat telegraphic, meaning the speech comes in short stucco bursts of words.

External decontamination Removal, often by dilution, of toxins on the body.

Extrapyramidal syndrome (EPS) A group of clinical disorders considered to be due to malfunctions in the extrapyramidal system (any of the brain structures affecting body movement other than the motor neurons, motor cortex, and pyramidal tract) that are characterized by abnormal involuntary movements.

Extremely low birth weight (ELBW) A neonate weighing less than 1 kilogram or 2.2 pounds.

Extrinsic Something originating outside a body or area.

Exudates A extra–vascular fluid containing protein and cellular debris.

Failure to thrive (FTT) A general delay in an infant's development, characterized by poor weight gain and growth during infancy.

Fasciculation Involuntary muscle twitching under the skin.

Febrile seizures A condition that occurs in children ages 3 months to 6 years old triggered by a rapid rise in body temperature, causing involuntary muscular contractions. Although scary to the patient, febrile seizures are usually benign and self-limiting.

Fenestrated tubes Tubes that have a hole in the cannula which allows air to flow outside the tracheostomy tube proximally up to the larynx. This allows the patient to speak with the tube in place and improve swallowing in patients requiring long-term tracheostomy.

Fetal alcohol spectrum disorders Behavioral and cognitive problems in children who were exposed to alcohol prenatally, which include fetal alcohol syndrome (FAS), fetal alcohol effects (FAE), alcohol-related neurodevelopmental disorder (ARND), and alcohol-related birth defects (ARBD).

Fetal alcohol syndrome A disease that affects unborn children of mothers who drink alcohol during pregnancy. Children with this disorder can be recognized by their wide-set eyes, flat bridge of nose, and small cheek bones. These children suffer from hyperactivity, mental retardation, and often have difficulty with social integration.

Fetal attitude The normal fetal attitude is the fetal position, in utereo, a position where fetus's head is either flexed or extended making delivery more difficult.

Fetal circulation The network of blood vessels between the pregnant woman and fetus that provides the fetus with all its necessary nutrients and substrates, including oxygen.

Fetal hydrops A condition seen in newborns characterized by generalized subcutaneous edema accompanied by ascites, pleural effusions, and/or pericardial effusions.

Fetal lie The way the long axis of the fetus corresponds in line with the long axis of the mother.

Fetus A developing human after the embryonic stage and before birth.

Fetor hepaticus A musty odor on a patient's breath caused by a mixture of ammonia, thiol, a sulfur compound, and volatile ketones secondary to liver failure.

Fibrinolytic system A process that plays a major role in hemostasis by dissolving existing blood clots and also slowing down the activation of several of the proteins in the coagulation system.

Fibromyalgia A painful syndrome that includes muscular pain, digestive disorders, chronic headaches, and even sleep disorders that may affect 3% to 6% of the population. The cardinal symptom of fibromyalgia is exhaustion that is coupled with muscle pain.

Fick equation A calculation of the amount of oxygen delivered to the body's tissues (VO_2), which equals the cardiac output (CO) times the arterial oxygen content minus venous oxygen content ($VO_2 = CO \times (CaO_2 - CvO_2)$).

First rank symptoms Those symptoms that distinguish schizophrenia from other mental illness, which can be remembered by the mnemonic ABC (auditory hallucinations, broadcasting, controlled thought).

Flashbacks Invasive thoughts of a traumatic event that can lead to sleep disturbances and nightmares in the patient with PTSD.

Flexor tenosynovitis An infection of the tendons in the hand and forearm, often caused by minor injury to the finger or hand, that causes significant injury.

Fluency disorders Difficulty speaking fluently with stuttering and inappropriate lapses and pauses in speech.

Focal atrial tachycardia Sometimes called ectopic atrial tachycardia, this condition is the result of an enhanced automaticity in the atrium, usually near the pulmonary veins proximal to the atrial septum, that creates very fast heart rates (around 150 bpm with a range of 100 to 250 bpm).

Foley catheters Urinary tube with inflatable balloon to hold the tube in place in the bladder which are easily placed in a nonsurgical fashion through the urethra and advanced into the urinary bladder.

Fomite An inanimate object that is capable of transmitting an infectious agent from one person to another and thus infect a person.

Fontanels Sometimes called soft spots, the openings between the skull's bones in the suture line seen in newborns.

Foramen ovale The opening between the right and left ventricle in the fetus.

Fragile X syndrome One of the most common forms of inherited mental retardation, caused by a mutation in a single gene called the *fragile X mental retardation 1 (FMR1) gene*.

Frank breech A situation during childbirth in which the newborn's buttocks present first, with the newborn's hips flexed and the knees extended backwards.

Fungi Eukaryotes, a group of microorganisms that contain a nucleus and reproduce by means of spores.

Gastric decontamination See Internal decontamination.

Gastritis An inflammation of the lining of the stomach that is caused by bacterial infections, NSAIDs, alcohol abuse, steroids, radiation, and a host of other causes.

Gastroenteritis Often called the stomach flu, a viral or bacterial illness that causes abdominal cramping, nausea, vomiting, and diarrhea.

Gastroesophageal reflux disease (GERD) A disorder characterized by reflux of stomach acids on the lower third of the esophagus, sometimes called heart burn. This "backwash" can be the result of an incompetent cardiac valve that closes off the stomach from the esophagus or a hiatus hernia.

Gastrointestinal bleeding Bleeding into the GI tract that can be divided into two categories: upper gastrointestinal bleeding and lower gastrointestinal bleeding.

Gastroschisis Known as "split abdomen," a congenital defect in the abdominal wall allowing a loop of bowel to protrude from the belly. The congenital defect is typically lateral to the umbilicus, on the right side of the abdominal wall, and the bowel is external to the body without the covering membrane.

Gastrostomy tubes Also known as G tubes, feeding tubes that are placed in the stomach. These tubes are placed more easily than jejunostomy tubes, but patients using them have a higher risk of aspiration.

Generalized anxiety disorder An excessive or irrational fear of normal situations. The symptom pattern includes exaggerated worry and constant anxiety about facets of living such as finances, family matters, and health.

Geriatrics The study of all aspects of aging, including the psychological, pathological, economic, and sociological problems connected with aging.

German measles See Rubella.

Gestational diabetes An elevation in a woman's blood glucose levels that begins during pregnancy.

Gestational trophoblastic disease (GTD) A condition that may develop after a molar pregnancy is removed. GTD can be thought of as an abnormal tissue growth that can develop into cancer.

Giardia lamblia A protozoan parasite that reproduces in the small intestine and causes massive diarrhea.

Global aphasia A loss of all ability to communicate in either written or spoken word.

Glomerulonephritis (GN) An inflammation of the blood vessels within the glomerular process in the kidneys.

Glomerulosclerosis A scarring, or hardening, of the arteries within the glomeruli. Advanced glomerulosclerosis can lead to end-stage renal disease in the elderly.

Glucagon A hormone produced in alpha cells of the islets of Langerhans in the pancreas to break down glycogen, thereby increasing blood levels of glucose. It is secreted in response to low blood glucose levels (hypoglycemia).

Glucocorticoids Hormones that are responsible for the actions that assist the body in responding to stresses, whether physical, emotional, external (e.g., trauma), or internal (e.g., infection).

Glucometer A handheld device that requires less than a drop of blood to measure the patient's glucose level.

Gluconeogenesis The process of breaking down fat into free fatty acids and glucose which can provide energy to the body in times of prolonged starvation.

Glycogen A chemical compound composed of long chains of glucose molecules, a.k.a. polysaccharide connected together which are created from excess glucose in the body and stored in the liver and muscles for immediate use.

Glycogenolysis The process through which glucagon breaks down glycogen into its component glucose molecules in the liver and skeletal muscle.

Goiter An enlargement of the thyroid gland that may be caused by inflammation, cancer, or overproduction of hormone.

Gonorrhea A common sexually transmitted disease caused by the bacterium Neisseria gonorrhea which is characterized by inflammation of the mucous membranes in the genital region.

Goodpasture's syndrome An autoimmune disease which attacks the kidneys and causes blood to pass through the glomerular process and into the urine, causing hematuria.

Graft thrill A palpable pulsation in AV grafts as the blood flows through the graft.

Graves' disease Hyperthyroidism induced by autoimmune disease.

Gravida The number of times a woman has been pregnant. It does not matter if the pregnancy ended in an abortion, a miscarriage, or a living baby—each counts as one in the total number of pregnancies in this determination.

Gullain-Barré syndrome An autoimmune condition in which the body's immune system is triggered to attack the myelin sheath in peripheral motor nerve fibers, causing significantly slowed nerve conduction and can lead to paralysis.

Gummas A soft, non-cancerous growth, a.k.a. granuloma, occurring in tertiary syphilis.

Gynecomastia Breast enlargement.

Hallucinations Perceptions not associated with reality. Seeing pink elephants would be an example of a hallucination.

Hamman's crunch A crunching sound caused by subcutaneous emphysema which is most audible every time the heart beats. Paramedics often appreciate this sound while auscultating the patient's chest during auscultation.

Head bobbing A rhythmic nodding of the head as that the patient becomes somnolent secondary to hypercarbia.

Healthcare proxy An individual selected by a patient to make decisions if he or she becomes unconscious or mentally incapacitated.

Hebephrenic schizophrenia A mental disorder that typically manifests in a patient's adolescence. The symptom pattern includes regressive behaviors, inappropriate affect, and hypochondriac complaints, as well as isolation from peers and peculiar mannerisms.

HELLP syndrome An obstetric emergency; HELLP stands for hemolytic anemia, elevated liver enzymes, and low platelet count. The syndrome is characterized by malaise, upper abdominal pain, headaches, blurred vision, and nausea. Untreated HELLP syndrome can lead to widespread disseminated intravascular coagulation and acute renal failure.

Helminthes The scientific term for the microbe worms.

Hemarthrosis Bleeding into the body's larger joints (most commonly the knee).

Hematochezia Bright red blood in the stool, indicative of lower GI bleeding.

Hematuria The appearance of frank blood in the patient's urine.

Hemiparesis Weakness in one side of the patient's body.

Hemolytic uremic syndrome (HUS) A condition in which platelets clumping in the small blood vessels in the kidney cause localized ischemia within the kidney as well as a hemolytic anemia as the red blood cells have difficulty passing through the smaller blood vessels.

Hemophilia A A coagulation disorder caused by a deficiency in factor VIII which affects approximately 1 in 5,000 males.

Hemophilia B An inherited coagulation disorder caused by a deficiency in factor IX which is far less common than hemophilia A, a.k.a. Christmas disease.

Hemoptysis A cough producing either frank blood or bloody sputum, which may occur if small pulmonary vessels rupture.

Hemorrhagic strokes A loss of blood flow to the brain due to rupture of blood vessels (an aneurysm); 20% to 25% of strokes are hemorrhagic strokes.

Hemostasis Arrested bleeding typified by clot formation.

Heparin-induced thrombocytopenia (HIT) A common immune-related cause of thrombocytopenia (abnormal drop in number of blood cells). HIT occurs when a patient taking the anticoagulant heparin develops antibodies to heparin. These antibodies, in turn, activate platelets and encourage thrombosis.

Hepatic encephalopathy A potentially reversible metabolic derangement brought on by liver failure that affects brain function.

Hepatitis A series of liver diseases which are the result of a number of separate viral infections that have a similar impact on the liver, leading to the label hepatitis. During the early stage of hepatitis, the symptoms are nonspecific and include low grade fevers, diarrhea, and headache. As the disease progresses, the patient may experience anorexia, abdominal tenderness, and the characteristic jaundice.

Hepatomegaly Enlargement of the liver, often caused by liver cirrhosis secondary to alcohol abuse.

Hepatorenal syndrome A condition in which liver failure causes acute tubular necrosis in the kidneys, leading to acute renal failure (ARF).

Hernia A weakness (or an opening) in the muscular structure of the abdominal wall through which intestines can protrude. The hernia causes a bulging defect that is noticed by tightening the abdominal muscles or by bearing down (inguinal hernia).

Herniation A rupture of the material surrounding disks in the vertebrae, leading to bulging disks in the spine.

Herpes zoster See Shingles.

Hexaxial reference system An artificial construct used to help conceptualize the heart's normal electrical axis in the frontal plane and determine if there is any deviation.

Hiatus hernia An outpouching of the stomach through the cardiac opening and into the thoracic cavity.

Hirschsprung's disease A genetic mutation that causes a congenital absence of ganglia (nerves) in the bowel walls, resulting in megacolon.

Holter monitoring An ambulatory monitor that consists of a recorder capable of simultaneously recording two or three ECG leads for rate, rhythm, and rhythm disturbances. Patients may also complete a diary as part of the monitoring process.

Homans' sign Pain in the back of the knee with dorsiflexion of the foot on the affected side, which has long been considered a cardinal sign of DVT but recently has been questioned for specificity and sensitivity.

Homeostasis The body's ability to maintain a state of internal balance. This occurs through many complex mechanisms that maintain blood sugar, temperature, oxygen, and acid levels within a narrow physiologic range.

Homonymous hemianopia Loss of the same half of a visual field in both eyes (e.g., both right sides of the two visual fields), which is a typical sign of an occipital lobe stroke.

Hospice A place that provides holistic care for both the patient and the family through a multidisciplinary team of nurses, doctors, social workers, clergy, and counselors. Hospice care encompasses physical, mental, and spiritual care to manage the patient's distress and to decrease her suffering.

Hospice services An organization that provides patients with quality comfort care at the end of life.

Host resistance A patient's ability to withstand an infection.

Huber needle A non-coring needle with a 90-degree angle midshaft to permit easier entry into a venous access port surgically installed under the skin.

Human immunodeficiency virus (HIV) An RNA virus that is transmitted through sexual intercourse and shared drug needles that attacks the body's immune system.

Huntington's disease (HD) A genetic movement disorder that involves bizarre, uncontrolled movements and progressive dementia. Huntington's disease occurs due to a loss of neurons in the brain that help to control motion by inhibiting motor signals from the brain.

Hyaline membrane disease A respiratory distress syndrome in which the premature infant's lungs have not developed sufficient surfactant, a complex lipid-protein compound that reduces the surface tension of the fluid that covers the intra-alveolar space, so as to allow the lungs to inflate at birth.

Hydatidiform mole A mass (actually cysts) of grape-like tissue that forms in the uterus instead of a placenta in some women. Although the fetus cannot survive, the tissue continues to grow and stimulate all of the hormonal changes of pregnancy.

Hydrocephalus A condition in which an increased amount of fluid (spinal fluid) surrounds the brain.

Hydrophobia A fear of water.

Hyperacute transplant rejection A situation in which the body's immune system attacks a transplanted organ at the time of transplantation, which is usually a result of a mismatch of the major antigens.

Hyperacute T wave An increase in the amplitude of a T wave, which may be caused by a increase in potassium or early myocardial ischemia.

Hyperalgesia Pain that is out of proportion to the stimulus.

Hyperammonemia Elevated ammonia levels in the blood which can lead to cerebral edema, increased intracranial pressure, and death.

Hyperbaric chamber An enclosed device that increases pressure atmospheric pressure from standard atmospheric pressure.

Hyperbilirubinemia A condition that increases the levels of circulating bilirubin in the blood. It is caused by a combination of factors (malfunctioning Kupffer cells, the liver's impaired protein synthesis, sequestered bilirubin) that together increase bilirubin levels.

Hypercalcemia An elevated level of calcium in the blood.

Hypercarbia A situation in which a patient has a larger-than-normal amount of carbon dioxide in the blood.

Hypercholesterolemia The presence of an abnormal amount of cholesterol in the blood.

Hypercoagulability A state of increased tendency for thrombus formation.

Hyperemesis gravidarum Excessive vomiting of the pregnant woman leading to profound dehydration and a loss of as much as 20% of body weight.

Hyperglycemic hyperosmolar nonketotic syndrome (HHNS) See Hyperosmolar nonketotic syndrome (HONKS).

Hyperinsulinemia Increased levels of insulin circulating in the blood.

Hyperkalemia A higher-than-normal level of potassium in the blood.

Hypermagnesemia An elevated level of magnesium in the blood.

Hypernatremia A higher-than-normal serum concentration of sodium. Hypernatremia can be caused by either water loss or an increase in total sodium content.

Hyperopia Also called farsightedness, a progressive occurrence in which vision of things nearby begins to distort. The patient with hyperopia often requires prescription lenses that must be changed at regular intervals.

Hyperosmolar nonketotic syndrome (HONKS) A condition which results from gradual pancreatic failure coupled with renal insufficiency. Patients with HONKS have extremely high blood glucose levels (> 600) and profound dehydration (up to 9 L), but do not typically become acidotic or produce ketones.

Hyperresponsiveness The tendency of the bronchioles to narrow (bronchoconstrict) with the smallest of stimulus.

Hypersensitive carotid sinus syndrome Syncope caused by an exaggerated reflex response to carotid sinus stimulation.

Hypertensive emergency Severe hypertension (high blood pressure) that results in end-organ damage (e.g., the brain, heart, lungs, or kidneys).

Hypertensive encephalopathy Altered mental status, seizures, or visual disturbances caused by hypertension as a result of an abrupt increase in a patient's blood pressure, resulting in a lack of blood flow through the narrowed cerebral blood vessels.

Hypertensive urgency An acute hypertensive episode without evidence of end-organ damage, even though the patient has risk factors to develop acute end-organ damage. It is very difficult to distinguish this from an acute hypertensive episode in the field.

Hyperthyroidism An overactive thyroid gland that can occur for several reasons, including problems with the pituitary gland; inflammation of the thyroid gland that may be caused by radiation, infection, trauma, or autoimmune disease; or drug use.

Hypertrophic cardiomyopathy Hypertrophy of the myocardium, which impairs myocardial efficiency. Thought to be genetic in some cases.

Hypoadrenalism Decreased adrenal gland function.

Hypocalcemia An abnormally low level of calcium in the blood.

Hypokalemia A low serum potassium level in the blood.

Hypomagnesemia A state of low magnesium levels in the blood.

Hyponatremia A less-than-normal blood concentration of sodium, caused by either increasing the amount of water (drinking large amounts) or losing sodium faster than water (profuse or prolonged sweating).

Hypopituitarism A condition in which the pituitary gland does not produce some, or all, of its typical hormones.

Hypothyroidism A disorder in which there is a decreased amount of circulating thyroid hormone.

Hypoxemia A partial oxygen pressure (PaO_2) of less than 70 mmHg in the blood or an oxygen saturation of less than 90%.

Hypoxic-ischemic encephalopathy (HIE) Damage to the cells in the central nervous system that develops from inadequate oxygenation.

Iatrogenic disease Adverse effects or complications of treatment that develops because of the actions of a physician or healthcare provider.

Icterus A yellowish tinge to the skin and the whites of the eyes as a result of the accumulation of bilirubin (bile pigment).

Ideal body weight The weight at which a person is most healthful.

Idiopathic thrombocytopenic purpura (ITP) An autoimmune condition in which the body's immune system is triggered to develop an antibody to its own platelets, usually through infection or some other attack on the immune system.

Immune-mediated hemolytic anemias A condition involving the destruction of red blood cells due to antibodies that develop against either the red blood cells, with the end result being red blood cell destruction.

Immunity The body's defenses against infection.

Immunodeficiency The body's lack of immunologic response to stimulating antigens.

Implantable cardioverter–defibrillators (ICD) A medical device that detects and terminates potentially lethal tachydysrhythmia. This highly effective device is used to abort supraventricular tachycardia, ventricular tachycardia, and ventricular fibrillation by the delivery of a low energy countershock via internally placed electrodes.

Incompetent cervix Situation in which the cervix is weak and unable to contain the products of conception, caused by damage to the cervix during a previous difficult birth; a congenitally malformed cervix; previous trauma to the cervix, such as from a dilation and curettage (D&C); or previous surgery to the cervix (e.g., secondary to cervical cancer).

Incomplete abortion A condition in which some, but not all, of the products of conception are passed.

Incomplete breech A situation during childbirth in which either one of the newborn's legs (i.e., single footling) or both legs (double footling) presents first rather than the head.

Incubation period The time between contact with the infectious microbe and the appearance of the first symptoms of disease.

Independent living apartments A group living situation for the chronically ill and/or elderly where residents are independent. Although additional resources are available for their medical needs, they do not have the constant care provided in skilled nursing facilities.

Infection An attack of microorganisms upon the body that results in disease.

Infectivity A pathogen's ability to cause an infection.

Inflammation A process the body initiates to remove an irritant and start the body's healing.

Inflammatory bowel disease (IBD) A group of conditions, likely the result of an immune disorder, in which patients may have crampy abdominal pain as well as blood per the rectum.

Inoculation The injection of an attenuated infectious agent designed to let the body develop a resistance to it.

Inoculums The microbe introduced into the body.

Inotropy The force of the heart's contraction.

Insulin A hormone that helps transport glucose from the bloodstream into cells. Insulin does not physically transport glucose into the cell. Instead, insulin opens pores in the cell wall, which then allows glucose (a relatively large molecule) to pass into the cell.

Insulin pumps Small programmable pumps approximately the size of a cell phone which deliver a constant amount of insulin 24 hours a day, which is called the basal rate. The user can also administer additional boluses of insulin based on food intake.

Insulin resistance A situation in which the body produces insulin normally in response to elevated glucose, but the body cells are unable to use the insulin due to resistance at the cells' insulin receptors. In other words, patients produce sufficient amounts of insulin but are unable to use it.

Integrative medicine A blending of traditional and complementary medicine, with supportive measures like acupuncture and massage used as supplements to standard medical treatment.

Internal (gastric) decontamination Dilution of the effects of toxins taken into the body. In the prehospital environment, this will take the form of either administration of an emetic agent, such as ipecac, or an agent to prevent absorption of an ingested toxin, such as with activated charcoal.

Intimate partner violence (IPV) Also referred to as domestic violence (DV), abuse that can be described as violence between partners in an ongoing or past relationship regardless of marital status or sexual orientation.

Intra-aortic balloon pumps A device used in patients with cardiogenic shock to augment coronary artery filling and improve cardiac function.

Intraparenchymal bleeding Bleeding within the brain tissue.

Intrapartum history The patient's history of labor and delivery including contractions.

Intraventricular hemorrhage (IVH) A life-threatening complication of prematurity that occurs when fragile capillaries bleed in the fluid-filled ventricles of the brain, secondary to sudden increases in blood pressure.

Intrinsic Originating within the body.

Introitus Opening to a tube, for example the vaginal opening.

Intussusception A condition in which one section of the small bowel or large bowel telescopes into another section of bowel.

Inverted T waves A situation in which the normally upright T waves on an ECG become inverted in the ECG leads that overlay the ischemic area.

Involution A process of forceful contraction during labor while the uterus shrinks.

Irritable bowel syndrome (IBS) A common condition affecting the intestines that leads to crampy pain, bloating, gassiness, and changes in bowel habits. Around 30% of patients with IBS have blood in their stool.

Ischemia Insufficient supply of oxygenated blood to meet the metabolic demands of a tissue.

Ischemic patterns Changes in the ECG that occur as a result of myocardial ischemia.

Ischemic penumbra A process in which the area immediately distal to an occlusion becomes injured, then ischemic, and then infarction occurs or the ischemia cascades. As bordering tissue starts to become affected, increasing areas of hypoperfusion lead to a series of ring-like zones of damage.

Ischemic strokes A loss of blood flow to the brain due to an occlusion; 75% to 80% of strokes are ischemic strokes.

Jacksonian march The progressive spread of convulsions from one point across the body, which suggests the spread of the electrical storm from one point of the cerebral cortex across the entire brain.

Jaundice The yellowish color in the skin and sclera of the eyes, a.k.a. icterus.

Jejunostomy tubes Also known as J tubes, these are feeding tubes placed in the jejunum, the second section of the small bowel. They are often used in patients who have problems with either poor stomach emptying or who are at risk of aspiration.

J point The start of the ST segment found at the juncture of the QRS and ST segment where the QRS angle changes.

Junctional ectopic tachycardia (JET) A rare dysrhythmia thought to be due to increased automaticity of an ectopic focus, probably outside of the AV node and near the bundle of His.

Junctional tachycardia An accelerated heart rate, arising from the AV node, in which the P waves may be found inverted, as a result of retrograde depolarization, in front of the QRS complex.

Kernig's sign An indication of meningeal irritation in which the patient cannot completely extend the knee without pain in the neck.

Ketogenic pathway The use of glucagon to help convert free fatty acids into ketoacids and other ketonic bodies, which in turn are metabolized in the liver into energy.

Kinin system A continuation of the inflammatory response that involves maintaining the body's vasodilation, specifically the polypeptide bradykinin.

Koplik's spots Clusters of irregularly shaped red spots with white centers that resemble a bull's eye which are the distinguishing rash of measles.

Korsakoff's syndrome Also known as Korsakoff's psychosis, a disorder involving behaviors that can be attributed to a lack of vitamin B1 (thiamine) secondary to alcoholism.

Kussmaul's sign An increase in jugular venous distention (JVD) noted with each inspiration in a patient with pericardial tamponade.

Kyphosis An increase of the normal forward curve of the thoracic spine, which can result from a number of processes, including normal loss of muscle tone, osteoporosis, arthritis, ankylosing spondylitis, and tumors.

Labyrinthitis An inflammatory response in the inner ear causing rapid onset of vertigo symptoms that slowly resolve within a few hours to days.

Lacunar infarct An occlusion of a penetrating artery in the cerebral cortex which cause a stroke but that often causes no apparent neurological damage.

Language disorders A sluggish ability to understand speech accompanied by slow growth in vocabulary and sentence structure.

Large bowel obstruction Condition that occurs when something blocks the bowel's ability to reabsorb fluids that were mixed with food in the intestine.

Large volume nebulizer A stream of fluid crashes with a sphere in the device which aerosolizes the solution in the container, creating a mist that is administered to the patient.

Laryngeal nerve injury A type of birth trauma involving unilateral laryngeal nerve paralysis and subsequent difficulties with swallowing characterized by a hoarse cry or respiratory stridor.

Laryngotracheobronchitis The medical name for croup, an infection starting from the larynx and ending in the lungs (the upper airway).

Lead pipe rigidity Increased muscle tone in the extremities that resists movement. Seen in Parkinson's disease.

Left ventricular hypertrophy (LVH) An increase in the left ventricle's muscle mass due to increased resistance against which the left ventricle must contract to expel blood.

Length-based tape A tool used to help the Paramedic determine the approximate weight of a child in order to decide treatment. The length-based tapes, which are laid beside the supine patient and have sections for determining the child's weight range, typically include dosing information for common resuscitation medications as well as airway equipment.

Lentigines Also called liver spots, age spots, or sun spots, small discolorations on the skin which are named for their liver-like color. True lentigines are not related to liver problems and do not require treatment.

Leukocytopenia A decline in the number of circulating white blood cells. As a result, the patient with leukocytopenia is unable to effectively combat infection.

Ligamentum arteriosum A strip of connective tissue (which develops from the ductus arteriosus) which tethers the newborn's heart to the aorta.

Lightening The descent of the uterus deeper into the pelvis, which usually occurs one to two weeks before the onset of labor in the first-time mother, i.e., the fetus has dropped.

Lipogenesis The body's creation of triglycerides from fatty acids and glycerol.

Liver cirrhosis A chronic degenerative disease of the liver that interferes with the liver's metabolism of fats, proteins, and carbohydrates. The resultant damage to the hepatocytes leads to inflammation, scarring, and fibrosis of the liver.

Liver flap A muscular tremor, which appears to be a flapping motion, seen in the patient's wrists when the arms are extended outward and the wrists extended.

Living will An advance directive a person completes to make known their wishes regarding life-prolonging medical treatments.

Livor mortis The pooling of blood in dependant portions of the body, leaving a reddish-blue discoloration.

Locked-in syndrome A condition in which a patient has an active and intact brain that is housed inside a body that is completely paralyzed from head to toe. This patient is capable of sensing and understanding what is going on around him, but is incapable of movement.

Lown-Ganong-Levine (LGL) syndrome A congenital disorder that uses a pre-excitation accessory pathway that bypasses the AV node.

Long QT syndrome A hereditary disorder of the heart's electrical rhythm characterized by delayed repolarization following depolarization.

Loose association A string of topics in a conversation that do not appear related to one another.

Los Angeles Stroke Scale (LASS) A prehospital stroke scale used in the field that considers the patient's age, prior history of seizure, new onset of neurologic symptoms in the past 24 hours, if patient was ambulatory prior to the event, blood glucose levels, facial smile, grip, and arm weakness.

Lovset's maneuver A technique used during childbirth if both arms are above the newborn's head. Holding the newborn by the hips, the Paramedic turns the newborn in a one-half circle, like a corkscrew, while applying downward pressure. This allows the formerly posterior arm to deliver anteriorly and to pass under the pubis. The Paramedic then reverses the corkscrew maneuver and delivers the other arm.

Lower gastrointestinal bleeding Blood loss (passage of blood) from the bowel distal to the ligament of Treitz, the suspensory muscle of the duodenojejunal flexure.

Ludwig's angina A severe complication of dental infections that causes swelling of the floor of the mouth and neck and potential airway compromise. This condition involves the spread of bacteria from the infected tooth or teeth along the tissue planes in the floor of the mouth, and can extend down to the larynx.

Lymphadenopathy A chronic, abnormal enlargement of the lymph nodes, typically due to infection.

Lymphangitis Inflammation of the lymph nodes as noted by streaking redness that occurs in a proximal direction from the area of infection, indicating its lymphatic spread.

Macrocircuit A large pathway for conduction of an impulse, such as may exist between the atria and ventricles through the AV node.

Macrosomia Fetal growth in excess of normal rates, resulting in newborns weighing over 4,000 grams.

Malaise A general physical discomfort associated with being unwell.

Mallory-Weiss tear A longitudinal tear in the esophageal or stomach wall. These tears, which usually occur in people who have been forcefully vomiting or retching, can lead to significant bleeding from the submucosal arteries.

Manic-depressive illness See Bipolar disease.

Mason-Likar modification A method to minimize ECG distortion from artifact in which the leads are moved more centrally to the shoulders and hip.

Mass vaccination A general vaccination of a population to prevent the spread of an infectious disease.

Mauriceau maneuver A technique used to deliver the newborn's head during a breech delivery in which the newborn's body is supported by the Paramedic's right forearm while traction is made upon the shoulders with the left hand. The Paramedic raises the newborn's body until the nose and mouth deliver.

McBurney's point A location two-thirds of the distance on an imaginary line drawn from the umbilicus to the right anterior superior iliac crest under which the appendix lies in the majority of patients. The Paramedic may press in this location when evaluating for appendicitis.

McRoberts maneuver A technique used to assist with shoulder dystocia in which the mother pulls her knees to her chest, along each side of the abdomen, to maximize the pelvic opening. This maneuver can increase the diameter of the pelvic opening by 30%. The Paramedic then applies suprapubic pressure while another Paramedic applies gentle downward pressure to free the newborn's shoulder.

Mean arterial pressure (MAP) The average blood pressure. A mathematical average of the systolic and diastolic pressure.

Measles A highly contagious viral disease characterized by cough, coryza (head cold with runny nose), and conjunctivitis (eye irritation). Following the prodromal symptoms, a raised flat (maculopapular) rash appears that starts at the head and proceeds in a cephalic-to-caudal fashion (head to toe).

Mechanical capture A pacer spike and its corresponding QRS complex, as seen on the ECG, are followed by a cardiac contraction. The presence of mechanical capture is assessed by palpating a pulse that corresponds to the set rate of the pacer.

Meconium The infant's first bowel movement.

Meconium aspiration syndrome A condition that occurs when an infant inhales its first feces. The syndrome consists of airway obstruction, disruption of the surfactant fluid coating that helps keep the alveoli open, a chemically induced inflammation of the lungs, and pulmonary hypertension.

Medically fragile Those who have a strong tendency to develop complications as a result of a chronic disease process because the balance that exists in their baseline status is easily tipped by relatively minor illnesses and trauma.

Medical Orders for Life-Sustaining Treatment (MOLST) A form completed by a patient and their physician that provides healthcare providers with the patient's wishes regarding life-sustaining treatment.

Medical restraint A medically necessary restriction of the patient's freedom so that he cannot harm himself or others.

Megacolon An enlargement of the colon as the result of its inability to contract normally and move its contents.

Melanoma Skin cancer that results from prolonged exposure to the sun.

Melena Dark tarry stool that has a dark color due to digested of blood from upper GI bleeding.

Ménière disease Vertigo, tinnitus (ringing in the ears), and hearing loss due to an abnormality in the circulation of fluid in the inner ear, which may occur up to several times per week.

Meningeal signs The clinical symptoms, such as headache, photophobia, and neck stiffness, that serve as manifestations of meningitis.

Meningocele Also called meningeal cyst, a bony defect of the spinal cord where the meninges protrude through an opening in the newborn's spinal column, typically proximal to the sacrum.

Menorrhagia Heavy menstrual flow.

Mental illness A departure from the normal patterns of behavior that characterize human interaction. These patterns of behavior demonstrate a loss of contact with reality, or a distorted perception of reality, which results in loss of control and affects the patient's activities of daily living.

Mental status examination (MSE) A systematic assessment of the patient's psychiatric status that creates a symptom complex, a list of psychiatric signs that can be used to derive a diagnosis.

Metastasis The spread of disease from one organ to another, often associated with the spread of cancer.

Metered dose inhaler (MDI) A device, first launched in 1956, that holds medication suspended in an aerosol inside a pressurized canister.

Methemoglobinemia A form of hemoglobin that is not able to carry oxygen. The condition often occurs after there has been a stressor on the red blood cells from medications, toxins, or chemicals.

Metromenorrhagia A combination of both heavy and irregular menstrual bleeding.

Metrorrhagia Irregular uterine bleeding, whether due to hormonal imbalance or other conditions that produce irregular menses.

Miami Emergency Neurologic Deficit (MEND) Exam A stroke assessment that includes a quick review of the patient's mental status, cranial nerves, and extremities as well as prompts for treatment and an abridged fibrinolytic checklist.

Microangiopathic A condition narrowing smaller blood vessels where they leak; seen in diabetes.

Microbes A microorganism that causes disease. There are six general classifications of microbes, from largest to smallest—worms, fungus, protozoa, bacteria, viruses, or prions.

Microcircuit A small pathway for conduction of an impulse such as may exist within either the atrium or the ventricles.

Mineralocorticoid Hormones, such as aldosterone, that are secreted by the adrenal cortex and regulate the balance of water and electrolytes in the body.

Missed abortion The death of the embryo or fetus before 20 weeks' gestation with no loss of any of the products of conception.

Mobitz type I See Type I second degree block.

Mobitz type II See Type II second degree block.

Monomorphic ventricular tachycardia A potentially lethal tachydysrhythmia whose ventricular origin is a single ectopic focus that creates a classic sine wave configuration on the ECG.

Monoparesis A weakness in just one of the patient's limbs.

Monosyllabic answers Simple one-word responses uttered by a patient in respiratory distress when answering a Paramedic's question.

Morbidity The incidence of a disease in a population.

Morbidity and Mortality Weekly Report (MMWR) A weekly dissemination of epidemiological information regarding diseases affecting Public Health, provided by the Centers for Disease Control.

Mortality The number of deaths that occur from a disease.

Mucokinetics Drugs or medications that thin and liquefy viscous phlegm for removal by suctioning or expectoration.

Mucolytics Also called expectorants, drugs that can help to dissolve mucus, promote coughing, and allow for better pulmonary toilet by the Paramedic.

Multifocal Premature beats in a sinus rhythm that have different morphologies, or shapes, and arise from different ectopic foci.

Multifocal atrial tachycardia (MAT) A tachydysrhythmia created by at least two ectopic atrial foci. The resultant rhythm appears like paroxysmal atrial tachycardia, but is irregular as a result of the competing ectopic foci.

Multigravida A woman who has been pregnant more than one time.

Multiple-resistant Staphylococcus aureus (MRSA) A multiple antibiotic resistant infection that colonizes the nostrils, open wounds, intravenous sites, and urinary catheters and is easily transmitted, by contact, from person to person.

Multiple sclerosis (MS) A chronic and progressive disorder that involves the destruction of the nerve myelin sheath, thought to be triggered by either a viral or environmental cause. The syndrome has scattered neuron demyelination in discrete areas (as opposed to the generalized demyelination along the entire neuron that characterizes Guillain-Barré syndrome).

Mumps A highly contagious disease characterized by fever, headache, sore throat, and the distinctive swollen parotid glands in about 50% of cases.

Munchausen Syndrome by Proxy (MSP) A form of child abuse where an attention-seeking parent may either fabricate or induce an illness in their child so that medical professionals will have to treat the child.

Mural thrombi A blood clot formed in atria of the heart during atrial fibrillation.

Murphy's sign A test for cholecystitis in which the Paramedic and asks the patient to exhale and then places a hand over the patient's right upper quadrant at the midclavicular line and then the patient is asked to inhale. If the patient stops inhaling due to pain in the right upper quadrant, but not the left upper quadrant, then the patient has a positive Murphy's sign.

Myasthenia gravis An autoimmune disease that affects the neuromuscular junction. Antibodies attack the acetylcholine receptors at the motor end plate, resulting in a decrease in the number of receptors at the neuromuscular junction and causing patient fatigue and progressive weakness.

Myasthenic crisis A situation in which a patient develops profound motor weakness to the point where the patient cannot maintain a gag reflex and needs emergent intubation to control the airway.

Myelomeningocele A birth defect in which the spinal cord is encased in an external sac, most often in the area of the lumbar spine or sacrum.

Myocardial ischemia Situation that occurs when myocardial cells are deprived of oxygen, usually due to a blocked coronary artery, and hypoxia ensues. During this phase, myocardial cells convert to anaerobic metabolism to conserve energy.

Myocarditis An inflammation of the myocardial tissue which can occur from an infectious cause as well as rheumatological and autoimmune disorders.

Myxedema coma A severe and rare form of hypothyroidism, in which the patient develops altered mental status, hypothermia, hypoglycemia, and bradycardia.

Myxoma An intracardiac, unusually noncancerous, tumor in the heart.

Narcolepsy A focal motor seizure characterized by excessive daytime sleepiness, uncontrollable sleep attacks and cataplexy.

Narcosis Use of a drug to anesthetize the brain, particularly the reticular activating system of the brainstem, to induce a state of impaired consciousness ranging from stupor to coma.

Nasal flaring The exaggeration of the nostrils (alae nasi).

National Institutes of Health Stroke Scale (NIHSS) A 15-item stroke assessment that focuses on six areas concerning the patient suspected of having a stroke: level of consciousness, visual fields, facial palsy, speech, motor function, and thought processes.

Near-syncope See Pre-syncope.

Necrosis The irreversible death of cells, tissues, and organs.

Negative symptoms The absence of emotions at times when emotions would be expected. They can be summarized as the three A's: alogia, affective flattening, and avolition.

Neglect A form of child abuse that occurs when an adult with custodial responsibilities fails to provide legally mandated care for the child (food, clothing, shelter, and medical, surgical, and dental care as well as compulsory education).

Neisseria meningitidis The gram-negative bacterium meningococcus and associated with meningitis.

Neonatal respiratory distress syndrome See Hyaline membrane disease.

Nephrolithiasis Kidney stones which form either due to a super saturation of the urine, which encourages the formation of crystals, or an infectious foci.

Nerve stimulators Implanted devices that provide electrical pulsations to certain nerves in an effort to control epilepsy as well as treat chronic pain.

Neural adaptation A situation that occurs whenever a neuron is constantly stimulated. As a result, the neuron becomes less responsive to the stimulus over time.

Neurocardiogenic syncope Sometimes called vasovagal syncope, a sudden loss of consciousness caused by simultaneous withdrawal of sympathetic stimulation, resulting in vasodilation, and an increase in parasympathetic stimulation, i.e., increased vagal tone.

Neuroglycopenia Inadequate blood sugar to the brain with resulting alterations in cerebral function.

Neuroleptic malignant syndrome (NMS) A potentially life-threatening adverse reaction to psychotropic medications. Symptoms include muscular rigidity, high fever, and labile blood pressure, which are suggestive of autonomic nervous system dysfunction.

Neurosyphilis An infection of the brain or spinal cord that affects people with untreated syphilis 10 to 20 years after the disease is contracted. The central nervous system's involvement causes headaches, meningeal signs such as nuchal rigidity, and cranial nerve involvement. Perhaps the most telling sign of neurosyphilis is the psychotic features including personality changes, insomnia, and paranoia.

Neutral thermal environment Where an incubator or isolette keeps the neonate's body temperature within the normal range, thereby reducing oxygen demand, decreasing glucose consumption, and maintaining a minimum metabolic demand.

Night sweats Sweat that drenches the patient's bedding and night clothes, thought to be due to infection, cancer and tuberculosis, for example.

Nocturia To awaken from sleep to urinate.

Noncephalic Breech position.

Noncompensatory pause A situation in which a premature depolarization reaches the SA node, causing the entire sinus node rhythm to be reset, and the underlying rhythm begins from a premature beat. The R-R-R rhythm—which includes a normal beat, a premature beat, and another normal beat—will be shorter than a sinus node rhythm containing three normal beats.

Nonconducted PACs A premature atrial complex that occurs when the ventricle is in a refractory period and is unable to be conducted down the bundle of His. They are recognizable on an ECG by the pause that is created following the QRS, as the PAC interrupts the sinus rhythm, and by the peaked T wave.

Nonconsensual A lack of permission to engage in some activity, often associated with unwanted sexual intercourse.

Non-invasive pressure support ventilation The standard in the treatment of patients with APE and many other respiratory diseases like COPD. There are two types of non-invasive pressure support ventilation: continuous positive airway pressure (CPAP) and bi-level positive airway pressure (Bi-PAP).

Nonspecific ST changes ST segment changes on an ECG that do not fit a pattern of ischemia or are not contributory to another diagnosis, caused by improper lead contacts, electrolyte abnormalities, drug-induced changes, or hyperventilation, for example.

Non-ST elevation myocardial infarction (NSTEMI) Permanent damage to myocardial cells that does not show ST segment elevations on a typical 12-lead ECG. This condition is sometimes seen in patients who have had intermittent severe symptoms over several hours or less than a complete occlusion.

Nuchal cord An umbilical cord wrapped around the neck.

Nuchal rigidity Neck stiffness.

Nulligravida A woman who has never been pregnant.

Nystagmus A twitching extraocular eye movement (EOM) observed when assessing the patient's cardinal gazes, suggestive of intoxication or neurological disorder.

Obese A classification given when a patient's BMI exceeds 30, indicating the person's weight is above overweight.

Obsessive–compulsive disorder (OCD) An anxiety disorder consisting of recurring thoughts (obsession) and repetitive behaviors (such as compulsions that manifest themselves as rituals). Repetitive behaviors, such as excessive hand washing and cleaning, are the hallmarks of a patient with this condition.

Obturator sign In this test for appendicitis, the patient lies supine with the right knee bent and right hip flexed 90 degrees. The Paramedic then takes the right ankle and gently rotates the hip away from the body. If the obturator (muscle proximal to the appendix) is inflamed, then the patient will experience pain.

Occult blood The microscopic amount of blood in urine or feces discovered by laboratory testing.

Ocular migraines A condition characterized by intense headache, nausea, and vomiting along with blurred vision or even blindness.

Oculogyric crisis A condition in which the patient's eyeballs appear to have an involuntary rotational movement, and may have other symptoms (clenched teeth, a protruding tongue, and/or facial grimacing); a dystonic reaction to neuroleptics and psychotropic medications in some cases.

Ogilvie syndrome An acute pseudo-obstruction of the colon, which is thought to be due to an autonomic nervous system imbalance.

Oligohydramnios A disorder of pregnancy characterized by a insufficient amniotic fluid to protect the fetus.

Oliguria A decrease in urine output, a sign of dehydration, urinary obstruction or kidney failure.

Omphalocele A mid-abdominal wall defect characterized by an abdominal organ, such as the bowel or liver, protruding through a defect in the abdominal wall. This defect is covered by a membrane.

Open mouthed breathing A form of exaggerated ventilation used by patients who may be in pain, have fear, or have air hunger in which the patient breathes through the mouth rather than the nose.

Ophthalmoscope An instrument used to examine the posterior wall of the eye, which contains a series of different magnifying lenses on a disc through which the examiner can view the retina at different degrees of focus.

Opiates Drugs that are derived from opium, a product of the poppy plant. The opium alkaloids, such as morphine, are used as painkillers and rank among the most commonly prescribed drugs in the United States today.

Opisthotonus A massive skeletal muscle contraction that causes the entire body to arch, or "bridge" and can be caused by traumatic brain injury, cerebral palsy and tetanus.

Opsonization The process of coating invading microbes to help antibodies identify them.

Organophosphates A group of commonly used pesticides, insecticides and nerve gas agents, that can produce a cholinergic toxidrome.

Orthodromic conduction Conducting impulses in the normal direction as a result of one branch conducting the impulse forward and the other conducting the impulse backward.

Orthopnea Difficulty breathing while lying flat. A situation that occurs when a patient with heart failure lies down and fluid returns to the pulmonary capillaries, decreasing the patient's ability to diffuse gasses. The patient usually needs to sit upright to properly breath.

Osteogenesis imperfecta A congenital medical condition where improperly formed bones are easily fractured, often from no apparent trauma.

Osteomyelitis An infection of the bone.

Otitis externa An outer ear infection.

Otitis media A middle ear infection.

Otoscope An instrument used to evaluate the inside of the ear canal.

Ovarian cysts Fluid-filled sacs that develop on the surface of the ovaries.

Ovarian torsion An uncommon but serious medical condition that occurs when the ovary twists on the ovarian ligament attaching the ovary to the uterus.

Overdrive pacing An attempt to gain control of over a tachydysrhythmia by increasing the rate of a transcutaneous pacer (TCP) until the TCP takes dominence and then gradually slow the pacemaker to a tolerable range.

Oversensing A situation in which the heart's pacemaker picks up artifact (termed noise) and the inhibition prevents the pacemaker from pacing.

Pacemaker syndrome A number of physiologic impacts (vertigo, syncope, and hypotension) caused as a result of in appropriate A/V stimulation resulting in dysynchrony.

Palliative care Treatments provided to patients who have a terminal illness which reduces suffering and improves the quality of life without prolonging life (i.e., comfort measures).

Palliative care facility An organization whose purpose is to treat a dying patient's pain and administer comfort measures rather than extend life.

Palmar erythema Redness of the palms, characterized by mottling of the palms which blanches under pressure.

Palpitation The sensation of one's heart beating in the chest, typically felt with tachydysrhythmia.

Pancreatitis An inflammation of the pancreas typified by a sudden severe pain in the epigastric area that radiates to the back, which commonly occurs anywhere from one to two hours to several days after a bout of drinking.

Pancytopenia A deficiency of red blood cells (anemia), white blood cells (leukocytopenia) and platelets (thrombocytopenia) associated with bone marrow disorders.

Pandemic An infectious disease that is contagious (easily spread) and affects a wide geographical area.

Panic attack A sudden brief overwhelming feeling of fear that is part of the panic disorder.

Panniculus A large, dense layer of fatty tissue over the abdomen.

PaO$_2$ The percentage of oxygen dissolved into the blood's plasma and the value is of the partial pressure of oxygen in the blood.

Papillary muscles The muscles that secure the chordae tendineae (heart strings) which open the two leaflets of the mitral and tricuspid valve.

Parity The number of pregnancies that ended in the birth of a baby that reached the point of viability, which is often defined as 26 weeks of age or 1,000 grams.

Paracentesis A surgical procedure that may be performed to drain fluid from the abdomen.

Paradoxical pulse A pulse that decreases during inhalation and increases as one exhales, in contrast to a normal pulse.

Paralytic ileus A condition in which peristalsis does not move the fecal material through the intestine because of uncoordinated or absent nerve impulses within the colon.

Paraneoplastic syndrome Physical signs that are the result of the cancer's effect on the nervous system: cachectic appearance, tremors, difficulty walking, wasting of limbs, and neurological signs (slurred speech, difficulty swallowing, memory loss, visual problems, sleep disturbances, dementia, seizures).

Paranoid schizophrenia A mental disorder with abnormalities of the perception of reality and characterized by a patient experiencing delusions and hallucinations.

Paresthesia Either an abnormal feeling, like "pins and needles," or a lack of feeling, like the extremity is "asleep."

Parkinson's disease A movement disorder that produces muscle rigidity, slow movements, and classic motor findings on physical examination. Parkinson's disease develops due to a lack of dopamine in the substantia nigra part of the brain, a key area for regulating motor movement.

Paronychia A cutaneous abscess located around a nail bed, most often in the hand. Bacteria are transmitted to the cuticle from individuals who bite their fingernails or cuticles.

Paroxysmal atrial tachycardia A dysrhythmia that arises from errors of conduction in a micro re-entry circuit located in the atrial wall that creates a sustained tachycardia.

Paroxysmal nocturnal dyspnea (PND) A situation in which patients with heart failure awaken from sleep or rest short of breath, caused by an increase in the return of fluid to the lungs in the supine patient.

Patent ductus arteriosus (PDA) A complication of prematurity characterized by abnormal blood flow between the aorta and pulmonary artery, leading to heart failure and hypoglycemia, thrombocytopenia, and sepsis in a neonate.

Pathogen A microbe that produces disease.

Pathogenesis The ability of a pathogen to cause an infection.

Pediatric Assessment Triangle (PAT) A tool developed to assist the Paramedic in rapidly identifying pediatric patients who require immediate intervention.

Pediculosis capitis The common louse found on a patient's head.

Pediculosis corporis The common louse found on a patient's body.

Pediculosis pubis Sometimes referred to as crabs, the common louse found on a patient's genitals.

Pedophile An adult who is sexually attracted to a child.

Pelvic inflammatory disease (PID) An infection of the cervix, most commonly caused by sexually transmitted bacterial infections, that extends up into the uterus, fallopian tubes, and occasionally into the abdomen.

Penumbra If hypoperfusion is uncorrected, the predictable pathway from cell injury to necrosis to infarction. Often concentric expanding rings exist as penumbra expands over an area of cells or tissue.

Primary atypical pneumonia (PAP) An incessant lung infection that is not so debilitating as to require bedrest, although it is incapacitating, has a protracted recovery, and is often resistant to antibiotic therapy. It is often due to an infection of mycoplasma pneumoniae and affects primarily young adults.

Primigravida A woman who is pregnant for the first time.

Primipara A woman who delivered a viable neonate for the first time.

Prion Perhaps the smallest infective agent, a protein which infects cells in a manner similar to virion but lacking nucleic acid and tends to affect nerve cells.

Probiotics Beneficial or "good bacteria. These competitive bacteria, such as lactobacillus found in active culture yogurt, help to restore the intestinal flora and create a competitive inhibition of C. difficile.

Prodromal phase The early period in a disorder when symptoms begin to develop.

Prodrome The period of incubation preceding an infection.

Prognosis The predicted outcome of a disease on a patient.

Prolonged twilight An extended state of semi-consciousness in a patient with epilepsy during which the seizure has not yet ended.

Protozoa A mobile unicellular eukaryote, typically via amoeboid action or with a tail (flagella) to propel them, that has an ability to form a protective layer to protect itself from harsh conditions.

Prurigo A condition of the skin, sometimes seen in pregnancy, characterized by pruritus and soft papular lesions on the hands and feet.

Pruritus An itch sensation that can be secondary to the buildup of bile salts under the skin (which is often worse on the hands and feet).

Pseudoseizures A physical manifestation of what appears to an epileptic seizure, but is psychogenic.

Psychogenic A psychological disorder with which focuses on a person's emotions, rather than a physiologic origin.

Pthirus pubis See Pediculosis pubis.

Ptosis A condition of drooping upper eyelid.

Puerperium The period from the birth of the baby to six weeks postpartum.

Pulmonary edema An accumulation of fluids in the lungs, starting in the interstitial spaces of the lungs.

Pulmonary embolism (PE) An occlusion of the pulmonary artery, usually by a blood clot originating outside the lungs.

Pulmonary hypertension An elevated pressure in the pulmonary vascular system.

Pulmonary toilet The combination of deep breathing, coughing, medications to reduce secretions, and respiratory treatments with bronchodilators that

result in a productive cough, thus clearing the airway and improving ventilation.

Pulse deficit A situation in which the cardiac output is strong enough to create a central pulse, but is not strong enough to create a peripheral pulse. Therefore, there is a difference between central pulses, and the peripheral pulse (e.g., a radial pulse).

Pulseless electrical activity (PEA) Formerly called electromechanical dissociation (EMD), an organized non-perfusing rhythm.

Pulsus paradoxus A drop in systolic pressure that is most notable during inspiration. It occurs when the intrathoracic pressures increase, secondary to air trapping and hyperinflation, causing the venous return to the heart to decrease. Without adequate preload, the heart's cardiac output is diminished.

Purpura A condition that occurs in cases of end-stage sepsis, in which the integrity of blood vessels is lost and blood collects under the skin.

Purpura fulminans Widespread arterial and venous thrombosis and occlusion that produce pooling of blood and a purplish discoloration on the affected areas. Purpura fulminans is most often associated with sepsis.

Pursed lip breathing A self-rescue technique taught to patients with respiratory disease that utilizes partially closed lips to slow exhalation and increase the time of exhalation to approximately two to three times longer than normal.

Purulent sputum Infectious phlegm expelled from the lungs.

Pyelonephritis Inflammation of the kidney from a bacterial infection.

Pyonephrosis An infection in an obstructed kidney that can lead to acute kidney failure, urosepsis, and systemic sepsis.

Pyrogens Fever-producing substances released within the body, for example endotoxins.

Quadrageminy A sinus rhythm sequence in which every fourth complex is a premature ectopic beat.

Quadriparesis A weakness in all four of the patient's extremities.

Quickening The mother's initial awareness of the unborn baby's movements, usually at about 20 weeks and at about the point of viability.

Q waves Pathologic signals on an ECG that indicate electrical silence (no depolarization) in a portion of a ventricular wall due to cell death, i.e., infarction.

Radiation The heat transfer of energy without direct contact through emission of electromagnetic waves such as infrared rays.

Radiotherapy The use of focused energy to kill cancer cells in a specific area (target tissue) while sparing the rest of the body. Radiotherapy can be used alone (as a curative treatment), in conjunction with other

treatments (as an adjunctive treatment), or for symptomatic relief (or palliative care).

Rales Described as crackles, these soft, short, high-pitched sounds are usually heard in the late-inspiratory phase of breathing in the lower, or dependent, lung fields. They signify opening of the small airways and alveoli against fluid.

Rape trauma syndrome (RTS) The temporary loss of ability to cope with life situations related to overwhelming stress. RTS is further defined as the behavioral, somatic, and psychological reactions that occur as a result of rape or attempted rape.

Receptive aphasia Also called Wernicke's aphasia, the patient's inability to comprehend the spoken word. Receptive aphasia is also called fluent aphasia, meaning that the patient's speech is clear and understandable—just incomprehensible, producing a sort of word salad.

Reciprocal changes Concomitant ST segment depressions seen on the 12-lead ECG in leads that face the wall opposite the ST segment elevation.

Rectal fissures Tears in the rectal lining, which may occur due to passage of hard stool or insertion of objects into the rectum.

Reed switch A magnet switch that turns certain functions of a pacemaker on or off. A donut-shaped magnet is applied to the body of the pacemaker and turned 90 degrees to turn the Reed switch off.

Re-entry phenomena The return passage of a depolarization wave through a structure, such as the AV node, that the wave has passed through once already.

Referred pain Discomfort felt in one particular area by the patient even though the actual pathology is in another area.

Reflex sympathetic dystrophy (RSD) See Complex regional pain syndrome (CRPS).

Regional enteritis See Crohn's disease.

Regurgitation The backward flow of blood in the heart due to an incompetent valve.

Relative refractory period The period during the second half of a T wave in which some of the ventricular mass is able to sustain a depolarization. Depolarization during this time tends to lead to fibrillation.

Remission A disease-free state following a disease (e.g., cancer) in which there is a possibility that the disease may return at a later time.

Renal colic The pain that occurs from the passage of a kidney stone, often characterized as a constant pressure that builds up until it becomes a severe unremitting pain.

Reportable disease Diseases considered to be of great public health importance and whose existence must be reported to the health department, by law.

Residuals Remnants of an infection or disease after convalescence is complete, such as a pox mark following chickenpox.

Respiratory distress syndrome A condition that primarily occurs in preterm neonates as well as adults and is characterized by increased respiratory difficulty, leading to hypoxia and hypoventilation. This syndrome leads to progressive atelectasis.

Respiratory sinus arrhythmia A slight variation in cardiac rhythm and output due to changes of intrathoracic pressure—compressing and releasing the great vessels and in particular the vena cava.

Respiratory syncytial virus (RSV) A respiratory infection that is a major cause of lower airway infection in children. Can mimic the common cold, characterized by wheezing, sneezing, a low-grade fever, runny nose, and a cough.

Resuscitation Attempts made to revive someone from apparent death or from unconsciousness.

Reticular activating system (RAS) An area located in the brainstem between the medulla oblongata and the midbrain which is responsible for wake-sleep cycles.

Retinopathy of prematurity (ROP) A complication of prematurity leading to blindness in some cases due to oxygen toxicity.

Retrograde Moving or extending backward.

Retrograde conduction On an ECG, an impulse that occurs after the QRS as an inverted P wave that represents reverse depolarization backward through the atrium.

Retropharyngeal abscess A bacterial infection located in the soft tissue between the pharynx and vertebrae.

Return of spontaneous circulation (ROSC) The return of a self-sustaining rhythm that creates a pulse and blood pressure, often following defibrillation and/or advanced cardiac life support.

Reverse or protective isolation Measures that a healthcare provider takes to prevent an infection from reaching an immune-deficient patient, such as wearing gloves or a mask.

Reverse R wave progression (RRWP) The loss of an R wave progression in an ECG, which is suggestive of an anterior wall myocardial infarction.

Rhabdomyolysis A condition caused by the breakdown of muscle that is most often associated with crush injury, electrical injury, excessive exercise or prolonged soft tissue compression (e.g., the elderly patient who is found after lying on the floor of his apartment for several days after a fall).

Right atrial enlargement (RAE) An increase in the size of the right atrium, which commonly accompanies right ventricular hypertrophy and is often secondary to pulmonary hypertension.

Right chest leads A repeated ECG taken with leads placed at the fifth right intercostal space for midclavicular (V4R), fifth right intercostal space anterior axillary line (V5R), and fifth right intercostal space at midaxillary (V6R) to observe the right ventricle.

Rigor mortis The classic sign of death, characterized by stiffening of muscles as the result of biochemical changes which makes the body rigid.

Ring vaccination Administering vaccinations to the persons immediately at risk of acquiring a disease due to their proximity with the infected or ill people (the "ring" around the infected population), even if they haven't had direct contact with them.

Risus sardonicus A contortion of the face, with raised eyebrows and a twisted grimace, likened to an evil sneer due to tetanus toxin.

Ritgen maneuver A delivery technique in which the Paramedic should allow the newborn's head to gradually extend, by exerting gentle control on the newborn's chin, to decrease injury to the perineum, while being careful not to impede the progress of the head with overly aggressive counterpressure.

Romano-Ward syndrome (RWS) A genetic abnormality that causes long QT syndromes where the heart rhythm degenerates into torsades de pointes (TdP).

Romberg test An assessment of cerebellar function that tests the patient's ability to stand in a steady upright position with the eyes closed. A positive Romberg test occurs when the patient starts to sway, demonstrating truncal instability.

Roseola A highly contagious childhood infection caused by the herpes virus characterized by one of an unexplained fever followed by a truncal rash.

Rovsing's sign Pain in the right lower quadrant when the left lower quadrant is palpated; a sign of appendicitis.

Rubella Sometimes referred to as German measles, a mild, short-lived infection that typically occurs in childhood characterized by a distinctive red rash, low grade fever, and swollen glands.

Rubeola The paramyxovirus that causes measles, sometimes called hard measles.

Runs of ventricular tachycardia See Salvos.

R wave progression A series of changes in the primary deflection of the QRS from negative in V1 to positive in V6 seen in the precordial leads of a normal 12-lead ECG.

Saddle anesthesia A numbness or "pins and needles" sensation located in the perineum, the area between the legs, the external genitalia, and the anus.

Saddle embolism A large embolus, most often a systemic thrombus, that straddles the bifurcation of the pulmonary artery. As a result, there is a sudden loss of venous return, loss of preload, and a dramatic drop in cardiac output that frequently results in sudden cardiac death.

Salvos PVCs that occur more than two at a time, but are not sustained and self-terminate after a few beats. Often a precursor to ventricular tachycardia.

Scabies Mites that burrow under the skin, causing pruritis. These are transmitted from person-to-person contact.

Schizophrenia A mental disorder that gets its name from the Greek word meaning "split mind." The disorder impairs the patient's perception of reality and, as a result, the patient separates from reality.

Sclera The whites of the eyes.

Sclerotherapy A process of injecting a vein with a caustic substance that causes blood clot formation or thrombosis.

Scotomata A visual disorder that involves diminished or loss of an area of vision.

Secondary apnea A breathing disorder in premature newborns in which gasping breaths due to hypoxia become agonal, after which breathing ceases altogether and is unresponsive to oxygen.

Sedative-hypnotics Drugs used primarily for treatment of anxiety and sleep disorders, although they have also been used to treat muscle spasm, seizures, and alcohol withdrawal. The two main classes are (1) benzodiazepines, which include diazepam and midazolam; and (2) barbiturates, such as pentobarbital and phenobarbital.

Seizure An involuntary contraction of voluntary muscles (sometimes called a fit or convulsion) caused by a disorder in the brain.

Senile keratosis A small rough spot on skin chronically exposed to the sun, precancerous, that can develop into a skin cancer.

Sepsis A state of systemic inflammation or shock.

Septicemia A systemic blood infection that may be categorized by the appearance of purpura and is due to microvascular bleeding under the skin secondary to endotoxins.

Sequelae A pathological condition left after a disease has run its course. The post-polio paralysis is an example of the sequela of the disease poliomyelitis.

Serotonin syndrome A condition that occurs when a patient takes an antidepressant medication, such as a SSRI, MAOI, or TCA, and has excessive levels of serotonin in the body.

Sexual abuse Non-consensual sexual activity. When this occurs between a parent or caregiver and a child it is often called molestation.

Sexual assault (SA) Any crime in which the offender subjects the victim to sexual contact that is unwanted and offensive. Sexual assault encompasses rape and includes nonconsensual sexual intercourse that is committed by physical force, or the threat of injury.

Sexual assault forensic examination (SAFE) centers An area that provides victims of sexual assault with access to trained staff 24 hours per day 7 days per week to obtain appropriate forensic evidence for use in the prosecution of a sexual assault.

Sexual assault nurse examiner (SANE) A registered nurse who has undergone additional intensive classroom and clinical training to treat the sexual assault victim.

Sexual exploitation A situation that occurs when an adult uses a child in a sexual performance or in the production of pornography. Sexual exploitation also occurs when an adult uses a child for purposes of, or to obtain, sexual arousal.

Sexually transmitted diseases (STD) Formerly known as venereal disease (VD), infections that are passed from person to person through intimate contact.

Sexually transmitted infection (STI) An infection passed from person to person through intimate contact. HIV would be an example of an STI (asymptomatic infection), whereas AIDS would be an STD (full-blown disease).

Sexual molestation Sexual acts that are performed for the sexual gratification of the perpetrator, who may be the child's caregiver which may or may not involve penetration. Examples of sexual molestation include permitting a child to watch adults having intercourse, masturbating in front of a child, or having a child touch an adult's genitals.

Shaken baby syndrome (SBS) A condition in which an infant is violently shaken to and fro, resulting in shearing forces during acceleration and deceleration. These forces tear fragile bridging veins in the skull and cause subsequent subdural bleeding, as well as cause metaphyseal fractures and retinal hemorrhage.

Shaver's syndrome See Hypersensitive carotid sinus syndrome.

Shigellosis An infection with the bacteria shigella, characterized by cramping, vomiting, dysentery, tenesmus, and fever.

Shingles A viral disease caused by a reactivation of the varicella zoster virus responsible for chickenpox. The patient with this disease will have a painful skin rash with blisters over the reddened areas.

Shoulder dystocia A rare situation in which the newborn's shoulders will fail to deliver through the pelvic outlet.

Shunting A process of diverting flow from one area to another.

Sickle cell disease An inherited condition in which a percentage of the normal hemoglobin in the red blood cells is replaced by a different form of hemoglobin. When this form of hemoglobin, called HbS, is deoxygenated, it deforms the red blood cell into the characteristic sickle shape.

Sick sinus syndrome A condition that can cause a profound bradycardia, which may be the result of natural fibrosis of the SA node that occurs with aging, or pathological conditions such as acute myocardial infarction and subsequent ischemia of the SA node.

Simple schizophrenia The most subtle form of schizophrenia, which starts insidiously with socially dysfunctional behaviors that progressively lead to an inability to perform the activities of daily living. The key clinical feature of simple schizophrenia is the blunting of the patient's affect and the other negative symptoms.

Sinoatrial node re-entry tachycardia A relatively rare tachydysrhythmia that results from a re-entry circuit around the SA node.

Sinus bradycardia A slow sinus rhythm, with a heart rate less than 60 beats per minute.

Sinus pause Often termed a sinus arrest, a situation that occurs when the sinus node fails to initiate an impulse due to a change in automaticity.

Sinus tachycardia A situation in which the heart's sinus rhythm exceeds 100 beats per minute.

Situs inversus A condition in which the body's organs are the mirror opposite of normal position.

Skilled nursing facilities A group living situation for the chronically ill and/or elderly that provides ongoing medical care for the residents.

Slipped capital femoral epiphysis (SCFE) An injury affecting adolescents, particularly males and obese children, that produces leg pain when the proximal end of the femur becomes displaced from the femoral shaft at the growth plate.

Small bowel obstructions (SBO) A blockage of the small bowel, caused by postoperative adhesions, cancer, Crohn's disease, foreign bodies, hernias, and more.

Small volume nebulizer (SVN) A device that takes a small volume of solution and creates a medical aerosol via mist formation.

Social distancing A technique used to prevent the spread of communicable disease by banning public gatherings (i.e., limiting access to places where groups of people congregate, such as theaters and schools).

Social phobia A condition in which patients have overwhelming anxiety during social encounters. At its mildest, patients may have a fear of public speaking. In extreme cases, a patient may be so fearful that he will not seek medical attention, preferring to die rather than be embarrassed or humiliated.

Somatic pain Discomfort that, in the case of the abdomen, comes from the parietal peritoneum, which is innervated by somatic nerves. These pain receptors, or nociceptors, are sensitive to heat and cold, as well as inflammation and ischemia.

Somatizing A manifestation of mental pain as pain in one's body.

Somatogenic A theory on mental illness that accepts psychotic behavior as a malfunction of the central nervous system.

Space-occupying lesions Any lesion in the brain, including cancer or hematoma, that places pressure onto adjacent brain tissues, crushing those tissues as well as compromising adjacent structures.

Spacer A reservoir that allows the mist from an MDI to be suspended until the patient is ready to inhale. When properly used, a spacer can increase the MDI's efficiency by as much as 20%.

Spina bifida A birth defect that involves incomplete closure of the unborn child's spine during pregnancy.

Spinal stenosis A narrowing of the spinal canal caused by degeneration of the disks and the vertebral joints as people age.

Spontaneous abortion A situation in which a pregnancy ends before 20 weeks' gestation, often due to a genetic issue with the fetus.

Spores A means of reproduction used by fungus. Spores must have a host that provides nutrition in order to grow, and tend to survive for long periods of time—even under unfavorable conditions—until they germinate.

Spotting Breakthrough vaginal bleeding a woman may experience as her hormonal levels adjust to her pregnancy. Spotting may also be an early sign of miscarriage, ectopic pregnancy, or simply the result of intercourse.

Stable angina Cardiac pain that occurs with exertion and goes away with rest.

Staghorn stones A large struvite stone that grows within the renal pelvis, occupying a large area, and blocks urine flow, leading to hydronephrosis.

Status asthmaticus A severe prolonged asthma attack with significant air trapping and respiratory distress that does not respond to usual treatment aimed at bronchodilation and decreasing inflammation.

Status epilepticus One continuous seizure that lasts for greater than 30 minutes.

Steatorrhea Foul-smelling diarrhea caused by fats that often occurs with excessive alcohol use.

Steatosis A process in which globules of fat become stored in vacuoles within the liver cells, distending the hepatic cells.

ST elevation myocardial infarction (STEMI) Complete occlusion of the coronary artery in which the 12-lead ECG reveals at least 1 mm elevation of the ST segments in at least two contiguous anatomical leads.

Stenosis Scarring of a cardiac valve, commonly due to endocarditis or rheumatic fever.

Steroids A lipid substance which controls glucose production, protein, and fat metabolism. It also maintains salt balance, vascular tone, cardiac contractility, and reproductive cycles.

S3 gallop An extra heart sound caused by the splitting of the sound of ventricle contraction, normally S2, which is suggestive of a heart going into failure. Also called a ventricular gallop.

Stilted speech The use of extremely formal terminology in everyday conversation. Such speech is generally inappropriate to the setting.

Stokes–Adams attack A cardiac issue characterized by a sudden loss of consciousness, without warning, while seated or standing, which may be followed by a convulsion. It is thought to occur because of ventricular asystole, such as what occurs in a prolonged sinus arrest.

Stridor A high-pitched sound that occurs when the upper airway is narrowed.

Stroke An interruption of blood flow to a portion of the brain, resulting in loss of function. This loss of function can result in permanent disability.

Struvite stone An infectious stone created when chemicals such as magnesium, ammonium, and phosphate (struvite) form around bacteria.

ST segment depression A drawing down of the ST segment below the J point on an ECG, often caused by injured endocardial cells.

ST segment elevation A rise in the ST segment on an ECG, above the J point on an ECG, often caused by a full thickness (transmural) injury.

Subarachnoid hemorrhage (SAH) Bleeding that occurs in the subarachnoid space around the brain.

Subendocardial ischemia Restriction of blood flow in the deeper myocardial tissues that prolongs repolarization as represented by a prolonged QT interval.

Subphrenic abscess A collection of pus just below the diaphragm, which can cause pain in either upper abdominal quadrant.

Sudden infant death syndrome (SIDS) The unexplained and sudden death of an infant at less than 1 year of age, a.k.a. crib death.

Sudden onset asthma (SOA) A rare form of asthma in which the patient rapidly deteriorates into respiratory arrest despite aggressive medical treatment, sometimes seen in steroid dependent patients with sudden withdrawal of steroids.

Superinfections A situation in which, either a patient becomes reinfected with a drug resistant infection or a secondary bacterial infection concomitant with another infection, often viral.

Supine hypotensive syndrome A condition that commonly occurs when a pregnant woman lies in the supine position. The weight of the uterus and its contents compresses the inferior vena cava, decreasing venous return to the heart, which in turn decreases venous return and lowers cardiac output causings arterial hypotension.

Suprapubic catheters Devices that drain urine from the bladder that are surgically placed through the lower abdominal wall just superior to the pubic symphysis.

Supraventricular tachycardias (SVT) Accelerated heart rates that originate above the ventricles.

Surfactant A phospholipid that reduces surface tension in the alveoli of the lungs.

Surge capacity A hospital's or EMS system's ability to handle a large influx of new patients should a widespread medical emergency occur.

Symbiotic relationship A mutually beneficial association between two parties.

Sympathomimetics Drugs that stimulate the sympathetic nervous system, commonly referred to as the fight or flight syndrome. They are often called rescue drugs because of their effectiveness.

Syncope The brief sudden loss of consciousness and postural tone.

Syncytium The concept that the atria and ventricles beat as one in synchrony; a multinucleated mass of cytoplasm that is not separated into individual cells.

Syndactyly Fused digits or webbed fingers.

Syndrome of inappropriate sinus tachycardia (SITS) Condition that results from dysautonomia in which the heart rate suddenly increases to 140 or 150 beats per minute for no apparent reason.

Syphilis A sexually transmitted disease that passes from person to person by micro-tears of genital mucosa and exchange of blood occurs during intercourse. The disease progresses from the appearance of chancres to development of a rash to final neurological deterioration.

Systemic inflammatory response syndrome (SIRS) A pathological condition that arises when cytokine levels become elevated (e.g., during a cytokine storm, because of unchecked T cell and macrophage activity) that the inflammatory response has a negative effect on the body.

Systolic dysfunction Low cardiac output that occurs when the impaired ventricle is unable to produce adequate pressures to expel its end-diastolic volume, i.e., reduced ejection fraction resulting in reduced cardiac output.

Tachydysrhythmia A rapid and abnormal cardiac rhythm.

Tactile fremitus Vibrations felt on the chest wall when the patient speaks because of consolidation or fluids in the lungs.

Targeted vaccination A vaccination given to the population of an area after those directly in contact with the disease have been vaccinated, in an attempt to stop the disease from spreading further.

Technology dependent A situation in which patients rely on advancing medical technologies (ventilators, left ventricular assist devices, insulin pumps, syringe infusion pumps, etc.) to allow them to undergo long-term treatment at home.

Tendonitis An inflammation of a tendon often caused by either injury or repetitive motion of a joint. The tendon swells within its sheath, causing it to rub against the inner surface of the sheath, producing pain with movement of the affected joint.

Tenesmus A feeling of incomplete bowel emptying or persistent need for a bowel movement.

Teratogen Any substance, agent, or environmental factor that causes birth defects. This may include alcohol, occupational exposures, cytomegalovirus, prescribed medications, and toxoplasmosis (a parasitic disease).

Tetralogy of Fallot The congenital condition, which consists of four congenital abnormalities (ventricular septal defect, i.e., a hole in between the ventricles, pulmonary stenosis resulting in obstruction of blood flow from the right ventricle to the lungs, overriding aorta, i.e., the aorta lying directly over the ventricular septal defect, and hypertrophy in the right ventricle).

TET spells Condition seen in infants with Tetralogy of Fallot in which the infant suddenly becomes cyanotic and has a syncopal episode. The child may be observed to squat, reducing blood flow the heart, to prevent syncope.

Therapeutic hypothermia Treatment of patients with return of spontaneous circulation through actively induced hypothermia (body cooling) to improve neurological outcome.

Thermogenesis The body's ability to make heat.

Thermoregulation The body's ability to control its temperature within a narrow physiologic range.

Third spacing Increased interstitial fluid leading to edema.

Thoracic outlet syndrome (TOS) A group of disorders that affect the upper extremity, causing neurological

deficits, as well as effects upon the blood vessels. The syndrome is caused by intermittent compression of the brachial nerve plexus and/or the subclavian and vertebral artery.

Thought blocking Condition in which an interruption in the patient's stream of thought occurs and the patient restarts her conversation on an entirely different topic.

Threatened abortion Heavy vaginal bleeding in a pregnant patient who has not yet passed the fetus, but may spontaneously terminate the pregnancy.

Thrombocytopenia An acquired coagulation disorder that involves decreased levels of circulating platelets in the body.

Thrombotic thrombocytopenic purpura (TTP) A condition in adults in which platelets clump together and partially occlude the small blood vessels. When this occurs, the red blood cells are damaged and break apart, producing the hemolytic anemia.

Thunderclap headache A sudden, severe headache—often starting in the back of the head—which is often described by patients as the worst headache they have ever experienced. This is a classic sign of a subarachnoid hemorrhage.

Thyroid-stimulating hormone (TSH) Hormone that controls the thyroid gland.

Thyroid storm A life-threatening elevation in thyroid hormones which is often precipitated by a specific event, such as surgery or an infection.

TICLS (Tone, Interactivity, Consolability, Look/ Gaze, Speech/Cry) A mnemonic Paramedics use to recall the important factors in assessing the child's appearance.

Tinnitus A ringing in the ears, which may be a sign of trauma, medication overdose, or increased pressure from fluid in the middle ear.

Tocolysis Use of drugs to suppress/slow labor.

Tonic—clonic seizures Formerly known as grand mal seizures, a series of involuntary contractions that have four distinct phases: aura, tonic, clonic, and postictal.

Tonic phase The second phase of a tonic—clonic seizure in which all of the body's muscles contract and the body appears to get stiff. At this point, the patient has lost consciousness and is unresponsive to verbal stimuli.

Torsades de pointes (TdP) A subset of polymorphic ventricular tachycardia that occurs with patients who either have congenital prolonged QT syndromes or who have a drug-induced QT interval prolongation.

Toxic megacolon A condition in which a patient has an enormously distended and dilated colon due to bacteria, which becomes dysfunctional. This causes abdominal distention and systemic infection.

Toxicology A branch of pharmacology that studies the harmful effects that poisons have upon the body.

Toxidromes Certain classes of toxins that produce a series of classic physical exam findings. Four classic toxidromes are sympathomimetics, anticholinergics, cholinergic toxidromes, and opiates.

Transcutaneous external pacemaker (TEP) A pacemaker applied to the chest during a cardiac emergency that electronically stimulates the heart to maintain a perfusing rhythm.

Transient ischemic attack (TIA) Known to the lay public as a "mini-stroke," a temporary cessation of blood flow in the brain that leads to a temporary focal neurological deficit.

Transmural ischemia Restriction of blood flow that affects the entire thickness of the myocardium, from the endocardium to the epicardium.

Transthoracic impedance The electrical resistance of the chest wall to the passage of electricity.

Transudate Low protein plasma-like fluid that has passed through a membrane.

Trigeminy A sinus rhythm sequence in which every third complex is a premature ectopic beat.

Trimesters The three subdivisions of the antenatal period, each consisting of a roughly three-month period.

Tripod position A method of body positioning used to improve breathing in which the patient leans forward with hands on the knees allowing the lungs to be suspended.

Trismus A spasm of the jaw muscles; clenched teeth.

Tumors Small masses of abnormal tissue. They may be benign (noncancerous) or malignant (cancerous).

Turbidity Cloudiness or haziness of a liquid.

Twiddler's syndrome A manipulation of the pulse generator buried just under the skin which causes coiling of the leads in the process by the patient. This can result in lead displacement or problems with connection of the lead and the pacemaker.

Type I first degree heart block A rhythm that starts with sinus bradycardia. Cellular hypoxia, in the AV node, does not allow the pacemaker cells to depolarize and repolarize as quickly as normal, resulting in bradycardia. Eventually the hypoxic AV node develops ischemia and the PR interval lengthens.

Type I second degree block Sinus rhythm in which, as the cellular damage progresses, the AV node starts to become ischemic. These changes (increased AV node refractoriness) are evidenced by a lengthening PR interval until the impulse is blocked by a refractory AV node, represented on the ECG as a dropped beat.

Type I third degree block A sinus rhythm that occurs when the injured AV node starts to infarct. The necrotic tissue of the infarcted AV node is unable to propagate the impulse to ventricles, establishing a complete heart block and an escape pacemaker below the AV node takes dominance.

Type II first degree block When the left coronary artery becomes occluded, the septal wall (and specifically, the bundle of His and/or the bundle branches) develops an ischemia that could affect two fascicles of the left bundle or one fascicle of the left bundle and the right bundle, a.k.a. bundle branch block.

Type II second degree block As the hypoxia continues, and the injury results within the bundle of His, the patient may start to experience dropped beats. Unlike type I dropped beats, these give no indication of an impending dropped beat. However, if the number of dropped beats is so high that the patient experiences a bradycardia, then the block is referred to as a high degree block.

Type II third degree block As the hypoxia from coronary occlusion continues the bundle branches infarct and a complete heart block occurs. An escape pacemaker below the bundle branches, i.e., the purkinje fibers takes dominance. The rhythm of the idioventricular pacemaker is not compatible with life.

Ulcerative colitis (UC) An inflammatory bowel disease that commonly affects the end of the colon (i.e., the rectum). Patients with ulcerative colitis can have crampy abdominal pain associated with diarrhea, along with intermittent rectal bleeding.

Undersensing A situation in which the pacemaker fails to sense the heart's underlying or native rhythm due to a faulty connection, lead failure, improper lead position, or electrolyte abnormalities.

Unifocal Situation in which premature ectopic beats originate from a single source and present with identical morphologies, or shapes.

Unifocal PVC Premature ventricular complexes originating from a single ectopic focus that are uniform in shape or morphology.

Unipolar lead A single positive electrode used as an "exploring" lead that can be placed anywhere on the thorax to view any angle of the heart.

Unstable angina Cardiac pain that may occur at rest, or is increasing in frequency or intensity or duration or persists despite treatment, a.k.a. pre-infarction angina.

Upper gastrointestinal bleeding Bleeding which originates above the ligament of Treitz and may occur between the esophagus extending to the middle of the intestines. The upper gastrointestinal tract is very vascular and therefore can be the source of devastating bleeding.

Uremia A syndrome caused by loss of kidney function, both as an excretory organ and as an endocrine organ. Excessive accumulation of nitrogenous waste, i.e., urea, that leads to electrolyte abnormalities and systemic neurologic and muscular dysfunction.

Uremic frost A condition in which nitrogenous wastes are excreted through the sweat glands, particularly on the face, and form crystals on the skin after the sweat evaporates.

Urinary frequency The need to urinate often.

Urinary hesitancy Difficulty beginning to urinate.

Urinary tract infections (UTI) A bacterial infection that may occur anywhere in the urinary tract (bladder, urethra, kidneys, ureters).

Urinary urgency A sudden, compelling urge to urinate. One of the three signs of a UTI; frequency, hesitancy, and urgency.

Urticaria A pruritic (itchy), red, raised rash commonly seen in allergic reactions, a.k.a. hives.

Uterine atony A condition in which a woman's muscular uterus loses the ability to contract following childbirth.

Uterine prolapse A condition that occurs when the cervix and part of the uterus protrude from the vaginal opening.

Uterine rupture A catastrophic condition that may be represented by a weak spot in the uterine wall that may tear open, spilling the fetus and placenta into the mother's abdomen. Signs and symptoms of this uterine separation vary and may include mild or severe third trimester vaginal bleeding, intense abdominal pain, or the complete cessation of pain after an intense period of pain.

Vagal maneuvers Methods used to evaluate and treat tachydysrhythmia such as bearing down and breath-holding.

Vaginal foreign bodies Items that become lodged in the vagina and/or cannot be retrieved. Examples of foreign bodies include tampons and sexual gratification objects.

Vagus nerve stimulator A device that periodically sends electrical stimulus to the brain, via the vagus nerve, to discharge and neutralize irritable sites in the brain that could induce a seizure.

Valsalva maneuver A method of vagal stimulation using forceful exhalation against a closed glottis. that increases the intrathoracic pressure and reducing venous return. Upon exhalation the volume returns and the heart reflexively lowers the heart rate; stroke volume times heart rate equals cardiac output.

Varicella zoster virus (VZV) The disease-causing organism that causes chickenpox.

Vascular bypass A procedure in which a vascular surgeon takes a blood vessel and bypasses a blocked extremity artery.

Vascular resistance The force that must be overcome to push blood through the circulatory system.

Vasodepressor effect Stimulation of the carotid sense that leads to a decrease of sympathetic tone. The sympathetic nervous system maintains peripheral vascular tone and a loss of sympathetic stimulation causes vasodilation, significant venous pooling, and subsequent hypotension.

Vasodilatation Widening of blood vessels.

Vector The sum of electrical events on an ECG that indicates the common direction of the electrical wave front; also, an organism that indirectly transmits a pathogen from its reservoir to another person.

Venothromboembolus (VTE) A pooling of blood in an extremity that puts the patient at risk for developing a clot or thrombus in that extremity that can travel to other organs of the body.

Ventricular assist devices Implanted "mechanical hearts" that augment coronary artery filling during diastole and are generally reserved for patients who have end-stage heart failure and are awaiting transplant.

Ventricular flutter A form of extreme ventricular tachycardia that cannot be tolerated. Ventricular flutter is said to occur when the monitor complexes exceed 200 complexes per minute. Preexists before ventricular fibrillation.

Ventricular hypertrophy Ventricular muscle enlargement.

Ventricular premature beat (VPB) See Premature ventricular complex (PVC).

Ventricular remodeling Numerous changes that happen following an injury or chronic hypertension. It develops over time as a result of an increased hemodynamic load and/or neurohormonal activation.

Ventriculoperitoneal (VP) shunt An implanted tube that is placed inside the ventricle in the brain, exits the skull, and runs under the skin to the abdomen. The purpose of the VP shunt is to divert cerebrospinal fluid (CSF) from the brain to the peritoneum in patients who produce CSF at a faster than it can be reabsorbed, resulting in hydrocephalus or water on the brain.

Verbigeration The obsessive repetition of meaningless words or phrases.

Vertex delivery A normal, head-first childbirth.

Vertigo A feeling of things spinning around which is often dismissed as a disorder of the inner ear.

Vesicles Raised lesions that appear like a tiny blister and contain a clear, serous fluid that is loaded with virus.

Virchow's triad The collective name for the factors thought to contribute to the formation of venous thromboembolism: venous stasis (stagnant blood), a state of hypercoagulability, and inflammation or injury of the endothelial wall inside a vein.

Virulence The fitness of the microbe to survive and thrive in the host, determined by such factors of pathogenesis as ease of entry, route of entry, dose, and host defense.

Virus A small infectious agent that, unlike the fungus and bacterium, is not an independent life form and requires a host in order to be able to grow and reproduce.

Visceral pain Discomfort that comes from the abdominal organs, or viscera, which are innervated by the autonomic nerve fibers.

Visual language A communication technique used by those with hearing impairments that takes a variety of forms. Some persons use finger spelling, others use a combination of finger spelling and body movements (including facial expressions and mime), and still others use American Sign Language.

Voice production disorders Vocal abnormalities exhibited by inappropriate pitch, tone, volume, or quality, resulting from conditions affecting the vocal cords, hormonal or psychiatric disturbances, and severe hearing loss.

Volvulus An abnormal twisting of the gut, causing an acute loss of blood supply and bowel obstruction, with subsequent gangrene, perforation, and peritonitis.

Von Willebrand disease A hereditary coagulation disorder that results in a lack of von Willebrand factor (vWf), an essential factor for primary hemostasis, in the inner lining of the blood vessels.

VO_2 max The body's maximum oxygen consumption.

V-$\dot{Q}$ match A one-to-one relationship between the alveoli and the pulmonary capillaries (ventilation to perfusion). If there is a mismatch, either due to less ventilation or loss of perfusion, then the patient is said to have a V-$\dot{Q}$ mismatch.

Vulnerable period See Relative refractory period.

Vulvovaginitis An inflammation of the vulva and vagina that usually presents with vaginal discharge associated with itching or pain. It is primarily caused by infections but can also result from an irritant, allergic response, or from insertion of a foreign body into the vagina.

Walking pneumonia See Primary atypical pneumonia (PAP).

Wandering atrial pacemaker (WAP) A benign rhythm change in which the pacemaker site shifts from the sinus node into the atrial tissues. The ectopic foci within the atria start to compete with the SA node in a subtle manner whereby some sinus impulses may create depolarizations and others may not. Defined as three or more P waves of differing morphology.

Watershed strokes An interruption of blood flow to the distal portions of the brain which is a direct result of hypoxia, hypoglycemia, or hypoperfusion.

Wenckebach's phenomena See Type I second degree block.

Wernicke-Korsakoff syndrome (WKS) The loss of specific brain functions which can be attributed to thiamine deficiency.

Wharton's jelly A protective gel that surrounds the blood vessels carrying nutrients to the fetus.

Wolfe—Parkinson—White syndrome (WPW) The best known pre-excitation disorder in which an extra conduction pathway or accessory pathway allows the electrical signal to arrive at the ventricles too soon.

Word clusters Choppy bursts of words a patient in respiratory distress may use when answering a Paramedic's question.

Wound identification The determination if an injury is defined as a break or interruption in the continuity of tissue and if it is caused by physical or mechanical means.

Xanthine stone A kidney stone formed by the nitrogen compound xanthine, found in coffee, tea, and chocolate. It develops as a result of a rare genetic disorder, hereditary xanthine oxidase deficiency.

Yersinia pestis Also known as the plague, a disease with three forms, pneumonic, bubonic, and septicemic or blood poisoning. Symptoms including headache, lethargy, and bloody sputum.

Youth violence The intentional use of physical force or power (threatened or actual) exerted by or against children, adolescents, or young adults ages 10-19 which results in (or has a high likelihood of resulting in) injury, death, psychological harm, maldevelopment, or deprivation.

Zollinger—Ellison syndrome A disorder of the production of gastrin, which in turn produces excessive stomach acid. Those with this syndrome may be at risk for peptic ulcer disease.

Zoonoses A natural animal reservoir in which an infectious agent may exist.

Zoonotic disease Any disease that is transmitted from an animal (a vector) to humans.

INDEX